VOLUME TWO

Neurosurgery

Editors

Robert H. Wilkins, M.D.
*Professor and Chief
Division of Neurosurgery
Duke University Medical Center
Durham, North Carolina*

Setti S. Rengachary, M.D.
*Professor, Section of Neurological Surgery
University of Kansas Medical Center
Kansas City, Kansas;
Chief, Neurosurgery Section
Veterans Administration Medical Center
Kansas City, Missouri*

McGraw-Hill Book Company
New York St. Louis San Francisco Auckland Bogotá Guatemala Hamburg
Lisbon London Madrid Mexico Montreal New Delhi Panama
Paris San Juan São Paulo Singapore Sydney Tokyo Toronto

Notice

Medicine is an ever-changing science. As new research and clinical experience broaden our knowledge, changes in treatment and drug therapy are required. The editors and the publisher of this work have checked with sources believed to be reliable in their efforts to provide drug dosage schedules that are complete and in accord with the standards accepted at the time of publication. However, readers are advised to check the product information sheet included in the package of each drug they plan to administer to be certain that the information contained in these schedules is accurate and that changes have not been made in the recommended dose or in the contraindications for administration. This recommendation is of particular importance in connection with new or infrequently used drugs.

Neurosurgery

Copyright © 1985 by McGraw-Hill, Inc. All rights reserved. Printed in the United States of America. Except as permitted under the United States Copyright Act of 1976, no part of this publication may be reproduced or distributed in any form or by any means, or stored in a data base or retrieval system, without the prior written permission of the publisher.

4567890 HALHAL 89

ISBN 0-07-079790-0

This book was set in Plantin by York Graphic Services, Inc.; the editors were Robert E. McGrath and Stuart D. Boynton; the production supervisor was Avé McCracken; the designer was Caliber Design Planning.
Halliday Lithograph Corporation was printer and binder.

Library of Congress Cataloging in Publication Data
Main entry under title:

Neurosurgery.

   Includes bibliographies and index.
   1. Nervous system—Surgery. I. Wilkins, Robert H.
II. Rengachary, Setti S. [DNLM: 1. Neurosurgery.
WL 368 N4951]
RD593.N417   1985   617'.48   84-17188
ISBN   0-07-079790-0 (set)

*This book is dedicated to
our wives and children:*

*Gloria Wilkins and
Michael, Jeffrey, and Elizabeth Wilkins;*

*and Dhanalakshmi Rengachary and
Dave Anand and Usha Rengachary*

CONTENTS

List of Contributors　xiii
Foreword　xxvii
Preface　xxix

VOLUME I

Part I　Historical Aspects of Neurosurgery

1. History of Neurosurgery　*Robert H. Wilkins*　3
2. Two Giants: Harvey Cushing and Walter Dandy　*Paul C. Bucy*　16
3. History of Microneurosurgery　*R. M. Peardon Donaghy*　20

Part II　Clinical Examination of the Nervous System and Correlative Neuroanatomy

4. The Art of History Taking　*Barrie J. Hurwitz*　29
5. Clinical Examination of Cognitive Functions　*Samuel H. Greenblatt*　32
6. Psychological Assessment of Intelligence and Personality　*Patrick E. Logue, Frederick A. Schmitt*　42
7. Cranial Nerve Examination　*Setti S. Rengachary*　50
8. Neuro-ophthalmology　*Michael Rosenberg*　71
9. Nystagmus and Related Ocular Movements　*Nancy M. Newman*　102
10. Neurotology　*Robert W. Baloh*　111
11. Gait and Station; Examination of Coordination　*Setti S. Rengachary*　117
12. Examination of the Motor and Sensory Systems and Reflexes　*Setti S. Rengachary*　122

Part III　Ancillary Diagnostic Tests

Section A　Cerebrospinal Fluid Examination

13. Techniques of Ventricular Puncture　*Timothy B. Mapstone, Robert A. Ratcheson*　151
14. Intracranial Pressure Monitoring　*Gerald D. Silverberg*　156
15. Cerebrospinal Fluid: Techniques of Access and Analytical Interpretation　*James H. Wood*　161

Section B　Electrodiagnostic Tests

16. Electromyography　*Didier Cros, B. Shahani*　174
17. Electroencephalography　*William P. Wilson*　184
18. Electronystagmography　*Robert A. Schindler, Vivian D. Weigel*　196
19. Evoked Potentials from the Visual, Auditory, and Somatosensory Systems　*C. William Erwin, Andrea Brendle, Miles E. Drake*　211

Section C　Some Evolving Neurodiagnostic Tests

20. Computed Tomography: Recent Trends　*Burton P. Drayer, G. Allan Johnson, C. Roger Bird*　224
21. Positron Emission Tomography　*Myron D. Ginsberg*　255
22. Single Photon Tomography　*Allan H. Friedman, Burton P. Drayer, Ronald J. Jaszczak*　265
23. Brain Imaging with Nuclear Magnetic Resonance　*Michael Brant-Zawadzki*　268
24. Ultrasonic Brain Imaging in Pediatric Neurosurgery　*Philip R. Weinstein, Kai Haber*　274
25. Digital Subtraction Angiography　*Meredith A. Weinstein, Michael T. Modic, Anthony J. Furlan, William Pavlicek, John R. Little*　280

Section D　Brain Biopsy

26. Diagnostic Brain Biopsy　*Howard H. Kaufman, Peter T. Ostrow, Ian J. Butler*　289

Part IV　General and Perioperative Care

27. Evaluation of the Patient in Coma　*Allen D. Roses*　297
28. Seizure Disorders and Their Medical Management　*J. Scott Luther*　304
29. Evaluation of the Patient with Dementia and Treatment of Normal Pressure Hydrocephalus　*Robert G. Ojemann, Peter McL. Black*　312
30. Blood-Brain Barrier; Cerebral Edema　*Michael Pollay*　322
31. Increased Intracranial Pressure, Brain Herniation, and Their Control　*Donald O. Quest*　332
32. Induced Barbiturate Coma　*Warren Selman, Robert Spetzler, Joseph Zabramski*　343
33. Pseudotumor Cerebri　*Frederick H. Sklar*　350
34. Neurourology　*George D. Webster, Jorge L. Lockhart*　354
35. Preoperative Evaluation of a Neurosurgical Patient　*Ted S. Keller*　366
36. Blood Coagulation　*Salvatore V. Pizzo*　369
37. Blood Transfusion　*Fred V. Plapp, William L. Bayer*　372
38. Neuroanesthesia　*Maurice S. Albin*　384
39. Intensive Care　*Allan B. Levin*　396
40. Prevention and Treatment of Thromboembolic Complications in a Neurosurgical Patient　*Stephen K. Powers, Michael S. B. Edwards*　406
41. Spasticity and Spasm　*Wesley A. Cook, Jr.*　411
42. Principles of Rehabilitation of the Disabled Patient　*E. Wayne Massey*　416

Part V　Neurosurgical and Related Techniques

43. Principles of Neurosurgical Operative Technique　*Robert H. Wilkins*　427
44. Instrumentation for Microneurosurgery　*John M. Tew, Jr., Hans Jacob Steiger*　439
45. Prophylactic Antibiotics　*Stephen J. Haines*　448
46. Patient Positioning　*Donald H. Stewart, Jr., John Krawchenko*　452
47. Intraoperative Diagnostic Ultrasound　*George J. Dohrmann, Jonathan M. Rubin*　457
48. Self-Retaining Retractors　*I. M. Greenberg*　463
49. Automated Cutting and Suction　*Martin L. Lazar*　473
50. Ultrasonic Dissection　*Fred Epstein*　476
51. Application of the Laser to Neurological Surgery　*Leonard J. Cerullo*　478

52 Interventional Neuroradiology *Fernando Viñuela, Allan J. Fox* 484

Part VI Neuro-oncology

Section A Neuro-oncology: An Overview
53 Genetic Factors in Brain Tumors *Robert L. Martuza* 505
54 Neurofibromatosis and Other Phakomatoses *Robert L. Martuza* 511
55 Virus-Induced Brain Tumors *Jeffrey S. Walker, Darell D. Bigner* 522
56 Radiation-Induced Brain Tumors *Jeffrey S. Walker, Darell D. Bigner* 525
57 Chemically Induced Brain Tumors, Primary and Transplanted *Jeffrey S. Walker, Darell D. Bigner* 528
58 Cell Kinetics of Brain Tumors *Takao Hoshino* 531
59 Biochemistry of Brain Tumors *C. J. Cummins, B. H. Smith, P. L. Kornblith* 535
60 Immunology of Brain Tumors *Michael L. J. Apuzzo* 538
61 Tissue Culture Techniques in the Study of Human Gliomas *Joseph Bressler, Barry H. Smith, Paul L. Kornblith* 542
62 Tumor Markers *Dennis E. Bullard, S. Clifford Schold, Jr.* 548

Section B Gliomas
63 Gliomas: Pathology *Peter C. Burger* 553
64 Supratentorial Gliomas: Radiology *Kenneth R. Maravilla* 564
65 Supratentorial Gliomas: Clinical Features and Surgical Therapy *Michael Salcman* 579

Section C Metastatic Brain Tumors
66 Factors That Govern the Metastatic Process *Leonard Weiss* 591
67 Metastatic Brain Tumors *Joseph H. Galicich, Narayan Sundaresan* 597
68 Meningeal Carcinomatosis *John R. Little, Maurice R. Hanson* 610

Section D Meningiomas
69 Meningiomas: Pathology *Venkata R. Challa, William R. Markesbery* 613
70 Meningiomas: Radiology *Dixon M. Moody* 623
71 Meningiomas: Clinical Features and Surgical Management *Robert G. Ojemann* 635

Section E Epidermoid and Dermoid Tumors
72 Epidermoid and Dermoid Tumors: Pathology *Jere W. Baxter, Martin G. Netsky* 655
73 Epidermoid and Dermoid Tumors: Radiology *Dennis R. Osborne* 662
74 Epidermoid and Dermoid Tumors: Clinical Features and Surgical Management *Frances K. Conley* 668

Section F Tumors in the Region of the Pineal Gland
75 Pineal Tumors: Classification and Pathology *Maie Kaarsoo Herrick* 674
76 Pineal Region Masses: Radiology *Robert A. Zimmerman* 680
77 Pineal Masses: Clinical Features and Management *Henry H. Schmidek, Alan Waters* 688

Section G Cerebellopontine Angle Tumors
78 Tumors of the Cerebellopontine Angle: Pathology *F. Stephen Vogel* 694
79 Tumors of the Cerebellopontine Angle: Neurotologic Aspects of Diagnosis *Patrick D. Kenan* 698
80 Tumors of the Cerebellopontine Angle: Radiology *Philip Dubois* 704
81 Tumors of the Cerebellopontine Angle: Clinical Features and Surgical Management *William A. Buchheit, Tomas E. Delgado* 720

Section H Posterior Fossa Tumors
82 Radiology of Posterior Fossa Tumors *Shelley B. Rosenbloom, Arthur E. Rosenbaum* 730
83 Cerebellar Astrocytomas *David G. McLone* 754
84 Medulloblastomas *Luis Schut, Derek A. Bruce, Leslie N. Sutton* 758
85 Brain Stem Gliomas *Mark S. O'Brien, Mary M. Johnson* 762
86 Ependymomas *George J. Dohrmann* 767
87 Hemangioblastomas *Setti S. Rengachary* 772
88 Choroid Plexus Papillomas *Hector E. James* 783
89 Chemodectomas *James T. Robertson* 785

Section I Sellar and Parasellar Tumors
90 Hypothalamic Control of Anterior Pituitary Function: Surgical Implications *Robert B. Page* 791
91 Anatomy and Physiology of the Neurohypophysis *William A. Shucart, Ivor M. D. Jackson* 805
92 Microsurgical Anatomy of the Sellar Region *Albert L. Rhoton, Jr.* 811
93 Radiology of Sellar and Parasellar Lesions *James C. Hoffman, Jr.* 822
94 Classification and Pathology of Pituitary Tumors *Kalman Kovacs, Eva Horvath, Sylvia L. Asa* 834
95 Endocrine Diagnosis in Neurosurgery *Nicholas T. Zervas* 843
96 Prolactinomas *George T. Tindall, Daniel L. Barrow* 852
97 Cushing's Disease and Nelson's Syndrome *James E. Boggan, Charles B. Wilson* 859
98 Acromegaly and Gigantism *Edward R. Laws, Jr.* 864
99 Perioperative Endocrine Management of Patients with Pituitary Tumors *Kalmon D. Post, William Cobb* 868
100 Bromocriptine *William S. Evans, Michael O. Thorner* 873
101 Pituitary Apoplexy *Richard L. Rovit* 879
102 Empty Sella Syndrome *Peter W. Carmel* 884
103 Trans-sphenoidal Approach to the Pituitary Gland *J. Hardy* 889
104 Stereotactic Treatment of Pituitary Tumors *Robert W. Rand* 899
105 Subfrontal Approach to the Pituitary Gland *Russel H. Patterson, Jr.* 902
106 Craniopharyngiomas *Peter W. Carmel* 905
107 Optic Gliomas *Edgar M. Housepian, Merlin D. Marquardt, Myles Behrens* 916
108 Suprasellar Germinomas *John W. Walsh* 921
109 Diencephalic Syndrome *John E. Kalsbeck* 925
110 Cranial Chordomas *Edward R. Laws, Jr.* 927
111 Parasellar Granular Cell Tumors *Dennis H. Becker* 930
112 Benign Pituitary Cysts *Howard M. Eisenberg, Richard L. Weiner* 932

Section J Third Ventricular Tumors
113 Masses of the Third Ventricle *J. Lobo Antunes* 935
114 Operative Approaches to the Third Ventricle *Albert L. Rhoton, Jr., Isao Yamamoto* 938

Section K Tumors of the Orbit
115 Radiology of the Orbit and Its Contents *Richard E. Latchaw, William E. Rothfus* 952
116 Tumors of the Orbit *Joseph C. Maroon, John S. Kennerdell* 964

Section L Tumors of the Scalp and Skull
117 Noninvasive Tumors of the Scalp *B. Thomas Harter, Jr., Kathleen C. Harter, Donald Serafin* 977
118 Tumors of the Skull *Rand M. Voorhies, Narayan Sundaresan* 984
119 Craniofacial Resection for Advanced Head and Neck Cancers *James P. Neifeld, Harold F. Young* 1002

Contents

120 Surgical Resection of Tumors of the Skull Base
Leonard I. Malis 1011

Section M   Miscellaneous Intracranial Tumors
121 Primary Lymphoma of the Central Nervous System
Milam E. Leavens, John T. Manning, Sidney Wallace, Moshe H. Maor, William S. Velasquez 1022
122 Intracranial Sarcomas J. F. Ross Fleming, John H. N. Deck, Mark Bernstein 1030
123 Lipoma of the Corpus Callosum Doyle G. Graham 1036

Section N   Spinal Tumors
124 Radiology of Spinal Canal Neoplasia Andrew L. Tievsky, David O. Davis 1039
125 Spinal Intradural Tumors Bennett M. Stein 1048
126 Spinal Epidural Tumors Perry Black 1062
127 Spinal Chordomas Narayan Sundaresan, Ralph C. Marcove 1069
128 Vertebral Hemangiomas David C. Hemmy 1076
129 Masses of the Sacrum Setti S. Rengachary 1079

Section O   Adjunctive Therapy of CNS Tumors
130 Principles of Radiotherapy of CNS Tumors
K. Thomas Noell, Arnold M. Herskovic 1084
131 Conventional Radiotherapy of Specific CNS Tumors Steven R. Plunkett 1096
132 Heavy Particle Irradiation of Intracranial Lesions
John H. Lawrence, Cornelius A. Tobias, John A. Linfoot, Joseph R. Castro, William M. Saunders, George T. Chen, J. Michael Collier, Devron Char, Grant Gauger, Kay Woodruff, Sandra Zink, Jacob I. Fabrikant, John T. Lyman, Yoshio Hosobuchi 1113
133 Fast Neutron Irradiation of Malignant Gliomas Alexander M. Spence 1132
134 Interstitial Brachytherapy of Primary Brain Tumors Philip H. Gutin 1136
135 Immunotherapy of Human Gliomas
Michael L. J. Apuzzo 1139
136 Chemotherapy of Primary Brain Tumors
S. Clifford Schold, Jr., J. Gregory Cairncross, Dennis E. Bullard 1143
137 Blood-Brain Barrier Modification in Delivery of Antitumor Agents Edward A. Neuwelt 1153
138 Hyperthermia in the Treatment of Intracranial Tumors Robert G. Selker 1159

VOLUME II

Part VII   Vascular Diseases of the Nervous System

Section A   Occlusive Cerebrovascular Disease
139 Cerebral Blood Flow Thomas W. Langfitt, Walter D. Obrist 1167
140 Measurement of Cerebral Blood Flow Howard Yonas 1173
141 Normal Cerebral Energy Metabolism
Michael J. O'Connor, Steven J. Barrer, Frank A. Welsh 1179
142 Pathophysiological Consequences of Brain Ischemia
Jewell L. Osterholm 1185
143 Atherosclerosis Jack C. Geer, Julio H. Garcia 1189
144 Pathology of Ischemic Cerebrovascular Disease
John Moossy 1193
145 Clinical Syndromes of Brain Ischemia
David G. Sherman, J. Donald Easton 1199
146 Noninvasive Tests in the Diagnosis of Carotid Vascular Disease Robert M. Crowell, J. Philip Kistler 1212
147 Radiology of Ischemic Cerebrovascular Disease
Herbert I. Goldberg 1219
148 Extracranial Carotid Artery Atherosclerosis
Robert G. Ojemann 1236

149 Vertebral Artery Atherosclerosis James I. Ausman, Fernando G. Diaz, R. A. de los Reyes 1248
150 Moyamoya Disease David G. Piepgras 1254
151 Medical Treatment of Ischemic Cerebral Vascular Disease H. J. M. Barnett 1258
152 Potential Role of Perfluorocarbons in Neurosurgery
S. J. Peerless 1264
153 Surgery for Acute Brain Infarction with Mass Effect
Setti S. Rengachary 1267
154 Extracranial to Intracranial Bypass Grafting: Anterior Circulation Jack M. Fein 1272
155 Extracranial to Intracranial Bypass Grafting: Posterior Circulation Thoralf M. Sundt, Jr., David G. Piepgras 1281
156 Fibromuscular Dysplasia L. N. Hopkins, James L. Budny 1293
157 Arterial Dissections Allan H. Friedman 1297
158 Nonseptic Venous Occlusive Disease John P. Kapp 1300

Section B   Intracranial Aneurysms
159 Intracranial Aneurysms and Subarachnoid Hemorrhage: An Overview Bryce Weir 1308
160 Microsurgical Anatomy of Saccular Aneurysms
Albert L. Rhoton, Jr. 1330
161 Radiology of Intracranial Aneurysms Eugene F. Binet, Edgardo J. C. Angtuaco 1341
162 Intracranial Arterial Spasm Robert R. Smith, Junji Yoshioka 1355
163 Timing of Aneurysm Surgery Neal F. Kassell, David J. Boarini 1363
164 Patients with Ruptured Aneurysm: Pre- and Postoperative Management Neal F. Kassell, David J. Boarini 1367
165 Aneurysm Clips John M. Tew, Jr., Hans Jacob Steiger 1372
166 Middle Cerebral Artery Aneurysms Roberto C. Heros 1376
167 Distal Anterior Cerebral Artery Aneurysms
Alan S. Fleischer, Daniel L. Barrow 1383
168 Carotid-Ophthalmic Artery Aneurysms
Gary G. Ferguson 1385
169 Aneurysms of Internal Carotid and Anterior Communicating Arteries Eugene S. Flamm 1394
170 Giant Intracranial Aneurysms Yoshio Hosobuchi 1404
171 Carotid Ligation Richard A. Roski, Robert F. Spetzler 1414
172 Posterior Circulation Aneurysms S. J. Peerless, Charles G. Drake 1422
173 Surgery for Unruptured Intracranial Aneurysms
Duke Samson 1437
174 Inflammatory Intracranial Aneurysms John G. Frazee 1440
175 Aneurysm Treatments Other Than Clipping
John F. Alksne 1444

Section C   Vascular Malformations and Fistulas
176 Intracranial Arteriovenous Malformations
H. D. Garretson 1448
177 Vein of Galen Aneurysms A. Loren Amacher 1459
178 Other Cranial Intradural Angiomas Setti S. Rengachary, Uma P. Kalyan-Raman 1465
179 Dural Arteriovenous Malformations Alfred J. Luessenhop 1473
180 Surgical Anatomy of the Cavernous Sinus
Dwight Parkinson 1478
181 Carotid-Cavernous Fistulas and Intracavernous Aneurysms Sean Mullan 1483
182 Spinal Arteriovenous Malformations Ayub Khan Ommaya 1495
183 Spontaneous Intraspinal Hemorrhage Hugh S. Wisoff 1500

Section D Hypertension
184 Neurogenic Hypertension *Jack M. Fein* 1505
185 Spontaneous Intracerebral Hemorrhage
     Thomas B. Ducker 1510

Section E Coagulopathies and Vasculopathies
186 Coagulopathies Causing Intracranial Hemorrhage
     Justin W. Renaudin, Ralph P. George 1518
187 Vasculopathies *Setti S. Rengachary* 1521

Part VIII Trauma

Section A Cranial Trauma
188 Biomechanics of Head Injury *Thomas A. Gennarelli, Lawrence E. Thibault* 1531
189 Pathophysiology of Head Injury *A. John Popp, Robert S. Bourke* 1536
190 Pathology of Closed Head Injury *William F. McCormick* 1544
191 Neurological Evaluation of a Patient with Head Trauma: Coma Scales *Victoria Neave, Martin H. Weiss* 1570
192 Computed Tomography in Head Trauma *Chi-Shing Zee, Hervey D. Segall, Jamshid Ahmadi, Michael L. J. Apuzzo, Steven L. Giannotta* 1578
193 Resuscitation of the Multiply Injured Patient *Paul R. Cooper* 1587
194 Intensive Management of Head Injury *Donald P. Becker, Stephen Gardner* 1593
195 Pediatric Head Injury *Derek A. Bruce, Luis Schut, Leslie N. Sutton* 1600
196 Outcome Prediction in Severe Head Injury *Lawrence F. Marshall, Sharon A. Bowers* 1605
197 Minor Head Injury: Management and Outcome *Rebecca W. Rimel, John A. Jane* 1608
198 Scalp Injuries *William J. Barwick* 1612
199 Cephalhematoma and Subgaleal Hematoma *Derek A. Bruce, Luis Schut, Leslie N. Sutton* 1622
200 Skull Fractures *L. M. Thomas* 1623
201 Growing Skull Fractures of Childhood *Timothy B. Scarff, Michael Fine* 1627
202 Facial Fractures *Ronald Riefkohl, Gregory S. Georgiade, Nicholas G. Georgiade* 1629
203 Cerebrospinal Fluid Fistula *Ayub Khan Ommaya* 1637
204 Cranial Defects and Cranioplasty *Donald J. Prolo* 1647
205 Traumatic Intracranial Hematomas *Paul R. Cooper* 1657
206 Delayed and Recurrent Intracranial Hematomas and Post-Traumatic Coagulopathies *Michael E. Miner* 1666
207 Penetrating Wounds of the Head *Griffith R. Harsh, III, Griffith R. Harsh, IV* 1670
208 Vascular Lesions with Head Injury *Steven L. Giannotta, Jamshid Ahmadi* 1678
209 Sequelae of Head Injury *Byron Young* 1688

Section B Spinal Trauma
210 Experimental Spinal Cord Injury *Arthur I. Kobrine, Jerald J. Bernstein* 1694
211 High Cervical Spine Injuries *Richard C. Schneider* 1701
212 Mid- and Lower Cervical Spine Injuries *Martin H. Weiss* 1708
213 Psychological Aspects of Whiplash Injury *Henry Berry* 1716
214 Cervical Traction *Albert B. Butler* 1719
215 Halo Immobilization of Cervical Spine Injuries *William T. Hardaker, Jr.* 1723
216 Anterior Approach in Cervical Spine Injuries *Edward L. Seljeskog* 1727
217 Diaphragm Pacing *Ronald F. Young* 1733
218 Injuries to the Thoracic and Lumbar Spine *Wesley A. Cook, Jr., William T. Hardaker, Jr.* 1735
219 Injuries to the Sacrum and Pelvis *Barth A. Green, Ignacio Magana* 1744
220 Penetrating Wounds of the Spine *Carole A. Miller* 1746
221 Posterior Lumbar Spinal Fusion *J. Leonard Goldner* 1749
222 Post-Traumatic Syringomyelia *Joseph H. Piatt, Jr.* 1761

Part IX Disorders of Peripheral and Cranial Nerves and the Autonomic Nervous System

Section A Entrapment Neuropathies
223 Thoracic Outlet Syndromes *Russell W. Hardy, Jr., Asa J. Wilbourn* 1767
224 Entrapment Neuropathies *Setti S. Rengachary* 1771

Section B Acute Nerve Injuries
225 Anatomy and Physiology of Peripheral Nerves *Robert M. Worth* 1796
226 Peripheral Nerve Injuries: Types, Causes, Grading *F. Gentili, Alan R. Hudson* 1802
227 Pathophysiology of Peripheral Nerve Trauma *Thomas B. Ducker* 1812
228 Brachial Plexus Injuries *Alan R. Hudson, B. Tranmer* 1817
229 Diagnostic Approach to Individual Nerve Injuries *David G. Kline* 1833
230 Surgical Exposure of Peripheral Nerves *Charles L. Branch, Jr., David L. Kelly, Jr., George C. Lynch* 1846
231 Management of the Neuroma in Continuity *David G. Kline, Earl R. Hackett* 1864
232 Techniques of Nerve Repair *John E. McGillicuddy* 1871
233 Clinical Signs of Peripheral Nerve Regeneration *Irvine G. McQuarrie* 1881
234 Painful Neuromas *Suzie C. Tindall* 1884
235 Causalgia; Sympathetic Dystrophy (Sudeck's Atrophy) *William H. Sweet* 1886

Section C Nerve Tumors
236 Neoplasms of Peripheral Nerves *Humberto Cravioto* 1894
237 Ganglion Cysts of Peripheral Nerves *Suzie C. Tindall* 1900

Section D Neurovascular Compression Syndromes
238 Posterior Fossa Neurovascular Compression Syndromes Other than Neuralgias *Peter J. Jannetta* 1901

Section E Miscellaneous
239 Techniques of Diagnostic Nerve and Muscle Biopsies *Edward S. Connolly* 1907
240 Nontraumatic Brachial Plexopathy *E. Wayne Massey* 1909
241 Surgical Sympathectomy *Janet W. Bay, Donald F. Dohn* 1912

VOLUME III

Part X Infections

Section A Bacterial Infections
242 Acute Bacterial Meningitis *David T. Durack, John R. Perfect* 1921
243 Brain Abscess *Richard H. Britt* 1928
244 Inflammatory Thrombosis of Major Dural Venous Sinuses and Cortical Veins *Frederick S. Southwick, Morton N. Swartz* 1956
245 Cranial Epidural Abscess and Subdural Empyema *Justin W. Renaudin* 1961
246 Infections of the Scalp and Osteomyelitis of the Skull *Stephen J. Haines, Shelley N. Chou* 1964
247 Pituitary Abscess *James E. Boggan, Charles B. Wilson* 1967
248 Spinal Cord Abscess *Arnold H. Menezes, John C. VanGilder* 1969

Contents

249 Spinal Epidural and Subdural Abscesses
    Marshall B. Allen, Jr., Wayne D. Beveridge   1972
250 Osteomyelitis of the Spine   *Donald E. McCollum*   1975
251 Chronic Granulomatous Lesions: Tuberculosis, Leprosy, Sarcoidosis   *Mark L. Rosenblum*   1980

Section B   Viral Infections
252 *Herpes simplex* Virus Infections   *Richard J. Whitley, Richard B. Morawetz*   1987
253 Creutzfeldt-Jakob Disease   *Clarence J. Gibbs, Jr.*   1994

Section C   Fungal and Parasitic Infections
254 Fungal Infections   *Allan H. Friedman, Elizabeth Bullitt*   2002
255 Parasitic Infestations   *W. Eugene Stern*   2010

Part XI   Developmental Anomalies and Neurosurgical Diseases of Childhood

256 Neurological Evaluation of the Newborn and Child   *Andrew K. Hodson*   2019
257 Genetics of Developmental Defects   *David D. Weaver*   2025
258 Spinal Dysraphism   *Robin P. Humphreys*   2041
259 Occult Spinal Dysraphism and Related Disorders   *Larry K. Page*   2053
260 Diastematomyelia   *A. Norman Guthkelch*   2058
261 Intraspinal Cysts   *Robert H. Wilkins*   2061
262 Lateral and Anterior Spinal Meningoceles   *Robert H. Wilkins*   2070
263 Sacral Agenesis   *Dachling Pang*   2075
264 Sacrococcygeal Teratomas   *Howard C. Filston*   2077
265 Congenital Dermal Sinus   *J. Gordon McComb*   2081
266 Congenital Defects of the Scalp and Skull   *Dan Fults, David L. Kelly, Jr.*   2084
267 Encephaloceles   *E. Bruce Hendrick*   2087
268 Craniopagus Twins   *Theodore S. Roberts*   2091
269 Craniovertebral Junction Anomalies   *John C. VanGilder, Arnold H. Menezes*   2097
270 Chiari Malformations, Hydromyelia, Syringomyelia   *W. Jerry Oakes*   2102
271 Physiology of Cerebrospinal Fluid   *Humbert G. Sullivan, Jerry D. Allison*   2125
272 Hydrocephalus: Pathophysiology and Clinical Features   *Thomas H. Milhorat*   2135
273 Hydrocephalus: Treatment   *David C. McCullough*   2140
274 Double Compartment Hydrocephalus   *Eldon L. Foltz*   2151
275 Dandy-Walker Syndrome   *Robert L. McLaurin*   2153
276 Antenatal Diagnosis and Treatment of Hydrocephalus   *Robert A. Brodner*   2156
277 Intracranial Arachnoid and Ependymal Cysts   *Setti S. Rengachary*   2160
278 Craniosynostosis   *Ken R. Winston*   2173
279 Craniofacial Anomalies   *Harold J. Hoffman*   2192
280 Neonatal Intracranial Hemorrhage   *Herbert Lourie*   2203
281 Strokes in Children   *Mel H. Epstein*   2205
282 Subdural Hematomas and Effusions in Children   *Robert L. McLaurin*   2211
283 Control of Increased Intracranial Pressure in Reye's Syndrome   *Joan L. Venes*   2215

Part XII   Intervertebral Disc Disease and Selected Spinal Disorders

284 Biomechanics of the Spine   *Manohar M. Panjabi, Richard R. Pelker, Augustus A. White, III*   2219
285 Osteoporosis   *John M. Harrelson*   2228
286 Cervical Disc Disease and Cervical Spondylosis   *Julian T. Hoff*   2230
287 Rheumatoid Arthritis of the Cervical Spine   *Chitranjan S. Ranawat*   2240
288 Ossification of the Posterior Longitudinal Ligament   *Louis Bakay*   2243
289 Thoracic Disc Disease   *Phanor L. Perot, Jr.*   2245
290 Lumbar Disc Disease   *Frederick A. Simeone*   2250
291 Chemonucleolysis   *Clark Watts*   2260
292 Lumbar Intradural Disc Rupture   *Charles J. Hodge, Jr.*   2264
293 Postoperative Intervertebral Disc Space Infections   *Charles E. Rawlings, III, Robert H. Wilkins*   2266
294 Lumbar Spondylosis and Spinal Stenosis   *Joseph A. Epstein, Nancy E. Epstein*   2272
295 The Lateral Recess Syndrome   *Ivan Ciric, Michael A. Mikhael*   2279
296 Redundant Nerve Root Syndrome of the Cauda Equina   *Setti S. Rengachary*   2283
297 Lumbar Spondylolisthesis   *John M. Cuckler, Richard H. Rothman*   2285
298 The Failed Back   *Charles V. Burton*   2290
299 Postlaminectomy Kyphosis   *Eben Alexander, Jr.*   2293
300 Neurological Complications of Scoliosis   *Shelley N. Chou*   2298
301 Spinal Bracing   *James M. Morris*   2300
302 Neural Dysfunction in Paget's Disease of Bone   *Henry H. Schmidek, Alan Waters*   2305

Part XIII   Pain

Section A   Basic Science
303 Anatomy and Physiology of Pain   *Donlin M. Long*   2313
304 Gate Control Theory   *Ronald Melzack, Patrick D. Wall*   2317

Section B   Clinical Evaluation
305 Psychological Factors in the Assessment and Management of Chronic Pain   *Randal D. France*   2320
306 Multidisciplinary Pain Clinic   *Bruno J. Urban*   2323

Section C   Certain Specific Pain Syndromes
307 Craniofacial Pain Syndromes: An Overview   *Robert E. Maxwell*   2327
308 Trigeminal Neuralgia: Introduction   *Robert H. Wilkins*   2337
309 Trigeminal Neuralgia: Treatment by Percutaneous Electrocoagulation   *G. Robert Nugent*   2345
310 Trigeminal Neuralgia: Treatment by Glycerol Rhizotomy   *L. Dade Lunsford*   2351
311 Trigeminal Neuralgia: Treatment by Microvascular Decompression   *Peter J. Jannetta*   2357
312 Glossopharyngeal Neuralgia   *Burton M. Onofrio*   2363
313 Postherpetic Neuralgia   *Allan H. Friedman, Blaine S. Nashold, Jr.*   2367
314 Pain Following Spinal Cord Injury   *Charles H. Tator*   2368
315 Phantom Limb Pain   *John D. Loeser*   2371

Section D   Management of Chronic Intractable Pain
316 Drug Therapy of Chronic Pain   *Nelson Hendler*   2374
317 Diagnostic and Therapeutic Nerve Blocks   *Bruno J. Urban*   2382
318 Intraspinal Infusion of Narcotic Drugs   *Dennis W. Coombs, Richard L. Saunders*   2390
319 Physical Medicine and Physical Therapy   *John Mennell*   2397
320 Conservative Management of Lumbar and Cervical Pain   *Marcia Sirotkin-Roses*   2404
321 Acupuncture   *Terence M. Murphy*   2408

Section E   Electrical Stimulation
322 Transcutaneous Electrical Stimulation for Pain Relief   *Donlin M. Long*   2410
323 Peripheral Nerve Stimulation for Pain Relief   *James Gardner Wepsic*   2415

324 **Percutaneous Spinal Epidural Stimulation for Pain Relief** *Bruno J. Urban* 2417
325 **Deep Brain Stimulation for Pain Relief** *Donald E. Richardson* 2421

Section F Ablative Procedures
326 **Percutaneous Radio-Frequency Denervation of Spinal Facets** *Douglas E. Kennemore* 2427
327 **Dorsal Rhizotomy** *A. Basil Harris* 2430
328 **Dorsal Root Entry Zone Lesions for Pain Relief** *Blaine S. Nashold, Jr., Alfred C. Higgins, Bennett Blumenkopf* 2433
329 **Commissural Myelotomy for Pain Relief** *Robert B. King* 2438
330 **Open Surgical Cordotomy** *Bruce L. Ehni, George Ehni* 2439
331 **Percutaneous Spinothalamic Cordotomy** *Hubert L. Rosomoff* 2446
332 **Medullary Tractotomy for Pain Relief** *Robert B. King* 2452
333 **Stereotactic Ablative Procedures for Pain Relief** *Ronald F. Young, Luciano M. Modesti* 2454
334 **Hypophysectomy** *George T. Tindall, Suzie C. Tindall* 2458

Part XIV Stereotactic and Functional Neurosurgery
335 **Stereotactic Surgery: Principles and Techniques** *Ronald R. Tasker* 2465
336 **CT Stereotactic Guidance Systems** *M. Peter Heilbrun, Theodore S. Roberts* 2481
337 **Methods of Making Nervous System Lesions** *Eric R. Cosman, Bernard J. Cosman* 2490
338 **Medical Therapy of Movement Disorders** *C. Warren Olanow* 2499
339 **Surgical Therapy of Movement Disorders** *Philip L. Gildenberg* 2507
340 **Surgical Treatment of Epilepsy** *George A. Ojemann* 2517
341 **Neurosurgery for Behavioral Disorders** *H. Thomas Ballantine, Jr.* 2527
342 **Chronic Cerebellar Stimulation in Humans** *Richard D. Penn* 2537
343 **Neural Prostheses** *John P. Girvin* 2543
344 **Central Nervous System Grafting** *Richard Jed Wyatt, William J. Freed* 2546

Part XV Miscellaneous Topics
345 **Practice Management** *Phillip Earle Williams, Jr.* 2555
346 **Disability Evaluation** *Byron C. Pevehouse* 2561
347 **The Informed Consent** *William E. Hunt* 2569
348 **The Professional Liability Insurance Crisis** *William H. Mosberg, Jr.* 2571
349 **Clinical Research** *Donlin M. Long* 2579
350 **The Medical Determination of Death** *Roy Selby* 2585
351 **Transplantation of Cadaver Tissues and Organs** *Donald J. Prolo* 2598
352 **Methods and Techniques of Intraoperative Microphotography** *Ronald I. Apfelbaum* 2601

Part XVI Appendix

Appendix A Drugs Commonly Used in Neurological Surgery
Table A1 Drug Dosages 2611
Table A2 Drug Dosage Adjustments in Renal Insufficiency 2634
Table A3 Therapeutic and Toxic Dosage Ranges of Commonly Used Drugs 2636

Appendix B Range of Values for Commonly Performed Laboratory Tests
Table B1 Reference Ranges: Hematologic, Serologic, and Coagulation Studies 2637
Table B2 Reference Ranges: Clinical Chemistry 2638

Index 2643

LIST OF CONTRIBUTORS

Jamshid Ahmadi, M.D.
Assistant Professor, Department of Radiology, University of Southern California School of Medicine, Los Angeles, California

Maurice S. Albin, M.D., M.Sc. (Anes.)
Professor, Department of Anesthesiology and Director, Neuroanesthesia Service, University of Texas Health Science Center at San Antonio, San Antonio, Texas

Eben Alexander, Jr., M.D.
Professor, Section on Neurosurgery, Bowman Gray School of Medicine, Winston-Salem, North Carolina

John F. Alksne, M.D.
Professor and Chairman, Division of Neurological Surgery, University of California, San Diego, San Diego, California

Marshall B. Allen, Jr., M.D.
Professor and Chief, Section of Neurosurgery, Medical College of Georgia, Augusta, Georgia

Jerry D. Allison, Ph.D.
Assistant Professor, Department of Radiology, Medical College of Georgia, Augusta, Georgia

A. Loren Amacher, M.D., F.R.C.S.(C)
Associate Professor, Division of Neurosurgery, University of Connecticut, Hartford, Connecticut

Edgardo J. C. Angtuaco, M.D.
Department of Radiology, University of Arkansas for Medical Sciences, Little Rock, Arkansas

J. Lobo Antunes, M.D.
Professor and Chairman, Department of Neurological Surgery, University of Lisbon, Lisbon, Portugal

Ronald I. Apfelbaum, M.D.
Associate Professor, Leo M. Davidoff Department of Neurological Surgery, Albert Einstein College of Medicine, Bronx, New York

Michael L. J. Apuzzo, M.D.
Professor, Department of Neurosurgery, University of Southern California School of Medicine, Los Angeles, California

Sylvia L. Asa, M.D.
Department of Pathology, St. Michael's Hospital, University of Toronto, Toronto, Ontario, Canada

James I. Ausman, M.D., Ph.D.
Chairman, Department of Neurological Surgery, Henry Ford Hospital, Detroit, Michigan

Louis Bakay, M.D.
Professor and Chairman, Department of Neurosurgery, School of Medicine, State University of New York at Buffalo, Buffalo, New York

H. Thomas Ballantine, Jr., M.D.
Clinical Professor of Surgery Emeritus, Harvard Medical School, and Senior Neurosurgeon, Massachusetts General Hospital, Boston, Massachusetts

Robert W. Baloh, M.D.
Professor of Neurology and Surgery (Head and Neck), Department of Neurology, University of California Center for the Health Sciences, Los Angeles, California

H. J. M. Barnett, M.D., F.R.C.P.(C), F.R.C.P.
Richard and Beryl Ivey Professor, Department of Clinical Neurological Sciences, University of Western Ontario, London, Ontario, Canada

Steven J. Barrer, M.D.
Assistant Professor, Division of Neurosurgery, School of Medicine, University of Pennsylvania, Philadelphia, Pennsylvania

Daniel L. Barrow, M.D.
Resident, Division of Neurological Surgery, Emory University School of Medicine, Atlanta, Georgia

William J. Barwick, M.D.
Assistant Professor, Division of Plastic and Maxillofacial Surgery, Duke University Medical Center, Durham, North Carolina

Jere W. Baxter, M.D.
Assistant Professor, Department of Pathology, Vanderbilt University School of Medicine, Nashville, Tennessee

Janet W. Bay, M.D.
Department of Neurological Surgery, Cleveland Clinic Foundation, Cleveland, Ohio

William L. Bayer, M.D.
Community Blood Center of Greater Kansas City, Kansas City, Missouri

Dennis H. Becker, M.D.
Chief, Division of Neurosurgery, Santa Clara Valley Medical Center, San Jose, California

Donald P. Becker, M.D.
Professor and Chairman, Division of Neurological Surgery, Medical College of Virginia, Virginia Commonwealth University, Richmond, Virginia

Myles Behrens, M.D.
Associate Professor of Clinical Ophthalmology, College of Physicians & Surgeons, Columbia University, New York, New York

Jerald J. Bernstein, Ph.D.
Chief, Laboratory of Central Nervous System Injury and Regeneration, Veterans Administration Medical Center, Washington, District of Columbia

Mark Bernstein, M.D.
Division of Neurosurgery, University of Toronto, Toronto, Ontario, Canada

Henry Berry, M.D., D.Psych., F.R.C.P.(C)
Head, Department of Neurology, St. Michael's Hospital, Toronto, Ontario, Canada

Wayne D. Beveridge, M.D.
Associate Professor, Section of Neurosurgery, Medical College of Georgia, Augusta, Georgia

Darell D. Bigner, M.D., Ph.D.
Professor, Department of Pathology, Duke University Medical Center, Durham, North Carolina

Eugene F. Binet, M.D.
Professor and Vice Chairman, Department of Radiology, University of Arkansas for Medical Sciences, Little Rock, Arkansas

C. Roger Bird, M.D.
Assistant Professor, Department of Radiology, Stanford University Medical Center, Stanford, California

Perry Black, M.D., C.M.
Professor and Chairman, Department of Neurosurgery, Hahnemann University School of Medicine, Philadelphia, Pennsylvania

Peter McL. Black, M.D., Ph.D.
Assistant Professor of Surgery, Harvard Medical School; Assistant Visiting Neurosurgeon, Massachusetts General Hospital, Boston, Massachusetts

Bennett Blumenkopf, M.D.
Major, Medial Corps, U. S. Army; Assistant Chief, Neurosurgery Service, Brooke Army Medical Center, Fort Sam Houston, Texas

David J. Boarini, M.D.
Resident, Division of Neurosurgery, University of Iowa, Iowa City, Iowa

James E. Boggan, M.D.
Assistant Clinical Professor, Department of Neurological Surgery, School of Medicine, University of California, San Francisco, San Francisco, California

Robert S. Bourke, M.D.
Professor and Chairman, Division of Neurosurgery, Albany Medical College, Albany, New York

Sharon A. Bowers, B.S.N.
Division of Neurological Surgery, University of California, San Diego, San Diego, California

Charles L. Branch, Jr., M.D.
Resident, Section on Neurosurgery, Bowman Gray School of Medicine, Winston-Salem, North Carolina

Michael Brant-Zawadzki, M.D.
Associate Professor, Department of Radiology, School of Medicine, University of California, San Francisco, San Francisco, California

Andrea Brendle, B.A.
Evoked Potential Laboratory, Duke University Medical Center, Durham, North Carolina

Joseph Bressler, Ph.D.
Surgical Neurology Branch, National Institute of Neurological and Communicative Disorders and Stroke, Bethesda, Maryland

Richard H. Britt, M.D., Ph.D.
Assistant Professor, Division of Neurosurgery, Stanford University Medical Center, Stanford, California

Robert A. Brodner, M.D.
Assistant Professor, Department of Neurosurgery, Hahnemann University School of Medicine, Philadelphia, Pennsylvania

Derek A. Bruce, M.B., Ch.B.
Division of Neurosurgery, Children's Hospital of Philadelphia, Philadelphia, Pennsylvania

William A. Buchheit, M.D.
Professor and Chairman, Department of Neurosurgery, Temple University Health Sciences Center, Philadelphia, Pennsylvania

Paul C. Bucy, M.D.
Clinical Professor Emeritus of Neurology and Neurological Surgery, Bowman Gray School of Medicine, Winston-Salem, North Carolina

James L. Budny, M.D.
Dent Neurologic Institute, Buffalo, New York

Dennis E. Bullard, M.D.
Assistant Professor, Division of Neurosurgery, Duke University Medical Center, Durham, North Carolina

Elizabeth Bullitt, M.D.
Clinical Instructor, Department of Neurological Surgery, University of Cincinnati Medical Center, Cincinnati, Ohio

Peter C. Burger, M.D.
Associate Professor, Department of Pathology, Duke University Medical Center, Durham, North Carolina

Charles V. Burton, M.D.
Medical Director, Institute for Low Back Care, Minneapolis, Minnesota

Albert B. Butler, M.D.
Professor and Chairman, Department of Neurological Surgery, Health Sciences Center, State University of New York at Stony Brook, Stony Brook, New York

Ian J. Butler, M.B., F.R.A.C.P.
Professor, Department of Neurology, University of Texas Medical School at Houston, Houston, Texas

J. Gregory Cairncross, M.D.
Assistant Professor, Departments of Clinical Neurological Sciences and Radiation Oncology, University of Western Ontario, London, Ontario, Canada

Peter W. Carmel, M.D., D.Med.Sci.
Associate Professor, Department of Neurological Surgery, College of Physicians & Surgeons, Columbia University, New York, New York

Joseph R. Castro, M.D.
Lawrence Berkeley Laboratory and Donner Laboratory, University of California, Berkeley, Berkeley, California

Leonard J. Cerullo, M.D.
University Neurosurgeons, Chicago, Illinois

Venkata R. Challa, M.D.
Assistant Professor, Department of Pathology, Bowman Gray School of Medicine, Winston-Salem, North Carolina

Devron Char, M.D.
Lawrence Berkeley Laboratory and Donner Laboratory, University of California, Berkeley, Berkeley, California

George T. Chen, Ph.D.
Lawrence Berkeley Laboratory and Donner Laboratory, University of California, Berkeley, Berkeley, California

List of Contributors

Shelley N. Chou, M.D. Ph.D.
Professor and Chairman, Department of Neurosurgery, University of Minnesota Medical School, Minneapolis, Minnesota

Ivan Ciric, M.D.
Department of Neurosurgery, Evanston Hospital, Evanston, Illinois

William Cobb, M.D.
Assistant Professor, Department of Medicine, Tufts University School of Medicine, Boston, Massachusetts

J. Michael Collier, Ph.D.
Lawrence Berkeley Laboratory and Donner Laboratory, University of California, Berkeley, Berkeley, California

Frances K. Conley, M.D.
Associate Professor, Division of Neurosurgery, Stanford University Medical Center, Stanford, California

Edward S. Connolly, M.D.
Head, Department of Neurosurgery, Ochsner Clinic and Alton Ochsner Medical Foundation, New Orleans, Louisiana

Wesley A. Cook, Jr., M.D.
Associate Professor, Division of Neurosurgery, Duke University Medical Center, Durham, North Carolina

Dennis W. Coombs, M.D.
Assistant Professor of Surgery (Anesthesiology), Dartmouth-Hitchcock Medical Center, Hanover, New Hampshire

Paul R. Cooper, M.D.
Associate Professor, Department of Neurosurgery, New York University Medical Center, New York, New York

Bernard J. Cosman, M.S.
Radionics, Inc., Burlington, Massachusetts

Eric R. Cosman, Ph.D.
Department of Physics, Massachusetts Institute of Technology, Cambridge, Massachusetts

Humberto Cravioto, M.D.
Professor, Department of Pathology, New York University Medical Center, New York, New York

Didier Cros, M.D.
Assistant Professor, Department of Neurology and Psychiatry, Tulane Medical Center, New Orleans, Louisiana

Robert M. Crowell, M.D.
Professor and Head, Department of Neurosurgery, University of Illinois at Chicago, Chicago, Illinois

John M. Cuckler, M.D.
Clinical Assistant Professor of Orthopaedic Surgery, School of Medicine, University of Pennsylvania, Philadelphia, Pennsylvania

C.J. Cummins, Ph.D.
National Institute of Neurological and Communicative Disorders and Stroke, National Institutes of Health, Bethesda, Maryland

David O. Davis, M.D.
Professor and Chairman, Department of Radiology, The George Washington University Medical Center, Washington, District of Columbia

John H. N. Deck, M.D., F.R.C.P.(C)
Associate Professor, Division of Neuropathology, University of Toronto, Toronto, Ontario, Canada

Tomas E. Delgado, M.D.
Assistant Professor, Department of Neurosurgery, Temple University Health Sciences Center, Philadelphia, Pennsylvania

R. A. de los Reyes, M.D.
Department of Neurological Surgery, Henry Ford Hospital, Detroit, Michigan

Fernando G. Diaz, M.D., Ph.D.
Department of Neurological Surgery, Henry Ford Hospital, Detroit, Michigan

Donald F. Dohn, M.D.
Singing River Neurological Surgery, Pascagoula, Mississippi

George J. Dohrmann, M.D., Ph.D.
Associate Professor, Section of Neurological Surgery, University of Chicago Medical Center, Chicago, Illinois

R. M. Peardon Donaghy, M.D.
Professor Emeritus, Division of Neurosurgery, College of Medicine, University of Vermont, Burlington, Vermont

Charles G. Drake, M.D., F.R.C.S.(C)
Professor and Chairman, Department of Surgery, University of Western Ontario, London, Ontario, Canada

Miles E. Drake, M.D.
Assistant Professor, Department of Neurology, Ohio State University College of Medicine, Columbus, Ohio

Burton P. Drayer, M.D.
Associate Professor, Section of Neuroradiology, Department of Radiology, Duke University Medical Center, Durham, North Carolina

Philip Dubois, M.B., B.S., F.R.C.R., F.R.A.C.R.
Department of Radiology, Mater Misericordiae Private Hospital, South Brisbane, Queensland, Australia

Thomas B. Ducker, M.D.
Clinical Professor, Division of Neurological Surgery, University of Maryland School of Medicine, Baltimore, Maryland

David T. Durack, M.B., B.S., D.Phil., F.R.C.P.
Professor and Chief, Division of Infectious Diseases, Duke University Medical Center, Durham, North Carolina

J. Donald Easton, M.D.
Professor and Chief, Division of Neurology, University of Texas Health Science Center at San Antonio, San Antonio, Texas

Michael S. B. Edwards, M.D.
Associate Professor, Departments of Neurological Surgery and Pediatrics, School of Medicine, University of California, San Francisco, San Francisco, California

Bruce L. Ehni, M.D.
Clinical Instructor, Department of Neurosurgery, Baylor College of Medicine and Affiliated Hospitals, Houston, Texas

George Ehni, M.D., M.S.
Professor, Department of Neurosurgery, Baylor College of Medicine and Affiliated Hospitals, Houston, Texas

Howard M. Eisenberg, M.D.
Professor and Chief, Division of Neurosurgery, University of Texas Medical Branch, Galveston, Texas

Fred Epstein, M.D.
Professor, Department of Neurosurgery, New York University Medical Center, New York, New York

Joseph A. Epstein, M.D.
Professor of Clinical Surgery (Neurosurgery), State University of New York at Stony Brook, Stony Brook, New York

Mel H. Epstein, M.D.
Associate Professor, Department of Neurological Surgery, Johns Hopkins University School of Medicine, Baltimore, Maryland

Nancy E. Epstein, M.D.
Lecturer in Neurosurgery, New York University Medical Center, New York, New York

C. William Erwin, M.D.
Professor, Division of Biological Psychiatry, Department of Psychiatry, Duke University Medical Center, Durham, North Carolina

William S. Evans, M.D.
Research Assistant Professor, Department of Internal Medicine, University of Virginia Medical Center, Charlottesville, Virginia

Jacob I. Fabrikant, M.D., Ph.D.
Lawrence Berkeley Laboratory and Donner Laboratory, University of California, Berkeley, Berkeley, California

Jack M. Fein, M.D.
Associate Professor, Leo M. Davidoff Department of Neurological Surgery, Albert Einstein College of Medicine, Bronx, New York

Gary G. Ferguson, M.D., Ph.D., F.R.C.S.(C)
Professor, Division of Neurosurgery, University of Western Ontario, London, Ontario, Canada

Howard C. Filston, M.D.
Professor, Departments of Surgery and Pediatrics, Duke University Medical Center, Durham, North Carolina

Michael Fine, M.D.
Associate Professor, Department of Radiology, Loyola University Medical Center, Maywood, Illinois

Eugene S. Flamm, M.D.
Professor and Vice Chairman, Department of Neurosurgery, New York University Medical Center, New York, New York

Alan S. Fleischer, M.D.
Professor and Chief, Section of Neurosurgery, University of Arizona Health Sciences Center, Tucson, Arizona

J. F. Ross Fleming, M.D., M.S., F.R.C.S.(C)
Associate Professor, Division of Neurosurgery, University of Toronto, Toronto, Ontario, Canada

Eldon L. Foltz, M.D.
Professor, Division of Neurological Surgery, University of California, Irvine Medical Center, Orange, California

Allan J. Fox, M.D., F.R.C.P.(C)
Associate Professor, Departments of Diagnostic Radiology and Clinical Neurological Sciences, University of Western Ontario, London, Ontario, Canada

Randal D. France, M.D.
Assistant Professor, Department of Psychiatry, Duke University Medical Center, Durham, North Carolina

John G. Frazee, M.D.
Assistant Professor, Division of Neurosurgery, University of California Center for the Health Sciences, and Wadsworth Veterans Administration Hospital, Los Angeles, California

William J. Freed, Ph.D.
Adult Psychiatry Branch, National Institute of Mental Health, Saint Elizabeth's Hospital, Washington, District of Columbia

Allan H. Friedman, M.D.
Assistant Professor, Division of Neurosurgery, Duke University Medical Center, Durham, North Carolina

Dan Fults, M.D.
Resident, Section on Neurosurgery, Bowman Gray School of Medicine, Winston-Salem, North Carolina

Anthony J. Furlan, M.D.
Director, Cerebrovascular Program, The Cleveland Clinic Foundation, Cleveland, Ohio

Joseph H. Galicich, M.D.
Chief, Neurosurgery Service, Memorial Sloan-Kettering Cancer Center, New York, New York

Julio H. Garcia, M.D.
Professor, Department of Pathology, University of Alabama in Birmingham, Birmingham, Alabama

Stephen Gardner, M.D.
Head Injury Fellow, Division of Neurological Surgery, Medical College of Virginia, Virginia Commonwealth University, Richmond, Virginia

H. D. Garretson, M.D., Ph.D.
Professor and Director, Division of Neurological Surgery, University of Louisville School of Medicine, Louisville, Kentucky

Grant Gauger, M.D.
Lawrence Berkeley Laboratory and Donner Laboratory, University of California, Berkeley, Berkeley, California

Jack C. Geer, M.D.
Professor and Chairman, Department of Pathology, University of Alabama in Birmingham, Birmingham, Alabama

Thomas A. Gennarelli, M.D.
Associate Professor, Division of Neurosurgery, School of Medicine, University of Pennsylvania, Philadelphia, Pennsylvania

F. Gentili, M.D., M.Sc., F.R.C.S.(C)
Assistant Professor, Division of Neurosurgery, University of Toronto, Toronto, Ontario, Canada

Ralph P. George, M.D.
Associate Clinical Professor, Department of Medicine, University of California, San Diego, San Diego, California

Gregory S. Georgiade, M.D.
Assistant Professor, Divisions of General and Cardio-thoracic Surgery, Duke University Medical Center, Durham, North Carolina

Nicholas G. Georgiade, D.D.S., M.D.
Professor and Chief, Division of Plastic and Maxillofacial Surgery, Duke University Medical Center, Durham, North Carolina

Steven L. Giannotta, M.D.
Assistant Professor, Department of Neurological Surgery, University of Southern California School of Medicine, Los Angeles, California

Clarence J. Gibbs, Jr., Ph.D.
Laboratory of Central Nervous System Studies, National Institute of Neurological and Communicative Disorders and Stroke, National Institutes of Health, Bethesda, Maryland

Philip L. Gildenberg, M.D., Ph.D.
Clinical Professor, Division of Neurosurgery, University of Texas Health Science Center at Houston, Houston, Texas

Myron D. Ginsberg, M.D.
Professor, Department of Neurology, School of Medicine, University of Miami, Miami, Florida

List of Contributors

John P. Girvin, M.D., F.R.C.S.(C)
Professor and Chairman, Department of Clinical Neurological Sciences, University of Western Ontario, London, Ontario, Canada

Herbert I. Goldberg, M.D.
Professor, Department of Radiology and Division of Neurosurgery, School of Medicine, University of Pennsylvania, Philadelphia, Pennsylvania

J. Leonard Goldner, M.D.
James B. Duke Professor and Chief, Division of Orthopaedic Surgery, Duke University Medical Center, Durham, North Carolina

Doyle G. Graham, M.D., Ph.D.
Associate Professor, Department of Pathology, Duke University Medical Center, Durham, North Carolina

Barth A. Green, M.D.
Associate Professor, Department of Neurological Surgery, University of Miami School of Medicine, Miami, Florida

I. M. Greenberg, M.D.
Associate Professor of Clinical Neurosurgery, Department of Neurological Surgery, State University of New York at Stony Brook, Stony Brook, New York

Samuel H. Greenblatt, M.D.
Associate Professor, Division of Neurological Surgery, Department of Neurosciences, Medical College of Ohio, Toledo, Ohio

A. Norman Guthkelch, F.R.C.S.(Eng)
Professor, Department of Neurological Surgery, School of Medicine, University of Pittsburgh, Pittsburgh, Pennsylvania

Philip H. Gutin, M.D.
Assistant Professor, Department of Neurological Surgery, School of Medicine, University of California, San Francisco, San Francisco, California

Kai Haber, M.D.
Professor, Department of Radiology, University of Arizona Health Sciences Center, Tucson, Arizona

Earl R. Hackett, M.D.
Professor and Head, Department of Neurology, Louisiana State University Medical Center, New Orleans, Louisiana

Stephen J. Haines, M.D.
Assistant Professor, Department of Neurosurgery, University of Minnesota Medical School, Minneapolis, Minnesota

Maurice R. Hanson, M.D.
Department of Neurology, Cleveland Clinic Foundation, Cleveland, Ohio

William T. Hardaker, Jr., M.D.
Assistant Professor, Division of Orthopaedic Surgery, Duke University Medical Center, Durham, North Carolina

Jules Hardy, M.D., F.R.C.S.(C)
Professor and Chairman, Division of Neurosurgery, Faculty of Medicine, University of Montreal, Montreal, Quebec, Canada

Russell W. Hardy, Jr., M.D.
Department of Neurological Surgery, Cleveland Clinic Foundation, Cleveland, Ohio

John M. Harrelson, M.D.
Associate Professor, Division of Orthopaedic Surgery, Duke University Medical Center, Durham, North Carolina

A. Basil Harris, M.D.
Professor, Department of Neurological Surgery, University of Washington School of Medicine, Seattle, Washington

Griffith R. Harsh, III, M.D.
Professor and Director, Division of Neurosurgery, University of Alabama in Birmingham, Birmingham, Alabama

Griffith R. Harsh, IV, M.D.
Resident, Department of Neurological Surgery, School of Medicine, University of California, San Francisco, San Francisco, California

B. Thomas Harter, Jr., M.D.
Resident, Division of Plastic and Maxillofacial Surgery, Duke University Medical Center, Durham, North Carolina

Kathleen C. Harter, M.D.
Division of Plastic and Maxillofacial Surgery, Duke University Medical Center, Durham, North Carolina

M. Peter Heilbrun, M.D.
Professor and Chairman, Division of Neurosurgery, University of Utah School of Medicine, Salt Lake City, Utah

David C. Hemmy, M.D.
Associate Professor, Department of Neurosurgery, Medical College of Wisconsin, Milwaukee, Wisconsin

Nelson Hendler, M.D., M.S.
Clinical Director, Mensana Clinic, Stevenson, Maryland

E. Bruce Hendrick, M.D., F.R.C.S.(C)
Professor, Division of Neurosurgery, University of Toronto; The Hospital for Sick Children, Toronto, Ontario, Canada

Roberto C. Heros, M.D.
Director of Cerebrovascular Surgery, Massachusetts General Hospital, Boston, Massachusetts

Maie Kaarsoo Herrick, M.D.
Neuropathologist, Santa Clara Valley Medical Center, San Jose, California

Arnold M. Herskovic, M.D.
Associate Professor, Radiation Oncology Center, Wayne State University, Detroit, Michigan

Alfred C. Higgins, M.D.
Hickory, North Carolina

Charles J. Hodge, Jr., M.D.
Professor, Department of Neurological Surgery, State University of New York, Upstate Medical Center, Syracuse, New York

Andrew K. Hodson, M.B., Ch.B., M.R.C.P.(UK)
Chief, Division of Child Neurology, University Hospital of Jacksonville, Jacksonville, Florida

Julian T. Hoff, M.D.
Professor and Head, Section of Neurosurgery, University of Michigan Medical Center, Ann Arbor, Michigan

Harold J. Hoffman, M.D., F.R.C.S.(C)
Professor, Division of Neurosurgery, University of Toronto; The Hospital for Sick Children, Toronto, Ontario, Canada

James C. Hoffman, Jr., M.D.
Associate Professor, Department of Radiology, Emory University School of Medicine, Atlanta, Georgia

L. N. Hopkins, M.D.
Chairman, Department of Neurosurgery, Dent Neurologic Institute, Buffalo, New York

Eva Horvath, Ph.D.
Department of Pathology, St. Michael's Hospital, University of Toronto, Toronto, Ontario, Canada

Takao Hoshino, M.D., D.M.Sc.
Department of Neurological Surgery and Brain Tumor Research Center, School of Medicine, University of California, San Francisco, San Francisco, California

Yoshio Hosobuchi, M.D.
Professor, Department of Neurological Surgery, School of Medicine, University of California, San Francisco, San Francisco, California

Edgar M. Housepian, M.D.
Professor of Clinical Neurological Surgery, College of Physicians & Surgeons, Columbia University, New York, New York

Alan R. Hudson, M.B., Ch.B., F.R.C.S.(C)
Professor and Chairman, Division of Neurosurgery, University of Toronto, Toronto, Ontario, Canada

Robin P. Humphreys, M.D., F.R.C.S.(C)
Associate Professor, Division of Neurosurgery, University of Toronto; The Hospital for Sick Children, Toronto, Ontario, Canada

William E. Hunt, M.D.
Professor and Director, Division of Neurologic Surgery, Ohio State University College of Medicine, Columbus, Ohio

Barrie J. Hurwitz, M.B., M.R.C.P., F.C.P.(SA)
Assistant Professor, Division of Neurology, Duke University Medical Center, Durham, North Carolina

Ivor M. D. Jackson, M.D.
Professor, Department of Medicine, Tufts-New England Medical Center, Boston, Massachusetts

Hector E. James, M.D.
Associate Professor, Division of Neurological Surgery, and Department of Pediatrics, University of California, San Diego, San Diego, California

John A. Jane, M.D., Ph.D., F.R.C.S.(C)
Professor and Chairman, Department of Neurosurgery, University of Virginia Medical Center, Charlottesville, Virginia

Peter J. Jannetta, M.D.
Professor and Chairman, Department of Neurological Surgery, School of Medicine, University of Pittsburgh, Pittsburgh, Pennsylvania

Ronald J. Jaszczak, Ph.D.
Associate Professor, Department of Radiology, Duke University Medical Center, Durham, North Carolina

G. Allan Johnson, Ph.D.
Associate Professor, Department of Radiology, Duke University Medical Center, Durham, North Carolina

Mary M. Johnson, M.D.
Attending Neurosurgeon, Henrietta Egleston Hospital for Children and Scottish Rite Hospital for Children, Atlanta, Georgia

John E. Kalsbeck, M.D.
Professor, Section of Neurological Surgery, Indiana University School of Medicine, Indianapolis, Indiana

Uma P. Kalyan-Raman, M.D.
Associate Professor, Department of Pathology, University of Illinois College of Medicine at Peoria, Peoria, Illinois

John P. Kapp, M.D., Ph.D.
Professor, Department of Neurosurgery, University of Mississippi Medical Center, Jackson, Mississippi

Neal F. Kassell, M.D.
Professor, Division of Neurosurgery, University of Iowa, Iowa City, Iowa

Howard H. Kaufman, M.D.
Professor, Department of Neurosurgery, School of Medicine, West Virginia University, Morgantown, West Virginia

Ted S. Keller, M.D.
Assistant Professor, Division of Neurosurgery, University of Colorado Health Sciences Center, Denver, Colorado

David L. Kelly, Jr., M.D.
Professor and Head, Section on Neurosurgery, Bowman Gray School of Medicine, Winston-Salem, North Carolina

Patrick D. Kenan, M.D.
Associate Professor, Division of Otolaryngology, Duke University Medical Center, Durham, North Carolina

Douglas E. Kennemore, M.D.
Greenville, South Carolina

John S. Kennerdell, M.D.
Professor, Departments of Ophthalmology and Neurology, School of Medicine, University of Pittsburgh, Pittsburgh, Pennsylvania

Robert B. King, M.D.
Professor and Chairman, Department of Neurological Surgery, State University of New York, Upstate Medical Center, Syracuse, New York

J. Philip Kistler, M.D.
Associate Professor of Neurology, Harvard Medical School, Boston, Massachusetts

David G. Kline, M.D.
Professor and Chairman, Department of Neurosurgery, Louisiana State University Medical Center, New Orleans, Louisiana

Arthur I. Kobrine, M.D., Ph.D.
Professor, Department of Neurological Surgery, George Washington University Medical Center, Washington, District of Columbia

Paul L. Kornblith, M.D.
Chief, Surgical Neurology Branch, National Institute of Neurological and Communicative Disorders and Stroke, Bethesda, Maryland

Kalman Kovacs, M.D., Ph.D., F.R.C.P.(C)
Professor, Department of Pathology, St. Michael's Hospital, University of Toronto, Toronto, Ontario, Canada

John Krawchenko, M.D.
Clinical Assistant Professor, Department of Neurological Surgery, State University of New York, Upstate Medical Center, Syracuse, New York

Thomas W. Langfitt, M.D.
Charles Harrison Frazier Professor and Director, Division of Neurosurgery, School of Medicine, University of Pennsylvania, Philadelphia, Pennsylvania

Richard E. Latchaw, M.D.
Associate Professor, Departments of Radiology and Neurological Surgery, University of Pittsburgh Health Centers, Pittsburgh, Pennsylvania

John H. Lawrence, M.D.
Lawrence Berkeley Laboratory and Donner Laboratory, University of California, Berkeley, Berkeley, California

Edward R. Laws, Jr., M.D.
Professor, Department of Neurologic Surgery, Mayo Clinic and Mayo Medical School, Rochester, Minnesota

List of Contributors

Martin L. Lazar, M.D.
Department of Neurological Surgery, Texas Neurological Institute at Dallas, Dallas, Texas

Milam E. Leavens, M.D.
Associate Professor and Chief, Neurosurgery Service, M.D. Anderson Hospital and Tumor Institute, Houston, Texas

Allan B. Levin, M.D.
Associate Professor, Division of Neurological Surgery, University of Wisconsin Center for Health Sciences, Madison, Wisconsin

John A. Linfoot, M.D.
Lawrence Berkeley Laboratory and Donner Laboratory, University of California, Berkeley, Berkeley, California

Vicki Lea Linman, B.S., M.T.
Senior Medical Technologist, Duke University Medical Center Laboratories, Durham, North Carolina

John R. Little, M.D.
Department of Neurological Surgery, Cleveland Clinic Foundation, Cleveland, Ohio

Jorge L. Lockhart, M.D.
Associate Professor, Division of Urology, University of Miami School of Medicine, Miami, Florida

John D. Loeser, M.D.
Professor, Department of Neurological Surgery, University of Washington School of Medicine, Seattle, Washington

Patrick E. Logue, Ph.D.
Associate Professor, Division of Medical Psychology, Department of Psychiatry, Duke University Medical Center, Durham, North Carolina

Donlin M. Long, M.D., Ph.D.
Professor and Chairman, Department of Neurological Surgery, Johns Hopkins University School of Medicine, Baltimore, Maryland

Herbert Lourie, M.D.
Clinical Professor, Department of Neurological Surgery, State University of New York, Upstate Medical Center, Syracuse, New York

Alfred J. Luessenhop, M.D.
Professor and Chief, Division of Neurosurgery, Georgetown University Hospital, Washington, District of Columbia

L. Dade Lunsford, M.D.
Assistant Professor, Department of Neurological Surgery, School of Medicine, University of Pittsburgh, Pittsburgh, Pennsylvania

J. Scott Luther, M.D.
Assistant Professor, Division of Neurology, Duke University Medical Center, Durham, North Carolina

John T. Lyman
Lawrence Berkeley Laboratory and Donner Laboratory, University of California, Berkeley, Berkeley, California

George C. Lynch
Professor of Medical Illustration, Department of Audiovisual Resources, Bowman Gray School of Medicine, Winston-Salem, North Carolina

Ignacio Magana, M.D.
Fellow, Department of Neurological Surgery, University of Miami School of Medicine, Miami, Florida

Leonard I. Malis, M.D.
Professor and Chairman, Department of Neurosurgery, The Mount Sinai Medical Center, New York, New York

John T. Manning, M.D.
Assistant Professor, Department of Pathology, M.D. Anderson Hospital and Tumor Institute, Houston, Texas

Moshe H. Maor, M.D.
Associate Professor, Department of Radiotherapy, M.D. Anderson Hospital and Tumor Institute, Houston, Texas

Timothy B. Mapstone, M.D.
Assistant Professor, Division of Neurological Surgery, Case Western Reserve University School of Medicine, Cleveland, Ohio

Kenneth R. Maravilla, M.D.
Associate Professor, Department of Radiology, University of Texas Health Science Center at Dallas, Dallas, Texas

Ralph C. Marcove, M.D.
Orthopedic Service, Memorial Sloan-Kettering Cancer Center, New York, New York

William R. Markesbery, M.D.
Professor of Neurology and Pathology, University of Kentucky Medical Center, Lexington, Kentucky

Joseph C. Maroon, M.D.
Professor, Department of Neurological Surgery, School of Medicine, University of Pittsburgh, Pittsburgh, Pennsylvania

Merlin D. Marquardt, M.D.
Assistant Professor, Department of Pathology, College of Physicians & Surgeons, Columbia University, New York, New York

Lawrence F. Marshall, M.D.
Associate Professor, Division of Neurological Surgery, University of California, San Diego, San Diego, California

Robert L. Martuza, M.D.
Assistant Professor of Surgery, Harvard Medical School, and Director of the Neurofibromatosis Clinic, Massachusetts General Hospital, Boston, Massachusetts

E. Wayne Massey, M.D.
Assistant Professor, Division of Neurology, Duke University Medical Center, Durham, North Carolina

Robert E. Maxwell, M.D., Ph.D.
Associate Professor, Department of Neurosurgery, University of Minnesota Medical School, Minneapolis, Minnesota

Donald E. McCollum, M.D.
Professor, Division of Orthopaedic Surgery, Duke University Medical Center, Durham, North Carolina

J. Gordon McComb, M.D.
Associate Professor, Department of Neurological Surgery, University of Southern California School of Medicine; the Childrens Hospital of Los Angeles, Los Angeles, California

William F. McCormick, M.D.
Professor and Chief, Division of Neuropathology, University of Texas Medical Branch, Galveston, Texas

David C. McCullough, M.D.
Chairman, Department of Neurosurgery, Children's Hospital National Medical Center, Washington, District of Columbia

John E. McGillicuddy, M.D.
Associate Professor, Section of Neurosurgery, University of Michigan Medical Center, Ann Arbor, Michigan

Robert L. McLaurin, M.D.
Professor, Department of Neurological Surgery, University of Cincinnati Medical Center and Children's Hospital Medical Center, Cincinnati, Ohio

David G. McLone, M.D., Ph.D.
Chairman, Division of Pediatric Neurosurgery, Children's Memorial Hospital, Chicago, Illinois

Irvine G. McQuarrie, M.D., Ph.D.
Departments of Anatomy and Surgery (Division of Neurological Surgery), Case Western Reserve University School of Medicine, Cleveland, Ohio

Ronald Melzack, Ph.D.
Professor, Department of Psychology, McGill University, Montreal, Quebec, Canada

Arnold H. Menezes, M.D.
Associate Professor, Division of Neurosurgery, University of Iowa Hospitals and Clinics, Iowa City, Iowa

John Mennell, M.D.
Vero Beach, Florida

Michael A. Mikhael, M.D.
Department of Radiology, Evanston Hospital, Evanston, Illinois

Thomas H. Milhorat, M.D.
Professor and Chairman, Department of Neurosurgery, State University of New York, Downstate Medical Center, Brooklyn, New York

Carole A. Miller, M.D.
Associate Professor, Division of Neurologic Surgery, Ohio State University College of Medicine, Columbus, Ohio

Michael E. Miner, M.D., Ph.D.
Associate Professor and Chief, Division of Neurosurgery, University of Texas Health Science Center at Houston, Houston, Texas

Luciano M. Modesti, M.D.
Professor, Department of Neurological Surgery, State University of New York, Upstate Medical Center, Syracuse, New York

Michael T. Modic, M.D.
Division of Radiology, The Cleveland Clinic Foundation, Cleveland, Ohio

Dixon M. Moody, M.D.
Professor, Department of Radiology, Bowman Gray School of Medicine, Winston-Salem, North Carolina

John Moossy, M.D.
Professor, Departments of Pathology and Neurology, School of Medicine, University of Pittsburgh, Pittsburgh, Pennsylvania

Richard B. Morawetz, M.D.
Professor, Division of Neurosurgery, School of Medicine, University of Alabama in Birmingham, Birmingham, Alabama

James M. Morris, M.D.
Associate Professor, Department of Orthopaedic Surgery, School of Medicine, University of California, San Francisco, San Francisco, California

William H. Mosberg, Jr., M.D.
Clinical Professor, Division of Neurological Surgery, University of Maryland School of Medicine, Baltimore, Maryland

Sean Mullan, M.D., D.Sc., F.R.C.S.(Eng)
Professor and Chairman, Section of Neurological Surgery, University of Chicago Hospitals, Chicago, Illinois

Terence M. Murphy, M.D., F.F.A.R.C.S.
Professor, Department of Anesthesiology, University of Washington School of Medicine, Seattle, Washington

Blaine S. Nashold, Jr., M.D.
Professor, Division of Neurosurgery, Duke University Medical Center, Durham, North Carolina

Victoria Neave, M.D.
Resident, Department of Neurological Surgery, University of Southern California School of Medicine, Los Angeles, California

James P. Neifeld, M.D.
Associate Professor, Division of Surgical Oncology, Medical College of Virginia, Virginia Commonwealth University, Richmond, Virginia

Martin G. Netsky, M.D.
Professor, Department of Pathology, Vanderbilt University School of Medicine, Nashville, Tennessee

Edward A. Neuwelt, M.D.
Associate Professor, Division of Neurosurgery, The Oregon Health Sciences University, Portland, Oregon

Nancy M. Newman, M.D.
Associate Professor and Chief, Neuro-ophthalmology Division, Department of Ophthalmology, Pacific Medical Center, San Francisco, California

K. Thomas Noell, M.D.
Ramagosa Radiation Oncology Center, Lafayette, Louisiana

G. Robert Nugent, M.D.
Professor and Chairman, Department of Neurosurgery, West Virginia University School of Medicine, Morgantown, West Virginia

W. Jerry Oakes, M.D.
Assistant Professor, Division of Neurosurgery, Duke University Medical Center, Durham, North Carolina

Mark S. O'Brien, M.D.
Professor, Division of Neurological Surgery, Emory University School of Medicine, Atlanta, Georgia

Walter D. Obrist, Ph.D.
Professor of Research in Neurosurgery and Neurology, University of Pennsylvania, Philadelphia, Pennsylvania

Michael J. O'Connor, M.D.
Associate Professor, Division of Neurosurgery, School of Medicine, University of Pennsylvania, Philadelphia, Pennsylvania

George A. Ojemann, M.D.
Professor, Department of Neurological Surgery, University of Washington School of Medicine, Seattle, Washington

Robert G. Ojemann, M.D.
Professor of Surgery, Harvard Medical School and Visiting Neurosurgeon, Massachusetts General Hospital, Boston, Massachusetts

C. Warren Olanow, M.D.
Assistant Professor, Division of Neurology, Duke University Medical Center, Durham, North Carolina

Ayub Khan Ommaya, M.D., F.R.C.S.
Clinical Professor, Department of Neurological Surgery, George Washington University Medical Center, Washington, District of Columbia

Burton M. Onofrio, M.D.
Professor, Department of Neurologic Surgery, Mayo Clinic and Mayo Medical School, Rochester, Minnesota

Dennis R. Osborne, M.D.
Associate Professor, Department of Radiology, Duke University Medical Center, Durham, North Carolina

List of Contributors

Roger H. Ostdahl, M.D.
Camp Hill, Pennsylvania

Jewell L. Osterholm, M.D.
Professor and Chairman, Department of Neurosurgery, Jefferson Medical College of Thomas Jefferson University, Philadelphia, Pennsylvania

Peter T. Ostrow, M.D., Ph.D.
Associate Professor, Department of Pathology, The University of Texas Medical School at Houston, Houston, Texas

Larry K. Page, M.D.
Professor, Department of Neurological Surgery, University of Miami School of Medicine, Miami, Florida

Robert B. Page, M.D.
Associate Professor, Division of Neurosurgery, Milton S. Hershey Medical Center of the Pennsylvania State University, Hershey, Pennsylvania

Dachling Pang, M.D., F.R.C.S.(C)
Assistant Professor, Department of Neurological Surgery, School of Medicine, University of Pittsburgh, Pittsburgh, Pennsylvania

Manohar M. Panjabi, Ph.D., D.Tech.
Professor and Director, Biomechanics Research, Section of Orthopaedic Surgery, Yale University School of Medicine, New Haven, Connecticut

Dwight Parkinson, M.D.
Professor and Chairman, Section of Neurosurgery, University of Manitoba Health Sciences Centre, Winnipeg, Manitoba, Canada

Russel H. Patterson, Jr., M.D.
Professor and Chief, Division of Neurosurgery, The New York Hospital-Cornell Medical Center, New York, New York

William Pavlicek, M.S.
Diagnostic Physicist, The Cleveland Clinic Foundation, Cleveland, Ohio

S. J. Peerless, M.D., F.R.C.S.(C)
Professor and Chairman, Division of Neurosurgery, University of Western Ontario, London, Ontario, Canada

Richard R. Pelker, M.D., Ph.D.
Assistant Professor, Section of Orthopaedic Surgery, Yale University School of Medicine, New Haven, Connecticut

Richard D. Penn, M.D.
Associate Professor, Department of Neurosurgery, Rush Medical School, Chicago, Illinois

John R. Perfect, M.D.
Assistant Professor, Division of Infectious Diseases, Duke University Medical Center, Durham, North Carolina

Phanor L. Perot, Jr., M.D., Ph.D.
Professor and Chairman, Department of Neurosurgery, Medical University of South Carolina, Charleston, South Carolina

Byron C. Pevehouse, M.D.
Clinical Professor, Department of Neurological Surgery, School of Medicine, University of California, San Francisco, San Francisco, California

Joseph H. Piatt, Jr., M.D.
Resident, Division of Neurosurgery, Duke University Medical Center, Durham, North Carolina

David G. Piepgras, M.D.
Assistant Professor, Department of Neurologic Surgery, Mayo Clinic and Mayo Medical School, Rochester, Minnesota

Salvatore V. Pizzo, M.D., Ph.D.
Associate Professor, Department of Pathology, Duke University Medical Center, Durham, North Carolina

Fred V. Plapp, M.D., Ph.D.
Assistant Medical Director, Community Blood Center of Greater Kansas City, Kansas City, Missouri

Steven R. Plunkett, M.D.
Instructor, Section of Radiation Therapy, Bowman Gray School of Medicine, Winston-Salem, North Carolina

Michael Pollay, M.D.
Professor and Chief, Division of Neurosurgery, University of Oklahoma College of Medicine, Oklahoma City, Oklahoma

A. John Popp, M.D.
Associate Professor, Division of Neurosurgery, Albany Medical College, Albany, New York

Kalmon D. Post, M.D.
Associate Professor, Department of Neurological Surgery, College of Physicians & Surgeons, Columbia University, New York, New York

Stephen K. Powers, M.D.
Assistant Professor, Division of Neurological Surgery, School of Medicine, University of North Carolina at Chapel Hill, Chapel Hill, North Carolina

Donald J. Prolo, M.D.
Director, Neuroskeletal Transplantation Laboratory, Institute for Medical Research, San Jose, California

Donald O. Quest, M.D.
Associate Professor, Department of Neurological Surgery, Columbia University College of Physicians & Surgeons, New York, New York

Chitranjan S. Ranawat, M.D.
Professor of Orthopaedic Surgery, Cornell University Medical Center and the Hospital for Special Surgery, New York, New York

Robert W. Rand, Ph.D., M.D.
Professor, Division of Neurosurgery, School of Medicine, University of California, Los Angeles, Los Angeles, California

Robert A. Ratcheson, M.D.
The Harvey Huntington Brown, Jr. Professor and Chairman, Division of Neurological Surgery, Case Western Reserve University School of Medicine, Cleveland, Ohio

Charles E. Rawlings, III, M.D.
Resident, Division of Neurosurgery, Duke University Medical Center, Durham, North Carolina

Justin W. Renaudin, M.D.
Assistant Clinical Professor, Division of Neurological Surgery, University of California, San Diego, San Diego, California

Setti S. Rengachary, M.D.
Professor, Section of Neurological Surgery, University of Kansas Medical Center, Kansas City, Kansas; Chief, Neurosurgery Section, Veterans Administration Medical Center, Kansas City, Missouri

Albert L. Rhoton, Jr., M.D.
R. D. Keene Family Professor and Chairman, Department of Neurological Surgery, University of Florida College of Medicine, Gainesville, Florida

Donald E. Richardson, M.D.
Professor and Chairman, Department of Neurologic Surgery, Tulane University School of Medicine, New Orleans, Louisiana

Ronald Riefkohl, M.D.
Assistant Professor, Division of Plastic and Maxillofacial Surgery, Duke University Medical Center, Durham, North Carolina

Rebecca W. Rimel, B.S.N., M.B.A.
Assistant Professor, Department of Neurosurgery, University of Virginia Medical Center, Charlottesville, Virginia

Theodore S. Roberts, M.D.
Professor, Division of Neurosurgery, University of Utah School of Medicine, Salt Lake City, Utah

James T. Robertson, M.D.
Professor and Chairman, Department of Neurosurgery, University of Tennessee Center for the Health Sciences, Memphis, Tennessee

Arthur E. Rosenbaum, M.D.
Professor, Departments of Radiology and Radiological Science, and of Neurosurgery, The Johns Hopkins Medical Institutions, Baltimore, Maryland

Michael Rosenberg, M.D.
Associate Professor, Department of Ophthalmology, Northwestern University, Chicago, Illinois

Shelley B. Rosenbloom, M.D.
Assistant Professor, Department of Radiology and Radiological Science, The Johns Hopkins Medical Institutions, Baltimore, Maryland

Mark L. Rosenblum, M.D.
Associate Professor, Department of Neurological Surgery, School of Medicine, University of California, San Francisco, San Francisco, California

Allen D. Roses, M.D.
Professor and Chief, Division of Neurology, Duke University Medical Center, Durham, North Carolina

Richard A. Roski, M.D.
Assistant Professor, Division of Neurological Surgery, University of Louisville School of Medicine, Louisville, Kentucky

Hubert L. Rosomoff, M.D., D.med.Sc.
Professor and Chairman, Department of Neurological Surgery, University of Miami School of Medicine, Miami, Florida

William E. Rothfus, M.D.
Assistant Professor, Department of Radiology, University of Pittsburgh Health Centers, Pittsburgh, Pennsylvania

Richard H. Rothman, M.D., Ph.D.
Professor of Orthopaedic Surgery, School of Medicine, University of Pennsylvania, Philadelphia, Pennsylvania

Richard L. Rovit, M.D., M.Sc.
Director, Department of Neurological Surgery, St. Vincent's Hospital and Medical Center, New York, New York

Jonathan M. Rubin, M.D., Ph.D.
Assistant Professor, Department of Radiology, and Chief of Ultrasound Services, University of Chicago Medical Center, Chicago, Illinois

Michael Salcman, M.D.
Professor and Head, Division of Neurological Surgery, University of Maryland School of Medicine, Baltimore, Maryland

Duke Samson, M.D.
Associate Professor and Vice Chairman, Division of Neurological Surgery, University of Texas Health Science Center at Dallas, Dallas, Texas

Richard L. Saunders, M.D.
Associate Professor of Clinical Surgery and Chairman, Section of Neurosurgery, Dartmouth-Hitchcock Medical Center, Hanover, New Hampshire

William M. Saunders, M.D., Ph.D.
Lawrence Berkeley Laboratory and Donner Laboratory, University of California, Berkeley, Berkeley, California

Timothy B. Scarff, M.D.
Associate Professor, Division of Neurological Surgery, Loyola University Medical Center, Maywood, Illinois

Robert A. Schindler, M.D.
Associate Professor, Department of Otolaryngology-Head and Neck Surgery, School of Medicine, University of California, San Francisco, San Francisco, California

Henry H. Schmidek, M.D.
Professor and Chairman, Section of Neurosurgery, University of Vermont College of Medicine, Burlington, Vermont

Frederick A. Schmitt, Ph.D.
Center for the Study of Aging and Human Development, Duke University Medical Center, Durham, North Carolina

Richard C. Schneider, M.D.
Professor Emeritus, Section of Neurosurgery, University of Michigan Medical Center, Ann Arbor, Michigan

S. Clifford Schold, Jr., M.D.
Assistant Professor, Division of Neurology, Duke University Medical Center, Durham, North Carolina

Luis Schut, M.D.
Chief, Neurosurgical Services, Children's Hospital of Philadelphia, Philadelphia, Pennsylvania

Hervey D. Segall, M.D.
Professor, Department of Radiology, University of Southern California School of Medicine, Los Angeles, California

Roy Selby, M.D.
La Crosse, Wisconsin

Edward L. Seljeskog, M.D., Ph.D.
Professor, Department of Neurosurgery, University of Minnesota Medical School, Minneapolis, Minnesota

Robert G. Selker, M.D.
Professor, Department of Neurological Surgery, School of Medicine, University of Pittsburgh, Pittsburgh, Pennsylvania

Warren Selman, M.D.
Assistant Professor, Division of Neurological Surgery, Case Western Reserve University School of Medicine, Cleveland, Ohio

Donald Serafin, M.D.
Professor, Division of Plastic and Maxillofacial Surgery, Duke University Medical Center, Durham, North Carolina

Bhagwan T. Shahani, M.D., D.Phil.(Oxon)
Department of Neurology and Clinical Neurophysiology Laboratory, Massachusetts General Hospital, Boston, Massachusetts

David G. Sherman, M.D.
Associate Professor, Division of Neurology, University of Texas Health Science Center at San Antonio, San Antonio, Texas

William A. Shucart, M.D.
Professor and Chairman, Department of Neurosurgery, Tufts-New England Medical Center, Boston, Massachusetts

List of Contributors

Gerald D. Silverberg, M.D.
Associate Professor, Division of Neurosurgery, Stanford University Medical Center, Stanford, California

Frederick A. Simeone, M.D.
Professor, Division of Neurosurgery, School of Medicine, University of Pennsylvania, Philadelphia, Pennsylvania

Marcia Sirotkin-Roses, M.A., L.P.T.
Division of Neurology and Department of Physical Therapy, Duke University Medical Center, Durham, North Carolina

Frederick H. Sklar, M.D.
Director of Pediatric Neurosurgery, Children's Medical Center, Dallas, Texas

Barry H. Smith, M.D., Ph.D.
Surgical Neurology Branch, National Institute of Neurological and Communicative Disorders and Stroke, Bethesda, Maryland

Robert R. Smith, M.D.
Professor and Chairman, Department of Neurosurgery, University of Mississippi Medical Center, Jackson, Mississippi

Frederick S. Southwick, M.D.
Assistant Professor of Medicine, Harvard Medical School, Boston, Massachusetts

Alexander M. Spence, M.D.
Associate Professor, Department of Medicine (Neurology), University of Washington School of Medicine, Seattle, Washington

Robert F. Spetzler, M.D.
J. N. Harber Foundation Chairman of Neurological Surgery, Barrow Neurological Institute, Phoenix, Arizona

Hans Jacob Steiger, M.D.
Clinical Fellow, Department of Neurological Surgery, University of Cincinnati Medical Center, Cincinnati, Ohio

Bennett M. Stein, M.D.
Byron Stookey Professor and Chairman, Department of Neurological Surgery, Columbia University College of Physicians & Surgeons, New York, New York

W. Eugene Stern, M.D.
Professor of Neurosurgery and Chairman, Department of Surgery, School of Medicine, University of California, Los Angeles, Los Angeles, California

Donald H. Stewart, Jr., M.D.
Clinical Assistant Professor, Department of Neurological Surgery, State University of New York, Upstate Medical Center, Syracuse, New York

Humbert G. Sullivan, M.D.
Associate Professor, Section of Neurosurgery, Medical College of Georgia, Augusta, Georgia

Narayan Sundaresan, M.D.
Assistant Attending Surgeon, Memorial Sloan-Kettering Cancer Center, New York, New York

Thoralf M. Sundt, Jr., M.D.
Professor and Chairman, Department of Neurologic Surgery, Mayo Clinic and Mayo Medical School, Rochester, Minnesota

Leslie N. Sutton, M.D.
Division of Neurosurgery, Children's Hospital of Philadelphia, Philadelphia, Pennsylvania

Morton N. Swartz, M.D.
Professor of Medicine, Harvard Medical School, and Chief, Infectious Disease Unit, Massachusetts General Hospital, Boston, Massachusetts

William H. Sweet, M.D., D.Sc., D.H.C.
Senior Neurosurgeon, Massachusetts General Hospital, Boston, Massachusetts

Ronald R. Tasker, M.D., F.R.C.S.(C)
Professor, Division of Neurosurgery, University of Toronto, Toronto, Ontario, Canada

Charles H. Tator, M.D., Ph.D., F.R.C.S.(C)
Professor, Division of Neurosurgery, University of Toronto, Toronto, Ontario, Canada

John M. Tew, Jr., M.D.
Professor and Chairman, Department of Neurological Surgery, University of Cincinnati Medical Center, Cincinnati, Ohio

Lawrence E. Thibault, Sc.D.
Assistant Professor of Bioengineering, University of Pennsylvania, Philadelphia, Pennsylvania

L. M. Thomas, M.D.
Professor and Chairman, Department of Neurosurgery, Wayne State University School of Medicine, Detroit, Michigan

Michael O. Thorner, M.B., M.R.C.P.
Professor, Department of Internal Medicine, University of Virginia Medical Center, Charlottesville, Virginia

Andrew L. Tievsky, M.D.
Assistant Professor, Department of Radiology, The George Washington University Medical Center, Washington, District of Columbia

George T. Tindall, M.D.
Professor and Chief, Division of Neurological Surgery, Emory University School of Medicine, Atlanta, Georgia

Suzie C. Tindall, M.D.
Assistant Professor, Division of Neurological Surgery, Emory University School of Medicine, Atlanta, Georgia

Cornelius A. Tobias, Ph.D.
Lawrence Berkeley Laboratory and Donner Laboratory, University of California, Berkeley, Berkeley, California

B. Tranmer, M.D.
Resident, Division of Neurosurgery, University of Toronto, Toronto, Ontario, Canada

Bruno J. Urban, M.D.
Professor, Department of Anesthesiology, Duke University Medical Center, Durham, North Carolina

John C. VanGilder, M.D.
Professor and Chairman, Division of Neurosurgery, University of Iowa Hospitals and Clinics, Iowa City, Iowa

William S. Velasquez, M.D.
Associate Professor, Department of Medicine, M.D. Anderson Hospital and Tumor Institute, Houston, Texs

Joan L. Venes, M.D.
Assistant Professor, Section of Neurosurgery, University of Michigan Medical Center, Ann Arbor, Michigan

Fernando Viñuela, M.D., F.R.C.P.(C)
Assistant Professor, Departments of Diagnostic Radiology and Clinical Neurological Sciences, University of Western Ontario, London, Ontario, Canada

F. Stephen Vogel, M.D.
Professor, Department of Pathology, Duke University Medical Center, Durham, North Carolina

Rand M. Voorhies, M.D.
Department of Neurosurgery, Ochsner Clinic, New Orleans, Louisiana

Jeffrey S. Walker, M.D.
Chief Resident, Division of Neurosurgery, Duke University Medical Center, Durham, North Carolina

Patrick D. Wall, M.D.
Professor, Department of Anatomy, University College London, London, England

Sidney Wallace, M.D.
Professor, Department of Diagnostic Radiology, M.D. Anderson Hospital and Tumor Institute, Houston, Texas

John W. Walsh, M.D., Ph.D.
Associate Professor, Division of Neurosurgery, University of Kentucky Medical Center, Lexington, Kentucky

Alan Waters, F.R.C.S.
Senior Registrar in Neurosurgery, New Addenbrooke's Hospital, Cambridge, England

Clark Watts, M.D.
Professor and Chief, Division of Neurosurgery, University of Missouri-Columbia Health Sciences Center, Columbia, Missouri

David D. Weaver, M.D.
Associate Professor, Department of Medical Genetics, Indiana University School of Medicine, Indianapolis, Indiana

George D. Webster, M. B., F.R.C.S.
Associate Professor, Division of Urologic Surgery, Duke University Medical Center, Durham, North Carolina

Vivian D. Weigel, B.S.
Department of Otolaryngology-Head and Neck Surgery, School of Medicine, University of California, San Francisco, San Francisco, California

Richard L. Weiner, M.D.
Assistant Professor, Division of Neurosurgery, University of Texas Medical Branch, Galveston, Texas

Meredith A. Weinstein, M.D.
Section of Neuroradiology, Division of Radiology, The Cleveland Clinic Foundation, Cleveland, Ohio

Philip R. Weinstein, M.D.
Professor and Vice Chairman, Department of Neurological Surgery, School of Medicine, University of California, San Francisco, San Francisco, California

Bryce Weir, M.D., M.Sc., F.R.C.S.(C)
Clinical Professor and Director, Division of Neurosurgery, University of Alberta, Edmonton, Alberta, Canada

Leonard Weiss, M.D.
Director, Department of Experimental Pathology, Roswell Park Memorial Institute, Buffalo, New York

Martin H. Weiss, M.D.
Professor and Chairman, Department of Neurological Surgery, University of Southern California School of Medicine, Los Angeles, California

Frank A. Welsh, Ph.D.
Associate Professor of Biochemistry, Division of Neurosurgery, School of Medicine, University of Pennsylvania, Philadelphia, Pennsylvania

James Gardner Wepsic, M.D.
New England Baptist Hospital, Boston, Massachusetts

Augustus A. White, III, M.D., D.Med.Sci.
Professor of Orthopaedic Surgery, Harvard Medical School; Surgeon-in-Chief, Department of Orthopaedic Surgery, Beth Israel Hospital, Boston, Massachusetts

Richard J. Whitley, M.D.
Professor, Department of Pediatrics, School of Medicine, University of Alabama in Birmingham, Birmingham, Alabama

Asa J. Wilbourn, M.D.
Department of Neurology, Cleveland Clinic Foundation, Cleveland, Ohio

Robert H. Wilkins, M.D.
Professor and Chief, Division of Neurosurgery, Duke University Medical Center, Durham, North Carolina

Phillip Earle Williams, Jr., M.D.
Clinical Associate Professor, Division of Neurological Surgery, University of Texas Health Science Center at Dallas, Dallas, Texas

Charles B. Wilson, M.D.
Professor and Chairman, Department of Neurological Surgery, School of Medicine, University of California, San Francisco, San Francisco, California

William P. Wilson, M.D.
Professor, Department of Psychiatry, Duke University Medical Center, Durham, North Carolina

Ken R. Winston, M.D.
Senior Associate in Neurosurgery, The Children's Hospital, Boston, Massachusetts

Hugh S. Wisoff, M.D.
Associate Professor and Acting Chairman, Leo M. Davidoff Department of Neurological Surgery, Albert Einstein College of Medicine, Bronx, New York

James H. Wood, M.D.
Assistant Professor, Division of Neurological Surgery, Emory University School of Medicine, Atlanta, Georgia

Kay Woodruff
Lawrence Berkeley Laboratory and Donner Laboratory, University of California, Berkeley, Berkeley, California

Robert M. Worth, M.D.
Section of Neurological Surgery, Indiana University School of Medicine, Indianapolis, Indiana

Richard Jed Wyatt, M.D.
Chief, Adult Psychiatry Branch, National Institute of Mental Health, Saint Elizabeth's Hospital, Washington, District of Columbia

Isao Yamamoto, M.D.
Department of Neurosurgery, University of Florida Health Center, Gainesville, Florida

Howard Yonas, M.D.
Associate Professor, Department of Neurological Surgery, School of Medicine, University of Pittsburgh, Pittsburgh, Pennsylvania

Junji Yoshioka, M.D.
Mississippi Heart Association Fellow, University of Mississippi Medical Center, Jackson, Mississippi

Byron Young, M.D.
Professor and Chairman, Division of Neurosurgery, University of Kentucky Medical Center, Lexington, Kentucky

Harold F. Young, M.D.
Professor, Division of Neurological Surgery, Medical College of Virginia, Virginia Commonwealth University, Richmond, Virginia

List of Contributors

Ronald F. Young, M.D.
Professor, Division of Neurosurgery, School of Medicine, University of California, Los Angeles, Los Angeles, California

Joseph Zabramski, M.D.
Resident, Division of Neurological Surgery, Barrow Neurological Institute, Phoenix, Arizona

Chi-Shing Zee, M.D.
Assistant Professor, Department of Radiology, University of Southern California School of Medicine, Los Angeles, California

Nicholas T. Zervas, M.D.
Professor of Surgery, Harvard Medical School, and Chief, Neurosurgical Service, Massachusetts General Hospital, Boston, Massachusetts

Robert A. Zimmerman, M.D.
Professor, Department of Radiology, Hospital of the University of Pennsylvania, Philadelphia, Pennsylvania

Sandra Zink
Lawrence Berkeley Laboratory and Donner Laboratory, University of California, Berkeley, Berkeley, California

FOREWORD

Drs. Wilkins and Rengachary are neurosurgeons; they have written original papers; they have trained residents; and they keep up with current developments. I can think of no two better qualified to be the editors of this text.

Drs. Wilkins and Rengachary have obviously thought long and hard about this project, for they have covered all aspects of the field of neurosurgery in a comprehensive manner. Their talents for knowing the best authors to write the various sections, and for assembling and editing the material without incurring wrath, and for doing all that while remaining active in neurosurgery, are nothing short of impressive.

The introductory chapters dealing with neurosurgical history which begin this three-volume text, with the delightful authoritative section on Cushing and Dandy by Dr. Bucy (who was there), are themselves valuable contributions. But there is more, much more. Almost all details of neurosurgery and all of the neurosciences as they relate to neurosurgery are included. This text is not for the referring physician or the occasional surgeon. It is for the student, the graduate student, the neurosurgery resident, and the practicing neurosurgeon the world over. It will answer most questions on a given subject or refer the reader to the proper authority on that subject.

To have been asked to write this foreword is an honor, for this text is indeed an awesome compilation of neurosurgical knowledge.

Eben Alexander, Jr., M.D.

PREFACE

Advances in neurological surgery are occurring at such a rapid pace that attempts to capture a static image of the subject give a blurred picture at best. Ever-new diagnostic methodologies, advances in treatment, refinements in surgical technique, improvements in surgical instrumentation, and breakthroughs in the basic understanding of disease processes overwhelm even the most enthusiastic neurosurgeon. It has become impossible for any single individual to keep pace with all the advances and to be adept in all the techniques. We have thus resorted to a multiauthored text for a broad contemporary overview of the subject that is as up to date as we could make it.

The book is directed toward a wide readership, including residents in training in neurological surgery and neurosurgeons in an academic setting or in community practice. Since it is a reference text, medical students and specialists in related fields may find it useful as well.

Certain aspects of this text that reflect the philosophy of the editors deserve emphasis:

It deals with established as well as evolving aspects of neurological surgery. The reader will find such mundane topics as cranial nerve examination interspersed with esoteric ones like central nervous system grafting.

Subjects such as neuroradiology and neuropathology, which often are discussed in isolation in the beginning chapters of a text, are interwoven with related clinical material. This permits a meaningful correlation between clinical, radiographic, and pathological features instead of simply providing minitexts on neuroradiology or neuropathology.

An appropriate blend of "bench" and "bedside" is maintained. For example, in Part VI, which deals with neuro-oncology, each section begins with a discussion concerning the pathology of a tumor by a neuropathologist with particular interest in that area.

A judicious balance of basic and clinical sciences is kept throughout the book, and the historical aspects of neurological surgery are presented, especially in the beginning of the book. We hope that the historical material will be both informative and inspirational to our readers.

Clinical examination of the nervous system with correlated neuroanatomy is discussed in some depth, reflecting our conviction that newer diagnostic methodologies, however promising they may appear, will assist but can never replace the human mind.

To conserve space, the reference list at the end of most chapters is not comprehensive but contains the most pertinent and, to the extent possible, the most recent references. Any student exploring a particular topic in depth will be able to use the list as a good starting point for a search of the literature.

Important topics dealing with certain social, ethical, and legal issues, which are generally ignored in standard texts, are included in this work.

The contributors have been encouraged to follow their individual styles in writing and presentation to avoid monotony in exposition.

Finally, we have strived, wherever possible, to allow only healthy overlap, not undue repetition, throughout the text.

We thank all the contributors who volunteered to share their time, knowledge, and expertise, and especially Dr. Eben Alexander, Jr. who prepared the foreword and Dr. Eugene S. Flamm, who provided the historical woodcuts that introduce the various parts of the text. We also thank Mrs. Gloria K. Wilkins and Mrs. Yvonne Ellis for providing secretarial help, Mrs. Paula N. Ecklund for reading the proof, and Mrs. Elizabeth Adams and Mr. David K. Donlon for checking all of the references in the Duke Medical Center Library. Finally, we express our appreciation for the people at the McGraw-Hill Book Company, especially Mr. Stuart Boynton, Mr. Robert P. McGraw, and Mr. Robert E. McGrath, who enthusiastically supported this project from its very inception and worked very hard to complete it within the shortest possible time.

Robert H. Wilkins, M.D.
Setti S. Rengachary, M.D.

Part VII Vascular Diseases of the Nervous System

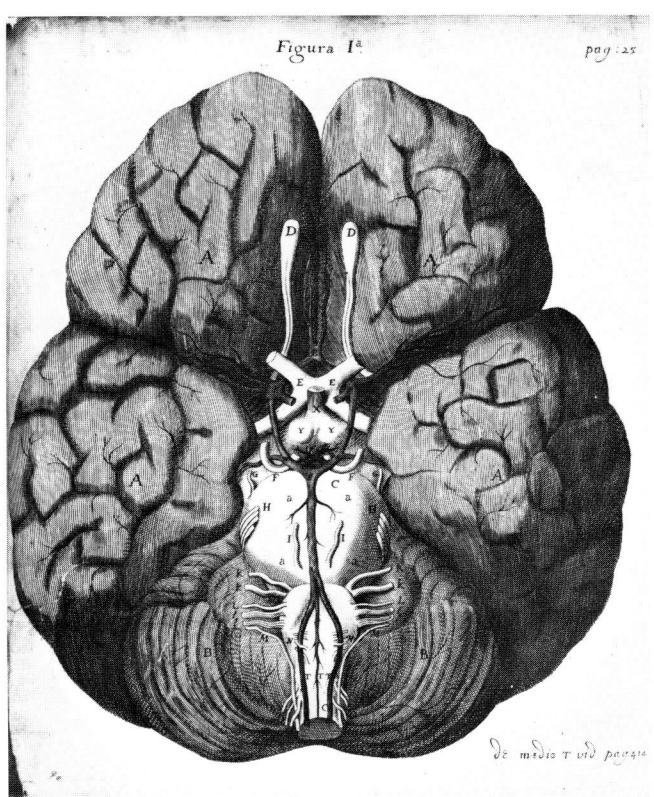

Willis T. *Cerebri Anatome*. London, Martyn & Allestry, 1664. An engraving of the base of the brain by Christopher Wren, illustrating the circle of Willis.

SECTION A
Occlusive Cerebrovascular Disease

139

Cerebral Blood Flow

Thomas W. Langfitt
Walter D. Obrist

Maintenance of adequate cerebral blood flow (CBF), globally or regionally, in patients with intracranial lesions is one of the major challenges of neurosurgery. In occlusive strokes, intracranial hemorrhage, head injury, and brain tumors, and in the course of intracranial surgery for most any condition, the final common pathway of irreversible brain damage is cerebral ischemia. Therefore, an understanding of the physiology of normal and impaired CBF is essential to proper understanding of the pathophysiology of most of the intracranial conditions that we are called upon to manage as neurosurgeons.

Control of CBF

Anatomy and Physiology of Cerebral Vessels

Large and medium-size arteries such as the intracranial carotid arteries and their branches are often referred to as *windkessel vessels*, which divide into the principal resistance vessels, the small arteries and arterioles. Together, all of these vessels constitute the precapillary resistance vessels, which with the capillary bed provide approximately 80 percent of the total resistance to blood flow through the intracranial space. The venules and veins provide the remaining 20 percent of the resistance. Precapillary sphincter vessels are primarily responsible for distributing blood to the capillary bed, and the true capillaries are the exchange vessels of the organ. The arteriole is 30 to 40 µm in diameter, is generally long and coiled, and gives off numerous side branches.

These branches are metarterioles, which are 20 to 30 µm in diameter and consist of an endothelial cell and a thin layer of smooth muscle. The muscle layer becomes discontinuous and disappears in the terminal arteriole. In many tissues, the terminal arteriole continues as a thoroughfare channel that can be followed through the capillary bed to the venous side. Side branches from terminal arterioles, metarterioles, and thoroughfare channels are of particular functional significance. They are 15 to 20 µm in diameter and branch off the parent vessel at acute angles. The region of the bifurcation is surrounded by smooth muscle and is called the *precapillary sphincter*. The sphincters are responsible for regulating the flow of blood to the capillary bed proper.

The capillaries are the principal exchange vessels of the microcirculation. The diameter of the capillary is about 6 µm, slightly smaller than a red blood cell. In the brain, the endothelial cells, which form the wall of the capillary, are tightly approximated to each other, forming a junction that does not permit even the smallest molecule to pass through. This junction constitutes the anatomical blood-brain barrier.

The fall in pressure from the cervical portion of the internal carotid artery to the origin of the middle cerebral artery is about 5 percent of the aortic pressure, and the fall in pressure across the middle cerebral artery from its origin to the larger pial arteries is 15 to 40 percent of aortic pressure. An additional fall in pressure of 15 to 20 percent of aortic pressure occurs from the larger pial arteries to arterioles 25 µm in diameter. This cascade of blood through the resistance vessels and the capillary bed results in a subarachnoid venous pressure of approximately 35 torr. In other studies in which techniques were used to measure pressure in the smallest elements of the microcirculation, the total vascular resistance between the aorta and the cerebral veins was shown to be divided into 39 percent resistance in the large arteries, 21 percent in the pial vessels, and the remaining 40 percent within the intracerebral vessels.[13]

Normally the cerebral vessels have a high degree of resting vasomotor tone. Maintenance of the tone is provided by the arterial CO$_2$ tension (Pa$_{CO_2}$) and by the normal extracellular potassium concentration of 3 mmol. In recent years much attention has been directed toward defining the importance of prostaglandin and arachidonic acid derivatives in the control of the cerebral vessels in normal and pathological circumstances.[9] Prostaglandins are synthesized from arachidonic acid, and the synthesis is inhibited by anti-inflammatory agents such as indomethacin and aspirin. The cyclic endoperoxides and thromboxane A$_2$ are short-lived derivatives of arachidonic acid. Cerebral arteries are capable of synthesizing large quantities of prostaglandins, and prostaglandins maintain the tone of several smooth muscle preparations. Tone is reduced by the addition of indomethacin. These observations on smooth muscle were supplemented by the demonstration that indomethacin reduces CBF without a change in cerebral metabolic rate of O_2 utilization ($CMRO_2$). Indomethacin also severely impairs the cerebral vascular response to changes in Pa_{CO_2}.

Autoregulation to Changes in Perfusion Pressure

When the systemic arterial pressure falls or when there is an occlusion, partial or complete, of a major cerebral artery, the cerebral resistance vessels dilate in an attempt to maintain normal blood flow in the face of the fall in perfusion pressure. When the systemic arterial pressure increases, cerebral vessels constrict in order to maintain blood flow constant. This phenomenon is termed *autoregulation* and is sometimes referred to as *pressure autoregulation*. It must be distinguished from the changes in CBF produced by changes in cerebral metabolism termed *metabolic regulation*.

If the systemic arterial pressure is lowered or raised quickly, cerebral blood flow falls or increases passively with the change in arterial pressure. Blood flow then returns to the control value within a few seconds when autoregulation is intact. When autoregulation is impaired, but still present, the adjustment of blood flow is slower and less complete, and when autoregulation is absent, blood flow passively follows changes in systemic arterial pressure. Thus, autoregulation is a quantitative, measurable variable in the control of the cerebral circulation and not an all-or-none phenomenon.

The lower limit of autoregulation to changes in mean systemic arterial pressure is approximately 50 torr; the upper limit is about 160 torr. This means that as the arterial pressure is decreased, the resistance vessels dilate until they are maximally dilated in response to the decreased perfusion pressure. At a mean pressure of about 50 torr, blood flow declines steeply with a further decrease in pressure. When arterial pressure is increased, the vessels constrict until the mean arterial pressure exceeds 160 torr, at which point the pressure head breaks through the vasoconstriction, causing passive dilatation and an increase in cerebral blood flow. Vital dyes usually enter the brain parenchyma at the moment of breakthrough, manifesting disruption of the blood-brain barrier. Presumably, this is a pressure phenomenon within capillaries and small veins: the barrier leaks because of a sudden distension of vessels within the microcirculation. If autoregulation is impaired by hypoxia, hypercarbia, or minimal blunt trauma to the exposed surface of the brain, and the blood pressure is then raised quickly, not only is there extravasation of protein-bound dyes into the brain, but the brain swells acutely and often massively.[3]

The term *autoregulation* implies that the mechanism is intrinsic to the vascular bed of the brain and suggests a smooth muscle reflex somewhere within the system of resistance vessels. According to this myogenic hypothesis, the resistance vessels have a high degree of resting vasoconstrictor tone due mainly to smooth muscle contraction of the walls. An increase in intraluminal pressure stimulates a further increase in tone by stretching the muscle and causing a reactive shortening of radial fibers and a reduction in vascular diameter. A decrease in intraluminal pressure has the opposite effect.

Figure 139-1, taken from a paper by Miller and colleagues,[6] demonstrates the normal curve of autoregulation in the dog and a population of abnormal autoregulatory responses in a series of dogs submitted to a period of cerebral hypoxia that had been demonstrated to impair autoregulation. In each instance CBF rises passively with increases in the systemic arterial pressure, but there are large differences, amounting to severalfold, in CBF at normal pressure. Thus, when autoregulation is impaired, not only does CBF

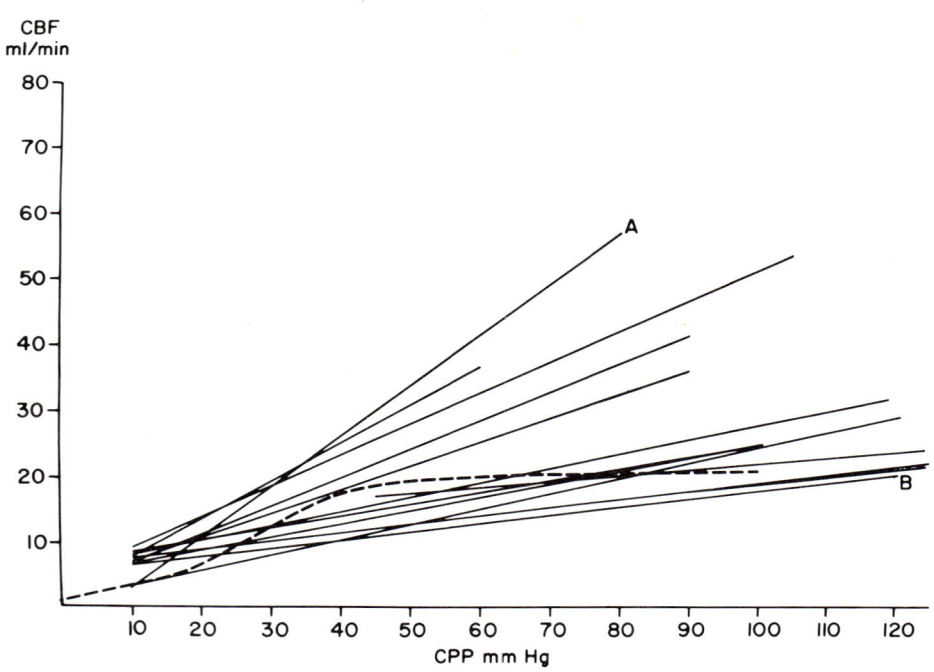

Figure 139-1 Plot of regression lines obtained from individual pressure/flow graphs obtained from animals with defective autoregulation (AR) to show the wide variation in CBF values with increased cerebral perfusion pressure (CPP). The dashed line indicates the mean flow for dogs with intact autoregulation. (From Miller et al.[6])

passively follow changes in perfusion pressure, the resting diameter of the resistance vessels is also altered. This point is particularly important because of its implications for therapy. Nearly always the CO₂ responsivity of cerebral vessels is still intact when autoregulation is impaired. Therefore, in the animals illustrated in Fig. 139-1, hyperventilation ought to cause a decrease in CBF, because the hypoxic insult was not very severe. Because the CBF in animal A at normotension is so high, even though autoregulation is grossly impaired, hyperventilation to very low levels of Pa_{CO_2} could be induced without risk of cerebral ischemia. In contrast, CBF at normotension is below normal in animal B, and therefore, even moderate hypocarbia might plunge the brain into ischemia. To summarize, the level of CBF at normal blood pressure is as important a determinant of the risk of brain ischemia when autoregulation is impaired as is the fact that autoregulation is defective.

According to the myogenic hypothesis, the stimulus to autoregulation is not, in fact, a change in intraluminal pressure but a change in the transmural pressure across the vasoactive vessels. It follows then that an alteration in transmural pressure produced by raising intracranial pressure (ICP) rather than lowering the intraluminal pressure ought to have the same effect.[6] Figure 139-2 illustrates the fact that the cerebral vessels do autoregulate with an increase in ICP in much the same way that they autoregulate with a decrease in systemic arterial pressure. In this series of experiments CBF did not begin to decline until the perfusion pressure, defined as the difference between the mean arterial pressure and mean ICP, had fallen to about 40 torr, compared with a threshold of about 50 torr when systemic arterial pressure was lowered.

Metabolic Regulation

A distinction must be made between alterations in the diameters of cerebral resistance vessels produced by changes in either intraluminal or extraluminal pressure and changes in vascular diameter produced by alterations in the demand of the cerebral tissue for oxygen and glucose. Normally there is tight coupling between the demands of cerebral tissue for oxygen and glucose and the volume of blood flowing through that tissue. As metabolism increases, during seizures, for example, local blood flow at the site of the seizure increases, and when metabolism decreases, as in hypothermia, blood flow decreases. This association is termed *metabolic regulation*. Although for many years there has been strong circumstantial evidence for the existence of metabolic regulation, it was not until the development of the [¹⁴C]-deoxyglucose method for measuring glucose uptake in autoradiographs of the brain, and subsequently the simultaneous measurements of glucose metabolism and local blood flow in the same region using the [¹⁴C]iodoantipyrine method, that this relationship was proven.[12]

There is general agreement that one or more chemical substances are responsible for the tight coupling between metabolism and flow. Most commonly the hydrogen ion has been held to be that substance. According to the hypothesis, increased metabolism results in the accumulation of hydrogen ions in the extracellular space, and this produces vasodilatation. When metabolism decreases to the prior level, the hydrogen ions are washed away and the cerebral vessels constrict to their former diameter. There is recent evidence, using pH microelectrodes, that the hydrogen ion may not be the only causal agent. Potassium and adenosine have also been invoked as causes.

Hypoxia and Changes in Pa_{CO_2}

Systemic hypoxemia causes dilatation of cerebral vessels and an increase in CBF. The purpose of the vascular dilatation is to increase blood flow to the brain at a time when the volume of oxygen per unit volume of blood has been reduced. As long as the increase in blood flow compensates for the reduction in the oxygen content of the blood, the oxygen needs of the brain are met, and the brain continues to metabolize normally. When Pa_{O_2} decreases to approximately 20 torr, the stimulus to vasodilatation has become maximum, and a further reduction of Pa_{O_2} leads to anaerobic glycolysis and a decrease in oxidative phosphorylation, the principal manifestations of metabolic derangement secondary to hypoxia or ischemia.[11]

The most common explanation for hypoxic vasodilatation has been chemical regulation through alterations in the composition of the extracellular space. According to this hypothesis, even a slight reduction in tissue P_{O_2} induces lac-

Figure 139-2 Effect of altering cerebral perfusion pressure (CPP) by decreasing arterial pressure (*open circles*) and by increasing intracranial pressure (*closed circles*) in dogs with intact autoregulation. Significance of variation between the changes was assessed by paired t test. (From Miller et al.[6])

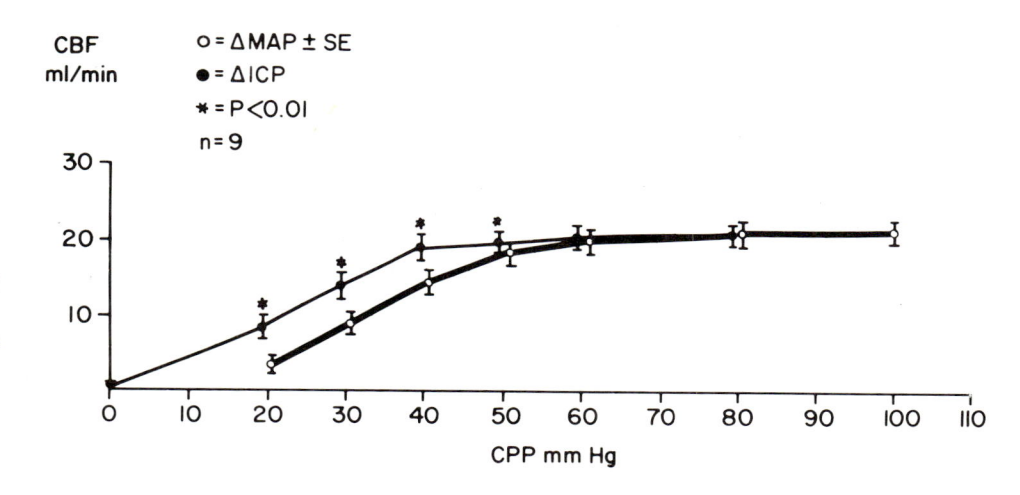

tic acidosis, which produces the dilatation. Although acidosis may contribute, it cannot be the primary cause of vasodilatation, because lactic acid does not appear until many seconds after CBF has increased. There is increasing evidence that adenosine is the substance most likely responsible for hypoxic vasodilatation.[14]

The most potent stimulus to cerebral vasodilatation is an increase in Pa_{CO_2}. Teleologically, the reason for the vasodilatation is to prevent the fall in extracellular pH that would be inevitable if CBF did not increase. The mechanism whereby changes in CO_2 alter vascular diameters is still not well understood. Since a change in Pa_{CO_2} is also detected by the peripheral arterial chemoreceptors, a reflex pathway could be the mediator. There have been several experimental observations to support this hypothesis, especially the finding that lesions in the tegmental reticular formation reduce or abolish the cerebral vascular response to changes in Pa_{CO_2}.[10] Alternatively, CO_2 and/or the hydrogen ion may act directly upon vascular smooth muscle.

Neurogenic Control

For a long time it has been known that the cerebral resistance vessels are densely supplied with sympathetic nerve endings. However, neither stimulation nor ablation of the sympathetic fibers has been demonstrated to have very much effect on CBF. Therefore, the conventional wisdom has been that CBF is almost entirely chemically controlled despite the presence of so many nerves on the cerebral vessels.

It is now clear that, in several circumstances, sympathetic nerves play a significant role in the control of the cerebral circulation. Stimulation of the superior cervical ganglion, the origin of the sympathetic innervation of the cerebral vessels, shifts the autoregulatory curve to the right. Thus, the ability of the resistance vessels to dilate when the intraluminal pressure is decreased is impaired by stimulation of the sympathetic nerves, and, of equal importance, sympathetic hyperactivity raises the threshold for the breakthrough of autoregulation that occurs with arterial hypertension. Since there is much evidence that the brain swelling characterized as hypertensive encephalopathy is due to a breakthrough of autoregulation and, probably, increased permeability of the blood-brain barrier, sympathetic hyperactivity protects against this complication of malignant hypertension. There is also evidence that in chronic hypertension the sympathetic discharge leads to cerebral vascular hypertrophy.

Cerebral vasodilator mechanisms are not as well understood as the sympathetic effects. In early studies, brain stem stimulation produced large increases in CBF that were still present when the arterial hypertension that usually accompanied the stimulation was abolished by sectioning the cervical spinal cord.[2] Also, the sites of stimulation were well removed from the facial nerve, which is known to carry some vasodilator fibers to the cerebral hemispheres.

There is evidence that cerebral arteries contain high levels of acetylcholine, but as was true with the sympathetic system until recent years, there still is not clear evidence that acetylcholine is an important transmitter for cerebral vasodilatation during neural stimulation. Altogether some 15 peptides have been found in cerebral vessels, but their contributions to the regulation of CBF are unknown.

Several studies have purported to demonstrate that vasomotor nerve fibers originating in the brain stem project diffusely to the cerebral hemispheres, then leave the brain parenchyma to innervate resistance vessels. The locus ceruleus has received particular attention as the source of these fibers. Despite the many reports on the subject, there is not clear morphological evidence for brain stem innervation of resistance vessels. The reader is referred to two reviews of the rapidly evolving field of neurogenic control of the cerebral circulation.[1,8]

Clinical Measurements of CBF and Brain Metabolism

Techniques for measuring CBF and the cerebral metabolic rates of O_2 ($CMRO_2$) and glucose (CMRGl) utilization are described in another chapter. The purpose of this section is to make some general comments about clinical CBF measurements and emphasize the importance of measuring $CMRO_2$ along with CBF whenever possible.

In the past 20 years the large majority of CBF studies of neurosurgical patients have been performed using the ^{133}Xe methodology developed by Lassen and Ingvar.[5] For many years the ^{133}Xe was administered by injection of a bolus of the isotope into a catheter in the internal carotid artery. The disadvantages of the technique were its invasiveness and the fact that CBF could be recorded from only one hemisphere at a time. Now most CBF laboratories around the world are using the inhalation or intravenous ^{133}Xe technique.[7]

The various systems available contain from a few to several hundred scintillation detectors. The isotope clearance curve from each detector is biexponential. The fast component is gray matter flow, and this is about four times the slower component, which is white matter flow. Usually CBF is expressed as mean flow, which in normal subjects is 53 ± 10 ml/100 g per minute, the same value obtained with the Kety-Schmidt nitrous oxide technique.

When highly oxygenated arterial blood enters the capillary bed, the amount of O_2 extracted is a function of the rate of metabolism of the brain cells supplied by that capillary bed. Therefore, the difference in O_2 content between the arterial and cerebral venous blood ($AVDO_2$) provides an estimate of $CMRO_2$. However, if $CMRO_2$ remains constant and CBF decreases, more O_2 will be extracted from each milliliter of blood passing through the capillary bed, and therefore, the O_2 content of cerebral venous blood falls, now because of a change in CBF rather than a change in $CMRO_2$. This means that when venous O_2 changes one cannot tell whether it is due to a change in metabolism or a change in flow without measuring CBF. It follows that $CMRO_2$, expressed as milliliters of O_2 utilized per hundred grams of brain per minute, can be calculated by multiplying mean CBF times $AVDO_2$. The range of normal for $CMRO_2$ in human beings is 3.0 to 3.5 ml/100 g per minute. In many clinical conditions that have been studied with CBF and $CMRO_2$ measurements, such as coma from head injury and other causes, $CMRO_2$ often remains quite constant over long periods of time whereas CBF changes frequently in response to a variety of stimuli, including various forms of therapy. In this circumstance measurements of AVDO$_2$, which can be performed in most any hospital, in contrast to CBF, which requires expensive equipment, provides a good estimate of CBF.

As noted in the previous section, when metabolic regulation is intact, CBF follows changes in CMRO$_2$. Metabolic regulation is impaired most notably in brain ischemia. Presumably products of the ischemic process, such as the H$^+$ ion or adenosine, produce vasodilatation that overrides the metabolic control of the cerebral vessels, resulting in hyperemia. The term *luxury perfusion*[4] is also used to describe this situation, meaning simply that the amount of blood flowing through the tissue is in excess of its metabolic needs.

The term *vasomotor paralysis*[3] was coined to describe the abnormal situation in which both autoregulation to changes in perfusion pressure and the responses of the vessels to changes in Pa$_{CO_2}$ are abolished. Metabolic regulation also disappears, and the normally vasoactive vessels are paralyzed to all stimuli. In addition, the cerebrovascular bed dilates passively because of loss of myogenic tone in the resistance vessels, and as the dilatation occurs, the arterial pressure head is transmitted downstream into the capillary bed and venous system. When dilatation of the cerebrovascular bed is maximum, the difference in pressure between the carotid artery and the dural sinuses may be only a few torr. The brain swells massively under these circumstances, resulting in a rise of ICP to the level of the cerebral venous pressure and, in the final stage of decompensation, to the level of the carotid artery pressure. CBF ceases because of collapse of the cerebral veins at their junction with the dural sinuses and, for the most part, of the sinuses themselves. The perfusion pressure across the intracranial space, from the carotid artery to the jugular vein, may be normal, but CBF ceases because the collapse of the cerebral veins creates an essentially infinite resistance to blood flow.

If a craniotomy is performed under these circumstances, the brain swells through the craniotomy defect, sometimes with rupture of the pia and extrusion of brain substance into the operative field. This malignant swelling that has plagued neurosurgeons since the earliest days of our specialty is the end stage of vasomotor paralysis, which can be initiated by ischemia, hypoxemia, or mechanical trauma to the brain.

In other pathological conditions, the response of the cerebral circulation is a decrease in CBF rather than hyperemia. In neurosurgery, a reduction in CBF resulting in cerebral ischemia occurs most notably in brain adjacent to an expanding mass lesion and globally throughout the brain when ICP exceeds the autoregulatory capacity of the cerebral vessels or when ICP increases only moderately but autoregulation is defective. When a mass lesion such as a subdural hematoma expands rapidly, tissue pressure in brain subjacent to the mass increases, and a pressure gradient is created across the brain. Blood flow through the compressed brain is now determined mainly by the difference between pressure in the small arteries supplying that region of brain and the tissue pressure, not ICP measured from a lateral ventricle or the subarachnoid space. Tissue pressure becomes the denominator in calculating the perfusion pressure. In the presence of a rapidly expanding mass, a large region of brain adjacent to the mass may be plunged into ischemia at a time when ICP is little elevated.

CBF and Metabolism in Head-Injured Patients

Among patients managed by neurosurgeons, CBF has been studied most frequently, in descending order, in occlusive stroke, head injury, subarachnoid hemorrhage, and brain tumors. For several years we and our colleagues have studied the cerebral circulation and brain metabolism in patients with acute, severe head injuries in an attempt to better understand the pathophysiology of head injury and to determine whether the studies could be used to guide treatment and to evaluate various forms of therapy.

To date we have measured CBF in over 100 patients, from shortly following admission to the hospital to death or maximum recovery, using the ^{133}Xe intravenous technique. CMRO$_2$ was measured in about two-thirds of the patients. It is calculated from the product of AVDO$_2$ (cerebral venous blood is obtained from a catheter in the jugular bulb) and the mean flow for sixteen probes, eight over each hemisphere. Following discharge from the hospital, patients were brought back on an outpatient basis for repeat CBF measurements, at which time they also received a neurological examination and a battery of neuropsychological tests.

Among a total of 112 patients studied, 37 patients were excluded because either they were not comatose (generally defined as a Glasgow coma score of more than 8), the first study occurred 96 h or more after the injury, the patient had a penetrating rather than a closed head injury, the patient was determined to be brain dead, or finally, the patient was already in deep barbiturate coma at the time of the first study. Among the remaining 75 patients included in the study, the average Glasgow coma score at the time of the first CBF measurement was 6.2 ± 1.7. Two-thirds of the patients were studied during the first 24 h following admission.

The CBF findings permitted division of the patients into two distinct and nearly equal categories. Just over half of the patients had hyperemia, defined as a mean CBF for all 16 detectors that was increased relative to the decreased metabolism of all the patients. Figure 139-3 illustrates the two groups. In patients with reduced flow there is a good correlation between CBF and CMRO$_2$, demonstrating essentially intact metabolic regulation. In contrast, in the patients with hyperemia there is no relationship between CBF and metabolism, and in some cases CBF is several times the metabolic needs of the tissue.

Table 139-1 demonstrates some of the consequences of hyperemia in head-injured patients. Diffuse cerebral swelling on CT scan, defined as slitlike or absent ventricles and perimesencephalic cisterns, was present in nearly half of the patients with hyperemia but only a fifth of the patients with reduced flow. We have postulated that the diffuse swelling is secondary to the hyperemia, the actual increase in brain bulk being due to either increased cerebral blood volume or to a combination of increased blood volume and superimposed edema. As might be expected from the relative incidence of diffuse swelling, ICP was elevated twice as often in the hyperemic patients as in those patients with reduced flow.

As a general statement, in head-injured patients global changes in CBF override regional changes. Also, improvements in CBF over time correlate well with clinical improve-

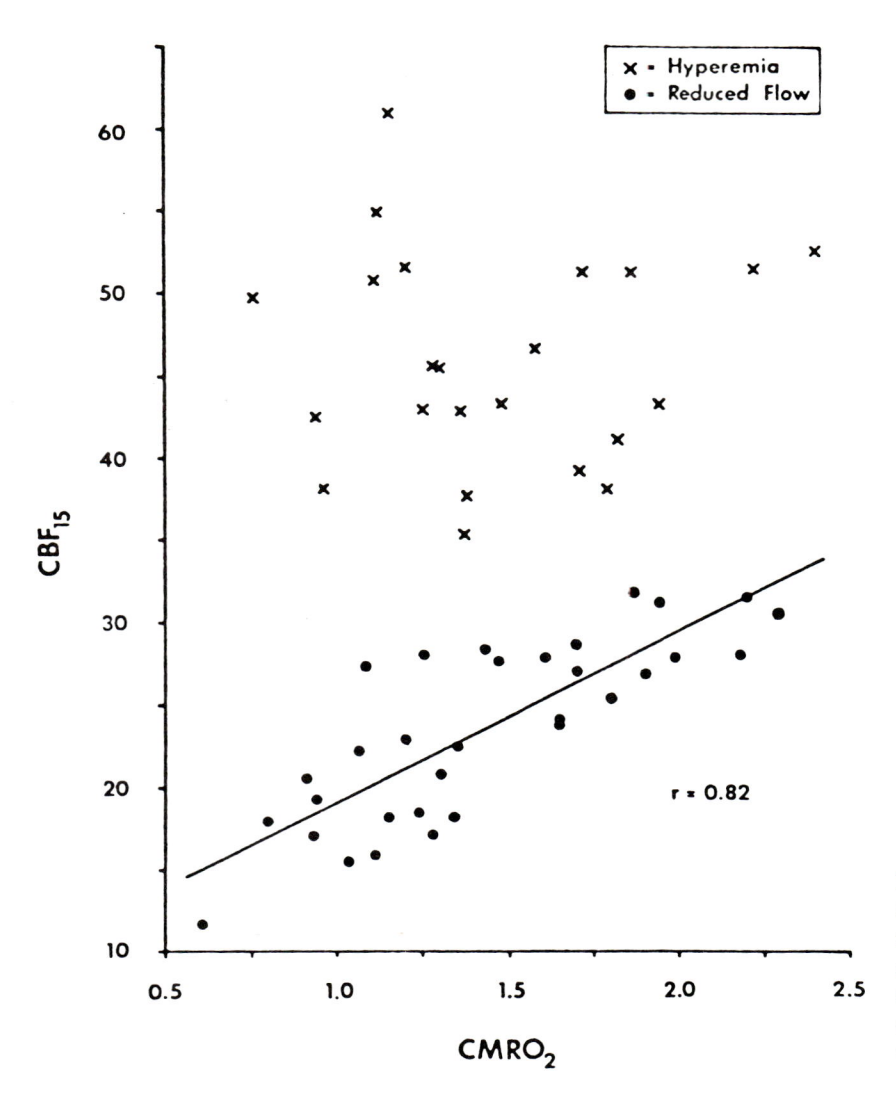

Figure 139-3 CBF plotted against CMRO$_2$ in a series of comatose head-injured patients. The reduced flow group shows coupling between CBF and metabolism ($r = 0.82$), which is absent in the hyperemic group ($r = 0.03$).

ment of the patient. These observations are summarized in Table 139-2. In 30 cases followed for a period of at least 6 months after injury, there were no instances of persistent hyperemia. One-quarter of the patients still had a generalized reduction in CBF, which correlated well with their neurological status. Some hemispheral or regional asymmetry was present in the majority of patients during the acute phase, but as noted above, generalized alterations in CBF were more prominent. The reason that the figures for hyperemia and CBF reduction add up to more than 100 percent is because many patients pass through periods of both increased and decreased flow during the first week of their illness. Normally blood flow in the frontal lobes is higher than in the occipital lobes, but during coma the anterior-posterior gradient was reversed in a number of the patients.

TABLE 139-1 Incidence of Elevated Intracranial Pressure and Diffuse Cerebral Swelling: Comparison of Two Groups Classified by Cerebral Blood Flow

	Percent of Cases*	
CBF Group	ICP > 20 mmHg	Diffuse Swelling (CT)
Acute hyperemia ($N = 28$)	57%	46%
Reduced flow ($N = 30$)	23%	23%
Total sample ($N = 58$)	40%	34%

*The groups differed significantly in both ICP elevation ($p < 0.01$) and diffuse swelling ($p < 0.05$).

Conclusion

Under normal conditions the cerebral circulation is exquisitely regulated to the metabolic needs of the brain. That metabolic linkage is severed by changes in Pa$_{CO_2}$, by the sympathetic nervous system in select circumstances, by hypoxia and ischemia, which produce hyperemia, and by brain compression and increased intracranial pressure. Regional hyperemia is often accompanied by brain swelling in that region, and global hyperemia may lead to diffuse brain swelling and intracranial hypertension. The ratio of CBF to CMRO$_2$ ought to be an important guide to therapy in patients with intracranial hypertension. For example, hyperventilation is a more logical treatment of hyperemia than is

TABLE 139-2 Regional Cerebral Blood Flow Analysis of Severely Head-Injured Patients

CBF Findings*	Percent of 30 Cases	
	Acute and Subacute	6- to 12-Month Follow-Up
Generalized hyperemia	57	0
Generalized CBF reduction	90	27
Hemispheral or regional asymmetry	70	17
Reverse anterior-posterior gradient	37	10
Focal CBF reduction	33	10
Overall incidence of abnormality	100	47

*Criteria for interpretation of CBF findings were derived from 22 healthy subjects of comparable age.

hypertonic mannitol, but mannitol ought to be the agent of choice if CBF is reduced because hyperventilation might lower CBF enough to produce cerebral ischemia.

Much has been learned about the control of the cerebral circulation under normal and pathological circumstances. A major issue now is whether this information can be used to better manage neurosurgical patients with head injuries, subarachnoid hemorrhage, occlusive vascular disease, and other disorders.

References

1. Heistad DD: Summary of symposium on cerebral blood flow: Effect of nerves and neurotransmitters. J Cereb Blood Flow Metab 1:447–450, 1981.
2. Langfitt TW, Kassell NF: Cerebral vasodilatation produced by brain-stem stimulation: Neurogenic control vs. autoregulation. Am J Physiol 215:90–97, 1968.
3. Langfitt TW, Weinstein JD, Kassell NF: Cerebral vasomotor paralysis produced by intracranial hypertension. Neurology 15:622–641, 1965.
4. Lassen NA: The luxury-perfusion syndrome and its possible relation to acute metabolic acidosis localised within the brain. Lancet 2:1113–1115, 1966.
5. Lassen NA, Ingvar DH: Regional cerebral blood flow measurement in man. Arch Neurol 9:615–622, 1963.
6. Miller JD, Stanek A, Langfitt TW: Concepts of cerebral perfusion pressure and vascular compression during intracranial hypertension. Prog Brain Res 35:411–432, 1971.
7. Obrist WD, Thompson HK Jr, King CH, Wang HS: Determination of regional cerebral blood flow by inhalation of 133-xenon. Circ Res 20:124–135, 1967.
8. Owman C, Edvinsson L (eds): *Neurogenic Control of the Brain Circulation.* Oxford, Pergamon Press, 1977.
9. Pickard JD: Role of prostaglandins and arachidonic acid derivatives in the coupling of cerebral blood flow to cerebral metabolism. J Cereb Blood Flow Metab 1:361–384, 1981.
10. Shalit MN, Shimojyo S, Reinmuth OM: Carbon dioxide and cerebral circulatory control: I. The extra-vascular effect. Arch Neurol 17:298–303, 1967.
11. Siesjö BK, Plum F: Cerebral energy metabolism in normoxia and in hypoxia. Acta Anaesthesiol Scand [Suppl] 45:81–101, 1971.
12. Sokoloff L: Influence of functional activity on local cerebral glucose utilization, in Ingvar DH, Lassen NA (eds): *Brain Work: The Coupling of Function, Metabolism and Blood Flow in the Brain.* Copenhagen, Munksgaard, 1975, pp 385–398.
13. Stromberg DD, Fox JR: Pressures in the pial arterial microcirculation of the cat during changes in systemic arterial blood pressure. Circ Res 31:229–239, 1972.
14. Winn HR, Rubio GR, Berne RM: The role of adenosine in the regulation of cerebral blood flow. J Cereb Blood Flow Metab 1:239–244, 1981.

140
Measurement of Cerebral Blood Flow
Howard Yonas

An early attempt at the understanding of the nature of cerebral blood flow (CBF) was made in the late 1770s when Monro proposed that the quantity of blood flow within the head must be the same or nearly so at all times. He believed that because the brain is enclosed in bone and it is incompressible, the volume of blood within the cranium also has to be constant. Although this is basically correct, a false assumption was also made: that the vasculature is passive and incapable of actively changing its diameter. The later work of Roy and Sherrington in the late 1800s established an active role for the vasculature following observations of the pial vasculature through cranial window preparations.

A major step toward quantitation of cerebral blood flow was made in the 1920s with the capability of obtaining jugular bulb blood samples, which in turn made possible a measure of the arterial to jugular venous O_2 difference. This approach subsequently laid a solid scientific foundation for our current understanding of cerebral blood flow physiology and established the dominant role of CO_2 as a regulator of cerebral blood flow.

The description in 1945 by Kety and Schmidt of a method of quantifying cerebral blood flow in humans based on the Fick principle established the modern era of CBF measurement.[4] Kety and Schmidt mathematically characterized the Fick principle and utilized nitrous oxide, a metabolically inert and highly lipid soluble gas, as the tracer of blood flow. The Fick principle had stated that the quantity of a gas taken up by a tissue per unit of time (Q_i) is equal to the quantity entering it via the arterial blood minus the quantity leaving in the venous blood: $dQ_i/dt = F_i(C_a - C_v)$ where F_i is equal to blood flow and C_a and C_v are equal to the arterial and venous concentrations, respectively. Knowing the time course of the changes in the inert gas concentrations in the arterial blood flowing into the brain and the venous blood leaving it, and knowing the blood/brain partition coefficient, enables one to calculate the average cerebral blood flow. The governing relationship as characterized by Kety and Schmidt for a single tissue compartment, i, is

$$C_i(T) = \lambda_i k_i C_a(\mu) e^{-k_i(T-\mu)} d\mu$$

where flow is $F_i = \lambda_i k_i$. The input functions for this equation are the partition coefficient (λ_i), the flow rate constant (k_i), the time-dependent tracer concentration in the arterial blood $C_a(\mu)$, and the time-dependent tracer concentration in the venous blood. For this relationship the tissue concentration (C_iT) is assumed to be equal to the venous blood content divided by λ. This equation is then valid for saturation or desaturation studies depending on the boundary conditions that are set. This measurement of global cerebral blood flow with nitrous oxide required the following assumptions: (1) blood flow is in a steady state during the period of study and is not affected by the tracer, (2) the venous blood from the superior internal jugular vein is representative of the mixed cerebral venous blood with no contamination from extracerebral blood, (3) the period of measurement is long enough to allow equilibration of gas in the brain with the cerebral venous blood, (4) no significant arterial-venous shunts are present in the brain, and (5) the value of the partition coefficient of the inert gas is representative of the entire brain. The initial studies with nitrous oxide demonstrated that blood flow studies with this tracer did meet the above assumptions under most situations with the exception being in a region of disturbed physiology, where arteriovenous shunting may be significant and where the partition coefficient is likely to be altered.

A major advance toward the broad clinical application of cerebral blood flow measurement came with the substitution of radiolabeled [85]Kr for nitrous oxide and scintillation counting as the direct measure of tracer movement within the tissue, the latter measure being substituted for the difference of the arterial and venous concentrations of the tracer. This approach provided a regionality of blood flow determination that was lacking in the global blood flow measures provided by nitrous oxide, but this was significantly hampered by contamination from extracranial emissions. Initially this was experimentally dealt with by the injection of [85]Kr directly into the internal carotid artery and by scintillation counting over the exposed cortex. Subsequently with the substitution of the gamma emitter, ^{133}Xe, for [85]Kr, higher and more adequate counting rates were obtained through the skull. The application of this technique with internal carotid artery injection then became widely utilized both clinically and experimentally as a means of obtaining regional CBF measurements (Fig. 140-1). Because this approach requires an internal carotid artery catheter, its application has generally remained limited to situations where patients were undergoing angiography and already required the placement of such a catheter.

A more broad approach became possible, however, with the work of Obrist, who, utilizing a multicompartmental analysis of the Kety equation, was able to separate the washout curve into three components, the extracranial contamination appearing as a well-defined, late washout (Table 140-1). If this contamination is subtracted from the remaining fast (gray matter) and slow (white matter) curves, an analysis of flow can then be done, with an additional correction being made for the recirculation of gas. The later measure was made by a separate recording of the end tidal ^{133}Xe concentration as an indirect measure of the capillary and therefore arterial concentration of the gas. As a "noninvasive" inhalation study, ^{133}Xe inhalation flow determinations have been shown to maintain the numerical reliability of the intracarotid injection method.[6] Refinements have permitted relatively short periods of data acquisition (10 min) during the clearance phase in which only the fast "gray matter" flows are extracted, again without significant loss of validity against the intracarotid technique. Commercially available units utilizing this methodology commonly incorporate about 16 individual NaI scintillation counters, which are ideally placed about both hemispheres, so that each is perpendicular to the surface of the brain. The ultimate in collimation was developed in Lassen's laboratory, where 254 independent collimators were made into a unilateral array.[5] Elegant studies of regional flow disturbance in disease and during activation studies of physiological stimulation have been demonstrated with this technique. The Anger camera, using a single crystal and sequential sampling from multiple portals as a recording system, has also been shown to be able to provide useful cerebral blood flow information from either a lateral or vertex view.

The ^{133}Xe methodology, however, suffers from a number of significant limitations. Counts arising from extracranial tissues still provide a signal contamination, as do emissions arising from the opposite hemisphere. This technique is dependent on the use of "normal" partition coefficients, which in diseased states can vary by as much as 50 percent. Although a careful analytic approach to data analysis with this technique has been able to positively identify the side of a cerebral infarction in 80 percent of the cases in which a stroke was evident on computed tomography, regions of slow flow tend to be inadequately taken into account while small regions of no flow may be totally missed.[3] This technique may detect a raised or normal flow in a region of infarction because counts from the hyperemic rim numerically overshadow the area of low or no flow just below it. As a major limitation of this technique, this "look through" phenomenon has prompted the development of a tomographic imaging system for [133]Xe.[5] A tomographic imaging device is now commercially available, but it is also limited because of the dependence on "normal" partition coefficient values. Currently only limited resolution is provided because of a relatively limited signal produced by ^{133}Xe, which may be improved with the substitution of stronger gamma emitter tracer gases and a greater number of detectors used for the tomographic reconstruction of the image.

Additional quantitative and regionally specific tomographic techniques for blood flow determination are being

TABLE 140-1 Methods of Measuring Cerebral Blood Flow

Method	Description	Provides	Theoretical Limit of Resolution	Advantages	Disadvantages
Clinical and Laboratory: Quantitative					
^{133}Xe	Gamma scintillation counting on NaI crystals with IA, IV, or inhalation of ^{133}Xe	Regional flow		Simplicity Availability Reproducibility	Signal contamination "Look through" phenomenon "Normal" λ values
	Rotational single photon emission tomography with ^{133}Xe inhalation	Local flow	11+ mm	Simplicity	"Normal" λ values
Positron emission tomography	Coincident positron counting, tomographic reconstruction from positron-emitting tracer	Local flow	4+ mm	Studies flow and metabolism	Major scientific effort
Stable xenon enhanced CT	CT enhanced by inhalation of 30–40% xenon-oxygen mixture	Local flow	2+ mm	Availability λ, K calculated	Xenon anesthetic effect
Pulsed Doppler	Doppler measure of carotid diameter and velocity	Global flow		Noninvasive	Indirect index of CBF
Clinical and Laboratory: Qualitative					
Isotope transit	Anger camera and sequential 4-s imaging of ^{99m}Tc transit	Regional blood flow pattern		Simplicity Availability	Poor spatial resolution
CT-iodine transit	Rapid sequential CT scanning and IV iodine bolus	Local blood pattern		Simplicity Availability	Limited to one CT level Requires IV bolus
Laboratory: Quantitative					
Autoradiography	Approximation of thin brain sections with photographic plate following iodo[^{14}C]antipyrine	Local flow	<1 mm	High resolution	One point in time Animal killed
Radiolabeled microspheres	Microspheres with different energy-emitting isotopes	Local flow	8 × 8 × 8 mm	Can provide up to five flow measurements in each region	Animal killed
Hydrogen clearance	Electrical potential measured in reference to an implanted polarized electrode following IV bolus or inhalation of H_2	Local flow	5 × 5 × 5 mm	Multiple in situ CBF determinations Simplicity Availability	Requires passage of probe into region of interest

A B

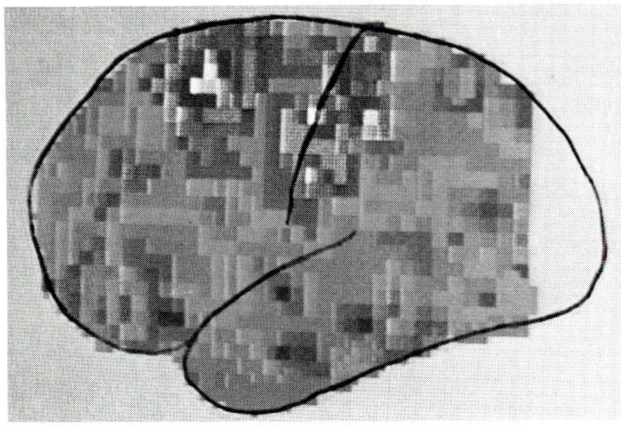

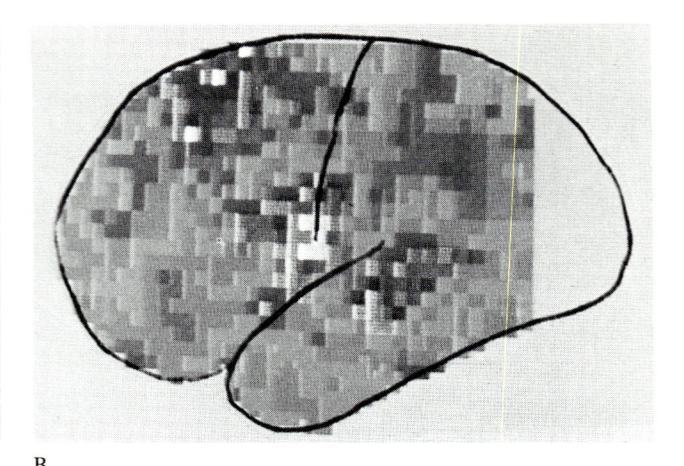

Figure 140-1 These are cerebral blood flow studies utilizing ^{133}Xe introduced by intracarotid injection with imaging through an array of 254 externally placed scintillation detectors. Each detector is collimated to scan approximately 1 cm^2 of the brain surface. Lightest shades of gray indicate rates of flow up to 20 percent above baseline; the darkest shades indicate 20 percent below baseline. *A.* This study demonstrates an enhanced focal pattern which accompanies hand movements of the opposite side. *B.* This study demonstrates the flow pattern that accompanies counting out loud. Note enhanced flow values not only in the area of the cortex thought to cause mouth motions, but also in the supplemental motor area and the auditory cortex. (Courtesy of Drs. N. A. Lassen, D. H. Ingvar, and E. Skinhøj, Bispebjerg Hospital, Copenhagen, Denmark, and University Hospital, Lund, Sweden.)

actively developed. These are positron emission tomography and stable xenon enhanced transmission tomography. One approach utilizes a mathematical image reconstruction technique of positron-emitting markers to evaluate cerebral blood flow.[1] This approach provides regionally specific information of flow, which, coupled with studies of metabolism, provides a highly useful and potent instrument for the study of normal and altered physiological states. Three approaches are currently being investigated as a means for appraising flow. The first is a clearance technique of a bolus injection of ^{15}O-labeled H$_2$O. The second is the buildup of scintillation counts following continuous inhalation of ^{15}O-labeled CO$_2$ with the conversion to ^{15}O-labeled H$_2$O by pulmonary carbonic anhydrase (Fig. 140-2). The third technique utilizes a "microsphere" approach in which ^{13}N-labeled ammonia is used as a marker that becomes fixed within the brain at a relatively high percentage during a single pass through the vasculature. Although it is a new and exciting approach to brain imaging, this is a major new technology that demands the effort of a team of scientists. The flow data provided by this technique are locally specific and provide a resolution that is theoretically limited to about 4 mm.

Another tomographic approach for acquiring local cerebral blood flow information involves the use of stable xenon as a marker of tissue flow combined with transmission computed tomography (Figs. 140-3 and 140-4).[2] For this technique, CT scans obtained during and/or after a 4- to 6-min inhalation of nonradioactive xenon-oxygen gas mixtures are utilized to record the movement of this lipid-soluble and radiodense gas into the brain substance. Because the relatively slow process of diffusion of this agent is being characterized, scans obtained at 1-min intervals provide the required data. Rapid scanning techniques with incremental table movements permit data acquisition at three to five additional levels during each inhalation sequence. The end tidal xenon concentration measured by a thermoconductivity analyzer or a mass spectrophotometer is utilized to indirectly record the arterial concentration during the buildup and/or washout of xenon. This information, plus the degree of image enhancement, is then used to derive the partition coefficient (λ) and the local cerebral blood flow by multivariable analysis. A major advantage to this approach is that both λ and local cerebral blood flow are derived for each specific tissue of interest. Recent experimental studies with concurrent radiolabeled microsphere injections suggest that xenon blood flow values are reproducible and within reasonable expected limits. Anatomical resolution appears to be high and theoretically could approach the resolution of the CT scanners. Current experimental and clinical studies suggest that this methodology has the potential for broad utilization as a noninvasive, reproducible, and generally available means of obtaining local cerebral blood flow information. Although it has been shown that 30 to 35 percent xenon concentrations do not significantly alter cerebral blood flow or significantly alter the sensorium of most individuals, its sedative effect may cause patient movement, which does make cerebral blood flow determinations either very difficult or impossible.

Qualitative information about cerebral blood flow is also being provided by two simple and readily available approaches. Clearance curves of ^{99m}Tc-labeled technetium pertechnetate combined with rapid data acquisition on a single-crystal Anger camera has been utilized for a decade to

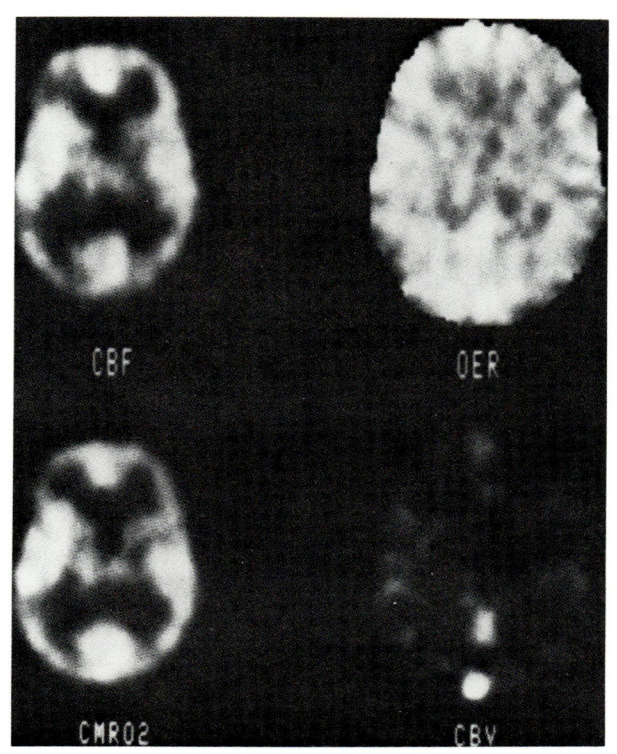

Figure 140-2 Normal cross-sectional images demonstrating cerebral blood flow (CBF), oxygen metabolism (CMRO$_2$), oxygen extraction ratio (OER), and cerebral blood volume (CBV). These studies were obtained with the ECAT II PCT system using the $^{15}O_2$ steady-state inhalation technique. In these images white is the highest value in the gray scale. (Courtesy of Drs. R. S. J. Frankowiak, A. A. Lammertsma, G. L. Lenzi, and T. Jones, MRC Cyclotron Unit, Hammersmith Hospital, London.)

provide information about the movement of blood within comparative blood pools. The same type of data, but with better localization, is also being provided by rapid CT scanning following an intravenous iodine bolus. Studies at the level of the middle cerebral arteries or at the level of the brain stem have been shown to provide a readily accessible means of evaluating regional asymmetries of movement within blood pools. Although fourth-generation scanners can provide sequential 1-s scans and better definition of the time course of contrast movement, this technique thus far has been unable to provide quantitative information due to the inability to characterize the time course of the arterial concentration following an intravenous bolus injection. Because of the broad availability of this technology and the possible importance of flow asymmetries, however, this technique should have a broad application for the evaluation of regional blood flow pattern abnormalities.

Three additional approaches to cerebral blood flow measurement are applicable only in the laboratory. These are autoradiography with iodo[^{14}C]antipyrine,[7] sequential injections of different radiolabeled isotope microspheres, and hydrogen clearance techniques.[8]

Autoradiography utilizing iodo[^{14}C]antipyrine as a dif-

fusible indicator of flow has proven to be a highly quantitative means of obtaining data concerning flow with a high degree of spatial resolution. For this study the animal needs to be sacrificed shortly after the intravenous injection of iodo[^{14}C]antipyrine. The brain is then removed and frozen to −70°, followed by thin sectioning and application of tissue slices to radiographic plates for 5 to 6 days. Multiple sequential arterial blood samples are used to provide the arterial input function. The emission densities on the photographic plates are then interpretable as measures of blood flow which contain a high degree of spatial resolution. The major limitation of this approach is that it permits a measure of flow at only one point in time, although recent work has suggested that two isotopes with differential counting can be used to record flow at two points in time.

Radiolabeled microspheres measuring 6 to 8 μm in diameter provide a nondiffusible means of measuring flow. Microspheres of this size are extracted into the microcirculation at a rate of over 90 percent for a single pass through the cerebral circulation. By recording the rate of extraction of radiolabeled isotopes from the arterial circulation and then directly counting the number of counts in each tissue volume, blood flow data are obtained. Currently up to five independent isotope injections (^{141}Ce, ^{133}Sn, ^{85}Sr, ^{95}Nb, ^{46}Sc) and therefore blood flow determinations can be made after isotope separation utilizing a matrix algebra approach for the

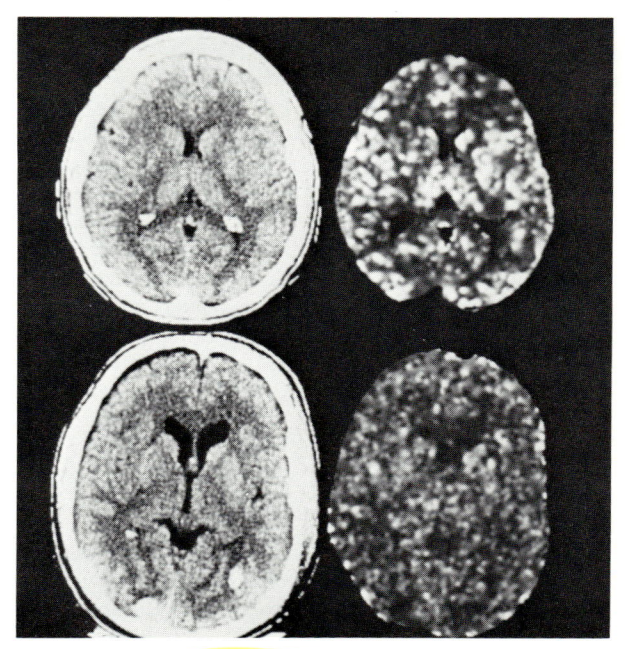

Figure 140-3 Two cerebral blood flow studies with stable xenon and computed tomography. The top left CT scan is of a normal individual breathing 35 percent xenon, 65 percent oxygen. The flow map on the top right depicts flows on a scale of 0 to 80 ml/100 g per minute. Note the elevated flow pattern in the basal ganglia in clear distinction from the surrounding white matter tracts. The lower set of studies is of a 40-year-old individual following a closed head injury and while receiving barbiturate therapy. Flow values are diffusely reduced into the 20 to 40 ml/100 g per minute range.

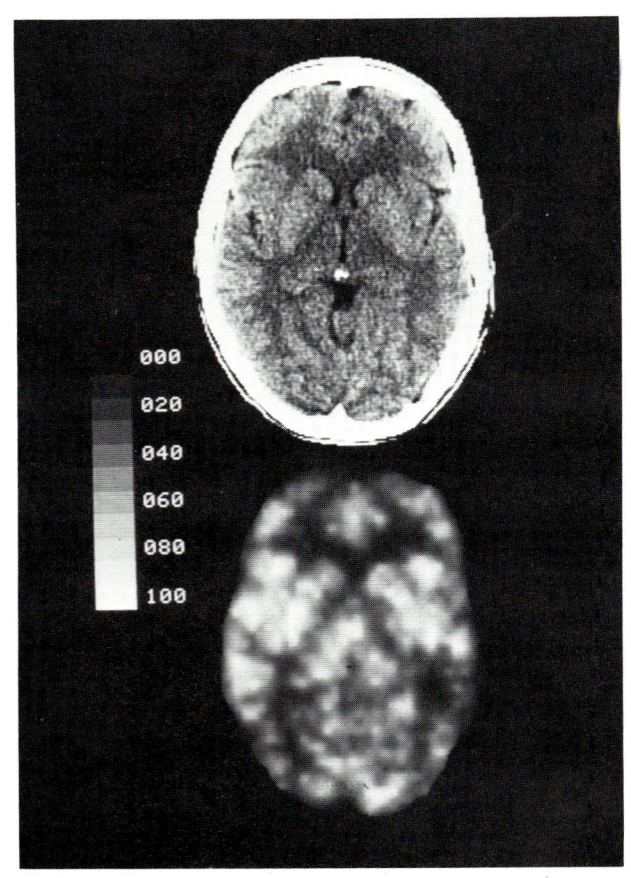

Figure 140-4 The single-level blood flow map below is derived from the above baseline CT image and the four enhanced images that followed while the patient inspired a mixture of 33 percent xenon and 67 percent oxygen. This normal study was obtained on a woman 23 years of age with a history suggestive of multiple sclerosis. A clear distinction between flow values from the fast-flow (gray matter) and slow-flow (white matter) regions is apparent. The scale on the left is in milliliters per 100 g per minute.

solution of simultaneous equations. The major disadvantage of this approach in a laboratory is that a volume of 8 × 8 × 8 mm is typically required to obtain adequate counts for reliable statistical determinations.

The third approach involves measuring the clearance of hydrogen gas from about a reference platinum-iridium probe previously placed within the brain substance. Fine probe diameters (0.01 in.) with exposure of only the terminal 2 mm are commonly being utilized. An array of as many as six simultaneous probes are currently being used, and this approach has been shown to provide a highly reproducible and locally specific means of repeatedly determining local cerebral blood flow. This technique has the advantage of repeatability with the opportunity to make flow calculations every 10 to 15 min for days or even weeks. A recent critical review of this topic has suggested that the tissue volume of study may be 5 × 5 × 5 mm.[8] The only major limitation to this approach is that the data acquisition is limited to only the immediate region about the tip of the probe, which does require disturbance of the tissue to be studied by its placement.

Two additional techniques also warrant mention. Although heat dilution in reference to an intraparenchymal probe has been utilized for a number of years for flow determinations, a superficial cortical probe is now available and has been utilized to evaluate flow alterations during experimental and clinical procedures in which the cortex is exposed. Recent reports have also described the use of a range-gated Doppler flowmeter to measure the extracranial blood flow through major vessels. This instrument directly measures both the diameter of the vessel and the velocity of the fluid within it. Blood flow in the vessel is directly calculated from these two parameters. Carotid artery studies of flow have been found to be in reasonable agreement with concurrent measurements made with ^{133}Xe CBF studies.

References

1. Ackerman RH, Subramanyam R, Correia JA, Alpert NM, Taveras JM: Positron imaging of cerebral blood flow during continuous inhalation of C^{15}O$_2$. Stroke 11:45–49, 1980.
2. Gur D, Good WF, Wolfson SK, Yonas H, Shabason L: In vivo mapping of local cerebral blood flow by xenon-enhanced computed tomography. Science 215:1267–1268, 1982.
3. Halsey JH Jr, Nakai K, Wariyar B: Sensitivity of rCBF to focal lesions. Stroke 12:631–635, 1981.
4. Kety SS, Schmidt CF: The determination of cerebral blood flow in man by the use of nitrous oxide in low concentrations. Am J Physiol 143:53–66, 1945.
5. Lassen NA, Henriksen L, Paulson O: Regional cerebral blood flow in stroke by ^{133}xenon inhalation and emission tomography. Stroke 12:284–288, 1981.
6. Obrist WD, Thompson HK Jr, King CH, Wang HS: Determination of regional cerebral blood flow by inhalation of 133-Xenon. Circ Res 20:124–135, 1967.
7. Sakurada O, Kennedy C, Jehle J, Brown JD, Carbin GL, Sokoloff L: Measurement of local cerebral blood flow with iodo[^{14}C]antipyrine. Am J Physiol 234:H59–H66, 1978.
8. Young W: H$_2$ clearance measurement of blood flow: A review of technique and polarographic principles. Stroke 11:552–564, 1980.

141

Normal Cerebral Energy Metabolism

Michael J. O'Connor
Steven J. Barrer
Frank A. Welsh

The complex behavior of the simplest living organism will convince the most casual observer that a highly organized system must control this behavior. The degree of organization of the neuropil that can be visualized on an electron micrograph will, however, astound even the most sophisticated investigator. Given this degree of organization and the second law of thermodynamics defining entropy, it comes as no surprise that maintenance of this degree of organization in the adult human brain accounts for 25 percent of the body's oxygen consumption. Actually, when one takes into consideration the remarkably high surface/volume ratio and steep chemical gradient across membranes, one may wonder how such a system is kept organized at such a small energy expenditure (about 18 W based on complete glucose oxidation and 12 W based on maximum ATP production). This very consideration led Dr. Ling to conclude that the complex organelles that we can visualize are not bags of chemicals and ions that are dissolved in free water, but rather that much of the water is bound, the surrounding membrane playing a relatively unimportant role. Although in recent years it has been shown that to some degree his conclusions are correct, it is still the general consensus that the semipermeable cell membrane, with its selective ion pores, is the container of free water with dissolved ions and molecules within. Given this conclusion then, a major use of energy metabolism must be for the transport of ions across these membranes. In addition, the amount of energy required to reconstitute these membranes, although not known, may be significant, especially in the developing human brain, which accounts for 50 percent of the body's oxygen consumption.

Regardless of how this energy is used, it is clear that brain function is highly dependent on its continuous supply. Failure occurs within 10 s of cessation of blood flow, and this failure becomes irreversible in 5 to 30 min of complete flow failure.

Recently, it has been found that partial interruption of oxygen supply or blood flow may result in functional failure, but not irreversible damage.[2] This is most apparent when there is regional failure of blood flow. A number of approaches have been tried to minimize the adverse effects of restriction or interruptions of the supply of blood flow or energy. In our efforts to minimize structural or functional failure, a better understanding of the metabolism of the normal brain should be of some help. The purpose of this chapter is to briefly update the reader on the what, how, where, and why of normal cerebral energy metabolism. The effects of a few common clinical manipulations will be reviewed. Finally, comments will be made on new methods that are being used or are likely to be used in the future.

Current View of Cerebral Energy Metabolism

What: Major Sources of Metabolic Energy

The primary source of energy for the brain is the oxidation of glucose. Theoretically, 1 mol of glucose is oxidized by 6 mol of oxygen to 6 mol of carbon dioxide and water, 38 mol of ATP and 934 kJ. In fact, the respiratory quotient (RQ = AVDCO$_2$/AVDO$_2$) for brain in the normally fed human is about 0.98. A small amount of lactate and pyruvate may be released; however, this is somewhat controversial and energetically insignificant. Ketone bodies substitute for glucose after just a 12- to 16-h fast and may account for 60 percent of O$_2$ consumption after a 30-day fast. The four carbons of β-hydroxybutyrate are normally oxidized by 4.5 molecules of O$_2$ whereas acetoacetate has an RQ of 1.[28] Normally, the nitrogen balance of the brain is near zero. There may, however, be a net uptake of branched chain and dibasic amino acids.[17]

Kety and Schmidt in 1946 first quantitated cerebral metabolism in humans, reporting consumption of 46 ml of O$_2$ per minute.[13] This work has been confirmed many times, and their method is probably still the best available for measurement of the cerebral metabolic rate of oxygen (CMRO$_2$). However, no regionalization or lateralization is possible. The CMRGl, CMRLac and CMRO$_2$ are about 0.30 μmol/g per minute; 0.02 μmol/g per minute; and 1.7 μmol/g per minute, respectively. The oxygen-glucose index, OGI = (AVDO$_2$/6 × AVDG1) 100, is often reported to be 90 to 95 percent.[28]

Adequate O$_2$ supply is critical to brain function, and with decreased cerebral blood flow (CBF), O$_2$ deficit is apparent before glucose deficit. Therefore, it is not surprising that arterial oxygen tension (Pa$_{O_2}$) is a major regulator of CBF.[12] Patients with primary decreases in inspired oxygen concentration will have increased cerebral blood flow despite the decreasing Pa$_{CO_2}$ caused by tachypnea. In cases in which there is both a decrease in arterial oxygen content and hypercarbia, there is a marked increase in cerebral blood flow. Neither of these conditions, however, has been shown to be associated with a change in the cerebral metabolic rate for oxygen in normal people. Primary hypocarbia is also thought to be associated with a constant CMRO$_2$,[28] even though Kety and Schmidt found a significant increase with spontaneous hyperventilation.[13] This observation, if it were true, would indicate a critical balance between Pa$_{O_2}$ and

How: Metabolic Pathways

There is facilitated transport of glucose across the blood-brain barrier.[23] Once in the cell, glucose is metabolized irreversibly in the cytoplasm along the glycolytic pathway. The major controlling enzyme is phosphofructokinase, which converts fructose-6-phosphate to fructose-1,6-diphosphate (FDP). This enzyme's activity is inhibited by ATP and citrate and stimulated by ADP and AMP. FDP is subsequently split into two 3-carbon fragments, which are further metabolized from glyceraldehyde-3-phosphate to pyruvate. It requires the conversion of two ATP to two ADP molecules to form glyceraldehyde phosphate (GAP) from glucose (one ATP if glycogen is used instead of glucose). In the conversion of each glyceraldehyde phosphate to pyruvate, two ATP and one NADH are formed. If oxygen is not available for the conversion of the NADH back to NAD, then it is necessary for pyruvate to be converted to lactate with the associated oxidation of NADH back to NAD. However, under normal circumstances, pyruvate is further metabolized in the mitochondria and cytoplasm, since NADH cannot cross the mitochondrial membrane.

Pyruvate enters the mitochondria as a 3-carbon fragment and loses one carbon as CO_2 with the associated formation of the high-energy compound NADH. This 2-carbon fragment enters the tricarboxylic acid cycle (TCA or citric acid cycle) and is then condensed with the 4-carbon oxaloacetate to form citrate. This reaction seems to be almost irreversible. It should be noted also that the intermediate acetyl Co A is a final common pathway not only for pyruvate but also for ketone bodies and many amino acids. Two more carbons are removed and four dehydrogenase steps occur with the resulting formation of three more NADH molecules and one FADH. The net result is 4 NADH + 1 FADH + GTP and one oxaloacetate. The reduced high-energy NADH can each be oxidized by the cytochrome chain with the resultant formation of three ATP, whereas the FADH is oxidized with the formation of two ATP. This oxidative phosphorylation occurs in a tightly coupled group of enzymes, which are also physically close to the enzymes of the citric acid cycle. These enzymes, called the *cytochrome chain*, transfer reducing equivalents from NADH to oxygen resulting in the formation of water. In most cases, three ADP are converted to three ATP. It is clear that at the substrate end of the cytochrome chain the degree of reduction is much greater than at the oxygen end (cytochrome oxidase, also known as cytochrome aa_3). There is, however, some debate as to whether the cytochrome oxidase is normally 99 percent oxidized or 70 to 90 percent oxidized as has been reported by Jöbsis.[11] If the latter situation is true, then thermodynamic considerations of the cytochrome chain will predict that the partial pressure of oxygen would have a significant effect on the rate of electron transport and oxygen consumption. Thus, not only would the rate of electron transport be controlled by ADP, ATP, and inorganic phosphate (P_i) concentration[28] but also by the oxygen tension. Thus, the complex topic of control of energy production by the cell is not clear. There is evidence at this time that energy supply is controlled not only by energy needs but also by oxygen supply even in the normal brain at standard oxygen pressures.

There are several points that deserve special consideration. The pathway followed by glucose from entry into the cell to leaving as CO_2 is well established and is as outlined above. A small percentage (1 percent) of the glucose may pass through the pentose shunt for RNA, DNA, and other nucleotide synthesis. Ten percent of the pyruvate may be used to replenish TCA cycle intermediates via CO_2 fixation and be used for protein synthesis.[28] With these few exceptions the path is fairly predictable. However, the driving force for many of the reactions is uncertain. Since most of the reactions that involve a large change in energy have NAD^+ and NADH + H^+ as substrate or product, knowledge of the NAD^+/NADH ratio and H^+ concentration is critical to understanding the thermodynamics of these reactions. The NAD^+/NADH ratio defines the oxidation-reduction (redox) state of the medium in which the reaction is occurring, and a great deal of effort has been devoted to measuring this ratio in the cytoplasm and in the mitochondria. Knowledge of these ratios is critical to understanding the coupling between the cytoplasm and the mitochondria as well as the events within each.

For example, in brain the malate oxaloacetate shuttle is thought to transfer reducing equivalents from the cytoplasm to the mitochondria, thus oxidizing the cytoplasmic NADH and reducing the mitochondrial NAD. Since examination of cytoplasmic (lactate-pyruvate) and mitochondrial (β-hydroxybutyrate-acetoacetate) redox couples has led to the conclusion that the cytoplasmic NAD/NADH ratio is 100 to 500 times greater than the mitochondrial ratio, it has been proposed that aspartate is actively transported out of the mitochondria in exchange for glutamate.[5] An active mechanism such as this is needed to explain the apparent difference in the cytoplasmic and mitochondrial redox state since these compartments should be in equilibrium through the couples. Unfortunately, interpretation of the redox couples has led to conflicting reports,[19,29] which indicates that this interpretation is possibly subject to error. A report by Laman et al. indicates that even in the relatively simple system of a red blood cell, the expected effect of pH on the NAD/NADH ratio might be just the opposite of the measured effect.[15] The interpretation of these couples in a multicompartment system might be even more hazardous. On careful examination of the constraints under which these redox couples are calculated,[19] it seems that most constraints are not met in brain mitochondria. Most commonly used couples have both the substrates and the enzyme in the mitochondria and cytoplasm, and the substrates are even in the blood and extracellular fluid. The activities in the mitochondria and the effect of substrate binding seem almost impossible to evaluate. There are no independent indicators of intramitochondrial pH; and therefore, the hydrogen ion concentration must be assumed in the calculation of the equilibrium for a single substrate couple. Also, the effect of pH on equilibrium constants cannot be included. Based on all of these considerations, it seems that the substrate couple cannot be used to evaluate intramitochondrial NAD/NADH ratio in the brain. The mitochondrial redox state can be evaluated qualitatively by recording the fluorescence of

NADH.[7] This method does not permit a calculation of the NAD/NADH ratio, and therefore a description of neither the precise thermodynamics of the reactions within the mitochondria nor of the redox couple between the cytoplasm and the mitochondria is possible at this time.

The nervous system may have a unique feedback mechanism that permits control of energy demand by energy supply.[34,35] Several of the TCA cycle intermediates can be converted to putative neurotransmitters. α-Ketoglutarate (α-KG) conversion to glutamate then glutamine or δ-aminobutyric acid (GABA) is a good example. The flux of these neurotransmitters could be controlled by a number of mechanisms,[27] the redox state of the mitochondria (NAD/NADH) being an obvious direct mechanism. If flux through the GABA shunt (an alternate route off the TCA cycle from α-KG to succinate, which is slightly less energy-efficient and coupled to both GABA and NH_4 detoxification) were controlled by tissue redox state and if this flux in turn controlled activation metabolism, then when O_2 supply was limited, ATP demand could be reduced by reducing neuronal discharges. This mechanism is speculative, but it is clear that many of the TCA cycle intermediates or their metabolites have profound excitatory, inhibitory, or even toxic effects.[18,22,27] Therefore, these provide an excellent potential feedback path of metabolism on neuronal activity.

Where: Sites of Metabolism

At the subcellular level, it is well established that the oxidative pathways for glucose metabolism are located in mitochondria. It is not possible to measure the metabolic rate of one region of a cell compared with another. However, it is possible to evaluate the location of the oxidative enzymes that would be required for the metabolism. Histochemical stains have clearly demonstrated that the citric acid cycle enzymes are associated with mitochondria. The cytochrome chain has also been clearly demonstrated to lie within the mitochondria. There is some speculation that the number of cristae in mitochondria is related to the enzyme concentration. This, in general, correlates with the size of mitochondria; however, there can be a closer packing of the cristae and, presumably, an increase in the enzyme concentration (see references in Ref. 21).

Although the metabolic rate at the subcellular level cannot be evaluated directly, it seems reasonable to estimate the maximum metabolic rate by evaluating the enzyme concentration within various portions of the cell or by comparing the enzyme concentration of one cell type with that of another. For the nervous system, this has been done in a quantitative level in the cell body. It has been found that the neuron has a higher concentration of mitochondria than does the astroglial cell by a factor of 2. In nonquantitative ways, it has also been observed that the concentration of mitochondria increases in dendritic processes of neurons whereas in astrocytes and glial sheets, in general, the concentration of mitochondria drops (see references in Ref. 21). Since the greatest part of the gray matter is made up of neuropil, rather than cell bodies, it is necessary to assay the concentration of mitochondria and to try to identify the type of process that the mitochondria are in. This has been done in layer 4 of the cat visual cortex, and it was found that 91 percent of the mitochondria by volume were located in neurons or their processes. The remaining 9 percent were in unidentified processes, but not necessarily glial.[20] In a nonquantitative study Blackstead[21] found that about 95 percent of the mitochondria were in neurons or their processes in the hippocampus. Based on these studies, it seems that in normal gray matter the vast majority of oxidative metabolism occurs in neurons or their processes. It should be pointed out that in reactive glial tissue or in glial tissue in tissue culture, the histological stains have demonstrated a much increased oxidative enzyme concentration.[21] Based on the results of these studies, it can be further hypothesized that energy-requiring processes are not normally present in glial cells or their processes. However, the capability to support energy-requiring processes develops in reactive tissue, as occurs in gliosis and presumably low-grade tumor formation.

Enzyme concentration is probably more representative of maximum metabolic rate than typical metabolic rate. Therefore, it may be incorrect to conclude that the vast majority of oxidative metabolism occurs in neurons. Glial cells with a fixed metabolic rate near their maximum capability may account for a surprisingly high proportion of metabolic activity. Although this may be true for reactive glial tissue, it seems unlikely to be the case in normal brain since most techniques lead to the same conclusion: Neurons account for a high percentage of oxidative metabolism.[28]

Considering regional variations in metabolic rate at higher than the cellular level, a great deal of knowledge has been gained by the deoxyglucose technique. This technique has a resolution of approximately 100 μ.[31] The gray matter metabolic rate is two to four times that of white matter. CMRGl is strongly dependent on functional activity. A small column of cells at the cortical level can be stimulated by stroking the whisker of a cat. An epileptic focus and the regions it affects have a markedly increased metabolic activity, but there is no appreciable change in white matter metabolic rate. Conversely, anesthetic agents decrease gray matter metabolic rate. It seems safe to conclude that the gray matter's metabolic rate varies widely depending on functional state, whereas white matter metabolism continues at a relatively fixed rate. It has been found that mild ischemia actually results in higher lactate and lower phosphocreatine levels in the white matter than in gray matter.[32] This might be a result of the white matter's relatively fixed metabolic rate and, therefore, its inability to adjust function to supply, whereas the gray matter seems to be able to modulate functional demands in response to variations in metabolic supply.

Why: Purpose of Brain Energy Metabolism

It is generally thought that most of the brain's energy metabolism is devoted to supporting ion pump activity, mainly the sodium pump. The transient increase in oxidative metabolism during seizures is essentially all related to ion pumping.[20] Astrup concluded that 75 percent of metabolism supports sodium pump activity based on the effects of lidocaine and ouabain on in vivo $CMRO_2$ measurements.[1,3] Estimates of this pump-related fraction are, however, subject to significant error since quantification of this fraction in whole brain seems virtually impossible.[11,28] It seems reasonable to conclude that between 50 and 95 percent of the brain's oxidative metabolism is devoted to ion pumping. Neurotransmitter metabolism probably accounts for about 1 percent of total metabolism. However, rapid protein turnover may account for a relatively high percentage.[28] The sodium pump is a membrane-bound enzyme (Na-K-ATPase) that is in high concentration in nerve cell bodies and their dendrites, especially around synapses. It is also found in the cell membrane around synapses. Although serial sections have not been done, these membranes are thought to be glial.[33] Based on this report, it would be concluded that neurons and glial cells have high sodium pump activity even though the glial processes have a low concentration of mitochondria.

Na-K-ATPase has been isolated, and its activation by Na^+, K^+, and Mg^{2+} outlined.[30] It is likely that this enzyme not only maintains an intracellularly high $[K^+]$ and low $[Na^+]$, but also is electrogenic and therefore interacts with neurons functionally.[16] Coupling of function and metabolism has been demonstrated in preparations ranging from isolated nerve fibers to brain.

From these studies, it is clear that function of nervous tissue defined in terms of electrical activity is tightly coupled to oxidative metabolism. Regional blood flow studies by Lassen and others have demonstrated an increase in blood flow associated with neuropsychological tasks.[10] Positron emission tomography has made it possible to measure regional changes in glucose metabolism during neuropsychological testing, and it is clear that visual and auditory tasks are associated with appropriate regional increases in metabolism.[20,25,31] The degree of intellectual function or activation associated with a task seems to be coupled to the energy metabolism associated with the neuropsychological tasks. This is best demonstrated by the example of the marked increase in oxidative metabolism that occurs when a trained musician listens to classical music versus the change that occurs when the naive listener hears the same music.[24] This coupling of oxidative metabolism and function is not only confined to the physical and intellectual functions of the brain but also to the subject's affect.

Clinical Manipulations of Metabolism

Effects of Changes in Pa_{CO_2} in Metabolism

Hypercapnea has been found to be associated with a decrease in both lactate and pyruvate (the lactate/pyruvate ratio increases) as well as the TCA cycle intermediates. There is also an increase in glucose-6-phosphate and glucose. These effects can be explained by a decrease in phosphofructokinase activity, which would cause an increase in metabolites before this enzyme step and a decrease in those coming after. The increased lactate/pyruvate ratio and the decrease in phosphocreatine with hypercapnea may not reflect hypoxia but could be due to the associated acidosis. There does not seem to be a clear effect of hypercapnea on $CMRO_2$ except at very high levels of Pa_{CO_2}, which result in a decrease in $CMRO_2$.[28] Conversely, hypocapnea is associated with an increase in the concentration of TCA cycle intermediates as well as an increase in the lactate and pyruvate concentrations. The lactate/pyruvate ratio decreases. It is postulated that the increase in TCA cycle intermediates is a result of the increased pyruvate concentration. The increase in pyruvate and lactate concentrations could be the result of the known direct stimulating effect of alkalosis on glycolysis.[28]

The changes in metabolism that occur with either hypo- or hypercarbia have the effect of tending to keep the intracellular pH constant. That is, hypocarbia would make the intracellular and extracellular fluid alkalotic, but the increase in lactate concentration minimizes the pH shift. Conversely, with hypercarbia there is a decrease in the tissue concentrations of citric acid cycle intermediates and of amino acids such as glutamate and aspartate.[28] These metabolic changes start to occur within 15 min of the change in Pa_{CO_2}, and they are near maximal by 3 h.

The metabolic effects of low Pa_{CO_2} in the normal brain are likely to have beneficial effects during oligemia. Since the effects of hypocarbia seem to be overridden by the effects of hypoxia, areas that are not hypoxic will have an increase in cerebrovascular resistance, whereas hypoxic areas will be unresponsive to the hypocarbia and will not increase cerebrovascular resistance. The effect of such changes should be to improve the flow to the poorly perfused areas. It is generally thought that changes in Pa_{CO_2} do not affect $CMRO_2$, even though the initial report of the changes in CO_2 on the $CMRO_2$ in human beings demonstrated an increase in $CMRO_2$ with mild voluntary hypocapnea.

The Effect of Temperature on Metabolism

Enzyme-catalyzed reactions are affected to a much greater extent by temperature than are passive reactions. Since most of the enzyme-catalyzed reactions that can control the rate of a series of reactions usually have a maximum rate far in excess of what is normally required, the estimation of effect of temperature on metabolic activity cannot be calculated merely by assaying the change in reaction rate per 10°C change in temperature (Q10) of one or several reactions. Instead, it is likely that the metabolic rate is largely controlled by the metabolic demand. Thus, the rate at which ATP is made available is probably to a large degree responsible for the metabolic rate until the electrical activity of the brain is essentially eliminated. The major determinant of metabolic demand at that point would be the passive process of sodium leakage out of and potassium leakage into the cell. At these very low temperatures the enzyme-catalyzed reactions are affected much more and result in an accumulation of intracellular sodium and extracellular potassium. However, above these extreme low temperatures, the flux of ions across membranes is affected by the change in membrane permeability resulting from synaptic activity. This is not likely to have a simple relationship to temperature. Therefore, the log linear relationship between $CMRO_2$ and absolute temperature that can be predicted from thermodynamic considerations of temperature on rate constants is not likely to accurately describe the relationship between $CMRO_2$ and temperature.[28] Somewhat surprisingly, Bering reported such a relationship in monkeys and found a Q10 of 3.5 over the range 19 to 37°C.[4] The relationship between temperature and $CMRO_2$ can be better approximated by a 5 percent reduction of $CMRO_2$ for each degree Celsius.[28] This decrease in metabolic rate would presumably be associated with a decrease in ATP concentration if viewed in a simplistic fashion. No such change has been reported; however, several investigators have found increases in phosphocreatine with hypothermia. The decreased metabolic rate does not lead to increased tissue storage of either glycogen or glucose, and, in fact, at mild hypothermia the glucose and glycogen concentrations were found to be decreased. At more severe hypothermia (22 to 27°C) the substrate flux through phosphofructokinase seems to be decreased as glucose-6-phosphate and citrate concentrations are increased. All other metabolites measured were found to be decreased.[9]

The effects of hyperthermia seem to be part of the continuum from those of normothermia. The data are not precisely quantitative, and there are differences in various laboratories. However, it seems likely that from 37 to 42°C there is an increase in $CMRO_2$ that may be as high as 50 percent, and might also be approximated by 5 percent per degree Celsius. At about 42 to 43°C the $CMRO_2$ decreases, and it is at this level that irreversible damage and severe toxic effects of hyperthermia, including convulsions, become apparent.[28]

Barbiturates

The $CMRO_2$ can be reduced to about 25 to 30 percent of normal with barbiturates.[1] The CMRGl seems to be decreased slightly more that the $CMRO_2$ during deep pentobarbital anesthesia. This effect is possibly due to mobilization of endogenous glucose stores. The utilization of high-energy phosphate during pentobarbital anesthesia is decreased by as much as 60 percent, as shown by an increased phosphocreatine and decreased ADP and AMP concentrations.[28]

Lidocaine

Astrup reported that 160 mg/kg of lidocaine decreased cerebral metabolic rate for oxygen and glucose 15 to 20 percent in animals that had already been rendered in deep coma with deep pentobarbital anesthesia.[1] He also reported a further 20 to 25 percent reduction in $CMRO_2$ with blockage of the sodium pump with ouabain.

Presumably, the effect of lidocaine is due to the decreased permeability of the membrane to sodium. Therefore, even though synaptic events were probably, to a large degree, blocked by the deep barbiturate anesthesia, the lidocaine further reduced membrane permeability with further reduction in sodium pump activity. The addition of ouabain, according to Astrup, further blocked sodium pump activity, as was evidenced by a rise in the extracellular potassium. The doses of lidocaine used in this study were much higher than is routinely used, but were reasonably well tolerated. The doses of ouabain used resulted in severe systemic toxicity.

New Techniques

PET: Positron Emission Tomography

Positron emission tomography has high resolution because doublet emission permits precise localization of the site of emission, especially if time of flight is taken into consideration. However, the emitted particle, a positron, which has the opposite charge and the same weight of an electron, travels a mean path length of 2 to 4 mm prior to collision with an electron. This mean path length in brain varies depending on the isotope used. This unchanging physical property determines the theoretical resolution of the PET (4 to 8 mm). The restrictions that are encountered with PET regarding interpretation of the chemical data are similar to those encountered in autoradiography. Many of these problems stem from the use of a tagged analogue rather than an isotope of the chemical normally metabolized by the brain. The analogue is used for a number of reasons, but primarily because it permits trapping of the metabolite and, therefore, separation of the rapid kinetics that might be encountered with the native molecule. When an analogue such as deoxyglucose is used, difficulties arise with the rate of reaction of the enzymes with the analogue, as well as with the distribution of the analogue. In the case of deoxyglucose, the differences in metabolism that might be detected because of the use of this analogue have been for the most part resolved.[24,31] The extensive work that was required to define its rate constant and the lump constant—parameters that take into account the differences stemming from the use of the analogue—would be required for other analogues that are of potential use. These problems do not occur, however, when an isotope of the parent molecule is used (e.g., oxygen 15). The physical problems, however, remain.[8]

NMR: Nuclear Magnetic Resonance

Atomic nuclei that possess a magnetic moment (for example, ^1H, ^2H, ^{13}C, ^{15}N, ^{19}F, ^{23}Na, ^{31}P, and ^{39}K) will absorb and emit a radio frequency when aligned by placing them in a strong, uniform, and constant magnetic field. The nuclei precess about this constant field at a fixed rate with a resultant radio-frequency signal emission that has a frequency that is determined by the magnetic field strength, the makeup of the atomic nucleus, and the atomic environment. In order to detect this signal, the nuclei must be synchronized. This is done with a short pulse of radio-frequency magnetic field oscillation near the frequency of the nuclei to be detected. The major determining factor of the resonant frequency is the atomic nucleus itself and the field in which it is placed. However, small shifts in frequency occur as a result of the surrounding molecules. For example, the alpha phosphate that is closest to the nucleotide of ATP has a different frequency than does the gamma phosphate. The gamma phosphate is farthest from the nucleotide in ATP. Also, changes in the environment of the molecules can result in a shift of the frequency emitted. Therefore, it is possible to detect a change in pH by measuring the difference in frequency between inorganic phosphate and phosphocreatine. Also, the proportion of bound water in a tissue changes the length of time that the nuclei will remain synchronous.

It is also possible to detect this. It is this property that is used to generate the anatomical pictures of proton NMR.

A major problem with NMR is that the signal is small and dependent on concentration of the nuclei under study. Since hydrogen is in high concentration in biological systems, an identifiable signal can be obtained from even a few cubic millimeters. The concentration of ^{31}P or ^{13}C, however, is much lower. As a result, spatial resolution is greatly reduced.[6,26]

Noninvasive Monitoring of Cerebral Oxidative Metabolism

Hemoglobin and the cytochrome chain have characteristic absorption spectra that extend into the near infrared. These spectra change depending upon the redox state of the molecule in question. The near infrared has a relatively low absorption by tissue. Jöbsis reports that changes in the absorption spectra of cerebral hemoglobin and cytochrome aa_3 can be recorded through the intact human skin and skull.[11] There is some debate about the validity of some of the observations because, thus far, they cannot be confirmed in vitro.

References

1. Astrup J: Energy-requiring cell functions in the ischemic brain: Their critical supply and possible inhibition in protective therapy. J Neurosurg 56:482–497, 1982.
2. Astrup J, Siesjö BK, Symon L: Thresholds in cerebral ischemia: The ischemic penumbra. Stroke 12:723–725, 1981.
3. Astrup J, Sørensen PM, Sørenson HR: Oxygen and glucose consumption related to NA^+-K^+ transport in canine brain. Stroke 12:726–730, 1981.
4. Bering EA Jr: Effect of body temperature change on cerebral oxygen consumption of the intact monkey. Am J Physiol 200:417–419, 1981.
5. Bremer J, Davis EJ: Studies on the active transfer of reducing equivalents into mitochondria via the malate-aspartate shuttle. Biochim Biophys Acta 376:387–397, 1975.
6. Burt CT, Cohen SM, Bárány M: Analysis of intact tissue with ^{31}P NMR. Annu Rev Biophys Bioeng 8:1–25, 1979.
7. Chance B, Cohen P, Jöbsis F, Schoener B: Intracellular oxidation-reduction states in vivo. Science 137:499–508, 1962.
8. Frackowiak RSJ, Lenzi GL, Jones T, Heather JD: Quantitative measurement of regional cerebral blood flow and oxygen metabolism in man using ^{15}O and positron emission tomography: Theory, procedure, and normal values. J Comput Assist Tomogr 4:727–736, 1980.
9. Hägerdal M, Harp JR, Siesjö BK: Effect of hypothermia upon organic phosphates, glycolytic metabolites, citric acid cycle intermediates and associated amino acids in rat cerebral cortex. J Neurochem 24:743–748, 1975.
10. Ingvar PH, Lassen NA (eds): *Brain Work: The Coupling of Function, Metabolism and Blood Flow in the Brain*. Copenhagen, Munksgaard, 1975.
11. Jöbsis FF: Oxidative metabolic effects of cerebral hypoxia. Adv Neurol 26:299–318, 1979.
12. Kety SS: Circulation and metabolism of the human brain in health and disease. Am J Med 8:205–217, 1950.
13. Kety SS, Schmidt CF: The effects of active and passive hyperventilation on cerebral blood flow, cerebral oxygen consumption, cardiac output, and blood pressure of normal young men. J Clin Invest 25:107–119, 1946.
14. Kreisman NR, Sick TJ, LaManna JC, Rosenthal M: Local tissue oxygen tension: Cytochrome a,a_3 redox relationships in rat cerebral cortex in vivo. Brain Res 218:161–174, 1981.
15. Laman D, Theodore J, Robin ED: Steady state adenine dinucleotide metabolism and the use of substrate redox pair analysis, in Robin ED (ed): *Extrapulmonary Manifestations of Respiratory Disease*, vol 8: *Lung Biology in Health and Disease*. New York, Marcel Dekker, 1978, pp 47–61.
16. Lewis DV, O'Connor MJ, Schuette WH: Oxidative metabolism during recurrent seizures in the penicillin treated hippocampus. Electroencephalogr Clin Neurophysiol 36:347–356, 1974.
17. Lying-Tunell U, Lindblad BS, Malmlund HO, Persson B: Cerebral blood flow and metabolic rate of oxygen, glucose, lactate, pyruvate, ketone bodies and amino acids: I. Young and old normal subjects. Acta Neurol Scand 62:265–275, 1980.
18. Meldrum BS: Epilepsy and δ-aminobutyric acid–mediated inhibition. Int Rev Neurobiol 17:1–36, 1975.
19. Miller AL, Hawkins RA, Veech RL: The mitochondrial redox state of rat brain. J Neurochem 20:1393–1400, 1973.
20. O'Connor MJ: Origin of labile NADH tissue fluorescence, in Jöbsis FF (ed): *Oxygen & Physiological Function*. Dallas, Professional Information Library, 1977, pp 90–99.
21. O'Connor MJ, Herman CJ, Rosenthal M, Jöbsis FF: Intracellular redox changes preceeding onset of epileptiform activity in intact cat hippocampus. J Neurophysiol 35:471–483, 1972.
22. Olney JW: Neurotoxicity of excitatory amino acids, in McGeer EG, Olney JW, McGeer PL (eds): *Kainic Acid as a Tool in Neurobiology*. New York, Raven Press, 1978, pp 95–121.
23. Pardridge WM, Oldendorf WH: Transport of metabolic substrates through the blood-brain barrier. J Neurochem 28:5–12, 1977.
24. Phelps ME, Huang SC, Hoffman EJ, Selin C, Sokoloff L, Kuhl DE: Tomographic measurement of local cerebral glucose metabolic rate in humans with (F-18)2-fluoro-2-deoxy-D-glucose: Validation of method. Ann Neurol 6:371–388, 1979.
25. Phelps ME, Mazziotta JC, Kuhl DE, Nuwer M, Packwood J, Metter J, Engel J, Jr: Tomographic mapping of human cerebral metabolism: Visual stimulation and deprivation. Neurology (NY) 31:517–529, 1981.
26. Roberts JKM, Jardetzky O: Monitoring of cellular metabolism by NMR. Biochim Biophys Acta 639:53–76, 1981.
27. Shank RP, Campbell GL: Glutamate, in Lajtha AJ (ed): *Handbook of Neurochemistry*, 2d ed, vol 3. New York, Plenum, 1983, pp 381–404.
28. Siesjö BK: *Brain Energy Metabolism*. New York, Wiley, 1978.
29. Siesjö BK, Berntman L: Cytoplasmic and mitochondrial redox changes in the brain during hypoxia. Adv Neurol 26:319–323, 1979.
30. Skou JC: Enzymatic basis for active transport of Na^+ and K^+ across cell membrane. Physiol Rev 45:596–617, 1965.
31. Sokoloff L: Localization of functional activity in the central nervous system by measurements of glucose utilization with radioactive deoxyglucose. J Cereb Blood Flow Metabol 1:7–36, 1981.
32. Welsh FA, O'Connor MJ, Marcy VR, Spatacco AJ, Johns RL: Factors limiting regeneration of ATP following temporary ischemia in cat brain. Stroke 13:234–242, 1982.
33. Wood JG, Jean DH, Whitaker JN, McLaughlin BJ, Albers RW: Immunocytolochemical localization of the sodium, potassium activated ATPase in knifefish brain. J Neurocytol 6:571–581, 1977.
34. Wood JD, Watson WJ: The effect of hyperoxia and hypoxia on free and bound δ-aminobutyric acid in mammalian brain. Can J Biochem 47:994–997, 1969.
35. Wood JD, Watson WJ, Ducker AJ: Oxygen poisoning in various mammalian species and the possible role of gamma-aminobutyric acid metabolism. J Neurochem 14:1067–1074, 1967.

142
Pathophysiological Consequences of Brain Ischemia

Jewell L. Osterholm

There are a number of diseases that may result in ischemia of the brain. Although stroke is usually first to come to mind, other emergency clinical syndromes such as cardiac arrest, severe shock, cerebral or subarachnoid hemorrhage, cerebral trauma, and elevated intracranial pressure due to a neoplasm may all result to some degree in cerebral ischemia. Common to all of these clinical abnormalities is a reduction of cerebral blood flow below levels that are sufficient to maintain normal cerebral metabolic function.

In the conditions mentioned above, the ischemia may affect blood flow to the whole brain, and therefore is called global ischemia, or it may affect blood flow to a localized area, in which case it is termed focal ischemia. In addition, the ischemic insult may be characterized by the degree to which blood flow to the brain is reduced. For example, in incomplete ischemia the brain circulation is not totally abolished, resulting in a hypoxic state, whereas complete ischemia implies a total absence of cerebral circulation, resulting in an anoxic state. Another important factor is the duration of ischemia; if prolonged, it may cause irreversible damage. It is important to recognize that the duration of ischemia, the degree of reduced blood flow, and the magnitude of the area of the brain affected are all pertinent variables in this discussion of altered metabolic responses following the insult of cerebral ischemia.

The final outcome of ischemic insult is often unpredictable.[19] There are certain neurophysiological changes, however, that have been found to regularly occur following decreases in cerebral blood flow.[13] The normal cerebral blood flow ranges from 45 to 60 ml per 100 g per minute. The blood flow may be reduced to a threshold level of 20 to 25 ml per 100 g per minute without affecting EEG activity in a normothermic, lightly anesthetized individual. Below that threshold level, the EEG activity gradually disappears, and at a blood flow of 15 ml per 100 g per minute, the evoked electrical cortical response disappears. At cerebral flow rates of approximately 5 ml per 100 g per minute, there is a massive release of potassium ions from the neurons into the extracellular space.

From several experimental observations there may be two pathophysiological steps or thresholds in response to ischemia.[2] Ischemia at the first threshold, which is generally reversible, induces inhibition of synaptic transmission as a result of neurotransmitter depletion. In order to restore the transmitter materials into the synaptic granules, ATP is required. Energy depletion therefore results in reuptake failure and synaptic arrest. The second threshold of ischemia is associated with structural changes of neuronal membranes in which high-energy phosphates are depleted and intracellular ionic balances cannot be maintained. This has been viewed as an irreversible state.

Under conditions of rapid circulatory arrest, the brain is more susceptible to injury than other organs because the brain has a high energy requirement, and a relatively low store of high-energy phosphates and oxygen. With a sudden decrease in blood flow to the brain, there is an immediate cessation of oxidative phosphorylation, resulting in a rapid depletion of mitochondrial ATP.[5] The first metabolic response to ischemia is an activation of cerebral glycolysis, and the available stores of glucose are rapidly utilized. Increased glucose utilization appears to occur even before overt anaerobic metabolism can be detected following mild ischemia. The metabolic trigger for glycolysis, which may reach levels greater than tenfold, is unknown. Some evidence has been presented to implicate an elevated activity of phosphofructokinase, as this enzyme is regulated by accumulating levels of ADP. With increases in cerebral norepinephrine levels, as governed by the locus ceruleus, there is a rise in cyclic AMP, which stimulates glycogenolysis. Glycogen is rapidly broken down, as are the available stores of pyruvate NADH, ketone bodies, and α-ketoglutarate. The remaining mitochondrial stores of cellular oxygen are depleted.

A predictable series of other biochemical changes occur with continuing ischemia.[12,13,22] These changes include a rapid decrease in tissue levels of phosphocreatine and adenosine triphosphate. The $NADH^+/NAD$ ratio increases, ADP and AMP contents rise, and there is an attendant loss of the cellular energy charge. Following these metabolic adjustments pyruvate declines rapidly and then disappears. At this point phosphocreatinine and ATP levels fall toward zero.

As a consequence of primarily anaerobic metabolism, lactate accumulates. There is an increased intracellular hydrogen ion concentration because of the excessive lactate presence. All available glucose, glycogen, and other suitable materials are metabolized to lactate. The actual degree of glycolysis under different ischemic conditions has been related to pathological, metabolic, and structural reactions.

Experimental animals that were rendered hyperglycemic prior to stroke production did not fare as well as their normoglycemic mates.[20,21] In the high glucose group, the intracellular pH dropped to 6.1 compared with 6.6 for the others. The pH difference between the two groups was associated with a disparity in recovery of the EEG, which was substantially delayed in the hyperglycemic group.

A destructive effect has been noted if tissue concentrations of lactate exceed 20 to 25 μg per gram of tissue. Animals that had cerebral cortex lactate of either 15 or 35 mm per liter were studied. In animals with lower lactate levels, there was considerable recovery of the cellular energy state and electrical activity during recirculation after ischemia.

1185

The animals with higher lactate levels, however, had persistent energy failure with no return of electrical activity. The low lactate specimens had minor structural alterations, but in the high lactate group there was extensive and severe tissue damage evident. There is, therefore, considerable evidence to implicate the degree of tissue lactic acidosis as a prime feature associated with the progressively worsening cellular effects and in development of irreversible ischemic nerve cell injury.[17]

A significantly increased uptake of [^{14}C]deoxyglucose was seen during ischemia of the hippocampus, globus pallidus, and substantia nigra compared with other brain areas.[7] These regions are well known for their sensitivity to oxygen lack, and their selective and excessive glucose utilization may contribute to the early structural damage that was observed.

The relationship between pH changes and structural damage requires comment. It has been shown that ultrastructural and metabolic changes following total ischemia are less severe than those that occur under conditions of partial blood flow. This apparent contradiction has been explained by the fact that the pH fall is abrupt but not sustained after the tissue glucose pool is exhausted in global ischemia. Partial ischemia, however, provides some glucose trickle so that there is continued lactate accumulation and hydrogen ions, which reach levels that are incompatible with cellular survival.

Another sequence of events that occurs with severe ischemia is loss of membrane integrity. Membranes are disturbed both at the intracellular and axonal level. Under normal circumstances, a large amount of total brain energy production is consumed in re-establishing ionic gradients of Na$^+$ and K$^+$ after axonal depolarization. ATP is required to pump the ions against a gradient under the influence of the membrane-bound Na$^+$,K$^+$-ATPase. The rapid decline of ATP following ischemia makes it impossible to re-establish normal ionic movements and gradients. Brain cells leak K$^+$ almost immediately after ischemia.[3] Extracellular K$^+$ rises from 3.0 mM to 28.5 mM after 4 min of ischemia, and 48.1 mM in 8 min.[23] Extracellular acidosis is evident at both time points. As potassium leaves the cell, sodium and water enter. The glia are also involved in this pathophysiological process for it has been found that glial nuclei are significantly depleted of sodium and potassium as early as 15 s after an ischemic insult.[10] This change is associated with a concomitant and significant drop in high-energy substrates in the glial nuclei as well as the total brain. These observations have important implications in terms of glial swelling, which is commonly associated with postischemic states.

Electron transport and oxidative phosphorylation occur at the inner mitochondrial membrane. An important ionic disruption after ischemia is inhibition of energy-linked calcium ion accumulation by the mitochondria. This phenomenon was found to be very severe in moribund animals. The inability of mitochondria to accumulate calcium may be used as an indicator of irreversible damage to the organelles during the course of ischemia. In terms of energetics calcium accumulation is competitive with phosphorylation at the mitochondrial membrane level.

Ischemia causes substantial disruption of amino acid metabolism.[15,18] During the first minute of ischemia there is an accelerated α-ketoglutarate consumption, and a marked increase in γ-aminobutyric acid (GABA) levels. Within 4 min pyruvate levels are decreased, which subsequently affects the glutamate and alanine levels. Glutamate is remarkably increased during anoxia. This accumulation can be explained in the following way:

1. The utilization of glutamate as an oxidative substrate may be inhibited during ischemia.
2. Nucleotides may stimulate the synthesis of glutamate using the increased levels of ammonia available.
3. Glutamate content may be increased as a result of enhanced glutamine decay.

There is a late accumulation of cystine, proline, methionine, cystidine, tryptophan, and tyrosine while lysine and phenylalanine decline. A hallmark chemical change in ischemia is an increased ammonia production in cerebral tissue. The ammonia may originate from glutamine, nucleotide, or protein amide groups. It is theorized that a decrease in the amount of glutamine early in ischemia is caused by a deamidation of this product.

Regional protein synthesis was measured at intervals of up to 48 h after cerebral ischemia of 10 or 30 min duration.[8] One hour following the 10-min ischemia period protein synthesis, as measured by incorporation of [^{14}C]valine into protein, was inhibited by 67 percent. However, protein synthesis at normal rates was achieved within 4 h of recirculation. In animals subjected to longer ischemic periods, protein synthesis was inhibited by 83 percent during the first hour. Thereafter protein synthesis recovery was slow and required 25 to 48 h for restitution. ^{14}C autoradiography revealed that pyramidal neurons and neurons in the hippocampus and caudate nucleus failed to recover normal protein synthesis rates even after 48 h of recovery.

The extensive surface area of excitable and intracellular membranes contains a wide variety and quantity of phospholipids. It has been found that immediately after interrupting the blood supply to the brain, a strikingly rapid increase of free fatty acids (FFA) takes place.[4] The rate of production of the cerebral FFA is of the same order of magnitude as that observed in adipose tissue under maximal lipolytic hormonal stimulation. It has been postulated that the cascade regulatory process of producing FFA may act on membrane-bound phospholipase A$_2$. This enzyme is responsible for production of arachidonic acid, docosahexanoic acid, and other unsaturated fatty acids. Also elaborated under this stress are palmitic, stearic, and oleic acids. In the course of experiments using electroshock, FFA are produced in the brain in a fashion similar to that observed attending ischemia. These data suggest that membrane lipids in the central nervous system actively deacylate and reacylate long-chain unsaturated fatty acids. An analysis of myelin and mitochondrial lipids from ischemic brain showed a decrease in fatty acid content. The components of decreased fatty acids fractions corresponded well to the types and amounts of FFA accumulating in the ischemic brain. An important consequence of the increased FFA production is an impairment of cerebral energy functions.[14] These materials play an important role in uncoupling oxidative phosphorylation at the respiratory chain. Active ionic transport across plasma membranes is deeply affected by the FFA. It has been found that the addition of FFA, glycerol, glycerol phospholipids, and deoxycholate in low concentrations inhibit calcium accumulation in the mitochondria.[24] The accumulation of calcium ions in the brain mitochondria is decreased by 35 percent after ischemia. Thus, increased FFA impairs brain function by:

1. Disturbing ionic transport across plasma membranes
2. Uncoupling oxidative phosphorylation at the respiratory chain level

The FFA can also induce structural changes. If ischemia is reversed before accumulation of free fatty acids surpass certain critical concentrations, no damage may occur. If these derivatives continue to increase, they can reach harmful and toxic levels where cellular damage may occur, since the accumulating free fatty acids can be involved in instituting irreversible cellular damage. The main FFA thought to have toxic properties is arachidonic acid. Increased arachidonic acid leads to increased production of prostaglandins E_2 and $F_{2\alpha}$. Prostaglandin formation requires a precursory fatty acid to be in free form and not esterified.

Some of the more important biochemical alterations in ischemia occur in the oxygen-mediated reactions in the electron transport chain.[19] During normal electron transport various partial oxidation productions possessing single unpaired electrons, termed *free radicals*, are formed through the action of molecular oxygen on membrane proteins. A constant level of free radical oxidation reactions, or peroxidation, is normally maintained in the cell through a delicate balance of activators to inhibitors of these reactions. A major peroxidation activator is molecular oxygen, but the partially reduced superoxide, perhydroxyradicals also contribute to peroxidation, as do the partially degraded fatty acid moieties. Endogenous peroxidation inhibitors include certain intracellular enzymes, such as catalase and superoxide dismutase as well as antioxidants such as ubiquinone, ascorbic acid, α-tocopherol, and glutathione. A change in the relationship of the optimum ratio of catalyst to inhibitors leads to development of pathological changes. An example of this would be a marked decrease in antioxidant tissue ability, since this would cause an accumulation of free radicals and specific degradation products of peroxidation that constitute disruptive influences.

Associated with ischemia there is an alteration in the proteins of the electron transport chain, producing a state of excessive reduced membrane proteins capable of reacting pathologically with residual tissue oxygen to produce additional free radicals. Membrane disruption also follows as the pathologically free radicals react with the unsaturated fatty acid moieties of the phospholipids making up the major portions of the cellular membranes, particularly those of cellular organelles such as mitochondria. Neurochemical disruptions of the membrane phospholipids may sufficiently damage the physiochemical state so as to alter ion selectivity and disturb functional capability of the membrane itself. An end result of this pathological chain reaction is an irreversible injury of the inner membrane of mitochondria. The mitochondria are the anatomical power locus for aerobic metabolism. With pH decreased because of increases in acidic metabolites and the breakdown of functional proteins, ATP net synthesis is no longer possible.

The neurotransmitters have not been identified in major pathological actions after ischemia. Serotonin (5-hydroxytryptamine) is implicated in cerebral edema, as shall be discussed below. Dopamine and norepinephrine have been reported to have an increased turnover during the first 2 h following ischemia.[6] Norepinephrine probably activates adenyl cyclase to elevate cyclic AMP, resulting in early metabolic changes in ischemia. It has been found that electrical stimulation of the locus ceruleus triggers an induction of cyclic AMP throughout the ipsilateral hemisphere.[9] At least one important function of cyclic AMP under these conditions is to stimulate glycogen breakdown and hence initiate improved glycolysis as the first line of metabolic defense against ischemia. Dopamine fibers have been found to be most sensitive to ischemia and are damaged by mild degrees of ischemia that are well tolerated by other cells.

A major pathophysiological change that occurs after ischemia is tissue edema.[1] Cerebral edema has been categorized into cytotoxic and vasogenic types, and defined by an abnormal water accumulation associated with increase in brain tissue volume.[11] Cytotoxic edema involves primarily the parenchymal structural elements that are affected directly by noxious chemical factors, resulting in intracellular swelling, while vasogenic edema causes an increase mainly in extracellular water content. Early in the course of ischemia the predominant edema type is almost purely cytotoxic. Cytotoxic edema is associated with sodium entering the cell and potassium escaping into the extracellular compartment. Water follows the intracellular movement of sodium, resulting in tissue edema. Vasogenic edema becomes prominent at a later stage of cerebral ischemia and coincides primarily with the reflow period. During restoration of the cerebral blood flow there is an accelerated leakage of plasma constituents from the blood due to damage of the blood-brain barrier. After short periods of ischemia a prompt restoration of cerebral blood flow drastically reduces the degree of brain edema. Following longer periods of ischemia, however, the return of cerebral blood flow enhances greatly the degree of vasogenic cerebral edema.

A better understanding as to the mechanism of cerebral edema that occurs after ischemic insult has been obtained through biochemical investigations.[16] Na^+, K^+-ATPase, cyclic AMP, and serotonin have been identified as principal factors responsible for the production of brain edema. The reduction of Na^+, K^+-ATPase activity at the capillary level is the triggering mechanism for the leaky capillaries that exist at the reflow period. The fall in Na^+, K^+-ATPase impairs the capillary's ability to restore proper ionic balance, and hence the vessels are leaky. Following ischemia a rise of cyclic AMP that is induced by released serotonin increases the outward flux of potassium from the cells into the extracellular space. A combined effect of serotonin release along with the impairment of vessel wall Na^+, K^+-ATPase are major factors responsible for the development of the severe postischemic vasogenic edema. The liberation of free fatty acids from nervous tissue has also been linked with tissue edema in postischemic states.[4] Experimental studies involving intracerebral injection of various polyunsaturated fatty acids indicate that these substances are capable of producing tissue edema. When injected into the brain, arachidonic acid, which has been identified in the brain after ischemia, can result in severe edema similar to that seen after stroke.

A complex cascade of pathophysiological events attending cerebral ischemia has been described. During the initial ischemia stages glycolysis is preserved through the breakdown of glycogen to glucose under the influence of catecholamines and cyclic AMP. Ketone bodies may also be utilized during this period. Under these anaerobic conditions the end metabolic product is lactate. The prolongation of glycolytic anaerobic metabolism is detrimental as a result of the formation of lactate. The high tissue lactate level lowers intracellular pH and may be the cause of irreversible cerebral injury following an ischemic insult. The continued progress of glycolysis obtained during incomplete ischemia is more harmful to the cerebral tissues than is complete circulatory arrest. In the latter conditions all the metabolites are utilized quickly, thereby preventing the accumulation of the excessive lactate and the decline of intracellular pH. After cellular energy stores are exhausted, ionic membrane pumps fail, with an attendant dislocation of ionic components and the production of edema. Fatty acids accumulate as degradation materials from the phospholipid membrane walls. In the presence of large quantities of fatty acids the pathological changes that occur include the formation of edema, increased synthesis of the prostaglandins, and disturbances of the mitochondrial membranes. There are also changes in the physical state of the proteins themselves. Lipid peroxidation can, under some circumstances, be initiated, and the consequences of this reaction have been discussed. The central issue of reversibility versus irreversibility probably hangs upon a complex number of factors. The factors that have been identified as most important are the degree of intracellular acidosis, the presence or absence of continued anaerobic metabolism, and the relative integrity of the mitochondrial and cellular membranes.

At this time there is extensive experimental evidence to support the contention that neurons can survive ischemia for extended time periods under very specific conditions. Resuscitation has been obtained in vivo after global ischemia of 1-h duration. We found that in brain sliced in vitro following ischemia, the brain slices would reinitiate uptake of glucose and norepinephrine after as long as 4 h of ischemia when they were resupplied with glucose and oxygen. Stroke therapy will be improved when methods are designed that effectively control intracellular pH levels and resupply the neurons within their limits of ischemia tolerance.

References

1. Abe K, Abe T, Klatzo I, Spatz M: Effect of endogenous central nervous system depressants in ischemic cerebral edema of gerbils. Adv Neurol 28:429–441, 1980.
2. Astrup J: Energy-requiring cell functions in the ischemic brain: Their critical supply and possible inhibition in protective therapy. J Neurosurg 56:482–497, 1982.
3. Astrup J, Rehncrona S, Siesjö BK: The increase in extracellular potassium concentration in the ischemic brain in relation to the preischemic functional activity and cerebral metabolic rate. Brain Res 199:161–174, 1980.
4. Bazan NG, Rodriguez de Turco EB: Membrane lipids in the pathogenesis of brain edema: Phospholipids and arachidonic acid, the earliest membrane components changed at the onset of ischemia. Adv Neurol 28:197–205, 1980.
5. Benzi G, Dagani F, Arrigoni E: Acute model for the estimation of the cerebral energy state during or after hypoxia and complete or incomplete ischaemia. Eur Neurol 17 (Suppl I):87–96, 1978.
6. Bralet J, Beley P, Bralet AM, Beley A: Catecholamine levels and turnover during brain ischemia in the rat. J Neural Transm 48:143–155, 1980.
7. Diemer NH, Siemkowicz E: Increased 2-deoxyglucose uptake in hippocampus, globus pallidus and substantia nigra after cerebral ischemia. Acta Neurol Scand 61:56–63, 1980.
8. Dienel GA, Pulsinelli WA, Duffy TE: Regional protein synthesis in rat brain following acute hemispheric ischemia. J Neurochem 35:1216–1226, 1980.
9. Harik SI, Busto R, Martinez E: Norepinephrine regulation of cerebral glycogen utilization during seizures and ischemia. J Neurosci 2:409–414, 1982.
10. Ignelzi RJ: Sodium, potassium, and metabolic studies of glial, liver, and kidney nuclei under anoxic-ischemic conditions. Neurol Res 2:35–46, 1980.
11. Ito U, Ohno K, Nakamura R, Suganuma F, Inaba Y: Brain edema during ischemia and after restoration of blood flow: Measurement of water, sodium, potassium content and plasma protein permeability. Stroke 10:542–547, 1979.
12. Keykhah MM, Welsh FA, Miller AS, Harp JR, DeFeo SP: Cerebral energy metabolite levels and survival following exposure to low inspired oxygen concentration. Crit Care Med 6:330–334, 1978.
13. Kogure K, Scheinberg P, Utsunomiya Y, Kishikawa H, Busto R: Sequential cerebral biochemical and physiological events in controlled hypoxemia. Ann Neurol 2:304–310, 1977.
14. Kuwashima J, Nakamura K, Fujitani B, Kadokawa T, Yoshida K, Shimizu M: Relationship between cerebral energy failure and free fatty acid accumulation following prolonged brain ischemia. Jpn J Pharmacol 28:277–287, 1978.
15. Melitauri NN, Chikvaidze VN, Nikolaishvili LN: Change in the content of free amino acids in the brain of rabbits under circulatory hypoxia (ischemia). Neuropatol Pol 3:379–389, 1979.
16. Mršulja BB, Djuričić BM, Cvejić V, Mršulja BJ, Abe K, Spatz M, Klatzo I: Biochemistry of experimental ischemic brain edema. Adv Neurol 28:217–230, 1980.
17. Rehncrona S, Rosen I, Siesjö BK: Excessive cellular acidosis: An important mechanism of neuronal damage in the brain? Acta Physiol Scand 110:435–437, 1980.
18. Rossowska M, Zalewska T: Effect of hypoxia and ischemia on the distribution of protein in brain cellular fractions. Neurochem Res 4:15–23, 1979.
19. Shaller CA, Jacques S, Shelden CH: The pathophysiology of stroke: A review with molecular considerations. Surg Neurol 14:433–443, 1980.
20. Siemkowicz E, Gjedde A: Post-ischemic coma in rat: Effect of different pre-ischemic blood glucose levels on cerebral metabolic recovery after ischemia. Acta Physiol Scand 110:225–232, 1980.
21. Siemkowicz E, Hansen AJ: Brain extracellular ion composition and EEG activity following 10 minutes ischemia in normo- and hyperglycemic rats. Stroke 12:236–240, 1981.
22. Siesjö BK: *Brain Energy Metabolism.* New York, Wiley, 1978.
23. Silver IA: Changes in PO_2 and ion fluxes in cerebral hypoxia-ischemia. Adv Exp Med Biol 78:299–312, 1977.
24. Strosznajder J: Role of phospholipids in calcium accumulation in brain mitchondria from adult rat after ischemic anoxia and hypoxic hypoxia. Bull Acad Pol Sci [Biol] 27:683–692, 1980.

143

Atherosclerosis

Jack C. Geer
Julio H. Garcia

The average age at which atherosclerotic lesions are first evident in craniocervical arteries is greater than that at which they are first evident in the aorta and coronary arteries. Fatty streaks (sessile lipid-containing intimal streaks or dots) are first evident in the cerebral arteries during the second decade of life. These lesions do not cause symptoms. They probably are the early stage of the atherosclerotic fibrous plaque, which is the raised mass lesion protruding into the vascular lumen made up of a core of lipid debris, atheroma, and cap of fibromuscular tissue. Fibrous plaques are first evident in the third decade of life in carotid arteries, and in the fourth decade in vertebral and intracranial arteries. The extent (percent intimal surface affected) of atherosclerotic lesions (fatty streaks and plaques) generally is less than that seen in the aorta or coronary arteries. With advancing age the extent of lesions increases in the cerebral arteries, parallel to the increases seen in the aorta and coronary arteries.[7]

Studies of arterial lesions and their association with disease have shown that it is the plaques that cause symptoms. These studies have disclosed no evidence to suggest that the pathogenesis of cerebral arterial lesions differs from that in other arteries. We may infer that etiologic factors for atherosclerotic lesions also do not differ, but such factors could have greater or lesser effects in the various arterial beds. That atherosclerotic lesions develop in cerebral arteries later in life (one to two decades) than they do in coronary arteries or aorta has been documented but not explained. A practical implication of this observation is that when extensive or occlusive atherosclerosis is present in cerebral arteries, severe atherosclerosis can be expected to exist in other arteries.

Atherosclerotic plaques cause clinical disease by two mechanisms: (1) obstruction of blood flow to the peripheral tissue; and (2) ulceration or fissuring in the surface of plaques (Fig. 143-1) with subsequent platelet and fibrin deposition resulting in peripheral tissue ischemia or necrosis by either embolism from the forming thrombus, vasoactive substances released by aggregating platelets, or total thrombotic vascular occlusion. Basic questions in atherogenesis are: How do plaques form and grow? Why do some plaques ulcerate or fissure?

Atherogenesis

Atherogenesis is a process characterized by intimal thickening with focal deposition of lipid derived from the blood plasma, smooth muscle cell proliferation, influx of blood monocytes, and connective tissue formation. Two theories attempt to account for the above. The thrombogenic hypothesis states that thrombi form on the vascular surface, presumably in response to endothelial injury; subsequently, these thrombi become incorporated into the intima by endothelial overgrowth. The thrombotic material degenerates in the intima, releasing bound lipids and lipid from lipoproteins, thereby yielding the lipid component of the lesion. Smooth muscle cells in the adjacent intima or media proliferate and synthesize connective tissues (collagen and glycosaminoglycans), which are characteristic of the organization (scarring) process. Cholesterol is the predominant lipid constituent of atherosclerotic lesions at all stages of development. If an organizing thrombus is a common pathogenetic pathway, it must be assumed that the phospholipids and triglycerides derived from cellular or lipoprotein degeneration are catabolized by smooth muscle cells or blood monocytes that have migrated into the developing lesion. Cholesterol cannot be catabolized by these cells, and thus it represents, in a sense, a "foreign body" that must be physically removed from the tissue or sequestered. Most students of atherosclerosis do not believe that mural thrombosis and organization represents a common or major mechanism for the fatty streak lesions of atherosclerosis. Few question,

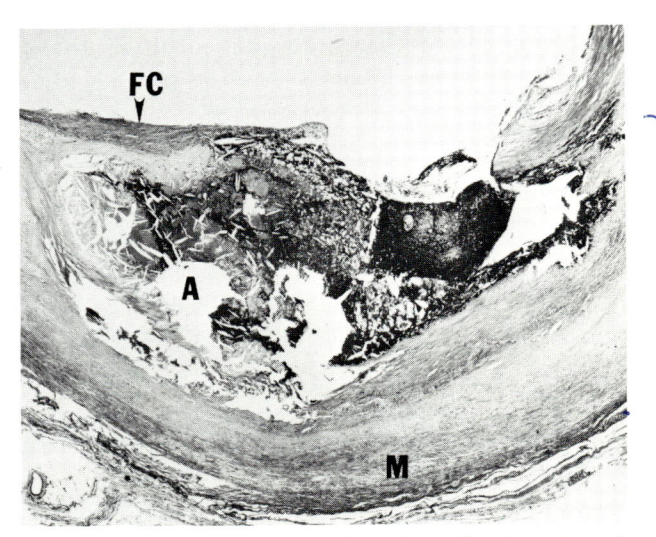

Figure 143-1 Histological section of the distal portion of the carotid bulb of a 72-year-old man dying with extensive neoplasm and pulmonary embolism. He had no clinical symptomatology related to the central nervous system, and no embolic lesions were found at autopsy. Shown is an ulcerated atheromatous plaque that had caused an approximately 40 percent stenosis of the lumen. Rupture of the fibrous cap (FC) is evident to the right of center, with hemorrhage into the atheroma (A). There is no evidence of thrombus formation. M, media.

however, that plaque lesions commonly increase in mass by this mechanism.

The dominant theory for the initiation and progression of early atherosclerotic lesions is the filtration or insudation hypothesis. This hypothesis states that blood plasma constituents traverse the endothelium into the intima wherein they stimulate cellular proliferative and connective tissue responses that characterize the lesions.[4]

Diffuse Intimal Thickening

Compositional-structural changes in the arterial intima may be prerequisite to the deposition of blood plasma constituents that are the supposed stimuli for lesion formation. The intima of human arteries progressively thickens with age up to the fourth decade of life. The components of the thickened intima are smooth muscle cells, glycosaminoglycans, collagens, and elastin. One or more of these components may trap blood plasma constituents that eventually produce the atheromatous core of the lesion and stimulate the cellular and connective tissue reaction. Intimal thickening (commonly referred to as diffuse intimal thickening) has been observed in all human populations examined. If intimal thickening is requisite for development of atherosclerosis, we can hypothesize that all population-race groups are susceptible to atherosclerosis and will develop such if the necessary etiologic factors are imposed. This hypothesis is supported by epidemiologic observations; a population-race group that migrates from an area or environment with a low incidence of atherosclerotic diseases to one with a high incidence subsequently manifests an increased incidence of atherosclerotic diseases.[4–7] Present evidence indicates that all populations of human beings exposed to the known risk factors for atherosclerosis will develop plaque lesions and atherosclerotic diseases; however, within any population there is wide individual variability for the extent to which such lesions develop. Individual variability probably is both genetically and environmentally determined.

Plasma Lipids

Cholesterol is the predominant lipid constituent of the lesions and is derived from the blood plasma exclusively, or at least nearly so. Thus, the amount of cholesterol in the blood may be an etiologic factor for atherogenesis. Epidemiologic studies have shown that the plasma cholesterol level correlates positively with atherosclerotic disease. This correlation has stimulated a vast amount of research on lipoprotein metabolism and diet, which indicates that low-density lipoprotein cholesterol level and dietary cholesterol and saturated fat are significant etiologic factors for atherogenesis. High-density lipoprotein, particularly HDL2, appears to have a negative correlation, affording some measure of protection against atherosclerosis. The mechanism for HDL protection remains to be proved. HDL may play a role in removal of cholesterol from tissue, which, as stated previously, must be accomplished physically, as arterial wall cells are not capable of catabolizing cholesterol. Critics of the hypercholesterolemia cause for atherogenesis call attention to the large number of persons with atherosclerotic diseases who do not have hypercholesterolemia or hyperlipidemia of any recognized type. Remnant or variant lipoproteins that are atherogenic exist and are not measured by the commonly used methods for assay of lipoproteins. These lipoproteins include remnant chylomicrons; partially delipidated, very low density lipoprotein; and heavy low-density lipoprotein. Low level of the putative protective high-density lipoprotein also could be a factor in subjects with plasma total cholesterol levels in the normal range. Research currently underway should clarify the role of remnant or variant lipoproteins in atherogenesis and their possible relation to established risk factors for atherosclerosis: diet, smoking, hypertension, diabetes mellitus, and obesity.[8,11]

Endothelium

The filtration hypothesis requires movement of plasma constituents from the blood compartment across the endothelium into the intimal compartment. Endothelial injury causing increased permeability may be a factor in atherogenesis by increasing influx into the intima of plasma constituents that in turn stimulate the cellular and connective tissue responses. Most attention has been directed to lipid influx because of the large amount of lipid that accumulates in the lesions. Other plasma constituents have been identified in the lesions that also may contribute to the intimal cellular and connective reaction. These constituents include albumin, fibrinogen, apolipoproteins, and globulins.[4,10]

The mechanism for transport of plasma constituents across the endothelium remains to be elucidated. Endothelial injury and resultant increased permeability could have several causes, among which are hemodynamic stress and vasoactive substances. The injury could alter the endothelial glycocalyx and cause platelet adhesion. Platelets may then aggregate and release vasoactive substances, such as thromboxane A_2, serotonin, or cationic protein, that increase endothelial permeability. Endothelial cell injury also could decrease prostacyclin formation, which would permit platelet adhesion and aggregation.[9] These possible mechanisms are all speculative and must be substantiated. A curious phenomenon occurs in an experimental model where the vascular endothelium is removed by balloon catheter; in the presence of induced hyperlipidemia, arterial intimal lipid deposition occurs only after the endothelium regenerates.

Infectious-immune causes for endothelial or intimal cellular reactive changes have been suggested. Chickens with Marek virus infection develop arterial lesions. Hyperlipidemic rabbits with serum sickness develop arterial plaques that closely resemble those of human beings. Vasectomized monkeys develop more arterial lesions than do normal monkeys. Transplanted hearts are more susceptible to arterial lesion development than are normal hearts. These observations suggest the possibilities of virus-induced cellular change and immune complex injury. Immune complexes may fix complement on the endothelium, thereby causing increased cellular permeability or cell death. That infectious-immune mechanisms are major and common etiologic factors for atherogenesis is difficult to reconcile with available epidemiologic data for atherosclerosis unless infection

Smooth Muscle Cells

Smooth muscle cells, monocyte-derived macrophages, and mast cells are found in atherosclerotic lesions. Smooth muscle cells are the predominant cell in most human lesions. Mast cells are present in small number. The role of mast cells in atherogenesis is unknown. Smooth muscle cells present in diffuse intimal thickening, fatty streaks, and plaques are thought to be derived from medial smooth muscle cells that have migrated into the intima. Smooth muscle cells in the intima increase in number by mitotic division. Intimal smooth muscle cells accumulate cytoplasmic lipid and synthesize connective tissues.[4]

Stimuli for smooth muscle cell proliferation in vitro include a platelet-derived growth factor and low-density lipoprotein. Whether these substances react similarly in vivo remains to be determined. It is quite possible that yet to be identified plasma- and cell-derived mitogenic substances are involved.[10]

Smooth muscle cells in atherosclerotic lesions perform at least two functions: intracellular lipid storage and connective tissue synthesis. Smooth muscle cells may acquire numbers of cytoplasmic lipid inclusions that presumably contain cholesteryl esters. Cellular and extracellular lipid accumulation suggests the possibility of abnormal lipid metabolism in the artery wall as an etiologic or pathogenetic factor for atherogenesis. Esterification of cholesterol appears to be a normal or protective reaction by cells in the artery wall; potentially membrane-damaging nonesterified cholesterol is changed to biologically inert cholesteryl esters. Lipid composition studies of atherosclerotic lesions have provided little support for the abnormal metabolism hypothesis.[1] Future studies may, however, reveal effects on cellular integrity and function by lysosomal enzymes, hydroxy fatty acids, prostaglandins, oxidant injury, or leukotrienes.

Monocyte-Macrophage Foam Cell

The role of the monocyte-macrophage in atherogenesis has received much attention recently. Foam cells (cells laden with cholesteryl esters) have long been recognized in atherosclerotic lesions. The foam cell is derived from blood monocytes that migrate into the intima and are activated by unknown mechanisms to become macrophages. The identity of the foam cell as a monocyte-macrophage has been established by the demonstration of C3 and Fc membrane receptors which smooth muscle cells do not possess. The macrophage probably plays a major role in atherogenesis and regression of lesions. The stimulus for its migration from the blood into the intima is not known. The activated monocyte (macrophage) has, in addition to its phagocytic property, the capacity to synthesize a wide range of substances, including collagenase, elastase, and platelet-activating factor, that very likely are involved in atherogenesis. Foam cells in experimental lesions induced by diet hyperlipidemia show a marked reduction in number in lesions that have been allowed to regress by removing the diet stimulus to hyperlipidemia. Normalization of blood lipid level is associated with a marked reduction in the number of intimal foam cells and a sharp reduction in the cholesteryl ester content of the lesion. It is assumed that foam cells migrate from the intima into the blood.[2,3]

Connective Tissues

Smooth muscle cell–derived connective tissues are major constituents of atherosclerotic lesions. These connective tissues, particularly collagens, are scar tissue presumably stimulated by intimal deposition of plasma constituents. Connective tissues probably are also involved in binding plasma constituents in the intima. Lipid deposition in the intima could result from increased endothelial permeability (increased load) or impaired transport through the intima. As stated previously, glycosaminoglycans and elastin bind lipoproteins.[5] Binding (trapping) of lipid or other plasma constituents may be a major causative factor for the cellular reactions in the intima. This hypothesis differs in no substantial way from that proposed by Virchow over 100 years ago. The probable role of remnant or variant lipoproteins may be related to connective tissue binding. Future studies of binding of lipoproteins, molecular structure of connective tissues, and cellular reactions to bound lipoproteins should materially advance our knowledge of atherogenesis. Presently developed cell culture, lipoprotein isolation, and connective tissue isolation methods make such studies feasible.

Fibrous Plaques

Causes for and mechanisms by which fatty streak lesions transform into plaques are unknown. Indeed, some do not believe that fatty streaks are the early plaque lesion. We believe that some fatty streaks progress to plaque lesions whereas others remain static or regress. Structural and biochemical studies of fatty streaks have disclosed no differences between fatty streaks from various anatomical locations or population groups that might explain differences in potential. The basic question is: What are the stimuli for plaque formation and increase in plaque mass once the lesion is formed? Previous considerations of atherogenesis all obtain to some degree, but which are the most and least important is unknown. A hypothetical stimulus for plaque formation is necrosis of lipid-laden intimal cells, releasing lipid and other cellular contents into the interstitial space and thus forming the atheroma that somehow stimulates smooth muscle cell proliferation and connective tissue synthesis in the adjacent tissue. Cellular necrosis can be demonstrated in human lesions, but the role of such in plaque formation is conjectural. Another hypothesis is smooth muscle transformation, that is, monoclonal proliferation. Studies of glucose-6-phosphate dehydrogenase isozymes in human plaques have shown a single isozyme in the lesions, suggesting monoclonal proliferation, a neoplastic transformation. This interpretation has been questioned and an alternative explanation proposed, that of selective growth potential.

Selective growth potential means that cells with one isozyme are more likely to proliferate and thus survive than those with the other isozyme, thus the monoclonicity is apparent but not real.[1,7,12]

Once formed, the plaque lesion can increase in volume by several mechanisms. One mechanism is connective tissue synthesis. Plaques may be composed largely of collagen with little or no apparent atheroma. Whether such a plaque is due primarily to connective tissue synthesis or represents a lesion in which the atheromatous debris has been removed by macrophages is unknown. Mural thrombosis and organization are observed frequently in plaque lesions, and unquestionably represent a common mechanism for increasing plaque volume. The causes for the injury that stimulates thrombus formation are unknown. Hemodynamic stresses on the endothelium produced by the mass lesion protruding into the lumen may be a cause for the injury. Lipid accumulation from the blood plasma is another mechanism for plaque growth. Foam cells are observed frequently in the fibrous cap of a plaque lesion, suggesting lipid deposition. Alternatively, these foam cells could reflect lipid transport from the lesions to the blood. There is no way at present to know which role these cells play, and indeed, both processes could operate simultaneously. Lipid composition studies demonstrate clearly that the apparently inert atheroma lipid is in fact turning over. Another mechanism by which plaques may increase in volume is hemorrhage into the lesion. Hemorrhage may be due to focal rupture (ulceration, fissure) of the fibrous cap of the lesion (Fig. 143-1) or rupture of vasa vasora, which are small blood vessels that proliferate through the tunica media into the base of the lesion. It is not possible with present information to state which of the mechanisms presented above is the most common one. Observation of human lesions suggests that mural thrombosis and lipid accumulation are the most common mechanisms for plaque growth.[4]

Total thrombotic occlusion of an artery associated with atherosclerosis is almost invariably if not invariably associated with rupture of a plaque. Atheroma material is a strong procoagulant. For a totally occlusive thrombus to form, it is necessary that, in addition to plaque rupture and procoagulant activation of the coagulation system, blood flow be slowed. Evidence for the previous statement is indirect but substantial. Endarterectomy, balloon angioplasty, or experimental balloon de-endothelialization results in minimal thrombus formation if blood flow is rapid. Reduced blood flow in arteries with ruptured plaques may be due to distal occlusive atheromatous plaques or vasospasm.

References

1. Cornwell DG, Geer JC, Panganamala RV: Development of atheroma and the lipid composition of the deposit, in Masoro EJ (ed): *Pharmacology of Lipid Transport and Atherosclerotic Processes.* Oxford, Pergamon, 1975, pp 445–483.
2. Gerrity RG: The role of the monocyte in atherogenesis: I. Transition of blood-borne monocytes into foam cells in fatty lesions. Am J Pathol 103:181–190, 1981.
3. Goldstein JL, Hoff HF, Ho YK, Basu SK, Brown MS: Stimulation of cholesteryl ester synthesis in macrophages by extracts of atherosclerotic human aortas and complexes of albumin/cholesteryl esters. Arteriosclerosis 1:210–226, 1981.
4. Haust MD: The morphogenesis and fate of potential and early atherosclerotic lesions in man. Hum Pathol 2:1–29, 1971.
5. Hollander W, Paddock J, Colombo M: Lipoproteins in human atherosclerotic vessels: 1. Biochemical properties of arterial low density lipoproteins, very low density lipoproteins, and high density lipoproteins. Exp Mol Pathol 30:144–171, 1979.
6. Keys A: Coronary heart disease: The global picture. Atherosclerosis 22:149–192, 1975.
7. McGill HC (ed): *The Geographic Pathology of Atherosclerosis.* Baltimore, Williams & Wilkins, 1968.
8. McGill HC Jr: The relationship of dietary cholesterol to serum cholesterol concentration and to atherosclerosis in man. Am J Clin Nutr 32:2664–2702, 1979.
9. Moncada S: Prostacyclin and arterial wall biology. Arteriosclerosis 2:193–207, 1982.
10. Ross R, Glomset JA: The pathogenesis of atherosclerosis. N Engl J Med 295:369–377, 420–425, 1976.
11. Segrest JP, Chung BH, Cone JT, Hughes TA: Coronary heart disease risk: Assessment by plasma lipoprotein profiles. Ala J Med Sci 20:76–83, 1983.
12. Thomas WA, Reiner JM, Janakidevi K, Florentin RA, Lee KT: Population dynamics of arterial cells during atherogenesis: X. Study of monotypism in atherosclerotic lesions of black women heterozygous for glucose-6-phosphate dehydrogenase (G-6-PD). Exp Mol Pathol 31:367–386, 1979.

ID
144
Pathology of Ischemic Cerebrovascular Disease

John Moossy

Ischemic cerebrovascular disease may be of two types, *global ischemia* and *focal or regional ischemia*[6,16]

Global ischemia refers to the condition in which blood flow to the entire brain is suddenly reduced as a result of the failure of the heart as a perfusion pump, or to the development of severe, increased intracranial pressure.[6] Cardiac arrest due to a variety of causes, cardiac arrhythmias, shock, or intermittent, severe episodes of hypotension may all be associated with global cerebral ischemia. The most common clinical example of brief, completely reversible global cerebral ischemia is syncope. More grave, prolonged derangements of the total cerebral circulation, such as occur with cardiac arrest, may produce some degree of bilateral, multifocal, relatively symmetrical brain damage, usually microinfarcts and laminar cortical necrosis. These lesions are sometimes extensive, and at other times crudely limited to the arterial border zones. The degree and extent of brain damage correlate with the duration of ischemia, the adequacy of collateral circulation, pre-existing disease of the blood vessels, such as atherosclerosis, the age of the patient, and the efficacy of reperfusion.

Focal (or regional) cerebral ischemia is due to interruption or diminution of the blood supply to neural tissue in a specific arterial or venous territory. Arterial lesions are the most common clinically and at autopsy. The interruption or diminution of blood flow is usually due to occlusive lesions such as thrombi and emboli. When there is an abundant collateral circulation, lack of intrinsic vessel disease, and efficient reperfusion of tissue, occlusive lesions do not necessarily produce infarction, or even symptoms. Occlusive venous lesions, in particular, must be extensive before infarction occurs. With either type of occlusive lesion, arterial or venous, the production of ischemia, or reduced blood flow, is heralded first by functional changes at the electrophysiological level.[10] Then, well before significant tissue damage or infarction, symptoms occur. Not all neurons die within an area of persistent focal ischemia, and death or survival of cells is attributed to some intrinsic cellular differences as indicated by the concept of selective neuronal necrosis.[2,22] Although somewhat vague and purely descriptive, the term *selective neuronal necrosis* implies functional molecular differences in morphologically similar neurons and in different neuronal aggregates to account for their greater susceptibility or resistance to ischemic damage.

When focal ischemia is severe and persistent, and reperfusion is faulty, then necrosis of all neural elements—neurons, neuropil, glia, and even a few blood vessels—may occur, and this state is referred to as *infarction*. At the microscopic level, infarcts have the same cellular events whether due to focal ischemia or global ischemia.[6] In the former case they are circumscribed infarcts, confined to the territory of specific vessels (usually arterial) and grossly visible; in the latter case they are usually multifocal infarcts, often bilaterally symmetrical and microscopic in size, and therefore, not impressive in the early stages.

This chapter will deal with those varieties of ischemia severe enough to produce cerebral infarction: atherosclerosis and the complicated lesions leading to cerebral infarcts; cerebral thrombosis and embolism due to diverse causes; the gross and microscopic features of cerebral infarcts; and some important secondary complications such as brain edema and herniations.

Intracranial and Extracranial Atherosclerosis

The complicated lesions of atherosclerosis are the major intrinsic vascular factors responsible for ischemic cerebrovascular disease and cerebral infarction.[14,15] Atherosclerosis in its basic aspects is the subject of another chapter in this volume. In this section only the lesions of the intracranial and extracranial arteries supplying the brain will be considered. The gross and histopathological features of atherosclerosis differ little, if at all, in various parts of the body. Generally, extracranial cerebral atherosclerosis, chiefly in the carotid arteries, will evolve in the same manner and share the same risk factors as coronary artery atherosclerosis. However, there appear to be differences in the age of onset of the disease, its quantitative severity, the sites of lesion localization, and some risk factors when the intracranial arteries and the extracranial vertebral arteries are compared with the extracranial carotid and coronary arteries.[5]

The lesions of intracranial atherosclerosis usually appear a decade after those in coronary arteries and two decades after aortic lesions in autopsy populations. The early lesions (fatty streaks) are small, flat, sudanophilic, intimal foci and, of themselves, are of no known clinical significance. After adolescence, all arterial segments show a different lesion (or, more likely, an altered fatty streak) known as the fibrous plaque. This lesion, with its abundant connective tissue as well as lipid, may remain relatively static with no clinical consequences, or it may become complicated by stenosis, ulceration, thrombosis, calcification, ectasia, fusiform aneurysm formation, or hemorrhage within the plaque. It is these complicated fibrous plaques that may have clinical concomitants, including ischemia and infarction in the neural tissue supplied by the affected vessels. What causes some fibrous plaques in the cerebral circulation to become complicated remains unknown, but there are certain obvious risk factors,

1193

of which hypertension is the most important, followed by coronary artery disease, diabetes mellitus, and possibly the familial hyperlipidemias, although the data are not yet clear on the last point. Except for hypertension, these risk factors seem to be more significant for extracranial carotid atherosclerosis than for that in the intracranial arteries. There also appear to be differences due to sex and race. Women less often have severe extracranial carotid bifurcation disease in the form of complicated lesions compared with men. Blacks[9,23] and Japanese[19] have been reported to have more severe intracranial atherosclerosis likely to result in complicated lesions than do whites in whom both extracranial carotid artery lesions and intracranial disease are conspicuous components of cerebrovascular disorders.

Thrombosis and Other Complicated Lesions of Atherosclerosis

The major, clinically pertinent, complicated lesion of atherosclerosis is thrombosis. It is likely that all three elements of Virchow's triad—abnormality of blood flow, injury to the blood vessel lining, and alteration in the blood constituents—are important in cerebrovascular thromboses. The thrombotic process responsible for cerebrovascular ischemia is most directly documented in all its phases in carotid endarterectomy specimens. A full range of pathological changes have been described in various reports, but the apparent sequence of events appears to be as follows. Fatty streaks and then fibrous plaque formation begin in the tunica intima of the carotid bifurcation about the same time as coronary artery lesions appear, i.e., the second and third decades of life. In individuals with the appropriate risk factors, and for other reasons as yet unknown, there is progressive enlargement of the plaque as a result of increasing amounts of connective tissue and of degenerative changes with the plaque, the so-called atheromatous degeneration or atheroma formation. Atheromas are soft, necrotic foci within the fibrous plaque filled with cellular debris, lipid, cholesterol, and variable amounts of fibrin. As the plaque enlarges, a significant degree of luminal stenosis (greater than 75 percent of the luminal cross-sectional area) may occur and occasionally be productive of intermittent, brief, focal ischemic symptoms or transient ischemic attacks (TIAs), particularly if some other factor such as hypotension is present. More often, some injury (possibly related to hemodynamic stress to the endothelial cell lining over the plaque) takes place, such as ulceration or fissuration, and platelet aggregation and adhesion begins on the injured intimal surface. Exposed collagen and atheromatous debris powerfully attract platelets presumably because of their content of adenosine diphosphate (ADP). The adherent platelets release ADP, and additional platelet aggregation and adherence occurs.

Concurrent or rapidly evolving biochemical events, often referred to as the *coagulation cascade,* begin. This cascade is an exceedingly complex, still incompletely understood, process that involves plasma proteins, factor VIII, arachidonic acid, prostaglandins, thromboxane A_2, thrombin, fibrinogen, and ultimately fibrin. The aggregated and adherent platelets serve as a nidus for increasing amounts of fibrin deposition, and as the aggregate projects into the lumen, these small, mural fibrin-platelet thrombi entrap increasing numbers of white blood cells, then red blood cells, in roughly alternating layers (lines of Zahn). These are the basic cellular events in the formation of small (fibrin-platelet, white) thrombi and the larger, occlusive (red-white) thrombi.

A number of events may take place thereafter, if there is an adequate collateral circulation; the thrombus may be organized and fibrosed, and the entire process may remain clinically silent even if the vessel becomes completely occluded. In one study only about one-third of surgically occluded carotid arteries in the neck produced neurological sequelae.[13] Furthermore, clinically asymptomatic carotid occlusions are often documented when angiography is done for some reason other than ischemic cerebrovascular disease. Another possible sequel of thrombosis is fibrinolytic dissolution, although the larger the thrombus the less likely this is to occur with complete resolution. A third possibility is fragmentation of the thrombus with distal embolization of the fragments with, or without, symptoms of ischemia. A fourth possibility is that ischemia and then infarction occur as soon as blood flow through the affected vessel is restricted to a critical level, or abruptly shut off, by the thrombus. Although it is an inference rather than a direct observation, as in the carotid endarterectomy specimens, it is presumed that most of these events in the thrombotic process evolve in a similar fashion in severely atherosclerotic intracranial arteries when thrombosis takes place there.

Although atherosclerosis is the chief vascular lesion leading to thrombosis, other causes should be briefly mentioned that may affect both arteries and veins. Increased blood viscosity, as in polycythemia, in the puerperal period, with certain types of cyanotic congenital heart disease such as the tetralogy of Fallot, with fever and dehydration, and in a variety of other complex clinical disorders, may also be associated with the thrombosis of intracranial vessels, both arteries and veins.

Embolism

Cerebral embolism remains one of the major problems in clinical medicine. In various studies, emboli account for 20 to 30 percent of the instances of cerebral infarction at autopsy. Emboli may be of cardiac or extracardiac origin, the former being more common. The only pathognomonic morphological evidence of embolism is the presence of some material foreign to the blood stream within the lumen of a vessel, and a variety of such substances have been documented, such as atheromatous debris (Fig. 144-1), fat, bone marrow, fibrocartilage, air, and cotton fibers.[3] In most cases of embolism the occlusive material is one or more fragments of a thrombus (thromboembolism) dislodged from a distant site, usually the heart, but occasionally another vessel such as the carotid artery or the arch of the aorta (artery-to-artery embolization). Since the platelets and red and white blood cells that make up a thrombus are not foreign to the blood, the diagnosis of embolism clinically and at autopsy is most frequently inferential. The strength of the inference is based on the multiplicity of infarcts in the brain, the presence of visceral infarcts, especially in the kidneys, spleen, intes-

Pathology of Ischemic Cerebrovascular Disease

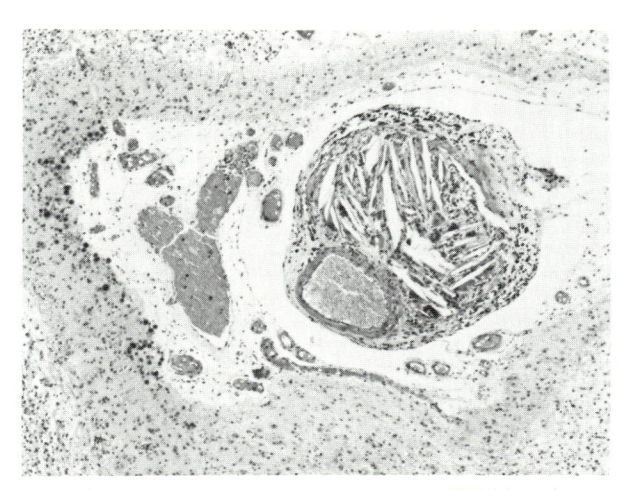

Figure 144-1 An atheromatous embolus within a leptomeningeal artery; the adjacent cortical tissue is infarcted. (H & E, ×25.)

tines, and peripheral arteries of the limbs,[1] and the frequent demonstration of one or more arterial occlusions in appropriate sites.

Cerebral embolism is most often of cardiac origin; the embolic material includes that derived from (1) a mural thrombus of the left ventricle accompanying myocardial infarction; (2) left atrial thrombi formed during atrial fibrillation; and (3) valvular thrombi formed as "vegetations" or excrescences on the mitral and aortic valves. These valvular lesions usually, but not invariably, form on valves damaged by rheumatic fever or otherwise altered. These lesions may be septic, as in bacterial endocarditis, or bland, as in the nonbacterial endocardiosis (marantic endocarditis) associated with the hypercoagulable state in patients with visceral cancer. Left atrial myxoma is a less frequent cause of cerebral embolism, but it should be considered in special cases of recurrent cerebral and systemic embolization because it is potentially curable.[18]

Extracardiac sources of cerebral emboli include artery-to-artery embolism, as in the case of extracranial carotid artery thrombosis at the bifurcation and subsequent embolization of small fibrin-platelet thrombi (white thrombi), fragments of larger red-white thrombi, or atheromatous debris derived from an ulcerated atherosclerotic plaque. Fibrin-platelet thrombi appear to be the most frequent type of embolic material and probably are responsible for most TIAs and episodes of amaurosis fugax so characteristic of extracranial carotid artery disease. An uncommon extracardiac source of cerebral emboli may be thrombi in the leg and pelvic veins if a cardiac septal defect exists, permitting a right-to-left shunt (this is referred to as *paradoxical embolism*).

Structural Aspects of Cerebral Infarction

When ischemia has been severe enough to produce infarction, macroscopic changes and cellular events take place in a patterned sequence that depends on a number of variables, some known and some unknown. These variables include the age of the patient, the type of affected vessel (i.e., artery or vein), the type and rapidity of occlusion, the location of the infarct in the brain, the adequacy of collateral circulation, the time of onset and pattern of reperfusion, and the presence of concurrent visceral and metabolic complications in the patient. Therefore, a description of the gross features and cellular elements must necessarily be preceded by the cautionary statement that individuals will vary in their cellular response to cerebral infarction. The following statements about the macroscopic features and cellular events in cerebral infarction are eclectic and drawn from a variety of published accounts and personal observations.

Cerebral infarcts of all sizes are more frequent in the carotid arterial distribution than in the vertebrobasilar system. About 80 percent of cerebral infarcts are in the distribution of the internal carotid arteries and their branches.[12,17] Within the carotid system, the parenchymal sites most frequently involved include the corpus striatum (especially the putamen) and internal capsule and portions of the cerebral cortex within the distribution of the middle cerebral artery (Figs. 144-2 and 144-3). In the vertebrobasilar territories, infarcts most often occur in the thalamus, pontine base, cerebellum, midbrain, and lateral medulla, roughly in that order. The small "lacunar" infarcts are most prevalent in the putamen, thalamus, pons (Fig. 144-4), cerebellar white matter, and cerebral hemispheric white matter and are most often associated with parenchymal arteriolar lesions.[4,5]

Okazaki follows the traditional manner of distinguishing three phases in the evolution of morphological changes

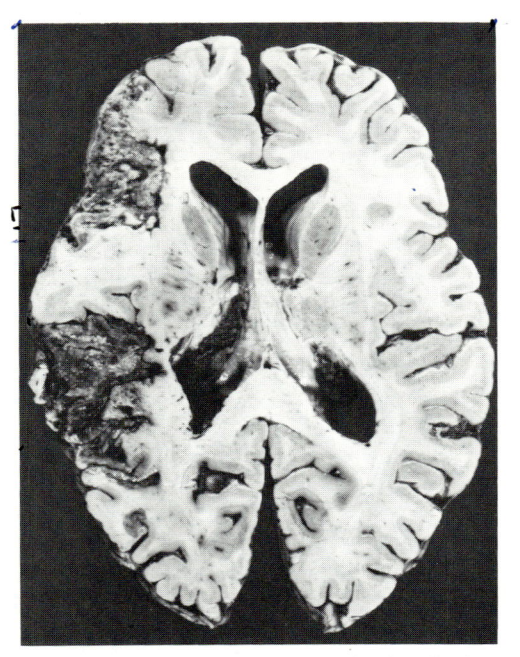

Figure 144-2 A recent infarct in the distribution of the left middle cerebral artery; the patient was a 78-year-old man with atrial fibrillation; the lesion was presumably embolic, although no visceral emboli were found. The infarcted tissue is largely hemorrhagic, but pale (or anemic) areas make up about 25 percent.

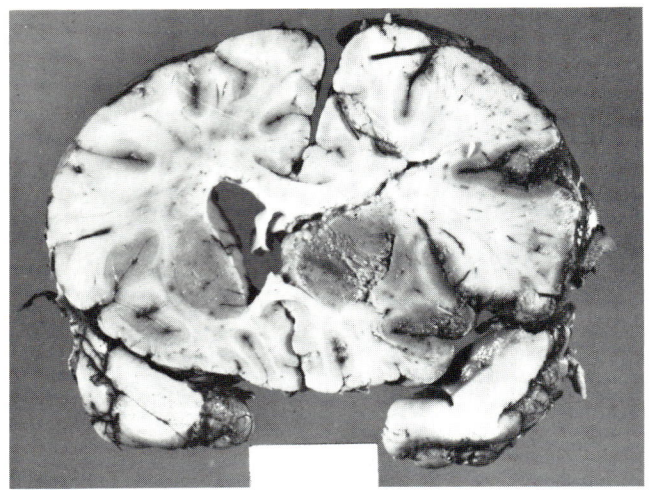

Figure 144-3 A recent infarct in the distribution of the left internal carotid artery after severe trauma to the neck. Thromboembolism to the left middle cerebral artery also occurred. In addition to thrombosis after trauma, there was severe carotid atherosclerosis and hemorrhagic dissection of the vessel wall. The infarct is both pale and hemorrhagic, involves the anterior and middle cerebral arterial territories, and is associated with a mass effect as indicated by ventricular compression and shift.

within an infarct: coagulation necrosis, liquefactive necrosis, and cavitation.[20] Those infarcts that are grossly visible, and most are, are initially (within the first 3 days of occurrence) pale and slightly swollen zones of parenchyma within a specific vascular territory, usually arterial (Figs. 144-2 and 144-3). Most cerebral infarcts, particularly those due to atherosclerotic thrombosis, are mixtures of pale (anemic) and slightly hemorrhagic infarction, the latter being a few petechiae scattered in a few foci of gray matter. Floridly hemorrhagic infarcts are often the result of multiple venous

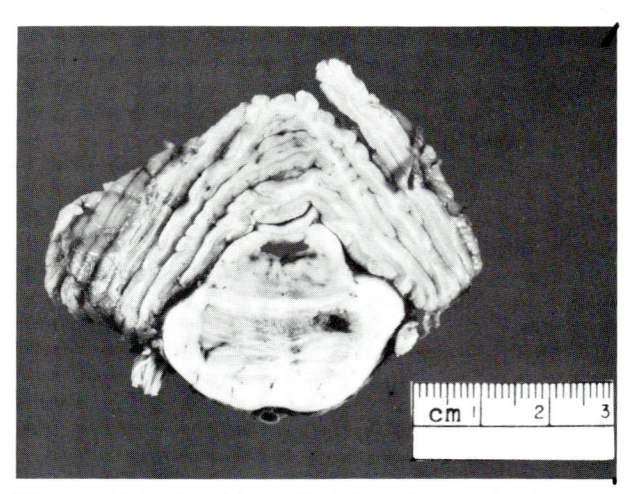

Figure 144-4 An old, small, infarct (lacune) in the pontine base; the patient was a 57-year-old black man with severe hypertension and atherosclerosis. There were similar lacunar infarcts in the thalamus and frontal white matter.

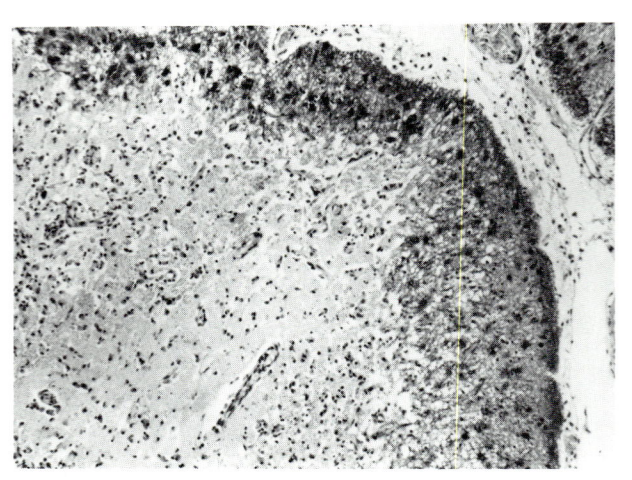

Figure 144-5 A recent cortical infarct with the reactive and marginal zones illustrated; the marginal zone is the dark periphery in which numerous, darkly stained fibrillary astrocytes are present. (Glial fibrillary acidic protein; immunoperoxidase technique, ×25.)

occlusions or of the type of external arterial occlusion seen with transtentorial herniation and compression of the posterior cerebral artery with a resultant occipital lobe infarction. Older infarcts, e.g., those a week to 10 days old, are soft and slightly friable. Those 2 to 3 weeks old are friable and mushy and show small foci of cavitation. After about 3 weeks, numerous cavitations are evident in the affected parenchyma. Infarcts 6 to 8 weeks old, and thereafter, are predominantly cavitary, irregular in shape, and sharply demarcated (Fig. 144-3).

The cytopathological and histopathological features are complex and vary slightly, especially in human beings, so that some of the most definitive studies of pattern come from experimental studies of cerebral infarction in primates.[8] Garcia and Kamijyo distinguish three zones (Fig. 144-5) of histological alteration within an infarct: *a central* zone within which there is poor staining of all cellular elements, and various forms of neuronal necrosis ranging from pale, swollen "ghost" cells to shrunken neurons with pyknotic nuclei (Fig. 144-6); *a reactive* zone at the periphery of the central zone and within which there is also neuronal necrosis, vacuolization of the neuropil, neutrophilic leukocyte infiltration, axonal spheroids, phagocytes (Fig. 144-7), and neovascularization; and *a marginal* zone peripheral to the reactive zone and within which there are shrunken neurons (Fig. 144-6) and swollen astrocytes in various stages of hyperplasia and hypertrophy. The appearance of some of the major cellular elements within infarctions of various ages is indicated in Table 144-1. Ultrastructural changes of several types are detectable within minutes and include changes in the Golgi apparatus, endoplasmic reticulum, and mitochondria of neurons, swelling of dendrites, and swelling of astrocytic processes in various phases.[6,7,21] In the earliest stages of ischemia there appear to be mainly neuronal and astroglial alterations with less effect on oligodendrocytes and capillaries.[6]

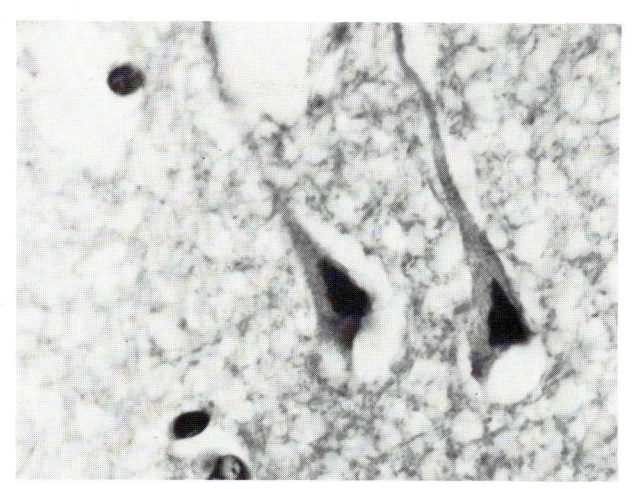

Figure 144-6 Ischemic neuronal necrosis in its early phases. The two neurons are shrunken, the Nissl substance is absent, and the nuclei are pyknotic. The perineuronal spaces are enlarged, and the neuropil is extensively vacuolated. (H & E, ×400.)

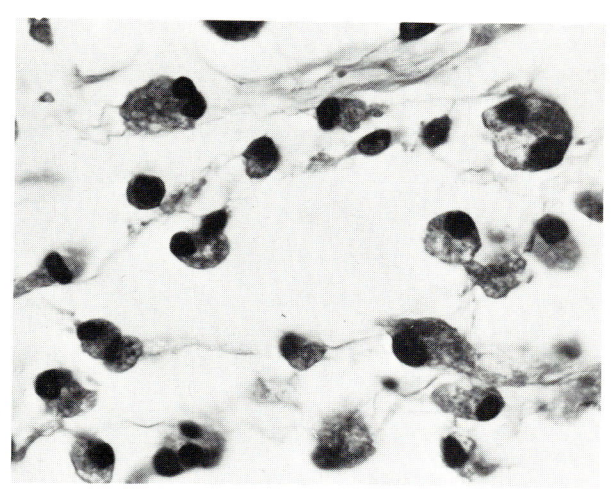

Figure 144-7 Phagocytes, chiefly mononuclear, within an infarct 4 weeks old. (H & E, ×400.)

Ischemic Cerebral Edema and Brain Herniations

The initial swelling in ischemic brain edema noted after experimental infarction appears to be restricted to the astrocytic processes, especially those around blood vessels. This intracellular phase is followed by the presence of extracellular fluid, possibly related to rupture of the membranes of some swollen astrocytes,[6,7] although other factors later enter the picture, including increasing capillary permeability due to various degrees of endothelial cell alteration ranging from purely functional changes, such as increased pinocytosis and changes in electric charge, to frank necrosis in some areas.

When infarcts are small, e.g., less than 1 to 2 cm³ in volume in the cerebral hemispheres, the accompanying edema is not likely to produce significant displacement of tissue and brain herniation. However, the larger the infarct, the more likely the mass effect, depending on its location; for example, larger infarcts significantly affecting the temporal lobe and the cerebellum are more likely to be associated with enough edema to produce brain herniations. If an infarct is large enough, e.g., in the middle cerebral artery territory, signs of transtentorial herniation do not become clinically evident until 3 to 5 days after the onset of infarction. The early phase of intracellular edema evolves in 18 to 24 h, but later phases with massive swelling, capillary leakage, and extracellular fluid accumulation develop over a 3- to 5-day period depending on infarct size and location. Because of the clinical frequency of carotid distribution infarctions, it follows that transtentorial hippocampal herniation occurs most frequently. Alterations in consciousness, ipsilateral pupillary dilatation, and other signs of upper brain stem compression due to hippocampal herniation may occur in the first week after a massive cerebral infarct. With such large infarcts, ischemic brain edema and herniation may be the cause of death. Cerebellar tonsillar herniation with dorsolateral compression of the medulla can be expected with

TABLE 144-1 Ischemic Cerebrovascular Disease: Microscopic Cellular Events in Infarcts

Time Elapsed	Neurons	Oligo	Astro	Phagocytes NL	M	C	Cav
3–6 h	++	±	+	0	0	0	0
24 h	+++	+	+	+	0	±	0
48 h	++++	+++	++	++	+	+	0
7 days	+++	++++	++	±	++	+++	0
14 days	++	+	++++	0	+++	++++	+
21 days	+	0	++++	0	++++	+++	++
30–60 days	0	0	++++	0	++	++	++++

Astro, astrocytes; C, capillary and small vessel reactions (hyperplasia and neovascularization); Cav, cavitation; M, monocytes and microglia; NL, neutrophilic leucocytes; 0, absent; oligo, oligodendrocytes and myelin; ±, questionable; +, minimal; ++, moderate; +++, severe or excessive; ++++, maximal.

large cerebellar infarcts and constitutes a major reason for the current interest in the surgical evacuation of some cerebellar infarcts (and hematomas).[11] The clinical concomitants of other forms of brain herniation often found at autopsy, such as subfalcial herniation of the cingulate gyrus, are less understood.

References

1. Askey JM: *Systemic Arterial Embolism: Pathogenesis and Prophylaxis.* New York, Grune & Stratton, 1957.
2. DeGirolami U, Crowell RM, Marcoux FW: Selective necrosis and total necrosis in focal cerebral ischemia: Neuropathologic observations on experimental middle cerebral artery occlusion in the Macaque monkey. J Neuropathol Exp Neurol 43:57–71, 1984.
3. Feigen I, Budzilovich GN: The general pathology of cerebrovascular disease, in Vinken PJ, Bruyn GW (eds): *Handbook of Clinical Neurology,* vol. 11, Part I. Amsterdam, North Holland, 1972, pp 128–167.
4. Fisher CM: Lacunar strokes and infarcts: A review. Neurology (NY) 32:871–876, 1982.
5. Fisher CM, Gore I, Okabe N, White PD: Atherosclerosis of the carotid and vertebral arteries: Extracranial and intracranial. J Neuropathol Exp Neurol 24:455–476, 1965.
6. Garcia JH: Ischemic injuries of the brain: Morphologic evolution. Arch Pathol Lab Med 107:157–161, 1983.
7. Garcia JH, Conger KA, Lossinsky AS: The cellular pathology of ischemic stroke, in Trump BF, Laufer A, Jones RT (eds): *Cellular Pathobiology of Human Disease.* New York, Gustav Fischer, 1983, pp 351–367.
8. Garcia JH, Kamijyo Y: Cerebral infarction: Evolution of histopathological changes after occlusion of a middle cerebral artery in primates. J Neuropathol Exp Neurol 33:408–421, 1974.
9. Gorelick PB, Caplan LR, Hier DB, Parker SL, Patel D: Racial differences in the distribution of anterior circulation occlusive disease. Neurology (Cleveland) 34:54–59, 1984.
10. Heiss WD, Rosner G: Functional recovery of cortical neurons as related to degree and duration of ischemia. Ann Neurol 14:294–301, 1983.
11. Heros RC: Cerebellar hemorrhage and infarction. Stroke 13:106–109, 1982.
12. Jörgensen L, Torvik A: Ischemic cerebrovascular diseases in an autopsy series: Part I. Prevalence, location and predisposing factors in verified thromboembolic occlusions, and their significance in the pathogenesis of cerebral infarction. J Neurol Sci 3:490–509, 1966.
13. Landolt AM, Millikan CH: Pathogenesis of cerebral infarction secondary to mechanical carotid artery occlusion. Stroke I:52–62, 1970.
14. Moossy J: Morphology, sites and epidemiology of cerebral atherosclerosis, in Millikan CH (ed): *Cerebrovascular Disease.* Proceedings of the Association Dec. 8 and 9, 1961, New York, N.Y. Research Publications, vol. 41. Assoc Res Nerv Ment Dis. Baltimore, Williams and Wilkins, 1966, pp 1–22.
15. Moossy J: Cerebral atherosclerosis: Intracranial and extracranial lesions, in Minckler J (ed): *Pathology of the Nervous System, Volume II.* New York, McGraw-Hill, 1971, pp 1423–1432.
16. Moossy J: Formal discussion, in Whisnant JP, Sandok BA (eds): *Cerebral Vascular Diseases: Ninth Conference.* New York, Grune & Stratton, 1975, pp 323–325.
17. Moossy J: Anatomy and pathology of the vertebrobasilar system, in Berguer R, Bauer RB (eds): *Vertebrobasilar Arterial Occlusive Disease.* New York, Raven Press, 1984, pp 1–13.
18. Moossy J, Wisotzkey H: Cerebral embolism with cardiac myxoma: Clinicopathological aspects, in Trufant SA (ed): Trans Am Neur Assoc 1971, vol. 96. New York, Springer, 1972, pp 286–288.
19. Nishimaru K, McHenry LC Jr, Toole JF: Cerebral angiographic and clinical differences in carotid system transient ischemic attacks between American caucasian and Japanese patients. Stroke 15:56–59, 1984.
20. Okazaki H: *Fundamentals of Neuropathology.* New York, Igaku-Shoin, 1983, pp 25–85.
21. Petito CK, Pulsinelli WA: Sequential development of reversible and irreversible neuronal damage following cerebral ischemia. J Neuropathol Exp Neurol 43:141–153, 1984.
22. Scholz W: Selective neuronal necrosis and its topistic patterns in hypoxemia and oligemia. J Neuropathol Exp Neurol 12:249–261, 1953.
23. Solberg LA, McGarry PA: Cerebral atherosclerosis in negroes and caucasians. Atherosclerosis 16:141–154, 1972.

145
Clinical Syndromes of Brain Ischemia

David G. Sherman
J. Donald Easton

Stroke is a common cause of death and disability. Each year in the United States approximately 140 persons of every 100,000 people suffer an initial stroke, and one-third of these individuals die as a consequence of their stroke and its attendant complications. Of those who survive beyond the first few weeks, the majority carry a persistent neurological deficit. A cost of over 1 billion dollars annually is incurred in addition to incalculable human suffering. Unfortunately, the treatment of most strokes is woefully inadequate. Good supportive medical care and intensive rehabilitation have, however, improved the lot of many patients with stroke.

Preventive measures such as control of hypertension, cerebral vascular surgery, and platelet antiaggregation therapy have an important role in reducing the likelihood of a stroke in the population at risk. Nevertheless, irreversible infarction occurs within minutes of a loss of blood flow to the brain, eliminating opportunities for prevention and setting into motion potentially devastating metabolic events.

Ischemic Stroke Syndromes

The clinical syndromes developing from focal brain ischemia are defined in terms of the arterial circulation involved and the time course of the resultant symptoms and signs. A patient's symptoms and signs (e.g., aphasia, amaurosis fugax, internuclear ophthalmoplegia) are the major testimony to the arterial circulation involved. This clinical assessment may be corroborated by diagnostic studies such as computed tomography (CT) scanning or cerebral angiography. However useful these and other diagnostic techniques may be, the stroke syndrome continues to be characterized by the nature and time course of the patient's clinical findings.

Within 10 s of a diminution in blood flow below about 15 ml/100 g per minute to an area of the brain, the affected neurons cease to function. This lack of metabolic reserve is the basis for the observation that clinical ischemic syndromes are almost invariably sudden in onset. If blood flow is re-established promptly, neuronal function recovers and neurological abnormalities resolve within a few minutes or hours. This brief disruption of function is termed a *transient ischemic attack* (TIA) if it is focal, or *syncope* if it is generalized. If perfusion is not restored, metabolic collapse occurs and ischemic infarction results in a clinical stroke. Thus the nature and time course of cerebral ischemic symptoms imply a particular underlying pathophysiology, which may in turn be linked to a presumed cause, prognosis, and therapeutic strategy.

Cerebral arterial occlusion or reduced flow may be the end result of a number of pathophysiological processes culminating in focal brain ischemia (Fig. 145-1). Disease of the artery, whether atherosclerosis, arteritis, or trauma, may cause a flow-restricting stenosis or promote thrombus formation. A number of disorders of the cardiac rhythm, heart valves, and the myocardial muscle itself may also promote thrombus formation with the risk of systemic embolization, often to the cerebral vessels. Focal ischemic symptoms also occur associated with the cerebral arterial vasospasm of subarachnoid hemorrhage and possibly migraine. In addition, the production of vasoconstricting substances in an area of ischemic brain may accentuate and widen the ischemic injury produced by a thrombotic or embolic occlusion. Similarly, changes in the blood constituents, as seen in polycythemia and hyperviscosity states, may produce focal ischemia or cause deterioration of already ischemic brain by impairing flow in the microcirculation. It is testimony to the effectiveness of the brain's collateral circulation that many, if not most, patients with stenotic or occlusive arterial lesions do not suffer a brain infarction. Even when cerebral blood flow is further reduced by transient systemic hypotension, symptoms of global brain ischemia (presyncope or syncope), rather than focal ischemia, generally develop.[4]

Transient Ischemic Attacks

Transient ischemic attacks are episodes of focal neurological dysfunction that result from ischemia and resolve completely within 24 h. Most TIAs last less than 10 to 15 min. One rarely has the opportunity to examine a patient during a TIA and therefore is dependent on the history for diagnosis. The onset of symptoms is sudden and focal in character. Monocular blindness, dysphasia, localized sensory loss, and hemiparesis are some of the symptoms that strongly suggest a focal ischemic episode, and the nature of the symptoms define the vascular distribution of the ischemia (Table 145-1).[15] Many other transient symptoms are far less specific and should not with confidence be attributed to focal brain ischemia (Table 145-2).[15] Still other symptoms are even less specific and are usually not symptoms of TIA (Table 145-3).[15]

TIAs may occur as a consequence of any of the potential causes of focal ischemia, i.e., extracranial arterial disease, cardiac embolization, migrainous "vasospasm," etc. (Fig. 145-1). However, specific pathophysiologies are suggested by certain features of a TIA. Carotid system TIAs of short duration (i.e., less than 10 to 15 min) are more likely to occur from atheroembolic disease of the internal carotid artery, and those of an hour or more are more likely the result

Abrupt Focal Cerebral Deficit

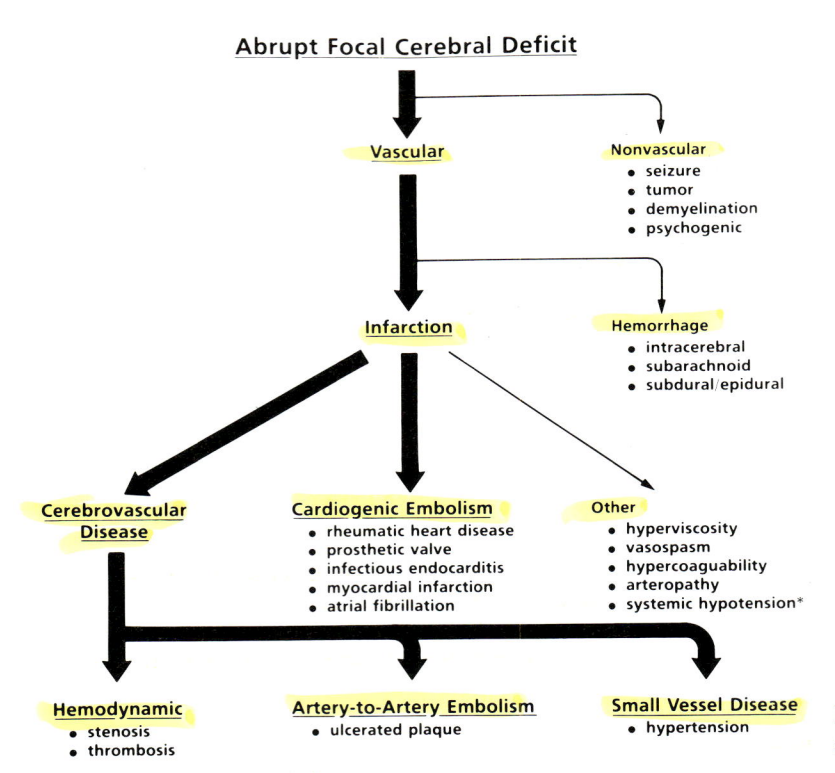

- Vascular
  - Infarction
    - Cerebrovascular Disease
      - Hemodynamic
        - stenosis
        - thrombosis
      - Artery-to-Artery Embolism
        - ulcerated plaque
      - Small Vessel Disease
        - hypertension
    - Cardiogenic Embolism
      - rheumatic heart disease
      - prosthetic valve
      - infectious endocarditis
      - myocardial infarction
      - atrial fibrillation
    - Other
      - hyperviscosity
      - vasospasm
      - hypercoaguability
      - arteropathy
      - systemic hypotension*
  - Hemorrhage
    - intracerebral
    - subarachnoid
    - subdural/epidural
- Nonvascular
  - seizure
  - tumor
  - demyelination
  - psychogenic

Figure 145-1 Pathophysiology of ischemic stroke.

of a cardiac embolus. Transient ischemia producing prominent visual scintillations and the slow buildup and march of paresthesias over 5 to 30 min without major paralysis after the spell is typical of late-life migraine accompaniments. These transient migraine accompaniments are disturbing, but unlike TIAs they appear to be relatively harmless.[8] Sud-

TABLE 145-1 TIA Symptoms

Carotid System	Vertebrobasilar System	Either System
Motor defect (paralysis, weakness, or clumsiness) of one extremity or of both extremities on the contralateral side	Motor defect (paralysis, weakness, or clumsiness) of any combination of extremities up to quadriplegia, sometimes changing from one side to another in different attacks	Dysarthria, if it occurs alone
Sensory defect (numbness, including loss of sensation, or paresthesias) involving one or both extremities on the contralateral side	Sensory defect (numbness, including loss of sensation, or paresthesias) in any combination of extremities including all four or involving both sides of the face or mouth; frequently bilateral; sometimes changes from side to side in different attacks	Homonymous hemianopsia, if it occurs alone
Aphasia (language disturbance that may be only a minor defect or may be global)	Loss of vision, complete or partial in both homonymous fields (bilateral homonymous hemianopsia)	
Loss of vision in one eye or in part of one eye (amaurosis fugax)	Homonymous hemianopsia	
Homonymous hemianopsia	Ataxia, imbalance, unsteadiness, or dysequilibrium not associated with vertigo	
Combinations of the above	Either vertigo (with or without nausea and vomiting), diplopia, dysphagia, or dysarthria not considered as a TIA when any of these symptoms occurs alone; but in combination with one another or with any of the first four items above, the attacks should be considered a TIA	
	Combinations of the above	

Clinical Syndromes of Brain Ischemia

TABLE 145-2 Uncertain TIA Symptoms

Vertigo alone	Dysphagia alone
Dysarthria alone	Diplopia alone

den transient numbness of the face, arm and leg on one side in the absence of weakness, homonymous hemianopsia, and aphasia is typically due to hypertensive arteriolar changes in small penetrating vessels, rather than to disease of the large vessels. It is sometimes the prelude to a lacunar infarct.[9]

The importance of TIAs lies in their role as harbingers of brain infarction. In some studies the incidence of TIA preceding cerebral infarction has been in the 10 to 20 percent range, while others have found an incidence as high as 80 percent.[2] Forty to fifty percent is quoted by most authors. It is quite likely that this variability is dependent on the type and location of the causative lesion (i.e., left atrial thrombus; internal carotid artery stenosis, ulceration, occlusion, plaque hemorrhage, dissection; carotid siphon disease; and small penetrating artery lipohyalinosis or arteriosclerosis). For carotid lesions amenable to carotid endarterectomy the incidence is probably 40 to 50 percent. Some patients experience multiple TIAs over an extended period of time and never suffer a brain infarction. However, most patients have fewer than four TIAs prior to their stroke. The period of greatest risk is the first hours and days following a first TIA, with about one-half of the strokes occurring within the first month. The risk is sustained, however, such that by 5 years approximately 35 percent of patients experiencing a TIA will have suffered a completed stroke.[6a,14] Many clinicians view "crescendo TIAs" with particular alarm. This term describes a cluster of TIAs occurring at increasing frequency or duration over a few hours or days. Patients with crescendo TIAs are considered particularly unstable neurologically and at risk of imminent brain infarction.

Reversible Ischemic Neurological Deficit

Reversible ischemic neurological deficit (RIND) is the term used to describe a focal ischemic event lasting longer than 24 h but with complete resolution of the deficit within 3 weeks. These episodes are also referred to as *stroke with recovery* or *stroke with full recovery*. Greater diagnostic certainty exists with a RIND than a TIA because one can substantiate the focal neurological findings on physical examination.

From a management perspective a TIA and a RIND are

TABLE 145-3 Non-TIA Symptoms

Unconsciousness including syncope
Tonic and/or clonic activity
March of a sensory defect
Incontinence of bowel or bladder
Dizziness or wooziness alone
Loss of vision associated with alteration of consciousness
Focal symptoms associated with migraine
Scintillating scotomata
Confusion alone
Amnesia alone

viewed similarly, even though a RIND, like a completed stroke, is somewhat more likely to have a stuttering or gradual onset compared with the abrupt onset of a TIA. Some authors have found that cerebral angiograms are more often normal in RIND patients than in those with either TIA or completed stroke, suggesting that cardiogenic cerebral embolism, or some mechanism other than cervical artery atherosclerosis, is more likely to be causative in RINDs. It has also been suggested that compared with patients with TIA, those with a RIND are less liable to a subsequent stroke. Other authorities believe that TIA, RIND, and completed stroke are all on a continuum of worsening cerebral vascular disease and that the risk of subsequent stroke is substantial for all of them. Most experts manage all of these patients similarly, as threatening stroke patients, unless they have already suffered a major completed stroke.

It seems likely that the risk for having a completed stroke in the future is about the same for the TIA, RIND, and completed stroke patients. The incidence is approximately 5 to 9 percent per year after the initial ischemic event.[13,14] The TIA patient is the least stable and will have the highest incidence in the first month following the initial ischemic event.

Progressing Stroke

The term *progressing stroke*, or *stroke in evolution*, describes the progression of focal ischemic symptoms over many minutes to several hours. The nature of the new neurological deficit suggests extension of the area of ischemia to encompass areas of brain immediately adjacent to the already involved area. Neurological worsening from ischemic edema should not be confused with progressing stroke. Hemispheric edema in the ischemic brain causes gradual worsening of the deficit from 48 h to 96 h after onset, whereas most progressing infarctions in the carotid territory have completed their evolution within 24 h, or occasionally 48 h.[11]

About 20 percent of patients with acute carotid system cerebral infarction experience clear progression within the first 48 h (Table 145-4).[11] Less than 5 percent show ischemic worsening after a stable period of 48 h or more. Progressing stroke appears to be more common in the vertebrobasilar territory where early progression occurs in about 40 percent of patients (Table 145-4).[12] In addition, there appears to be a longer period of risk for progression in vertebrobasilar strokes, with 15 to 20 percent of patients worsening between 48 to 96 h after onset.[12]

Worsening of an existing deficit may also arise from hypoxia or other metabolic disturbances and may be difficult to differentiate from a stroke in evolution. Consequently, in comparison to a TIA, RIND, or completed stroke, a progressing stroke conveys somewhat greater diagnostic uncertainty, and a neoplasm, or a subdural or intracerebral hematoma, is more often a real differential diagnostic consideration in progressing stroke than in the other ischemic syndromes.

A progressing stroke appears to forebode the gravest consequences of any of the ischemic syndromes. As many as one-half of patients with an evolving stroke in the vertebrobasilar distribution will die if untreated. The prognosis is better when the carotid distribution is involved.

TABLE 145-4 Temporal Profile of Cerebral Infarction
(Clinical Course over 7 Days)

Course	Carotid, %	Vertebrobasilar, %
Stable (unchanged)	39	11
Improving	35	35
Progressing	19	43
Remitting-relapsing	3	11
Late worsening (> 48 h)	4	0
Death	10.6	27

SOURCE: Adapted from Refs. 11 and 12.

Completed Stroke

A completed stroke is a stable, focal ischemic neurological deficit. Most embolic strokes have their maximal deficit appear suddenly and then stabilize or progressively improve over the subsequent hours, days, and months. Thrombotic infarctions may be just as sudden, but more commonly they evolve rapidly, over several minutes or a few hours, to a completed stroke. The commonest presentation is for the patient to awaken from sleep with a complete focal neurological deficit that remains stable or progressively improves. If one sees a patient during the early hours following a cerebral infarction, it is important to observe the patient closely to determine whether one is dealing with a progressing stroke or a completed stroke. The earlier it is after the onset of an ischemic deficit, the less certainty there is that the stroke is complete. An apparent stable deficit observed at 4 to 6 h from onset may resolve by 24 h, proving to be a TIA, or it may suddenly worsen into a stroke in evolution.

Syndrome of Cardiogenic Embolic Occlusion[6,6a,7,10]

Possibly 20 to 30 percent of ischemic strokes originate from a cardiogenic embolus. The determination that a stroke is embolic in origin generally results from the demonstration of an appropriate cardiac abnormality in a patient with a stroke featuring characteristics suggestive of an embolus.

Certain cardiac abnormalities are widely incriminated as sources of systemic and cerebral emboli (Table 145-5). Rheumatic mitral valvular disease with atrial fibrillation, prosthetic valves, infectious endocarditis, and intracardiac tumor are universally recognized causes of emboli. The role of disorders such as nonvalvular atrial fibrillation, myocardial infarction, and mitral valve prolapse is less clear. These latter abnormalities are relatively common, and although they are capable of producing systemic emboli, the frequency with which they do so remains unclear. The difficulty in identifying the role of the heart is magnified further when the cardiac abnormality may be episodic (e.g., atrial fibrillation) and perhaps not be recognized by either the patient or the physician.

Certain clinical features of a stroke suggest a possible cardiac embolic origin. Embolic strokes are usually sudden in onset with their maximal neurological deficit appearing immediately. A headache or seizure at the onset is more common with an embolic than a thrombotic stroke. Most cardiogenic emboli lodge in the stem or a branch of the middle cerebral artery with perhaps as few as one out of ten cardiac emboli coming to rest in a branch of the anterior cerebral or basilar artery. Thus, an infarction in the anterior cerebral artery distribution or in the brain stem is less likely due to a cardiogenic embolus than is an ischemic stroke in the middle cerebral artery distribution. Multifocal cerebral infarctions, especially in a patient with an associated systemic arterial occlusion, e.g., renal or limb, strongly suggest an embolic source. Additionally, certain radiological and laboratory findings may corroborate the clinical suspicion of embolic infarction. The CT scan may demonstrate an infarct in the middle cerebral artery distribution, it may reveal multiple infarcts, and it may demonstrate a hemorrhagic infarct. While hemorrhagic infarcts are infrequently demonstrated by CT scan, their presence strongly suggests a cardiac embolic source. A hemorrhagic infarct presumably develops when blood flow is re-established to an area of ischemia after the occluding embolus lyses. Cerebral angiography often shows an embolic occlusion of the stem or a branch of the middle cerebral artery within the first few hours or days, but it may show no occlusion thereafter. Also there may be no cerebrovascular atherosclerosis.

Specific Vascular Syndromes[1]

Stroke syndromes are defined not only by their temporal profile, e.g., TIA, progressing stroke, etc., but also by the vascular supply to the area of ischemic brain. The amount of brain rendered ischemic by a particular vascular occlusion is very much dependent on the nature of collaterals to the affected region. An occlusion of the internal carotid artery may result in infarction of the entire cerebral hemisphere in one patient and cause no symptoms in another. In general, the more distally an occlusion occurs, the greater the likelihood an infarct will result. This must be partially explained by the diminishing opportunity for collateral circulation as one moves distal to the carotid bifurcation, the ophthalmic artery origin, and the circle of Willis. Thus, in order to be

TABLE 145-5 Commonest Causes
of Cardiogenic Cerebral Embolism

Rheumatic heart disease
   Mitral stenosis ± atrial fibrillation
Coronary heart disease
   Myocardial infarction
Nonvalvular atrial fibrillation
Prosthetic valve
Other
   Cardiomyopathy
   Infectious endocarditis
   Nonbacterial thrombotic endocarditis
   Mitral valve prolapse
   Congenital heart disease
   Venous clots and intracardiac shunt
   Mitral annulus calcification
   Atrial myxoma
   Fat emboli

certain of the significance of a particular vascular lesion in a patient with an area of regional ischemia, one must visualize the relationships of several vessels to one another and to the area of ischemia.

Internal Carotid Artery Occlusion

An occlusion of the internal carotid artery (ICA) characteristically causes ischemia in the middle cerebral artery (MCA) territory. Areas of the brain supplied by the anterior cerebral artery (ACA), anterior choroidal artery (AchA), or posterior cerebral artery (PCA) are often involved in addition.

Symptoms of retinal and optic nerve ischemia are important clues to ICA disease. The ophthalmic artery is the first major branch of the ICA, and retinal ischemia may occur in response to diminished flow from an ICA stenosis or occlusion, or as a consequence of microemboli arising from an ulcerated ICA plaque. Episodic and transient monocular visual loss (amaurosis fugax) is the usual clinical correlate of ophthalmic artery ischemia. This transient loss of vision usually progresses from the periphery toward the center of vision. The visual loss often develops like a dark curtain descending from above or ascending from below, and it often abates in the reverse manner. The complete or partial blindness evolves over a few seconds and lasts only 1 to 5 min, rarely longer. Vision is usually back to normal within 5 to 15 min. While migraine, polycythemia, and other disorders may cause transient monocular blindness, most authorities believe that the majority of such episodes in patients over 40 years old is due to atherosclerosis at the origin of the internal carotid artery. These plaques may produce hemodynamic changes or emboli that cause the episodes of distal ischemia. Occasionally patients with an ICA occlusion may complain of transient, ipsilateral, monocular visual blurring following exposure to bright sunlight. This rare complaint presumably arises because of a limited retinal metabolic reserve on an ischemic basis.

Middle Cerebral Artery Occlusion

Ischemia to regions of the cerebral hemisphere supplied by one or more of the penetrating or cortical branches of the MCA is the basis for the most common stroke syndromes. The superior division of the MCA supplies the frontal and anterior parietal cortex (Fig. 145-2). Its several branches nourish the motor and sensory cortex about the central sulcus. Ischemia here produces a contralateral weakness of the face, hand, and arm. Sensory loss in a similar distribution may accompany the motor deficit. A nonfluent aphasia results when the frontal branches of the dominant cerebral hemisphere are involved. If only the more posterior parietal branches of the superior division are occluded, motor abnormalities may be limited primarily to limb apraxias, or a conduction aphasia if the dominant hemisphere is affected.

The inferior division of the MCA nourishes the posterior parietal and temporal cortex (Fig. 145-2). Occlusion of one of its branches may produce a Wernicke's aphasia in the dominant hemisphere, left-sided neglect in the nondominant hemisphere, and associated agnosias, apraxias, or visual disturbances including a contralateral homonymous hemianopsia.

Several small penetrating arteries arise from the proximal portion of the MCA and supply the internal capsule and parts of the basal ganglia (Fig. 145-3). Occlusion of these vessels, usually associated with hypertension, produces small infarcts called *lacunes*.[9] The commonest stroke syndrome arising from these 1- to 5-mm lacunes is a *pure motor hemiplegia*.[9] Typically a hypertensive patient notes the stuttering onset of paralysis of the face, arm, and leg without accompanying sensory loss, aphasia, or hemianopsia. Striking recovery often occurs in the ensuing weeks. Other penetrating arteries arise from the circle of Willis, the stem of the anterior cerebral artery, the posterior cerebral artery, and the basilar artery. Occlusion of these vessels can also lead to lacunar infarction, producing a variety of other lacunar stroke syndromes.[9] A *pure sensory stroke* occurs with a lacunar infarct in the ventral posterior thalamus. Numbness and paresthesias affect one side of the body without motor, language, or visual abnormalities. A stroke syndrome consisting of slurred speech and clumsiness of one hand occurs with lacunar infarction and has been termed the *dysarthria–clumsy hand* syndrome. *Homolateral ataxia and crural paresis* is the designation for the occurrence of arm and leg ataxia with weakness of the foot and ankle. Both of these latter two syndromes have been attributed to lacunar infarctions of the brain stem or posterior limb of the internal capsule.

Anterior Choroidal Artery Occlusion

The anterior choroidal artery (AchA) arises from the ICA or proximal MCA and sweeps posteriorly to supply the medial temporal lobe, the internal capsule, and the geniculocalcarine tract (Fig. 145-3). Ischemia in the distribution of the AchA may produce contralateral hemiparesis, hemihypesthesia, or hemianopsia.

Anterior Cerebral Artery Occlusion[16]

The anterior cerebral arteries (ACAs) supply the medial portions of the frontal and anterior parietal lobes (Fig. 145-4). Collateral flow from the anterior communicating artery and the cortical branches of the MCA are variable from one person to the next and assume a pivotal role in determining the extent of infarction occurring after ACA occlusion. The characteristic pattern of an ACA infarct is paralysis of the opposite leg and foot with lesser weakness of the shoulder and arm. The face muscles are usually spared. Sensory loss over the leg and foot may accompany the weakness. Bilateral ischemia may produce paraplegia, urinary incontinence, and an apathetic, mute, "lobotomized" patient.

Heubner's artery arises from the proximal ACA and nourishes the anterior hypothalamus, a portion of the internal capsule and the anterior portions of the caudate and putamen. Occlusion of Heubner's artery may produce a contralateral hemiparesis involving the face, arm, and leg. When the dominant hemisphere is affected, a transcortical

Figure caption labels (as shown on diagram):

- AREA FOR CONTRAVERSION OF EYES AND HEAD
- MOTOR • SENSORY
- Rolandic A
- BROCA'S AREA (MOTOR APHASIA)
- HIP, TRUNK, ARM, HANDS, FINGERS, THUMB, FACE, LIPS, TONGUE, MOUTH
- Ant. parietal A
- Post. parietal A
- Angular A
- Prerolandic A
- Sup. division of middle cerebral A
- Lateral orbito-frontal A
- Inf. division of middle cerebral A
- Middle cerebral stem
- Temporal polar A
- Ant. temporal A
- Post. temporal A
- Lateral geniculate body
- AUDITORY AREA
- VISUAL RADIATION
- VISUAL CORTEX
- CENTRAL SPEECH AREA (CENTRAL APHASIA)
- PO = PARIETAL OPERCULUM (CONDUCTION APHASIA)
- PPR = POST. PARIETAL REGION (ALEXIA WITH AGRAPHIA)

Signs and symptoms	Structures involved
Paralysis of the contralateral face, arm, and leg	Somatic motor area for face and arm and the fibers descending from the leg area to enter the corona radiata
Sensory impairment over the contralateral face, arm, and leg (pinprick, cotton touch, vibration, position, two-point discrimination, stereognosis, tactile localization, barognosis, cutaneographia)	Sensory cortex and connections, analogous to motor areas
Motor speech disorder	Broca's area of the dominant hemisphere
"Central" aphasia, word deafness, anomia, jargon speech, alexia, agraphia, acalculia, finger agnosia, right-left confusion (the last four comprise the Gerstmann syndrome)	Central language area and parietooccipital cortex of the dominant hemisphere
Apractagnosia (amorphosynthesis), anosognosia, hemiasomatognosia, unilateral neglect, agnosia for the left half of external space, "dressing apraxia," "constructional apraxia," distortion of visual coordinates, inaccurate localization in the half field, impaired ability to judge distance, upside-down reading, visual illusions	Usually nondominant parietal lobe. Loss of topographic memory is usually due to a nondominant lesion, occasionally to a dominant one.
Homonymous hemianopia (often superior homonymous quadrantanopia)	Optic radiation deep to second temporal convolution
Paralysis of conjugate gaze to the opposite side	Frontal contraversive field or fibers projecting therefrom
Avoidance reaction of opposite limbs	Parietal lobe
Miscellaneous: frontal ataxia Loss or impairment of optokinetic nystagmus Limb-kinetic apraxia Mirror movements Cheyne-Stokes respiration, contralateral hyperhidrosis, mydriasis (occasionally)	– Frontopontine tract (?) – Supramarginal or angular gyrus – Premotor or parietal cortical damage – Precise location of responsible lesions not known
Capsular (pure motor) hemiplegia	Upper portion of the posterior limb of the internal capsule and the adjacent corona radiata.

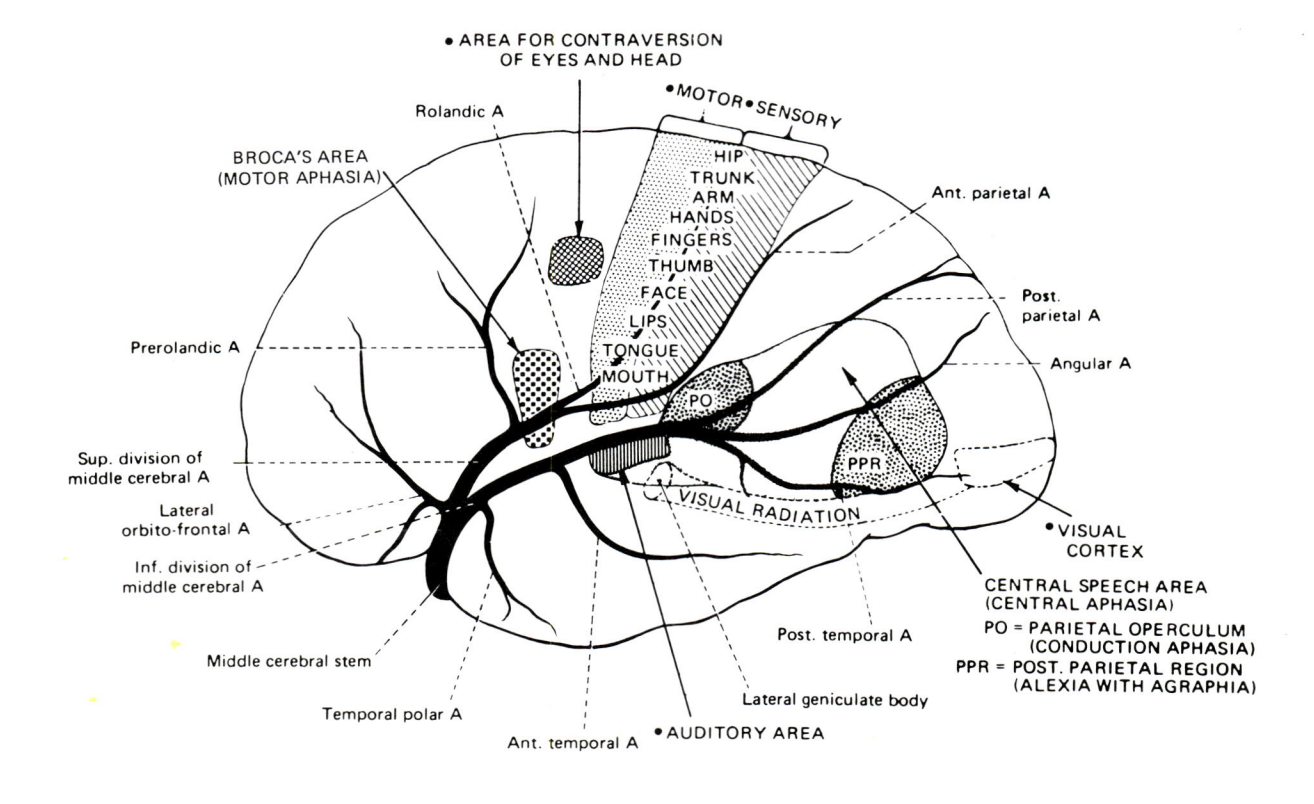

Figure 145-2 Diagram of a cerebral hemisphere, lateral aspect, showing the branches and distribution of the middle cerebral artery and the principal regions of cerebral localization. Below the diagram is a list of the clinical manifestations of infarction in the territory of the middle cerebral artery and the corresponding regions of cerebral damage. (From Adams and Victor.[1])

motor aphasia may also result. This language disorder is characterized by nonfluent speech with retained comprehension and speech repetition.

Posterior Cerebral Artery Occlusion[17]

The posterior cerebral arteries (PCAs) usually arise as the terminal branches of the basilar artery. However, about 25 percent of the time one or both PCAs are supplied by the ICA via the posterior communicating artery. Small penetrating arteries originate from the proximal PCA and supply the midbrain, subthalamus, and the thalamus (Fig. 145-3). Cortical branches supply the parietal and occipital cortex and the inferior temporal regions (Fig. 145-4). A contralateral homonymous hemianopsia develops with unilateral cortical branch occlusion and the resultant ischemia of the ipsilateral calcarine cortex or optic radiation. Bilateral occipital infarction produces cortical blindness usually accompanied by the patient's denial of visual impairment (Anton's syndrome). Visual defects may take the form of illusions or unformed or simply formed imagery. More complex visual hallucinations usually arise from temporal lobe lesions. Dominant hemisphere parieto-occipital ischemia may produce reading impairment (alexia with or without agraphia) and defects of color naming. Transient or persistent memory loss has been attributed to bilateral ischemia of the inferomedial temporal lobes. Episodes of memory loss lasting several hours have been ascribed to this mechanism and designated *transient global amnesia*.[10]

Several neurological abnormalities may emerge from occlusion of the penetrating arteries originating from the proximal PCA. Infarction of the thalamus produces contralateral sensory impairment. This sensory loss may partially recover but be replaced after several weeks or months by pain and hyperpathia in the affected limbs. This *thalamic pain syndrome* of Dejerine and Roussy is often extremely difficult to treat.

Unilateral midbrain and subthalamic ischemia may produce a number of signs singly or in combination. These include an ipsilateral oculomotor paralysis and contralateral hemiparesis, ataxia, or hemiballismus. Bilateral infarction of the central reticular formation may produce stupor or coma.

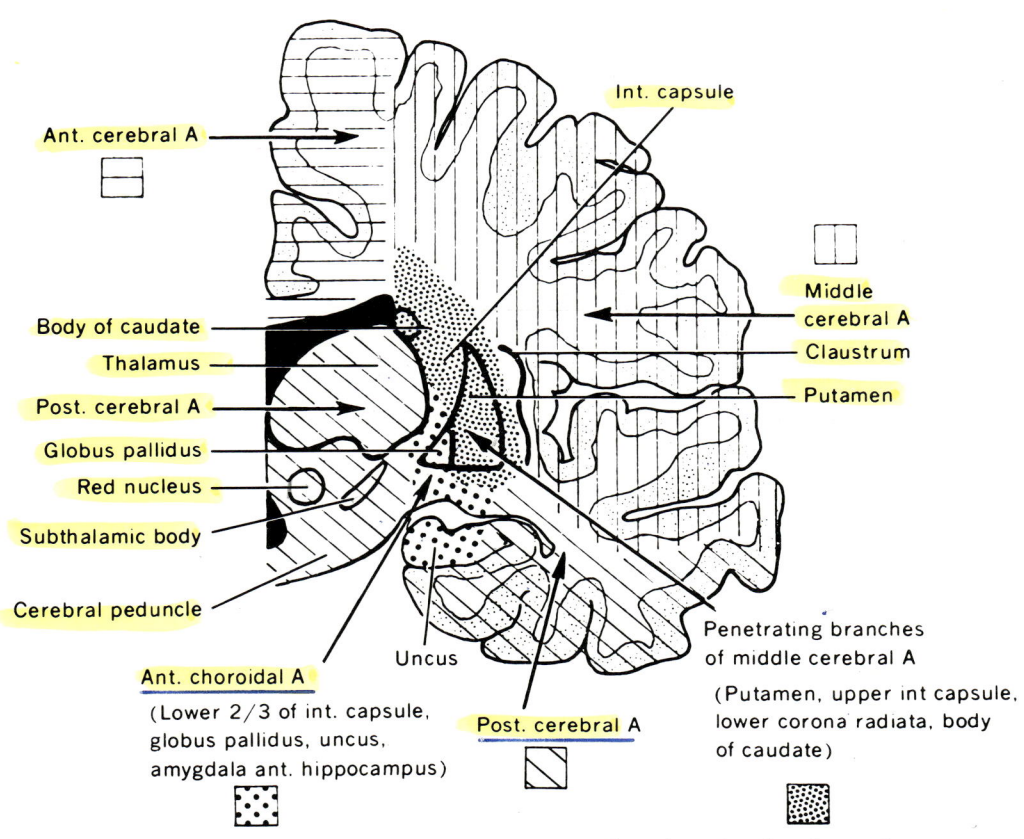

Figure 145-3 Diagram of a cerebral hemisphere, coronal section, showing the territories of the major cerebral vessels. (From Adams and Victor.[1])

Anterior Cerebral Artery Territory

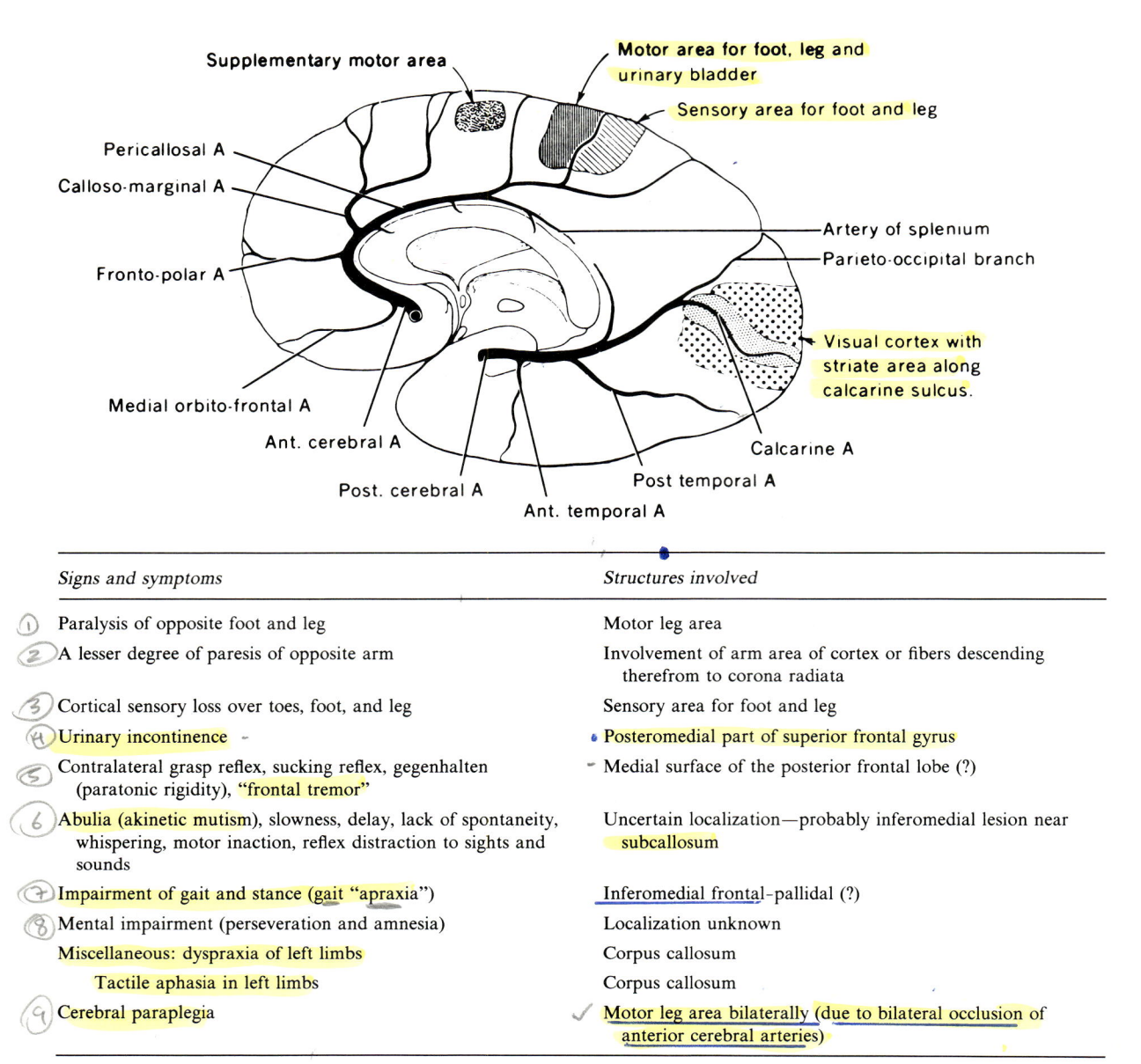

Signs and symptoms	Structures involved
1. Paralysis of opposite foot and leg	Motor leg area
2. A lesser degree of paresis of opposite arm	Involvement of arm area of cortex or fibers descending therefrom to corona radiata
3. Cortical sensory loss over toes, foot, and leg	Sensory area for foot and leg
4. Urinary incontinence	Posteromedial part of superior frontal gyrus
5. Contralateral grasp reflex, sucking reflex, gegenhalten (paratonic rigidity), "frontal tremor"	Medial surface of the posterior frontal lobe (?)
6. Abulia (akinetic mutism), slowness, delay, lack of spontaneity, whispering, motor inaction, reflex distraction to sights and sounds	Uncertain localization—probably inferomedial lesion near subcallosum
7. Impairment of gait and stance (gait "apraxia")	Inferomedial frontal-pallidal (?)
8. Mental impairment (perseveration and amnesia)	Localization unknown
Miscellaneous: dyspraxia of left limbs	Corpus callosum
Tactile aphasia in left limbs	Corpus callosum
9. Cerebral paraplegia	Motor leg area bilaterally (due to bilateral occlusion of anterior cerebral arteries)

Note: Hemianopia does not occur; transcortical aphasia occurs rarely.

Figure 145-4 Diagram of a cerebral hemisphere, medial aspect, showing the branches and distribution of the anterior cerebral artery and the principal regions of cerebral localization. Below the diagram is a list of the clinical manifestations of infarction in the territory of the anterior cerebral artery and the corresponding regions of cerebral damage. (From Adams and Victor.[1])

Basilar Artery Occlusion

The basilar artery (BA) is formed by the two vertebral arteries (VA) at the pontomedullary junction. It ascends anterior to the base of the pons and bifurcates into the two PCAs. Deviations from this "normal" relationship of the basilar artery to the VAs and PCAs are common. Penetrating paramedian branches of the BA supply the medial pons, short circumferential branches nourish the anterolateral pons, and the superior and anterior inferior cerebellar arteries supply the posterolateral pons and much of the cerebellar hemispheres. These multiple branches supplying the many structures traversing the pons cause a variety of neurological signs with BA ischemia. If the rostral BA is occluded, there may be ischemia to the midbrain, subthalamus, thalamus, and portions of the temporal and occipital lobes. The resulting neurological abnormalities have been designated the *top of the basilar syndrome*.[5] This syndrome includes visual field defects, disorders of vertical gaze and convergence, slow deviation of the eyes, pupillary constriction, somnolence, and hallucinations in addition to bilateral weakness, ataxia, and sensory loss of the extremities.

Occlusion of the BA or one or more of its paramedian or short circumferential branches can lead to a wide variety of

Clinical Syndromes of Brain Ischemia

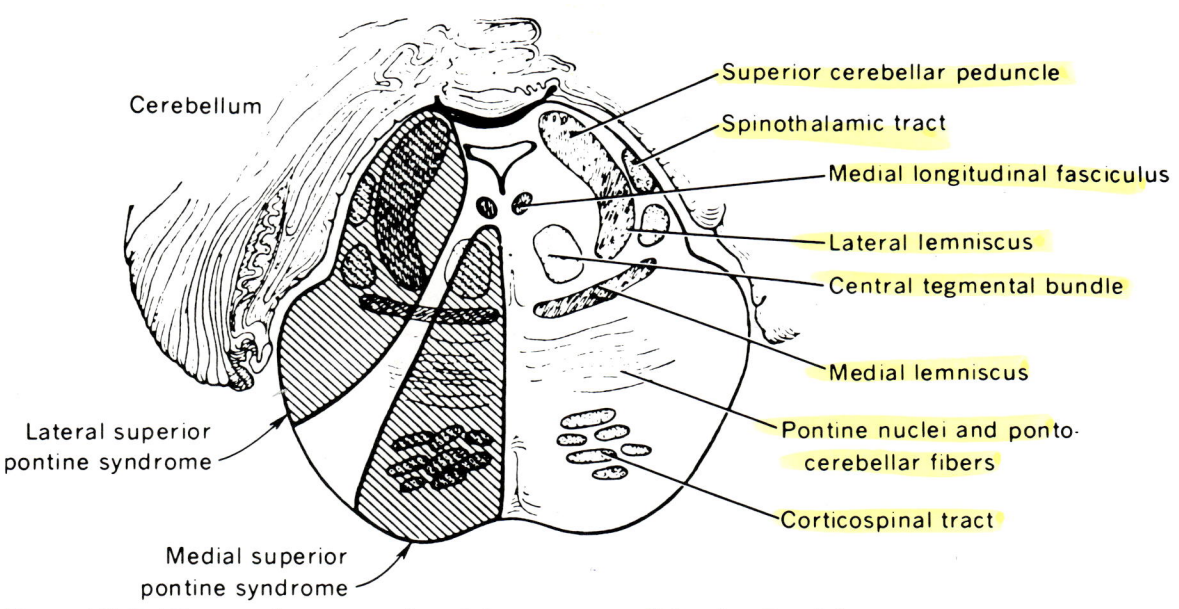

Figure 145-5 Diagram of a cross section of the upper pons. Below is a list of the clinical manifestations of medial and lateral superior pontine infarction and their corresponding regions of damage. (From Adams and Victor.[1])

Signs and symptoms	Structures involved
1. Medial superior pontine syndrome (paramedian branches of upper basilar artery	
a. On side of lesion	
(1) Cerebellar ataxia	Superior and/or middle cerebellar peduncle
(2) Internuclear ophthalmoplegia	Medial longitudinal fasciculus
(3) Rhythmic myoclonus of palate, pharynx, vocal cords, respiratory apparatus, face, oculomotor apparatus, etc.	Central tegmental bundle
b. On side opposite lesion	
(1) Paralysis of face, arm, and leg	Corticobulbar and corticospinal tract
(2) Rarely touch, vibration, and position senses are affected	Medial lemniscus
2. Lateral superior pontine syndrome (syndrome of superior cerebellar artery)	
a. On side of lesion	
(1) Ataxia of limbs and gait, falling to side of lesion	Middle and superior cerebellar peduncles, superior surface of cerebellum, dentate nucleus
(2) Dizziness, nausea, vomiting	Vestibular nucleus
(3) Horizontal nystagmus	Vestibular nucleus
(4) Paresis of conjugate gaze (ipsilateral)	Uncertain
(5) Loss of optokinetic nystagmus	Uncertain
(6) Skew deviation	Uncertain
(7) Miosis, ptosis, decreased sweating over face (Horner's syndrome)	Descending sympathetic fibers
b. On side opposite lesion	
(1) Impaired pain and thermal sense on face, limbs, and trunk	Spinothalamic tract
(2) Impaired touch, vibration, and position sense, more in leg than arm (there is a tendency to incongruity of pain and touch deficits)	Medial lemniscus (lateral portion)

(Territory of descending branch to middle cerebellar peduncle from superior cerebellar artery)

stroke syndromes. Some of the ocular abnormalities seen are nystagmus, internuclear ophthalmoplegia, gaze paresis, abducens palsy, ocular bobbing, and constricted pupils. Somnolence or coma occurs with reticular formation ischemia. Transient loss of consciousness in the absence of associated brain stem ischemic symptoms is rarely caused by vertebrobasilar ischemia. Weakness and hypesthesia of the face may be accompanied by similar impairment of the contralateral limbs, or all four limbs. Ischemia of the vestibular nuclei or pathways produces vertigo, nausea, vomiting, and nystagmus. Limb and gait ataxia occur following ischemia of the superior or middle cerebellar peduncles or cerebellar

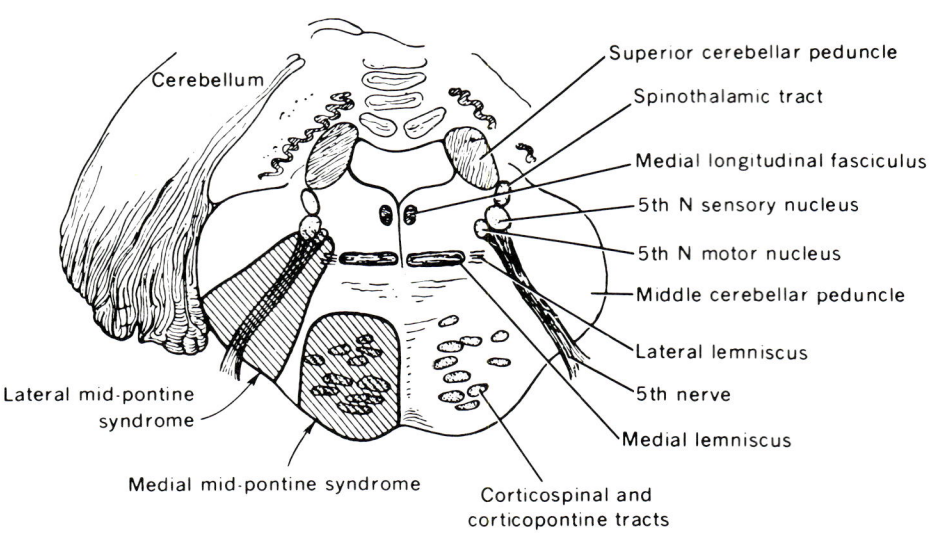

Figure 145-6 Diagram of a cross section of the pons at the level of the fifth nerve. Below is a list of the clinical manifestations of medial and lateral midpontine infarction and their corresponding regions of damage. (From Adams and Victor.[1])

Signs and symptoms	Structures involved
1. Medial midpontine syndrome (paramedian branch of midbasilar artery)	
a. On side of lesion	
(1) Ataxia of limbs and gait (more prominent in bilateral involvement)	Middle cerebellar peduncle
b. On side opposite lesion	
(1) Paralysis of face, arm, and leg	Corticobulbar and corticospinal tract
(2) Deviation of eyes	
(3) Variably impaired touch and proprioception when lesion extends posteriorly. Usually the syndrome is purely motor.	Medial lemniscus
2. Lateral midpontine syndrome (short circumferential artery)	
a. On side of lesion	
(1) Ataxia of limbs	Middle cerebellar peduncle
(2) Paralysis of muscles of mastication	Motor fibers or nucleus of fifth nerve
(3) Impaired sensation over side of face	Sensory fibers or nucleus of fifth nerve

hemispheres. TIAs in the vertebrobasilar circulation are subject to greater diagnostic uncertainty than are those in the carotid circulation. This difference is easily appreciated in light of the varied symptoms of brain stem ischemia (Table 145-1). Dizziness, vertigo, light-headedness, loss of consciousness, and visual blurring represent some of the commonest symptoms attributed incorrectly to vertebrobasilar ischemia (Tables 145-2 and 145-3). These symptoms occurring without other more definite symptoms of brain stem ischemia have such ubiquitous origins that they should not be attributed ipso facto to focal cerebrovascular disease.

The most characteristic syndromes resulting from basilar artery branch occlusions are the medial and lateral superior pontine syndromes, the medial and lateral midpontine syndromes, and the medial and lateral inferior pontine syndromes (Figs. 145-5 to 145-7). Each syndrome may be more or less complete. The usual artery involved in producing each of the syndromes is noted in the figure legends.

When all of the symptoms and signs of a posterior circulation ischemic episode can be accounted for by involvement of a single branch artery, the ischemic event can usually be attributed to occlusion of that specific artery. However, when the clinical features suggest multiple branch artery involvement, it is likely that the primary lesion is in the more proximal parent vessel, and one should be concerned about the possibility of a devastating basilar artery thrombosis (Table 145-6).[1,3]

Vertebral Artery Occlusion

The two vertebral arteries (VAs) ascend from the foramen magnum to nourish the rostral cervical spinal cord, the medulla, and the posterior inferior cerebellum before uniting to form the BA. There is considerable congenital variability in the diameter of the VAs. This fact, combined with the variability of collateral anastomoses from the external carotid and other neck arteries, the circle of Willis, and the BA, accounts for the diversity of neurological manifestations of VA disease. A VA occlusion may be asymptomatic, or it may

Clinical Syndromes of Brain Ischemia

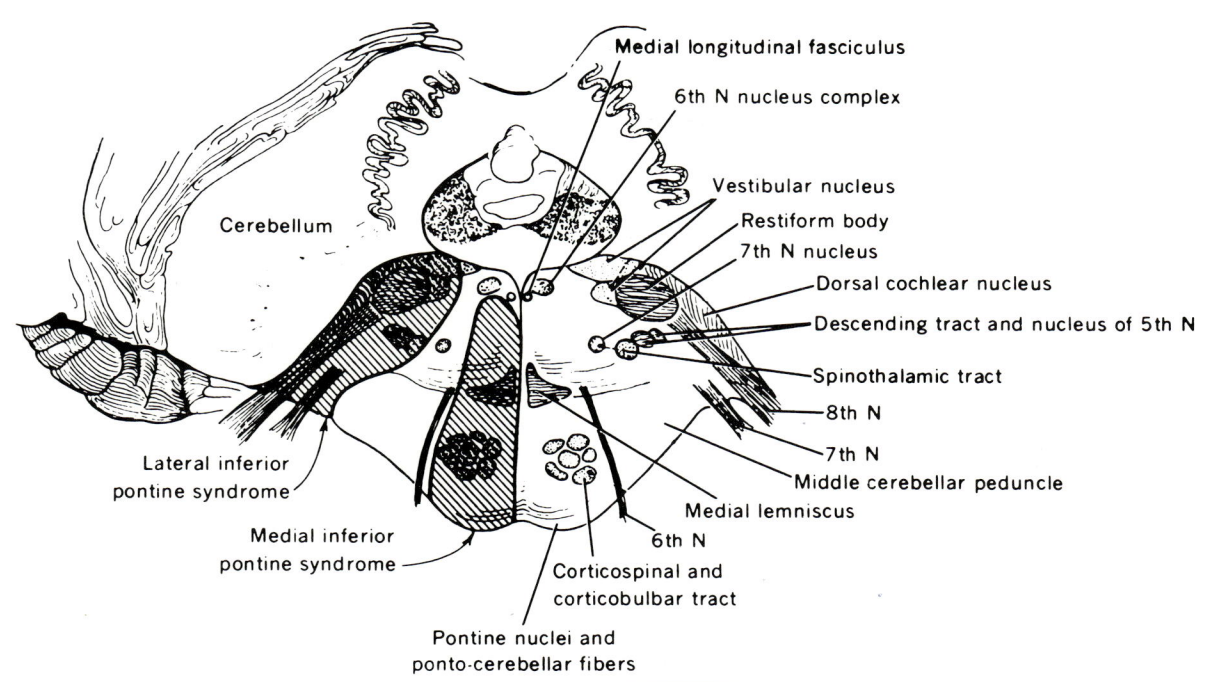

Figure 145-7 Diagram of a cross section of the pons at the level of the sixth and seventh nerve nuclei. Below is a list of the clinical manifestations of medial and lateral inferior pontine infarction and their corresponding regions of damage. (From Adams and Victor.[1])

Signs and symptoms	Structures involved
1. Medial inferior pontine syndrome (occlusion of paramedian branch of basilar artery)	
a. On side of lesion	
(1) Paralysis of conjugate gaze to side of lesion (preservation of convergence)	Paraabducens "center" for lateral gaze
(2) Nystagmus	Vestibular nuclei and connections
(3) Ataxia of limbs and gait	Middle cerebellar peduncle (?)
(4) Diplopia on lateral gaze	Abducens nerve
b. On side opposite lesion	
(1) Paralysis of face, arm, and leg	Corticobulbar and corticospinal tract in lower pons
(2) Impaired tactile and proprioceptive sense over half of the body	Medial lemniscus
2. Lateral inferior pontine syndrome (occlusion of anterior inferior cerebellar artery)	
a. On side of lesion	
(1) Horizontal and vertical nystagmus, vertigo, nausea, vomiting, oscillopsia	Vestibular nerve or nucleus
(2) Facial paralysis	Seventh nerve
(3) Paralysis of conjugate gaze to side of lesion	Paraabducens "center" for lateral gaze
(4) Deafness, tinnitus	Auditory nerve or cochlear nucleus
(5) Ataxia	Middle cerebellar peduncle and cerebellar hemisphere
(6) Impaired sensation over face	Descending tract and nucleus fifth nerve
b. On side opposite lesion	
(1) Impaired pain and thermal sense over half the body (may include face)	Spinothalamic tract
3. Total unilateral inferior pontine syndrome (occlusion of anterior inferior cerebellar artery); lateral and medial syndromes combined	

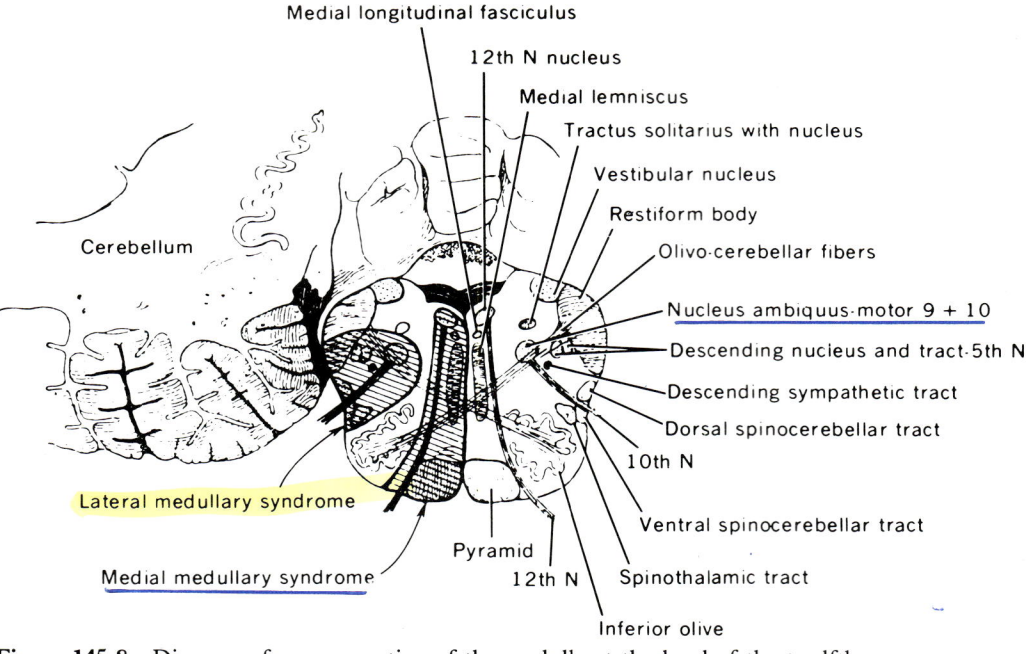

Figure 145-8 Diagram of a cross section of the medulla at the level of the twelfth nerve. Below the diagram is a list of the clinical manifestations of medial and lateral medullary infarction and their corresponding regions of damage. (From Adams and Victor.[1])

Signs and symptoms	Structures involved
1. Medial medullary syndrome (occlusion of vertebral artery or branch of vertebral or lower basilar artery)	
a. On side of lesion	
(1) Paralysis with atrophy of half the tongue	— Issuing twelfth nerve
b. On side opposite lesion	
(1) Paralysis of arm and leg sparing face	— Pyramidal tract
(2) Impaired tactile and proprioceptive sense over half the body	— Medial lemniscus
2. Lateral medullary syndrome (occlusion of any of five vessels may be responsible—vertebral, posterior inferior cerebellar, or superior, middle, or inferior lateral medullary arteries)	
a. On side of lesion	
(1) Pain, numbness, impaired sensation over half the face	— Descending tract and nucleus of fifth nerve
(2) Ataxia of limbs, falling to side of lesion	— Uncertain—restiform body, cerebellar hemisphere, olivocerebellar fibers, spinocerebellar tract (?)
(3) Vertigo, nausea, vomiting	— Vestibular nuclei and connections
(4) Nystagmus, diplopia, oscillopsia	— Vestibular nuclei and connections
(5) Horner's syndrome (miosis, ptosis, decreased sweating)	— Descending sympathetic tract
(6) Dysphagia, hoarseness, paralysis of vocal cord, diminished gag reflex	— Issuing fibers ninth and tenth nerves
(7) Loss of taste (rare)	— Nucleus and tractus solitarius
(8) Numbness of ipsilateral arm, trunk, or leg	— Cuneate and gracile nuclei
(9) Hiccup	— Uncertain
b. On side opposite lesion	
(1) Impaired pain and thermal sense over half the body, sometimes face	— Spinothalamic tract

3. Total unilateral medullary syndrome (occlusion of vertebral artery); combination of medial and lateral syndromes
4. Lateral pontomedullary syndrome (occlusion of vertebral artery); combination of medial and lateral syndromes
5. Basilar artery syndrome (the syndrome of the lone vertebral artery is equivalent); a combination of the various brainstem syndromes plus those arising in the posterior cerebral artery distribution. The clinical picture comprises bilateral long-tract signs (sensory and motor) with cerebellar and cranial nerve abnormalities.

   a. Paralysis or weakness of all extremities, plus all bulbar musculature — Corticobulbar and corticospinal tracts bilaterally
   b. Diplopia, paralysis of conjugate lateral and/or vertical gaze, internuclear ophthalmoplegia, horizontal and/or vertical nystagmus — Ocular motor nerves, apparatus for conjugate gaze, medial longitudinal fasciculus, vestibular apparatus
   c. Blindness, impaired vision, various visual field defects — Visual cortex
   d. Bilateral cerebellar ataxia — Cerebellar peduncles and the cerebellar hemispheres
   e. Coma — Tegmentum of midbrain, thalami
   f. Sensation may be strikingly intact in the presence of almost total paralysis. Sensory loss may be syringomyelic or the reverse or involve all modalities — Medial lemniscus, spinothalamic tracts or thalamic nuclei

cause a medullary infarction or ischemic symptoms throughout the BA or PCA distribution.

Infarction of the lateral medulla is usually caused by VA or posterior inferior cerebellar artery (PICA) occlusion, and it produces the Wallenberg syndrome, one of the commonest ischemic syndromes of the vertebrobasilar circulation (Fig. 145-8). The syndrome may be more or less complete. Involvement of the spinothalamic tract and the descending tract and nucleus of the trigeminal nerve produces a loss of pain and temperature sensation in the ipsilateral face and contralateral body and limbs. Ischemia of the vestibular nuclei causes vertigo, nausea, vomiting, oscillopsia, and nystagmus. Ischemia of the cerebellum or its connections yields ataxia of the ipsilateral limbs. A Horner's syndrome arises from descending sympathetic tract involvement. Inclusion of the lower cranial nerve nuclei and nerves produces dysphagia, hoarseness, a diminished gag reflex, hiccups, and rarely loss of taste.

Infarction of the medial medulla is rare but produces paralysis of the contralateral arm and leg because of pyramidal tract involvement (Fig. 145-8). Loss of touch and proprioceptive sensation in a similar distribution arises from medial lemniscus ischemia. Ipsilateral tongue paralysis occurs when the hypoglossal nerve is injured.

The subclavian steal syndrome is discussed elsewhere in this text.

References

1. Adams RD, Victor M: *Principles of Neurology*, 2d ed. New York, McGraw-Hill, 1981.
2. Barnett HJM: Progress towards stroke prevention: Robert Wartenberg lecture. Neurology (NY) 30:1212–1225, 1980.
3. Biemond A: Thrombosis of the basilar artery and the vascularization of the brain stem. Brain 74:300–317, 1951.
4. Byer JA, Easton JD: Therapy of ischemic cerebrovascular disease. Ann Intern Med 93:742–756, 1980.
5. Caplan LR: "Top of the basilar" syndrome. Neurology (NY) 30:72–79, 1980.
6. de Bono DP, Warlow CP: Potential sources of emboli in patients with presumed transient cerebral or retinal ischaemia. Lancet 1:343–346, 1981.
6a Easton JD, Hart RG, Sherman DG, Kaste M: Diagnosis and management of ischemic stroke: Part I. Threatened stroke and its management. Cur Prob Cardiol 8:1–76, 1983.
7. Easton JD, Sherman DG: Management of cerebral embolism of cardiac origin. Stroke 11:433–442, 1980.
8. Fisher CM: Late-life migraine accompaniments as a cause of unexplained transient ischemic attacks. Can J Neurol Sci 7:9–17, 1980.
9. Fisher CM: Lacunar strokes and infarcts: A review. Neurology (NY) 32:871–876, 1982.
10. Fisher CM, Adams RD: Transient global amnesia. Acta Neurol Scand [Suppl] 9:1–83, 1964.
10a Hart RG, Sherman DG, Miller VT, Easton JD: Diagnosis and management of ischemic stroke: Part II. Selected controversies. Cur Prob Cardiol 8:1–80, 1983.
11. Jones HR, Millikan CH: Temporal profile (clinical course) of acute carotid system cerebral infarction. Stroke 7:64–71, 1976.
12. Jones HR Jr, Millikan CH, Sandok BA: Temporal profile (clinical course) of acute vertebrobasilar system cerebral infarction. Stroke 11:173–177, 1980.
13. Marquardsen J: The natural history of acute cerebrovascular disease: A retrospective study of 769 patients. Acta Neurol Scand [Suppl] 38:1–192, 1969.
14. Millikan CH: Transient cerebral ischemia: Definition and natural history. Prog Cardiovasc Dis 22:303–308, 1980.
15. National Institute of Neurological and Communicative Disorders and Stroke: A classification and outline of cerebrovascular diseases, II. Stroke 6:564–616, 1975.
16. Ostrowski AZ, Webster JE, Gurdjian ES: The proximal anterior cerebral artery: An anatomic study. Arch Neurol 3:661–664, 1960.
17. Symonds C, Mackenzie I: Bilateral loss of vision from cerebral infarction. Brain 80:415–455, 1957.

146
Noninvasive Tests in the Diagnosis of Carotid Vascular Disease

Robert M. Crowell
J. Philip Kistler

Occlusive disease of the internal carotid artery is an important cause of ischemic stroke.[5] Carotid endarterectomy may remove carotid plaques to minimize the threat of stroke. Cerebral arteriography is a definitive method for visualizing the carotid circulation, but this test carries a small but definite risk, even in the best of hands. The need to evaluate the carotid circulation atraumatically and repeatedly before the onset of irreversible stroke has led to the development of noninvasive vascular tests.

Noninvasive tests assess circulatory parameters to detect hemodynamically significant carotid stenosis. Carotid arterial anatomy may be imaged by ultrasound techniques. Carotid artery physiology can be assessed to calculate residual lumen diameter. Instrumentation can measure velocity, volume, pressure, or pattern of flow at the common carotid bifurcation or in distal vessels. Multiple features of single physiological events may be monitored. For example, the ocular pulse wave can be examined for five different types of information pertinent to carotid disease. With these permutations, it is not surprising that over 20 types of noninvasive tests have been developed for clinical use (Table 146-1).[1] Investigators have described a host of combinations of tests. Hundreds of publications describe developments in this rapidly expanding field.

Little wonder that the clinical neurosurgeon may be baffled in this area. Which test is best? What are the indications? Can it replace angiography?

What follows is a neurosurgical perspective on noninvasive diagnosis developed by a group of clinicians dedicated to the management of cerebrovascular disease. Over a 5-year period, we have developed a personal experience with a broad range of noninvasive examinations. Some tests impressed us; others did not. We have developed a reliance on some examinations for neurosurgical decision making. Other approaches may be equally valid; we present here a neurosurgical utilization of noninvasive techniques that we have found helpful and reliable.

Ideal noninvasive tests for carotid occlusive disease should possess several key attributes. The tests should be such that a technician could perform them quickly and repeatedly in patients who may not be entirely cooperative. The tests should be risk-free and painless. A noninvasive examination should provide assessment of hemodynamically significant stenosis, with quantitative estimation of residual lumen diameter. In addition, ulcerated plaques should be detected. The data should not be clouded by the presence of bilateral or external carotid occlusive disease. Both anatomical and physiological changes should be assessed. The test should be inexpensive.

A review of existing tests reveals that no single examination is self-sufficient for the diagnosis of extracranial carotid occlusive disease. Direct tests examine the carotid bifurcation, but may overlook lesions beyond the field of the transducer and those that do not reflect echos or produce bruits. Some of these lesions may be detected by indirect tests of the distal circulation, if the lesions produce hemodynamically significant stenosis. On the other hand, some carotid occlusive and ulcerative lesions that produce no distal hemodynamic change will be missed by indirect tests but can be identified by direct tests.

Therefore, a combination of tests is needed for a spectrum of diagnosis of carotid occlusive disease. Tests may be selected to supplement limitations. Tests may be chosen to characterize pathological changes in both anatomy and physiology. The effectiveness of a battery of six tests, including an ultrasonic B-mode scanning device, was assessed

TABLE 146-1 Noninvasive Tests

Direct Tests	Indirect Tests
Carotid palpation	Cerebral circulation
Bruit auscultation	EEG with carotid compression
Carotid phonoangiography	Radionuclide angiography
Spectral quantitative phonoangiography	Superficial orbital circulation
Range-gated Doppler imaging	Dynamic palpation of facial pulses
Continuous wave Doppler imaging	Opacity pulse propagation time
B-scan ultrasonography	Thermography
Radionuclide angiography	Supraorbital photoplethysmography
Xerography	Supraorbital Doppler ultrasonography
	Deep orbital circulation
	Ophthalmodynamometry
	Arm-to-retina circulation time
	Oculoplethysmography (two types)
	Oculotonography
	Oculosonography
	Ocular pulse analysis

SOURCE: After Ackerman.[1]

in 500 consecutive patients. This approach was 90 percent effective in identifying carotid stenosis with a residual lumen of 2 mm or less. The false-positive rate was 3 to 5 percent. On the basis of theoretical considerations and relying on personal experience, Ackerman has recommended as a practical modern battery indirect tests of both the superficial and deep orbital circulations and a direct physiological monitor.[1]

Some tests are superior for specific problems. For the asymptomatic carotid bruit, quantitative spectral phonoangiography seems the most useful single test. For internal carotid artery occlusion, oculoplethysmography is 95 percent accurate. B-mode ultrasonography may detect minimal atherosclerotic changes. A combination of complementary tests comes closest to the ideals of noninvasive diagnosis. The nature of the tests selected depends on the indications for study. A group of tests, carefully chosen for specific indications, can help the neurosurgeon manage patients with carotid occlusive disease.

Direct Tests

Carotid Palpation and Auscultation

Assessment of abnormality near the carotid bifurcation begins at the bedside. Though evaluation of carotid pulses is unrewarding because of external carotid pulsation, palpation of a local thrill is highly suggestive of marked stenosis, usually in the internal carotid artery. Palpation should be gentle, for local atheroma may be dislodged by vigorous palpation. Bruit auscultation using a bell stethoscope is useful in the detection of stenosis. Careful auscultation over the entire course of the carotid artery from the clavicle to the angle of the jaw can often determine the point of maximum intensity, which thus suggests the origin of the bruit. In general, the higher the pitch, the tighter the stenosis. When a bruit extends into diastole, a marked stenosis is suggested. The examiner can be duped, however, by radiated murmurs, and in up to one-third of cases of significant carotid stenosis, there is no bruit for assessment.

Many laboratory tests have been devised for direct assessment of the carotid bifurcation. These techniques include spectral quantitative phonoangiography, qualitative bruit analysis, direct Doppler imaging, and B-mode ultrasonography. Of these methods, spectral quantitative phonoangiography provides the most useful information, a reliable quantitative assessment of residual lumen diameter. Direct Doppler imaging, which assesses flow velocity, also seems reliable, but it gives only a qualitative assessment of carotid stenosis. Other direct tests include xerography and radionuclide angiography, but these tests have not provided information adequate for neurosurgical decision making.

Spectral Phonoangiography

For carotid bruits, spectral (frequency) analysis can provide an accurate quantitative estimate of residual lumen diameter. This technique, developed by Lees, Duncan, and Kistler, provides a relatively inexpensive noninvasive method for the sequential follow-up of asymptomatic carotid bruit.[4,10]

A piezoelectric transducer is used to make recordings along the course of the common carotid artery (CCA) and the internal carotid artery (ICA) to the angle of the mandible (Fig. 146-1). The signal is amplified, stored on magnetic tape, and analyzed by a microprocessor-based system. By plotting bruit intensity against frequency, the frequency of maximum intensity (a characteristic "break frequency") can be determined. The residual lumen diameter is calculated as a function of the break frequency. A commercially produced instrument for performing this analysis is available for about $15,000 (Spectraview, Edwards Laboratories, Santa Ana, Calif.).

The results of quantitative spectral phonoangiography have been validated by comparison with carotid angiography.[4] For 60 carotid bruits, phonoangiography was compared with angiography. Fifty of the 60 bruits (83 percent) had characteristics of turbulent blood flow, and a residual lumen diameter could be calculated. The residual lumen diameter estimated from phonoangiography differed from the radiographic value by less than 1 mm in 83 percent and less than 1.5 mm in 92 percent of the studies.

Recently, spectral phonoangiography was correlated with surgical pathology for the estimation of residual lumen diameter in carotid stenosis.[10] Thirty-nine carotid bifurcations were studied. In six studies, the bruit was too faint to analyze. In 31 studies, the phonoangiogram predicted the residual lumen diameter to within 0.5 mm of the measured pathological value. In this study, spectral phonoangiography was as accurate as carotid angiography for the evaluation of carotid stenosis in patients with carotid bruit. Sequential studies, done over intervals of time, have documented progressive carotid stenosis.

There are limitations to spectral phonoangiography.[10] A

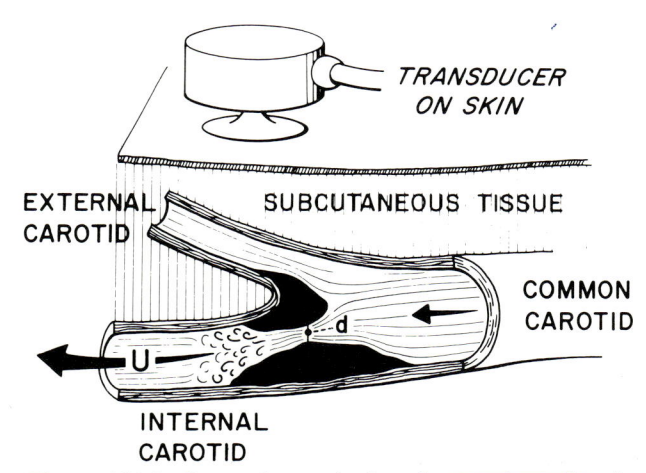

Figure 146-1 Spectral quantitative phonoangiography. A piezoelectric transducer detects turbulent flow (U) beyond an internal carotid stenosis with a residual lumen diameter (d). Bruit intensity is plotted against bruit frequency (f) to identify the maximal or "break" frequency (f_0). Residual lumen diameter (d) is calculated by dividing f_0 into U, which is assumed to be 500 mm/s.

bruit must be present for the technique to be used. A bruit may be too faint to give an accurate sound spectrum. This is particularly likely when the residual lumen diameter is less than 1 mm. Unsuitable bruits may also occur when the stenosis is so slight that disturbed flow is just beginning. The system for bruit analysis used in phonoangiography assumes peak systolic flow velocity of 500 mm/s, but flow velocity probably changes in relation to physiological alterations. The sound spectrum of some bruits may not have a clear break frequency. Bruits arising from external carotid stenosis may mimic those that arise from internal carotid artery lesion. The bruit of external carotid artery stenosis generally decreases markedly on compression of the superficial temporal artery.

Quantitative spectral phonoangiography provides accurate assessment of the extent of carotid stenosis. Since spectral phonoangiography is both quantitative and noninvasive, it will be useful in ascertaining the natural history of carotid stenosis. Since the technique can be used repetitively, it is helpful in identifying severe or progressive carotid stenosis that may warrant surgery for asymptomatic carotid bruit (Fig. 146-2).

Qualitative carotid phonoangiography is another method for assessing carotid bruits.[9] A microphone detects the signal, which is amplified for display on an oscilloscope screen. The device plots amplitude versus time for several locations in the neck. A rough estimate of bruit frequency is possible. Bruits loudest at the base of the neck are considered radiated, while bruits loudest over the carotid bifurcation are considered to represent internal carotid stenosis. The advantages of qualitative carotid phonoangiography are simplicity, low cost, and ability to localize the site of origin of many cervical bruits. Disadvantages include lack of quantitation and poor specificity.[7]

Direct Doppler Imaging

When ultrasound is reflected from a moving column of arterial blood and its echo recorded, features of the Doppler shift may be used to characterize flow in the studied vessel. A Doppler instrument may transmit continuous wave or range-gated (pulsed) signals. The continuous wave Doppler signals sample average flow velocity in arteries beneath the probe. Range-gated Doppler signals sample flow velocity in discrete volumes of blood within a single lumen. Detailed evaluation of the velocity waveform may provide several types of useful data, including mean velocity, peak systolic velocity, and systolic acceleration. Evaluation of the frequency content may augment the characterization of occlusive carotid disease.

Recently, the continuous wave Doppler technique has been used for simultaneous imaging of vessels and estimation of flow velocity.[15] These parameters may permit detection of carotid stenosis.

The Doppler probe records on a storage oscilloscope the probe position in two dimensions, as well as the flow velocity detected by the probe. Flow velocity is color-coded for three ranges (low, medium, and high). The probe is passed up and down the course of the cervical carotid artery, slowly building an image of arterial anatomy and flow velocity. A Polaroid photograph is a permanent copy of the image. Stenosis is seen as a zone of increased flow velocity. Subclavian and vertebral arteries may also be imaged. Commercial instruments for direct Doppler imaging are available for about $30,000.

Impressive statistics have been reported for identification of hemodynamically significant ICA stenosis. Major disadvantages are the extensive operator training required to obtain reliable results and the qualitative nature of the system.

When flow is reduced to a trickle, the instrument may not detect echos and therefore cannot differentiate between a marked stenosis and occlusion. After occlusion of the internal carotid artery, the image of two external carotid branches can be mistaken for the common carotid bifurcation.

B-Scan Ultrasonography

Ultrasound may be used to depict arteries in two dimensions.[14] Instruments termed B-scanners, after the mode of signal processing employed, generally employ a linear array of multiple ultrasonic transducers of 5- to 10-MHz frequency. The transducers are driven sequentially to produce an ultrasound signal that covers the sector of tissue beneath the transducer. These systems, which display arterial anatomy in real time, may have resolutions as high as 0.5 to 0.8 mm.[3]

The prospect of high-resolution imaging of the carotid bifurcation has excited great interest and commercial activity. The potential of the technique has thus far exceeded its utility. A number of limitations mar B-scan assessment of carotid occlusive disease. Lesions may lie above the mandible beyond the field of the ultrasound transducer. Some carotid plaques have no detectable echo (sonolucent plaques). In some atheromatous lesions, a calcific plaque nearer to the transducer casts an acoustic shadow obscuring the deeper portion of the lesion. The B-scan image does not routinely provide data from which residual lumen diameter may be determined. Ulcerations in plaques are not reliably identified. Occlusion and tight stenosis cannot be differentiated. Real-time B-scan imaging of the carotid bifurcation requires considerable skill on the part of the examiner. False-negative rates up to 59 percent have been reported. An additional disadvantage of the instrument is its high cost (about $100,000).

B-scan systems may provide useful information as part of a battery of noninvasive examinations. An estimate of the severity of disease can be provided, with a good correlation to angiography in 80.4 percent, moderate correlation in 10.3 percent, and poor correlation in 9.3 percent of cases. When the indirect tests suggest a hemodynamically significant lesion of the carotid-ophthalmic system, a B-scan indicating severe atheromatous change can localize the lesion to the bifurcation. An abnormal B-scan with negative indirect tests suggests the need for standard angiography. With negative indirect examination, B-scan evidence of moderate to severe atheromatous change at the bifurcation suggests the possibility of an ulcerated plaque.

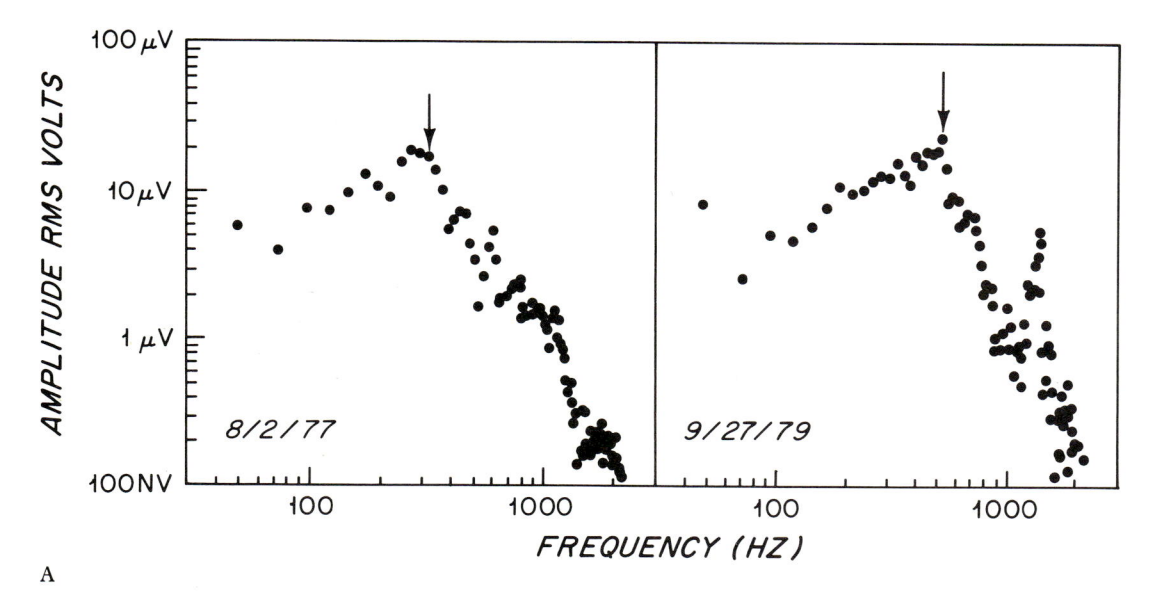

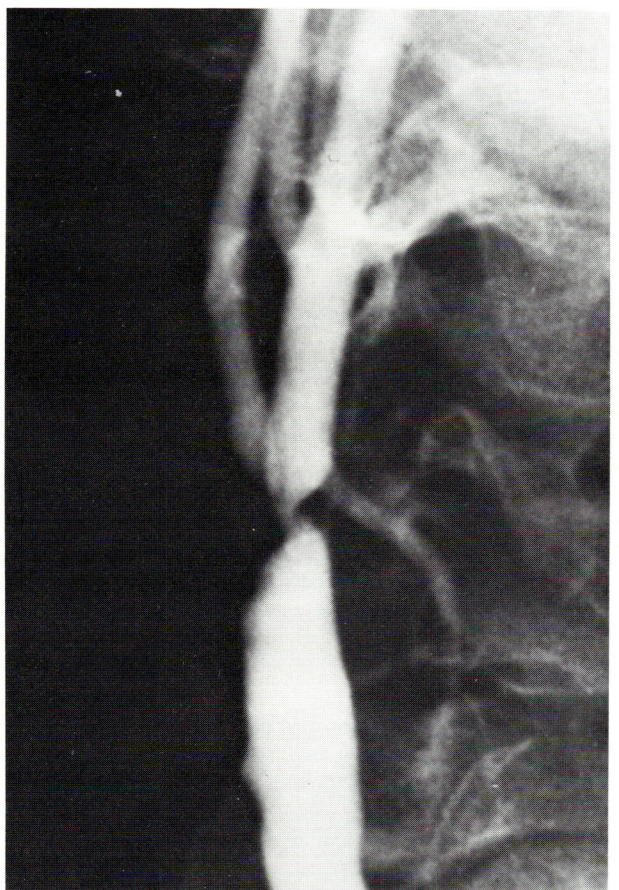

Noninvasive Tests in the Diagnosis of Carotid Vascular Disease

Figure 146-2 Spectral phonoangiography identifies progressive asymptomatic stenosis. *A.* The bruit break frequency rose from 300 Hz in 1977 to 500 Hz in 1979, at which time the residual lumen diameter was estimated at 1.5 mm. *B.* Angiographic confirmation of tight stenosis of the right internal carotid artery. *C.* Transverse section of the surgical plaque specimen shows a pinhole residual lumen. The patient had a smooth postoperative course.

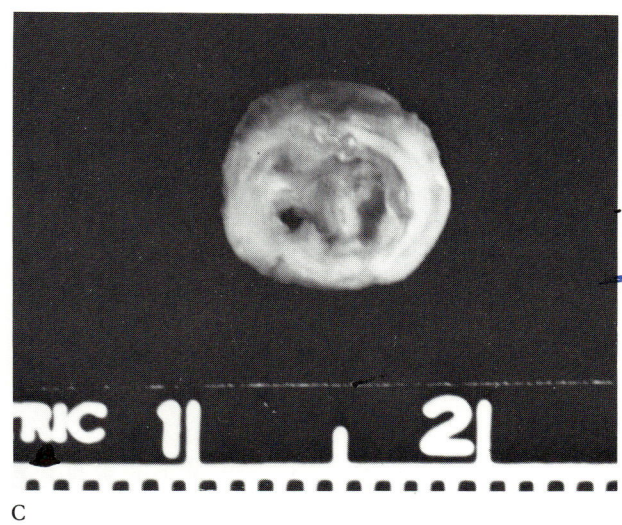

Indirect Tests

Dynamic Palpation of the Facial Pulses

Several authors have described methods for palpation of the facial pulses.[6] Elucidation of the functional anatomy of the periorbital collateral circulation in carotid occlusive disease has led to further development of these techniques. Dynamic palpation of the facial pulses, as described by Ackerman,[1] permits bedside assessment of periorbital collateral circulation. In this test, a brow artery is palpated with the index finger as the patient closes the eyes lightly. Concomitant compression of the superficial temporal artery may obliterate the brow pulsation. In this instance, the flow of blood must be from the external carotid circulation into the brow artery and thence retrograde via the ophthalmic artery to the carotid siphon. This finding strongly suggests virtual or complete occlusion of the internal carotid or ophthalmic artery. In some hypertensive patients the brow arteries can be reliably palpated, and the test is a useful bedside assessment. However, in up to 50 percent of the patients, we have been unable to palpate these brow arteries with confidence.

Ophthalmodynamometry

This test estimates the ophthalmic artery pressure in grams.[12] If the intraocular tension is known, the ophthalmic artery pressure in millimeters of mercury can be calculated. Ophthalmodynamometry (ODM) is best performed by two examiners, one applying the plunger at a point adjacent to the limbus, and the other recording ophthalmoscopically the change in the central retinal artery as the pressure increases. The onset of central retinal artery pulsation indicates the ophthalmic artery diastolic pressure. A cessation of pulsations in the ophthalmic artery indicates that the systolic pressure level has been exceeded. In addition, subjective loss of vision to the patient likewise demonstrates that systolic pressure has been exceeded. More than a 15 percent difference between diastolic pressure on the two sides is generally considered suggestive of abnormality. A 20 percent difference between the two sides is considered diagnostic. An absolute value of 30 g or less is diagnostic of virtual or complete occlusion of the carotid or ophthalmic arteries. Though it is cumbersome and uncomfortable for the patient, ophthalmodynamometry remains a useful bedside adjunct in the assessment of carotid occlusive disease. It may be a particularly handy examination in the postoperative assessment of carotid patency following carotid endarterectomy.

Oculoplethysmography

This approach is used to monitor flow and pressure in the ophthalmic artery. In the presence of occlusive disease of the internal carotid or ophthalmic artery, there are alterations in distal ophthalmic flow and pressure that may be detected by oculoplethysmographic assessment (OPG). Two types of OPG have been developed, both of which employ a suction device on the sclera. The Kartchner-McRae method monitors arrival time of the ocular pulse wave (OPG-Kartchner).[9] The Gee method estimates ophthalmic artery systolic pressure (OPG-Gee).[6] The OPG-Kartchner device employs just enough suction to the globe to hold the eye cup in place. The OPG-Gee technique increases intraocular pressure with scleral suction to a level above the ophthalmic artery systolic pressure. In this technique, the point at which ocular pulsation reappears is taken as the systolic pressure in the ophthalmic artery. A significant difference between the two sides is taken to indicate the presence of occlusive disease in the carotid-ophthalmic system.

In the OPG-Kartchner method, a comparison is made between the two sides of relative ophthalmic pressure, waveform, and pulse arrival time. Delayed pulse arrival suggests occlusive disease of the ipsilateral carotid-ophthalmic system. As compared with angiography, the test shows an accuracy of 89 percent in determining stenosis greater than 40 percent.[9] However, about 15 percent of patients with a positive OPG test have complete occlusion of the internal carotid artery on angiography. A false-negative rate of 7 to 10 percent is attributable to innominate or bilateral ICA occlusive disease. In the study of Ginsberg et al. OPG-Kartchner was normal in 95 percent of cases where the ICA lumen was less than 60 percent reduced on angiography.[7] The ocular pulse was delayed in 86 percent of cases where ICA stenosis was 60 percent or more. The diagnostic accuracy of OPG-Kartchner was 93 percent. In this study, OPG was as sensitive as supraorbital Doppler testing in detecting hemodynamically significant ICA stenosis without the unacceptable high false-positive rate observed in the supraorbital Doppler tests.

The advantage of the oculoplethysmographic methods are relative simplicity, an easily interpreted objective record, and relatively low cost of the equipment (under $5000). The primary limitation of OPG is the false-negative results recorded in the presence of bilateral disease.[7] Moreover, excellent cooperation from the patient is necessary for satisfactory examination. The assessment is qualitative, and the exact site of the occlusive process is not determined. One cannot distinguish between severe stenosis and total occlusion.

Periorbital Doppler Ultrasonography

A considerable area around the eye receives blood supply from the internal carotid artery via the brow branches of the ophthalmic artery. In the presence of severe internal carotid or ophthalmic artery stenosis or occlusion, the direction of flow in these facial vessels is usually reversed. Blood flows from the branches of the external carotid artery retrograde into the ophthalmic artery and thence into the carotid siphon. Periorbital directional Doppler ultrasonography may be used to determine the direction of flow in small brow arteries.[7,11] Compression of superficial temporal or facial artery branches may lead to diminution or reversal of brow vessel flow to an antegrade direction. Directional Doppler examination may be considered abnormal if resting flow is reversed, or if there is an abnormal response to compression of external carotid artery branches. Common carotid artery compression has been reported to enhance this evaluation, but in view of the potential for embolus, this maneuver is not recommended. The accuracy of the test is 85 to 90 percent.

In one careful study, supraorbital Doppler studies detected 88 percent of ICA stenoses, but there was a 13 percent false-positive rate and 12 percent false-negative rate with ICA stenosis of less than 60 percent.[7] Supratrochlear Doppler tests had only a 1 percent false-positive rate but detected only 48 percent of significant ICA stenoses. In this study, oculoplethysmography was as sensitive as supraorbital Doppler testing and did not have the high false-positive rate observed in supraorbital Doppler examinations. In another study, supraorbital artery flow reversal was seen in 59 percent of patients with ICA stenosis of 75 percent or greater. Experience in several laboratories indicates that this method can detect severe carotid stenosis or occlusion with as high as 95 percent sensitivity and specificity.[1]

The advantages of supraorbital Doppler studies are their simplicity, low cost, and relatively high sensitivity and specificity. Disadvantages of the test are its qualitative nature, the extensive operator experience required, and difficulties of the interpretation in the presence of external carotid or ophthalmic artery disease.[7]

Other Indirect Tests

Thermography and thermometry have been used to detect cool skin areas above the brow, which may indicate the presence of occlusive disease in the carotid-ophthalmic system. Unfortunately, the specificity of such changes and their sensitivity for diagnosis are low, and the techniques are qualitative only. Furthermore, thermographic cameras are expensive; so these methods are no longer in general use.

Carotid compression tonography monitors a pulse wave detected by a tonometer over the cornea. The relative amplitude of pulsation between the two sides is compared, and the slope of return of the pulse tracing is studied after carotid compression. There is a potential danger in carotid compression that could cause distal embolization.

In the opacity pulse propagation examination, photocells are used to evaluate changes in the opacity of periorbital tissues during the cardiac cycle. The pulse propagation time is prolonged ipsilateral to a hemodynamically significant lesion in comparison to the other side.

Radionuclide angiography is inaccurate for the diagnosis of carotid occlusive disease. A number of other tests have not had sufficient evaluation for present recommendation. These include supraorbital photoplethysmography, supraorbital fluorescein testing, arm-to-retina circulation time, ocular tonography, ocular sonography, and ocular pulse waveform analysis.

Digital Subtraction Angiography

The advent of computer technology has permitted reassessment of the role of intravenous angiography in the evaluation of cerebrovascular disease.[2] With intravenous digital subtraction angiography (DSA), extracranial and some intracranial arteries can now be visualized clearly on either an inpatient or outpatient basis. Techniques of DSA are described fully in another chapter.

DSA has proved in preliminary studies to be valuable in several settings of cerebrovascular illness. Internal carotid artery ulceration, stenosis, and occlusion can be visualized with a high degree of sensitivity and specificity of diagnosis. Subclavian artery stenosis has been visualized, and theoretically vertebral artery and basilar stenosis can be visualized with this technique. Intracranial studies have demonstrated internal carotid artery and middle cerebral artery occlusion, and moyamoya disease.

The quality of DSA images frequently approaches that of conventional angiography. In a recent investigation, 60 percent of extracranial cerebrovascular studies were classified as good to excellent bilaterally.[2] There was an excellent correlation between the DSA and conventional angiogram (sensitivity 95 percent, specificity 99 percent, accuracy 97 percent). When the carotid bifurcation is not well visualized by DSA, there is a substantial chance of misinterpretation.

Overall, DSA demonstrates the carotid bifurcation accurately in 71 percent of the arteries. A more recent study depicted the carotid bifurcation clearly in 88 percent of all studies.

Because DSA directly visualizes the extracranial-intracranial circulation, it has obvious advantages over noninvasive techniques that directly assess the status of the carotid bifurcation. Indirect noninvasive methods that assess the physiological significance of carotid occlusive disease may complement the DSA examination in some patients. The extracranial resolution of DSA is also superior to that achieved with direct noninvasive techniques such as Doppler scanning or B-mode ultrasonography. DSA can also visualize ulceration and mild stenosis while clearly separating total from subtotal internal carotid artery occlusion, tasks beyond the capability of noninvasive techniques at this time.

It must be noted, however, that DSA is not entirely noninvasive and innocuous. We have observed cerebral infarction due to dehydration after DSA, as well as hemothorax. The test cannot be recommended for patients with renal failure or hypersensitivity to the contrast agent. Moreover, DSA cannot reliably estimate residual lumen diameter in tight stenosis. For these reasons, serial phonoangiography is a good supplement to an initial DSA in the follow-up of patients with asymptomatic bruit.

Indications for Noninvasive Evaluation

Most patients with occlusive cerebral vascular disease are not candidates for noninvasive evaluation. Individuals with transient ischemic attacks or acute strokes should not be referred for noninvasive assessment. These individuals will require cerebral angiography or, perhaps in the future, digital intravenous subtraction angiography (DSA). Angiographic study will be required no matter what the noninvasive tests show. Patients with minor fixed deficits, or those with good recovery from a completed stroke, were formerly assessed by noninvasive testing, but DSA is likely more definitive for diagnosis in this group of patients. Demonstration of a tight carotid stenosis or deep ulcer might lead to surgery to prevent a further stroke. Patients with presentations equivocal for carotid disease have been evaluated with noninvasive tests. This practice may be superseded by DSA in view of its greater diagnostic specificity and sensitivity for the ulcerated plaque.

Asymptomatic Bruit A restricted group of patients with suspected cerebrovascular occlusive disease should be studied in the noninvasive laboratory. The prime indication is an asymptomatic carotid bruit. The natural history of this condition is uncertain. Fragmentary data, generally unsupported by clear-cut qualitative estimates of residual lumen diameter, have indicated a relatively benign prognosis. Other studies have indicated a much higher risk of stroke from asymptomatic carotid bruit. There is controversy as to whether asymptomatic carotid stenosis adds risks for patients undergoing major surgery of a type likely to produce intraoperative hypotension. In this uncertain setting, therapy remains uncertain. Some have recommended follow-up, others antiaggregant therapy, and others carotid endarterectomy.

Noninvasive testing can help evaluate the asymptomatic carotid bruit (Fig. 146-2). Quantitative methods, particularly spectral phonoangiography, can provide helpful information regarding residual lumen diameter. Serial studies with this test, complemented by DSA, could provide critical information on the natural history of asymptomatic carotid stenosis. Moreover, serial spectral phonoangiography can identify progressive carotid stenosis. We base our current management for asymptomatic bruit on the diagnostic accuracy of DSA and spectral phonoangiography, coupled with a 0 percent morbidity in 40 consecutive endarterectomies for asymptomatic stenosis. We recommend as initial evaluation the combination of DSA and spectral phonoangiography. If these tests demonstrate a residual lumen diameter of 2 mm or less, and the patient is medically stable, standard angiography is recommended, as is surgery if a tight stenosis is confirmed. Should the residual lumen diameter be greater than 2 mm, or in the case of an unstable medical status, we repeat spectral phonoangiography at 6-month intervals with intensive medical therapy. If the residual lumen diameter decreases below 2 mm, and the medical status stabilizes, angiography is recommended with potential endarterectomy. In this way, the bulk of patients with asymptomatic bruit are managed medically. For a small number with tight carotid stenosis and a stable medical condition, in whom the risk of the lesion likely outweighs that of surgery, angiography and surgery are recommended as prophylaxis for stroke.

Satisfactory DSA Unavailable For a variety of reasons, reliable DSA may be lacking for a given patient. In many hospitals, DSA is not available. In up to 30 percent of patients, largely because of poor cooperation, satisfactory DSA examinations of the carotid bifurcations cannot be obtained. In a small group of patients with renal failure, the iodine bolus required by DSA poses an unacceptable risk. In all of these settings, the noninvasive examinations play a valuable backup role. With no DSA, where transient monocular blindness or hemispheric ischemia are questionable, positive results in the noninvasive examination can help rule in cerebral angiography. Likewise, in patients with a minor deficit from a recent stroke or good neurological recovery after a completed stroke, in the absence of DSA, positive noninvasive studies urge standard angiography. If a tight carotid stenosis is identified and removed, recurrent stroke may be prevented. In those patients with clear-cut TIA or stroke, where angiography is indicated, other illness or patient refusal may preclude angiography. In such instances, positive noninvasive tests might help persuade patients or guide anticoagulant therapy.

Supplement to DSA For patients with stroke or TIA, DSA might be used as the initial examination. If an ulcerated lesion at the carotid bifurcation were disclosed, then indirect noninvasive testing (for example, OPG) if negative could go far toward excluding distal occlusive disease in the ICA. In this setting, conventional angiography might be omitted. In other patients where DSA left doubt regarding a carotid occlusive process, then noninvasive testing might help clarify the situation without conventional angiography.

Other Problems Internal carotid artery occlusive disease will be found in approximately 20 percent of patients with typical central retinal artery occlusion. It has been suggested that the noninvasive examination is highly accurate in this situation, and may be the sole determinant of cerebral angiography. DSA could be used in such cases.

Recommended Tests

For these indications, we recommend a combination of a direct and an indirect test. As a direct test, we have found spectral phonoangiography especially reliable for bruit analysis, but direct Doppler imaging also seems very reliable and requires no bruit. As an indirect test, we have found periorbital Doppler helpful, but OPG-Kartchner seems to provide similar (or better) results.

Future Prospects for Noninvasive Evaluation

The proliferation of noninvasive tests and laboratories will be restricted as digital subtraction angiography spreads. This method, which accurately depicts hemodynamically significant stenosis, as well as substantial ulceration, will supplant noninvasive testing in many clinical settings. For the asymptomatic carotid bruit, DSA and quantitative spectral phonoangiography may provide complementary assessment. When satisfactory DSA is unobtainable, noninvasive testing will maintain its role.

With regard to existing noninvasive techniques, ultrasound imaging will undoubtedly improve, both as regards resolution and evaluation of turbulence. The marriage of various existing systems as duplex units seems likely to flourish.[13] For example, a B-scanner may be combined with a range-gated Doppler instrument in such a way that the Doppler sampling volume can be placed in any desired location within the blood vessel imaged by the B-scanner.

Several entirely new approaches are in development. Radiolabeled platelets may be imaged as they aggregate within an ulcerated plaque. The rapid evolution of nuclear magnetic resonance imaging may bring this method into clinical use for accurate evaluation of arterial anatomy.[8] Nuclear medicine may develop techniques for the detection of early atherosclerotic lesions after injection of appropriate tracers into a peripheral vein.

The future will surely bring technological advances in noninvasive testing. These may supplement advanced DSA to restrict further the indications for conventional angiography. For the present, a combination of noninvasive tests assists the neurosurgeon in decision making for a limited number of patients with cerebrovascular disease.

References

1. Ackerman RH: A perspective on noninvasive diagnosis of carotid disease. Neurology (NY) 29:615–622, 1979.
2. Chilcote WA, Modic MT, Pavlicek WA, Little JR, Furlan AJ,

Duchesneau PM, Weinstein MA: Digital subtraction angiography of the carotid arteries: A comparative study in 100 patients. Radiology 139:287–295, 1981.
3. Cooperberg PL, Robertson WD, Fry P, Sweeney V: High resolution real-time ultrasound of the carotid bifurcation. J Clin Ultrasound 7:13–17, 1979.
4. Duncan GW, Gruber JO, Dewey CF Jr, Myers GS, Lees RS: Evaluation of carotid stenosis by phonoangiography. N Engl J Med 293:1124–1128, 1975.
5. Fisher M: Occlusion of the internal carotid artery. Arch Neurol Psychiatry 65:346–377, 1951.
6. Gee W, Smith CA, Hinsen CE, Wylie EJ: Ocular pneumoplethysmography in carotid artery disease. Med Instrum 8:244–248, 1974.
7. Ginsberg MD, Greenwood SA, Goldberg HI: Noninvasive diagnosis of extracranial cerebrovascular disease: Oculoplethysmography-phonoangiography and directional Doppler ultrasonography. Neurology (NY) 29:623–631, 1979.
8. Hinshaw WS, Andrew ER, Bottomley PA, Holland GN, Moore WS: Display of cross sectional anatomy by nuclear magnetic resonance imaging. Br J Radiol 51:273–280, 1978.
9. Kartchner MM, McRae LP: Noninvasive evaluation and management of the "asymptomatic" carotid bruit. Surgery 82:840–846, 1977.
10. Kistler JP, Lees RS, Miller A, Crowell RM, Roberson G: Correlation of spectral phonoangiography and carotid angiography with gross pathology in carotid stenosis. N Engl J Med 305:417–419, 1981.
11. Müller HR: The diagnosis of internal carotid artery occlusion by directional Doppler sonography of the ophthalmic artery. Neurology (Minneap) 22:816–823, 1972.
12. Paulson OB: Ophthalmodynamometry in internal carotid artery occlusion. Stroke 7:564–566, 1976.
13. Phillips DJ, Blackshear WM Jr, Baker DW, Strandness DE Jr: Ultrasound duplex scanning in peripheral vascular disease. Radiol Nucl Med Mag 5–10, 1978.
14. Strandness DE Jr, Sumner DS: *Ultrasonic Techniques in Angiology*. Bern, Hans Huber Publishers, 1975.
15. White DN, Curry GR: Color-coded differential Doppler ultrasonic scanning system for the carotid bifurcation: Results on 486 bifurcations angiographically confirmed, in Kurjak A (ed): *Recent Advances in Ultrasound Diagnosis*. Amsterdam, Excerpta Medica, 1978, pp 239–249.

147

Radiology of Ischemic Cerebrovascular Disease

Herbert I. Goldberg

Although various noninvasive tests are presently available for evaluation of cervical carotid artery occlusive disease in patients with transient cerebral ischemia, none is fully satisfactory either alone or in combination,[4] and cerebral angiography currently remains essential for study of the extra- and intracranial circulations before surgical intervention is undertaken. The noninvasive tests are discussed in another chapter. Each has its advantages and limitations. Current opinion suggests that such tests should be used for initial evaluation of patients who are asymptomatic with a carotid bruit, patients whose symptomatology is not localized to the carotid circulation or definitive for cerebrovascular disease, and patients in whom surgery would not be considered likely because of other serious medical problems or a probable nonsurgical cause for the transient ischemic attack (TIA), such as a cardiac embolus. Cerebral angiography should be the primary and probably the only diagnostic study needed for the evaluation of patients with localizing hemispheric or ocular ischemic symptoms who are surgical candidates. It alone currently provides the most accurate and complete method for evaluating both the extracranial and intracranial vasculature. Although noninvasive tests can detect the presence of significant carotid stenosis a high percentage of the time, they have great difficulty in differentiating very high grade stenosis from complete occlusion. Calcified plaques obscure visualization of the vascular lumen with B-mode scanning and create motion artifacts from pulsations that impair evaluation with intravenous digital subtraction angiography (IV-DSA). Ultrasound tests cannot determine the status of the vertebral arteries, the origins of the common carotid arteries, the cervical segment of the internal carotid artery above the angle of the mandible, or the intracranial circulation. Knowledge of possible arterial disease in these locations is vital for proper surgical management. Although IV-DSA has the potential for full evaluation of the cervicocranial vasculature, it currently cannot adequately study the intracranial circulation[46] and has difficulty in detecting severe carotid stenosis with only minimal distal flow (carotid pseudo-occlusion) and small carotid ulcerations. In addition, upward of 20 to 25 percent of the studies are either totally unsatisfactory, of suboptimal quality, or incomplete. Poor and failed DSA examinations may result from low contrast density secondary to decreased cardiac output, subtraction artifacts related to patient motion and swallowing,[16] vertebral artery superimposition on the carotid bifurcation, or obscuration of the bifurcation from positional variations at the origins of the internal and external carotid arteries.[35]

Plain Film Studies

Although currently not widely used because of their insensitivity, plain film roentgenograms of the head and neck may provide diagnostic information noninvasively on the status of both the extra- and intracranial vascular systems. When calcification detected at the common carotid bifurcation extends 1 cm or greater in length, about one-half of these arteries will have significant stenosis (Fig. 147-1).[58] However, minimal or absent calcification is frequently associated with severe occlusive disease. The parasellar segment of the internal carotid artery may demonstrate two types of calcification. The calcification of medial necrosis (Mönckeberg's sclerosis) that is not associated with stenosis is a dense uniform band that completely encircles this segment of the carotid artery. Atherosclerotic intimal disease may cause significant carotid siphon stenosis. The calcification it produces is usually thick, irregular, and scattered along the wall of the cavernous carotid artery.[14] There appears to be an association between the thickness of this calcification and the degree of stenosis. An atherosclerotic type of calcification may occasionally be seen in the supraclinoid segment of the internal carotid artery and the proximal middle cerebral artery as well as the vertebral and basilar arteries.

Cervical spine films may be helpful in the evaluation of vertebrobasilar TIA associated with head turning or flexion and extension of the neck. Vertebral artery compression may occur during these movements from Luschka joint osteophytes or anterior projecting facet joint osteophytes.[38] Vertebral angiography with head and neck turning to the symptomatic position is needed to substantiate this cause for vertebrobasilar TIA and localize the level and side of compression.[55]

Cerebral Angiography

Preparation

Prior to angiography, the patient should have a complete medical and neurological evaluation, including an electrocardiogram. A recent myocardial infarction would contraindicate the study. The following blood tests should be obtained.

1. Complete blood count (CBC), including platelet count
2. Blood urea nitrogen (BUN)
3. Creatinine
4. Prothrombin time (PT)
5. Partial thromboplastin time (PTT)

The CBC should be checked for evidence of polycythemia or an elevated platelet count, which could increase the risk of catheter thromboembolic complications. High BUN or creatinine levels would increase the risk of renal toxicity from the radiographic contrast material, and special precautions regarding the amount utilized would need to be observed if the study was critical. Prolongation of the PT and PTT times could result in difficulty obtaining hemostasis following catheter removal and rebleeding with hematoma formation at the catheterization site during the first 8 to 10 h after the procedure.

The patient should be well hydrated for the procedure, and clear fluids encouraged orally up to the time of the study. As discomfort from the procedure is usually very minimal, strong analgesics or sedation premedication should not be given as they may potentiate cardiovascular depression. Depending on the patient's level of anxiety and age, 5 to 10 mg of diazepam PO may be given 45 min before the study. Prior to the start of the procedure an intravenous line (preferably with a small catheter) should be inserted and maintained by the administration of a 0.5 normal saline, 5% glucose solution. This serves as a route for any drug administration and to maintain hydration.

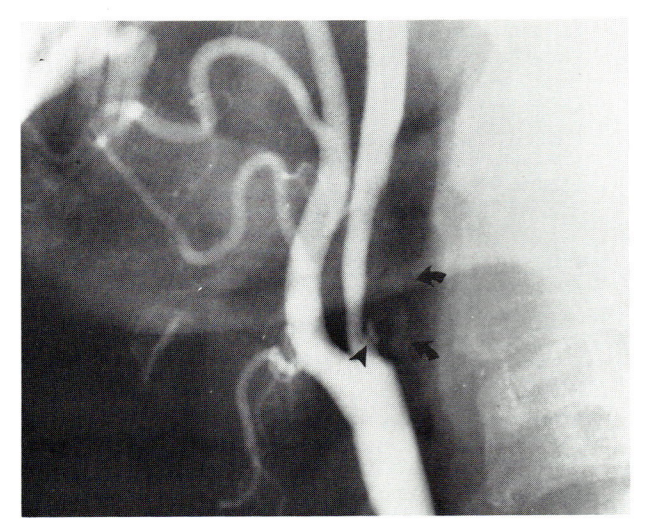

Figure 147-1 Lateral carotid angiogram reveals irregularly calcified (*arrows*) atheromatous plaque, with ulceration (*arrowhead*), at the origin of internal carotid artery. The plaque is causing significant stenosis.

Technique

Ideally the cerebral angiographic study should fully visualize with high detail the entire cervical-cranial vasculature from the aortic arch through its intracranial circulation.[11,56] Total visualization is essential since atherosclerotic disease is frequently widespread and may involve both the extracranial and intracranial arteries. The presence of a significant intracranial occlusive lesion in association with an extracranial stenosis, although not common, might dictate a change in surgical management of the patient. In addition, evaluation of the intracranial circulation occasionally reveals unsuspected nonocclusive vascular lesions, which could also alter therapy. Some, such as aneurysms, are encountered incidentally while others are disease processes that may mimic cerebral ischemic events such as subdural hematoma and tumor.

The cerebrovascular examination should not be limited to an aortic arch study. Contrast resolution is low with aortic arch injection, and even with subtraction roentgenograms there is poor visualization of the intracranial circulation and not infrequently suboptimal evaluation of the extracranial arteries.[11] Also, because of total vascular filling with aortography, imaging is impaired in many planes by superimposition of vessels. The lateral projection cannot be used, and with some oblique projections, there may be superimposition of the vertebral artery on the carotid bifurcation. The limited number of views that may be employed make it extremely difficult to achieve full visualization of the carotid bifurcation because of its frequent positional variations.[35] Subtraction film misregistration artifacts from patient motion may further degrade the images of the extracranial vessels. Ulcerations are difficult to identify, and there may be inaccuracy in the evaluation of the degree of stenosis.[11] In addition, a very high grade stenosis of the internal carotid artery may appear to represent a complete occlusion on aortic arch study.[21,62] The flow distal to a severe stenosis is very slow, and the carotid artery lumen constricts to a thin column because of the low pressure. Recognition of this "pseudo-occlusion" of the internal carotid artery requires the high contrast density obtained from selective common carotid injection, a prolonged serial filming sequence, and subtraction techniques (Fig. 147-2).

The angiographic study is best performed by percutaneous femoral artery catheterization, which permits both aortic arch and selective common carotid artery injections. If significant iliofemoral or abdominal aortic occlusive disease precludes this approach, right axillary artery catheterization can also achieve these objectives. Ordinarily the vertebral artery circulation is reviewed only on the aortic arch study unless specific symptoms dictate a more detailed examination. There is increased risk of neurological complication with direct catheterization of a diseased vertebral artery or when there is vertebrobasilar insufficiency symptoms.

The angiographic study should begin with selective visualization of the common carotid artery circulations. The common carotids are usually evaluated before the aortic arch since the arch study requires use of a no. 6 or no. 7 French catheter, and preferably a smaller no. 5 French catheter should be used for the selective common carotid injections. Bleeding would occur at the catheterization site if a smaller catheter was inserted after a larger one unless an exchange

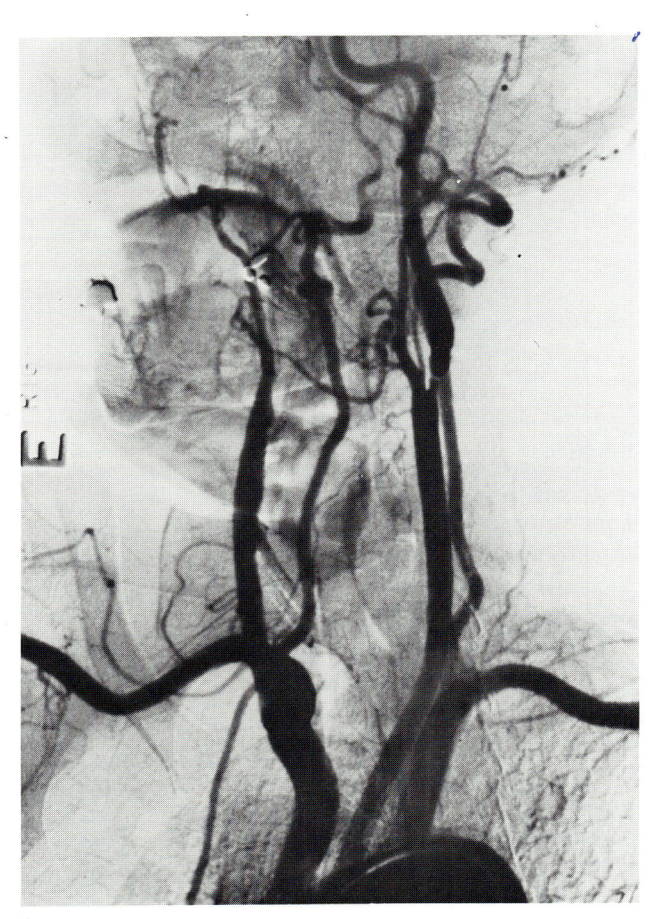

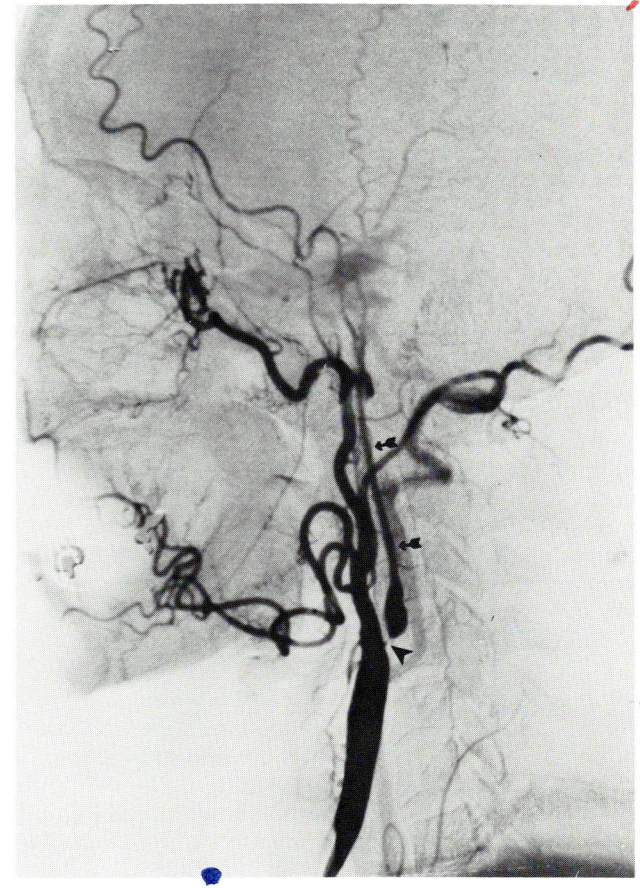

Figure 147-2 Pseudo-occlusion, right internal carotid artery. *A*. Aortic arch study, right posterior oblique view, fails to demonstrate the right internal carotid artery. *B*. Right common carotid injection reveals a severe stenosis at the origin of the right internal carotid artery (*arrowhead*), with slow flow beyond and low pressure collapse of the distal cervical segment of the internal carotid (*arrows*). A subsequent film revealed filling of the intracranial internal carotid and middle cerebral arteries.

sheath was utilized. However this in itself causes a larger hole in the artery and may result in a higher postremoval local bleeding complication rate. The incidence of neurological and local femoral artery complications are reduced with use of the smaller catheter size for selective carotid artery injections.[43] Initial visualization of the aortic arch is not necessary for successful and completely safe catheterization of the common carotid arteries.[26] The left carotid artery is ordinarily evaluated first. It has a more acute angular takeoff from the aortic arch than the right carotid artery, and this necessitates a tighter catheter curve configuration, which would be partially lost with a polyethylene catheter if the right carotid artery circulation was examined first.

Selective catheterization proceeds as follows. The position of the catheter tip is confirmed at the orifice of the left common carotid artery with a small puff of contrast material. A 0.035- to 0.038-in. flexible-tip guidewire with an 8-cm tapered mandrel is then carefully threaded up the common carotid artery. It should not be passed higher than the C5 level so as to stay below the bifurcation in most cases. Passage of the guidewire to a higher level increases the risk of dislodgement and embolization of atheroma or thrombus. It is important that the guidewire pass smoothly without any resistance so as to avoid an arterial wall dissection. With the guidewire held steady, the catheter is threaded into the common carotid artery with a twisting motion, with care not to pass it beyond the guidewire tip. The guidewire is then removed, and the catheter is flushed with heparinized saline (10 units per milliliter) after aspirating a few milliliters of blood to remove any clots that may have developed in the catheter during passage of the guidewire (when reflux of blood is likely to occur into its lumen). A 2-ml hand injection of the contrast agent is made into the common carotid artery to fluoroscopically evaluate the location of the catheter tip and flow dynamics.

Since atheromatous disease is frequently eccentrically situated on only one side of the artery lumen, it is essential that at least two views of the vessel be obtained at right angles to each other.[36,57] A significant stenosis or an ulceration could be missed or incompletely evaluated if the involved portion of the wall is not visualized tangential to the x-ray beam. All surfaces of the arterial wall are not fully visualized even with biplane projections. If there is a suspicious change on the symptomatic side at the common carotid bifurcation or if the bifurcation has not been fully profiled in two planes because of superimposition of the internal and external carotid arteries or tortuosity at the origin of the internal carotid artery, additional biplane oblique views should be obtained. These additional projections will provide more complete evaluation of the bifurcation and not infrequently will demonstrate significant disease not initially apparent.[10]

After selective study of the neck and head circulations of both common carotid arteries, the no. 5 French catheter is exchanged for a pigtail catheter with multiple side holes for the aortic arch study of the origins of the brachiocephalic vessels. We previously performed the aortic arch examination with a no. 7 French pigtail catheter utilizing an injection of 60 ml of 76% radiographic contrast material in 2 s. We now ordinarily image with a DSA system and need only inject 30 ml of a 60% contrast agent in 2 s, which can be delivered through a no. 5 French high-flow pigtail catheter to achieve excellent visualization of the origins of the brachiocephalic vessels. Not only is the amount of contrast reduced by over 50 percent, but use of this method permits the arch examination to be performed first if desired since the same size catheter is employed for both the arch and the selective carotid injections.

If difficulty is encountered in catheterizing the common carotid arteries with the no. 5 French polyethylene catheter because of an elongated aortic arch or marked tortuosity at the origins of the common carotid arteries, catheterization can usually be accomplished by using a Sims 3 sidewinder catheter. Imaging of the neck and brain vessels with a DSA system has also been useful in situations where the common carotid arteries could not be catheterized either because of technical difficulties or atheromatous disease at the carotid artery origins. Small injections with the catheter tip at or adjacent to the origins will usually result in sufficient contrast density with DSA imaging to adequately display the extra- and intracranial circulations. There is some reduction in spatial resolution with the usual 512 × 512 line DSA system compared with routine film screen angiography, and most units currently have only single-plane imaging capability. Aortic arch injections with a no. 5 French or even a no. 4 French pigtail catheter usually produce good contrast resolution of the extra- and intracranial vessels with DSA. However, vessel overlap problems and subtraction misregistration artifacts may impair consistent full evaluation with this technique.

Morbidity

There is an increased neurological complication rate from angiography, by a factor of around 4 to 1, in patients with cerebrovascular disease when compared with those not having ischemic neurological disease.[15] The overall incidence of neurological morbidity in the cerebrovascular disease group has ranged from 2.4 to 4.2 percent in several large series.[15,36,43] Permanent neurological complications occurred in from 0.15 to 0.6 percent and mortality in 0.15 to 0.5 percent of the cases. Older age, increased serum creatinine concentration, and the use of more than one catheter was found to be significantly associated with increased neurological complications in one recent series.[16]

Carotid Territory TIAs

Atherosclerotic Disease

The location and nature of the vascular disease causing both hemispheric and occular TIAs are for the most part the same. Symptoms may be either hemodynamic or embolic in origin.[2] Atherosclerotic narrowing and subintimal plaque hemorrhage are the usual cause of hemodynamic TIAs, whereas embolic TIAs develop from plaque ulceration with or without significant stenosis.[17,32,33,48] Although symptomatic vascular disease is usually located at the origin of the internal carotid artery, it may occur in any location from the origin of the common carotid artery through the intracranial branches. On occasion amaurosis fugax is caused by occlusive disease in the ophthalmic artery itself. Cardiac and aortic arch disease may also cause TIAs from emboli.

Significant inaccuracies may exist in the angiographic diagnosis of ulceration, depending on the strictness of one's criteria.[17-19] All apparent wall outpouchings are not ulcer craters. The appearance of an ulcer could be produced by the depression occurring between two adjacent atheromatous plaques or regions of plaque hemorrhage.[18,33] Ulcers that are smooth and broader on the lumen side are likely to be of such a nature. True plaque ulcerations tend to be wider on the arterial wall side (Fig. 147-1). They may also have an irregular-appearing base or are bootlike in shape with undercut edges (Fig. 147-3). Ulcers may not be imaged unless viewed tangentially.[10] Small ulcerations can be obscured by deposition of platelets or thrombus. A thrombus may occasionally be seen projecting into the arterial lumen. When it is small, a thrombus may be difficult to differentiate from a plaque. Larger thrombi have a polypoid appearance and project distally in the vessel (Fig. 147-4). Irregular-appearing plaques are probably those with superficial ulcerations.

Not infrequently the standard AP and lateral views of the head and neck do not fully profile both walls of the proximal internal carotid artery in each projection. This may occur because the course of the proximal internal carotid artery runs obliquely to one or both image planes or because of superimposition of the internal on the external carotid artery. In addition, with only biplane views a considerable portion of the lumen is not imaged tangentially even when both walls are seen on each view. Because of these factors, a

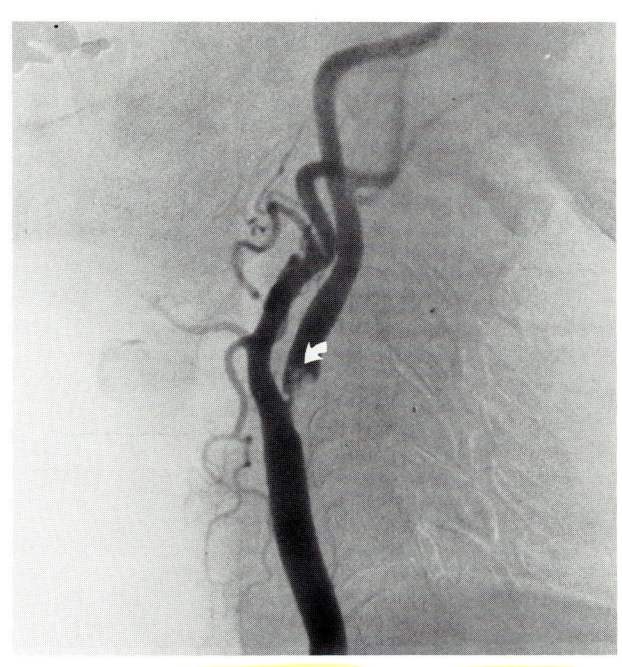

Figure 147-4 Irregular thrombus (*arrow*) extending into lumen from severely stenotic area caused by atheroma at origin of internal carotid artery.

significant stenosis or an ulceration could go undetected on one set of biplane images. Therefore, if the proximal internal carotid is poorly visualized or if a significant lesion is suspected but not clearly defined on the standard views, a second set of biplane images of the bifurcation should be obtained in the oblique projection. These additional views provide four additional tangential images of the vessel wall and frequently eliminate the visualization problems due to vessel overlap and obliquity. Also, a more reliable determination of the degree of stenosis is obtained because the initial biplane projections may not have accurately profiled the minimal residual luminal diameter since atheromatous plaques are frequently eccentrically situated in the arterial wall. Magnification and subtraction techniques further aid in detecting subtle arterial wall changes such as small ulcers and in making the measurements for determining the degree of stenosis.

There is some controversy as to the most appropriate method for evaluating the degree of stenosis in the proximal internal carotid artery. A common method is to determine the greatest percent reduction of the luminal diameter. Differences appear to exist in what measurement to take for the "normal" internal carotid artery diameter. Some have used the diameter of the carotid bulb, where the occlusive disease usually exists. Since the expected bulb diameter is frequently as much as 30 to 40 percent greater than the rest of the cervical segment of the internal carotid, which for the most part is relatively uniform in caliber throughout, a plaque narrowing the bulb diameter by this amount would in essence result in no narrowing of the bulb in relationship to the diameter of the distal cervical segment. Likewise a plaque producing a 60 to 70 percent bulb diameter stenosis,

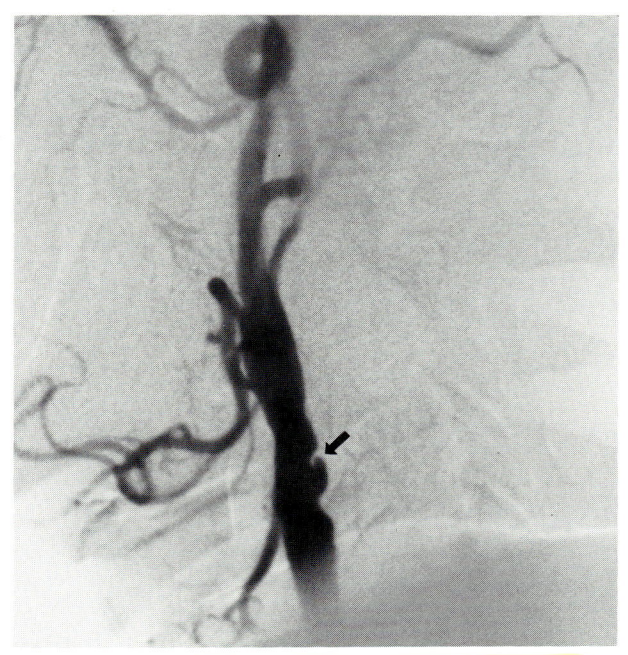

Figure 147-3 Atheromatous plaque with ulceration having an undercut edge (*arrow*) at the carotid bifurcation, as shown on a lateral carotid angiogram.

for instance, might result in only an inconsequential 30 to 40 percent stenosis in relationship to the distal cervical segment. Therefore, only the distal cervical segment diameter and not that of the bulb should be used for determining the percent stenosis of the proximal internal carotid artery.[33] Using the expected bulb diameter significantly overestimates the degree of effective carotid stenosis. In a paper using the distal internal carotid diameter as the normal reference diameter, a 60 percent stenosis was found to produce a highly consistent change in ophthalmic artery dynamics as measured by the oculoplethysmography technique.[25]

Others have suggested that the most appropriate method for evaluating the hemodynamic significance of a stenosis is determination of the minimal residual luminal diameter. A carotid artery with a residual diameter of less than 2 mm in absolute size is considered significantly stenosed.[57] In order to determine this measurement, a magnification correction factor must be employed. This varies somewhat with each study and is dependent on the radiographic technique and patient position. Since the injection catheter is usually visible along with the stenosis, the catheter's known outer diameter can be used for determination of the correction factor.

Another method for evaluating the significance of a carotid stenosis is to compare the circulatory dynamics of the internal and external carotid arteries. Normally the intracranial internal carotid branches in the high convexity region fill about 1 s before the filling of the superficial temporal artery branches over the same region of the head. If the external carotid artery terminal branches fill before or even simultaneously with the filling of the intracranial convexity arteries, an internal carotid artery stenosis should be considered hemodynamically significant. In order to utilize this evaluation, the external carotid artery must not have a significant stenosis.

Fibromuscular Dysplasia (FMD)

Internal carotid artery fibromuscular dysplasia is a condition predominantly affecting women of middle age. The disease, although usually asymptomatic, may cause ischemic symptoms. Symptoms result from FMD producing either a significant stenosis or a dissecting aneurysm.[24] Both are rare. Dissecting aneurysm may cause symptoms from increased luminal narrowing, occlusion, or emboli; the latter is a frequent occurrence with dissections.

FMD in the internal carotid artery develops in its mid- and upper cervical segments, usually around the C2 level, and frequently extends for several centimeters along the vessel, although it may be more focal.[30,32] It just about always spares the first few centimeters above the bifurcation. Carotid involvement is bilateral about 75 percent of the time, and the vertebral artery is simultaneously affected in about 15 percent of the cases.[31] The characteristic appearance of FMD is that of a "string of beads" configuration with an irregular wall (Fig. 147-5). There are alternating zones of ring-like luminal constriction with 3- to 7-mm-long segments of widening where the vessel caliber is commonly slightly larger than normal. Only rarely do the zones of constriction produce a significant stenosis. Most of the time the narrowings cause about a 40 percent or less diameter stenosis. Oc-

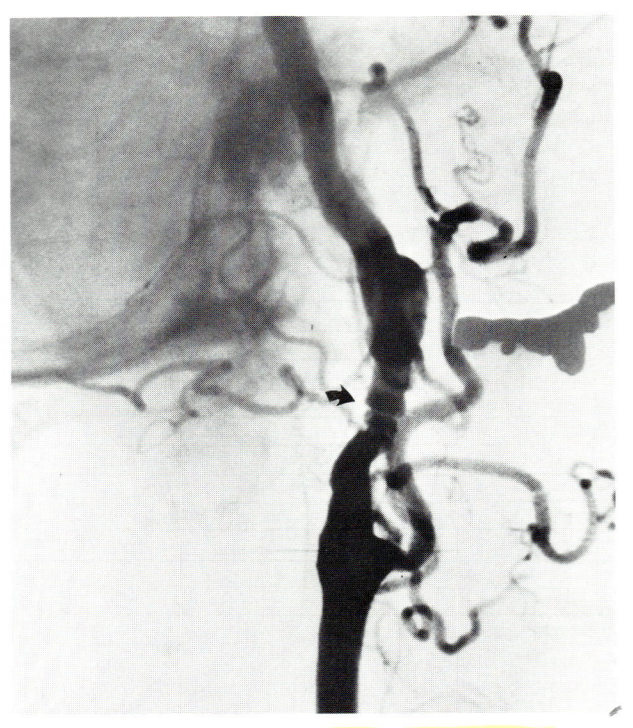

Figure 147-5 Fibromuscular dysplasia of the internal carotid artery in its midcervical segment, demonstrating the typical "string of beads" appearance (*arrow*).

casionally FMD appears atypically as a long or short segment of diffuse narrowing involving one or both walls. When one wall is narrowed or normal, the opposite wall may show ovoid dilatation. The proximal and distal ends of this lesion may reveal tubular constriction.

Dissecting Aneurysm

Dissecting aneurysm of the internal carotid artery may develop from penetrating or blunt trauma to the neck, spontaneous or forced rapid neck rotation causing carotid artery impingement on the C1 transverse process, fibromuscular dysplasia, congenital aneurysm, atheromatous plaque ulceration, or from unknown cause. The dissection may begin at or near the origin of the internal carotid artery, but more frequently it starts in the mid- and upper cervical portion. The internal carotid artery will usually demonstrate a tapered narrowing extending to the skull base or beyond, producing the so-called string sign (Fig. 147-6). The narrowing may begin and remain along one wall of the artery, giving a flattened ribbon-like appearance, but usually it extends around the entire vessel circumference more distally. The stenosis may not be uniform throughout. The luminal surface is usually smooth, but occasionally there is beading either as a result of infolding of the intima or fibromuscular dysplasia. The lumen of the dissection rarely opacifies. It may become evident if the dissection re-enters the lumen more distally. Occasionally a small subintimal contrast collection is present at the origin of the dissection.

Dissecting internal carotid aneurysm may cause cerebral ischemia by decreasing blood flow from the stenosis it pro-

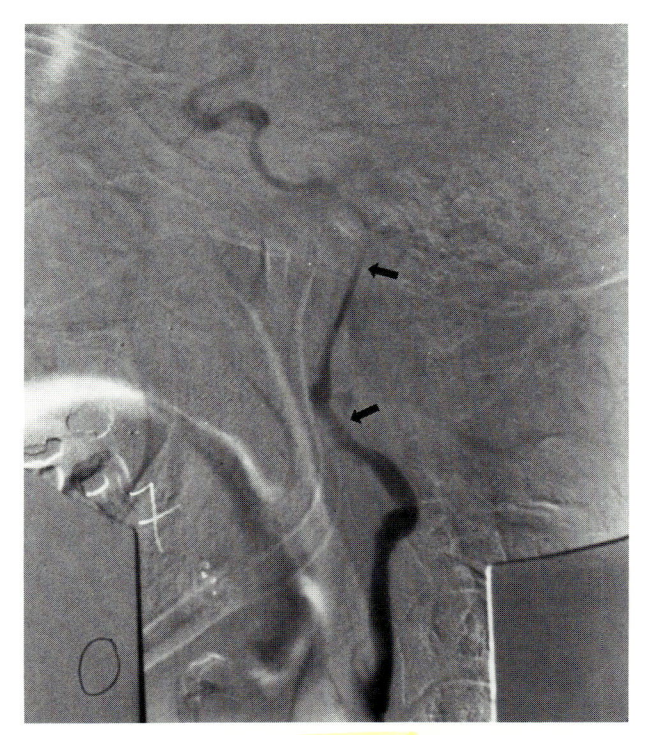

Radiology of Ischemic Cerebrovascular Disease

Figure 147-6 Dissecting aneurysm of the mid and upper cervical segments of the internal carotid artery. A lateral angiogram reveals irregular ribbon-like narrowing of the upper half of the cervical internal carotid segment (*arrows*).

duces, but probably more commonly symptoms are due to emboli developing on the exposed intima and media.[45]

The arteriographic abnormalities will frequently have completely resolved on follow-up study performed 6 to 8 weeks after the institution of conservative management with anticoagulation. Occasionally an aneurysm develops or there is a variable degree of persisting stenosis.

Takayasu's Arteritis

This condition is a panarteritis affecting mainly young women that involves the large arteries arising from the aorta, particularly the brachiocephalic and upper limb branches. There is progressive arterial narrowing secondary to round cell infiltration of the adventitia. Generalized constitutional symptoms may be present, including fever and myalgias. Pulse and blood pressure are usually decreased in the upper extremities and occasionally in the lower.

Radiologically, plain x-ray films may demonstrate calcification of the aortic arch and at the origins of the brachiocephalic branches. Aortic arch angiography usually demonstrates fusiform narrowing at the origins of the cerebral and limb arteries that extends for a variable distance along their length. The degree of narrowing is not uniform for all the vessels, and there may be complete occlusion. Atherosclerotic disease may also cause narrowing and occlusion at the origins of the brachiocephalic vessels; however, it has a more irregular contour than Takayasu's arteritis and occurs in an older age group. In Takayasu's disease, fusiform aneurysmal dilatation may develop in the aortic arch or at the origins of

its branches. This occurs when the disease involves the internal elastic lamina and is associated with atrophy of the media.

Arterial Kinking

The internal carotid artery may normally demonstrate considerable looping and tortuosity that does not cause any reduction in blood flow. In older patients with atherosclerotic disease, however, elongation of the internal carotid can result in acute bending with a kink stenosis. The kink frequently occurs about 3 to 5 cm beyond the origin of the internal carotid artery (Fig. 147-7). Significant narrowing may occasionally be caused by a kink, giving rise to clinical symptoms. Certain head and neck positions may increase the kink, resulting in intermittent flow reduction.

Embolic Disease

Emboli from the heart are a not infrequent cause for TIAs. They may develop from a mural thrombus in the left ventricle resulting from recent myocardial infarction or endocarditis, a thrombus in the left atrium occurring with fibrillation, a left atrial myxoma, an acute or subacute valvulitis, or a mitral valve prolapse. Cardiac septal defects and a patent foramen ovale may lead to paradoxical emboli from the venous system.

Cerebral emboli from atherosclerotic disease in the common and internal carotid arteries probably account for the majority of TIAs and strokes.[2,52] Emboli may develop from nonstenotic atheromata, particularly in the presence of plaque ulceration.[18] They may also occur at the time of carotid occlusion[20,51] and occasionally from the internal ca-

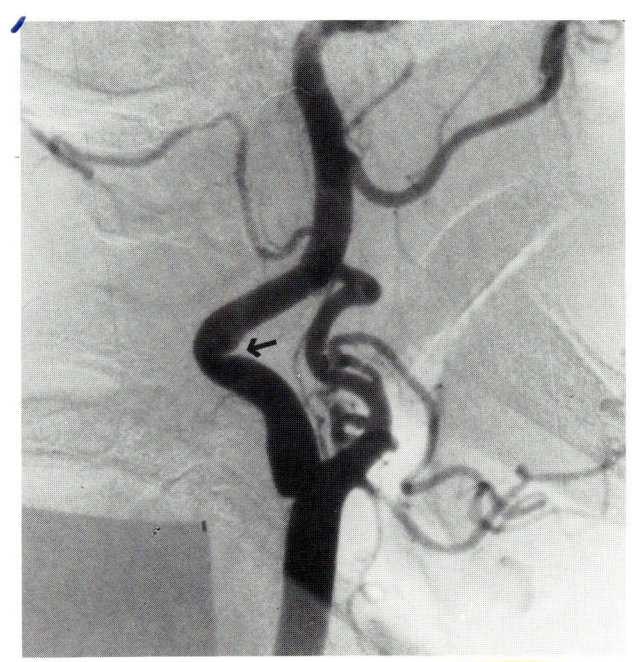

Figure 147-7 Kinking of the internal carotid artery. Nonhemodynamic web narrowing (*arrow*) from acute bending in the midcervical portion.

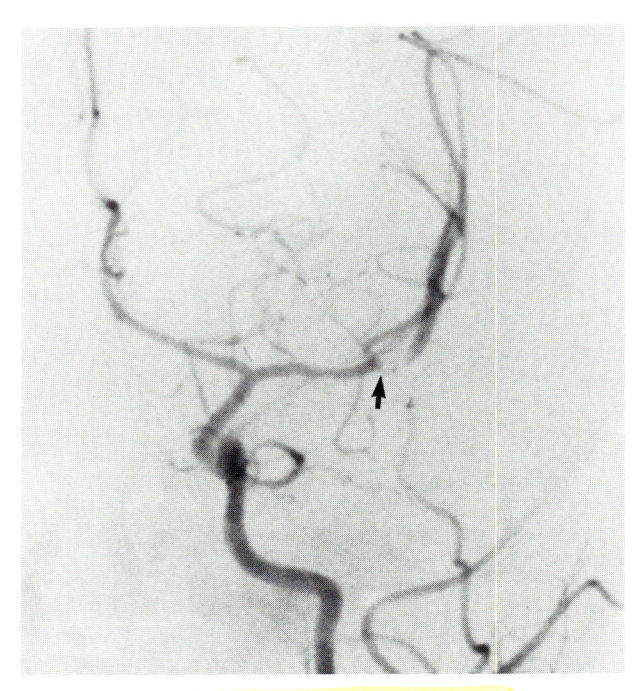

Figure 147-8 Middle cerebral artery embolus. Anteroposterior carotid angiogram showing meniscus-like proximal margin of embolus (*arrow*) at middle cerebral artery trifurcation. Embolus does not completely occlude the lumen and its intraluminal filling defect can be seen to extend 1 cm distally.

rotid stump[3] or from external carotid atherosclerosis following internal carotid artery occlusion.[5] Thrombus formation may occasionally be identified at the carotid bifurcation (Fig. 147-4). Emboli produce a characteristic appearance in both the large and small arteries. They tend to lodge at vessel bifurcations, producing a saddle-like filling defect within the lumen. One of the branches may be completely occluded by the embolus, or they both may be partially patent. Occasionally the embolus will extend fully into only one branch, producing a meniscus-like obstruction (Fig. 147-8). The proximal stump of the artery will be fully patent. Embolic occlusions usually undergo fragmentation and lysis, with the smaller residual portions then flowing distally to occlude more peripheral branches. Complete fragmentation and lysis may occur in less than 1 day for a small embolus or take several days for larger emboli. If angiography is performed 3 or more days after the initial ischemic event, the study could be normal or could reveal one or more small peripheral branch occlusions or occlusion of a larger proximal trunk. Occasionally angiography at an even later time may reveal an embolic fragment that is organized, partially or completely occluding a proximal or distal branch.

Large cardiac emboli will frequently initially lodge extracranially at the common carotid bifurcation. Mild ischemic symptoms may develop at this stage, with more severe symptoms developing several days later after passage of the partially lysed embolus into intracranial branches. Most emboli that enter the internal carotid artery will flow into the middle cerebral artery.

If no embolus is identified at angiography because of early lysis, secondary hemodynamic effects reflecting the prior ischemic insult may still be evident. The ischemic injury causes a variable degree of loss of autoregulation in the territory of the artery for several days to weeks. Angiographically this is revealed as an arteriolar-capillary vascular blush usually confined to the cerebral cortex, producing a gyriform appearance. The vascular blush becomes evident in the late arterial phase and is associated with early filling of local cortical veins (Fig. 147-9). This hyperemic reaction has been termed *luxury perfusion* by Lassen.[40] It may also develop in the basal ganglia region with the shunting of contrast material into the internal cerebral vein or basal vein of Rosenthal.

Vertebrobasilar TIAs

In the evaluation of transient ischemia in the vertebralbasilar territory it is usually safer to study this circulation without directly catheterizing the vertebral arteries. The origin of the vertebral artery is a frequent location for occlusive vascular disease, and direct catheterization carries a much higher risk for an angiographic complication. This might occur from dislodging of atheromatous debris or from plugging of an already stenosed lumen by the catheter. A recent vertebrobasilar TIA or a brain stem or cerebellar infarct within the past 2 to 3 months also increases the risk of neurological worsening because of the greater toxic effect of the contrast material on a disturbed blood-brain barrier. When flow is reduced by the catheter in the vertebral artery, contrast toxicity is increased. Therefore, it is usually best to evaluate the vertebrobasilar circulation indirectly.

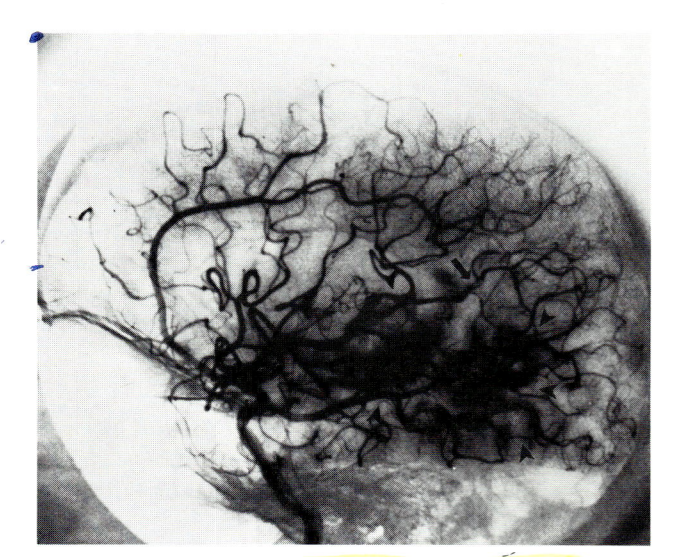

Figure 147-9 Postembolic "luxury perfusion" hyperemia, shown on a lateral carotid angiogram. There is a diffuse gyriform blush in the temporoparietal region in the midarterial phase (*arrowheads*). Subsequent films revealed early venous filling from this region. A small residual embolic clot is present in a parietal middle cerebral artery branch (*arrow*).

An aortic arch study with both oblique projections may adequately show the origins and cervical portions of both vertebral arteries. Visualization, however, is not infrequently suboptimal by this method because of poor contrast density, vessel overlap, and patient motion. A more detailed, successful, and relatively safe method for study of the vertebral circulation is by making the contrast injection into the subclavian artery at or near the origin of the vertebral artery. This may be accomplished via femoral or axillary artery catheterization or by a retrograde brachial artery injection. With catheterization, injections of 15 ml of 60% contrast material at the rate of 7 to 10 ml/s with blood pressure cuff occlusion of the brachial artery runoff will provide high contrast visualization of the vertebral artery and its intracranial circulation. Basilar artery imaging will be less optimal because of a variable degree of dilution from the unopacified contralateral vertebral artery. The amount of dilution will depend on the relative size of the vertebral arteries and the presence or absence of occlusive disease in one or the other artery. The two vertebral arteries are normally not of equal caliber, with the left being larger in the majority of cases. Occasionally, one of the vertebral arteries is very small with none of its circulation entering the basilar artery. If normal, however, it will supply the ipsilateral posterior inferior cerebellar artery. If full and detailed visualization of the basilar artery circulation is required for important clinical considerations and this is not accomplished by indirect vertebral artery opacification, then simultaneous high contrast opacification of both subclavian arteries might be considered by catheter and retrograde brachial techniques if direct catheterization of the vertebral artery appears contraindicated or very risky.

The retrograde brachial method for vertebral artery opacification is accomplished by countercurrent injection into the brachial artery utilizing an 18-gauge thin-walled needle or short Teflon cannula. Use of flow rates of 20 to 25 ml/s for a total of 45 ml of contrast results in excellent opacification of the vertebral artery circulation. In about 6 percent of individuals, the left vertebral artery arises directly from the aortic arch. In this situation, subclavian artery injection will not demonstrate the left vertebral artery. A diagnosis of vertebral artery occlusion should not be made unless a residual stump is identified at its origin or there is collateral filling of its cervical or intracranial segment. This distal reconstitution may arise from ascending cervical branches of the subclavian artery, the occipital branch of the external carotid artery, or the contralateral vertebral artery at its junction with the basilar artery.

All the same conditions that may cause carotid artery TIAs can be etiologic for vertebrobasilar TIAs. Probably the most frequent cause for nonfocal vertebrobasilar TIAs is hemodynamic fluctuation brought about by cardiac and vasomotor alterations. Vertebral artery circulation might also be compromised by intermittent artery compression from osteophytes originating at the Luschka and articular facet joints of the cervical vertebrae during head and neck turning.[38,55] These osteophytes compress the vertebral artery in its transverse foramen. A vertebral artery might also be significantly narrowed or occluded by compression from a normal C1–2 articulation during lateral neck rotation to the opposite side.[8] Vertebrobasilar ischemia will not develop unless the other vertebral artery is congenitally small or has a significant stenosis. Rarely an embolic stroke might develop because of thrombus formation from prolonged asymptomatic stagnation of vertebral artery flow as a result of head turning.[27] To evaluate if neck turning compromises vertebral artery flow, aortic arch or subclavian artery angiography should study vertebral artery circulation with the head and neck in both neutral and rotated positions.

Computed Tomography of Cerebral Infarction

Computed tomography (CT) is the most accurate method of identifying and localizing cerebral infarctions. The CT scan has been reported to be positive in from 66 to 98 percent of cerebral infarcts.[6,9,34] The percentage of positive cases increases when serial CT scans are obtained and intravenous contrast material is given.

The CT scan is usually normal in patients having TIAs. Several reports, however, have noted infarction in up to 20 percent of patients having only a history of TIAs.[9,39] These infarcts no doubt are related to small vaso-occlusive events in relatively silent areas of the brain. It is therefore prudent in the overall evaluation of TIA patients to obtain a CT scan to determine if old or recent cerebral infarction has occurred. In addition, the CT scan will demonstrate nonvascular lesions that may occasionally clinically simulate ischemic events. These include subdural hematoma and primary and metastatic brain tumors.

The CT appearance of cerebral infarctions may be very different at different times depending on the temporal relationship of the scan to the ischemic event, and its etiology, severity, size, and location. When evaluating a CT scan for possible ischemic alterations, all of these factors must be considered in the interpretation. The administration of intravenous contrast material may permit the detection of up to 13 percent of infarcts that reveal no abnormality on noncontrast scans.[44,59] In addition, contrast enhanced scans frequently help in evaluating the nature of the underlying vascular event causing the infarction. The temporal evolution of the CT alterations on plain and enhanced scans during the first 2 to 3 weeks frequently permits differentiation of infarction caused by embolic or primary cerebrovascular occlusive disease.

There are five main types of vaso-occlusive hemodynamic events that may occur with cerebral ischemic episodes. These are:

1. Permanent complete obstruction of anterograde flow into a large cerebral territory usually caused by atherosclerotic occlusion
2. Temporary complete blockage of anterograde circulation to a major cerebral territory usually caused by an embolus
3. Temporary reduction of anterograde flow to a hemisphere or to the whole brain
4. Permanent reduction in anterograde circulation to one cerebral hemisphere

5. Permanent complete occlusion of a penetrating cerebral arteriole

Each variety may reveal a relatively distinctive CT appearance.

Permanent Complete Obstruction of Anterograde Flow into a Large Cerebral Territory (Type 1)

Permanent occlusion of major intracranial branches usually results from atherosclerotic disease. Diabetes and hypertension predispose to this variety of occlusive disease. The infarction that frequently occurs has a typical CT evolution.

Depending on the severity and size of the ischemic insult, the CT may reveal changes as early as 6 to 8 h following the onset of symptoms.[34,59] The earliest changes consist of slight brain swelling evidenced by obliteration of sulci and cisterns in the infarct territory and a slight reduction in the size of the ipsilateral ventricle. A poorly marginated inhomogeneous region of mild hypodensity involving the cortex and underlying white matter may or may not be evident (Fig. 147-10). By 24 h the cortical and white matter hypodensity becomes more distinct, homogeneous, and sharply marginated. It assumes either a triangular or rectangular configuration extending from the brain surface down to the ventricular margin. The brain hypodensity is sharply confined within one vascular territory (Fig. 147-11). When the proximal middle cerebral artery trunk is occluded, the hypodensity will involve a large portion of the basal ganglia and internal capsule region that are supplied by the lenticulostriate branches arising from this segment of the middle cerebral artery. The degree of hemispheric infarction depends on the immediate adequacy of pial collateral circulation. More distal middle cerebral occlusion will spare the basal ganglia–capsular region.

The infarct hypodensity remains sharply confined to the involved vascular territory since it results mainly from tissue necrosis with intracellular (cytotoxic) edema.[1] This appears different from edema occurring with a brain tumor or abscess that is poorly marginated, has a pseudopod appearance, involves mainly white matter and spares the gray matter, and extends across vascular boundaries. Tumor edema is caused by disruption of the blood-brain barrier with leakage of protein and fluid from capillaries into the extracellular space. It is referred to as *vasogenic edema*.[37] Although the capillaries within the infarct may lose the integrity of their blood-brain barrier after 24 h, the vasogenic edema pattern does not develop. This is probably related to the markedly decreased blood flow and perfusion pressure within the infarcted tissue, which inhibits significant leakage of protein from the capillaries. If blood flow increases somewhat, capillary leakage will become evident at a certain critical level, which may be around 17 to 20 ml/100 g per minute.[54] Be-

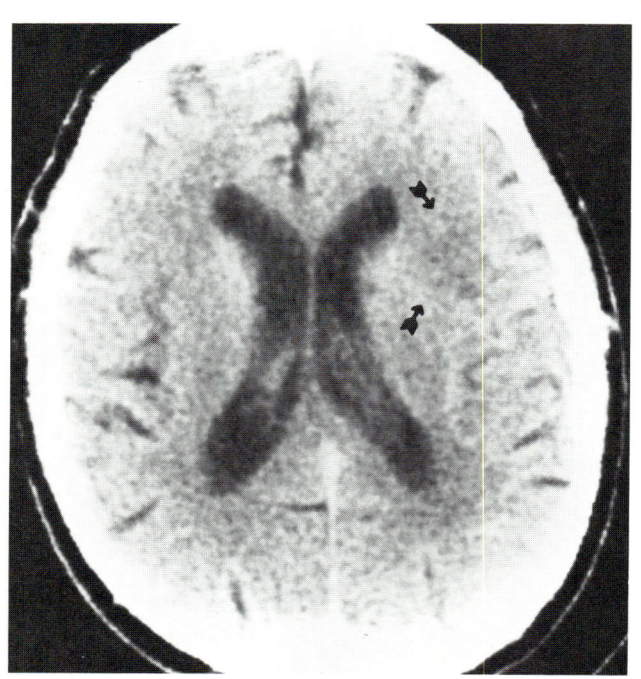

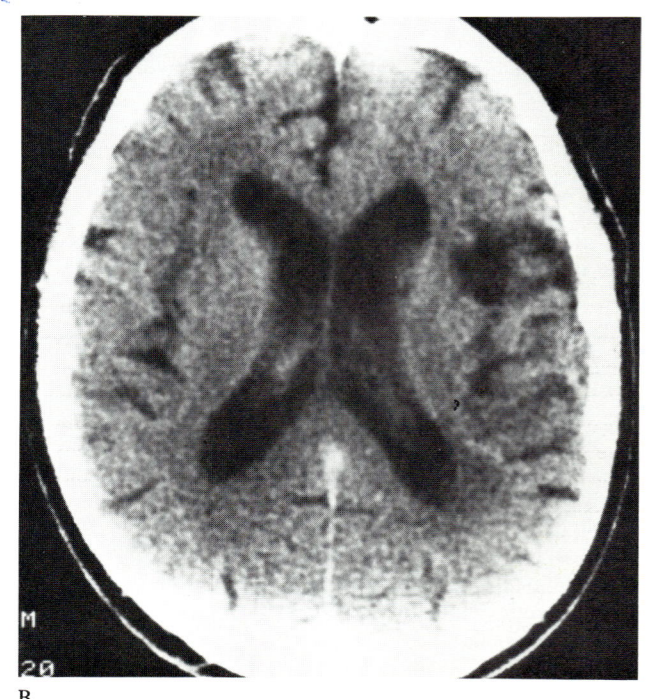

Figure 147-10 CT evolution of middle cerebral artery infarct. *A*. Early changes (about 15 h) include a mild ill-defined hypodensity in left posterior frontal region (*arrows*) with partial effacement of sylvian cistern and regional sulci (compare with contralateral hemisphere). *B*. Chronic changes at 9 months. Note the well-defined hypodensity close to that of CSF in same posterior frontal region, also involving the overlying cortex. The sylvian cistern and sulci in the region are prominent.

Radiology of Ischemic Cerebrovascular Disease

tween the third and fifth day, cytotoxic edema is most marked and the infarct hypodensity becomes very clearly defined and homogeneous. Local brain swelling is maximum at this time, and depending on the size of the infarct, a slight or considerable degree of ventricular compression and midline shift may be present. Large infarcts may cause massive midline displacement and transtentorial herniation.[49] The intravenous administration of a contrast agent will usually not demonstrate any uptake in the infarct at this time. After the first week, brain swelling begins to diminish and will usually be completely resolved by 14 to 21 days.

Cortical hypodensity frequently disappears around day 14, becoming isodense with adjacent normal cortex (Fig. 147-12). This results from a rich neovascular capillary ingrowth and improved collateral circulation. The increased blood volume in the involved cortex related to the above factors accounts for the development of the higher cortical density. Similarly, infarct hypodensity in the basal ganglia may clear at this time. The cortical hyperemia causes the margins of the infarct to become less sharply defined. Little increase in density occurs in the white matter region of the infarct. White matter hypodensity may even increase at this time because of the presence of abundant fat-laden phagocytic cells.

Contrast Enhancement

Contrast enhancement usually first appears around days 10 to 14 of the infarct. It reaches its maximum intensity during the third and fourth weeks, after which it declines.[34] Enhancement generally continues to the sixth or seventh week. With large infarcts it has been reported to persist for up to 12 weeks and rarely for a longer period of time. Upward of 88 percent of infarcts evaluated between the second and fourth week will reveal contrast enhancement.[41,50] Enhancement develops primarily within the cortical and deep gray matter region of the infarct. It occurs principally as a result of a defective blood-brain barrier in the neocapillaries growing into the infarct and in any persisting original capillaries and because of improved collateral circulation. Contrast material leaves the altered capillaries to enter the extracellular space. Even though enhancement reflects a blood-brain barrier abnormality, a typical tumor-like vasogenic edema pattern does not develop. This may be related to persisting low perfusion pressure, which limits edema formation. Very little of the contrast enhancement is due to the increased tissue blood volume. White matter regions do not usually demonstrate contrast enhancement at standard dosage of 28 to 42 g.

The enhancement of the cortex appears as a ribbon-like or gyriform pattern (Fig. 147-12B) that may have a heterogeneous or homogeneous appearance. A basal ganglia infarct will also demonstrate enhancement. Its pattern may be either uniform, heterogeneous, or ring-like in character (Fig. 147-13). Ring enhancement develops because of neovascularization of the ganglionic gray matter surrounding a central necrotic region. The ring enhancement pattern occurs commonly with infarcts in the basal ganglia since the supplying lenticulostriate arteries are essentially end arteries and their occlusion not infrequently results in central necrosis. Neovascularization with its contrast enhancement de-

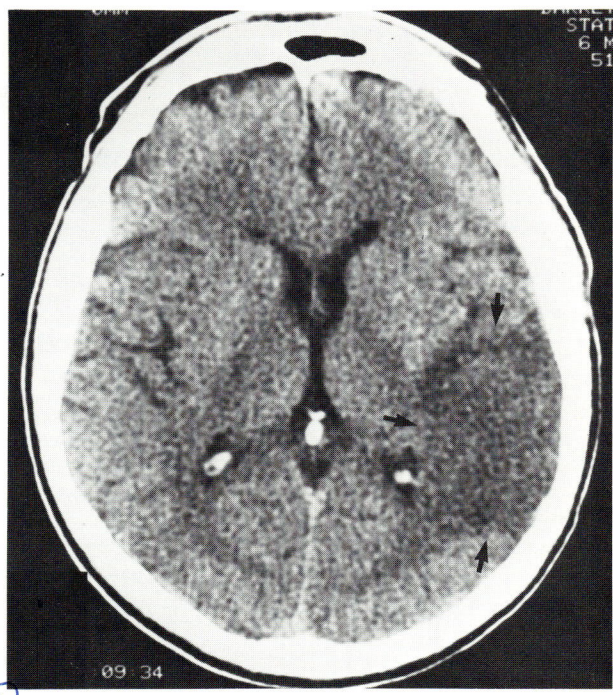

Figure 147-11 Middle cerebral territory infarct at about 36 h. Well-defined rectangular hypodensity involves the cortex and underlying white matter and extends down to the ventricular margin. Hypodensity is restricted to the destribution of the posterior temporal artery branch of the middle cerebral artery (*arrows*). There is effacement of the regional sulci and slight medial displacement of the atrium.

velops in the non-necrotic gray matter that surrounds the centrally necrotic portion of the infarction. True ring enhancement rarely occurs with convexity infarcts since the deep margin is necrotic white matter, which is very avascular and appears not capable of developing a prominent neovascular capsule. However, a pseudo enhancing ring is occasionally seen with certain patterns of cortical enhancement and is usually related to the CT section cutting across the deep extensions of adjacent enhancing gyri.

After 4 weeks, the infarct again becomes more sharply outlined and more uniformly hypodense as the isodense enhancing cortical bands begin to revert back to low density regions because of the resolution of the neovascular capillary hyperemia. The evolution of the pathological absorptive-reparative process is usually complete by the end of the third month, at which time the infarct consists of a cystic cavitation with gliotic bands. The density of the infarct at this time approaches that of the cerebrospinal fluid, and there is a contraction of the infarct volume. The portion of the lateral ventricle adjacent to the infarct dilates, and there may be a mild to moderate midline shift of the brain toward the infarct (Fig. 147-10). The CSF spaces over the infarction may dilate as a result of atrophy and necrosis of the cortex. Focal enlargement of sulci may be the only residual CT alteration with some varieties of infarcts that affect mainly the cerebral cortex. (See section on hemodynamic infarcts.)

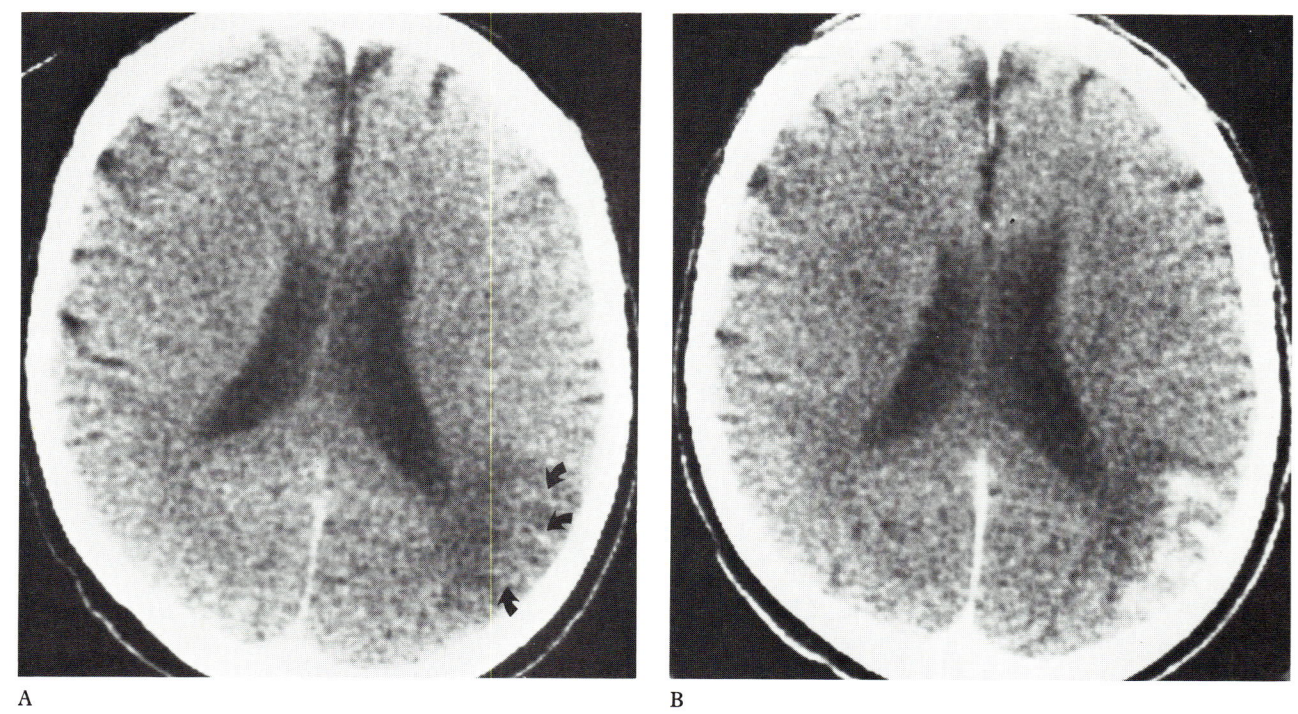

Figure 147-12 Middle cerebral territory infarct at 2 weeks. *A.* Noncontrast CT scan demonstrates isodense bands extending centrally from the surface into the underlying hypodensity to about the depth of the convolutions (*arrows*). *B.* Contrast-enhanced CT scan at same time as *A.* Enhancement of the isodense bands identified in *A* produces a gyriform pattern.

Embolic Infarcts (Type 2)

The incidence of embolic infarction is probably considerably higher than the 8 to 10 percent given by some clinical studies. A recent study that included four-vessel cerebral angiography, CT, and CSF examination reported a 31 percent incidence of embolic infarcts.[47] An autopsy study found that 68 percent of middle cerebral artery territory strokes were embolic in origin.[42]

Occasionally, the embolus may be directly identified on the unenhanced CT scan. Atheromatous emboli are frequently calcified and may be identified as a very high density nodule along the course of the anterior and middle cerebral arteries.[61] Pure thrombus emboli may also be identified within the intracranial arteries.[22] Fresh thrombus is slightly higher in density than flowing blood, and may occasionally be identified in large arterial trunks by comparison of the density of similar arteries on each side (Fig. 147-14). Visualization of a clot embolus may only be possible for a very short period of time (?1 to 5 days) after the infarct because of its early fragmentation, lysis, and distal migration. In addition, the breakdown of the hemoglobin molecule in the clot, which may occur in a few days, reduces its density.

The initial CT parenchymal alterations of embolic infarction are identical to those occurring with atherosclerotic occlusion infarction. With a cardiac source for the embolus, there may be multiple infarcts that are relatively close in age involving different vascular territories on the same or opposite sides of the brain.

After the usual dissolution of the embolus between 1 and 5 days after the stroke, anterograde flows return to the infarct territory. This circulatory change alters the usual evolution of the CT alterations observed with type 1 atherosclerotic occlusive infarcts. As the arterioles in the infarct territory have loss of their normal autoregulation ability and also because of vasomotor paralysis, the return of a high perfusion pressure and flow at this early stage leads to hyperemia[12] and a luxury perfusion[40] reaction localized mainly to infarcted gray matter. In addition, these hemodynamic alterations cause CT changes related to breakdown of the blood-brain barrier. The hyperemia results in increased CT density in the cortex and the basal ganglia. These areas become isodense or hyperdense in comparison to normal gray matter (Fig. 147-15). The density increase is mainly due to a larger blood pool in dilated capillaries resulting from the hemodynamic and autoregulatory changes. It may also be partly the result of some petechial hemorrhage in these tissues.[34] A more marked increase (>10 HU) above the normal cortical density would indicate the development of a frank hemorrhagic infarct (Fig. 147-16). Hemorrhagic infarction is usually the result of an embolus[28] after reperfusion occurs, and it may develop if reperfusion pressure becomes very high, when there is extensive infarct necrosis, or when blood coagulation is altered. When the gray matter hemorrhage is

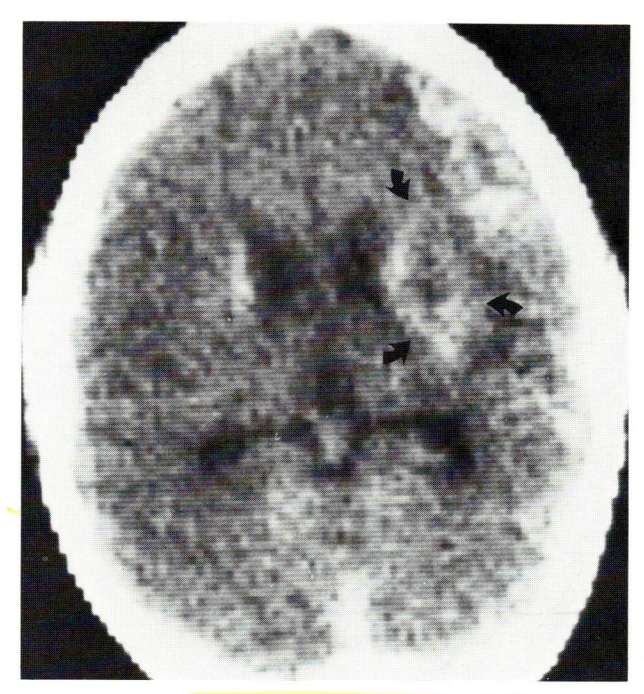

Figure 147-13 Ring enhancement of a basal ganglia infarct 3 weeks following middle cerebral artery embolic occlusion. Peripheral enhancement is present, surrounding a central low density necrotic region in the lateral basal ganglia region (*arrows*). Gyriform lateral frontal lobe enhancement is also evident on the same side, reflecting the distal middle cerebral territory infarct.

severe, it may extend into the white matter, making the hemorrhagic infarct appear very similar to an intracerebral hematoma.

The white matter hypodensity may become more marked and enlarge following clot lysis. This may be associated with clinical worsening related to the increased edema and mass effect. The new edema is now vasogenic in origin. It develops because with clot lysis there is considerable elevation of perfusion pressure, which in association with the blood-brain barrier loss causes increased capillary leakage of protein and fluid.

For reasons similar to the increased edema formation, contrast enhancement develops at this time and occurs predominantly in the involved gray matter (Fig. 147-15). Very little of the enhancement is secondary to the hyperemia by itself.[23] Enhancement also occurs with hemorrhagic infarction. High-dose (80 mg) contrast administration may demonstrate, on 2-h delayed scans, enhancement occurring also in the white matter. This may indicate the imminent development of a hemorrhagic infarction.[29]

Hemodynamic and Watershed Infarcts (Types 3 and 4)

Hemodynamic infarcts occur from a temporary decrease in cerebral blood flow caused mainly by an alteration in general circulatory dynamics. Generalized or focal symptoms may develop. Those individuals who develop focal symptoms usually have a pre-existing arterial stenosis or occlusion in the affected territory that may have been silent at their usual blood pressure.[60] Autoregulation may have been significantly altered by pre-existing arterial occlusive disease such that even a mild decrease in blood pressure could reduce cerebral blood flow in a region below the critical level needed for maintenance of brain tissue viability. Hypertension predisposes to hemodynamic ischemia, which might result from cardiac arrhythmias or prolonged blood pressure depression caused by certain medications or a marked diurnal depression occurring usually during the night.

Hemodynamic infarcts affect mainly the watershed or border zone territories of the cerebral circulation. These are located at the junctional regions between the anterior, middle, and posterior cerebral artery circulations.[7] Another border zone is in the deep white matter adjacent to the outer superior margin of the lateral ventricle and is the terminal zone of circulation for the penetrating arteries from the three main arterial trunks.[13] The cortical gray matter in the watershed region appears to be affected more severely with temporary hemodynamic alterations than the white matter. Conversely, with chronic ischemia the white matter, particularly in the periventricular watershed, may be the principal area affected (Fig. 147-17). The white matter may also be involved along with cortical zones when temporary hemodynamic ischemia is more severe or occurs in the presence of chronic hemispheric ischemia (Fig. 147-18). This may occur in individuals with long-standing carotid artery occlusion

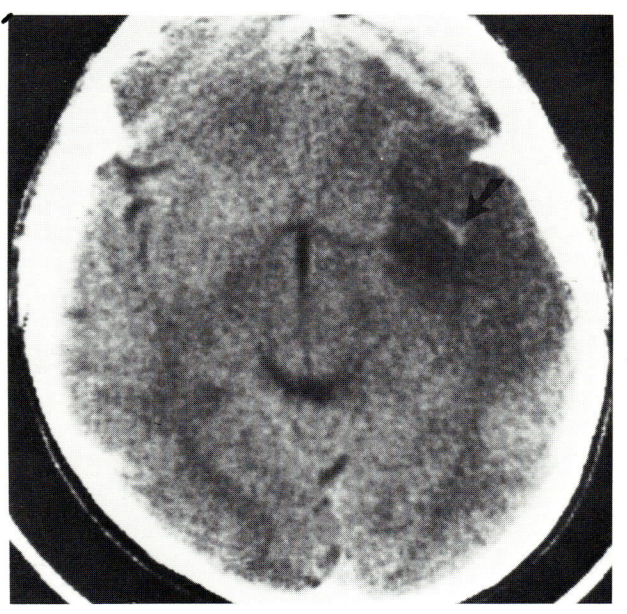

Figure 147-14 Hyperdense middle cerebral artery embolus, as shown by curvilinear hyperdensity in region of middle cerebral artery trifurcation (*arrow*). The adjacent superior section demonstrated peripheral extension of the linear hyperdensity along the course of the insular segment of the middle cerebral artery. The embolus is surrounded by a large acute infarct hypodensity involving the temporal and posterior frontal territory of the occluded middle cerebral artery.

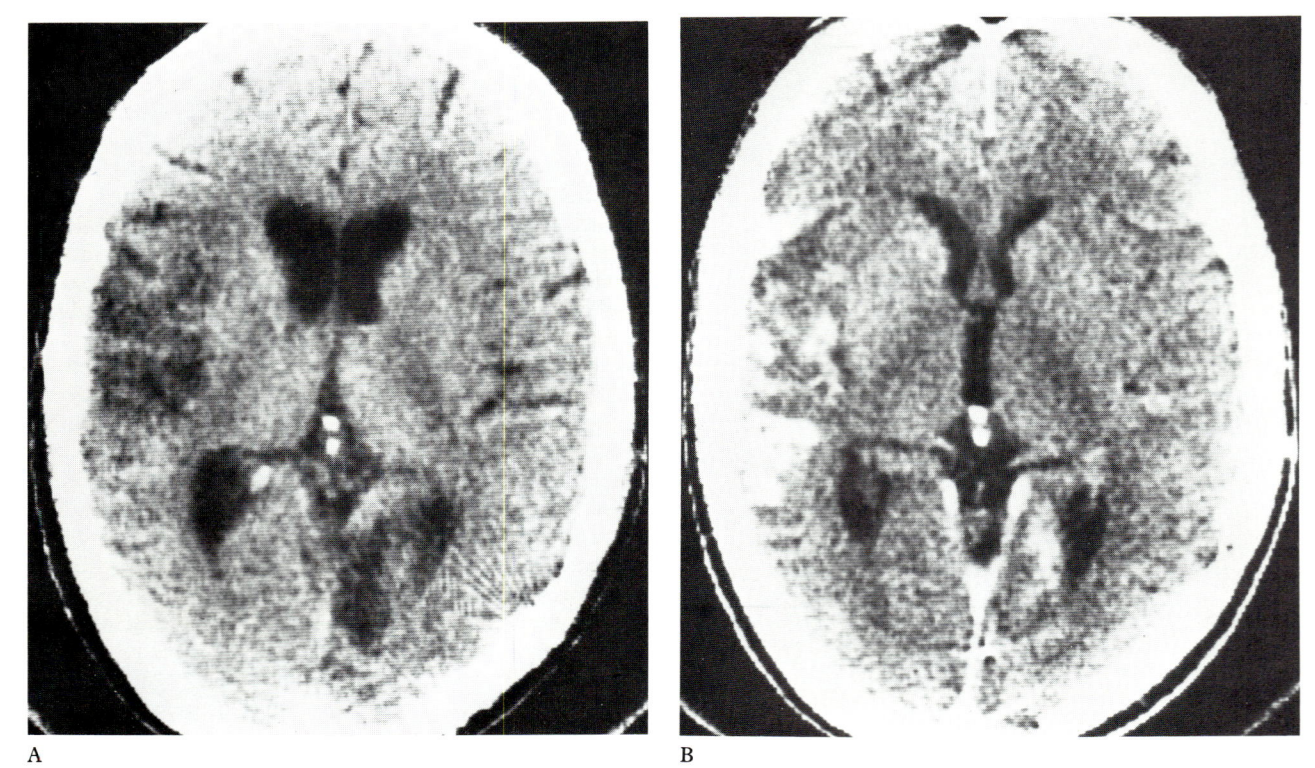

Figure 147-15 Embolic infarcts. Studies performed 4 days following left posterior cerebral and right middle cerebral artery territory embolic infarcts. *A.* Noncontrast CT scan demonstrates hypodensity in anterior aspect of left occipital lobe and right perisylvian region. *B.* CT scan after contrast reveals gyriform enhancement in region of right perisylvian hypodensity, right posterior temporal region, and medial aspect of left occipital horn. Enhancement occurs in regions of isodense to slightly hyperdense cortical bands as revealed in noncontrast CT scan (*A*).

and poor collateral circulation to the involved hemisphere.

The unenhanced CT scan may be completely normal with some hemodynamic strokes, particularly those resulting from temporary hemodynamic alterations. This occurs because the circulation to the affected brain region has in most cases returned to a normal level at the time of the CT and because the loss of autoregulation results in dilatation of the cortical arterioles and capillary hyperemia. This increased vascularity raises the density of the involved cortex. The blood-brain barrier is also abnormal, and therefore contrast enhancement occurs, demonstrating a gyriform cortical pattern. White matter areas, even if involved, will not show enhancement.

Lacunar Infarcts (Type 5)

Lacunar infarcts result from occlusive disease in the small penetrating arteries to the cerebrum, thalamus, and brain stem. They develop primarily in individuals with chronic hypertension because of the predominant occurrence of arteriolosclerosis with this condition, which frequently causes small artery occlusion. Infarction usually results from occlusion of a single penetrating artery since such vessels are essentially end arteries with only minimal potential for collat-

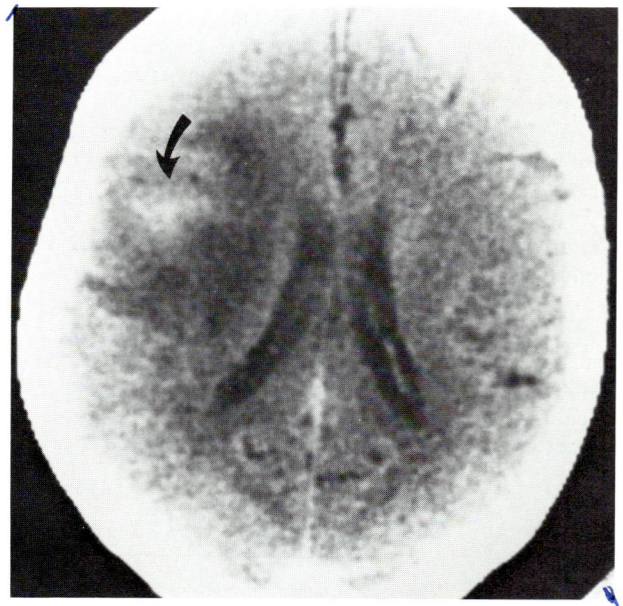

Figure 147-16 Hemorrhagic infarct with hyperdensity in range of blood (*arrow*) in cortical zone overlying hypodensity of infarcted white matter.

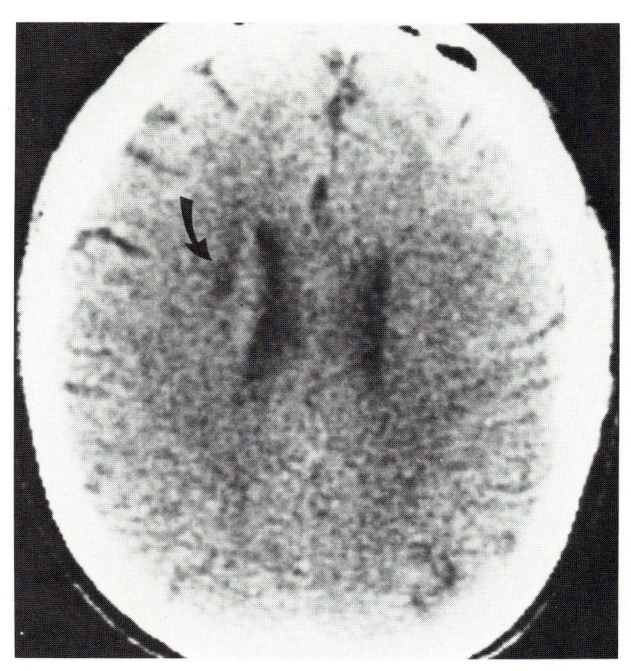

Figure 147-17 Terminal field infarct. A hypodense band is adjacent to upper outer margin of right lateral ventricle (*arrow*).

eral circulation into their territory. Lacunar infarcts range in size from 0.5 to 2.5 cm in maximum diameter. The variation in infarct size is related to anatomical differences in the territory supplied by the occluded penetrating artery and where along its course the occlusion occurs. The more proximal the occlusion, the larger the infarct size.

The most prevalent location for lacunar infarcts is within the territory of the lenticulostriate arteries which arise from the proximal middle cerebral artery and supply the basal ganglia–internal capsule region. Other affected locations are the brain stem and thalamus supplied by penetrating branches from the basilar artery. The cerebral white matter, particularly in the periventricular region, may also be involved. It is supplied by the transmedullary arterioles arising from the small arteries on the brain surface. When there is prominent white matter involvement from arteriolosclerosis, progressive dementia will usually be the main clinical manifestation. The condition is referred to as *Binswanger's disease* (subcortical arteriosclerotic encephalopathy).[53]

The lenticulostriate arteries are the largest of the penetrating vessels. They range in diameter at their origin from 0.2 to 0.8 mm. Occlusion of even a small lenticulostriate branch can result in a severe neurological deficit since the vessel may supply a critical motor or sensory pathway in the internal capsule region. However many silent lacunar infarcts in the lenticulostriate and other territories are seen on CT, most commonly in the head of the caudate nucleus, the anterior limb of the internal capsule, the putamen, and the thalamus. Lacunar infarcts in the brain stem and thalamus tend to be smaller than those in the basal ganglia–internal capsule region because of size differences of the penetrating arteries.

Identification of lacunar infarcts during the first few weeks after the stroke is very difficult, even for those involving the basal ganglia–capsular region, unless a large striate artery is affected. Small lacunar infarcts that are frequently not recognized during the acute phase may become evident in 4 to 6 weeks after the development of a well-defined lucent cystic encephalomalacic cavity. Basal ganglia lacunar infarcts that are larger than 1 cm in diameter may be demonstrated by CT after 24 to 48 h as an ill-defined oval region of decreased density oriented in the anterior-posterior plane (Fig. 147-19). The infarct frequently involves only one CT section, but it may extend more superiorly into the base of the corona radiata in the periventricular region. Since the hypodensity is very mild and ill defined initially, detection is helped by careful comparison of the basal ganglia density in both hemispheres. A slight mass effect may develop between the third and fifth days with mild compression of the adjacent portion of the lateral ventricle. Contrast enhancement may develop during the second week and last for 3 to 4 weeks. It may appear as a ring pattern. Brain stem lacunes in the acute phase are rarely identified because of their small size and the frequent transverse CT artifacts from the petrous ridges.

After several weeks, a lacunar infarct becomes more hypodense and better defined as phagocytosis removes the necrotic debris, leaving a small lucent cavitation. Brain stem lesions may even be seen. Thin CT sections (5 cm or less) will further improve identification, especially of the smaller lesions, because of less volume averaging with adjacent normal brain areas.

In Binswanger's disease, the CT reveals patchy or diffuse hypodensity in the periventricular white matter of both cerebral hemispheres (Fig. 147-20).[53,63] The involvement is usually not symmetrical. Occasionally there is extensive diffuse white matter hypodensity. Usually one or more lacunar infarcts are evident in the basal ganglia–internal capsular region or thalamus.

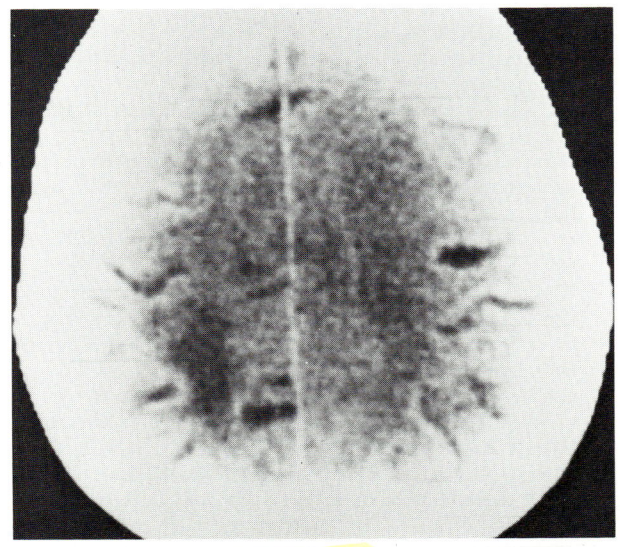

Figure 147-18 Watershed infarct. Note the hypodensity involving gray and white matter in the posterior parietal junction zone between the anterior, middle, and posterior cerebral artery territories.

A   B

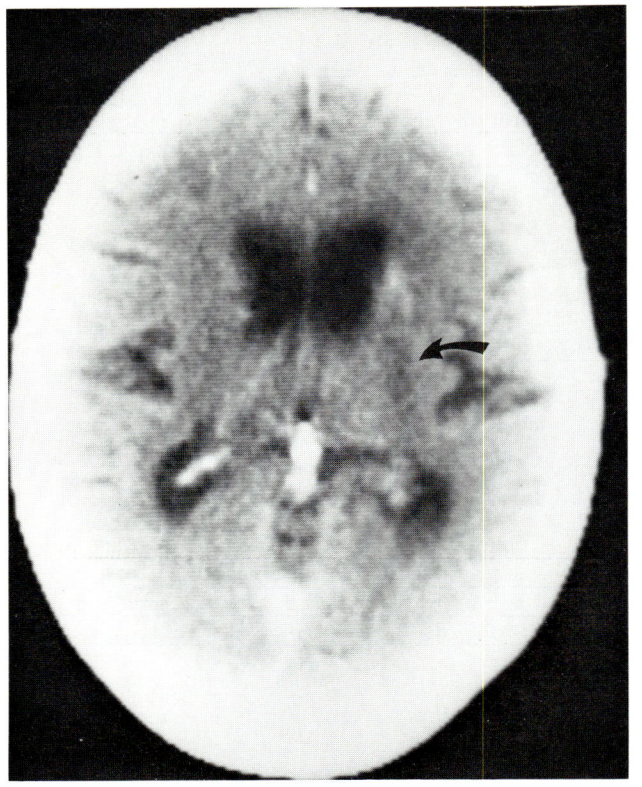

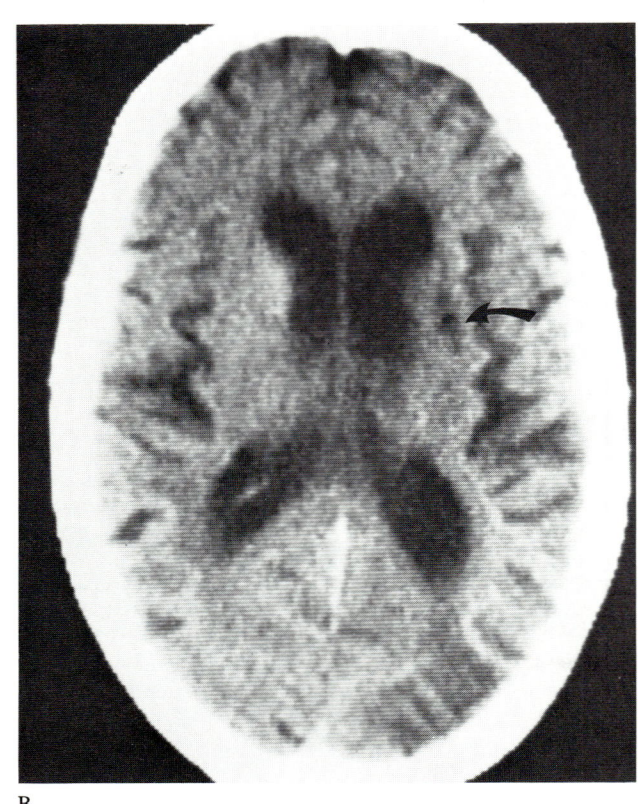

Figure 147-19 Lacunar infarct. *A*. Acute phase. There is a very slight, ill-defined hypodensity in the left internal capsule–putaminal region (*arrow*). *B*. Chronic phase after 3 months. Scan discloses a well-defined slit-like lucency of the left putamen (*arrow*).

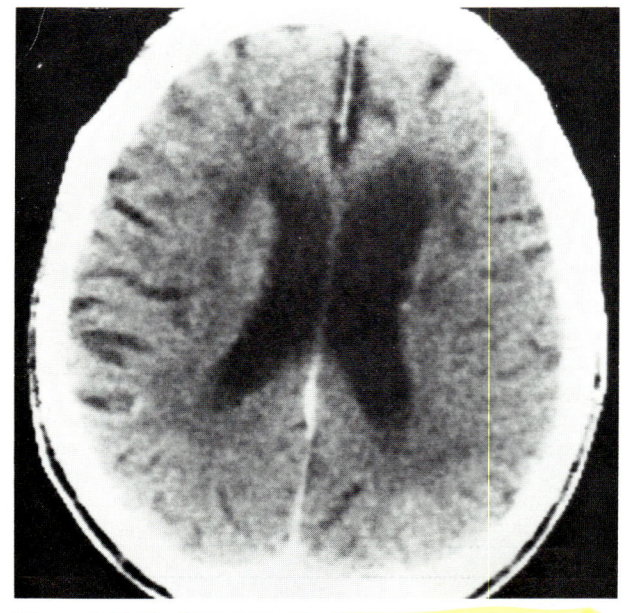

Figure 147-20 Binswanger's disease (subcortical arteriosclerosis). There are patchy bilateral periventricular hypodense regions. Lower sections through the basal ganglia demonstrated several lacunar infarcts.

References

1. Alcalá H, Gado M, Torack RM: The effect of size, histologic elements, and water content on the visualization of cerebral infarcts. Arch Neurol 35:1–7, 1978.
2. Barnett HJM: Progress towards stroke prevention: Robert Wartenberg lecture. Neurology (NY) 30:1212–1225, 1980.
3. Barnett HJM, Peerless SJ, Kaufmann JCE: "Stump" of internal carotid artery: A source for further cerebral embolic ischemia. Stroke 9:448–456, 1978.
4. Berguer R: Carotid artery noninvasive testing is being overused. Stroke 14:819–821, 1983.
5. Bogousslavsky J, Regli F, Hungerbühler JP, Chrzanowski R: Transient ischemic attacks and external carotid artery: A retrospective study of 23 patients with an occlusion of the internal carotid artery. Stroke 12:627–630, 1981.
6. Bradac GB, Oberson R: CT and angiography in cases with occlusive disease of supratentorial cerebral vessels. Neuroradiology 19:193–200, 1980.
7. Brierley JB: Cerebral hypoxia, in Blackwood W, Corsellis JAN (eds): *Greenfield's Neuropathology*. London, E. Arnold, 1976, pp 43–85.
8. Brown BSJ, Tatlow WFT: Radiographic studies of the vertebral arteries in cadavers: Effects of position and traction on the head. Radiology 81:80–88, 1963.
9. Buell U, Kazner E, Rath M, Steinhoff H, Kleinhans E, Lanksch W: Sensitivity of computed tomography and serial

scintigraphy in cerebrovascular disease. Radiology 131:393–398, 1979.
10. Chikos PM, Fisher LD, Hirsch JH, Harley JD, Thiele BL, Strandness DE: Observer variability in evaluating extracranial carotid artery stenosis. Stroke 14:885–892, 1983.
11. Cronqvist S: Total angiography in evaluation of cerebro-vascular disease: A correlative study of aorto-cervical and selective cerebral angiography. Br J Radiol 39:805–810, 1966.
12. Cronqvist S, Laroche F: Transient hyperaemia in focal cerebral vascular lesions studied by angiography and regional cerebral blood flow measurements. Br J Radiol 40:270–274, 1967.
13. De Reuck J: Arterial vascularisation and angioarchitecture of the nucleus caudatus in human brain. Eur Neurol 5:130–136, 1971.
14. Di Chiro G, Libow LS: Carotid siphon calcification and cerebral blood flow in the healthy aged male. Radiology 99:103–107, 1971.
15. Earnest F, Forbes G, Sandok BA, Piepgras DG, Faust RJ, Ilstrup DM, Arndt LJ: Complications of cerebral angiography: Prospective assessment of risk. AJNR 4:1191–1197, 1983.
16. Earnest F IV, Houser OW, Forbes GS, Kispert DB, Folger WN, Sundt TM Jr: The accuracy and limitations of intravenous digital subtraction angiography in the evaluation of atherosclerotic cerebrovascular disease: Angiographic and surgical correlation. Mayo Clin Proc 58:735–746, 1983.
17. Edwards JH, Kricheff II, Gorstein F, Riles T, Imparato A: Atherosclerotic subintimal hematoma of the carotid artery. Radiology 133:123–129, 1979.
18. Edwards JH, Kricheff II, Riles T, Imparato A: Angiographically undetected ulceration of the carotid bifurcation as a cause of embolic stroke. Radiology 132:369–373, 1979.
19. Eikelboom B, Riles TR, Mintzer R, Baumann FG, Defillip G, Lin J, Imparato AM: Inaccuracy of angiography in the diagnosis of carotid ulceration. Stroke 14:882–885, 1983.
20. Finklestein S, Kleinman GM, Cuneo R, Baringer JR: Delayed stroke following carotid occlusion. Neurology (NY) 30:84–88, 1980.
21. Gabrielsen TO, Seeger JF, Knake JE, Burke DP, Stilwill EW: The nearly occluded internal carotid artery: A diagnostic trap. Radiology 138:611–618, 1981.
22. Gacs G, Fox AJ, Barnett HJM, Vinuela F: CT visualization of intracranial arterial thromboembolism. Stroke 14:756–762, 1983.
23. Gado MH, Phelps ME, Coleman RE: An extravascular component of contrast enhancement in cranial computed tomography. Radiology 117:595–597, 1975.
24. Garcia-Merino JA, Gutierrez JA, Lopez-Lozano JJ, Marquez M, Lopez F, Liano H: Double lumen dissecting aneurysms of the internal carotid artery in fibromuscular dysplasia: Case report. Stroke 14:815–818, 1983.
25. Ginsberg MD, Greenwood SA, Goldberg HI: Noninvasive diagnosis of extracranial cerebrovascular disease: Oculoplethysmography-phonoangiography and directional Doppler ultrasonography. Neurology (NY) 29:623–632, 1979.
26. Goldstein SJ, Fried AM, Young B, Tibbs PA: Limited usefulness of aortic arch angiography in the evaluation of carotid occlusive disease. AJNR 2:559–564, 1981.
27. Grossman RI, Davis KR: Positional occlusion of the vertebral artery: A rare cause of embolic stroke. Neuroradiology 23:227–230, 1982.
28. Hakim AM, Ryder-Cooke A, Melanson D: Sequential computerized tomographic appearance of strokes. Stroke 14:893–897, 1983.
29. Hayman LA, Evans RA, Bastion FO, Hinck VC: Delayed high dose contrast CT: Identifying patients at risk of massive hemorrhagic infarction. AJNR 2:139–147, 1981.
30. Houser OW, Baker HL Jr: Fibromuscular dysplasia and other uncommon diseases of the cervical carotid artery: Angiographic aspects. AJR 104:201–212, 1968.
31. Houser OW, Baker HL Jr, Sandok BA, Holley KE: Cephalic arterial fibromuscular dysplasia. Radiology 101:605–611, 1971.
32. Imparato AM, Riles TS, Gorstein F: The carotid bifurcation plaque: Pathologic findings associated with cerebral ischemia. Stroke 10:238–245, 1979.
33. Imparato AM, Riles TS, Mintzer R, Baumann FG: The importance of hemorrhage in the relationship between gross morphologic characteristics and cerebral symptoms in 376 carotid artery plaques. Ann Surg 197:195–203, 1983.
34. Inoue Y, Takemoto K, Miyamoto T, Yoshikawa N, Taniguchi S, Saiwai S, Nishimura Y, Komatsu T: Sequential computed tomography scans in acute cerebral infarction. Radiology 135:655–662, 1980.
35. Kaseff LG: Positional variations of the common carotid artery bifurcation: Implications for digital subtraction angiography. Radiology 145:377–378, 1982.
36. Kerber CW, Cromwell LD, Drayer BP, Bank WO: Cerebral ischemia: I. Current angiographic techniques, complications, and safety. AJR 130:1097–1103, 1978.
37. Klatzo I: Neuropathological aspects of brain edema. J Neuropathol Exp Neurol 26:1–14, 1967.
38. Kovács A: Subluxation and deformation of the cervical apophyseal joints. Acta Radiol 43:1–16, 1955.
39. Ladurner G, Sager WD, Iliff LD, Lechner H: A correlation of clinical findings and CT in ischaemic cerebrovascular disease. Eur Neurol 18:281–288, 1979.
40. Lassen NA: The luxury-perfusion syndrome and its possible relation to acute metabolic acidosis localised within the brain. Lancet 2:1113–1115, 1966.
41. Lee KF, Chambers RA, Diamond C, Park CH, Thompson NL Jr, Schnapf D, Pripstein S: Evaluation of cerebral infarction by computed tomography with special emphasis on microinfarction. Neuroradiology 16:156–158, 1978.
42. Lhermitte F, Gautier JC, Derouesné C: Nature of occlusions of the middle cerebral artery. Neurology 20:82–88, 1970.
43. Mani RL, Eisenberg RL, McDonald EJ Jr, Pollock JA, Mani JR: Complications of catheter cerebral arteriography: Analysis of 5,000 procedures: I. Criteria and incidence. AJR 131:861–865, 1978.
44. Masdeu JC, Berhooz AK, Rubino, FA: Evaluation of recent cerebral infarction by computerized tomography. Arch Neurol 34:417–421, 1977.
45. McNeil DH Jr, Dreisbach J, Marsden RJ: Spontaneous dissection of the internal carotid artery: Its conservative management with heparin sodium. Arch Neurol 37:54–55, 1980.
46. Modic MT, Weinstein MA, Chilcote WA, Pavlicek W, Duchesneau PM, Furlan AJ, Little JR: Digital subtraction angiography of the intracranial vascular system: Comparative study in 55 patients. AJNR 2:527–534, 1981.
47. Mohr JP, Fisher CM, Adams RD: Cerebrovascular diseases, in Isselbacher KJ, Adams RD, Braunwald E, Petersdorf RG, Wilson JD (eds): *Harrison's Principles of Internal Medicine*, 9th ed. New York, McGraw-Hill, 1980, pp 1911–1942.
48. Moore WS, Hall AD: Importance of emboli from carotid bifurcation in pathogenesis of cerebral ischemic attacks. Arch Surg 101:708–716, 1970.
49. Plum F: Brain swelling and edema in cerebrovascular disease. Res Publ Assoc Res Nerv Ment Dis 41:318–348, 1961.
50. Pullicino P, Kendall BE: Contrast enhancement in ischaemic lesions: I. Relationship to prognosis. Neuroradiology 19:235–239, 1980.
51. Ring BA: Occlusio supra occlusionem: Intracranial occlusions following carotid thrombosis as diagnosed by cerebral angiography. Stroke 2:487–493, 1971.
52. Ringelstein EB, Zeumer H, Angelou D: The pathogenesis of

strokes from internal carotid artery occlusion: Diagnostic and therapeutic implications. Stroke 14:867–875, 1983.
53. Rosenberg GA, Kornfeld M, Stovring J, Bicknell JM: Subcortical arteriosclerotic encephalopathy (Binswanger): Computerized tomography. Neurology (NY) 29:1102–1106, 1979.
54. Sadoshima S, Fujishima M, Ogata J, Ibayashi S, Shiokawa O, Omae T: Disruption of blood-brain barrier following bilateral carotid artery occlusion in spontaneously hypertensive rats: A quantitative study. Stroke 14:876–882, 1983.
55. Sheehan S, Bauer RB, Meyer JS: Vertebral artery compression in cervical spondylosis: Arteriographic demonstration during life of vertebral artery insufficiency due to rotation and extension of the neck. Neurology 10:968–986, 1960.
56. Simmons CR, Tsao E, Smith LL, Hinshaw DB, Thompson JR: Angiographic evaluation in extracranial vascular occlusive disease. Arch Surg 107:785–790, 1973.
57. Spencer MP, Reid JM: Quantitation of carotid stenosis with continuous-wave (C-W) Doppler ultrasound. Stroke 10:326–330, 1979.
58. Taveras JM, Wood EH: *Diagnostic Radiology*. Baltimore, Williams & Wilkins, 1976, pp 861–862.
59. Wall SD, Brant-Zawadzki M, Jeffrey RB, Barness B: High frequency CT findings within 24 hours after cerebral infarction. AJNR 2:553–557, 1981.
60. Wodarz R: Watershed infarctions and computed tomography: A topographical study in cases with stenosis or occlusion of the carotid artery. Neuroradiology 19:245–248, 1980.
61. Yock DH Jr: CT demonstration of cerebral emboli. J Comput Assist Tomogr 5:190–196, 1981.
62. Yonas H, Meyer J: Extreme pseudo-occlusion of the internal carotid artery. Neurosurgery 11:681–686, 1982.
63. Zeumer H, Schonsky B, Sturm KW: Predominant white matter involvement in subcortical arteriosclerotic encephalopathy (Binswanger disease). J Comput Assist Tomogr 4:14–19, 1980.

148

Extracranial Carotid Artery Atherosclerosis

Robert G. Ojemann

The diagnosis of extracranial carotid artery stenosis offers the possibility of considering medical and surgical treatment to prevent a stroke. Symptoms in patients with carotid atherosclerosis and the noninvasive techniques and the radiographic studies used in evaluating these patients are discussed in other chapters in this textbook.

Incidence

There is good evidence that transient ischemic attacks (TIAs) that include either transient monocular blindness (TMB) or transient hemisphere attack (THA) are related to carotid atherosclerosis. Data from the Harvard Stroke Registry indicate that significant stenosis (lumen < 2 mm) or occlusion in the region of the common carotid artery bifurcation or proximal internal carotid artery is present in approximately 50 percent of the patients with transient ischemic attacks in the territory of the carotid artery while this is true in less than 10 percent of patients with stroke due to nonischemic cerebral disease.[15] Table 148-1 records the angiographic findings in 95 patients with TIAs. In addition to the 52 percent of patients with significant carotid stenosis or occlusion, six other patients (6 percent) had ulceration that may have been important in the symptomatology. When a patient has both THA and TMB, there is a very high probability of finding significant carotid atherosclerosis.

Pathogenesis

In patients with significant carotid atherosclerotic disease, TIAs may be caused by embolism arising from an atheromatous carotid lesion or from reduction in cerebral blood flow. Whether this latter cause relates to transient carotid occlusion, systemic reduction in blood pressure, or other factors has not been established.

When TMB is present it has been suggested that embolism is the cause because of the observation of embolic material in retinal vessels. This pathological mechanism can cause the wedge-shaped visual defects typical of central retinal artery branch occlusion, but this is an uncommon clinical finding. The common shade or curtain altitudinal symptoms suggest reduced circulation to the posterior ciliary arteries or circle of Zinn, an arterial network that could be occluded by emboli but is more likely to be susceptible to the effects of hypotension.[15]

The patient with a THA whose angiogram shows a normal carotid bifurcation or only minimal atherosclerosis and who has an intracranial branch occlusion is likely to have a cardiac embolic source. In the group of patients in the Harvard stroke study, 25 percent with THAs had intracranial branch occlusion on angiography.[15] The actual incidence might even be higher since embolic occlusions are often transient. When significant carotid artery stenosis is present, THA is probably due to inadequate distal perfusion in most cases, but what part emboli play has not been established.[7]

TABLE 148-1 Angiographic Findings in 95 Patients with Transient Ischemic Attacks*

Type of Attack	Carotid Occlusion	Severe[+] Stenosis (<2 mm)	Moderate[+] Stenosis	Minimal[+] Stenosis	Normal Carotid
Transient hemisphere attack (THA)	4	18	4	17	9
Transient monocular blindness (TMB)	5	14	1	5	8
Both THA and TMB	2	6	1	0	1
Total	11	38[+]	6	22[§]	18

*Thirteen patients had intracranial branch occlusion, and nine of these did not have significant carotid disease.
[+]This refers to the proximal portion of the internal carotid artery.
[+]Three patients also had an ulceration.
[§] Six patients had an ulceration.
SOURCE: Modified from Pessin et al.[15]

There is also the possibility that lacunar disease may be the cause of TIA. This diagnosis has been considered because of the pure motor or sensory character of some THAs, features characteristic of the lacunar stroke, and the finding that TIAs may precede pathologically documented lacunar infarction.[15]

Indications for Treatment

In this section I will consider the indications for treatment in patients with clinical syndromes due to carotid atherosclerosis and different combinations of angiographic abnormalities in the region of the carotid bifurcation. Previous publications have included an extensive review of the literature on this subject.[13,14] In the next section I will consider general risk factors that relate to planning surgical treatment.

TIAs with Unilateral Carotid Stenosis and/or Ulceration

Carotid endarterectomy is usually indicated for the patient with TIAs and severe stenosis (lumen < 2 mm in diameter), and/or severe ulceration in the common carotid artery bifurcation region or proximal internal carotid artery. These attacks are warnings of possible impending disaster. Removal of the pathological lesion not only stops the attacks but reduces the chance of a future stroke. Our results suggest that for the patient with severe carotid stenosis and TIAs, carotid endarterectomy is associated with less risk than the natural history of the disease or than medical therapy. However, statistical proof of this fact has not been presented.

If the angiogram shows severe stenosis with reduced flow in the internal carotid artery or a thrombus in the lumen, or if the clinical picture includes increasingly severe attacks in the preceding days, attention should be directed to performing the operation as soon as possible. If there is going to be a delay, the patient should be heparinized.

If ulceration is found with a nonobstructive plaque, a decision regarding surgical or medical therapy will be made based on the severity of the lesion. In the past, carotid endarterectomy has been recommended for patients with TIAs who were found to have an area of ulceration, even though the lumen diameter was greater than 2 mm. When the ulceration is deep, surgery is the recommended treatment. There is some evidence that a shallow ulcer associated with nonobstructive atherosclerosis may have a low risk of future stroke. Such patients may be treated with antiplatelet therapy and be followed with noninvasive studies of the carotid circulation. Should there be evidence of the development of stenosis or should TIAs continue, then surgery is indicated.

TIAs with Bilateral Carotid Stenosis

In some patients who are studied because of symptoms due to stenosis in one carotid artery, significant narrowing of the carotid artery is found on the opposite side. Occasionally a patient may present with a history of TIAs related to both carotid arteries. Noninvasive studies may be necessary to help decide the hemodynamic significance of the lesions.

When only one side is symptomatic, it is generally treated first unless the asymptomatic side has a tighter stenosis with a more severe hemodynamic lesion as demonstrated by angiography and noninvasive tests. If both sides are symptomatic, the side with the more severe hemodynamic lesion is operated upon first. The second side is usually done within 7 to 14 days. When the second stenosis is very severe, heparin therapy may be indicated until the second operation is performed.

TIAs with Ipsilateral Carotid Stenosis and Contralateral Occlusion

Most patients with this combination of lesions present with TIAs related to the internal carotid stenosis. Occasionally patients will have had neurological symptoms related to the contralateral carotid occlusion.

The indications for surgery are the same as for TIAs associated with unilateral carotid stenosis. The patient with a contralateral occlusion is more likely to have an EEG change and need a shunt at the time of the carotid occlusion for the endarterectomy than is the patient with an open contralateral internal carotid artery. However, our experience as well as that of others is that there is no increase in neurological complications in this group.[13,14]

TIAs with Tandem Stenosis

In a few patients with TIAs angiography will show the stenosis at the carotid bifurcation or proximal internal carotid artery and a second stenosis in the intracavernous or intracranial portion of the internal carotid artery. The occurrence of this problem emphasizes the importance of complete angiography. Usually the stenosis in the neck is more severe than that found in the more distal lesion. If the stenosis in the neck is less than 2 mm, carotid endarterectomy is indicated for TIAs even if the distal lesion is also severe. Postoperatively, a decision is made between anticoagulation or antiplatelet therapy and a bypass graft. A bypass graft may be followed by complete occlusion of the distal carotid stenosis. In general, our plan has been to use bypass surgery only if symptoms persist after carotid endarterectomy and a good program of medical treatment.

TIAs with Ipsilateral Internal Carotid Occlusion and the Problem of External Carotid Stenosis

TIAs can occur in the territory of a completely occluded internal carotid artery.[13] The cause of symptoms may be an embolus from the distal end of the occlusion, an embolus passing through the external carotid circulation from atheromatous stenosis of the external or distal common carotid artery or from the stump proximal to the occlusion in the internal carotid artery, or a reduction of flow to the eye and/or cerebral hemisphere.

Angiography should include the collateral circulation through the opposite carotid artery, in many cases the vertebrobasilar circulation, and lateral serial films of the head and neck for several seconds to determine the collateral flow and to see how far down the internal carotid artery the contrast agent flows. This is important in deciding about the cause of the symptoms and the probability of reopening the complete occlusion. If the angiogram shows retrograde flow below the carotid siphon, and especially if this is present to the base of the skull, there is a good chance of reopening the internal carotid artery with surgery.

If the occlusion of the internal carotid artery extends into the carotid siphon, a decision has to be made either to attempt to reopen the internal carotid artery, to use anticoagulation, or to perform a bypass graft. In general, patients with this angiographic finding will likely have had a carotid occlusion for some time, and we usually do not try to reopen the artery. Even if there is good collateral circulation, we have favored anticoagulation because of the risk of embolization.

If the angiogram shows a significant proximal stump in the occluded internal carotid artery in the neck and external carotid to ophthalmic artery collateral flow, this may be the source of embolus and should be treated with endarterectomy. If there is atherosclerosis with stenosis and/or ulceration at the origin of the external carotid artery, this may also be the source of emboli and ischemia and should be treated with surgery. When the internal carotid artery is open, external carotid stenosis or occlusion does not cause significant clinical symptoms.

Posterior Circulation TIAs with Carotid Stenosis

When there is evidence of carotid artery disease either from physical examination or noninvasive studies in a patient with posterior circulation TIAs, angiography is indicated. This should include both the carotid and posterior circulations. Carotid endarterectomy is usually indicated if the angiogram shows (1) filling of the posterior cerebral artery via the stenotic internal carotid artery, (2) filling of the posterior circulation from the internal carotid artery because of vertebral artery occlusive disease, or (3) a persistent hypoglossal or trigeminal artery. We have not been convinced that carotid endarterectomy will alter vertebrobasilar symptoms unless one of the conditions noted above is found on the angiogram. When severe carotid stenosis is present with no filling of the posterior circulation from that artery, one considers the problem as an asymptomatic carotid stenosis. The optimal treatment for this lesion is then correlated with management of the vertebrobasilar occlusive disease.

Established Stroke and Carotid Stenosis

In a group of patients we treated who had suffered a stroke and were found to have carotid disease, more than half had had a prior history of TIAs due to carotid stenosis that had not brought the patient to medical attention.[13] Since these patients are at risk for further stroke, they should be studied. A CT scan is done to define the extent of the infarction and to look for other lesions. If there is any suspicion of carotid occlusive disease, angiography is indicated.

In general, the presence of severe stenosis or a deep ulcer is an indication for surgical treatment. If the angiogram shows a thrombus in the lumen or a carotid occlusion that may be reopened, then surgery is performed promptly. In those patients with a recent stroke who are continuing to show improvement, and if prompt surgery is not indicated from the angiogram, operation may be delayed to allow recovery from cerebral ischemia. How long one should delay has not been established. Some have advocated waiting several weeks to reduce the possible chance of postoperative brain hemorrhage. If the neurological deficit is mild, we would operate within a few days. If the deficit is moderate to severe, the patient will usually have CT evidence of an infarct. In this circumstance, we would wait 2 to 3 weeks to allow maximum recovery. Surgery can then be done safely as long as there is careful control of the blood pressure postoperatively.

If the patient has had a massive stroke with a severe fixed deficit, only a CT scan may be done. These patients cannot be helped by carotid endarterectomy.

An occasional patient will have a slowly progressive neurological deficit due to chronic cerebral ischemia. A CT scan excludes an intracranial mass lesion. Angiography usually shows multiple vessel occlusion. A combination of endarterectomy and bypass procedures may need to be considered.

Acute Stroke with Carotid Stenosis or Occlusion

If the history and/or findings suggest carotid disease in a patient with increasing TIAs in preceding days, the sudden onset of a mild to moderate neurological deficit with or without prior TIAs, or a progressive or fluctuating neurological deficit, immediate angiography is indicated. If there is severe stenosis with delayed flow, a thrombus in the lumen distal to the stenosis, or carotid occlusion with reflux to the intrapetrous segment of the carotid artery, surgery should be done promptly to allow maximum blood flow to ischemic brain tissue, prevent extension of a thrombus, and remove a source of embolization. A stenosis with a residual lumen diameter greater than 2 mm (not hemodynamically significant) or ulceration in a plaque at the carotid bifurcation suggests an embolus as the cause of the problem, and the patient should be considered for anticoagulation. If an acute neurological deficit occurs with loss of a previously documented carotid bruit, emergency endarterectomy should be undertaken without CT scan or angiography. With the careful control of postoperative blood pressure, the risk of postoperative intracerebral hemorrhage is very low.[13]

When there is the sudden onset of a severe neurological deficit that persists, it is likely that significant infarction has occurred. This is almost certainly the case if there is a decreased level of consciousness. In this situation, restoration of blood flow by emergency carotid endarterectomy has generally not been beneficial.

Asymptomatic Carotid Stenosis

Reliable guidelines for the management of an asymptomatic carotid bruit have not been established. Consequently, controversies exist as to the value of antiplatelet or anticoagulant therapy and the indications for carotid endarterectomy. No data are available on the impact of antiplatelet or anticoagulant therapy on the eventual stroke rate in patients with asymptomatic bruit. Likewise, no statistical evidence has been presented that carotid endarterectomy improves the eventual outcome for patients with asymptomatic carotid stenosis.

At the present time, we recommend angiography in those medically stable patients with an asymptomatic carotid bruit who have a hemodynamically significant lesion or show definite evidence of progression of the stenosis on noninvasive studies of the carotid circulation. This usually means that the residual lumen diameter is 2 mm or less. Angiography usually confirms this finding, and surgery is recommended. If the noninvasive tests do not demonstrate a hemodynamic lesion and the clinical assessment of the bruit is not worrisome, it is recommended that the patient be followed and the noninvasive tests be repeated at 4- to 6-month intervals.

Preoperative Evaluation

Many patients with carotid artery atherosclerosis have significant medical risk factors. These include symptomatic coronary artery disease, myocardial infarction within 6 months, severe peripheral arterial disease, rheumatic heart disease, congestive heart failure, severe hypertension (blood pressure > 180/110 mmHg), and chronic obstructive pulmonary disease. Other factors to consider are diabetes, hyperlipidemia, and obesity. Previous publications have documented that the operative risks are higher in certain groups of patients with significant medical risk factors.[6,13,17] In patients without significant risk factors, the combined operative morbidity and mortality is 1 to 2 percent. The major medical risk relates to cardiac disease, and when this is present, the operative risk is significantly higher.

When there is a question about cardiac reserve, a treadmill ECG test is indicated. Failure to satisfactorily pass this test is taken as a relative contraindication to surgery. A history of myocardial infarction within 6 months or evidence of overt left ventricular failure are contraindications to the exercise stress testing and strong but not absolute contraindications to surgery.

Many patients will be on several drugs for treatment of the factors noted above. In general these drugs are continued. Patients receiving diuretic medication should have serum potassium checked prior to operation, and any deficiency should be treated. It is important that patients with severe hypertension be treated since the incidence of postoperative hypertension and morbidity are higher in this group. This is particularly true for those patients who have an associated cerebral infarction and are at risk to develop a cerebral hemorrhage.[6]

Indications for intraoperative monitoring with a pulmonary artery catheter include a failed treadmill ECG or stress test, left ventricular failure, a recent myocardial infarction, severe mitral valvular disease, and persistent angina after a coronary artery bypass. Patients with symptomatic heart block undergo placement of a temporary intravenous pacer.

Carotid Endarterectomy

Anesthetic Management

Preoperative medication is kept to a minimum because of the fragile cardiovascular state of many of these patients. We prefer general endotracheal anesthesia. This technique provides good airway control, maintenance of normal arterial blood gases, maximum patient comfort, optimal surgical exposure, and some protection against cerebral ischemia.

A radial intra-arterial cannula is inserted percutaneously for direct blood pressure recording and for blood gas measurement. The Pa_{CO_2} level is kept between 30 and 39 mmHg. If there is any indication of low blood volume or hypotension, central venous pressure (CVP) is recorded and the patient given fluid or colloid to raise the CVP to 8 to 10 cmH$_2$O. A vasopressor IV infusion is prepared, usually with 10 mg of phenylephrine hydrochloride (Neosynephrine,

Winthrop Laboratories, New York, N.Y.) in 250 ml of saline, and administered through a pediatric microdrip set as needed to maintain an adequate blood pressure.

Brain Protection and Monitoring

The best method of maintaining adequate cerebral circulation during the operation is to combine the benefits of general anesthesia with the maintenance of adequate blood volume and a normal or slightly elevated arterial pressure. At the time of carotid occlusion for carotid endarterectomy, the arterial pressure is elevated to an average systolic level of 170 mmHg if there is no cardiac contraindication.

The most effective method of monitoring the intracranial circulation during the time of vascular occlusion for the endarterectomy is continuous EEG recording with a full set of leads from both sides of the head.[2,13,14,18] A high degree of correlation has been found between cerebral blood flow measurements during carotid occlusion and changes in the EEG.[18] If a significant EEG abnormality occurs, with severe slowing or loss of amplitude, a shunt should be placed promptly.

The question of whether a temporary shunt is indicated during carotid endarterectomy has been the subject of several articles. Some surgeons routinely use a shunt for cerebral protection.[9] Others never use a shunt, and some use a shunt when monitoring indicates a need for it.[13,18] The use of a shunt carries with it a possible risk of embolization and of injury to the intima, although we have not seen this, and it does make the technical removal of the distal end of the plaque in the internal carotid artery a little more difficult. Everything should be done to reduce the morbidity of the operation to as low a level as possible. Every patient should be monitored. In only a small percentage of patients will a shunt be needed, but when it is indicated, it should be used. In some patients the surgeon will know preoperatively that a shunt will be needed. These include patients in whom the vertebrobasilar circulation depends on the carotid artery or in whom there are multiple occlusions of major extracranial vessels.

Operative Technique

Since the original report of our operative approach[14] we have gradually revised and refined the technique.[13] The general layout of the operating room is shown in Fig. 148-1. The patient is placed in the supine position with a thyroid bag inflated under the shoulders. The head is slightly extended and turned away from the side of the operation. The entire operation is done using a headlight and magnifying loupes.

The incision is made along the lower anterior border of the sternomastoid muscle and just below the level of the angle of the jaw and should be curved over the muscle posteriorly and superiorly toward the mastoid process (Fig. 148-2A). If necessary, this incision will allow maximum exposure to the base of the skull and helps avoid retraction on the lower branch of the facial nerve near the angle of the jaw.

After the skin incision is made, the platysma is incised. The external jugular vein is ligated, small transverse cervical nerves divided, and the great auricular nerve identified at the upper end of the exposure. Dissection is continued along the anterior border of the sternomastoid muscle.[13] Self-re-

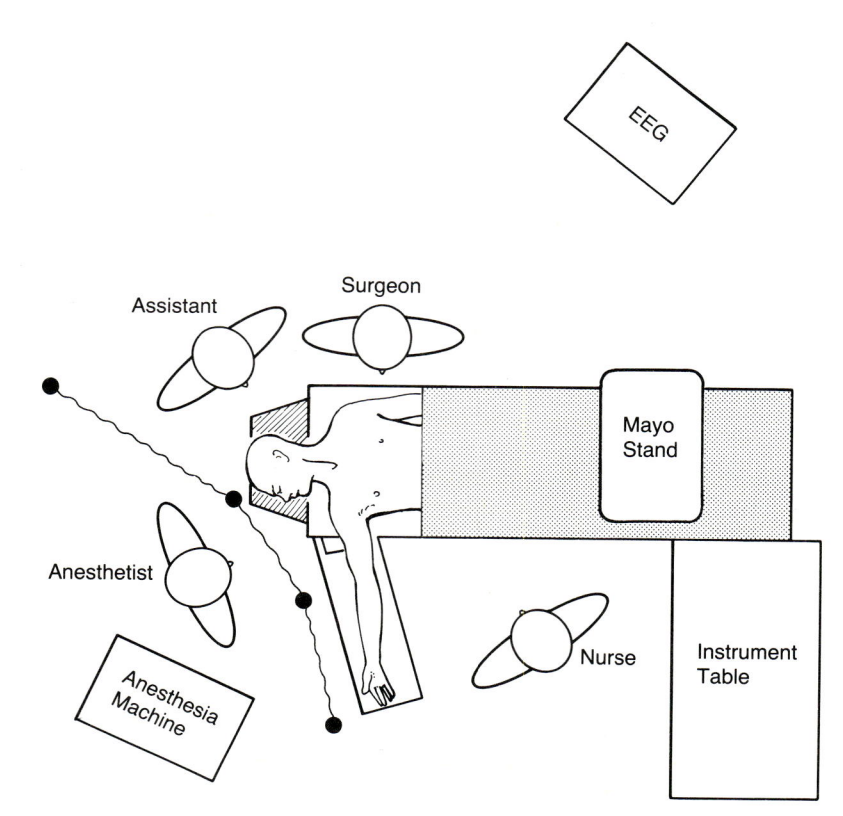

Figure 148-1 Operating room layout for a left carotid endarterectomy. We believe that it is helpful to have the scrub nurse stand across the table from the surgeon. (From Ojemann and Crowell.[13])

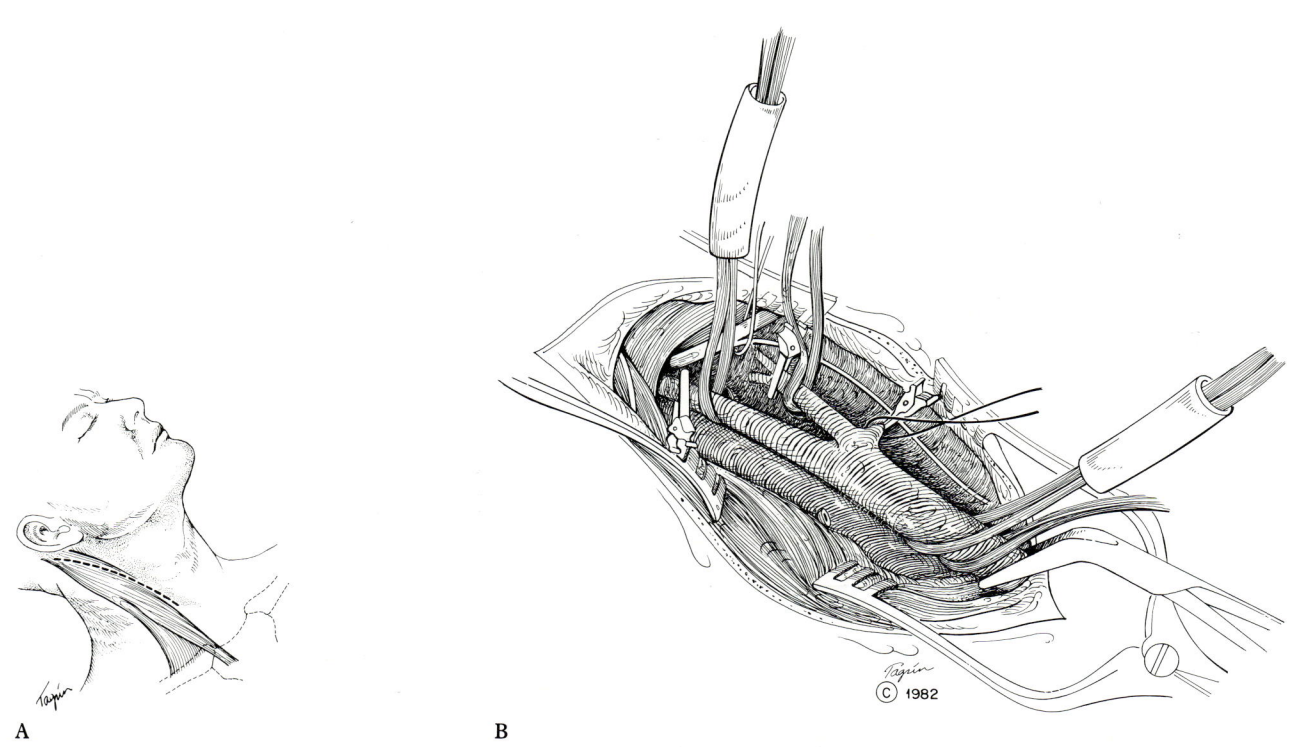

Figure 148-2 Exposure for a carotid endarterectomy. *A.* The incision begins along the lower anterior border of the sternomastoid muscle and curves over the upper portion of the muscle toward the mastoid process. *B.* The region of the carotid bifurcation has been exposed. Appropriate tapes and vascular occluding clamps have been placed. (From Ojemann and Crowell.[13])

taining retractors are used to aid the exposure. The medial blades must be kept on the subcutaneous tissue and platysma. If they are placed too deeply against the paratracheal muscles, there may be tracheal and nerve injury.

The internal jugular vein is identified just medial and deep to the sternomastoid muscle. The dissection then extends along the medial border of the internal jugular vein; medial draining branches are ligated as necessary. The descendens hypoglossi nerve is often seen in the tissue just medial to the internal jugular vein and overlying the common carotid artery. This nerve is reflected medially.

The common carotid artery is exposed medial to the internal jugular vein in the lower part of the incision. A tape is placed around this vessel, which maintains its exposure and facilitates the further dissection. On rare occasions the vagus nerve lies anteriorly on the common carotid artery, and one must be alert for this possibility.

The dissection is then extended superiorly along the medial border of the internal jugular vein. The descendens hypoglossi is kept medially and leads one to the hypoglossal nerve, which may swing low into the neck across the carotid bifurcation or lie high beneath the edge of the posterior belly of the digastric muscle. Often it lies just beneath the common facial vein and may be adherent to this vessel. In some patients, nerve branches will come around the lateral side of the common carotid artery to enter the descendens hypoglossi. Usually these branches are from the cervical plexus, but on rare occasions they seem to come from the vagus nerve. In most cases they can be divided to allow the descendens hypoglossi to be reflected medially. However, if the branch is large or is coming from the vagus nerve, the descendens hypoglossi is divided close to the hypoglossal nerve and the branch from the vagus nerve is reflected laterally. To give adequate exposure it may be necessary to remove a group of lymph nodes that are commonly present over the region of the carotid bifurcation. When the carotid bifurcation is exposed, the region of the carotid sinus is blocked with lidocaine hydrochloride (Xylocaine, Astra Pharmaceutical Products, Inc., Worcester, Mass.) to avoid a carotid sinus reflex bradycardia and hypotension. Care is taken to leave the region of the distal common carotid artery, carotid bifurcation, and proximal internal carotid artery adherent to the posterior tissue. This avoids undue manipulation of the area, reducing the possibility of dislodging an embolus, lessening the chance of carotid sinus stimulation, and avoiding possible injury to the superior laryngeal nerve.

The distal internal carotid artery is carefully exposed, staying in the tissue plane between the hypoglossal nerve or descendens hypoglossi medially and the internal jugular vein laterally (Fig. 148-2*B*). If one follows these guidelines, the distal internal carotid artery can be nicely exposed. As the hypoglossal nerve swings medially, an arterial branch often comes across the inner side of the curve of the nerve and passes posteriorly. This fairly constant sternocleidomastoid artery, often accompanied by a vein, is ligated. The hypoglossal nerve and, if necessary, the descendens hypoglossi are gently reflected medially with a soft rubber band tape. If the carotid bifurcation is located high in the neck, dissection is carried along the medial border of the internal jugular vein and beneath the parotid gland. It may be necessary to retract the posterior belly of the digastric muscle. On occasion the occipital artery must be divided to free the hypoglossal nerve in order to expose the distal internal carotid artery.

The superior thyroid artery is identified on the medial wall of the distal common or proximal external carotid artery, and a tape is placed around it. The external carotid artery is exposed to the level of the first major branching of this vessel, and a tape is placed at this point. If the arteriogram shows an ascending pharyngeal artery coming off the region of the bifurcation, this will have to be exposed and controlled separately. The exposure of the distal internal carotid artery is carried to a point at least 1 cm above the distal end of the plaque. In the majority of cases the atheromatous plaque extends several millimeters further up the posterior wall of the internal carotid artery than it does on the anterior wall. Great care is taken in exposing this vessel to avoid any undue pressure or manipulation of the artery. The vagus nerve may be closely adherent to the posterior wall of the artery; occasionally it will be lateral or superficial to the artery. It must be carefully dissected free before placing the tape around the vessel. Tourniquets are placed on the tapes on the common and internal carotid arteries to use in case a shunt is needed.

The patient is given an intravenous bolus of 5000 to 7000 units of heparin. The blood pressure is raised to at least 170 mmHg systolic.

The common carotid artery is then occluded with an appropriate vascular clamp, care being taken to avoid injury to the underlying vagus nerve. We prefer to use medium or long straight Heifetz aneurysm clips (Edward Weck and Co., Inc., Long Island City, N.Y.) to occlude the other arteries, but on occasion a large internal or external carotid artery will require the use of a small bulldog clamp. Care must also be taken to avoid injury to the vagus nerve at this point because it lies in the tissue adjacent to the internal carotid artery. The clip on the external carotid artery is also placed as far distally as possible, usually at or just below the first major bifurcation.

A longitudinal incision is made in the distal common carotid artery with a no. 15 knife blade (Fig. 148-3A). The incision is carried through the wall of the artery until the shiny yellow surface of the atheromatous plaque is seen. A Penfield no. 4 dissector is then used to separate the plane between the atheroma and outer arterial wall (Fig. 148-3B). Often the atheroma is adherent to a relatively thin outer wall at the bifurcation. It is best to separate the plaque for a few millimeters and then extend the incision superiorly with a Potts scissors before attempting further dissection. The distal end of the incision extends up the internal carotid artery to approximately the distal end of the plaque. The proximal extent of the incision can be estimated from the angiogram. The incision usually does not need to start more than 1 to 2 cm below the bifurcation. A thin layer of atheromatous plaque will usually extend proximally in the common carotid artery and does not need to be of concern as long as one is proximal to the stenosis.

The atheromatous plaque is then carefully separated from the outer arterial wall in the common carotid artery. A right angled clamp is placed around the plaque, and the plaque is cut off sharply at the proximal end of the arteriotomy in the common carotid artery (Fig. 148-3C). The plaque is kept intact and is removed first from the origin of the superior thyroid artery and the proximal external carotid artery. In some patients it is necessary to temporarily open the clamp on the external carotid artery to remove the plaque, which may extend quite far distally. Once this removal has been accomplished, the atheroma is carefully dissected from the outer wall of the internal carotid artery, keeping gentle traction on the intact plaque. Usually there is a very clean dissection plane. Great care is taken as the distal end of the plaque is reached (Fig. 148-3D). Usually the plaque will extend distally several millimeters further along the posterior wall of the artery. Care must be taken to remove this portion of the atheroma. Once the plaque has been separated, it usually comes away cleanly at the junction with normal intima and does not leave an intimal flap. Only on rare occasions is it necessary to suture the end of the plaque. The intima adjacent to and beyond the distal end of the plaque is usually of normal thickness and more firmly adherent to the media. Occasionally a very thin sheet of atheromatous material extends distally in the internal carotid artery but does not cause a problem.

The area of the endarterectomy is irrigated with heparinized saline and inspected with the help of the headlight and magnification. There are almost always some loose fragments adherent to the wall, which are picked up with a fine forceps or baby intestinal clamp and removed by peeling them in a circumferential fashion. The final inspection is made of the distal end of the endarterectomy in the internal and external carotid arteries, visualizing the area directly using a headlight and fine suction.

The arteriotomy is then closed with a continuous no. 5-0 Prolene (Ethicon, Inc., Somerville, N.J.) suture beginning at the distal end of the arteriotomy on the internal carotid artery and progressing down onto the common carotid artery (Fig. 148-4A). It is important that the sutures be placed just at the cut edge and not more than a millimeter apart. Magnification helps in placing these small sutures. Just before the final sutures are placed, back flow is allowed from both the external and internal carotid arteries so that air and any debris are flushed out of the area of the endarterectomy. If the back flow is poor, the arteriotomy is reopened and the problem corrected. In this situation there may be an intimal flap or narrowing at the distal end of the suture line. When the closure is completed, a rubber dam is placed over the suture line and held by a sponge with gentle pressure. Blood flow is allowed first into the external carotid artery to wash out any further residual debris and then into the internal carotid artery. Bleeding from the suture line is usually not a problem and is easily controlled by gentle pressure on the rubber dam. One should not be in any hurry to close small areas of leak from the suture line since most will clot with gentle pressure and patience. Surgicel (oxidized cellulose, Johnson and Johnson, New Brunswick, N.J.) is placed on the suture line. Rarely an area of persistent bleeding requires control by bringing across a flap of periarterial tissue or utilizing a small piece of muscle. Unless the hemorrhage persists, one

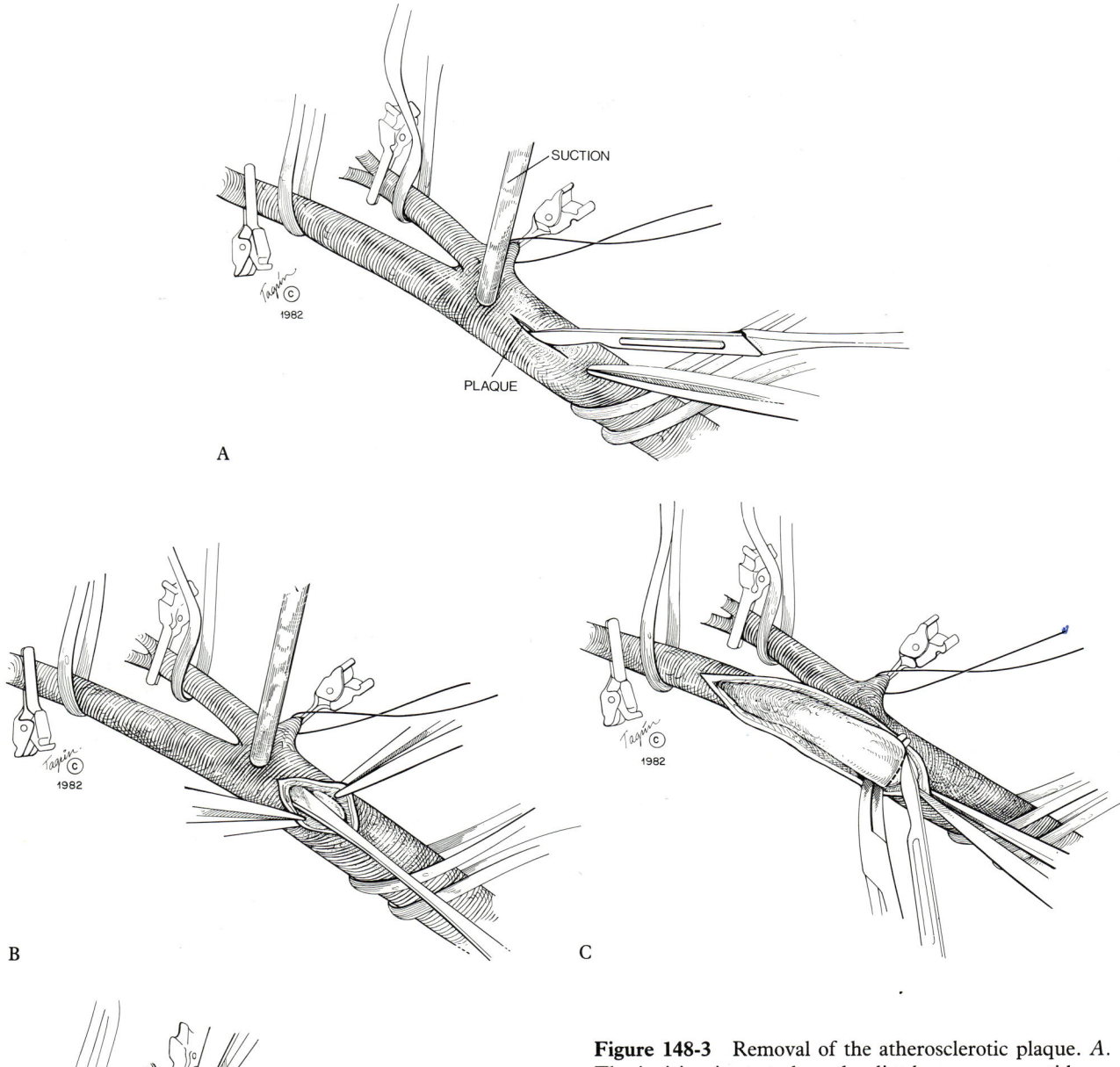

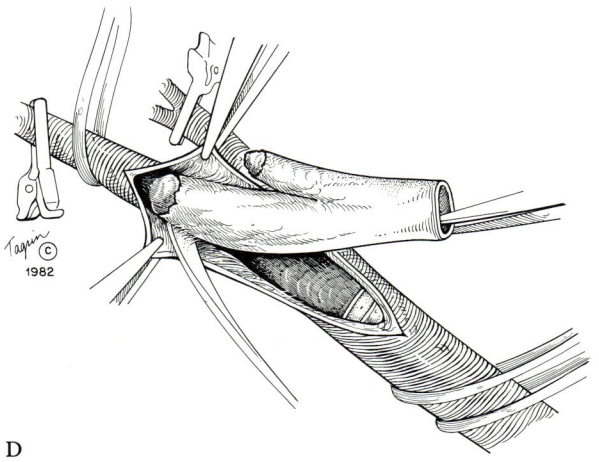

Extracranial Carotid Artery Atherosclerosis

Figure 148-3 Removal of the atherosclerotic plaque. *A.* The incision is started on the distal common carotid artery and carefully carried down to the surface of the plaque. *B.* The plaque is separated from the outer wall of the artery with a small dissector. *C.* The plaque is cut off cleanly in the distal common carotid artery. *D.* If possible the plaque is kept intact, which aids the dissection, and is removed first from the origin of the external carotid artery and then the internal carotid artery. (From Ojemann and Crowell.[13])

should avoid additional sutures into the arteriotomy incision.

Once flow has been re-established, the arteries are gently palpated. If there is a thrill in the internal carotid artery, the clamps are replaced and the artery reopened to correct the problem. If one is concerned about narrowing of the internal carotid lumen, a patch can be used. If there is a thrill in the external carotid artery, the vessel is occluded, maintaining internal carotid flow, and a separate incision is made on the proximal external carotid artery. Usually a flap of intima is the cause of the problem.

At this point a decision must be made regarding reversal of the heparin. There may be some advantage to not reversing the heparin since this may protect against thrombus formation, particularly during the first hour after the closure.[18] Therefore, if hemostasis is complete, no protamine sulfate (Eli Lilly and Co., Indianapolis, Ind.) is given.

The operative wound is irrigated with a bacitracin solution. Some surgeons prefer to leave a drain deep to the platysma for 12 to 24 h. This should always be done when anticoagulation is being continued in the immediate postoperative period. We prefer to use a small Hemovac drain (Snyder Laboratories, Inc., New Philadelphia, Ohio).

Special Technical Problems

Insertion of a Patch Graft

With the routine use of magnification for the endarterectomy, we have found that in most cases the arterial incision can be closed with a continuous no. 5-0 Prolene running suture. When the internal carotid artery appears to be too small for satisfactory closure or it appears that closure will compromise the lumen, we have no hesitation in using a patch graft.[13] In most patients with recurrent stenosis, a patch graft is used because of the scar formation in the wall of the artery. Some surgeons use a patch routinely.[18]

The patch graft can be made from either a saphenous vein taken from the ankle or a preclotted knitted Dacron fabric (USCI division of CR Bard Inc., Billerica, Mass.). We prefer the latter, and if there is any possibility that a patch will be needed it is prepared before the patient is heparinized. The patch is cut to fit the arteriotomy. The graft is usually 6 to 8 mm in width in the central portion and tapers to a rounded point at each end. Double-armed sutures of no. 5-0 Prolene are used at each end (Fig. 148-4B). One arm of the suture is placed through one end of the graft from the outer to the inner surface and then carefully placed at the distal end of the arteriotomy from inside the lumen to the outer wall. The other arm of the suture is placed in a similar fashion very close to the first, and the suture is then tied. The final length of the graft is determined, and another double-armed suture is placed in a similar fashion at the proximal end of the graft. One of the sutures is then used for a continuous closure on each side of the graft. The closure is done so that the knots can be tied away from the end of the graft. Just before the closure is completed, back flow is allowed, as is done in the usual endarterectomy closure.

Use of a Shunt

We use the Argyle (St. Louis, Mo.) carotid shunt catheters.[13] The advantage of these sterile polyethylene catheters is that the surgeon has four sizes (nos. 8, 10, 12, and 14 French) immediately available that are the correct length (15 cm) and have smooth ends. After arterial clamps and clips are placed, a rapid arteriotomy incision is made, including through the plaque, starting a few millimeters more proximally on the common carotid artery than one would nor-

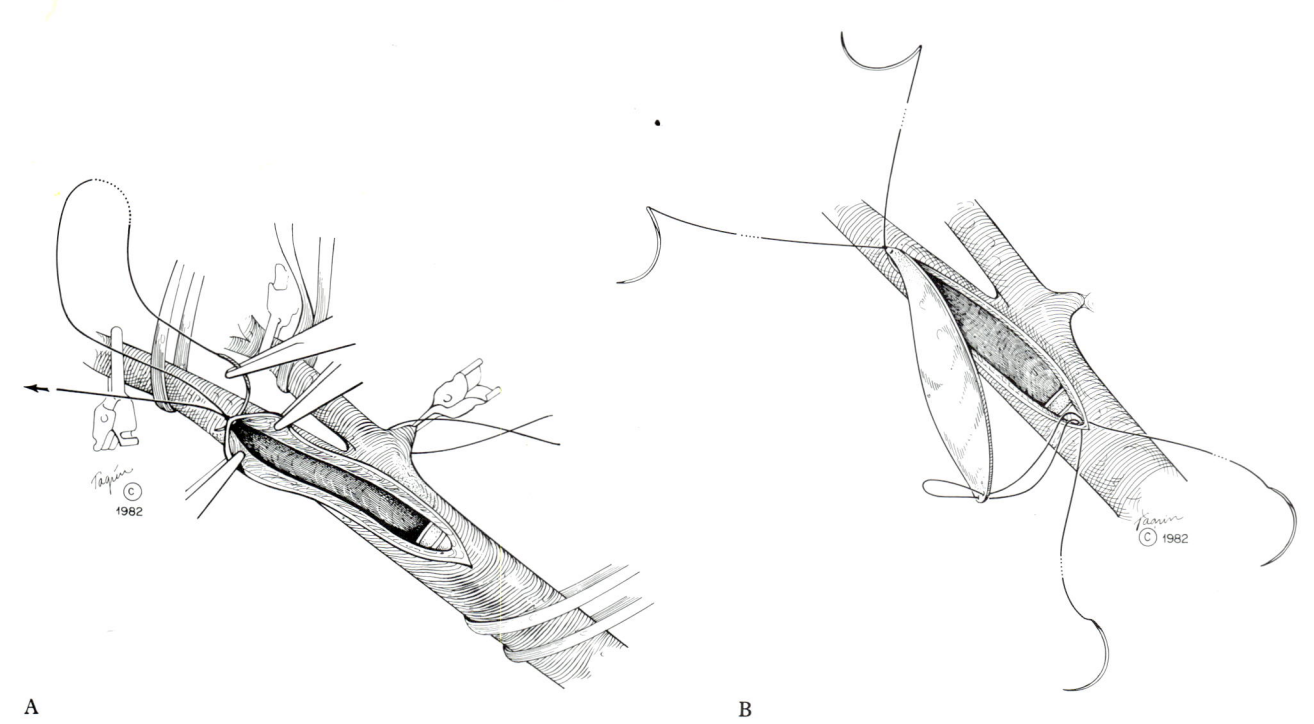

Figure 148-4 Closure of the arteriotomy. *A.* Usually the incision in the artery can be closed with a running suture. This is placed with the aid of magnification. *B.* Technique for placing a patch if it is needed. (From Ojemann and Crowell.[13])

mally start, and extending a few millimeters more distally on the internal carotid artery (Fig. 148-5). The shunt tube is first passed distally into the internal carotid artery; the surgeon visualizes the intima so that a flap is not dissected by the tip of the catheter. A tape and tourniquet gently keep the arterial wall snug around the shunt. The shunt is checked to be certain there is satisfactory back flow of blood. The catheter is temporarily occluded and is then passed proximally into the common carotid artery, and the tourniquet is tightened. The catheter usually remains outside the lumen at this point. The plaque can then be dissected and removed as previously described. The shunt tube is then placed in the lumen. All but about 3 mm in the central portion of the arteriotomy is closed. The catheter is clamped and removed, and the closure of the arteriotomy is completed.

Complete Internal Carotid Artery Occlusion

When the angiogram indicates a complete internal carotid occlusion, changes in the operative approach may be indicated. Great care is taken to avoid hypotension. An incision is made on the internal carotid artery distal to the plaque without occluding the common and external carotid arteries. In the majority of patients a thrombus will be found, but in a few the lumen of the internal carotid artery will be open distal to the atheromatous plaque. If there is a long-standing occlusion, the artery may be a firm fibrous cord and no further procedures are indicated.

If the thrombus can be removed and back flow established, the endarterectomy is completed as described. In some patients with complete occlusion of the internal carotid artery, the external carotid artery may supply significant collateral flow to the brain. In some of these patients, flow can be maintained in the external carotid artery by the application of a Satinsky clamp across the bifurcation at the origin of the internal carotid artery or by the use of a common to external carotid artery shunt.

Certain techniques may help in opening the completely occluded artery. If a thrombus is encountered in the internal carotid artery, an effort is made to withdraw it gradually with forceps using a hand-over-hand technique. Thrombi as long as 20 cm have been removed. If this technique fails, a smooth-ended suction catheter is introduced into the internal carotid lumen until resistance is felt. Suction is then applied, and this may withdraw the thrombus. If this method fails, a no. 3 Fogerty catheter is passed gently as far as the base of the skull, inflated, and withdrawn. Care is required to avoid injuring the distal internal carotid artery with subsequent development of a carotid-cavernous fistula. Measurements on the angiogram from the internal carotid bifurcation to the base of the skull may help in determining the safe length of catheter that may be inserted. An intraoperative angiogram is recommended to document restoration of flow without an intimal flap or distal thrombus. If good back flow with satisfactory angiography cannot be achieved, the internal carotid artery is doubly ligated with no. 0 silk sutures. When flow is re-established, anticoagulation should be continued in the postoperative period.

Postoperative Management

Systolic blood pressure is generally maintained in the range of 100 to 150 mmHg, with efforts to avoid both hypotension and hypertension. If hypotension develops, the ECG is checked. Mild hypotension will usually respond to the administration of fluid or colloid. The phenylephrine drip is available if needed. If the hypotension does not immediately respond to volume replacement, a CVP catheter is inserted. If the CVP is maintained in the range of 5 to 10 cm with judicious utilization of fluid, this problem will generally resolve. On occasion, bradycardia may develop and the administration of atropine may be necessary. The blood pressure and pulse usually return to normal level within a few hours.

Control of hypertension is also important. There is a significant incidence of postoperative hypertension.[3] Patients who develop postoperative systolic readings that are persistently above 170 mmHg require treatment with rapid-acting intravenous antihypertensive medication until long-acting medications become effective. We have encountered intracerebral hemorrhage with postoperative hypertension, as

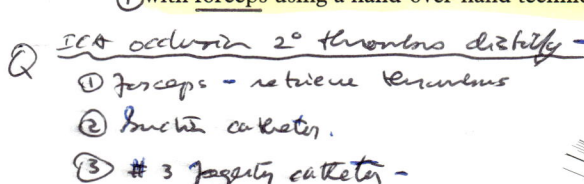

Figure 148-5 Placement of a shunt. The distal end of the catheter is placed first in the internal carotid artery. Then the proximal catheter is inserted into the common carotid artery. After the endarterectomy the shunt is placed internally until the closure is just about completed. (From Ojemann and Crowell.[13])

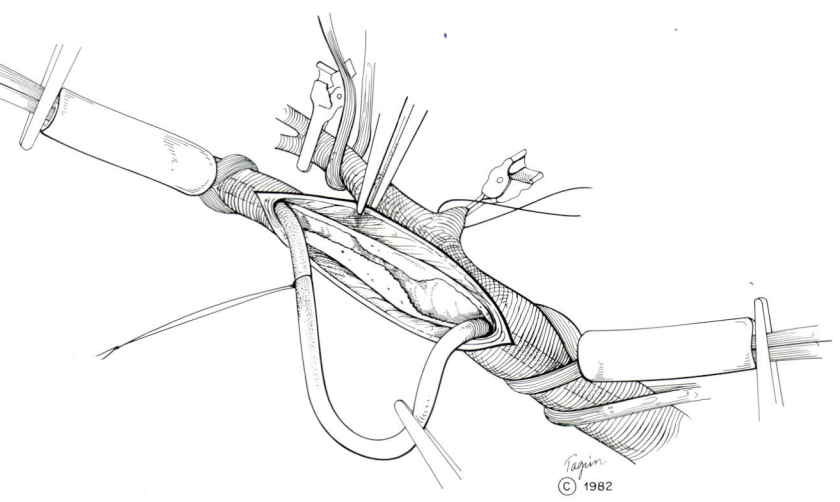

previously reported, but since the institution of careful postoperative blood pressure control, this complication has been rare.[3,14]

Generally we have not continued anticoagulation except in the circumstance when dissection was difficult, the endarterectomy plane seemed roughened, the plaque was particularly long, or a complete occlusion was reopened. A special circumstance where anticoagulation should probably be continued is when the patient has a severely stenotic contralateral internal carotid stenosis.

Results

Our results for carotid endarterectomies done for carotid stenosis and/or ulceration in patients with TIAs have been reported.[13,14] The mortality rate was 1 percent, the incidence of major stroke 1 percent, and the incidence of minor stroke 1 percent. Virtually all other patients returned to their previous level of activity. Several other reports of patients who have had elective carotid endarterectomies for TIAs have documented similar low morbidity and mortality rates when the operation is done by an experienced person in a center performing a significant number of operations.[1,2,5,6,9,16–19] For patients who have had a previous stroke there is a slight increase in risk.[14]

Reports of surgical treatment for asymptomatic carotid atherosclerosis include those of Thompson et al.,[20] who reported two strokes among 167 operations for asymptomatic bruit, and Moore et al.,[12] who reported no complications in 78 operations for asymptomatic carotid ulcerations. In our own series of 41 operations for asymptomatic carotid stenosis there was no morbidity or mortality.

Our results of operation for acute stroke in patients with carotid disease have been reported.[13] Among patients with worrisome TIAs, acute mild to moderate deficit, or fluctuating or progressive stroke, 29 enjoyed an excellent or good outcome. In this group there was one death; the patient had complete neurological recovery but then died of a cardiopulmonary complication. There were two occasions where the neurological deficit was worse after the operation, but there were also several spectacular recoveries in the immediate postoperative period after operation for both stenosis and occlusion. In another report of emergency carotid endarterectomy, 7 patients with crescendo TIAs all made a full recovery, and of 17 patients with stroke in evolution, none were worse, 4 were unchanged, 12 made a good recovery, and 1 died.[11] Encouraging results in selected cases have also been reported from other centers.[10,17]

Complications

Cerebral Ischemia

The EEG electrodes are left on the patient until the patient awakens in the recovery room. If a neurological deficit is found as the patient awakens and a significant EEG change has occurred after leaving the operating room, the patient is returned immediately for exploration of the artery. If the deficit is present with no change in the EEG, a measurement of retinal artery pressure is made immediately to look for occlusion and a CT scan is performed to look for hemorrhage. If these studies are normal, angiography is done. If studies show that the endarterectomy site is normal and that blood volume and blood pressure are maintained, a decision is made regarding anticoagulation. If the neurological deficit is mild and nonprogressive, usually no abnormality is found on angiography. In such patients it is assumed that an embolus was dislodged sometime during the dissection.

If the patient develops a neurological deficit after an initial good recovery, it often indicates occlusion at the site of the operation. If the superficial temporal pulse is lost or the retinal artery pressure is reduced, the patient should be taken immediately to the operating room to ascertain the status of the artery. In other cases a CT scan is done to look for hemorrhage, and if this study is normal, an angiogram is performed. The usual reason for postoperative carotid occlusion is a residual plaque or an intimal flap, but on rare occasions the problem may be associated with an unrecognized hypercoagulable state. In the future, digital subtraction angiography will be the procedure of choice to rapidly evaluate these postoperative neurological problems.

Transient Ischemic Attacks

A small number of patients will have one or more transient ischemic episodes in the postoperative period. Usually it is a single attack, but if there is more than one it usually does not recur after 10 to 14 days and does not signify a serious problem in the operated artery. None of our patients who experienced this has gone on to have a stroke.

Noninvasive studies are done to ascertain whether there is a hemodynamic lesion. In our experience most patients will not have evidence of stenosis. They are treated with antiplatelet or anticoagulant therapy and usually do not have further problems. If TIAs persist or a significant abnormality is present on the noninvasive tests, angiography is indicated and will probably demonstrate a lesion that needs reoperation.

Intracerebral Hemorrhage

Early in our series a typical hypertensive hemorrhage occurred in the basal ganglia 4 days after surgery when the patient's blood pressure was 200/100 mmHg. Since that time careful control of postoperative hypertension has reduced the incidence of this complication. However, occasionally even with a mild elevation in blood pressure, a hemorrhage may occur. This problem is also of concern when postoperative heparin or antiplatelet therapy is used and in patients who have had previous cerebral infarction.

Cranial Nerve Injury

If the incision is carried too near the angle of the jaw or retraction is too vigorous, the mandibular branch of the facial nerve can be stretched, causing weakness of the lower lip. This is an annoying problem; it causes a cosmetic change and may cause the patient to drool from the corner of the mouth. Spontaneous recovery almost always occurs. We have avoided this problem by curving the incision away from the angle of the jaw toward the mastoid process and being careful with placement of the self-retaining retractors. Injury to the vagus or recurrent laryngeal nerve with vocal cord paresis has been reported to occur in about 1 percent of patients undergoing carotid endarterectomy.[14,21] Traction or pressure on the nerve is the usual cause. As noted in the discussion of operative technique, the vagus nerve can lie on the anterior surface of the common carotid artery and may be encountered early in the dissection. Another area where the vagus nerve is susceptible to injury is in dissection of the internal carotid artery, to which surface it may closely adhere. The majority of patients will show spontaneous recovery within a year.

Injury to the hypoglossal nerve is generally avoided by following the steps outlined in "Operative Technique." When it does occur, it is usually due to excessive traction on the nerve. Nothing need be done. Usually there are no symptoms, and a majority of the patients will have a spontaneous recovery within a few months.

Other Complications

Cardiopulmonary complications have been reduced by following the guidelines described under "Preoperative Evaluation." Other neurological complications include seizures and headaches. When a headache occurs, it generally subsides in a day or so.

Recurrent Stenosis

Recurrent stenosis occurs in a small percentage of patients who have had a carotid endarterectomy.[4,8] There seem to be three groups of patients in which this problem arises:

1. Patients in whom surgical technique has contributed to the problem. This includes failure to remove the distal tongue of the plaque, narrowing of the lumen during the arteriotomy closure, and damage to the intima by vascular clamps.
2. Patients who have a tendency to excessive scar formation.
3. Patients in whom a combination of fibrosis, recurrent atherosclerosis, and at times associated thrombus formation develops.

Symptomatic stenosis may recur within a few months of the operation. This usually relates to one of the problems in surgical technique or to the thickened fibrosis of the arterial wall, which is grossly and histologically distinct from the typical atherosclerotic plaque. Fortunately, this tendency to excessive scar formation is a rare happening. Recurrent stenosis that occurs after 2 years usually has significant atheroma formation as well as fibrosis.

The operation is often difficult because of the dense periarterial scar and the fibrosis of the vessel wall. Great care is required to avoid injury to the internal jugular vein and the vagus and hypoglossal nerves. The thickened intima is often densely adherent to the other arterial wall, particularly in the region of the previous suture line. In most patients it is usually necessary to use a patch graft to repair the artery.

References

1. Bland JE, Lazar ML: Carotid endarterectomy without shunt. Neurosurgery 8:153–157, 1981.
2. Callow AD: An overview of the stroke problem in the carotid territory. Am J Surg 140:181–191, 1980.
3. Caplan LR, Skillman J, Ojemann R, Fields WS: Intracerebral hemorrhage following carotid endarterectomy: A hypertensive complication? Stroke 9:457–460, 1978.
4. Cossman D, Callow AD, Stein A, Matsumoto G: Early restenosis after carotid endarterectomy. Arch Surg 113:275–278, 1978.
5. Easton JD, Sherman DG: Stroke and mortality rate in carotid endarterectomy: 228 consecutive operations. Stroke 8:565–568, 1977.
6. Ennix CL Jr, Lawrie GM, Morris GC Jr, Crawford ES, Howell JF, Reardon MJ, Weatherford SC: Improved results of carotid endarterectomy in patients with symptomatic coronary disease: An analysis of 1546 consecutive carotid operations. Stroke 10:122–125, 1979.
7. Fisher CM: Clinical syndromes in cerebral thrombosis, hypertensive hemorrhage and ruptured saccular aneurysm. Clin Neurosurg 22:117–147, 1975.
8. French BN, Rewcastle NB: Recurrent stenosis at site of carotid endarterectomy. Stroke 8:597–605, 1977.
9. Giannotta SL, Dicks RE III, Kindt GW: Carotid endarterectomy: Technical improvements. Neurosurgery 7:309–312, 1980.
10. Goldstone J, Moore WS: A new look at emergency carotid artery operations for the treatment of cerebrovascular insufficiency. Stroke 9:599–602, 1978.
11. Mentzer RM Jr, Finkelmeier BA, Crosby IK, Wellons HA Jr: Emergency carotid endarterectomy for fluctuating neurologic deficits. Surgery 89:60–66, 1981.
12. Moore WS, Malone JM, Boren C, Roon AJ, Goldstone J: Asymptomatic ulcerative lesions of the carotid artery: Natural history and effect of surgical therapy compared. Stroke 10:96, 1979 (abstr).
13. Ojemann RG, Crowell RM: *Surgical Management of Cerebrovascular Disease.* Baltimore, Williams & Wilkins, 1983.
14. Ojemann RG, Crowell RM, Roberson GH, Fisher CM: Surgical treatment of extracranial carotid occlusive disease. Clin Neurosurg 22:214–263, 1975.
15. Pessin MS, Duncan GW, Mohr JP, Poskanzer DC: Clinical and angiographic features of carotid transient ischemic attacks. N Engl J Med 296:358–362, 1977.
16. Robertson JT, Auer NJ: Extracranial occlusive disease of the carotid artery, in Youmans J (ed): *Neurological Surgery,* Philadelphia, Saunders, 1982, pp 1559–1583.
17. Sundt TM Jr, Sandok BA, Whisnant JP: Carotid endarterectomy: Complications and preoperative assessment of risk. Mayo Clin Proc 50:301–306, 1975.
18. Sundt TM Jr, Sharbrough FW, Piepgras DG, Kearns TP, Messick JM Jr, O'Fallon WM: Correlation of cerebral blood flow and electroencephalographic changes during carotid endarterectomy: With results of surgery and hemodynamics of cerebral ischemia. Mayo Clin Proc 56:533–543, 1981.
19. Thompson JE, Garrett WV: Peripheral-arterial surgery. N Engl J Med 302:491–503, 1980.
20. Thompson JE, Patman RD, Talkington CM: Asymptomatic carotid bruit: Long-term outcome of patients having endarterectomy compared with unoperated controls. Ann Surg 188:308–316, 1978.
21. Wylie EJ, Ehrenfeld WK: *Extracranial Occlusive Cerebrovascular Disease: Diagnosis and Management.* Philadelphia, Saunders, 1970.

149

Vertebral Artery Atherosclerosis

James I. Ausman
Fernando G. Diaz
R.A. de los Reyes

Vertebrobasilar insufficiency (VBI) may result from atherosclerotic stenosis anywhere from the proximal subclavian artery to the distal basilar artery. This chapter will deal with those lesions of the vertebrobasilar system that are proximal to the origin of the posterior inferior cerebellar artery (PICA). We will thus focus on symptomatic structural lesions of the vertebrobasilar system, realizing that VBI may be secondary to or aggravated by extracerebrovascular causes such as cardiac dysrhythmias or hematologic causes, etc., which should be adequately worked up and ruled out. It is similarly important that the clinical diagnosis of VBI be based upon at least two separate symptoms indicative of posterior circulation ischemia, and not just dizziness alone.[3]

Anatomy

The vertebral artery is the first and usually the largest branch of the subclavian artery and may be anatomically divided into four segments. The first segment extends from the vertebral origin to its entry into the intravertebral foramen of the sixth cervical vertebra. The second portion runs through the foramina of C6 through C1 to become the third segment as it passes over the superior surface of the posterior arch of C1, behind the articular process, and enters the atlanto-occipital membrane to become the fourth segment. This latter segment is intracranial and courses anteriorly and superiorly giving rise to its largest branch (PICA) and joins the opposite vertebral artery in the midline on the ventral aspect of the pontomedullary junction, forming the basilar artery. It is worthy of note that the vertebrobasilar system is the only major arterial system in the body in which two arteries converge to form a third, single artery.

Incidence

There are few data regarding the incidence of intracranial occlusive disease of the posterior circulation. Autopsy studies on "random" populations seem to indicate the incidence of extracranial vertebral artery disease to be in the neighborhood of 5 percent. Clinical and angiographic studies demonstrate posterior circulation disease in 25 to 50 percent of all patients with cerebral vascular disease.

This apparent discrepancy can be explained, as in the case of anterior (carotid) circulation disease, by the fact that (1) not all lesions are symptomatic, and (2) not all patients with symptoms have corresponding structural lesions (e.g., patients with cardiac sources of emboli). This picture is further complicated by the peculiar anatomy of the vertebrobasilar system (see above) and the fact that ischemia from structural lesions may be the result of either decreased flow or embolism from atherosclerotic stenosis.[4]

Perhaps the best clinical study on the incidence and natural history of VBI is that by Cartlidge et al. in which the incidence of posterior circulation TIAs was found to be half that of anterior circulation TIAs and approximately 35 percent of these patients developed a cerebral infarction within 5 years.[3] It should be recalled, however, that this study was based on a nonangiogrammed population.

Diagnosis

The diagnosis of VBI should be entertained in any patient who complains of transient episodes of two or more symptoms that can be localized to the territory supplied by the posterior circulation. Thus brain stem symptoms such as diplopia, dysarthria, or dysphagia, cerebellar symptoms such as vertigo or ataxia, and occipital lobe symptoms such as bilateral amaurosis or hemianopsia with or without motor or sensory alterations involving any combination of the four extremities are consistent with this diagnosis.

The necessity to search for extracerebrovascular causes of VBI has already been discussed. Likewise, standard noninvasive neurological diagnostic studies, such as a CT scan, should be performed. The definitive diagnostic test, however, remains the cerebral angiogram. Cerebral angiography should include bilateral carotid and vertebral runs with visualization of the origins of all the vessels as well as assessment of collateral intracranial circulation. After all the diagnostic information is obtained, consideration can be given to the risks and benefits of all the available modes of therapy.

Therapy

Given a patient with symptoms of VBI and structural disease in the posterior circulation, one must then decide upon a course of therapy. The best available natural history study indicates a 35 percent incidence of cerebral infarction within 5 years.[3] Any treatment option must then be a significant improvement on this figure. There are to date no controlled randomized studies on an angiogrammed population with structural lesions in the posterior circulation to guide us in our choice of therapy, medical or surgical. It is evident then that this choice has to be made on an individual basis after obtaining a complete evaluation, including angiography, and weighing the potential risks and benefits of medical (anticoagulation, antiplatelet agents, etc.) versus surgical therapy. Clearly one must first decide what constitutes a significant structural lesion. Taking into account the above uncertainties, at present we believe that the following lesions of the vertebral system may result in VBI:

1. The subclavian steal syndrome (reversal of flow in a vertebral artery secondary to significant stenosis in the ipsilateral proximal subclavian artery)
2. Stenosis of one vertebral artery when the opposite vertebral artery is stenotic, occluded, or hypoplastic, or terminates in PICA
3. Single lesions in either vertebral artery causing stenosis and/or ulceration significant enough to cause decreased flow or embolism.

Beyond these general guidelines, the choice of therapy must be individualized. Certainly one would be more inclined to operate on a patient who has ongoing frequent episodes of vertebrobasilar insufficiency even while on anticoagulants, and who has angiographic demonstration of occlusion of one vertebral artery and severe stenosis of the distal portion of the remaining vertebral artery, than on a patient with infrequent episodes and a single lesion who has not been tried on antiplatelet therapy. We further believe that for surgery of the vertebrobasilar system to be considered, the patient should have ongoing episodes of VBI, since in our experience, patients who have had a single episode in the past and have been asymptomatic since have not significantly benefited from surgery, presumably because of the formation of adequate collateral circulation.

Surgical Therapy

Structural disease of the vertebral system may occur (1) in the subclavian artery proximal to the vertebral artery, causing the subclavian steal syndrome, (2) in the first portion of the vertebral artery, usually at the origin, (3) in the intraforaminal portion of the vertebral artery, and (4) in the third and fourth portions of the vertebral artery, from C1 to the origin of PICA or slightly beyond.

The Subclavian Steal Syndrome

The *subclavian steal syndrome* is the name commonly used to denote reversal of flow in a vertebral artery, usually secondary to stenosis in the ipsilateral subclavian artery proximal to the origin of the vertebral artery. This syndrome may not infrequently be angiographically demonstrated in otherwise asymptomatic patients. Symptomatic patients usually present with symptoms of neurological ischemia, most frequently in the posterior circulation, although a few patients may present with symptoms of brachial ischemia.[2] We refer here only to the symptomatic subclavian steal syndrome. Although a variety of operations have been designed to treat the subclavian steal syndrome (subclavian to subclavian artery bypass, axilloaxillary bypass, etc.), the principle for therapy of this condition should be that of restoration of antegrade flow to the cerebral circulation, or at least the prevention of retrograde flow therefrom. Because of a rich collateral supply, ischemic symptoms in the upper extremity are extremely rare during gradual occlusion of the subclavian artery by atherosclerosis.[2] While vertebral artery ligation at its origin is relatively simple, quick, and may be the procedure of choice in the patient who is at high risk for surgery due to other medical problems, it does not restore antegrade flow in the vertebral artery. In our experience (Table 149-1) the procedure of choice for this syndrome is vertebral artery to common carotid artery end-to-side anastomosis. Anastomosis of the subclavian artery to the common carotid is also an attractive approach, but we have had no experience with this procedure.

Surgical Technique

A vertical incision is made along the anterior border of the sternocleidomastoid muscle, extending from the sternoclavicular joint approximately 10 cm up the neck. The platysma is incised and the sternocleidomastoid is separated from the pretracheal fascia. The jugular vein is retracted laterally with the sternocleidomastoid muscle, and the carotid sheath is entered exposing the common carotid artery. The sternocleidomastoid muscles are then displaced laterally, and the posterior cervical fascia is exposed. The transverse process of the sixth cervical vertebra is identified by palpating the carotid tubercle on its anterolateral aspect, and the vertebral artery is identified by dissecting the space between the anterior scalene muscle insertion and the insertion of the longus coli muscle onto the carotid tubercle. The inverted V that is left by the insertion of these two muscles marks the location of the entry of the vertebral artery into the foramen transversarium. The vertebral artery is usually covered by a spiral of veins, necessitating careful electrocoagulation and incision during the dissection from the carotid tubercle to the origin of the vertebral artery. Care must also be taken to identify, ligate, or coagulate the lymphatic channels draining into the subclavian vein, particularly the thoracic duct on the left side. On the right side special care must be taken to avoid injuring the recurrent laryngeal

TABLE 149-1 Surgical Treatment of Subclavian Steal Syndrome

Operation	No. of Patients	Angiographic Patency	Postoperative Course	Permanent Complications
Vertebral-carotid transposition	5	5/5	Better	None
Vertebral artery ligation	1	—	?	Phrenic nerve injury; dysphagia

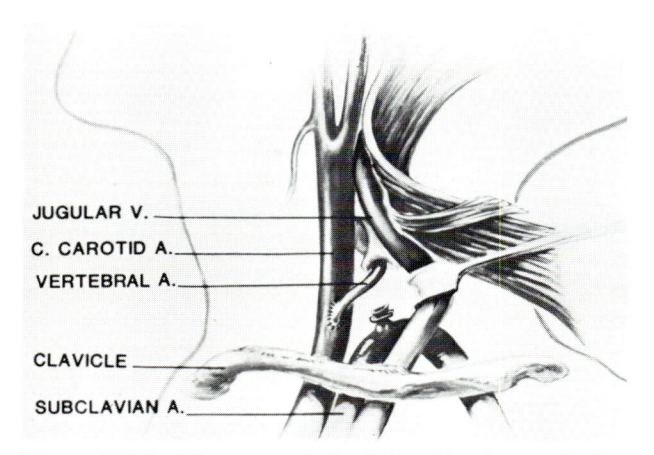

Figure 149-1 The anatomical relationships in vertebral-carotid transposition.

nerve, which is most frequently identified below the origin of the inferior thyroid vein. Once the vertebral artery has been completely dissected, the patient receives 5000 units of intravenous heparin. A ligature and silver clip are then placed at the origin of the vertebral artery, a temporary clip is placed on the vertebral artery at the level of the foramen transversarium, and the artery is then transected. If additional length of vertebral artery is needed in order to avoid a tense anastomosis, the anterior surface of the foramen transversarium may be removed with rongeurs. This is, however, usually not necessary. A fish-mouthed opening is then made at the origin of the vertebral artery. The site of anastomosis is then chosen on the common carotid artery, and the appropriate segment of the common carotid is isolated between two clamps, below the bifurcation. A 4- or 5-mm stoma is then made with an aortic punch in the common carotid artery, and an end-to-side anastomosis is performed using no. 7-0 monofilament nylon and the operating microscope (Fig. 149-1). The clamps are then removed and the flow is restored. Clamp time is usually in the range of 20 to 30 min. The incision is then closed in layers in the usual manner (Figs. 149-2 and 149-3).

Results

Our experience with five such patients is summarized in Table 149-1. All symptoms were either significantly improved or resolved completely. A sixth patient, who was at high risk for surgery because of severe cardiovascular instability, underwent vertebral artery ligation due to crescendo TIAs of the posterior circulation. Although his TIAs ceased postoperatively, he was left with a persistent dysphagia, as well as an elevated left hemidiaphragm, presumably due to intraoperative phrenic nerve injury.

Vertebral Origin Stenosis

Vertebrobasilar insufficiency may result from atherosclerotic stenosis at the vertebral origin if the opposite vertebral artery is stenotic, occluded, or hypoplastic or terminates in the PICA. The presumed mechanism here would be hemodynamic compromise of the posterior circulation due to stenosis of the remaining vertebral artery. Whether the same can occur from a single lesion in one vertebral origin with an angiographically normal contralateral vertebral is open to speculation. Only slightly less controversial is the matter of embolization from an atherosclerotic vertebral artery plaque. Atherosclerotic emboli in the distal basilar system have been found at autopsy in patients with vertebral artery plaques,[4] and our own intraoperative experience has shown us that ulceration can occur in vertebral artery plaques, but there are no available data regarding the frequency of VBI secondary to atherosclerotic emboli.

Our experience with 23 cases of vertebral origin stenosis, associated in most cases with compromise of the opposite vertebral artery, is summarized in Table 149-2. Experience with several different types of vertebral origin surgery has

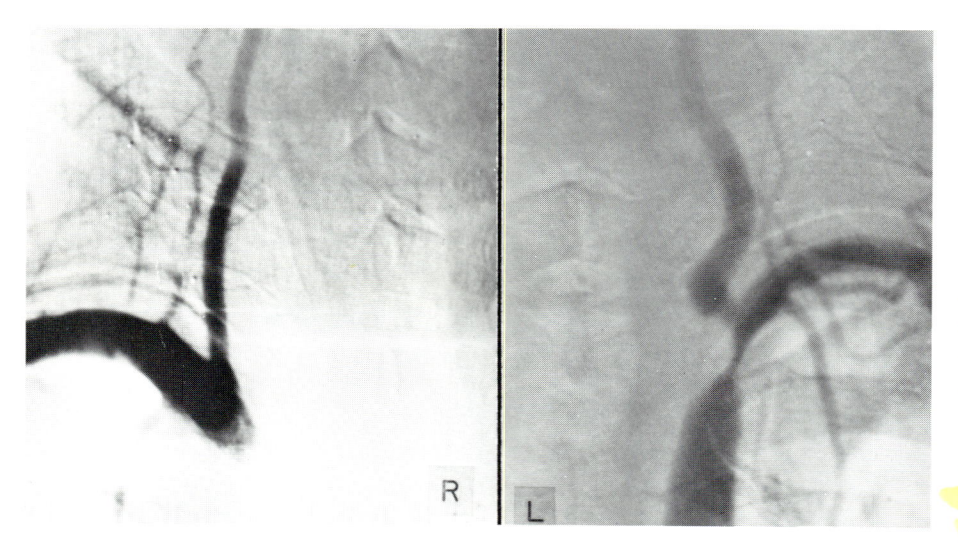

Figure 149-2 Preoperative bilateral subclavian-vertebral angiograms, demonstrating stenosis of the left subclavian artery proximal to the origin of the left vertebral artery. The patient had clinical as well as angiographic findings consistent with the subclavian steal syndrome.

Vertebral Artery Atherosclerosis

shown us that, in our hands, vertebral-carotid transposition is the operation of choice for this condition, because it avoids the torsion and double anastomosis necessary for subclavian to vertebral artery vein grafts. It also eliminates the tension on the anastomosis afforded by transposition of the vertebral to other sites on the subclavian artery. Most patient's symptoms have improved or disappeared, and morbidity has been limited for the most part to the development of Horner's syndrome, which in all but two cases was transient. We have, additionally, had experience with 13 patients who have ipsilateral vertebral and internal carotid artery stenosis (Table 149-3). In these cases we perform the vertebral-carotid transposition prior to proceeding with a standard carotid endarterectomy, as suggested by Bohmfalk et al.,[2] in order to restore antegrade flow in the vertebral artery prior to occluding the carotid artery.

Atherosclerotic stenosis in the second (intraforaminal) portion of the vertebral artery may result from intrinsic narrowing due to a plaque[5] or from extrinsic compression due to cervical spondylosis.[6] Symptomatic stenosis in this portion of the artery is, in our experience, much less frequent than that in the more proximal or distal portions. There have been case reports describing the resection of osteophytes[6] to relieve extrinsic compression or bypasses[5] for the treatment of intrinsic stenosis. Direct endarterectomy of intrinsic stenosis in this portion of the artery is another alternative. We have performed this twice in two patients with stenosis at C5, with patency of the endarterectomies (Table 149-4 and Figs. 149-4 and 149-5).

Distal Vertebral Stenosis

Atherosclerotic stenosis in the third and fourth portions of the vertebral artery may be either bypassed (occipital artery to PICA anastomosis) or dealt with directly (C1-intracranial vertebral endarterectomy). Those procedures are designed primarily to treat disease proximal to the origin of the PICA. The bypass procedure may be performed to treat either stenotic or occlusive disease proximal to PICA, and it is discussed elsewhere in the text. Direct intracranial vertebral endarterectomy can be used only for stenotic disease, but it has the advantages of providing a larger channel for blood

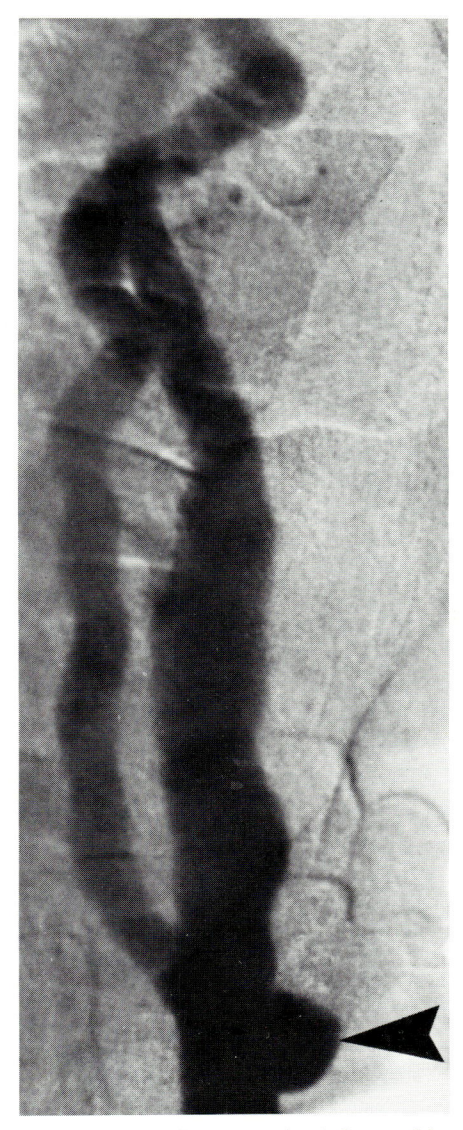

Figure 149-3 Postoperative left carotid angiogram (same patient as in Fig. 149-2) showing a patent vertebral-carotid transposition. The arrowhead points to the site of anastomosis.

TABLE 149-2 Surgical Treatment of Vertebral Origin Stenosis

Operation	No. of Patients	Angiographic Patency	Postoperative Course	Permanent Complications
Vertebral-carotid transposition	19	18/18	17 better 2 same	2 permanent Horner's syndrome
Vertebral-subclavian transposition	1	1/1	Better	None
Vertebral-thyrocervical transposition	1	0/1	Better	None
Vertebral origin endarterectomy	1	1/1	Better	None
Vertebral-carotid saphenous vein graft	1	1/1	Better	Transient upper brachial plexopathy

TABLE 149-3 Surgical Treatment of Vertebral Origin Stenosis and Ipsilateral Internal Carotid Stenosis

Operation	No. of Patients	Angiographic Patency	Postoperative Course	Permanent Complications
Vertebral-carotid transposition; carotid endarterectomy	13	13/13	13 better	1 recurrent laryngeal nerve injury 1 permanent Horner's syndrome

flow and removing the atheroma, with its (at least theoretical) potential for embolization.

Surgical Technique

The operation is done with the patient in the three-quarter prone position, with the involved side down to facilitate viewing the lumen of the artery after the arteriotomy is performed. A midline incision is made from the inion to the spinous process of C5 and carried down to expose the laminae of C2 and C1. Dissection is then carried out in the region of the foramen magnum, and extended laterally until the vertebral artery is palpated. The vertebral artery is then carefully dissected from the surrounding tissue and freed of its surrounding venous plexus. A suboccipital craniectomy is then performed on the involved side to expose the vertebral artery as it enters the posterior fossa. This allows exposure of the vertebral artery as it penetrates the dura next to the condyle. The dura is then opened from the point at which the vertebral artery penetrates it, thereby exposing the full length of the vertebral artery. The arachnoid is then opened. A vessel loop is placed around the vertebral artery for the purposes of retraction and, if necessary, temporary occlusion. Clips are placed at appropriate locations on either side of the plaque, and a longitudinal arteriotomy is performed. A no. 11 bladed knife is used for this, and the incision is extended with microscissors. The plaque is then dissected circumferentially using a Penfield dissector and microdissectors. The plaque may be cut flush using microscissors if necessary, and luminal tags are removed using a microbiopsy forceps. After adequate irrigation with heparin, the arteriotomy is closed with a running no. 7-0 Prolene suture (Ethicon Inc., Somerville, N.J.), and the incision is closed in layers in the usual manner.

Results

This operation was first reported by Allen et al. in 1981,[1] and experience with it has been limited to date. We have attempted four such endarterectomies and were able to complete three (Table 149-5; Figs. 149-6 and 149-7). The fourth resulted in ligation of the vertebral artery as a result of tech-

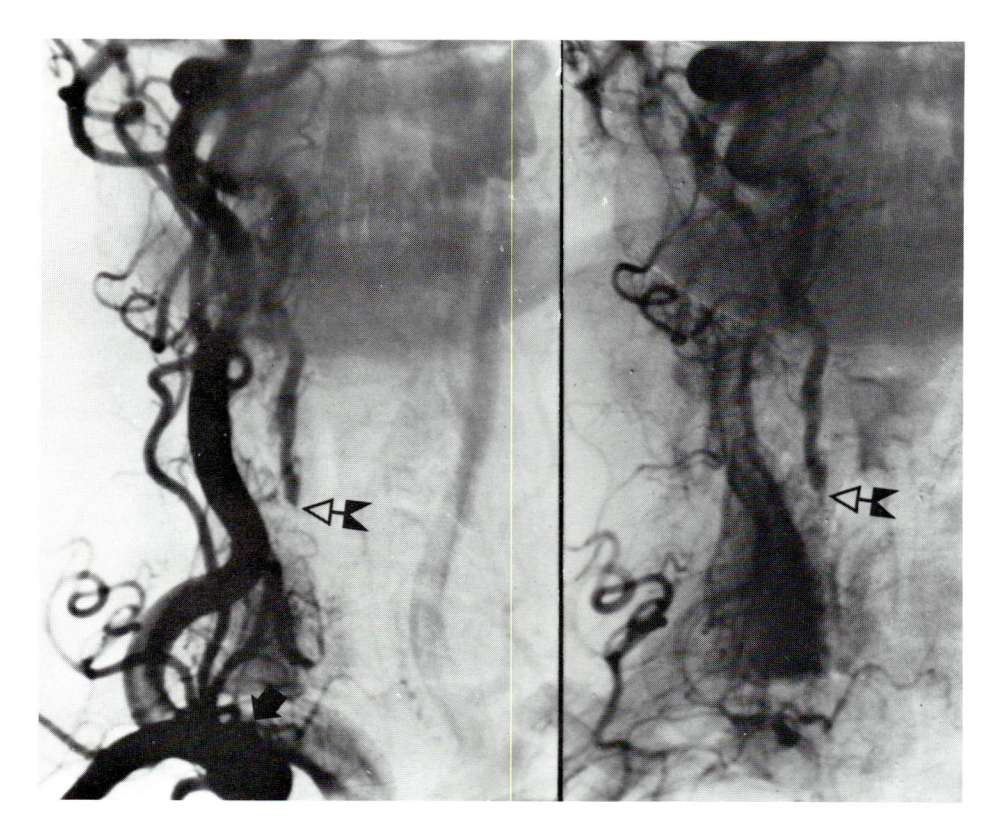

Figure 149-4 Right retrograde brachial cerebral angiograms demonstrating occlusion of the right vertebral artery at its origin (*solid arrow*) with reconstitution in the midcervical region (*open arrow*).

Vertebral Artery Atherosclerosis

TABLE 149-4 Surgical Treatment of Midvertebral Stenosis

Operation	No. of Patients	Angiographic Patency	Postoperative Course	Permanent Complications
Midvertebral endarterectomy	2	2/2	Better	None

nical factors in the dissection of the plaque. Of the three successful intracranial vertebral endarterectomies, two remained patent. Interestingly enough, however, all three patients were symptomatically improved, including the patient whose vertebral artery was not patent postoperatively, raising the possibility of an embolization as a possible cause of the patient's intermittent ischemic symptoms. Only further experience with this operation will determine whether this is a feasible surgical alternative to occipital artery to PICA anastomosis.

Conclusion

We have covered the surgical aspects of vertebral artery atherosclerosis. Although surgical procedures for the treatment of this disease have been performed since the late 1950s and early 1960s, it has only been with recent advances in neuroradiology and increased sophistication in diagnosis that adequate assessment of the entire vertebrobasilar system has been available on a routine basis. The indications for this type of surgery are, therefore, still in the stages of development. It is evident that full and complete diagnostic evaluation, including angiography, is essential before a rational management decision can be made for these patients. More data regarding the natural history of vertebral artery atherosclerosis in an angiogrammed population, as well as its course in populations treated medically and surgically, are needed. Pathological and physiological studies regarding the frequency of embolic versus hemodynamic causes of vertebrobasilar insufficiency are likewise necessary. In the meantime, however, one must make do with the available information when faced with a patient who meets the criteria for the diagnosis of vertebrobasilar insufficiency. Each case must be evaluated on an individual basis. Given a patient with vertebrobasilar insufficiency thought to be due to structural lesions in the vertebral system, the surgical choices include vertebral to carotid transposition for the subclavian steal syndrome and for vertebral origin disease, decompression or bypass for disease in the intraforaminal portion of the artery, and bypass or direct endarterectomy for lesions in the distal vertebral artery. Further experience will reveal whether these operations are reasonable therapeutic alternatives in the management of vertebrobasilar insufficiency due to vertebral artery disease.

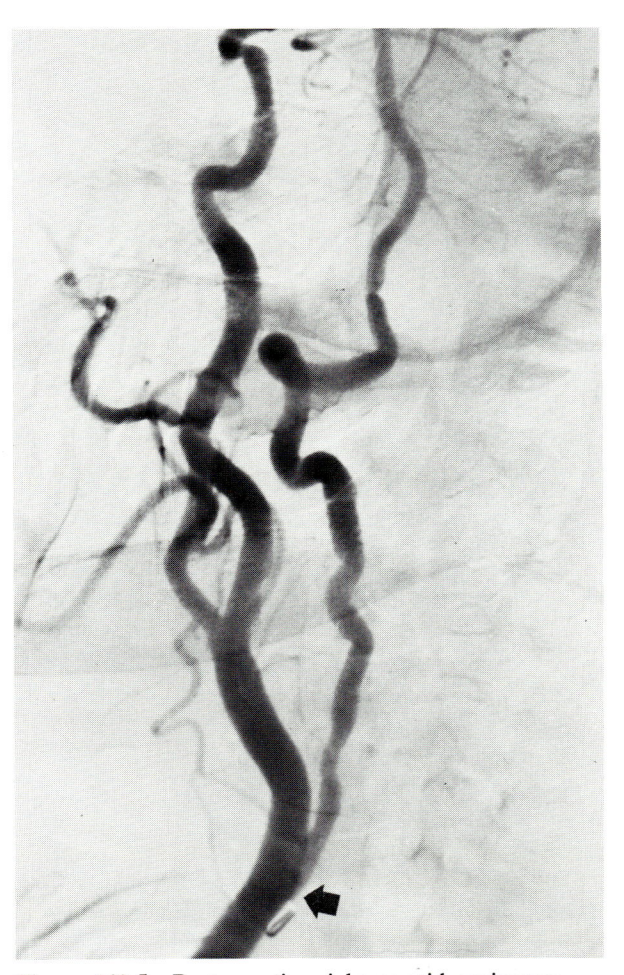

Figure 149-5 Postoperative right carotid angiogram (same patient as in Fig. 149-4) following endarterectomy of the right vertebral artery in the midcervical region and vertebral-carotid transposition. The arrow points to the site of anastomosis.

TABLE 149-5 Surgical Treatment of C1-Intracranial Vertebral Stenosis

Operation	No. of Patients	Angiographic Patency	Postoperative Course	Permanent Complications
Intracranial vertebral endarterectomy	3	2/3	3 better	None
Intracranial vertebral artery ligation	1	—	1 worse	Wallenberg syndrome

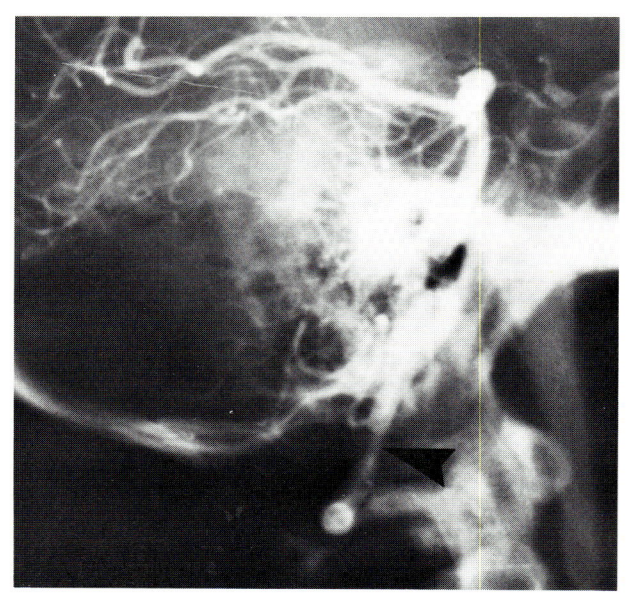

Figure 149-6 Preoperative right vertebral angiogram. The arrowhead points to the area of stenosis at the level of C1.

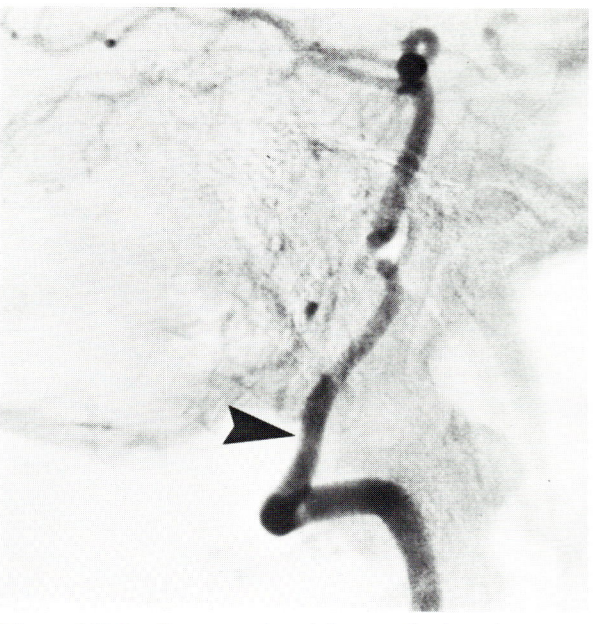

Figure 149-7 Postoperative right vertebral angiogram (same patient as in Fig. 149-6). The arrowhead points to the site of endarterectomy.

References

1. Allen GS, Cohen RJ, Preziosi TJ: Microsurgical endarterectomy of the intracranial vertebral artery for vertebrobasilar transient ischemic attacks. Neurosurgery 8:56–59, 1981.
2. Bohmfalk GL, Story JL, Brown WE Jr, Marlin AE: Subclavian steal syndrome: Part I. Proximal vertebral to common carotid artery transposition in three patients, and historical review. J Neurosurg 51:628–640, 1979.
3. Cartlidge NEF, Whisnant JP, Elveback LR: Carotid and vertebral-basilar transient cerebral ischemic attacks: A community study, Rochester, Minnesota. Mayo Clin Proc 52:117–120, 1977.
4. Castaigne P, Lhermitte F, Gautier JC, Escourolle R, Derouesné C, Der Agopian P, Popa C: Arterial occlusions in the vertebrobasilar system: A study of 44 patients with post-mortem data. Brain 96:133–154, 1973.
5. Corkill G, French BN, Michas C, Cobb CA, Mims TJ: External carotid-vertebral artery anastomosis for vertebrobasilar insufficiency. Surg Neurol 7:109–115, 1977.
6. Nagashima C: Surgical treatment of vertebral artery insufficiency caused by cervical spondylosis. J Neurosurg 32:512–521, 1970.

150

Moyamoya Disease

David G. Piepgras

In the early 1960s, Takeuchi and Suzuki et al. each described a cerebrovascular condition affecting Japanese patients, characterized by angiographic findings of intracranial carotid artery stenoses and occlusions and a fine network of vessels at the base of the brain.[8] The latter angiographic feature, and hallmark of the condition, was called moyamoya for its hazy, puff-of-smoke appearance. Subsequently, case reports, series analyses, and study of pathological material have led to a clearer, but as yet incomplete, understanding of this rare condition. It now appears that the radiographic moyamoya appearance, which is due to numerous dilated collaterals of the basal perforating arteries and arterioles, is nonspecific and may be seen with chronic occlusive processes of the intracranial carotid circulation that arise from a variety of causes, including atherosclerosis, meningitis, sickle cell anemia, and radiation therapy.[7] In addition, but most important, there does seem to exist a distinct entity, moyamoya disease, that occurs most frequently in Japanese people but affects other populations as well, both children and adults and seemingly females more than males. The cause of moyamoya disease remains unknown, and theories of inflammatory and immunologic pathophysiological mechanisms remain unproven. There is strong evidence for hereditary factors in the disease, with familial cases being reported especially among the Japanese but also from Europe and in identical twins.

Radiographic Features

The diagnosis of moyamoya disease is made on the basis of angiographic findings, the features and progression of which have been well described by Suzuki and Takaku.[8] In its earliest stage there is stenosis of the supraclinoid portion of the internal carotid artery, frequently bilaterally. With progression, there develops some dilatation of the main intracerebral arteries, and basal perforating vessels begin to enlarge to form the characteristic moyamoya. Carotid stenoses progress to occlusions, and there is extension of the occlusive process to the middle and anterior cerebral arteries with development of leptomeningeal collaterals and intensification of the moyamoya. This basal vascular network is contributed to by lenticulostriate, choroidal, thalamoperforating, premammillary, and thalamogeniculate arteries as well as by unnamed branches arising directly from the circle of Willis.

Later there may be extension of the occlusion into the posterior communicating and posterior cerebral arteries, with reduction of some of the moyamoya. Conversely, there is enlargement of extracranial transdural collaterals, including meningeal branches; superficial temporal, occipital, and internal maxillary arteries from the external carotid system; and ethmoidal, recurrent meningeal, and anterior falcine arteries from the ophthalmic circulation. Figures 150-1 and 150-2 show typical angiographic changes. In the late stages of the disease, there may be complete obliteration of the internal carotid artery intracranially, disappearance of the moyamoya, and complete dependence of the cerebral circulation on external carotid collaterals and the vertebrobasilar circulation.

Serial angiography in moyamoya disease has shown progressive changes in most childhood cases, whereas the process is less predictable in adults and may arrest itself at any stage or rarely show some spontaneous improvement.[8]

Although not diagnostic, computed tomography may show characteristic changes, including multiple low-density areas in the brain and more general atrophy. With contrast enhancement, tortuous curvilinear vessels in the basal ganglia and cortical surface may be seen corresponding to the moyamoya and leptomeningeal collaterals (Fig. 150-3). The proximal portions of the anterior and middle cerebral arteries are often poorly visualized.[9]

Pathology

The pathological changes of the stenotic and occluded vessels are nonspecific, the most prominent features being intimal thickening and hyperplasia and irregularities in the internal elastic lamina.[8] The moyamoya vessels appear to be markedly dilated intracerebral perforating arteries and arterioles, without abnormal histology,[10] although microaneurysm formation, fibrin deposition, and attenuation of the vessel wall have also been observed.[7]

Clinical Features

In most cases, patients with moyamoya disease present either with brain ischemia or hemorrhage. In children, the most typical symptoms are ischemic, producing recurrent, sometimes alternating episodes of focal cerebral deficit, especially hemiparesis but also speech and sensory disturbances. Seizures and involuntary movement disorders are also more common in children. It has been stated that the severity of moyamoya disease varies inversely with the age of onset; it is most severe in young children, in whom it may produce a progressive course of motor deficit and intellectual deterioration.[2]

In adult patients, intracranial hemorrhage, either subarachnoid or intracerebral and intraventricular, is the most common presenting event, although ischemic symptoms may also occur. Hemorrhages may occur from several different pathological processes. Two of them, moyamoya vessels and pseudoaneurysms, are peculiar to moyamoya disease. Bleeding may also occur from saccular aneurysms, which have a predilection for the vertebrobasilar circulation.

Until recently, the mechanism of hemorrhage in moyamoya disease was usually attributed to a breakdown of the greatly dilated perforating moyamoya vessels that form the extensive basal collateral network. In a survey by Nagamine et al., such a mechanism was identified in 6 of 20 cases.[6] Pseudoaneurysms have also been described in cases of hemorrhage, identified angiographically as discrete vascular dilatations typically arising from the peripheral portions of the perforating and anterior and posterior choroidal arteries in a paraventricular location.[4,6,7] It has been postulated that these pseudoaneurysms form along the abnormally dilated collaterals as a result of hemodynamic stress.[11] Commonly they will be shown to disappear on follow-up angiography.

Saccular aneurysms also have been demonstrated in association with moyamoya disease, with a significantly increased proportion on the basilar artery compared with other aneurysm series. This increased frequency of basilar artery aneurysms has also been attributed to hemodynamic factors of increased flow in the posterior circulation in these patients with compromised carotid arteries.

Therapy

Because of either limited experience or lack of success, there is little information regarding medical therapies for moyamoya disease, although Krayenbühl does allude to reported good results from vasodilator therapy.[5] It is clear, however, that at present no definitive treatment for moyamoya disease exists. Suzuki and Kodama have carried out perivascular sympathectomy and superior cervical ganglionectomy in the treatment of 48 patients, reporting "encouraging" results, with improvement in 61 percent of

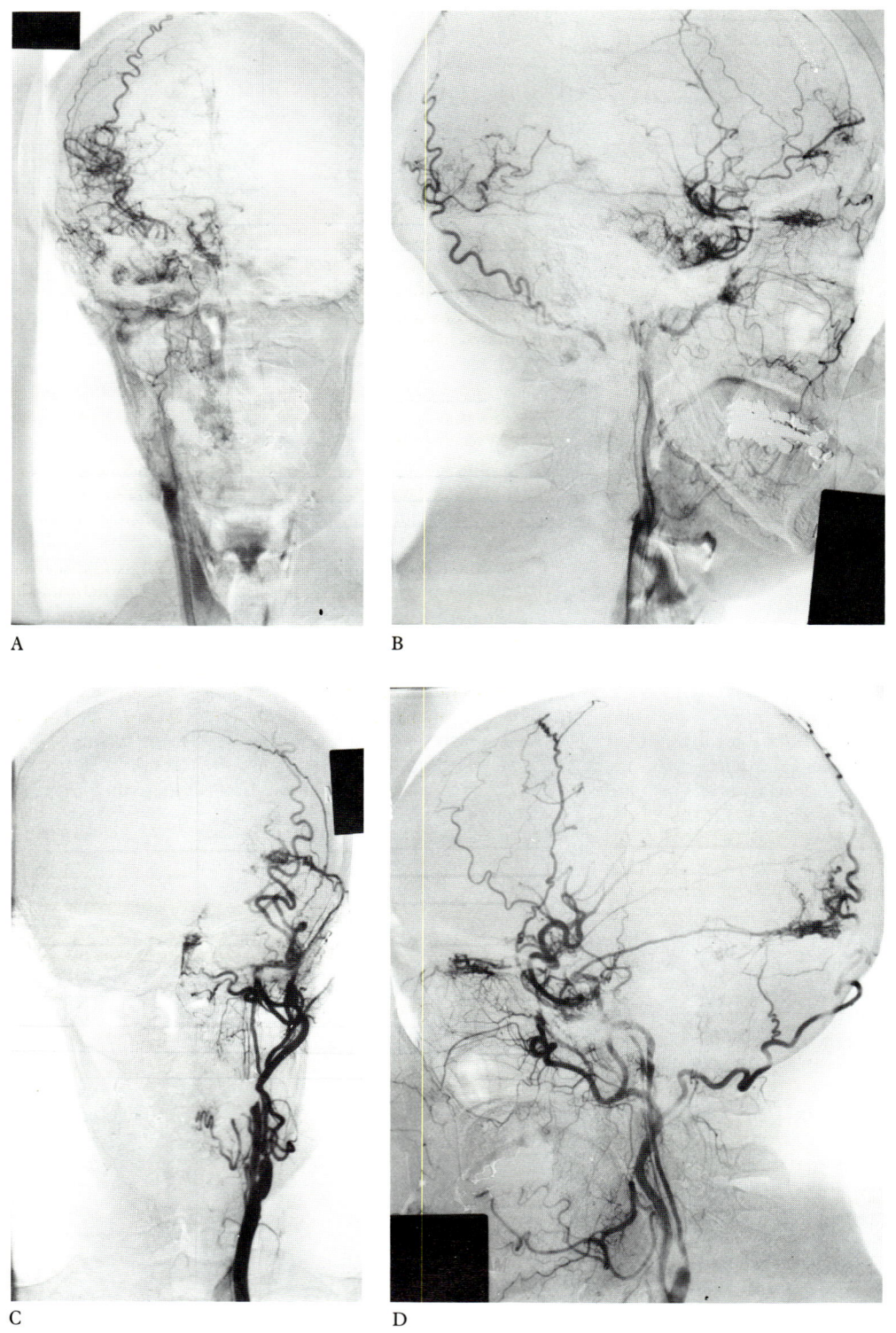

Figure 150-1 Bilateral carotid angiograms in a 52-year-old woman with moyamoya disease. The right carotid angiogram, anteroposterior (A) and lateral (B) views, shows occlusion of the entire right internal carotid artery and extensive external carotid and ophthalmic system collateralization. There is mild moyamoya development. The left carotid angiogram, anteroposterior (C) and lateral (D) views, shows left internal carotid occlusion at the level of the clinoid and similar extensive extracranial to intracranial collaterals.

Moyamoya Disease

children and 47 percent of adults.[7] Other authors have questioned the efficacy of these procedures.

Selected patients suffering from recurrent or progressive focal cerebral ischemic events in the distribution of an occluded or stenotic carotid artery have been successfully treated with superficial temporal to middle cerebral artery (STA-MCA) anastomosis. Boone and Samson reported dramatic resolution of ischemic symptoms in one patient treated with bypass. The improved venous drainage and decrease in the moyamoya disclosed on follow-up angiograms were attributed to improved cerebral perfusion as well.[1] Karasawa et al. reported a series of 23 STA-MCA anastomoses and 7 encephalomyosynangioses in the treatment of 17 patients, although 4 of these cases were probably not moyamoya disease.[3] An excellent outcome with recovery of neurological deficit and disappearance of transient ischemic attacks (TIAs) was found in nine cases, and a good outcome (improvement of neurological deficit and resolution or reduction of TIAs) in five more. Two patients were unchanged, and one had a fair result in a follow-up of 1 to 4 years. These authors also attributed a gradual reduction of basal moyamoya after the bypass to a decreased demand for these collateral channels, although this may also be seen in the course of the disease, as has already been mentioned.

Finally, neurosurgical intervention may be indicated in the treatment of intracranial hemorrhage. As in those patients without moyamoya disease, indications for evacuation of intracerebral hematomas and ventricular drainage should follow standard neurosurgical principles and guidelines.

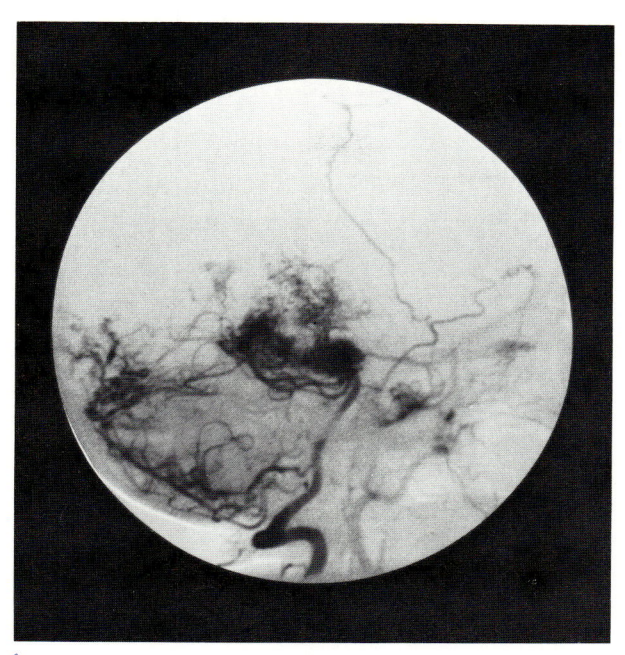

Figure 150-2 Vertebral angiogram, lateral view, of the patient shown in Fig. 150-1 showing normal vertebral and basilar arteries with extensive moyamoya development from the posterior choroidal and posterior perforating vessels.

A

B

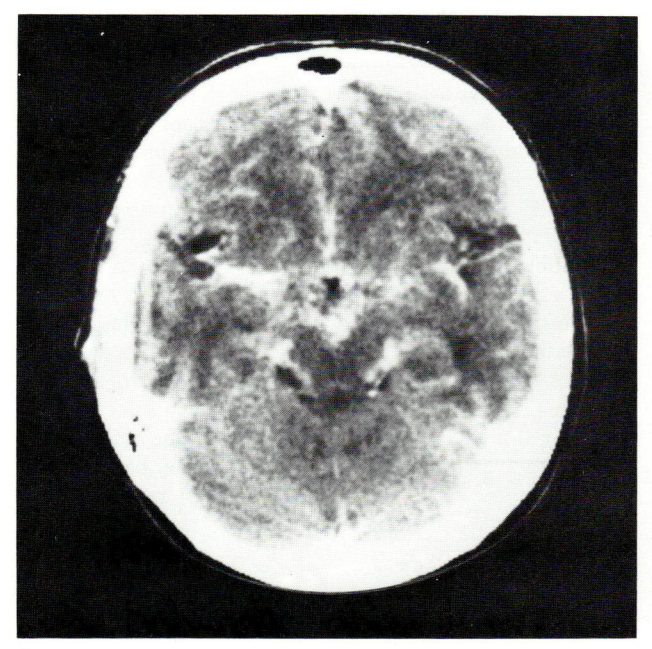

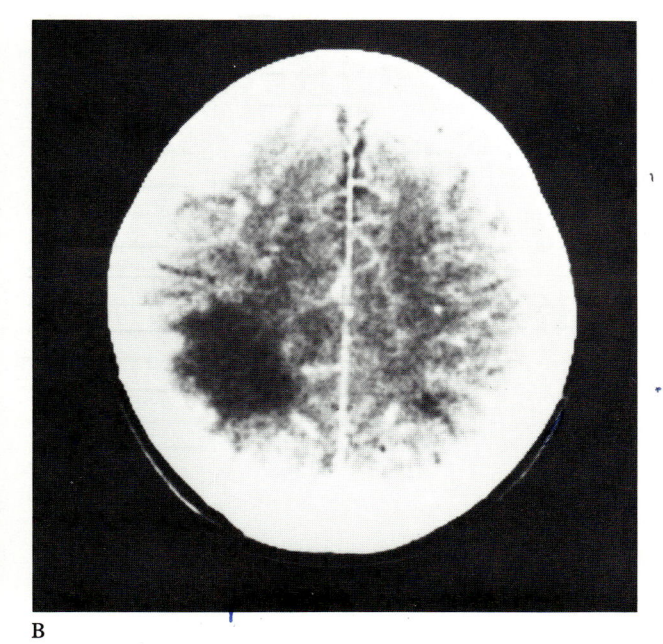

Figure 150-3 A contrast enhanced CT scan of the same patient shown in Figs. 150-1 and 150-2 showing extensive basal collateral (moyamoya) vessels on the lower cut (A). On the higher cut (B), large right and smaller left parietal infarcts are present and enlarged leptomeningeal collateral channels are visualized on the cortical surfaces.

Operations directed at pseudoaneurysms are rarely indicated, however, inasmuch as these lesions usually obliterate themselves, and follow-up angiography is advised in these cases.[4] Occasionally, patients with moyamoya disease will sustain subarachnoid hemorrhage due to a saccular aneurysm, and surgery directed at repair of these lesions, assuming the aneurysm is the likely source of hemorrhage, may be advisable. The surgeon must be aware, however, that the presence of moyamoya vessels may limit the exposure and increase the risks of ischemic complications.[6]

References

1. Boone SC, Samson DS: Observation on moyamoya disease: A case treated with superficial temporal-middle cerebral artery anastomosis. Surg Neurol 9:189–193, 1978.
2. Carlson CB, Harvey FH, Loop J: Progressive alternating hemiplegia in early childhood with basal arterial stenosis and telangiectasia (moyamoya syndrome). Neurology (Minneap) 23:734–744, 1973.
3. Karasawa J, Kikuchi H, Furuse S, Kawamura J, Sakaki T: Treatment of moyamoya disease with STA-MCA anastomosis. J Neurosurg 49:679–688, 1978.
4. Kodama N, Suzuki J: Moyamoya disease associated with aneurysm. J Neurosurg 48:565–569, 1978.
5. Krayenbühl HA: The moyamoya syndrome and the neurosurgeon. Surg Neurol 4:353–360, 1975.
6. Nagamine Y, Takahashi S, Sonobe M: Multiple intracranial aneurysms associated with moyamoya disease: Case report. J Neurosurg 54:673–676, 1981.
7. Suzuki J, Kodama N: Moyamoya disease: A review. Stroke 14:104–109, 1983.
8. Suzuki J, Takaku A: Cerebrovascular "moyamoya" disease: Disease showing abnormal net-like vessels in base of brain. Arch Neurol 20:288–299, 1969.
9. Takahashi M, Miyauchi T, Kowada M: Computed tomography of moyamoya disease: Demonstration of occluded arteries and collateral vessels as important diagnostic signs. Radiology 134:671–676, 1980.
10. Takeuchi K, Hara M, Yokota H, Okada J, Akai K: Factors influencing the development of moyamoya phenomenon. Acta Neurochir (Wien) 59:79–86, 1981.
11. Tanaka Y, Takeuchi K, Akai K: Intracranial ruptured aneurysm accompanying moyamoya phenomenon. Acta Neurochir (Wien) 52:35–43, 1980.

151

Medical Treatment of Ischemic Cerebral Vascular Disease

H. J. M. Barnett

Hemorrhagic and ischemic stroke have declined by an astonishing 45 percent in 25 years. A clear understanding of the exact reason(s) behind this decline would serve as a most useful guide in planning further preventive measures. Remarkably, the exact role of any of the possible causal factors is not readily identifiable. In vital statistics deaths attributed to hypertension and rheumatic heart disease, two conditions closely linked to stroke, have declined dramatically during this same period. Several other concomitant phenomena coincide with this record decline of the last decade. The number of carotid endarterectomies has increased threefold in the decade, and the sales of aspirin have gone up in North America by nearly 20 percent. Because the decline in stroke has been most steep during the last few years, the temptation is to claim that some or all of these developments and treatments have played a role. Caution must be exercised in assuming such a direct relationship. For example, the enthusiasm for endarterectomy in Europe has not been comparable to its increased performance in North America, and yet the decline is shared on the two continents. Endarterectomy is an uncommon procedure in Japan, but here too the stroke decline has begun to follow that in the other developed countries. No figures are available for aspirin usage in Europe or Japan. Lacking as well are sufficient details on the extent of changes in lifestyle, such as fat intake and cigarette smoking, to allow for any conclusions about their impact on the decline. The most important factor behind the reduced morbidity and mortality from vascular stroke appears on the surface to be improvement in the control of hypertension.

The effect of risk factors in stroke have been examined very carefully in the Framingham study.[20] The possibility of attending to risk factors in stroke prevention has been addressed by the same group, and will not be reviewed here. This chapter will concern itself with a review of the current knowledge regarding antithrombotic agents in stroke-threatened patients.

Antithrombotic Therapy

Antithrombotic agents, consisting of anticoagulants and platelet inhibitors, will be discussed here with certain mandatory rules concerning the source and the admissibility of the information:

1. An evaluation of any form of treatment to be used in stroke prevention requires a close scrutiny of the methodology used in every study purporting to claim or to deny a benefit.
2. An evaluation demands critical appraisal of the evidence or otherwise of skillful neurological input into the reported observations.
3. Evaluation of treatment by anecdotes or by nothing more than "clinical judgment" is of no value in chronic disease processes where the event-rate is low.
4. Comparison of results with historical controls is of little value in the light of the sharp decline of stroke; this changing baseline distorts comparisons in favor of any proposed treatment.
5. The reduction and even the cessation of transient ischemic attacks (TIAs) is of dubious value as a measure of successful treatment because not infrequently TIAs are known to cease spontaneously.
6. Laboratory data are of value in assessing treatment modalities only when they are correlated carefully with clinical results. Such data have been studied, for example, with attempts to record improved abnormalities of platelet function in the evaluation of platelet antiaggregant therapy and with the normalization of regional cerebral blood flow and oxygen extraction fractions recorded in the study of revascularization procedures. In none of these instances have impressive correlates with the real goal of stroke prevention emerged.

For all chronic diseases in which few end points occur on an annual basis and in which the disease is of protean nature, *the gold standard for evaluating therapy is the well-designed clinical trial.* A sufficient number of patients must be entered; a truly comparable, contemporary, and bias-free control group must be made available from the same population; and the randomization into treatment categories must be done in such a way as to avoid any hint of prejudice. The process is very consuming of time, energy, and money, but the alternatives yield vague and unconvincing results.

Good methodology by itself is not enough to ensure a believable study. *Sophisticated clinical input* into trials assessing therapy is obligatory. In the case of threatened stroke it is apparent that some reports overlook the fact that the term *TIA* describes not a single entity but a group of conditions (to be detailed below). It is not possible, for example, to compare results from one study confined to patients with atherothrombotic disease in the extracranial arteries to another study that includes patients with lacunar disease, cardiac emboli, spontaneous arterial dissection, fibromuscular dysplasia, and other entities. Some of these disorders, such as spontaneous dissection, are representative of low-risk categories in terms of prognosis and natural history. By contrast, others, such as cardiac embolic lesions, contribute high-risk categories of patients. Natural history studies and prognostic assessments are of importance in determining the sample-size requirements for studies designed to evaluate treatment. The relative risks of endpoints in particular populations are recognized, including the differential prognosis known to exist in the several varieties of pathogenic mechanisms producing TIA, in the different age groups, and in the sex distribution of the population under study.

Anticoagulants and platelet antiaggregants in stroke prevention will be reviewed in the light of these general principles.

Anticoagulants

Set against the background of modern biostatistics, methodological principles, and the need for expert clinical determination of the neurology of threatened stroke, it is fair to state that acceptable evaluation of anticoagulants has never been done. Using the randomized clinical trial as the gold standard, four reported clinical trials have addressed the question of the value of warfarin sodium for TIA patients.[3,4,14,19] The aggregate of patients in the control group was a mere 85, followed for an average of 21 months; the aggregate of patients in the active treatment group was only 93 with an average follow-up of 21 months. In the follow-up period 8 strokes occurred in the treatment groups and 10 in the control patients; 15 patients died in the treated groups compared with 10 in the control groups. The difference in mortality was related to the increase in deaths linked to hemorrhage in the patients receiving warfarin.

These data cannot be interpreted as showing that there is no value in giving warfarin sodium to patients with TIAs. The conclusion must be that adequate information on the subject is lacking because not a single study acceptable to modern critics has been carried out. The numbers were too small (even in aggregate), and the mix of patients is unknown. Patients with cardiac causes, as well as those with small hemorrhages detectable only by CT scanning and those with other types of ischemic lesions, some of lower risk, in all probability were unknowingly included. Risk factors were not recognized as being of such consequence as is the case today, were not known to be balanced in the treatment groups, and were not attended to in the baseline therapy. Finally, the scrupulous care with which warfarin must be administered was not always understood and could have unfavorably distorted the results compared with what might be obtained today, especially in terms of mortality. Added to this catalog of paucity and uncertainty of information is the knowledge that the use of warfarin carries a definite risk even when utilized with optimum care.

It is clear that decisions about the use of warfarin and heparin must be made on the basis of empiricism. Although empirical decisions are not ideal for any therapeutic strategy, they may be acceptable where no additional data are available for a treatment based on reasonably rational assumptions. It remains common practice to administer, empirically, warfarin and heparin under the circumstances outlined in Tables 151-1 and 151-2, where noncardiac and cardiac causes of cerebral ischemic events, respectively, are suspect. *It is emphasized that each case is different and all must be judged carefully on their own merits with as much knowledge as possible of causal mechanisms.*

It is not the purpose of this chapter to comment on the surgical management of cerebral arterial lesions. It is evident that some individuals with TIA, reversible ischemic neurological disability (RIND), and partial nonprogressing stroke (PNS) will not be, or may not consent to be, candidates for endarterectomy or a revascularization procedure. If such

TABLE 151-1 Empirical Indications for Anticoagulation in Cerebral Ischemic Events of Noncardiac Origin

A. Atherothrombotic or nonarteriosclerotic arterial lesions causing ischemic symptoms not responsive to platelet antiaggregants
B. Ischemic symptoms in conditions where coagulation abnormalities are known or suspected
C. Thrombi visualized in the poststenotic portion of carotid arteries
D. Venous origin
   1. Thrombi suspected in pulmonary veins
   2. Peripheral venous thrombosis with patent foramen ovale
   3. Cerebral vein and sinus thrombosis
E. Progressing stroke

---

individuals continue to have cerebral ischemic events despite the use of platelet antiaggregant therapy, it is common practice to administer warfarin to these individual patients. Because there is a tendency for TIA symptoms to come and go spontaneously, it is reasonable to utilize warfarin in this group of patients not responding to or unable to tolerate platelet antiaggregants. It should be given for a finite period, usually 3 months, and reinstituted later should a failure again attend a return to platelet inhibitors. This recommendation would be applicable whether or not the patient was admitted to the treatment regimen with a few or with many ischemic events. Patients experiencing a large number of TIAs at the beginning of therapy are just as likely to be responsive to antithrombotic therapy as those reporting a few or single episodes. There is no convincing support in any published data for the concept of "crescendo TIAs" as the neurological counterpart to "crescendo angina." Indeed there is as much or more danger in a single or a few retinal or cerebral TIAs as with a flurry of TIAs. The presence of many events, therefore, does not commend an immediate use of anticoagulants in preference to platelet antiaggregants.

Anticoagulants are more rational when thrombosis is suspected to have been induced by a triggering of the coagulation cascade, in contrast to a platelet-induced thrombogenesis. This applies for example to young individuals evidencing ischemic events while taking the contraceptive pill or in the postpartum period. It applies to individuals of any age with known cancer, with recognizable coagulation disturbances associated with thrombosis, or who develop ischemia after a general surgical procedure, or who have been subjected to trauma other than to the neck or head. In most of these individuals, a short period of 6 to 12 weeks on anticoagulants is indicated.

Stenosis in arteries is associated with poststenotic dilatation, and at times under these circumstances the poststenotic segment of a cervical carotid artery is the site of a radiologically recognized thrombus. At times, an arterial thrombus can be observed intracranially as well. In a similar way, trauma with or without dissection of a cervical carotid artery may be accompanied by visible thrombus formation in the neck and/or in the intracranial arteries. Some neurosurgeons are on record as regarding these individuals as candidates for emergency endarterectomy. In my experience, these patients are in a higher operative risk category than those without visible thrombi, and I recommend a 6- to 8-week period on anticoagulants, followed by further angiography as a prelude to consideration of surgery. Downstream thrombi must contribute to the fact that the risk to this group is high, and since the downstream lesions are inaccessible, the argument favoring a period of anticoagulant stabilization is strengthened.

Venous disease proceeding to thrombus formation is accompanied by a triggering of the coagulation cascade more than disorders of the faster-flowing arterial channels in which platelet-induced thrombogenesis is of greater importance. Thus, the use of anticoagulants, heparin followed by warfarin, is a rational but empirical therapy. Thrombi may be suspected in pulmonary veins in patients with prolonged pulmonary sepsis but also in patients who have experienced serious chest trauma. Other venous disorders, all of which are difficult at times to recognize, are listed in Table 151-1.

Progressing stroke, wherein a stepwise or (most uncommonly) an indolent progression of neurological disability is observed over a number of hours, may be due to recurrent thromboembolic phenomena or (rarely) to extension of an intraluminal thrombus into more distal parts of the arterial tree. These would be indications for such effective antithrombotic therapy as is available. Other phenomena related to the damaged brain may be of more consequence, however, in determining the neurological decline. Unfortunately, the distinction between a stroke worsening because of these thrombotic processes and one that is worsening as a result of spreading edema or because of the development of a hemorrhagic component to the infarction is difficult. Progressing stroke is identified in approximately 20 percent of patients. It is common custom in progressing stroke to institute anticoagulant therapy. The evidence upon which this therapy is based is scanty. Heparin administration followed in sequence by warfarin for 6 to 12 weeks appears to be a rational, albeit unproven, therapy. The need for a major study of this problem is very apparent.

Cardiac lesions are recognized with increasing frequency as important in cerebral ischemic lesions at all ages. They can be more readily identified as the main operative cause in younger patients. The offending thromboemboli vary in size because the origin may be from a very large thrombus, as in the atrium of a patient with mitral stenosis, or may be com-

---

TABLE 151-2 Empirical Indications for Anticoagulants in Cerebral Ischemic Events of Cardiac Origin

A. Myocardial infarction
   1. Recent—large, septal, with atrial fibrillation, with congestive failure
   2. Old—with akinetic segment
   3. Either, with thrombi visualized in heart chambers
B. Mitral stenosis
   1. With atrial fibrillation
   2. Without atrial fibrillation but symptomatic of thromboembolism
C. Atrial fibrillation, irrespective of cardiac cause with evidence of cerebral or retinal ischemia
D. Prosthetic heart valve
E. Miscellaneous valvular lesions, in the treatment of which platelet antiaggregants have failed
F. Other miscellaneous heart conditions

ing from a platelet-fibrin thrombus of less than 3 mm in size attached to an ulcerative lesion in myxomatous degeneration of the mitral valve (prolapsing mitral valve, PMV). In the case of cardiac lesions productive of cerebral emboli it is not possible to state that any of the indications (Table 151-2) has been unequivocally validated by acceptable trials. The best studies have been those in which episodes of thromboembolism from prosthetic heart valves have been reduced in number by anticoagulants with or without platelet antiaggregants.[17] However, empirical indications on reasonably rational grounds appear to exist to commend the use of anticoagulants in the conditions listed in Table 151-2.

Thromboembolism resulting from endocardial damage as a result of myocardial infarction is common, and in approximately 2 percent of patients affected with myocardial ischemia the clinical features of retinal or cerebral ischemia complicate their illness. The risk of stroke is increased if the myocardial infarct is a large one, if it involves the septum, or if there is coexisting congestive heart failure or atrial fibrillation. When any of these phenomena complicates a myocardial infarction, justification can be advanced for a period of 3 months on anticoagulant therapy. Similarly, a thrombus visualized by echocardiogram or wall motion study in the ventricle provides justification for this therapeutic decision. Such thrombi may occur in the weeks following a myocardial infarction or may develop in an akinetic segment. In the latter there may be no alternative to the prolonged use of warfarin. Opinion is divided as to whether or not surgical removal of these akinetic segments is an alternative strategy, but its discussion is beyond the scope of this chapter.

For the most part, the use of warfarin can be regarded as a finite procedure in the circumstances listed in Table 151-1 and in those related to myocardial infarction. The other indications listed in Table 151-2 present the disturbing possibility of a need for the prolonged usage of a hazardous medication. The administration of anticoagulants under these circumstances demands an accurate diagnosis and a rigid program for their usage. A search for alternative safer measures must be continued.

Hemorrhagic cerebral infarction is commonest when the origin is related to thromboembolism. The heart is often the source of the larger thrombi producing the larger areas of cerebral infarction, and these large lesions have a propensity to become visibly hemorrhagic. The use of the CT scan for the exclusion of hemorrhagic infarction is an acceptable alternative to withholding warfarin therapy for 48 to 72 h.

Platelet Antiaggregants

Sufficient information has been amassed about the use of platelet-inhibiting drugs to indicate that they have a role, for the time being, in stroke prevention. Yet they are imperfect:

1. A number of individuals progress to ischemia of minor and major degree despite their use.
2. A number of individuals cannot tolerate them largely because of gastrointestinal upset, including hemorrhage.
3. They have not been tested in a number of the varieties of threatened stroke.
4. Their use after the coagulation cascade has been triggered and in the presence of a substantial quantity of thrombus material is dubious.

There is no resolution as yet about the problems relating to the optimum dosage, the apparent difference of responsiveness between sexes, and the possibility that a combination of platelet antiaggregants is superior to the use of one alone. They should not be regarded as an alternative to all or any other therapeutic strategies, and should not preclude attention to the management of recognized risk factors nor consideration of potential surgical measures.

Two trials have had sufficiently large numbers of patients randomized into well-disciplined double-blind and placebo-controlled studies to qualify for acceptability by modern methodological and neurological standards. In my study, 585 patients followed for an average of 26 months were given 1300 mg of aspirin per day in divided dosage with a placebo, 800 mg of sulfinpyrazone per day with a placebo, both of these active treatments, or simply the placebo of both.[8] The results, which have been reported, involved patients with carotid or vertebral-basilar symptoms, with or without minor residual neurological deficit, and indicated a 30 percent reduction in stroke or death, but the reduction reached significance only in males, in whom a 50 percent reduction in stroke or death and in stroke or fatal stroke was achieved. There was no benefit from sulfinpyrazone and no significant difference between the groups that were given aspirin alone or aspirin with sulfinpyrazone. The collaborative trial from Paris compared 1200 mg of aspirin per day against placebo, entered 600 patients, followed them for an average of 36 months, and had a higher percentage of patients who at entry to the trial had some residual than in the Canadian study.[7] The results for stroke and stroke death in the aspirin-treated group indicated a 50 percent risk reduction, in both sexes, compared with the placebo group.

Two smaller placebo-controlled studies, one of 179 patients[11] and one of 58 patients,[16] yielded positive benefit for four tablets of aspirin per day compared with placebo. Two other studies, of medium size and duration, one with 203 patients studied in Copenhagen, and one with 302 patients from Toulouse, gave negative results for 1 g of aspirin per day.

In two large trials designed to assess the possible benefit in reducing recurrent myocardial ischemia use of aspirin was compared with placebo (AMIS trial),[2] and aspirin alone was compared with aspirin and dipyridamole, both controlled by placebo (PARIS trial).[15] In these studies, four aspirin tablets (1200 mg) per day were administered. Neither study revealed a benefit in risk reduction that was significant in terms of the prevention of recurrent myocardial infarction, but in both studies the number of strokes in the aspirin-treated groups were reduced by close to 50 percent compared with the placebo groups. Because there were too few patients with stroke as the endpoint (despite the fact that approximately 7000 patients entered the studies subsequent to myocardial infarction), the results were interesting but not quite statistically significant.

Only one small study, a negative one, has addressed the possible value of dipyridamole alone in stroke prevention.[1] This cannot be construed as the final answer here. There is an American-Canadian study nearing completion consisting of 900 patients who have received either four tablets of aspirin (1200 mg) or the same dose coupled with 300 mg of dipyridamole.[18] The results of this comparison will be available in early 1984.

There remain several burning issues yet to settle in terms of stroke prevention with aspirin and other platelet inhibitors. The first to consider is that a number of conditions have not yet been subjected to clinical trials to test the efficacy of these agents (Table 151-3). Some of these conditions are too uncommon for truly meaningful trials to be done, even on a multicenter basis.

The prognosis for patients who have suffered cerebral ischemia due to fibromuscular dysplasia or to spontaneous arterial dissection has been shown in recent studies to be good. It is evident that platelet inhibitors are a reasonably rational prophylaxis, but the disorders are sufficiently infrequent that a clinical trial is not likely to become available. The value of the therapy will remain speculative but its usage reasonable. After neck trauma from direct or indirect injury (e.g., manipulation), carotid and vertebral arteries suffer endothelial damage, dissection, and even occlusion. In all but the latter, a period on platelet antiaggregants is a reasonable therapy to consider for patients symptomatic from these conditions. In the instance of fibromuscular dysplasia, an indefinite usage of aspirin therapy, if tolerated, would be indicated. For dissections, spontaneous or otherwise, a 6-month period followed by digital angiography to reappraise the need would be recommended.

There is a clinical variety of postradiation arteriopathy in which the sclerosis of the carotid artery (common, internal, and external) produces a devastating constrictive effect and there are no indications of recurrent ischemic events suggestive of thromboembolism. On other occasions, repeated events proclaim the real possibility that there is endothelial damage with thrombi forming, and in these patients the use of aspirin will be a first therapeutic measure.

Clear evidence has been advanced in experimental studies that aspirin will diminish the platelet-fibrin thrombi that form on an intra-arterial catheter tip, at the site of direct arterial puncture, and in the area of endothelial damage produced by the catheter. Hence, the rationale has been established to utilize aspirin (and in some centers, for fear of an elevation in bleeding time initiated by its use, to utilize dipyridamole) for individuals to be subjected to arteriography. No studies have been done to support this prophylaxis, but in my center the administration of four tablets of aspirin in the 24 h before angiography is routine. It is coupled, of course with other precautions, including the careful administration of fluids, if necessary by intravenous route, to ensure adequate hydration prior to the procedure.

In experimental studies on dogs, endarterectomy has been followed by fewer thrombotic obstructions when aspirin has been administered. This use of platelet inhibitors has not been studied in an organized fashion in human subjects after surgery, but a recent randomized trial in coronary artery bypass surgery that utilized dipyridamole preoperatively and administered dipyridamole in conjunction with 1 g of aspirin postoperatively yielded very convincing and statistically significant information about the patency of the grafts in the treated group compared with those patients given placebo.[9] This was validated by postoperative angiograms, first of all in those done, on the average, on the eighth postoperative day, and was substantiated in over 300 patients when a further angiogram was carried out a year after the operative procedure.[10] It would appear very reasonable to recommend platelet antiaggregants before and as a sequel to carotid endarterectomy and superficial temporal to middle cerebral artery bypass procedures.

It is beyond the scope of this chapter to discuss cardiac valvular lesions in detail. Suffice it to say that in younger individuals there is unequivocal evidence that thromboembolism is associated with lesions on the atrial surface of a prolapsing mitral valve. Similarly there is indirect evidence that in an older individual the same valve that is the site of mitral annulus calcification (MAC) will be accompanied at times by cerebral and retinal ischemic events. Some of these events will be related to embolization from the fragmented caseating lesion on the surface, and others will be of thrombotic origin.[6] It is not possible to distinguish between them, nor is it possible to be sure when the ischemic events are related to coexisting arterial disease. Again, no definitive studies have been done, but platelet antiaggregants in the form of four aspirin tablets (approximately 1 g) per day are recommended as the initial therapy when these conditions are identified as the suspicious site of origin for the ischemic occurrences. In theory, if nonbacterial thrombotic endocarditis can be recognized in vivo, the platelet-fibrin thrombi that adhere to the valves in these conditions might be prevented from becoming thromboembolic with the use of aspirin. Most often this condition is a postmortem diagnosis. Prosthetic heart valves remain thrombogenic. Earlier studies have indicated that a combination of warfarin and a platelet inhibitor are better than an anticoagulant alone.[17] There is no evidence that platelet inhibitors alone have reduced the incidence of thromboembolism, and at this point in time this is not recommended. Although some reports have suggested that warfarin with aspirin can be utilized without hemorrhagic consequences, it has not been the general experience and is not recommended. Warfarin and dipyridamole (50 mg four times per day) are two substances that may be used together, with less risk of aggravated bleeding, and this would be a more acceptable recommendation.

Lacunar infarction, in the early descriptions of this entity, was associated with hypertensive arteriolar disease.

TABLE 151-3 Indications for Platelet Antiaggregants (No Clinical Trials)

A. Nonarteriosclerotic lesions of major arteries
  1. Fibromuscular dysplasia
  2. Postdissection aneurysms
  3. Post-traumatic arteriopathy
  4. Postradiation arteriopathy
B. Preangiogram prophylaxis
C. Prophylaxis after endarterectomy or extracranial-intracranial bypass
D. Cardiac valvular lesions
  1. Prolapsing mitral valve (PMV)
  2. Mitral annulus calcification (MAC)
  3. Nonbacterial thrombotic endocarditis (NBTE)
  4. Prosthetic valve
E. Lacunar infarction
F. Asymptomatic bruits and stenoses

When this is the case, the patients must be treated primarily with antihypertensive therapy. More recent descriptions have enlarged the scope of this disorder to include microemboli to the penetrating vessels supplying the pons, basal ganglia, and capsular regions. A condition of microatheroma in these small arteries has been postulated as well, but lacks adequate pathological definition. The ischemic events in the category described as lacunar infarction are reasonable considerations for the use of platelet inhibitors.

Asymptomatic carotid bruits and stenoses are the subject of considerable controversy. I am of the opinion that any evidence that they are best treated by surgery is totally unconvincing. No data exist comparing the benefit for such patients treated with platelet antiaggregants and those not treated at all. On an empirical basis, the use of platelet inhibitors is recommended, particularly when there is no question that the origin of the bruit is from the arteries and not from the heart and where it is certain that it is not of venous origin. Frequently this information will have been acquired by the use of noninvasive studies or digital venous angiography.

Controversy has developed regarding the optimum dosage of aspirin to be administered in stroke prevention since the determination that prostacyclin formed in the vessel wall exerts a protective benefit against intravascular thrombosis and has vasodilating properties. Its production is inhibited by the usual platelet antiaggregants through inhibition of the enzyme cyclo-oxygenase. This inhibition, theoretically, is undesirable, but at the same time the inhibition of the same enzyme in the membrane of the platelet and interference with thromboxane production has the desirable effect of producing a diminished tendency to thrombosis and to vasoconstriction. In vitro experiments indicate that it might be possible to reduce the effective interference with prostacyclin production by a small dose of aspirin and yet maintain the inhibition of the thromboxane production. The antithrombotic effect of one-half tablet (165 mg) per day in plastic tubes inserted for dialysis in subjects afflicted with renal failure has been shown to be effective.[12] No comparison has been made, however, with a similar placebo-controlled study utilizing four aspirin tablets per day, and there is no information as to whether or not one tablet is better than four with a similar placebo-controlled study utilizing four aspirins per day. Therefore, there is no information as to whether one tablet is better than four in these circumstances. Likewise, a single tablet of aspirin per day, when administered to patients afflicted with unstable angina, protected against death and myocardial infarction as compared with a placebo group.[13] Once again, no comparison was made between one and four tablets. These clinical (and in the case of the plastic tubes, artificial) circumstances cannot be interpreted as comparable to patients with stroke-threatening symptoms from cardiac or arterial causes. In vitro data and data from different disease processes may serve as a guide to future study but cannot be utilized as convincing evidence sufficient to initiate proven therapy. Fortunately, the British have a very large study nearing completion wherein 1500 patients have been given either placebo, one tablet of aspirin, or four tablets of aspirin per day. These TIA patients will be followed until 1985 when the analysis will determine whether one tablet is superior to four and whether either are superior to placebo in a major repetition of the Canadian and French trials (C. Warlow, personal communication).

The Canadian study found no substantial benefit for female patients taking aspirin.[8] On the other hand, a 50 percent reduction in male and female patients was found in TIA and minor stroke patients studied in the multicenter study conducted by Bousser et al. in Paris.[7] This conflicting evidence has emerged from two studies, into each of which only 200 female patients were entered. Because it is known now that females with TIA and minor stroke have a significantly better prognosis than do males,[5] it is evident that both the Canadian and French studies were directing attention in this subgroup to lower-risk patients. Conclusive evidence one way or the other cannot be drawn from these two small groups of females. Again, the final answer may come from the British study, where approximately 500 female patients will have been entered and followed for an average of greater than 4 years.

It is evident that antithrombotic agents have an important role to play in stroke prevention. It is equally evident that they are imperfect and that they should be used in conjunction with properly evaluated surgical measures and the careful attention to the management of risk factors.

References

1. Acheson J, Danta G, Hutchinson EC: Controlled trial of dipyridamole in cerebral vascular disease: Br Med J [Clin Res] 1:614–615, 1969.
2. Aspirin Myocardial Infarction Study Research Group: A randomized, controlled trial of aspirin in persons recovered from myocardial infarction. JAMA 243:661–669, 1980.
3. Baker RN, Broward JA, Fang HC, Fisher CM, Groch SN, Heyman A, Karp HR, McDevitt E, Scheinberg P, Schwartz W, Toole JF: Anticoagulant therapy in cerebral infarction: Report on cooperative study. Neurology 12:823–835, 1962.
4. Baker RN, Schwartz WS, Rose AS: Transient ischemic strokes: A report of a study of anticoagulant therapy. Neurology 16:841–847, 1966.
5. Barnett HJM: The Canadian Cooperative Study of platelet-suppressive drugs in transient cerebral ischemia, in Price TR, Nelson E (eds): *Cerebrovascular Diseases: Eleventh Princeton Conference.* New York, Raven Press, 1979, pp 221–236.
6. Barnett HJM: Heart in ischemic stroke—a changing emphasis. Neurol Clin 1:291–315, 1983.
7. Bousser MG, Eschwege E, Haguenau M, Lefaucconnier JM, Thibult N, Touboul D, Touboul PJ: "AICLA" controlled trial of aspirin and dipyridamole in the secondary prevention of athero-thrombotic cerebral ischemia. Stroke 14:5–14, 1983.
8. Canadian Cooperative Study Group: A randomized trial of aspirin and sulfinpyrazone in threatened stroke. N Engl J Med 299:53–59, 1978.
9. Chesebro JH, Clements IP, Fuster V, Elveback LR, Smith HC, Bardsley WT, Frye RL, Holmes DR Jr, Vlietstra RE, Pluth JR, Wallace RB, Puga FJ, Orszulak TA, Piehler JM, Schaff HV, Danielson GK: A platelet-inhibitor-drug trial in coronary-artery bypass operations: Benefit of perioperative dipyridamole and aspirin therapy on early postoperative vein-graft patency. N Engl J Med 307:73–78, 1982.
10. Chesebro JH, Clements IP, Fuster V, Elveback LR, Smith HC, Bardsley WT, Frye RH, Holmes DR, Pluth JR: Benefit of perioperative dipyridamole plus aspirin therapy for late postopera-

tive aortocoronary vein graft patency. Circulation 66 [Suppl 2]: II-94, 1982 (abstr).
11. Fields WS, Lemak NA, Frankowski RF, Hardy RJ: Controlled trial of aspirin in cerebral ischemia. Stroke 8:301–314, 1977.
12. Harter HR, Burch JW, Majerus PW, Stanford N, Delmez JA, Anderson CB, Weerts CA: Prevention of thrombosis in patients on hemodialysis by low-dose aspirin. N Engl J Med 301:577–579, 1978.
13. Lewis HD Jr, Davis JW, Archibald DG, Steinke WE, Smitherman TC, Doherty JE III, Schnaper HW, LeWinter MM, Linares E, Pouget JM, Sabharwal SC, Chesler E, DeMots H: Protective effects of aspirin against acute myocardial infarction and death in men with unstable angina: Results of a Veterans Administration Cooperative Study. N Engl J Med 309:396–403, 1983.
14. Pearce JMS, Gubbay SS, Walton JN: Long-term anticoagulant therapy in transient cerebral ischaemic attacks. Lancet 1:6–9, 1965.
15. Persantine-Aspirin Reinfarction Study Research Group: Persantine and aspirin in coronary heart disease. Circulation 62:449–461, 1980.
16. Reuther R, Dorndorf W, Loew D: Behandlung transitorisch-ischämischer Attaken mit Azetylsalizylsäure. Munch Med Wochenschr 122:795–798, 1980.
17. Sullivan JM, Harken DE, Gorlin R: Pharmacologic control of thromboembolic complications of a cardiac-valve replacement. N Engl J Med 284:1391–1394, 1971.
18. The American-Canadian Co-operative Study Group: Persantine-aspirin trial in cerebral ischemia. Stroke 14:99–103, 1983.
19. Veterans Administration Cooperative Study of Atherosclerosis, Neurology Section: An evaluation of anticoagulant therapy in the treatment of cerebral vascular disease. Neurology 11 (Part 2): 132–138, 1961.
20. Wolf PA, Kannel WB, Verter J: Current status of risk factors for stroke. Neurol Clin 1:317–343, 1983.

152
Potential Role of Perfluorocarbons in Neurosurgery
S. J. Peerless

In 1966, Gollan and Clark startled the scientific community by demonstrating that mammals could survive breathing fluorinated organic liquids and silicone oils.[5] The same workers demonstrated that the isolated rat heart continued to contract vigorously when perfused alternatively with oxygenated liquid fluorochemical and oxygenated diluted blood.

In 1967, Sloviter and Kamimoto showed that a liquid fluorocarbon with a high solubility for oxygen in a simulated blood plasma maintained the electrical activity of a perfused isolated rat brain.[13] They also showed that this compound was as effective as a suspension of erthyrocytes in the same simulated blood plasma. Sloviter also showed that mice, whose blood contained 10 to 20 percent of emulsified fluorocarbon, could survive longer than control animals in an atmosphere containing 4 percent carbon monoxide—conditions where the transport of oxygen by red cells is almost completely inhibited.[12]

In 1973, Geyer succeeded in effecting a total replacement of the blood of rats with a fluorocarbon emulsion containing 12 to 20 percent of fluorocarbon by volume with subsequent survival of the animals.[3] In these experiments, the hematocrit was brought down to less than 1 vol % and the animals appeared to function normally. The plasma protein and hematocrit levels were back to normal 7 to 10 days after this exchange transfusion, and the animals continued to grow and develop without any apparent abnormality and with a normal life span.

Since then, there have been many studies that have confirmed the feasibility of oxygenating the brain and, indeed, the whole animal, with perfluorochemical (PFC) emulsions.

Pharmacology of Perfluorochemicals

Highly fluorinated organic compounds are generally inert but are able to dissolve more oxygen and carbon dioxide than the parent hydrocarbons. A large number of these compounds have been made by two different methods: either by the substitution of hydrogen with fluorine on the carbon ring or by the synthesis from perfluorinated building blocks using a fully fluorinated starting material.

For these compounds to function as a blood substitute, three inherent properties of the compounds need to be modified. Fluorocarbons are not soluble nor miscible with water, and therefore the preparations need to be in the form of a stable emulsion. In addition, since many of the perfluorochemicals have a high vapor pressure, there exists a hazard of embolization caused by rapid vaporization of the material at body temperatures. Finally, fluorocarbons with low vapor pressures cannot be eliminated from animals by the usual route through the lung but are scavenged and retained, perhaps permanently, by the reticuloendothelial system (RES). Emulsions, like blood, are complex non-Newtonian fluids whose properties depend not only on the nature of the components (PFCs, saline, water, surfactants, etc.) but also on the mean particle size. Particle size and distribution are of particular importance in constructing blood substitutes in that they determine the surface area available for gaseous exchange, viscosity characteristics, intravascular persistence, toxicity, excretion, and the extent to which they are taken up by the reticuloendothelial system.

Of the many preparations available, the one most frequently used clinically, Fluosol-DA, contains two fluorocarbons, perfluorodecalin and perfluorotripropylamine, mixed with the surfactant Pluronic (Wyandotte Chemicals Corporation, Wyandotte, Mich.) and natural surfactants containing phospholipids from egg yolk. This material remains stable when stored frozen and has a particle size of 0.1 to 0.2 µm. To be administered as a blood substitute, the fluorocarbon emulsion is thawed and a concentrated salt solution is added. This forms a milky liquid with a viscosity of approximately one-half that of whole blood, with a large surface area for the uptake and release of oxygen at about the same rate as that of normal erythrocytes. Thus 20% Fluosol-DA, exposed to a P_{O_2} of 760 mm Hg at 37°C, will dissolve 5.6 ml/dl of oxygen.[11]

Physiology and Toxicity of Perfluorochemicals

The administration of perfluorochemical (PFC) blood substitutes represents both an artificial organ transplant and a whole body, multiple organ perfusion. Clinical use of these substances will be only as a temporary or supportive measure, and therefore adequate elimination of the PFC is necessary and desirable.

The lung is the key organ in PFC physiology. For PFCs to transport significant amounts of oxygen, the O_2 tensions in the alveoli must be well above normal physiological levels. An animal circulating PFCs and breathing air at ambient pressures will have a negligible increase in Pa_{O_2} (Fig. 152-1). However, when breathing 100 percent oxygen, a Pa_{O_2} of 500 to 600 mmHg can be obtained. This necessity to maintain artificially high concentrations of oxygen may limit the widespread application of PFCs as blood substitutes. But when blood is not available or is refused on religious grounds and oxygen is available, fluorocarbons may be important and useful alternatives. Similarly, since the altered ligands that form when hemoglobin is combined with carbon monoxide and cyanide are incapable of carrying oxygen, the administration of oxygen and fluorocarbons, which are unaffected by these toxins, may be life-saving. Excretion of PFCs injected intravenously occurs almost exclusively through the lung by exhalation and by transpiration. Trace amounts have been detected in bile, and apparently none is excreted by the kidney.

Infusion of the PFC emulsions causes a decrease in blood viscosity that will cause an increase in the cardiac output and a mild decrease in mean arterial blood pressure. Perfusion of the liver, heart, and brain increases significantly with an increase in the oxygen pressure in these tissues. These observations suggest that the PFC emulsions enhance the flow in the microcirculation.

The survival of animals after total exchange transfusion with pure PFC emulsion suggests the absence of an acute toxicity from their chemical characteristics. Toxicity, when seen, is more often the result of inadequate physical features such as gaseous embolism from excessive vapor pressure,

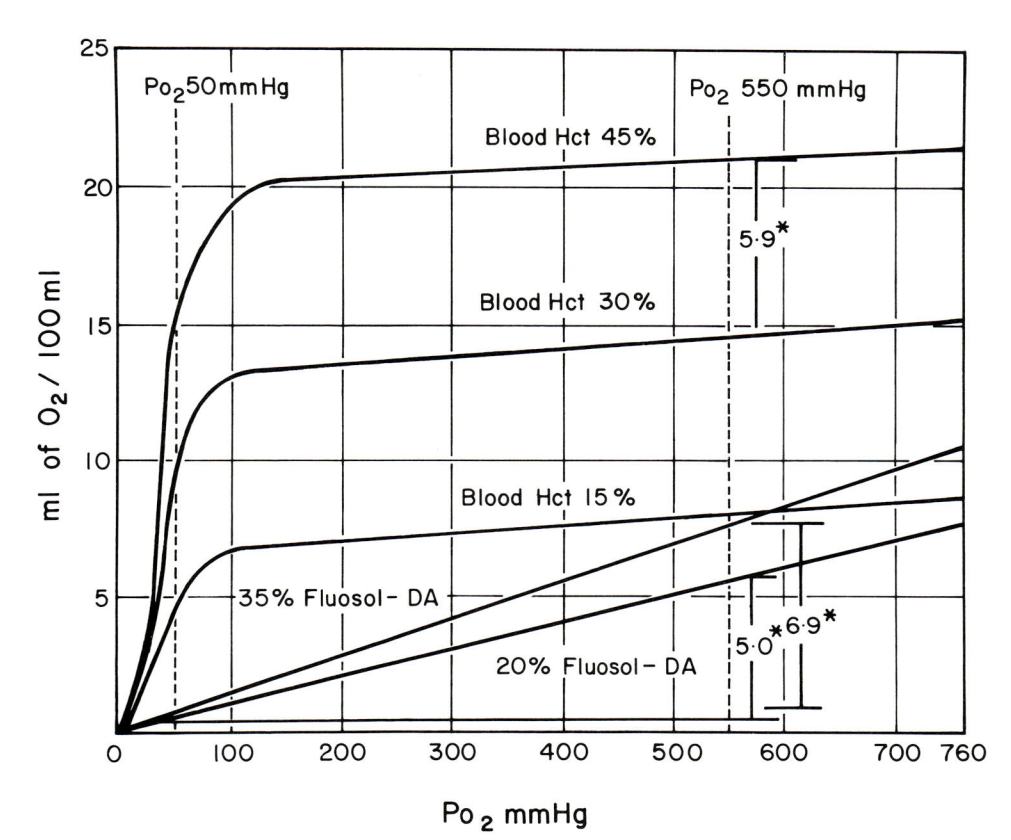

Figure 152-1 Oxygen dissociation curves of Fluosol-DA and whole blood. Numbers marked with an asterisk show the oxygen volume (ml O_2 per 100 ml) that can be released from Fluosol-DA and whole blood (hematocrit 45 percent) with a drop of P_{O_2} from 550 to 50 mmHg. (Modified from Naito R, Yokoyama K: *Perfluorochemical Blood Substitutes "Fluosol-43," "Fluosol-DA, 20% and 35%."* Technical Information Ser. No. 5. Osaka, Green Cross Corp., June 30, 1978.)

coarse particle size, excessive perfusion rate, or low osmotic pressure. There does not appear to be any specific chemical toxicity, although occasional acute activation of the complement system may result from impurities in the surfactant.

The life span of perfluorochemicals now available for administration to human beings is measured in hours to several days. PFCs, with vapor pressures between 5 and 20 mmHg, will have a half-life of 2 to 65 days, depending somewhat on particle size. PFCs are stored and excreted unchanged. Careful analysis for catabolites or free fluoride ions in blood, bile, urine, or exhaled gases have proved negative. Uptake of PFCs occurs rapidly in the RES, i.e., the spleen, liver, pancreas, adrenals, and bone marrow. The persistent half-life in these organs varies with the particular fluorocarbon, but for Fluosol-DA, this is 24 days. Prolonged tissue contact with a PFC does not appear to be carcinogenic or teratogenic nor does it cause inflammatory reactions, but blockage of the RES may alter the clearing function of this organ.[11]

Potential Uses in Neurosurgery

Perfluorochemical emulsions are effective in providing oxygen transport to the brain and seem capable of maintaining, for a limited time, normal cerebral metabolism and electrical activity. The small particle size and low viscosity suggest that a PFC may protect cerebral tissue from infarction in patients with vasospasm or cerebrovascular occlusion. In these clinical situations, where regional cerebral blood flow (rCBF) is reduced to critical levels, enrichment of the existing or collateral flow may be accomplished by the addition of oxygenated PFC. The evidence to support this hypothesis is compelling. It may be significant that oxygen delivery to the brain and spinal cord may be accomplished both by intravascular perfusion and by subarachnoid perfusion.

Doss et al., using a feline model, replaced the CSF with oxygenated perfluorochemical emulsion and then subjected the animal to inhalation of 100 percent nitrogen. They were able to demonstrate by O_2 electrodes in the cortex an elevation of the mean O_2 tension by a factor of 2 lasting for 11 min following a single bolus infusion.[2] Kontos et al. demonstrated that CSF perfusion with PFC emulsions equilibrated with 100 percent O_2 completely eliminated the expected reactive vasodilatation of the cerebral microcirculation induced by systemic hypoxia or hemorrhagic shock.[8] Similarly, Osterholm and his colleagues recently reported the apparent reversal of severe adverse metabolic effects and normalization of electrical activity in cats with severe total cerebral ischemia by ventriculosubarachnoid perfusion of an oxygenated perfluorocarbon emulsion.[9]

Hansebout and co-workers demonstrated significant modification of acute spinal cord injury in dogs treated by the subarachnoid perfusion of an oxygenated PFC as compared with animals receiving no treatment or only saline perfusion.[7] They not only postulated the value of increased oxygen delivery to the traumatized cord, but also raised the possibility that the fluorocarbon might scavenge noxious substances from the area of injury.

Dirks and co-workers extended Sloviter's original observations by perfusing isolated rat brains with an oxygenated PFC emulsion and demonstrated maintenance of the electrical and metabolic activity of the brain for up to 7 h.[1] Goldsmith et al. used a perfluorochemical emulsion to exchange-transfuse rats to a hematocrit of less than 12 percent; control animals had replacement with 3 percent albumin in saline.[4] There was a significant difference in the cerebral redox state between the two groups, with the treated group having higher mean arterial pressures and maintenance of metabolic cerebral function.

Studies in our laboratory demonstrated a protective effect of Fluosol-DA (both 35 percent and 20 percent) in cats subjected to middle cerebral artery occlusion as compared with control cats given mannitol or saline.[10] Significant modification of ischemic changes in cortical neurons and striking reductions in the size of infarctions were observed in the treated animals. These histological observations have been shown to be due to the PFC emulsion increasing CBF, supporting critical flow in the microcirculation, and enhancing collateral flow, thus permitting the oxygen-carrying particle to reach the ischemic area.

In their original observations, Handa et al. demonstrated that dogs and monkeys exchange-transfused with Fluosol-DA to hematocrits of 1 to 6 percent all survived with no observable alterations in the EEG or on detailed histological evaluation of the brain.[6] These encouraging results led them to a trial of 20 % Fluosol-DA in the treatment of humans suffering from ischemic deficits secondary to subarachnoid hemorrhage and vasospasm. In their original report, 12 of 20 patients showed a dramatic reversal of signs of neurological dysfunction.[6] Handa has accumulated experience with a larger series of patients suffering from vasospasm, and has noted overall good or excellent results in 65 percent of the patients so treated (Handa H: Personal communication).

It is evident that perfluorochemical emulsions are able to dissolve and off-load O_2 and CO_2 in biologically significant amounts. To be useful to neurosurgeons, a commercial product with a high perfluorocarbon content, small particle size, and low viscosity is necessary to enhance oxygen transport and flow to the microcirculation of the brain. The compound will have to be proved safe, with a negligible acute or chronic toxicity and minimal tissue retention. It should be stable and capable of prolonged storage. Products meeting these specifications will soon be available. Although the biological data supporting the clinical value of these new emulsions are preliminary, the evidence accumulated to date is exciting and promising. In the next decade, one might expect readily available perfluorochemical emulsions that will protect the brain from potential infarction and will resuscitate ischemic neuronal tissue.

References

1. Dirks B, Krieglstein J, Lind HH, Rieger H, Schütz H: Fluorocarbon perfusion medium applied to the isolated rat brain. J Pharmacol Methods 4:94–108, 1980.
2. Doss LL, Kaufman N, Bicher HI: Protective effect of intrathecal oxygenated fluorocarbon injection on the fall of cerebral TpO2 induced by anoxic anoxia. Bibl Anat 15:412–415, 1977.
3. Geyer RP: Fluorocarbon-polyol artificial substitutes. New Engl J Med 289:1077–1082, 1973.

4. Goldsmith MM, Palladino GW, Proctor HJ: Cerebral cortical ATP and lactate concentrations after exchange transfusion with fluosol (F-43). Surg Forum 32:16–19, 1981.
5. Gollan F, Clark LC Jr: Organ perfusion with fluorocarbon fluid. Physiologist 9:191, 1966 (abstr).
6. Handa H: Effect of fluosol-DA on cerebral circulation in human, in Frey, Beisbarth, Stosseck (eds): *Oxygen Carrying Colloidal Blood Substitutes*. Munich, West Germany, W. Zuckschwerdt Verlag, 1981, pp 204–207.
7. Hansebout RR, Van der Jagt RHC, Sohal SS, Little JR: Oxygenated fluorocarbon perfusion as treatment of acute spinal cord compression injury in dogs. J Neurosurg 55:725–732, 1981.
8. Kontos HA, Wei EP, Raper AJ, Rosenblum WI, Navari RM, Patterson JL Jr: Role of tissue hypoxia in local regulation of cerebral microcirculation. Am J Physiol 234:H582–H591, 1978.
9. Osterholm JL, Alderman JL, Triolo A, D'Amore BR, Williams H, Frazer G: Reversal of severe cerebral ischemia by ventriculo-subarachnoid perfusion with oxygenated fluorocarbon. Presented at the Annual Meeting of the American Association of Neurological Surgeons, Washington, DC, April 25, 1983.
10. Peerless SJ, Ishikawa R, Hunter IG, Peerless MJ: Protective effect of Fluosol-DA in acute cerebral ischemia. Stroke 12:558–563, 1981.
11. Riess JG, LeBlanc M: Artificial blood substitutes based on perfluorochemicals in Banks RE (ed): *Preparation, Properties and Industrial Applications of Organofluorine Compounds*. Chichester, England, Ellis Horwood Ltd, 1982, pp 83–138.
12. Sloviter HA: Perfluoro compounds as artificial erythrocytes. Fed Proc 34:1484–1487, 1975.
13. Sloviter HA, Kamimoto T: Erythrocyte substitute for perfusion of brain. Nature 216:458–460, 1967.

153

Surgery for Acute Brain Infarction with Mass Effect

Setti S. Rengachary

Many clinicians intuitively assume that brain infarcts are nonexpanding intracranial lesions. Indeed, this tenet forms the basis of differentiation of infarcts from expanding neoplastic lesions in brain imaging studies. Although this is true with old healed infarcts, some degree of brain swelling is present in the acute phase, the extent of the swelling depending upon the size of the infarct. It ranges from virtually no discernible swelling such as in a small capsular infarct to a massive hemispheric swelling due to multilobar infarction from internal carotid or middle cerebral artery thrombosis (Fig. 153-1). In the latter, there may be an increase in intracranial pressure and massive shift of structures across the midline, with intracranial pressure gradients and uncal or cingulate herniation. Because of the acute rise in intracranial pressure, the perfusion pressure is reduced, compounding brain ischemia. Distortion of the brain with obstruction of cerebrospinal fluid pathways further aggravates the problem.

Experimental studies indicate that following acute focal ischemia with subsequent tissue necrosis there is at first accumulation of intracellular fluid (cytotoxic edema).[8] At this stage the blood-brain barrier (BBB) is not yet disrupted. This is indicated by a negative radionuclide brain scan, an essentially normal computed tomogram with failure of enhancement (Fig. 153-1A), and a failure of extravasation of protein-bound dyes. Within a few hours to days, the BBB is disrupted with extravasation of plasma-like fluid into the interstitial space (vasogenic edema) (Fig. 153-1B). Ischemic edema due to focal brain ischemia thus begins as a cytotoxic

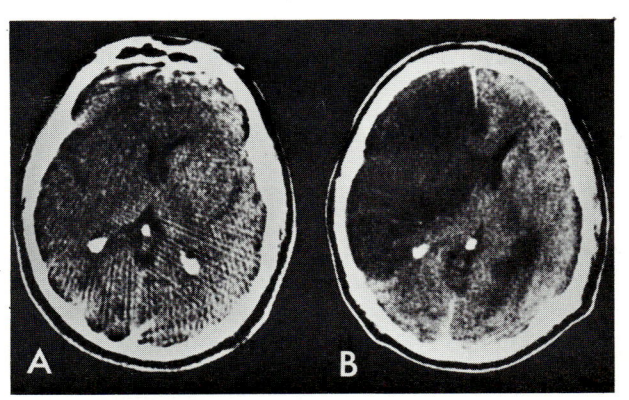

Figure 153-1 Axial computed tomograms of a patient with occlusion of the right internal carotid artery. *A*. This study, done on admission, is essentially normal. The ventricular system is in the midline. By retrospective analysis there is infarction of the right hemisphere, with cytotoxic edema, and no disruption of the blood-brain barrier (BBB). *B*. Four days later, with disruption of the BBB and superimposition of vasogenic edema, a large area of decreased density involving the frontotemporoparietal area has become evident. There is a massive shift of the midline structures. Note that the cortical mantle is involved but the thalamic area is spared (differentiation from neoplastic brain edema).

type, and the vasogenic component is superimposed on it subsequently.

Several clinical,[14,19] experimental,[9] and autopsy[1,12,16] studies have underscored the importance of brain swelling and herniation as a cause of death in the acute phase of ischemic stroke. Pressure gradients have been demonstrated in experimental models, the pressure being higher on the side of the infarct than on the opposite side, or the posterior cranial fossa.[13] In a study of 353 consecutive cases of supratentorial cerebral infarction, 45 (13 percent) showed severe brain swelling and marked herniation.[12] Brain swelling is maximal between the third and fifth days unless an extension of thrombus occurs later, with the delayed onset of signs of brain swelling and herniation.

Syndromes and Their Management

Supratentorial Compartment

Large cerebral hemispheric infarctions may present either as a syndrome simulating a brain neoplasm or a syndrome of uncal herniation. These two syndromes, of course, are not mutually exclusive.

Brain Infarction Simulating a Brain Tumor

Most neurosurgeons may be able to recount an occasional personal experience of operating upon a patient with a cerebral infarct with a mistaken preoperative diagnosis of brain tumor. In such instances, the onset of symptoms may not be apoplectic and the clinical course may be stuttering. The patient may not be able to relate an accurate history either because of dysphasia or an impaired sensorium. The patient may live alone and be brought to the emergency room with no reliable history. Brain imaging studies may be equally confusing. A bizarre enhancing pattern and a mass effect in a computed tomogram (Fig. 153-2) may mimic a primary neoplasm such as a malignant glioma or lymphoma. A radionuclide scan may show an irregularly rounded area of increased uptake rather than the diagnostic wedge-shaped area. Cerebral arteriography may show evidence of an avascular mass without definite occlusion of a major blood vessel.

If the diagnostic studies point to a tumor, it is inevitable that the patient will undergo an operative procedure, and the true diagnosis may not be established until after a biopsy. If a differential diagnosis of infarction is entertained based on diagnostic studies, then it would be prudent, if clinical circumstances permit, to wait 2 to 3 weeks then reassess the patient and repeat the diagnostic studies.

Numerous helpful features have been suggested to differentiate an infarct from a tumor on a CT scan, but none is absolute.[11] They include the following:

1. Neoplastic white matter edema spares the cortex, whereas the low density due to infarction includes the cortex as well (Fig. 153-1).
2. The thalamic area is spared in infarction, especially those infarcts occurring in the middle cerebral or internal carotid artery distribution; such sparing is rare with peritumoral edema (Fig. 153-1).
3. Ring enhancement of the white matter is common in glioma and is rarely observed in recent infarcts.
4. Intense gray matter enhancement occurs in infarct but not in tumor.

Brain Infarction with Uncal Herniation

This generally follows massive multilobar infarction of the cerebral hemisphere from thrombotic or embolic occlusion of the internal carotid or the middle cerebral artery (Fig. 153-1). The etiologic factor may be atherosclerosis, trauma to the extracranial or intracranial vessels, thromboembolic disease secondary to the use of contraceptives, or arterial spasm following aneurysm rupture or clipping. The patient may be obtunded and densely hemiplegic at the outset. More commonly, the patient is admitted with an intermittent or mild fixed neurological deficit that, over a period of a few hours to days, progresses to a profound deficit with progressive depression in the sensorium. Transtentorial herniation and rostral brain stem compression is manifest clinically as an ipsilaterally dilated, nonreactive or poorly reactive pupil; contralateral decorticate or decerebrate posturing in the previously flaccid and paralyzed limbs; bradycardia, increase in pulse pressure; and altered respiratory pattern. If this condition is not treated, medullary failure usually culminates in death.

Aggressive medical therapy should be instituted in patients with massive cerebral infarction with early brain stem compression. Therapy is monitored with intracranial pressure measurements. The patient is intubated and hyperventilated, maintaining a Pa_{CO_2} of 30 mmHg. Mannitol is given in an initial bolus of 1 g/kg and is then repeated at 0.3 g/kg every 6 h. Furosemide used concurrently with mannitol may have a synergistic effect. Induced barbiturate coma has not conclusively been shown to be effective in reversing the changes following massive focal brain ischemia. If the pa-

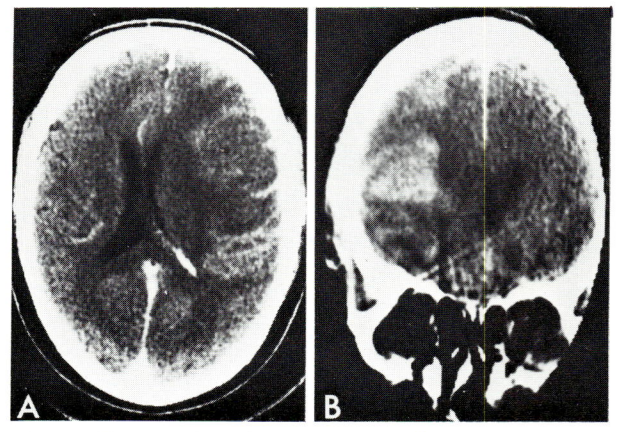

Figure 153-2 Axial (*A*) and coronal (*B*) views of a CT scan (after contrast enhancement), showing cerebral infarction with mass effect, marked ventricular displacement, and intense contrast enhancement. A diagnosis of neoplasm may be entertained, but the wedge shape of the lesion in the coronal view favors the diagnosis of infarction.

tient does not show a significant response to therapy within several hours, consideration should be given to decompressive craniectomy.[7,15,20] One of the key factors determining the success of a decompressive procedure is judicious timing. It should not be attempted without the patient receiving full benefits of nonoperative therapy; yet, it should not be postponed so long that irreversible brain stem changes (such as Duret hemorrhages) occur.

The decompressive procedure of choice is ipsilateral hemicraniectomy (Fig. 153-3). The size of the hemicraniectomy may be tailored to the size of the infarct, but it is better to err on the generous side (subtemporal decompression through a small temporal craniectomy is ineffective). As the dura is opened, the pale infarcted avascular brain herniates outward into the wound. One notes conspicuous absence of pial circulation. A cortical biopsy may be done to confirm the diagnosis; there is usually no bleeding from the biopsy site. It is not necessary to resect the infarcted tissue unless necrotic material extrudes out under pressure. Resection of the necrotic brain is not advisable for two reasons: First, cranial decompression itself is adequate in allowing outward migration of the swollen brain and relieving the pressure on the rostral brain stem; second, in the acute phase of stroke, the margins of the infarct are poorly defined—if resection is attempted there is the risk of removing viable but nonfunctioning neural tissue ("idling neurons") from the margins of the "ischemic penumbra." The dura is not closed. A Silastic sheet may be laid on the brain to prevent cortical adhesions. The bone flap is preserved frozen in an antibiotic solution, to be replanted about 3 to 6 months later. The scalp is closed in watertight fashion. The recovery from the surgery is prompt. There is usually a striking and rapid improvement in the sensorium, although the focal motor deficit remains unchanged.

Hemicraniectomy seems to be more appropriate for patients with unilateral hemispheric swelling from stroke than for patients with head injury for several reasons:

1. In head injury, the brain herniating through the cranial defect tends to become incarcerated outside the skull, leading to impediment of venous drainage and contusion of the cortex at the margin of the defect, further aggravating brain edema; in stroke, the necrotic herniated brain has sluggish or nonexistent venous outflow.
2. In patients with hemispheric stroke, because the mass effect is strictly unilateral, hemicraniectomy corrects the

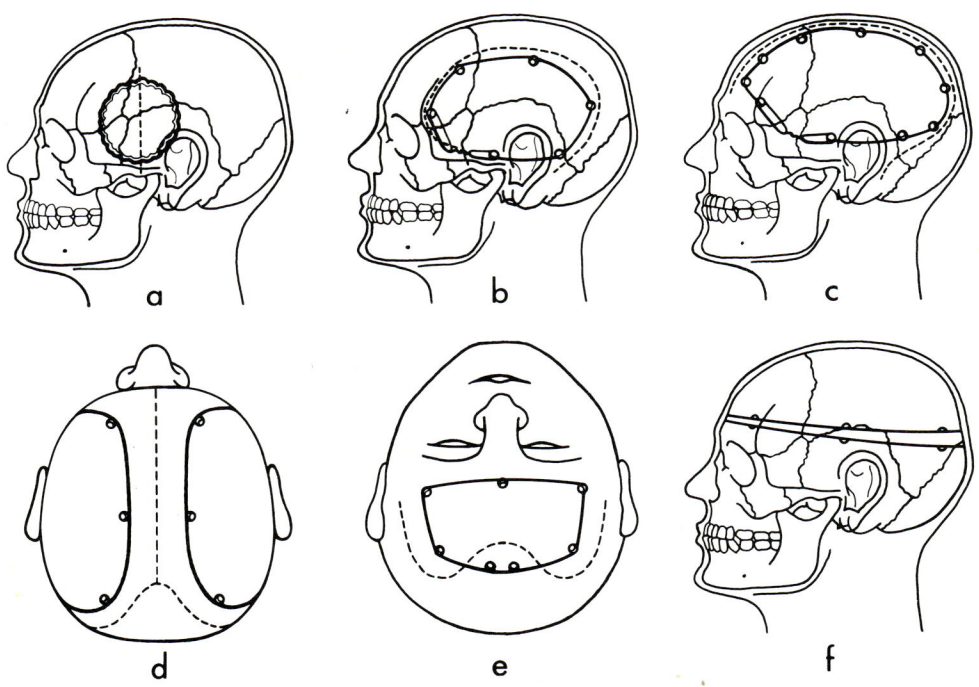

Figure 153-3 Cranial decompressive procedures for supratentorial masses: *a.* Subtemporal craniectomy: Popular in the Cushing era, this procedure is now of historic interest only. The size of the craniectomy is insufficient to alleviate increased intracranial pressure. Medium (*b*) and large (*c*) unilateral hemicraniectomy: This is ideally suited for patients with a large cerebral hemispheric infarct in whom medical therapy has failed. *d.* Bilateral hemicraniectomy: A bilateral decompressive procedure may be needed in situations where the brain swelling is diffuse and nonlateralizing, e.g., diffuse brain contusion, Reye's syndrome, lead encephalopathy, benign intracranial hypertension, etc. *e.* Bifrontal craniectomy: This procedure allows bifrontal decompression, but the temporal lobes are retained by the sphenoidal ridges and the anterior walls of the middle cranial fossa, preventing their forward migration. *f.* Circumferential craniectomy: This procedure carries the highest morbidity and mortality risk of all cranial decompressive procedures and should be avoided.

brain displacement to relieve the pressure on rostral midbrain structures; head-injured patients tend to have diffuse brain swelling requiring bilateral decompressive procedures.
3. The brain stem is quite viable in patients with stroke unless irreversible changes such as Duret hemorrhages occur from the presence of uncal herniation that is not corrected. This is reflected in improvement in consciousness almost immediately after hemicraniectomy. Patients who have sustained trauma from severe acceleration-deceleration injuries tend to have associated brain stem injuries as well, and this adversely affects the prognosis.
4. In patients with head injury, if there is significant trauma to the posterior fossa contents in addition to the supratentorial structures, there is risk of upward herniation of the posterior fossa contents through the tentorial notch toward the zone of least pressure after hemicraniectomy. This phenomenon carries as bad a prognosis as does rostrocaudal tentorial herniation. Upward transtentorial herniation does not occur in stroke patients because the posterior fossa contents are normal.

One must consider four goals in the management of a patient with ischemic stroke: (1) preservation of life, (2) prevention of extension of thrombosis and ischemic infarction, (3) prevention of systemic complications, and (4) long-term rehabilitation. Hemicraniectomy helps to realize the first objective if the patient's life is threatened from an increase in intracranial pressure. One may philosophically argue whether preservation of life is worthwhile in the face of a severe neurological deficit. Every case must be reviewed individually to resolve this question, and no general statement is possible. The factors to be taken into consideration in deciding to operate are:

1. The age of the patient—younger patients are more suitable candidates for surgery because of a reduced mortality risk, an increased likelihood of some neurological recovery, and a better potential for rehabilitation and vocational therapy.
2. Dominance of the hemisphere—stroke involving the nondominant hemisphere is more likely to have an acceptable neurological deficit because of the preservation of speech and other functions of communication.
3. Complicating illness—well-documented severe ischemic disease of the heart, uncontrolled diabetes mellitus, generalized arteriosclerosis, or dementing illness such as Alzheimer's disease, etc., will adversely influence prognosis.
4. The attitude of the immediate members of the family toward accepting attempts at preservation of life in the face of a severe neurological deficit.

Infratentorial Compartment: Cerebellar Infarction with Mass Effect

Since the initial description by Germain and Morvan in 1938[3] and with subsequent series of reports in the literature over the past four decades, cerebellar hemispheric infarction acting as an acute expansive process in the posterior cranial fossa with brain stem compression has come to be recognized as a clinically definable syndrome with a specific constellation of symptoms and signs.[5] The use of computed tomography has permitted easier recognition and has enhanced the accuracy in the diagnosis of this syndrome (Fig. 153-4).

The disease generally affects older hypertensive men with diffuse atherosclerotic cardiovascular disease with clinical evidence of previous myocardial or cerebral infarcts.[18] Embolic occlusion of the vertebral or ipsilateral posterior inferior cerebellar artery from a thrombus in the heart is thought to be the etiologic factor in about one-half of the patients. The superior cerebellar artery is an uncommon site of occlusion. Other causative factors include penetrating or blunt trauma to the vertebral artery in the neck from chiropractic manipulation, football injuries, calisthenics, yoga exercises, bow hunting, stab or gunshot wounds of the neck, cervical dislocation, or anterior cervical discectomy. Spontaneous forced rotation of the head with occlusion of the vertebral artery has been an occasional cause in infants. Rarer causes include basilar artery migraine, severe dehydration, congenital heart disease, sickle cell anemia, and (as a complication of) vertebral angiography. Cerebellar infarction in the pediatric age group is being recognized increasingly.[4]

The infarct is generally unilateral. The posteroinferior aspect of the cerebellar hemisphere in the territory of the posterior inferior cerebellar artery is the consistent site of softening.[10] Cerebellar infarctions sufficient enough to cause brain stem compression are always extensive, involving one-third to one-half of the hemisphere. In one-fourth of the cases, the infarction is hemorrhagic. A rich anastomotic network between the posterior inferior and the anterior inferior cerebellar arteries across the cerebellar hemispheric surface accounts for the rarity of cerebellar hemispheric infarction. The occurrence of infarction thus signifies poor development of this anastomotic network or spasm or atherosclerotic narrowing of the anastomotic vessels. The rapidity of embolic occlusion of the parent vessel may leave inadequate time for the collateral bed to expand sufficiently to carry the obligatory minimum volume of blood to sustain neural tissue. The cerebellar tonsil may undergo infarction as well and may herniate down to the level of C1. The ultimate cause of death is brain stem compression and medullary failure. Lateral medullary infarction may be associated with cerebellar infarction in about 15 percent of the cases.

The initial symptoms at onset may include dizziness or vertigo, nausea and vomiting, headache, ataxia of the limbs or trunk with inability to stand or walk, and dysarthria.[2] A history of transient ischemic attacks referable to the posterior circulation may be elicited in some patients. The subsequent clinical course is dependent upon the size of the infarct. If the infarct is small, no further progression may occur, the symptoms resolve, and a mistaken diagnosis of labrynthitis may be made. In massive infarction with brain stem compression and obstruction of the fourth ventricle, the patient progressively becomes obtunded. Horizontal nystagmus when present denotes involvement of the vestibular connections of the cerebellum. Pontine compression is denoted by pinpoint and sluggish pupils, ipsilateral abducens or facial (lower motor neuron type) weakness, and forced conjugate deviation of the eyes to the opposite side that does not revert with cold caloric stimulation as a result

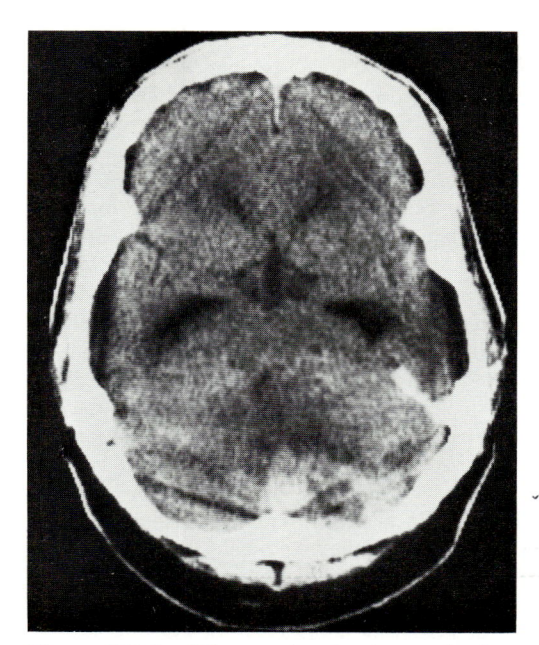

Figure 153-4 CT scan showing hemorrhagic cerebellar infarction with mass effect in the posterior cranial fossa. The fourth ventricle is compressed and there is early obstructive hydrocephalus. (Courtesy of Hilton I. Price, M.D.)

of pressure on the ipsilateral para-abducens nucleus and ipsilateral horizontal-gaze paresis. Respirations may be ataxic or there may be central hyperventilation. Ocular bobbing, skew deviation of the eyes, decorticate or decerebrate posturing, bilateral Babinski signs, and Cheyne-Stokes respirations may occur preterminally.

Therapy should be initiated promptly. As with massive cerebral infarction, medical therapy consisting of hyperventilation and the administration of osmotic agents and steroids should be instituted. If there is no improvement, consideration should be given to surgical therapy. The treatment options are external ventricular drainage or posterior fossa craniectomy and resection of infarcted cerebellar tissue.[6,17] The choice of therapy will depend upon the clinical status of the patient; if the patient has significant hydrocephalus with minimal signs of brain stem compression, ventricular drainage may be the procedure of choice. If there is not a prompt clinical improvement, then posterior fossa surgery should be undertaken without much procrastination. In patients with significant brain stem compression from massive infarction, one should proceed directly with posterior craniectomy. A rapidly done craniectomy along with resection of avascular cerebellar tissue with the patient in the prone position is a relatively simple and definitive procedure. It quickly relieves the direct pressure on the brain stem, which is virtually the sole cause of death. Improvement is quick and dramatic, provided the brain stem has not undergone permanent changes from extrinsic pressure, or has itself undergone infarction from occlusive vascular disease.

References

1. Adams JH, Graham DI: Twelve cases of fatal cerebral infarction due to arterial occlusion in the absence of atheromatous stenosis or embolism. J Neurol Neurosurg Psychiatry 30:479–488, 1957.
2. Feely MP: Cerebellar infarction. Neurosurgery 4:7–11, 1979.
3. Germain A, Morvan A: Ramollissement cérébelleux pseudotumoral. Ann Med Interne (Paris) 44:1695–1700, 1938.
4. Harbaugh RE, Saunders RL, Reeves AG: Pediatric cerebellar infarction: Case report and review of the literature. Neurosurgery 10:593–596, 1982.
5. Heros RC: Cerebellar hemorrhage and infarction. Contemp Neurosurg 2 (25):1–6, 1980.
6. Horwitz NH, Ludolph C: Acute obstructive hydrocephalus caused by cerebellar infarction: Treatment alternatives. Surg Neurol 20:13–19, 1983.
7. Ivamoto HS, Numoto M, Donaghy RMP: Surgical decompression for cerebral and cerebellar infarcts. Stroke 5:365–369, 1974.
8. Katzman R, Clasen R, Klatzo I, Meyer JS, Pappius HM, Waltz AG: Brain edema in stroke: Study group on brain edema in stroke. Stroke 8:512–540, 1977.
9. Laurent JP, Molinari GF, Moseley JI: Clinicopathological validation of a primate stroke model. Surg Neurol 4:449–455, 1975.
10. Lehrich JR, Winkler GF, Ojemann RG: Cerebellar infarction with brain stem compression: Diagnosis and surgical treatment. Arch Neurol 22:490–498, 1970.
11. Masdeu JC: Infarct versus neoplasm on CT: Four helpful signs. AJNR 4:522–524, 1983.
12. Ng LKY, Nimmannitya J: Massive cerebral infarction with severe brain swelling: A clinicopathological study. Stroke 1:158–163, 1970.
13. O'Brien MD, Waltz AG: Intracranial pressure gradients caused by experimental cerebral ischemia and edema. Stroke 4:694–698, 1973.
14. Plum F: Brain swelling and edema in cerebral vascular disease. Res Publ Assoc Res Nerv Ment Dis 41:318–348, 1961.
15. Rengachary SS, Batnitzky S, Morantz RA, Arjunan K, Jeffries B: Hemicraniectomy for acute massive cerebral infarction. Neurosurgery 8:321–327, 1981.
16. Shaw CM, Alvord EC Jr, Berry RG: Swelling of the brain following ischemic infarction with arterial occlusion. Arch Neurol 1:161–177, 1959.
17. Shenkin HA, Zavala M: Cerebellar strokes: Mortality, surgical indications, and results of ventricular drainage. Lancet 2:429–432, 1982.
18. Sypert GW, Alvord EC: Cerebellar infarction: A clinico-pathological study. Arch Neurol 32:357–363, 1975.
19. Van Trotsenburg L, Vinken PJ: Fatal cerebral infarction simulating an acute expanding lesion. J Neurol Neurosurg Psychiatry 29:241–243, 1966.
20. Young PH, Smith KR Jr, Dunn RC: Surgical decompression after cerebral hemispheric stroke: Indications and patient selection. South Med J 75:473–475, 1982.

154
Extracranial to Intracranial Bypass Grafting: Anterior Circulation

Jack M. Fein

Extracranial to intracranial bypass surgery, also known as EC-IC bypass, was developed to treat patients with arterial occlusive lesions that are not directly repairable. In the anterior circulation these procedures increase the collateral circulation in the distribution of the middle cerebral artery. EC-IC bypass has also been used to augment the distal circulation in patients who require deliberate arterial occlusion or trapping for the management of aneurysms.[6]

The diagnosis of carotid occlusive disease was made possible by the introduction of carotid arteriography in 1927. However, surgical procedures designed to re-establish flow in the occluded vessel were not attempted until 26 years later. Strully et al. first described the use of carotid thrombectomy,[26] but it was soon realized that this procedure was not successful in treating patients with complete occlusion of the internal carotid artery. A variety of other occlusive lesions of the anterior circulation are not amenable to direct repair. Stenotic lesions in the distal internal carotid artery and in the middle cerebral arteries were identified in a number of patients with cerebrovascular occlusive disease. Attempts at direct surgical treatment of these lesions were successfully made by Welch,[28] Scheibert,[23] and Chou[2] between 1954 and 1960. However, such approaches to the arteries at the base of the brain were technically difficult and were not demonstrably effective.

An alternative approach toward cerebral revascularization focused on methods of improving the collateral circulation distal to the obstructing lesion. In 1942 Henschen attempted to increase the collateral blood supply in a patient with bilateral carotid occlusion.[13] He transposed the temporalis muscle intracranially to stimulate extracranial to intracranial collateral flow. Since postoperative angiography was not carried out, it is unclear whether this was successful. Rather than stimulating collateral outgrowth from vascularized tissues, such as muscle or omentum, it was more practical to attempt anastomosis of collateral channels directly to intracranial arteries. In 1963, Woringer and Kunlin described a bypass procedure in which a saphenous vein graft was placed between the common carotid artery and the intracranial portion of the internal carotid artery in a patient with internal carotid occlusion.[29] Further experience with this approach has been limited by the necessity for brain retraction, the frequency of atherosclerotic involvement of the intracranial internal carotid artery, and the relatively low patency rate of free vein grafts. On the other hand, direct arterial anastomosis to the cortical circulation was beset by the problems of accurately manipulating arteries 1 mm in diameter and required major innovations in vascular surgical techniques, instrumentation, and suture materials. In 1960, Jacobson and Suarez described the application of microsurgical techniques used in other surgical disciplines to vascular surgical procedures.[16] The development of these microsurgical techniques for incision and repair of small arteries was a prerequisite for successful extracranial-intracranial microanastomosis. During the period between 1960 and 1967, adaptations were also made in microsurgical instruments, sutures, and the operating microscope for use in microvascular neurosurgery.[30]

Donaghy developed a microsurgical laboratory to foster the skills required for microvascular surgery.[4] Arteriotomy repair as well as end-to-end and end-to-side anastomoses were developed in arteries 1 to 2 mm in diameter, with patency rates of over 90 percent. Donaghy and Yasargil developed the procedure of superficial temporal artery to middle cerebral artery (STA-MCA) anastomosis and operated on the first two patients in Zürich, Switzerland and Burlington, Vermont in 1967 (see Chap. 3 for more details).

Hemodynamic Basis for Bypass Surgery

The mechanism by which vascular occlusive lesions produce ischemic symptoms is not well understood. However, hemodynamic insufficiency, thromboembolism to the distal arterial circulation, and viscosity changes in blood are the most likely factors responsible.

Gratzl et al. studied a group of patients with transient ischemic attacks with preoperative and postoperative measurement of regional cerebral blood flow (rCBF).[10] In patients with relative focal ischemia, the bypass was associated with significant improvement in postoperative rCBF. In another study the greatest increase in postoperative blood flow values was found in patients with the lowest preoperative flow values.[12] Intraoperative measurements of cortical artery pressure have been carried out in 92 patients with occlusive lesions of the internal carotid and middle cerebral arteries.[7] The decrease in cortical artery pressure was generally related to the severity and distribution of the cerebrovascular occlusive lesion. Patients with middle cerebral artery occlusive lesions had lower mean cortical artery pressures than those with internal carotid artery lesions, and those with multiple lesions had lower mean cortical artery pressures than those with single lesions. Hypoperfusion may therefore be an important mechanism for the production of symptoms and may be responsive to augmentation of blood flow.

However, volume flow in the superficial temporal artery (24 to 74 ml/min) is significantly less than that in the middle cerebral artery (120 to 170 ml/min), and this has caused concern regarding the ability of an STA-MCA bypass to augment flow significantly. Regional cerebral blood flow studies indicate that neurophysiological dysfunction does not occur until regional cerebral blood flow decreased to levels of 18 to 22 ml/100 g per minute. It may be necessary, therefore, only to keep regional blood flow values above a threshold to provide clinically effective augmentation of flow by bypass surgery. Cerebral blood flow measurements after bypass procedures have in fact shown variable increases in regional flow of up to 30 percent.[12]

Preoperative Evaluation

The management of any patient with cerebrovascular insufficiency begins with a detailed history of the onset, time course, and resolution of each ischemic event. In addition to a thorough neurological examination, neurovascular examination will elicit evidence of pulse asymmetry, bruits, or thrills in the carotid and scalp arteries. Careful general physical examination and review of systems will reveal evidence of cardiac, general circulatory, or respiratory problems. Coronary insufficiency, hypertension, and a history of smoking are common findings in patients with cerebrovascular insufficiency. An ECG examination should include a 24-h Holter monitor to rule out significant arrhythmias. Hematologic abnormalities and coagulopathies should be sought with a blood count, platelet studies, prothrombin time, and lipid and lipoprotein determinations.

Several relatively noninvasive studies are useful for evaluating patients with cerebral ischemia. These include CT scans, cerebral blood flow studies, and digital intravenous angiography. CT scanning is useful to determine the extent of cerebral infarction and the presence of areas of brain edema. If infarction is extensive, the value of any surgical procedure is questionable. If significant edema is present, it is best to delay surgery until this resolves. Regional cerebral blood flow studies using the inhalation of ^{133}Xe can identify asymmetric hemisphere perfusion, areas of relative focal ischemia, and evidence of loss of autoregulation. It should be recognized, however, that rCBF rates are often normal between episodes of transient ischemia.

Digital subtraction venous angiography (DIVA) is one of the more effective screening tests in patients with cerebrovascular disease. Stenosis or occlusion of the cervical carotid arteries as well as occlusive lesions of the largest intracranial arteries may be visualized. Once a significant lesion is found on the DIVA study, an arterial angiogram should be performed prior to operation in order to visualize details of the intracranial circulation that are not resolved adequately by DIVA.

Nuclear magnetic resonance (NMR) scanning is not widely available but is rapidly becoming a clinically useful imaging technique. In acute cerebral infarction changes may be seen within several hours on NMR, while such evidence may not be seen on CT scan for 24 to 48 h.

Arterial angiography is carried out by transfemoral selective catheterization to assess the presence of specific lesions of the internal carotid and middle cerebral arteries. If symptoms are clearly hemispheric in nature, selective injection of both carotid arteries and one vertebral artery is performed. High-quality serial studies are often necessary to visualize the contribution of ophthalmic collaterals to the carotid siphon area and the contribution of leptomeningeal collaterals to the middle cerebral areas. A transorbital oblique view will visualize the carotid siphon area, and a transorbital view will visualize the proximal portion of the middle cerebral artery.

Clinical Indications for Bypass Surgery

It has been suggested that revascularization during the course of a progressing stroke or within 8 to 10 h of onset of an acute stroke may favorably influence the outcome.[3] The neurological deficit associated with cerebral infarction may be related to a surrounding zone of ischemic but viable neural tissue. Augmentation of blood flow to these areas may improve the function of these so-called idling neurons. Several surgical series suggest that the recovery rate may be enhanced by this intervention. The efficacy of flow augmentation under these circumstances is unknown, however, and the risk of converting an ischemic infarct to a hemorrhagic infarct is significant. Management of such patients should be based primarily on providing optimal cerebral hemodynamics and arterial blood gas values. Cerebral edema is treated with steroids, and if this is severe and progressive, intracranial pressure monitoring in conjunction with intravenous mannitol is used.

Bypass grafting in patients with a chronic completed stroke in an effort to improve neurological function has generally been unrewarding. Several authors have described tests designed to predict which patients will improve after bypass grafting. Holbach et al. have suggested the use of hyperbaric oxygenation to determine whether clinical improvement occurs in response to increased tissue nutrition in such patients.[14] While the use of such a screening examination may theoretically identify patients who are suitable candidates for revascularization, the data to date are unconvincing, and bypass surgery is not recommended in this setting.

At present, the major goal of bypass surgery is to reduce the incidence of a new stroke in patients at risk. After a TIA in the anterior circulation the risk of a new completed stroke within 4 years of the first event varies from 32 to 43 percent.[19] The risk of a second stroke after a completed stroke may be as high as 67 percent within 24 months.[15] Because it was recognized that our knowledge of the natural history of TIAs and stroke was limited, tentative clinical and angiographic criteria were developed to select patients for bypass surgery. Candidates for surgery include patients who have experienced either recurrent transient ischemic attacks (TIAs), a reversible ischemic neurological deficit (RIND), or a nondebilitating completed stroke (CS).

Angiographic Indications

Angiography will demonstrate the presence of arterial occlusive lesions not amenable to direct repair in 20 to 30 percent of patients with cerebrovascular insufficiency. Internal carotid artery occlusion, found in approximately 16 percent of such patients, is usually inoperable by carotid endarterectomy (Fig. 154-2). Occasionally collateral circulation through the ophthalmic artery or through tympanic and cavernous branches shows reflux of contrast down to the petrous portion of the carotid artery. In my experience, in five such cases, back flow was re-established by carotid endarterectomy. Two of these patients, however, developed recurrent thrombosis within 3 days of operation. The majority of patients with internal carotid occlusion have some degree of collateral circulation to the ipsilateral hemisphere from the contralateral side across the anterior circle of Willis or from the posterior circulation through the posterior communicating artery. Visualization of these collaterals after the occlusion has progressed to completion, however, does not facilitate predictions of future risk since these collateral channels were inadequate to prevent the primary ischemic event. Most younger patients will tolerate unilateral internal carotid occlusion; however, in a postmortem series reviewed by Fisher, 67 percent of older patients with associated cerebrovascular disease were symptomatic. In the presence of collateral flow via the external carotid, internal maxillary, and ophthalmic arteries, embolization from the proximal stump of the internal carotid artery may be responsible for ischemic symptoms. Our current state of knowledge would dictate that patients who have recurrent ischemic episodes after internal carotid occlusion has been demonstrated on angiography should undergo an EC-IC bypass procedure, unless such collateral channels are already prominent.

Patients with segmental stenosis of the distal cervical or intracranial portions of the internal carotid artery are suitable for bypass surgery. The exposure for carotid endarterectomy is inadequate for stenotic lesions located more than 2 cm distal to the carotid bifurcation. The most distal of these lesions may interrupt collateral flow from the posterior communicating and anterior choroidal arteries. Low flow rates associated with any distal high-grade stenosis may produce a "slim" sign in the proximal internal carotid artery because of pooling of slowly flowing contrast in the supine position. This must be differentiated from longitudinal narrowing of the arterial walls seen with inflammatory processes or with a traumatic or spontaneous dissection. Similarly, low flow rates and a miniscule column of contrast distal to a high-grade stenosis at the origin of the internal carotid artery may give the appearance of a complete occlusion. The "pseudo-occlusion" should be suspected when a tapered narrowing of contrast is seen and can be better visualized with a larger dose of contrast coupled with a more rapid frame sequence. Endarterectomy rather than bypass surgery should be offered to such patients. Tandem lesions of the origin and distal segment of the internal carotid artery occurred in 8 percent of the patients in our series. Under such circumstances, poor back flow is seen during carotid endarterectomy and may lead to postoperative thrombosis at the arteriotomy site. The distal lesion is usually most critical, and patients with such lesions should be selected for bypass surgery. If symptoms recur and the proximal plaque shows ulcerative changes, an endarterectomy may be performed subsequently.

In North America stenosis or occlusion of the middle cerebral artery occurs in 7 percent of patients with cerebrovascular insufficiency, but it occurs more frequently in Japan. Lesions of the middle cerebral artery from its origin to the superior and inferior trunks in the Sylvian fissure are suitable for treatment with a bypass graft.

Patients with bilateral internal carotid occlusion or a combination of occlusion and contralateral stenosis may have severe postural symptoms. Patients with internal carotid occlusion ipsilateral to the symptoms and contralateral internal carotid stenosis may benefit from a bypass, particularly if cross flow is poor. In moyamoya disease, progressive occlusion of cerebral arteries evokes an exuberant proliferation of small intradural collateral channels at the base of the brain.[17] Persistent ischemic events may be benefited by additional collaterals constructed during a bypass.

Selection of patients for surgery should therefore be based on both clinical and angiographic criteria. Patients at risk for future strokes, as is evidenced by a history of ischemic events, may be suitable for bypass in the presence of complete internal carotid occlusion, distal internal carotid stenosis, middle cerebral stenosis, or middle cerebral occlusion.

In addition to its value in the treatment of atherosclerotic lesions, the bypass graft may be utilized in certain cases where ligation of the internal carotid or middle cerebral artery is planned. Large unclippable internal carotid aneurysms may be treated more effectively by internal carotid ligation than by common carotid ligation. The risks of a delayed hemispheric stroke attendant upon internal carotid ligation may be reduced by simultaneous EC-IC bypass grafting.[6,21] The bypass has also been employed in a few patients with basal tumors. The risks of trapping or ligating the internal carotid or middle cerebral artery during these resections may be reduced by increasing collateral blood flow.

The superficial temporal artery should be at least 1.2 mm in diameter at the point where the anastomosis will be created. The rate of technical failures or suboptimal bypass grafts will rise significantly with smaller diameter grafts.

Contraindications

Since bypass surgery is primarily a prophylactic procedure, it should not be used in severely debilitated patients. Patients with other diseases that limit their life expectancy to less than 5 years are also unsuitable candidates. Conditions that increase the perioperative risk such as severe coronary ischemia, acute or chronic pulmonary disease, or other advanced diseases are all relative contraindications to surgery. Prophylactic therapy for a future stroke should not be offered to a patient who is threatened by another more pressing disorder. Occlusive lesions caused by cardiac emboli and hemodynamic failure related to cardiac arrhythmias require attention to the source of the disorder.

Timing of Surgery

The timing of bypass surgery depends on the severity of the patient's symptoms. Transient ischemic attacks are associated with no residual deficit, and revascularization may take place any time thereafter. In the event that the attacks are frequent, an attempt should be made to control them with an intravenous heparin infusion; surgery may be planned after several symptom-free days.

If there is evidence on CT scan that infarction has occurred, it may be best to delay surgery for several weeks. After an ischemic infarction there is disruption of the blood-brain barrier, parenchymal softening, and cerebral edema. Revascularization procedures should be carried out only when the effects of the acute insult have resolved and 3 to 4 weeks have elapsed for healing. If revascularization is carried out within the first few weeks, there is an increased incidence of hemorrhagic complications.

Most of the patients selected for bypass surgery should be evaluated by a cardiologist to assess the risks of surgery. Twenty-five percent of the patients in our series had essential hypertension preoperatively. Decisions regarding the selection of antihypertensive medication and the management of the inevitable hypertensive swings immediately postoperatively should be discussed beforehand. Ten percent of my patients have had previous myocardial infarction and 15 percent have had cardiac arrhythmias.

Sequence of Procedures

A significant number of patients have multiple lesions. Each of these may require separate correction. The priority given each is dependent primarily on its relationship to the presenting symptoms. The most common combination of lesions is an internal carotid occlusion and a contralateral internal carotid stenosis. In the joint stroke study, approximately 55 percent of patients with this combination of lesions had symptoms referable to the occluded side, 10 percent had symptoms referable to the stenotic side, and 16 percent had bilateral symptoms.[9] In my series, 57 patients had this combination of lesions: 49 had symptoms referable to the occluded side, and 30 had bilateral symptoms. Thirty patients were treated by bypass grafting followed by endarterectomy. Eighteen patients were treated by bypass grafting alone, and nine patients were treated by contralateral endarterectomy alone. During endarterectomy the intraoperative EEG changes associated with carotid clamping were less prominent over the occluded side in patients who had had a previous bypass graft, whereas all nine patients who underwent primary endarterectomy had such changes and required an intraoperative shunt. After a mean follow-up of 3 years there was only one minor ischemic event in the ipsilateral hemisphere among the patients who had bypass surgery. However, three of the nine patients with primary endarterectomy had transient ischemic events referable to the occluded site after endarterectomy and subsequently required bypass grafting. In this setting, bypass grafting has the advantage of producing increased flow without the risks of temporary clamping of the major blood supply to the cerebral hemisphere. Contralateral carotid endarterectomy is then carried out for the treatment of symptoms in the contralateral hemisphere.

Fourteen of our patients with appropriate angiographic lesions also had stenosis of the origin of the external carotid artery. Prior to STA-MCA bypass grafting an external carotid endarterectomy was performed. In six patients, the external carotid artery appeared to be the source of collateral channels to the intracranial internal carotid circulation, and endarterectomy was performed with an intraluminal shunt and a patch graft angioplasty.

Technique of EC-IC Bypass Grafting

Different bypass procedures are possible in the anterior circulation and depend on the choice of extracranial and intracranial arteries. The most commonly performed procedure is a bypass between the superficial temporal artery and a cortical branch of the middle cerebral artery.

Anesthetic Technique

After induction with sodium thiopental and endotracheal intubation, a Foley catheter is placed into the urinary bladder and the head is shaved. The patient is placed in the three-quarter supine position with the head turned into the full lateral position (Fig. 154-1). Severe rotation of the cervical spine should be avoided. This is particularly important in patients with severe osteoarthritis or contralateral carotid or vertebral atherosclerosis. In that instance, the patient is placed in the full lateral decubitus position. The head is fixed in the pin head holder. An arterial catheter is placed percutaneously in the radial artery to monitor the blood gas concentration as well as the blood pressure. A high normal arterial P_{CO_2} (between 34 and 40 mmHg) and a high normal blood pressure are maintained throughout the procedure.

Surgical Technique (STA-MCA Bypass)

Magnification and illumination are provided by an operating microscope fitted with 12.5× eyepieces, an inclined binocular tube, and a 200-mm objective. A beam splitter is used to accommodate a television camera and a 35-mm camera. A binocular observer tube positioned on the right side is used by the first assistant.

The superficial temporal artery divides into a frontal and a parietal branch approximately 1 cm anterior and superior to the external auditory meatus. The position of the scalp artery is localized anterior to the tragus by palpation or with a Doppler stethoscope if necessary. With the microscope in position over the temporal region (with a magnification of 6×) an incision is made with a no. 15 scalpel blade directly over the proximal portion of the superficial temporal artery. The skin edges are retracted with an Alm self-retaining retractor to minimize bleeding. Subcutaneous bleeding ves-

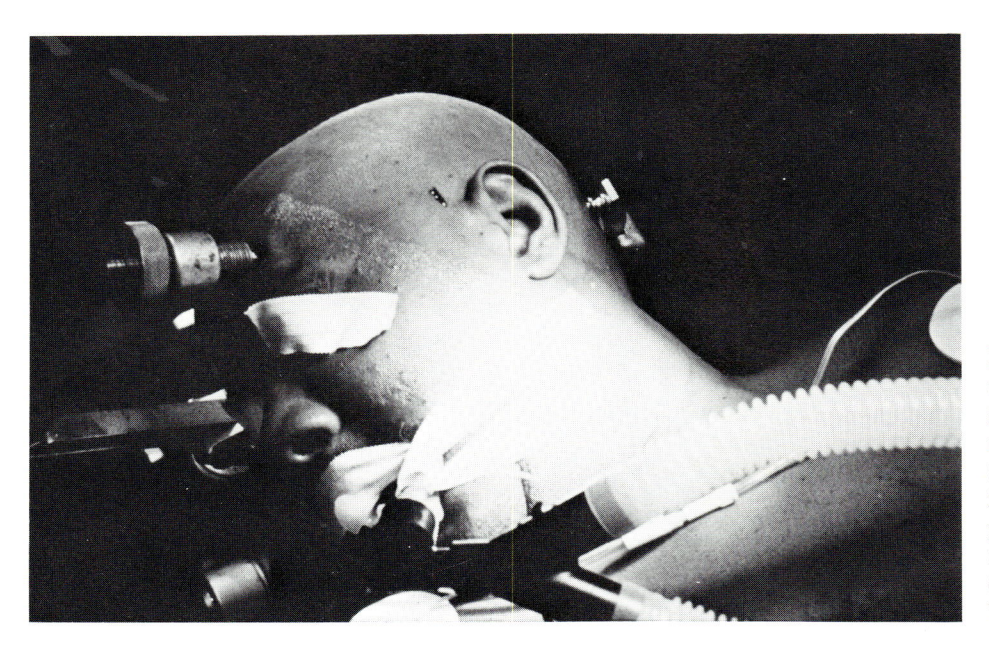

Figure 154-1 Patient positioned in the pin head holder for superficial temporal artery–middle cerebral artery (STA-MCA) anastomosis. The incision is started along the proximal segment of the STA. (From Fein JM, Flamm E: *Cerebrovascular Surgery.* New York, Springer-Verlag, 1983.)

sels are individually coagulated with an angled bipolar microcautery forceps. The scalp artery is exposed on its superficial aspect, but left undisturbed in its fascial bed (Fig. 154-2). The dissection continues in the plane between the adventitia and the overlying subcutaneous fascia. Although the frontal branch is usually larger than the parietal branch, this is not dissected if it provides collateral channels to the orbit. The appropriate branch is exposed progressively by sharp dissection of the skin and the fascia overlying the artery for 5 to 6 cm. This length is necessary, bearing in mind the new course of the vessel through the cranial layers and across the subdural space. Incisions are then made through the galea on either side of the artery and down to the temporalis fascia. This provides a cuff of fascia on three sides of the scalp artery. The distal 1 cm of the scalp artery is then prepared and cleaned of its surrounding fascia and fat by a sharp dissection technique.

The skin incision is then extended posteriorly approximately 3 cm above the ear. Scalp flaps are raised and held apart by dural hooks. A stellate incision is made in the muscle using the electrocautery. Muscle flaps are then elevated by subperiosteal dissection, but the muscle fascia should be preserved for later closure. A craniectomy 4 to 6 cm in diameter is made in the posterior temporal region using the craniotome. Unless the dura is tightly adherent to the inner table, the edges are lined with strips of Gelfoam and no. 4-0 tenting sutures are placed along the bone edge. The dura is then opened in stellate fashion, and the dural edges are thoroughly coagulated and held back with sutures. The subarachnoid space may bulge against the craniotomy edges, in which case the arachnoid is opened sharply to release cerebrospinal fluid. This is sufficient to relax the brain.

The angular artery is usually the largest cortical branch of the middle cerebral artery, with a mean diameter of 1.2 mm. The posterior temporal artery and the posterior parietal branches are also usually larger than 1.0 mm. When an appropriate recipient artery is selected, the investing arachnoid directly over the artery is elevated with Dumont forceps and cut sharply with a curved microscissor under 16× magnification. Traction on the periarterial chordae that suspend the arteries in the subarachnoid space should be avoided, as this will produce vasospasm. Further manipulation of the artery may then be more difficult. If vasospasm occurs, a few drops of papavarine solution may be applied to the vessel. The cortical artery is mobilized from the cortical surface by coagulating and cutting two to three penetrating branches. This should provide a 1.5 cm length of the cortical artery for bypass grafting. After the cortical artery is mobilized, a small rubber dam is cut and placed under the artery to protect the underlying cortex.

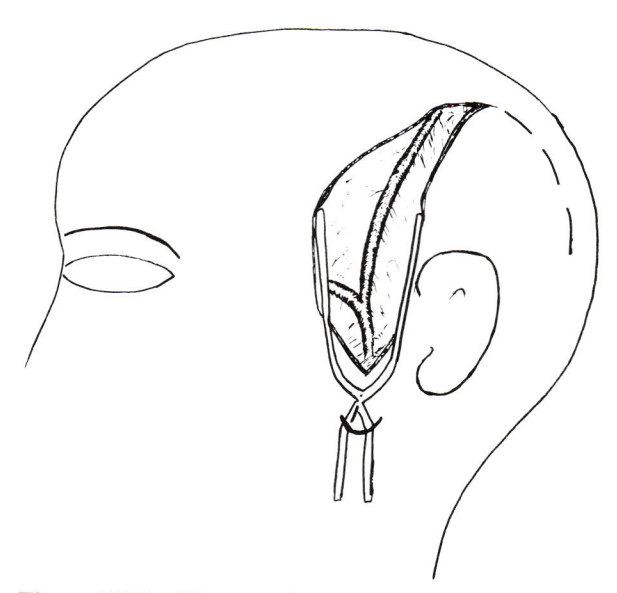

Figure 154-2 The operating microscope (6×) is used to expose the STA in the subcutaneous tissue. (From Fein JM, Flamm E: *Cerebrovascular Surgery.* New York, Springer-Verlag, 1983.)

The proximal portion of the STA is temporarily occluded with a long Biemer clip, and the distal portion is permanently occluded with a Weck clip. The distal STA is then transected on a bevel and transposed intracranially after it has been irrigated with heparinized saline. Small Biemer clips are then applied to the cortical artery. An elliptical arteriotomy incision two to three times the diameter of the artery is then made with a curved microscissors. This isolated arterial segment is cleansed of blood by irrigation with heparinized saline.

The STA should then be aligned with its leading edge directed toward the proximal segment of the cortical artery. The lumen of the STA and the lumen of the cortical artery should be perfectly opposed. The lumen of the STA can be enlarged by a simple extension of the incision along the shorter wall if necessary (fish-mouth opening). Separate tacking sutures (no. 10-0 Ethilon, Ethicon, Inc., Somerville, N. J.) are then placed 180 degrees apart and are used as a continuous suture on either side of the anastomosis. Each suture is tied to itself and remains independent of the other sutures. This partially continuous suture allows delayed expansion of the graft.

After the anastomosis is completed, the distal cortical clip is opened first to allow back bleeding at the anastomosis. The proximal cortical clip and finally the clip on the STA are then removed. Pulsations should progress from the STA toward the proximal portion of the cortical artery. There may be some persistent ooze from the fascia of the superficial temporal artery, and these points are identified with gentle irrigation and controlled with microbipolar cautery. Absolute hemostasis is required before closure. The dura is left open and a disc of Gelfoam is placed over the craniectomy defect. The temporalis muscle is partially closed so that the artery is not kinked. The galea is usually deficient where the STA was dissected, and special care is needed to close this layer with sutures of inverted polyglactin (Vicryl, Ethicon, Inc.) The skin edges are then gently opposed with a nylon suture.

Low molecular weight dextran is infused intravenously at a rate of 50 ml/h beginning about 2 h after the operation. This is maintained for the first 24 h postoperatively. The patient is observed in the intensive care unit to be certain that the blood pressure, pulse, and arterial blood gases are monitored frequently. Liberal fluid replacement at approximately 100 ml/h is employed. After 24 h the patient is gradually elevated and may sit out of bed with continuous blood pressure monitoring. Scalp sutures are removed 7 days postoperatively. Patency of the bypass can often be evaluated by palpating the pulse from the proximal segment of the STA to the edge of the craniectomy. The Doppler stethoscope is also used when necessary to assess patency.

Alternate Bypass Grafts

Other arteries or graft materials have been used for bypass grafting when the caliber of the STA has been inadequate. The occipital branch of the external carotid artery has been used by Spetzler and Chater[24] and others. The middle meningeal arteries were used by Nishikawa et al. in a patient with moyamoya disease.[20]

Lougheed et al. described the use of a free vein graft harvested from the leg and interposed between the common carotid and intracranial internal carotid artery in a patient with recurrent symptoms secondary to a right internal carotid occlusion.[18] Attempts in two other patients were unsuccessful because of atheroma in the intracranial internal carotid artery. Interposition free grafts have been employed by Ausman et al. in patients with common carotid artery occlusion. A long vein graft was placed from the ipsilateral subclavian artery to the external carotid artery followed by an STA-MCA bypass for retinal ischemia.[1] Radial artery grafts have been used between the external carotid artery and middle cerebral branches by a number of surgeons, but have been complicated by intimal hyperplasia. We have utilized long saphenous vein grafts to the cortical artery in five patients with inadequate superficial temporal arteries; a short saphenous vein graft was used between the proximal STA and the cortical artery in a patient with an STA that ramified into small branches that were inadequate for use. Synthetic materials have been used by other authors. For example, Story et al. described the use of expanded polytetrafluoroethylene.[25] The long-term patency rates using these materials are not as good as with the superficial temporal artery. All free grafts require both a proximal and a distal anastomosis and are devoid of an intrinsic blood supply. In addition, vein grafts tend to react to arterial blood pressure surges with intimal hyperplasia.

Results

There were 207 bypass procedures performed between 1972 and 1983. These procedures were evaluated by postoperative hemodynamic studies, and the patients were evaluated by serial clinical examinations. There are various techniques for measuring the quality and degree of cerebral perfusion achieved through the bypass graft; however, none is as reliable or informative at present as cerebral angiography. The results of various methods indicate that our patency rate immediately after surgery is excellent, with some decrease in the patency rate over long-term follow-up as a result of occasional graft occlusion.

Postoperative Angiography

Angiography provides detailed visualization of the bypass and its relative contribution to cerebral perfusion (Figs. 154-3 to 154-5). In our patients a single postoperative angiogram was performed between 1 week and 1 year after the operation. Sixty-four postoperative angiograms were performed during the original hospitalization. There was an overall patency rate of 96 percent. The STA was measurably larger on the first postoperative study in only five cases (8 percent). A second postoperative angiogram was performed in 59 cases between 6 months and 4 years after surgery. The patency rate decreased to 93 percent. However, enlargement of the bypass graft was seen in 41 patients, or 69 percent, of those restudied. An increase in the number of branches perfused through the graft was seen in 32 patients, or 54 per-

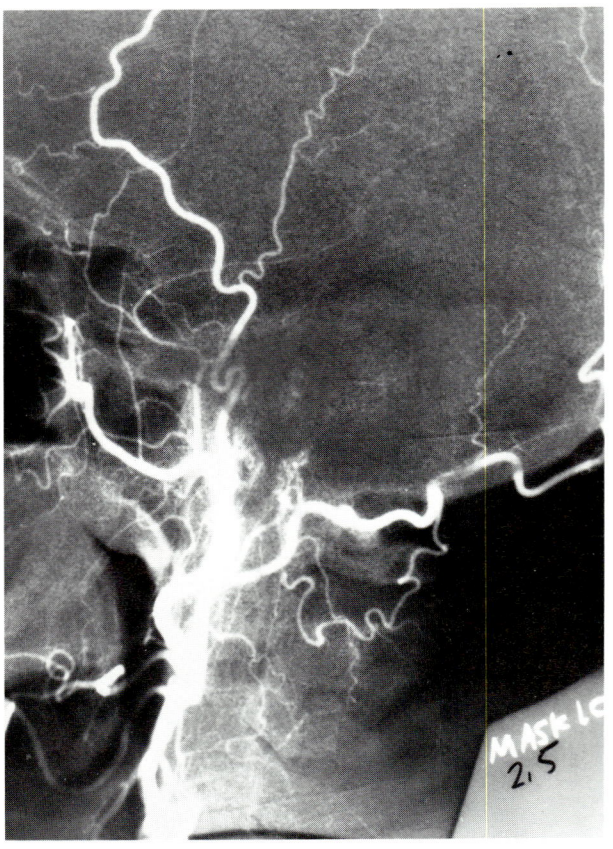

Figure 154-3 Preoperative left lateral carotid angiogram of a 58-year-old man with recurrent transient dysphasia. The angiogram disclosed complete occlusion of the left internal carotid artery. The frontal branch of the STA is prominent. (From Fein JM, Flamm E: *Cerebrovascular Surgery*. New York, Springer-Verlag, 1983.)

cent, of those studied. These studies indicate that both immediate and more delayed augmentation of flow through the bypass may be anticipated.

Digital Angiography

The patency rates determined by current generation DIVA studies and by arterial angiography are similar. However, the details of intracranial filling patterns are not as good with DIVA as with conventional arterial angiography. In 27 cases in which postoperative DIVA studies were performed, 22 showed a patent bypass. Three studies were equivocal, and two showed no intracranial filling. Arterial angiograms disclosed that 26 of the 27 bypass grafts were patent.

Regional Cerebral Blood Flow Studies

Regional cerebral blood flow studies using the ^{133}Xe inhalation method are subject to significant problems of interpretation. These are related to assumptions regarding the partition coefficient for ^{133}Xe in abnormal tissue and the nontomographic nature of most of the recording techniques. Studies by some authors[10,12] have demonstrated a significant increase in regional, hemispheric, and even contralateral blood flow, but this has not been confirmed by others.[11] An intracerebral steal favoring the ischemic area can be corrected.[5]

Clinical Results

The major goal of surgery is to reduce the risk of future ischemic events in patients with a history of TIA, RIND, or CS. In my series of 207 patients the frequency of ischemic

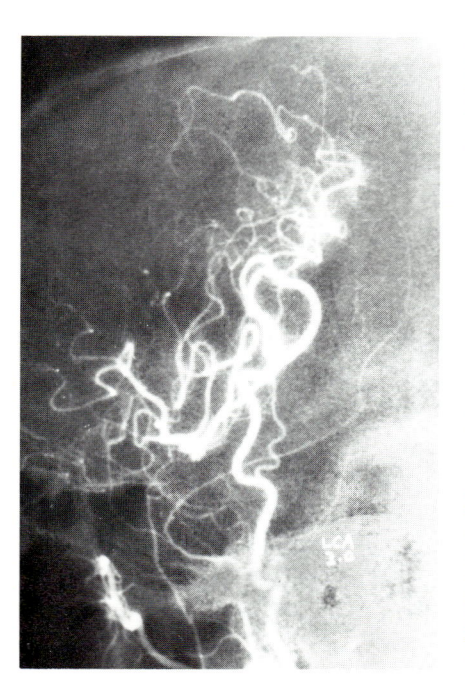

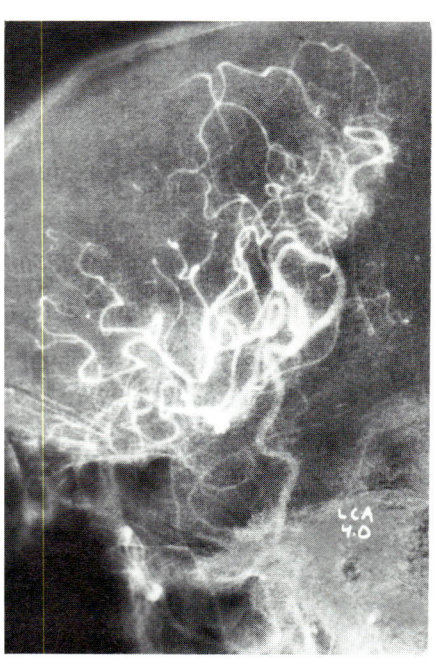

Figure 154-4 Same patient as in Fig. 154-3. Postoperative lateral angiogram views show excellent reflux into all of the branches of the MCA from the STA. (From Fein JM, Flamm E: *Cerebrovascular Surgery*. New York, Spring-Verlag, 1983.)

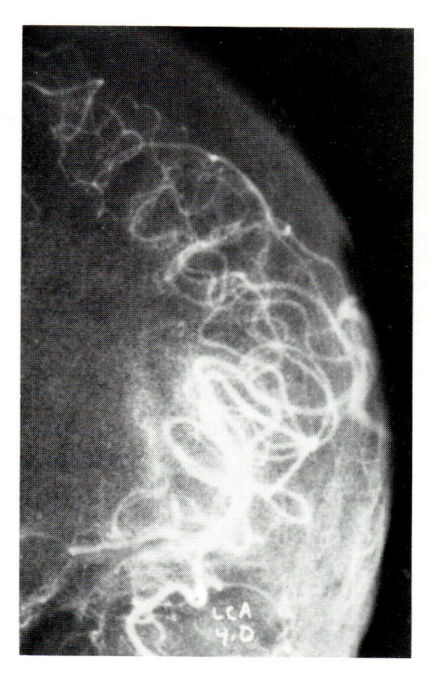

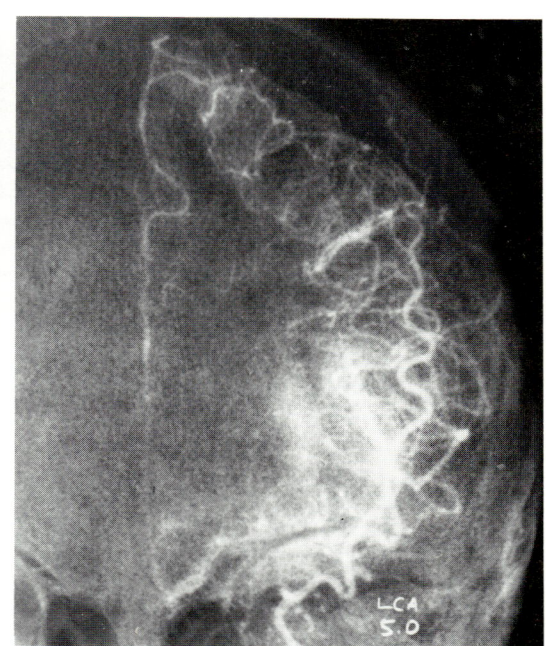

Figure 154-5 Same patient as in Figs. 154-3 and 154-4. Postoperative anteroposterior films of the left common carotid injection show intracranial filling of the middle cerebral artery group by the STA. (From Fein JM, Flamm E: *Cerebrovascular Surgery*. New York, Springer-Verlag, 1983.)

events was 1.2 percent per year and the frequency of new completed strokes was 0.04 percent per year over an average follow-up of 4.5 years. Occlusion of the graft was found in five of eight patients with new ischemic events.

In three patients a repeat angiogram disclosed poor graft function with a single cortical branch filling from the bypass. The bypass was probably occluded in three others, although this was not documented. The incidence of stroke in several large surgical series appears to be significantly lower than that expected in patients at risk.[8,27] Samson et al. found that patients with a completed stroke who subsequently develop TIA(s) in the territory of an occluded carotid artery have a lower incidence (7 percent) of subsequent stroke compared with the rate expected from previously published studies (40 percent).[22]

A cooperative randomized study to compare the frequency of future ischemic events in patients treated with aspirin and in those treated with aspirin and bypass grafting is in progress. The aim of the study is to see if there is a 50 percent reduction in the frequency of stroke. To date, no therapy used for the treatment of cerebrovascular disease has fullfilled this stringent criterion for effectiveness. It is unlikely that this degree of risk reduction can be found in a heterogeneous population of patients with a variable intrinsic risk for stroke. It is unclear whether trends could then be found in smaller subgroups of patients that might benefit from bypass surgery.

Complications

The EC-IC bypass is a low-risk procedure in properly selected patients. Surgical mortality rates have varied from 0 to 7.7 percent.[8,17,27] Ischemic complications are more frequent in patients operated on for stroke in evolution. The only stroke-related death in our series occurred in a 38-year-old woman with bilateral carotid occlusive disease who had surgery during a stroke in evolution. She developed a hemorrhagic infarction 24 h after the operation and rapidly deteriorated thereafter. The other surgical death was the result of an acute myocardial infarction that occurred 25 days postoperatively in a 72-year-old patient. In my series, the mortality rate was 0.9 percent.

Ischemic complications during surgery or immediately thereafter are unusual. None of the patients in my series had an intraoperative or perioperative stroke. The frequency of local complications was 7 percent. Scalp necrosis developed at the junction of the T-shaped incision in 14 patients. This most often involved only the skin, and it healed with no specific treatment. Surgical revision, consisting of debridement and reapproximation of the edges, was required in two patients. Since the muscle and dural closure is incomplete, a superficial infection may rapidly communicate with the subdural or subarachnoid compartments through the open dura. Subgaleal and subdural empyema was seen in two patients. Both patients developed fever and focal seizures. Both required reoperation, irrigation, and debridement followed by a single-layer closure of the scalp flap with nylon sutures. There were no long-term sequelae in these patients. Cellulitis of the skin overlying the bypass occurred in one patient and responded to intravenous penicillin and chloramphenicol. There were no lasting effects from this. Since a tight dural closure cannot be achieved, a very meticulous and complete closure of the galea is employed in anticipation of a CSF leak.

The rate of cardiac and systemic complications was low. Four patients developed new cardiac arrhythmias, and two had recurrence of perioperative arrhythmias, which were successfully treated. One patient had a myocardial infarction 2 weeks postoperatively with no sequelae. Three patients developed transient pneumonia, and 11 percent had transient urinary tract infections.

Future Prospects

The feasibility of using other techniques for bypass surgery is under study. Interposition vein grafts have the advantage of a greater flow capacity, but are technically more difficult to use and have a lower long-term patency rate. The limitation on their function is usually related to the small size of the distal anastomosis, which can only be partially overcome by the onlay graft technique described above. Anastomosis to one of the main divisions of the middle cerebral artery through the Sylvian fissure may be more successful. Preoperative and postoperative evaluations of these patients may be more fruitful with the development of tomographic techniques for studying CBF.

References

1. Ausman JI, Lindsay W, Ramsey RC, Chou SN: Ipsilateral subclavian to external carotid and STA-MCA bypasses for retinal ischemia. Surg Neurol 9:5–8, 1978.
2. Chou SN: Embolectomy of middle cerebral artery: Report of a case. J Neurosurg 20:161–163, 1963.
3. Diaz FG, Ausman JI, de los Reyes RA, Dujovny M: Successful application of acute cerebral revascularization to stroke in evolution. Presented at the 55th Scientific Session, American Heart Association, October 1982.
4. Donaghy RMP: Patch and bypass in microangional surgery, in Donaghy RMP, Yasargil MG (eds): *Microvascular Surgery*. St Louis, Mosby, 1967, pp 75–86.
5. Fein JM: Reversal of intracerebral nutrient steal phenomenon after extracranial-intracranial (EC-IC) bypass graft. Neurosurgery 2:158, 1978 (abstr).
6. Fein JM, Flamm E: Planned intracranial revascularization before proximal ligation for traumatic aneurysm. Neurosurgery 5:254–258, 1979.
7. Fein JM, Lipow KI: Cortical artery pressure measurements in cerebrovascular occlusive disease (in press).
8. Fein JM, Reichman OH (eds): *Microvascular Anastomoses for Cerebral Ischemia*. New York, Springer-Verlag, 1978.
9. Fields WS, Lemak NA: Joint study of extracranial arterial occlusion: X. Internal carotid artery occlusion. JAMA 235:2734–2738, 1976.
10. Gratzl O, Schmiedek P, Spetzler R, Steinhoff H, Marguth F: Clinical experience with extra-intracranial arterial anastomosis in 65 cases. J Neurosurg 44:313–324, 1976.
11. Halsey JH Jr, Morawetz RB, Blauenstein UW: The hemodynamic effect of STA-MCA bypass. Stroke 13:163–167, 1982.
12. Heilbrun MP, Reichman OH, Anderson RE, Roberts TS: Regional cerebral blood flow studies following superficial temporal-middle cerebral artery anastomosis. J Neurosurg 43:706–716, 1975.
13. Henschen C: Operative Revaskularisation des zirkulatorisch geschädigten Gehirns durch auflage gestielter Muskellappen (Encephalo-Myo-Synangiose). Langenbecks Arch Klin Chir 264:392–401, 1950.
14. Holbach KH, Wassmann H, Hoheluchter KL, Jain KK: Differentiation between reversible and irreversible post-stroke changes in brain tissue: Its relevance for cerebrovascular surgery. Surg Neurol 7:325–331, 1977.
15. Hutchison EC, Acheson EJ: *Strokes: Natural History, Pathology and Surgical Treatment*. London, Saunders, 1975.
16. Jacobson JH II, Wallman LJ, Schumacher GA, Flanagan M, Suarez EL, Donaghy RMP: Microsurgery as an aid to middle cerebral artery endarterectomy. J Neurosurg 19:108–115, 1962.
17. Kikuchi H, Karasawa J: Clinical experiences with STA-MCA anastomosis in 54 cases, in Fein JM, Reichman OH (eds): *Microvascular Anastomoses for Cerebral Ischemia*. New York, Springer-Verlag, 1978, pp 278–283.
18. Lougheed WM, Marshall BM, Hunter M, Michel ER, Sandwith-Smyth H: Common carotid to intracranial internal carotid bypass venous graft. J Neurosurg 34:114–118, 1971.
19. Millikan C: Treatment of occlusive cerebrovascular disease, in Siekert RG (ed): *Cerebrovascular Survey Report* (Joint Council Subcommittee on Cerebrovascular Disease, National Institute of Neurological and Communicative Disorders and Stroke). Bethesda, Md., National Institutes of Health, 1980, pp 244–289.
20. Nishikawa M, Hashi K, Shiguma M: Middle meningeal-middle cerebral artery anastomosis for cerebral ischemia. Surg Neurol 12:205–208, 1979.
21. Roski RA, Spetzler RF, Nulsen FE: Late ischemic complications of carotid ligation in the treatment of intracranial aneurysms. Presented at the 48th Annual Meeting, American Association of Neurological Surgeons, New York, April 21, 1980.
22. Samson D, Watts C, Clark K: Cerebral revascularization for transient ischemic attacks. Neurology 27:767–771, 1977.
23. Scheibert CD: Middle cerebral artery surgery for obstructive lesions. Presented at the 27th Annual Meeting, Harvey Cushing Society, New Orleans, May 1959.
24. Spetzler R, Chater N: Occipital artery-middle cerebral artery anastomosis for cerebral artery occlusive disease. Surg Neurol 2:235–238, 1974.
25. Story JL, Brown WE Jr, Eidelberg E, Arom KV, Stewart JR: Cerebral revascularization: Proximal external carotid to distal middle cerebral artery bypass with a synthetic tube graft. Neurosurgery 3:61–65, 1978.
26. Strully KJ, Hurwitt ES, Blankenberg HW: Thrombo-endarterectomy for thrombosis of the internal carotid artery in the neck. J Neurosurg 10:474–482, 1953.
27. Sundt TM Jr, Siekert RG, Piepgras DG, Sharbrough FW, Houser OW: Bypass surgery for vascular disease of the carotid system. Mayo Clin Proc 51:677–692, 1976.
28. Welch K: Excision of occlusive lesions of the middle cerebral artery. J Neurosurg 13:73–80, 1956.
29. Woringer E, Kunlin J: Anastomose entre la carotide primitive et la carotide intra-cranienne ou la sylvienne par greffon selon la technique de la suture suspendue. Neurochirurgie 9:181–188, 1963.
30. Yasargil MG: *Microsurgery Applied to Neurosurgery*. Stuttgart, Georg Thieme Verlag, 1969, pp 51–58.

155

Extracranial to Intracranial Bypass Grafting: Posterior Circulation

Thoralf M. Sundt, Jr.
David G. Piepgras

Ischemic symptomatology in the posterior circulation is very frequently related to vascular disease in the penetrating vessels with the production of lacunar infarcts. However, there does remain a large number of patients with symptomatology related to large vessel occlusive disease in the posterior circulation. Very commonly symptoms are caused by hemodynamic changes from high-grade stenotic lesions rather than from emboli. We will consider in this chapter the surgical approach to large vessel occlusive disease in the posterior circulation. It should be emphasized that these are major procedures and should not be undertaken unless it is clear that the patient's symptomatology is progressing on conservative management.

Vascular Anatomy and Blood Flow

The intracranial circulation is divided into conducting arteries and penetrating arterioles. The conducting vessels are the carotid, middle cerebral, anterior cerebral, vertebral, basilar, and posterior cerebral arteries in addition to their major (named) and minor (unnamed) branches on the surface of the brain. These branches form a vast network of interconnecting and anastomosing vessels on the surface of the brain. The conducting vessels may be regarded as nonresistance-type vessels because there is only a 10 percent drop in perfusion pressure from the aorta to major branches of the middle cerebral artery and a similar gradient from these large branches to the level of the penetrating arterioles. The latter enter the brain parenchyma at right angles to the surface vessels from which they are derived. The system of conducting vessels serves as a pressure head or pressure equalization reservoir to furnish an adequate perfusion pressure to the penetrating or nutrient arterioles wherein primary autoregulation probably resides. The conducting vessels, the recipients of emboli and the sites of primary atherosclerosis, form a low-resistance bed that is ideal for bypass surgery. The penetrating vessels, when involved with arteriolar sclerosis, cause lacunar infarcts.[6]

The rate of normal blood flow to the brain is about 50 to 55 ml/100 g per minute.[8] However, the brain can accommodate a substantial reduction in flow and still function. Laboratory and clinical studies indicate that the minimal amount of blood flow required to sustain normal electrical activity in the brain approximates 15 ml/100 g per minute.[2,7,10,13] Reductions of flow below this critical level are associated with physiological paralysis and, if prolonged, cerebral infarction. Ischemic tolerance of neural tissue depends both upon the duration and the severity of ischemia, but the elegant studies of Symon and co-workers have demonstrated that flows of 5 ml/100 g per minute are associated with electrolyte shifts and cellular membrane changes that are probably not reversible.[2] Fortunately, many patients with ischemic symptomatology have marginal flows that, although inadequate to sustain physiological function, are nevertheless adequate to prevent anatomical infarction.

Patterns of Large Vessel Occlusive Disease

Fisher and his colleagues[6] reported that, in contrast to the carotid arteries where symptomatic occlusions were often extracranial, in the vertebral arteries symptomatic occlusions were more often intracranial. This observation, later confirmed by other workers,[5] is of considerable importance because the commonest site for stenosis or occlusion of the vertebral artery is at its origin from the subclavian artery. However, stenotic lesions at this location are usually protected by a collateral system of vessels arising from deep muscular branches of the thyrocervical and costocervical arteries, so that brain infarction from this source is uncommon. Atherosclerotic plaques are diffusely distributed throughout the vertebral arteries, but ulceration of these plaques is not common.[5] Again this is in contrast to the carotid system where plaques are often near the bifurcation of the common carotid artery and ulceration with secondary embolization is common.

Emboli (from the heart or common carotid artery bifurcation) are thought to be the chief cause of occlusion of the major branches of the internal carotid artery intracranially. This does not seem to be the case in the vertebrobasilar system where Castaigne and associates found thrombosis on a pre-existing stenosis to be the cause of 90 percent of basilar artery occlusions and 70 percent of intracranial vertebral artery occlusions (the correlation of infarction with basilar artery occlusion was 100 percent and with vertebral artery occlusion, 50 percent).[5] These workers thought that occlusion on a pre-existing stenosis was uncommon in the extracranial vertebral artery but common in the intracranial portion of that vessel. In that study, occlusions of the posterior cerebral artery were thought to be embolic in origin in 94 percent of their cases; this finding indicated that these vessels, the terminal branches of the basilar artery, were the likeliest recipients of emboli and in this respect were similar to the major branches of the internal carotid artery.

Although the cause of infarction in the carotid and vertebrobasilar systems can be evaluated pathologically, the cause of transient ischemic attacks (TIAs) are more difficult to assess. Various causes have been proposed, but two are most often considered, namely, emboli from ulcerated plaques of large vessels to more distal arteries and hemodynamic changes distal to the site of stenosis or occlusion of an artery. The hemodynamic changes may result from either variations in systemic perfusion pressure or failure of collateral flow. The former seems to occur more often in the carotid circulation, the latter (in the authors' judgment) in the vertebrobasilar circulation.

Ischemic Syndromes

Correlation of clinical symptoms and signs with the results of angiographic and cerebral blood flow studies indicate that flow rates between 20 and 30 ml/100 g per minute are borderline.[7,13] Patients with flow rates this low are often neurologically unstable and particularly vulnerable to the effects of emboli. The development of infarction is related to both the degree and the duration of ischemia. It occurs within minutes in areas of zero flow, but may take hours in regions of marginal flow. Blood flow in zones of incomplete focal ischemia is nonhomogeneous with areas of reactive hyperemia and zones of decreased perfusion often being adjacent to infarcted tissue.

A transient focal neurological deficit due to ischemia less than 24 h in duration is considered to represent a transient ischemic attack. In the vertebrobasilar system, TIAs are less stereotyped than those in the carotid system. Vertigo is a common component of a TIA in the vertebrobasilar system; however, vertigo alone is most commonly a manifestation of a labyrinthine disorder and therefore, unless associated with some other manifestation of brain stem ischemia, should not be regarded as a TIA. A transient hemiparesis, hemisensory deficit, or homonymous hemianopsia can arise from ischemia in either the anterior or the posterior circulatory systems. However, they are usually considered to represent a carotid TIA unless symptoms occur on alternating sides in different episodes or there is a history of cranial nerve dysfunction or contralateral sensory dysfunction. The occurrence of alternating sides with ischemic events or a transient quadriparesis is most commonly of brain stem origin.

Dysarthria and dysphagia, which are symptoms of bulbar ischemia, may be seen in patients with pseudobulbar palsy from supratentorial lesions, but they are most commonly brain stem in origin. Transient impairment of function of the extraocular muscles may be of definite localizing value, but if diplopia is due to a TIA, it will usually be associated with other symptoms. Ataxia of gait or of the extremities is also of localizing value but must be distinguished from a transient paresis. This is often difficult to determine on the basis of a history alone. Nausea, vomiting, and vertigo may occur with a brain stem TIA, but this combination is not useful for distinguishing brain stem from labyrinthine dysfunction.

A reversible neurological deficit (RIND) is a neurological deficit that persists longer than 24 h but nevertheless is fully reversible. In the past this was considered to represent a small infarction, but in the light of laboratory studies it is probable that this is a prolonged ischemic event with a physiological paralysis that has not progressed to anatomical infarction.

A progressing stroke is a stepwise or gradually progressing neurological deficit evolving during hours or a few days. The dysfunction begins as a relatively minor deficit that culminates in a major deficit in the absence of treatment. Progressing strokes involving the vertebrobasilar system are often severe and may cause pronounced incapacity leading to death.

Primary orthostatic cerebral ischemia describes generalized, nonfocal, cerebral ischemia related to erect posture in a patient with multiple occlusions of major extracranial vessels. We described this in an earlier report, but the credit for the initial analysis of this syndrome goes to Caplan and Sergay.[4] Postural light-headedness or syncope, dimming or blurring of vision, and ataxia and altered mentation or memory are prominent symptoms.

Syncope alone is most commonly related to systemic orthostatic hypotension. However, patients with major extracranial vessel occlusions often have syncope associated with the upright position without a drop in the peripheral blood pressure. Perhaps this syndrome can arise from localized ischemia in the brain stem, but in general, syncope appears to represent a generalized or nonfocal form of cerebral ischemia.

Ischemic pain related to vertebrobasilar occlusive disease is most often referred to the occipital area. Obviously, headaches alone are more commonly due to causes unrelated to ischemia, so that one must be cautious in attributing this relatively common complaint to the relatively rare syndrome of vertebrobasilar occlusive disease. The mechanism of this complaint with ischemia in the posterior circulation remains obscure.

Indications for Angiography and Surgical Intervention

The patients on whom we have operated to date are either suffering from a progressing neurological deficit or have been disabled by the frequency and severity of transient ischemic events. Patients accepted for an occipital to posterior inferior cerebellar artery bypass procedure have had either bilateral intracranial vertebral artery occlusions proximal to the origins of the PICAs or unilateral vertebral artery occlusion in tandem with a high-grade intracranial stenosis of the opposite vertebral artery. Patients accepted for an interposition vein graft between the external carotid artery and the proximal posterior cerebral artery have had a high-grade stenosis of the basilar artery or a total occlusion of that vessel. In these patients the posterior communicating arteries are invariably absent or very small so that there has been no collateral flow from the carotid system to the basilar system.

Presenting complaints have included: ataxia, visual disturbances, altered mentation, and changes in sensorium with erect posture. Some patients had progressing strokes in the brain stem or cerebellum. Others had multiple TIAs not altered by anticoagulant therapy. No patients were evaluated who had only one or two TIAs of the posterior circulation. In our experience, angiograms in these patients are often normal or show only minimal large vessel disease.

Selected Cases

Occipital Artery Pedicle to PICA Bypass Procedure

A 55-year-old retired farmer came to our institution in February 1976 with complaints of "dizziness and roaring in the ears" of 14 months' duration. In January 1975, he had begun to experience intermittent vertigo associated with blurred vision and a sensation that he was losing consciousness. These episodes occurred daily and were usually associated with exercise or standing up from a sitting position. In April 1975, more severe vertigo developed together with the sensation of a "pounding" in his head. Symptoms progressed to the point where the patient was forced to retire from active employment. Anticoagulants and aspirin were unsuccessful in relieving the patient's symptomatology. Angiograms performed in his local hospital demonstrated symmetrically placed, high-grade stenotic lesions of both vertebral arteries just proximal to the origin of the posterior inferior cerebellar arteries.

At the time of medical and neurological examination at our clinic, loud systolic bruits were heard on auscultation over the mastoid processes bilaterally. Peripheral blood pressures were 136/82 mmHg; there was no orthostatic decrease. The results of the remainder of the examination were normal.

A relatively large occipital artery originating from the vertebral artery at the level of C1 rather than the external carotid artery was anastomosed to the left posterior inferior cerebellar artery in April 1976. The patient had an uncomplicated recovery. The pounding sensation ceased, and the bruits were no longer heard on auscultation. Postoperative angiography of the patient before dismissal demonstrated good patency of the graft.

Repeat angiography in September 1976 showed further enlargement of the bypass graft (Fig. 155-1). The vertebral artery stenotic lesions had progressed to total occlusion, and the entire posterior circulation filled through the bypass graft. The patient had returned to normal activities and was essentially asymptomatic.

Interposition Saphenous Vein Graft

A 69-year-old retired salesman was admitted to his local hospital on August 7, 1980 with a 1-week history of intermittent attacks of vertigo, light-headedness, diaphoresis, dysarthria,

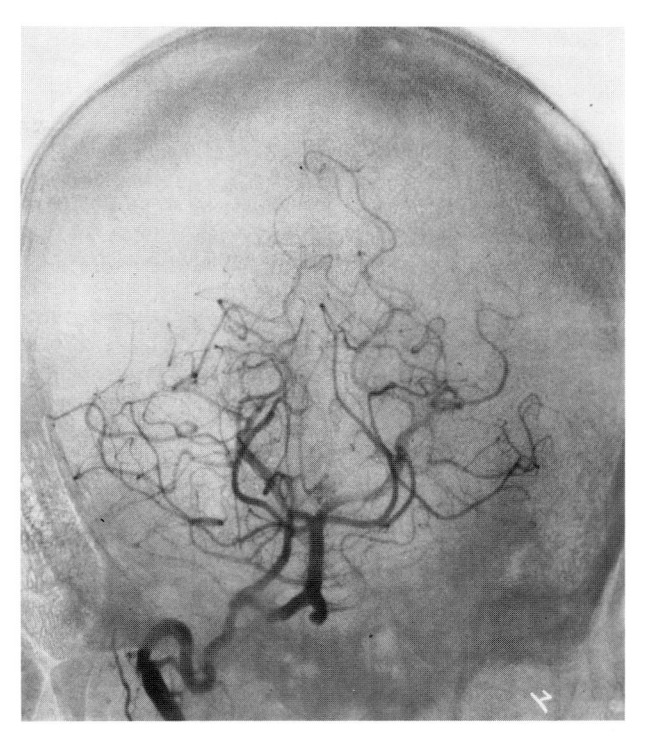

Figure 155-1 Postoperative angiogram 6 months after bypass graft in Patient 2. Further enlargement of the bypass graft and occlusion of the vertebral artery at the site of previous stenosis are seen. The entire vertebrobasilar system, together with the distal segment of the opposite vertebral artery (distal to the site of the opposite vertebral artery stenosis), fills from the occipital artery to PICA bypass graft.

right hemiparesis, right hemisensory deficits, and occasional diminution or loss of consciousness. These attacks were particularly associated with sitting up or standing up from the supine position, and lasted 30 to 45 min. He had no previous history of cerebral vascular insufficiency. He was not a diabetic. He had undergone a successful two-vessel coronary bypass procedure 7 years previously.

A computed tomography (CT) scan on admission was normal. The patient was placed on a course of heparin and bed rest. He continued to have two to three episodes per day consisting of several or all of the above symptoms. On at least one occasion he was noted to have a left hemiparesis rather than a right hemiparesis. The extreme orthostatic nature of his problem was noted on at least two occasions when he sat up for one reason or another in bed and promptly had an ischemic attack. Angiograms on August 18, 1980 identified total occlusion of the left vertebral artery up to the level of a small posterior inferior cerebellar artery. The right vertebral artery was small and ended in a large posterior inferior cerebellar artery. The carotid systems were essentially normal.

On August 19, the patient was transferred by air ambulance to our hospital, a distance of some 300 miles, without incident. However, it was necessary to keep him in the supine position on arrival, because his attempts to sit on the edge of the bed or assume the upright position resulted in ischemic events. The neurological examination revealed no major fixed deficit.

On August 22, surgery was performed under general anesthesia through a modified pterional approach. The right saphenous vein, which had been harvested between the groin and the knee, was anastomosed end to end between the resected stump of the right external carotid artery and the proximal posterior cerebral artery just distal to the third nerve. This graft was brought through a tunnel in the neck; it ran from the carotid bifurcation, through the subcutaneous tissue anterior to the ear, and then through the lower margin of the craniotomy in the inferior aspect of the temporal fossa just superior to the zygoma. The intracranial anastomosis was completed using a running no. 7-0 Prolene (Ethicon, Inc., Somerville, N.J.) suture, and the proximal anastomosis was constructed using interrupted no. 5-0 Prolene sutures. Blood flow through the graft was recorded at 140 ml/min.

The patient awoke from the operative procedure with no neurological deficit and had an uncomplicated postoperative recovery. He was discharged from the hospital on September 3, 1980. Postoperative angiograms (Fig. 155-2) demonstrated excellent flow through the bypass graft. He has remained well since discharge, and is taking aspirin and dipyridamole.

Surgical Technique

Occipital Artery Pedicle to Posterior Inferior Cerebellar Artery Bypass Procedure

The operative technique is illustrated in Fig. 155-3. The patient is placed in the sitting position with the head flexed anteriorly and secured in a pinion head holder.[11] A hockey-stick incision is preferred, with the longitudinal component of the incision positioned over the midline avascular plane. The musculature is swept unilaterally from the arch of C1 and the occiput. The cutting current is not used for the scalp incision but is useful to reflect the deep neck muscles from the occiput as far laterally as the mastoid process. The occipital artery is identified in its fascial plane, being located by palpation in the mastoid groove just posterior and medial to the mastoid process. This vessel is then dissected free from

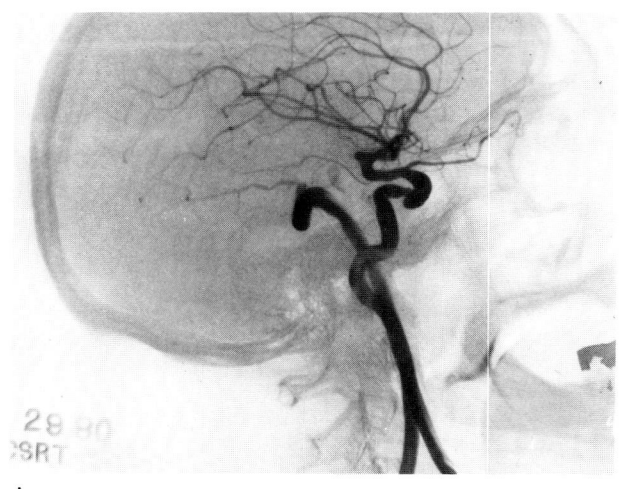

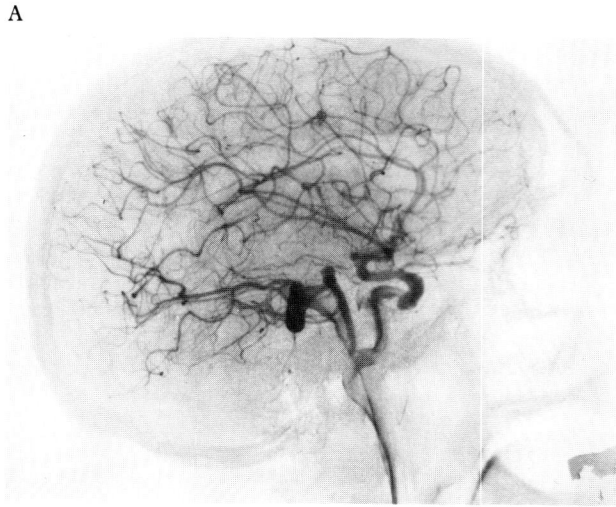

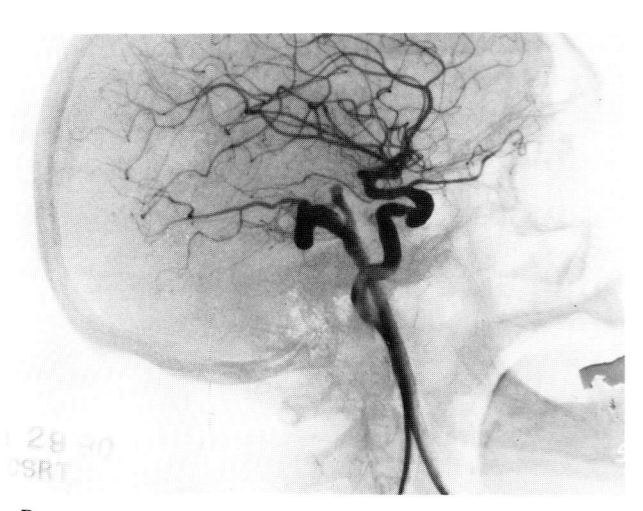

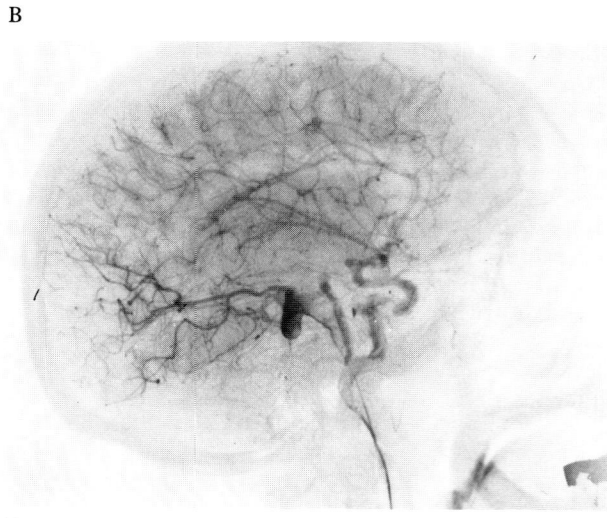

E F

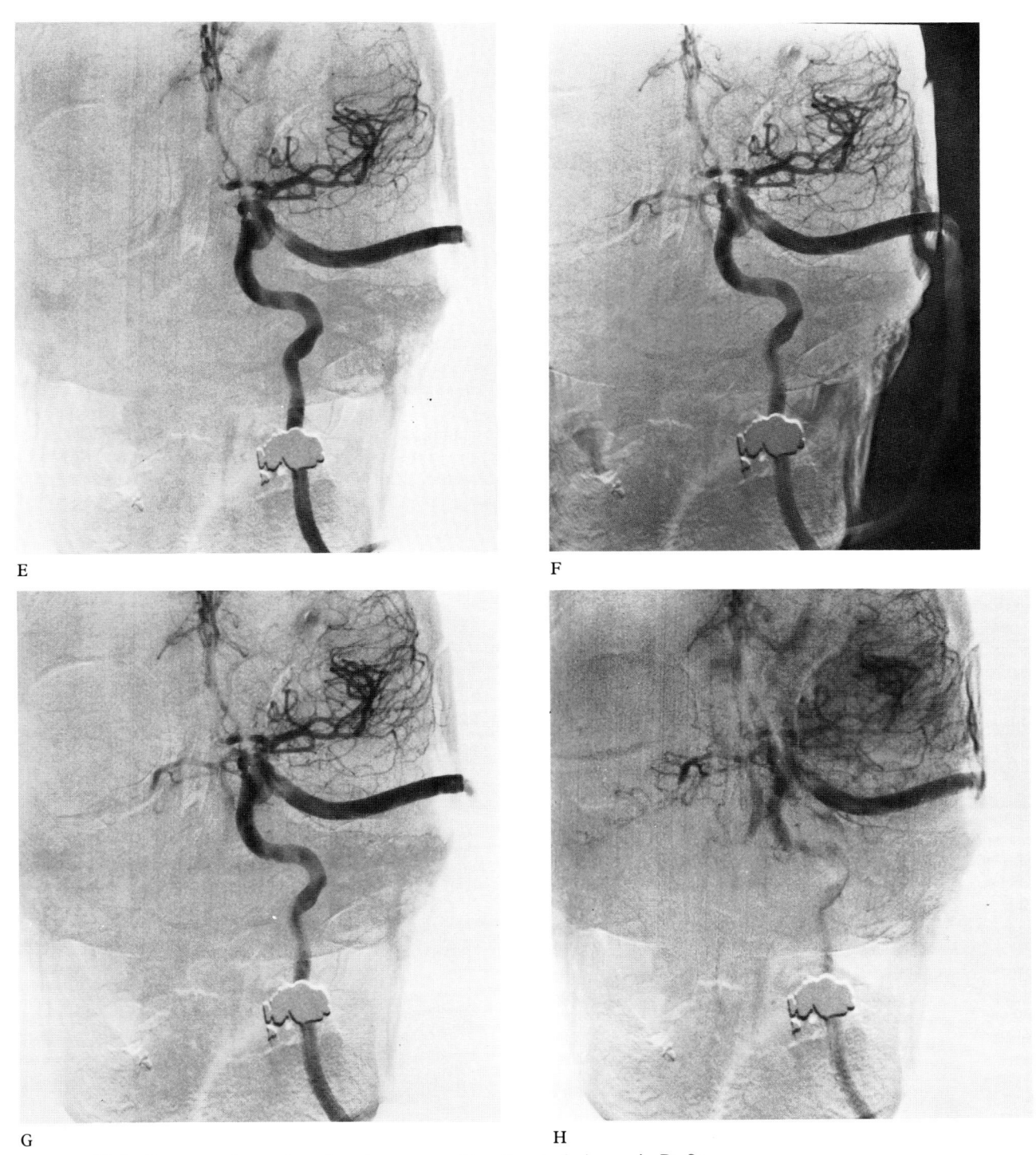

G H

Figure 155-2 Postoperative series of angiograms, subtraction technique. *A–D.* Serial lateral films revealing good flow through the bypass graft, with retrograde filling of the basilar artery to the point of its origin from the junction of the vertebral arteries. *E–H.* Serial anteroposterior films indicating the contour and shape of the saphenous vein bypass graft. There is filling of the opposite posterior cerebral artery. (From Sundt et al.[12])

the surrounding tissue using small blunt scissors. Small branching vessels are coagulated with the bipolar coagulator before division. This is perhaps the most difficult part of the operation as the vessel is intimately adherent to the surrounding tissue and is much more difficult to isolate than is the superficial temporal artery for anterior circulation bypass procedures. It is surrounded by a venous plexus and distally joins a fascial sheath shared by the occipital nerve. The vessel is followed to its point of entrance into the mus-

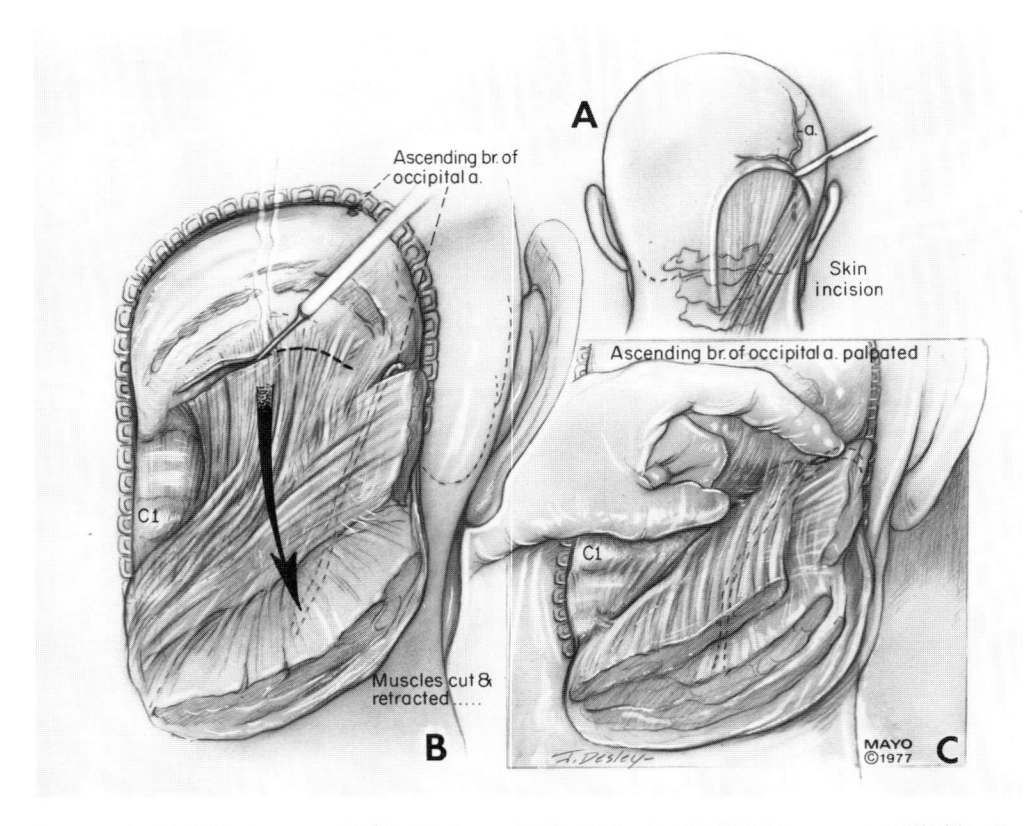

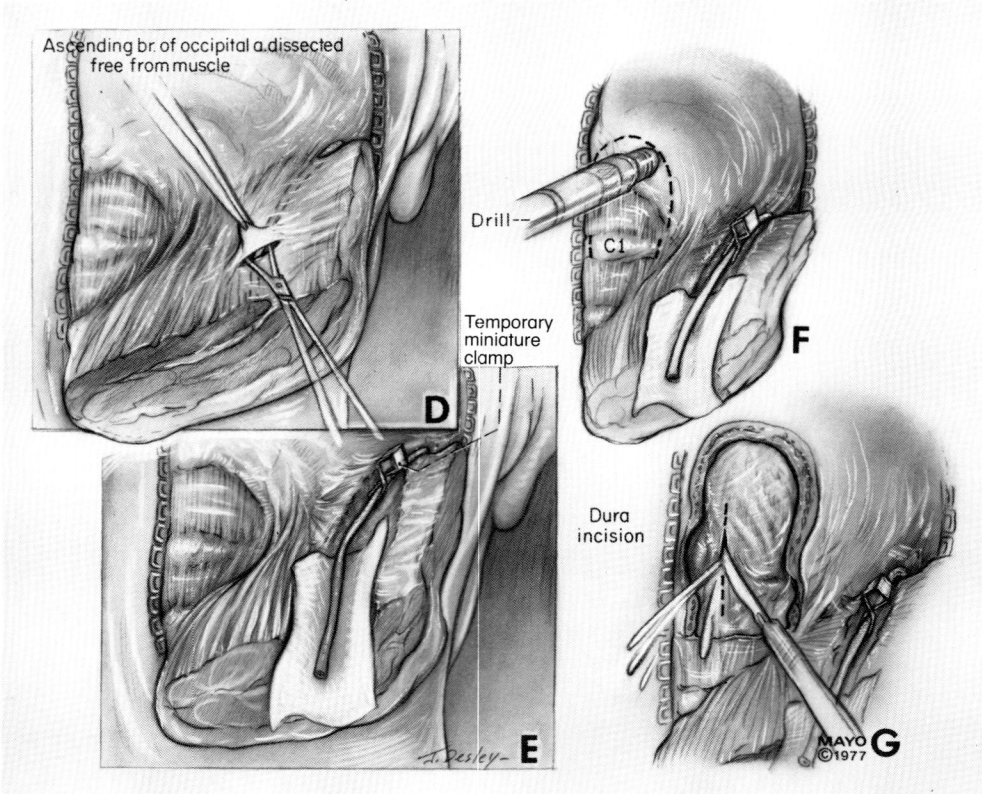

cular bed at the mastoid groove. In its transplanted course it lies at the base of the occiput and follows a straight path from the mastoid groove to the point of anastomosis. It is

Extracranial to Intracranial Bypass Grafting: Posterior Circulation

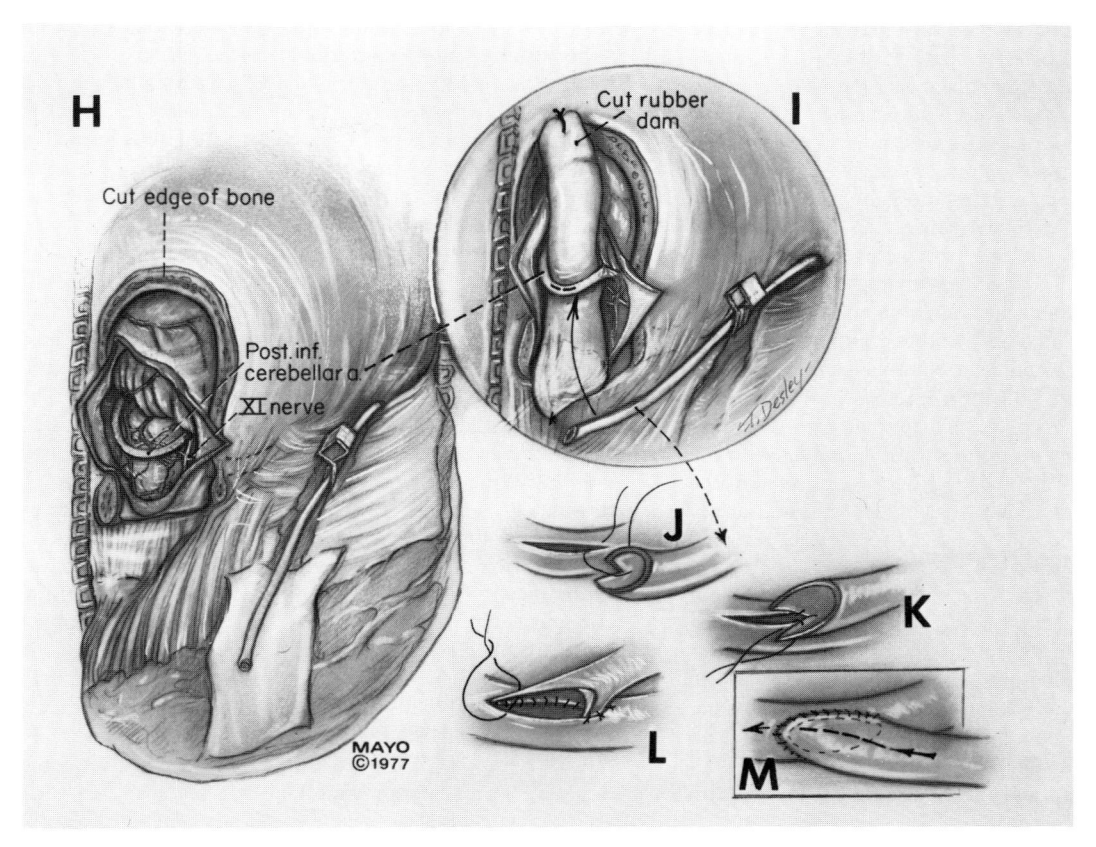

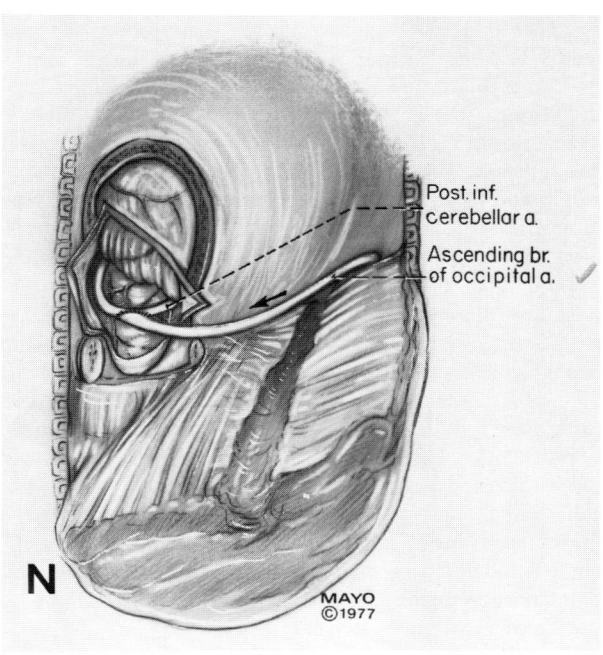

Figure 155-3 Sketches of the surgical procedure of an occipital artery to PICA bypass graft. *A.* Hockey-stick skin incision is made, extending above the level of the superior nuchal line. *B.* The deep neck muscles are cut from their insertion, leaving a cuff of tissue for closure. *C.* The occipital artery is identified in the mastoid groove posterior and superior to the mastoid process. *D.* The occipital artery is dissected free from the adjacent tissue; the vessel lies deep to the splenius capitis and longissimus capitis muscles; dissection is simplified by maintaining this tissue plane. *E.* The occipital artery is shown lying free in the muscle bed from which it was dissected. *F.* A small unilateral suboccipital craniectomy is made, with unilateral resection of the arch of C1. *G.* The dura is opened with a straight incision. *H.* The dura is sutured to the margins of the craniectomy, and the medullary loop of PICA is identified. *I.* PICA is elevated by a temporary rubber dam. *J.* PICA is opened with a linear incision, and the occipital artery is fish-mouthed. *K, L.* The anastomosis is performed with interrupted no. 9-0 monofilament nylon sutures. *M.* The completed anastomosis. *N.* The transplanted course of the occipital artery. (From Sundt and Piepgras.[11])

important to mobilize this vessel as far proximally as possible to obtain adequate length for the graft. Proximal dissection often permits the resection of the distal 1 to 2 cm of the graft, allowing one to use a larger component of the graft for the anastomosis.

A small unilateral suboccipital craniectomy is effected with a unilateral resection of the arch of C1. The dura is then opened in a linear fashion and the margins sutured to adjacent tissue. The medullary loop of the posterior inferior cerebellar artery is identified as this vessel passes around the brain stem on its way to the vermis. A small rubber dam is then temporarily placed deep to this artery and the vessel elevated by suturing the superior end of the rubber dam to the margin of the bone and the inferior end of the dam to muscle or reflected dura. Miniature Mayfield clips or temporary Sugita clips are placed on either side of the area selected for arteriotomy. A small linear incision is made in the posterior inferior cerebellar artery with a broken razor blade on an appropriate holder. The arteriotomy is extended in both directions with small microscissors. The donor vessel (previously prepared for the anastomosis by resection of excess length, removal of excessive soft tissue, and spatulation of the end) is sewn to the apex of the arteriotomy with a double-armed no. 9-0 monofilament nylon suture. This initial suture is an important one and is placed in both vessels from the inside to the outside. The remaining portion of the vessel is then anastomosed in a routine fashion by techniques previously described. Interrupted sutures are used in most cases, but on occasion we have used a running suture. The no. 9-0 monofilament nylon suture is preferred to the no. 10-0 monofilament nylon suture because the wall of the occipital artery is thicker than that of the temporal artery and tends to bend the smaller needles provided for no. 10-0 monofilament nylon suture.

Flow is restored by removing the clips on the recipient artery initially and the clip on the donor vessel last. Small bleeding points, if they occur, usually cease within a few minutes from light pressure with an absorbable gelatin sponge (Gelfoam; The Upjohn Company, Kalamazoo, Mich.). On occasion, however, it is necessary to place an additional suture if the bleeding does not terminate with light pressure. The temporary rubber dam is removed and the dural graft is then sewn into place. The dural closure is facilitated by a separate incision in the lateral wall of the dura for the entrance of the artery into the subarachnoid space. Nevertheless, a completely watertight closure is not possible because of the necessity of allowing adequate room for the occipital artery as it passes through the dural opening. Accordingly, a very tight muscle closure is necessary, which in turn is facilitated by retaining the muscular cuff in the transverse portion of the wound and taking the patient's head out of the flexed position. Sutures are left in place for 2 weeks. The transplanted occipital artery lies deep in the wound and follows a transverse course to the point of the anastomosis. However, it is still palpable posterior to the mastoid process.

Interposition Vein Graft from the External Carotid Artery to the Posterior Cerebral Artery

A subtemporal approach (Fig. 155-4) is used to expose the posterior cerebral artery. We routinely use both mannitol and cerebrospinal fluid drainage to achieve good exposure of the posterior cerebral artery so that there is a very modest amount of brain retraction. The Yasargil self-retaining retractor is essential (one blade is sufficient). The inferior aspect of the temporal lobe is covered with one large square of Surgicel (oxidized regenerated cellulose, Surgikos, New Brunswick, N.J.) before the cottonoids are placed for the brain retractor. The Surgicel is left in place and has prevented small bleeding points from developing when the cottonoid is removed from the wound. This is particularly important because the 4000 to 5000 units of heparin given just prior to posterior cerebral artery occlusion is not reversed.

Heparin is given in an effort to prevent thrombus formation in the posterior cerebral artery during the period of stagnant flow and to impede the formation of thrombus in the vein graft when flow is restored. In one case, early in the series and before we used heparin routinely, a thrombus formed in the vessel during a 20-min occlusion time. Just prior to temporary occlusion of the posterior cerebral artery the patient is also given 250 mg of pentobarbital.

The posterior cerebral artery is dissected free from the arachnoid as it courses around the peduncle (the P_2 segment of the posterior cerebral artery). The P_1 segment of the vessel is not exposed, and it is not necessary to disturb the third nerve. There is no need to identify the posterior communicating artery, which in these cases is always very small. The portion of the vessel that is isolated for temporary occlusion has been referred to by Zeal and Rhoton as the anterior half of the P_2 segment.[15] It measures approximately 25 mm long. Fortunately, in most instances, long and short circumflex thalamoperforating vessels arise either from the P_1 segment or the portion of the P_2 segment very close to the posterior communicating artery, and it is possible to place the first temporary clip distal to these vessels. The hippocampal, peduncular perforating, and medial posterior choroidal arteries are also seen to arise most commonly from the very anterior portion of this segment. The anterior temporal artery often arises in the field of occlusion, but bleeding from this vessel can be controlled readily with the self-retaining retractor. The posterior choroidal and posterior temporal branches arise distal to the site of the anastomosis. We have found considerable variation in the distribution of these branches along the segment that has been isolated for temporary ligation. Invariably, however, one is able to select a portion of the vessel about 1.5 cm in length, free of perforating vessels, that is suitable for receiving the anastomosis. The posterior cerebral artery at the point of the anastomosis has appeared to be slightly smaller than a middle cerebral trunk, and we estimate that the diameter approaches 3 mm in most instances. This compares favorably with the measured diameter in fixed specimens reported by Zeal and Rhoton.[15]

After the posterior cerebral artery has been exposed, the self-retaining retractor is partially removed from the wound and a saphenous vein graft, which has been exposed in the thigh or leg, is harvested. The distal end of the graft (the end toward the foot) is secured firmly with a ligature to a Shiley vein distender. Ice-cold heparinized saline is used to distend the graft and to identify leaks. With the use of a Shiley catheter having a 200-mm bulb, overdistension of the graft is prevented. This is important because if the graft is distended under too much pressure, small hemorrhages will develop subsequently in the wall of the vein, promoting thrombosis and graft failure.

A tunnel for the graft is created between the medial inferior surface of the temporalis muscle and the external carotid artery in the neck. This tunnel for the graft crosses the zygoma anterior to the ear and then follows a fascial plane deep to the parotid gland. It enters the neck at the apex of the cervical incision that has been used to expose the external carotid artery. A thoracotomy tube is brought through this tunnel and through an opening in the temporalis muscle created just above the zygoma in such a fashion that the vein

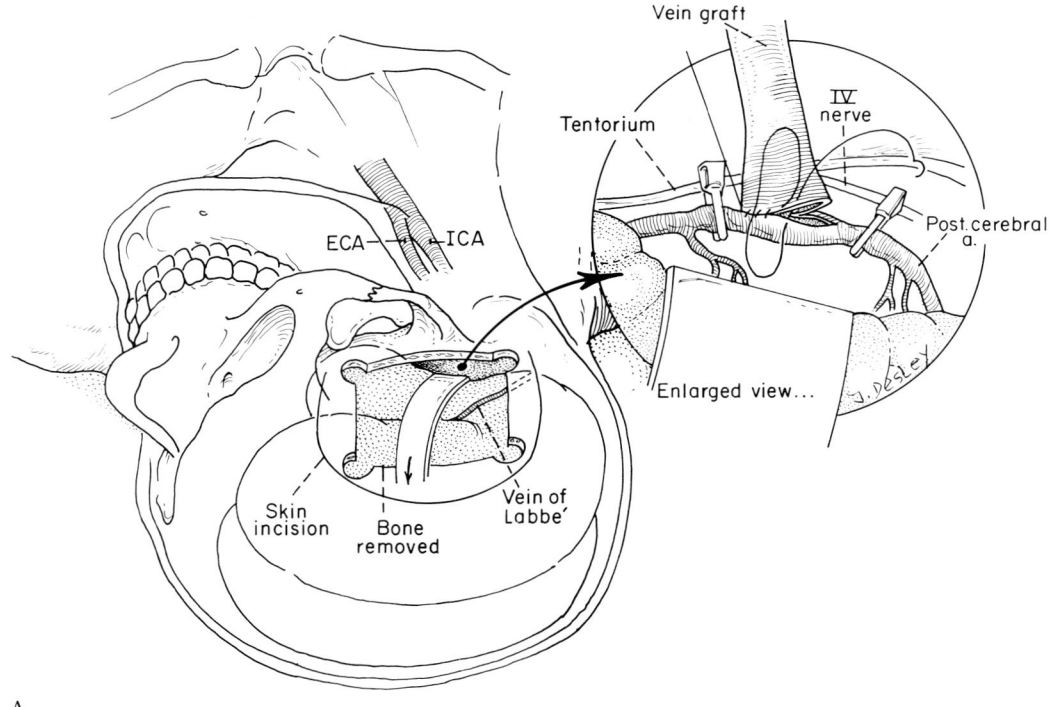

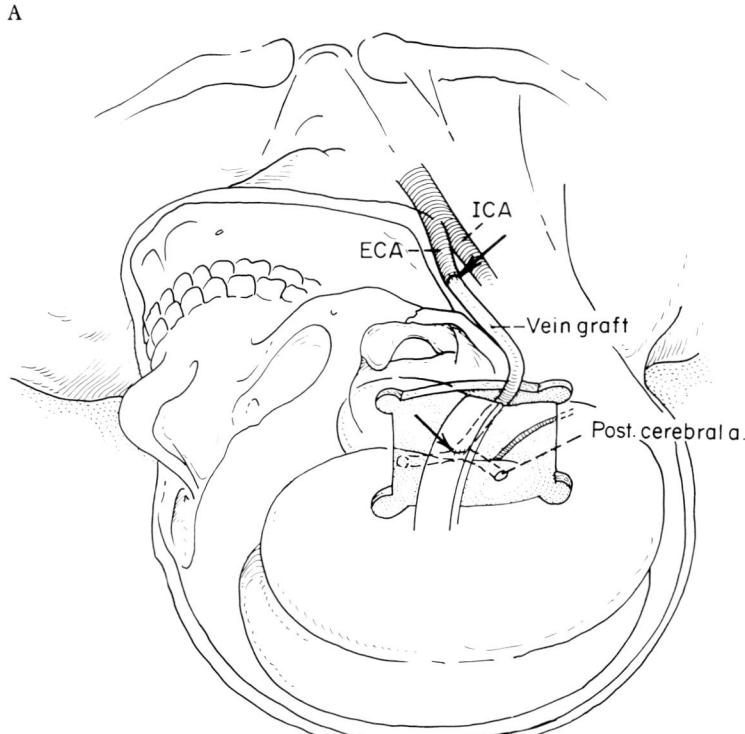

Extracranial to Intracranial Bypass Grafting: Posterior Circulation

Figure 155-4 *A.* Operative sketches of the subtemporal approach currently used for exposure of the posterior cerebral artery for bypass grafting. This approach minimizes brain retraction and yet provides an adequate space for suture manipulation with a single blade of the self-retaining retractor. *B.* Diagram of the vein following completion of the proximal and distal anastomoses. The tunnel for the vein passes from the medial aspect of the temporalis muscle to the subgaleal space over the zygoma, through the subcutaneous tissue anterior to the ear, and then through a fascial plane deep to the parotid gland to join the external carotid artery (ECA) at the level of the digastric muscle. ICA, internal carotid artery. (From Sundt et al.[12])

will not kink as it crosses the zygoma. The vein is then brought through the lumen of the thoracotomy tube, and the thoracotomy tube is removed. In this manner twisting and kinking of the vein is avoided. The vein is now distended with a temporary Sugita clip placed on the distal end of the vein, the end destined for anastomosis with the posterior cerebral artery. Throughout the remaining portion of the anastomotic procedure the vein is intermittently irrigated with heparinized saline through the Shiley distender. The free length of the vein graft approximates 20 to 25 cm. The distal segment of the graft is allowed to remain redundant in the middle fossa, as this facilitates the placement of the vein in various positions during the intracranial anastomosis. This is an important point as it enables the surgeon to work relatively free from obstruction created by the vein itself. Cotton balls work well to pack the vein into the anterior middle fossa during the initial part of the anastomosis. Before the vein is placed in the depths of the wound for the anastomosis, its end is prepared by making a horizontal cut across the vessel proximal to the site of the temporary clamping. Depending upon the size of the vein, it may either be spatulated or cut on an oblique angle. The distended saphenous vein in most instances approximates 7 mm in diameter at the site of the anastomosis.

The self-retaining retractor is then replaced and the posterior cerebral artery temporarily occluded after barbiturates and heparin have been administered. Temporary Sugita clips are useful for this temporary occlusion. The vessel is then opened with a broken razor blade secured in a microholder. On occasion it has been necessary to extend the suture line with microscissors. The apex suture is placed using no. 7-0 or no. 8-0 Prolene suture cut to a length of approximately 3 cm. The final tie in the suture line is completed between the cut stump end of the first knot and the free end of the running suture, so an adequate amount of suture should be left on the knot for this final tie. We have routinely closed the medial side initially and then reversed direction of the sutures at the opposite apex of the arteriotomy using a single backhanded suture. The distal temporary clip is removed first, and then the proximal temporary clip on the posterior cerebral artery is removed. There is no back bleeding out of the vein graft because of the valves. At this point the graft is thoroughly irrigated (as it has been intermittently during the procedure up to this point to prevent the entrapment of air in the lumen of the vein). The graft is then withdrawn further into the neck so that the appropriate length of the graft in the middle fossa can be measured and contoured to the shape of the middle fossa.

The external carotid artery is then doubly ligated distally and divided for the end-to-end anastomosis, or if an end-to-side anastomosis is preferred, it is only temporarily ligated distally with a vessel loop. The proximal external carotid artery can easily be occluded with a McFadden clip or a small vascular clamp. The end-to-end technique employs approximately 14 interrupted no. 5-0 Prolene sutures. The end-to-side technique uses a running no. 5-0 Prolene suture. For the end-to-end anastomosis the vein graft is fishmouthed; for the end-to-side anastomosis, the vein is cut on an oblique angle and spatulated. It is not necessary to isolate the common or internal carotid arteries for this anastomosis. It is, however, necessary to dissect the external carotid artery as far distally as possible in order to give adequate length to that vessel for the rotations that will be required for the placement of interrupted sutures in the end-to-end anastomosis. With greater experience in this operative procedure we have preferred the end-to-side anastomosis of the vein to the external carotid artery and commonly use a long arteriotomy in the external carotid artery approximating 15 mm.

Subdural hygromas are such a frequent complication of this procedure that we now routinely take precautions to treat this potential complication during the initial procedure. An atrial catheter is positioned in the inferior portion of the superior vena cava using ECG localization. This catheter is threaded through the resected stump of the common facial vein in the neck and threaded through the jugular vein. It is then connected through a low-pressure Hakim valve in a tunnel posterior to the ear to a Hakim ventricular catheter placed in the subdural space.

The wounds are then closed using a dural graft. Although we commonly use a subgaleal drain for aneurysm cases, it is not used in this procedure as it tends to promote the development of a subgaleal hygroma.

Operative Results

Occipital to Posterior Inferior Cerebellar Artery Bypass

Among the 20 patients who were disabled there were two deaths within 2 months from the date of the operative procedure. In both cases death resulted from a failure to provide adequate flow through the graft. In one case the graft occluded, and in another the graft simply could not carry the amount of flow demanded. The remaining 18 patients were improved by the operative procedure and virtually all resumed an ambulatory status, with 10 patients having an excellent result (meaning normal function) and 8 patients achieving a self-care status with no major fixed deficit other than ataxia. In the 19 patients not disabled prior to surgery, there were no deaths, but there were four occlusions in this group probably related to an insufficient gradient across the site of the anastomosis, implying that retrospectively the operation was ill-advised. There were 15 excellent results, with the patients returning to normal employment. There was no morbidity and no mortality. The four patients in whom the grafts occluded were unchanged following the operation.

Interposition Vein Grafts

Thirty-three cases were operated upon in this group. There were 19 excellent results, with patients resuming normal activities without a focal neurological deficit, and six good results, with patients achieving a vast improvement in clinical symptomatology but without the resumption of normal employment or activities. One patient remained unchanged from his condition prior to the operation with continued transient ischemic attacks (graft occluded). Two patients had a poor result, and there were five deaths. In these seven cases of poor results or death, four were attributable to progressing strokes not altered by the operative procedure and three to graft occlusions.

Analysis of Complications

Occipital Artery to Posterior Inferior Cerebellar Artery Bypass

Our primary problems in connection with this operative procedure are related to the marginal neurological status of these patients before surgery. Respiratory complications are frequent, and usually have resulted from previously impaired cranial nerve function that makes swallowing and handling of secretions difficult. Accordingly, we have followed the practice of leaving a nasotracheal tube in place in all patients in whom the preoperative neurological examination has revealed impairment in ninth and tenth nerve function.

Surgery with patients in the sitting position carries with it the potential risk of air emboli, hypotension, and convexity subdural hygromas or air accumulation. We feel, however, that these risks are well justified by the advantages achieved by this position. All patients should receive adequate blood volume replacement on a unit-for-unit basis. This helps to prevent air emboli by maintaining a high venous pressure and also avoids hypotension. These patients have areas in the brain in which autoregulation is no longer preserved, and they are extraordinarily vulnerable to fluctuations in perfusion pressure and cardiac output. Accordingly, it is imperative to maintain an adequate perfusion pressure throughout the operation.

Complications such as epidural hematoma and aseptic meningitis related to blood in the subarachnoid space are not unique to this type of procedure and can be prevented with appropriate measures.

Interposition Vein Grafts

Many of the complications in this procedure have also been related to the patient's marginal preoperative neurological function. However, there were two major types of technical complications in the series: graft occlusion and subdural hygroma. Graft occlusion appeared to be related to atherosclerosis in the recipient vessel with damage to atherosclerotic plaques from temporary clips, distal occlusions in the posterior cerebral arteries during the period of temporary occlusion (manifested by virtually no back flow from those vessels following release of the occluding clips), and technical or surgical errors in the suture lines or in procuring the saphenous vein graft. Although one cannot minimize the contribution that surgical errors or technical difficulties will make in an operation of this magnitude, we were impressed that the particular cases in which the graft became occluded were not clearly related to technical difficulties in either the proximal or distal anastomosis. One occlusion may have been attributable to overdistension of the graft in its period of preparation because the graft became hard and it became difficult to palpate a freely pulsatile pulse for several days before the graft became occluded, as measured by the Doppler flow probe. We have concluded that intraoperative heparinization is a risk that must be accepted in these cases as it appears that the posterior cerebral artery is more likely to undergo spontaneous thrombosis with stagnant flow than is a branch of the middle cerebral artery during temporal artery to middle cerebral artery bypass grafting. We have never failed to have a back flow out of one of these vessels in the middle cerebral artery distribution during a period of 20 to even 45 min of temporary occlusion. It is quite possible that the reaction of ischemia in larger vessels is more sensitive than that in the smaller arteries, and for this reason we strongly believe that intraoperative heparinization is necessary, without reversal.

Subdural hygromas have been such a frequent complication in this series that we now routinely place a subdural-atrial shunt at the time of the operation. The cause for the development of a subdural hygroma is not apparent, but curiously in one patient who had both a subdural hygroma and a late graft occlusion, the subdural hygroma resolved following the late graft occlusion. We believe that the combination of a pulsating graft through a small opening in the arachnoid at the base of the brain in the area of cerebrospinal fluid flow along with a pre-existing degree of cerebral atrophy predisposes these patients to this complication. Subdural hygromas are one of our most common complications after temporal artery to middle cerebral artery bypass procedures, but symptomatic subdural hygromas in this group are found in only 2 to 3 percent of surgically treated patients. However, in our group of patients with interposition vein grafts this frequency approaches 50 percent. In two cases the subdural hygromas became acutely symptomatic, producing a profound increase in intracranial pressure and occluding the vein graft.

A homonymous hemianopsia is a complication that one might expect to find not infrequently in this group of patients. It has proved to be relatively uncommon. Two patients had transient field defects that persisted for approximately 24 h, and one patient with a patent graft had a permanent homonymous field defect. This latter patient did not have evidence of a venous infarction on angiography or CT scanning. Drake has previously commented on the collateral flow to the distal posterior cerebral artery.

We have had one venous infarction with an associated intracerebral hematoma in the series that required reoperation and removal of the hematoma. Four patients had isolated small hematomas in the temporal lobe that did not require surgery.

Other Operative Procedures for Posterior Circulation Ischemia

The variety of atherosclerotic lesions in the posterior circulation and the unique characteristics of the frequently anomalous vasculature has made it necessary that a variety of approaches be developed for the surgical management of these cases.[3,9,11,12,14] Although major ischemic symptomatology in the posterior circulation, as indicated above, is usually related to intracranial large vessel disease, there is a role for vertebral artery transposition procedures at the origin of the vertebral artery with rotation of the vertebral artery and anastomosis of that vessel to the common carotid artery. Similarly, interposition vein grafts between the common carotid artery and the vertebral artery have been employed as well as onlay patch grafts of vertebral artery stenotic lesions.

We have performed intracranial vertebral endarterectomies and believe that this procedure has a definite role in selected patients who have a high-grade stenosis of the vertebral artery near the point where the vertebral artery pierces the dura to enter the posterior fossa.[1]

Intraluminal angioplasty[14] has a role in the management of very focal stenotic lesions of the basilar artery, but it is a procedure that carries with it considerable risk and, in our judgment, should only be used if one of the other procedures cannot be employed for one reason or another. We have had two excellent results with this operation but have had three deaths.

In our experience the use of the superficial temporal artery as a pedicle donor for a bypass procedure to the posterior cerebral or superior cerebellar artery has been unsuccessful. There were seven cases operated upon in this group, but only two of the seven patients maintained a good flow through the bypass graft. Typically a good pulse was palpable over the site of entry of the vessel into the middle fossa for the first several days following the operation, and thereafter the pulse progressively diminished. Postoperative angiography would demonstrate patency of the graft but very little flow through the anastomosis.

The intracranial side-to-side anastomosis between the posterior cerebral artery and the superior cerebellar artery is an operative procedure that is indicated in patients who have a fetal type of circulation and a proximal lesion in the basilar or vertebral artery.[12] In the five cases operated upon to date there has been no morbidity and no mortality. In our experience this is perhaps the best type of bypass graft available to us. The indications for this procedure are limited, but the results have been excellent.

References

1. Allen GS, Cohen RJ, Preziosi TJ: Microsurgical endarterectomy of the intracranial vertebral artery for vertebrobasilar transient ischemic attacks. Neurosurgery 8:56–59, 1981.
2. Astrup J, Symon L, Branston NM, Lassen NA: Cortical evoked potential and extracellular K$^+$ and H$^+$ at critical levels of brain ischemia. Stroke 8:51–57, 1977.
3. Ausman JI, Diaz FG, De Los Reyes RA, Pak H, Patel S, Mehta B, Boulos R: Posterior circulation revascularization: Superficial temporal artery to superior cerebellar artery anastomosis. J Neurosurg 56:766–776, 1982.
4. Caplan LR, Rosenbaum AE: Role of cerebral angiography in vertebrobasilar occlusive disease. J Neurol Neurosurg Psychiatry 38:601–612, 1975.
5. Castaigne P, Lhermitte F, Gautier JC, Escourolle R, Derouesné C, der Agopian P, Popa C: Arterial occlusions in the vertebrobasilar system: A study of 44 patients with post-mortem data. Brain 96:133–154, 1973.
6. Fisher CM, Gore I, Okabe N, White PD: Atherosclerosis of the carotid and vertebral arteries—extracranial and intracranial. J Neuropathol Exp Neurol 24:455–476, 1965.
7. Houser OW, Sundt TM Jr, Holman CB, Sandok BA, Burton RC: Atheromatous disease of the carotid artery: Correlation of angiographic, clinical, and surgical findings. J Neurosurg 41:321–331, 1974.
8. Kety SS, Schmidt CF: The nitrous oxide method for the quantitative determination of cerebral blood flow in man: Theory, procedure and normal values. J Clin Invest 27:476–483, 1948.
9. Khodadad G, Singh RS, Olinger CP: Possible prevention of brain stem stroke by microvascular anastomosis in the vertebrobasilar system. Stroke 8:316–321, 1977.
10. Sundt TM Jr, Grant WC, Garcia JH: Restoration of middle cerebral artery flow in experimental infarction. J Neurosurg 31:311–322, 1969.
11. Sundt TM Jr, Piepgras DG: Occipital to posterior inferior cerebellar artery bypass surgery. J Neurosurg 48:916–928, 1978.
12. Sundt TM Jr, Piepgras DG, Houser OW, Campbell JK: Interposition saphenous vein grafts for advanced occlusive disease and large aneurysms in the posterior circulation. J Neurosurg 56:205–215, 1982.
13. Sundt TM Jr, Sharbrough FW, Anderson RE, Michenfelder JD: Cerebral blood flow measurements and electroencephalograms during carotid endarterectomy. J Neurosurg 41:310–320, 1974.
14. Sundt TM Jr, Smith HC, Campbell JK, Vlietstra RE, Cucchiara RF, Stanson AW: Transluminal angioplasty for basilar artery stenosis. Mayo Clin Proc 55:673–680, 1980.
15. Zeal AA, Rhoton AL Jr: Microsurgical anatomy of the posterior cerebral artery. J Neurosurg 48:534–559, 1978.

156

Fibromuscular Dysplasia

L. N. Hopkins
James L. Budny

Fibromuscular dysplasia (FMD) is a multifocal angiopathy of unknown etiology most commonly affecting aortic branch arteries with multiple constrictions and aneurysmal dilatations. The diagnosis is usually made by angiography. It is most commonly found in the renal arteries. Surgical correction with transluminal angioplastic techniques has been shown to reverse renovascular hypertension.

In the mid-1960s various reports demonstrated FMD in most of the branches of the abdominal aorta and in the cervical portion of the internal carotid artery (ICA). In the past decade, FMD has been described in the vertebral and, more recently, the intracranial vessels, although the most common cerebral vessel involved is the ICA at the level of the second cervical vertebra.[3] Cerebral FMD is most often diagnosed in middle-aged females and is commonly associated with intracranial aneurysms. The diagnosis is usually made by angiography in patients being evaluated for ischemic, hemorrhagic, or nonspecific neurological symptoms. Two recent articles provide an excellent review and comprehensive bibliography of cerebral FMD.[6,7]

Pathology

Histological studies of FMD are somewhat limited in view of the fact that relatively few cases have been followed to autopsy, and surgical resection of the involved arteries is rarely indicated. The histological pattern originally described by Harrison and McCormack in the renal arteries and later modified by Stanley appears to be the same in all affected vessels.[10] There is a spectrum of lesions of mixed histological pattern based on the location of lesions within the vessel wall. The most common type (medial hyperplasia) consists of areas of deficient smooth muscle or internal elastic membrane in which alternating ridges of fibroproliferative tissue or collagen disrupt the smooth muscle layer and protrude as webs into the vessel lumen. Microaneurysms are also seen in areas of deficient smooth muscle or internal elastic membrane.[10] This histological pattern results in the angiographic "string of beads" pattern that is seen in 60 to 85 percent of the cases.[8] Other rare forms of FMD are seen, with dysplasia of intimal or adventitial layers predominating. Macroscopic aneurysms, outpouchings, and dissections probably represent complications of FMD and are not classified separately. Recent ultrastructural studies suggest that all forms of FMD are based on a uniform morphological process of fibroblastic transformation of smooth muscle cells.[7,9]

Etiology

The etiology of FMD is unknown. Recent studies suggest a multifactorial origin in which minor congenital lesions of the smooth muscle and internal elastic membrane predispose to an abnormal fibroproliferative response to mechanical and circulatory stimuli. Aneurysm formation and dissection probably result from defects in vessel walls caused by the disease. The characteristic location in the distal portion of the cervical ICA and associated findings of renal FMD in 15 percent and intracranial aneurysms in greater than 20 percent of patients along with occasional familial occurrence all suggest a congenital component. Hormonal, metabolic, and immunologic factors, in addition to vessel ischemia and repeated trauma, have all been implicated as etiologic factors.[6-8] FMD has been demonstrated to be progressive in some cases, which fits with the above hypothesis of mechanical and circulatory aggravation of congenital medial defects.[9] Mettinger's work with pedigrees of FMD patients shows a relatively high incidence of stroke, hypertension, and migraine and suggests that FMD is inherited as a dominant trait with reduced penetrance in males.[7]

Angiography

Angiographically, FMD is divided into three separate types (Fig. 156-1) based on Osborn and Anderson's classification.[8]

Type 1 The majority of FMD patients show an angiographic pattern of multiple, irregularly spaced, concentric constrictions alternating with normal or dilated intervening segments in the involved vessel described as the string of beads appearance (Figs. 156-1, and 156-2). Fibroplasia of the media is the histological type usually associated with this angiographic finding. The angiographic differential diagnosis includes stationary arterial waves or circular spastic contractions in which the constrictions are more regular and evenly spaced without the intervening segmental dilatation usually seen in FMD. FMD lesions can also be confused with atherosclerosis and arteritis. Type 1 lesions are seen in 80 to 100 percent of reported cases in the literature.[7-9]

Type 2 Focal tubular stenosis (Fig. 156-1) is a much less common pattern that is seen in approximately 7 percent of reported cases. The smooth concentric tubular narrowing is less specific than the string of beads appearance and can be associated with any histological type of FMD. The angiographic differential diagnosis includes Takayasu's or sclerosing arteritis, arterial hypoplasia, diminished vessel caliber

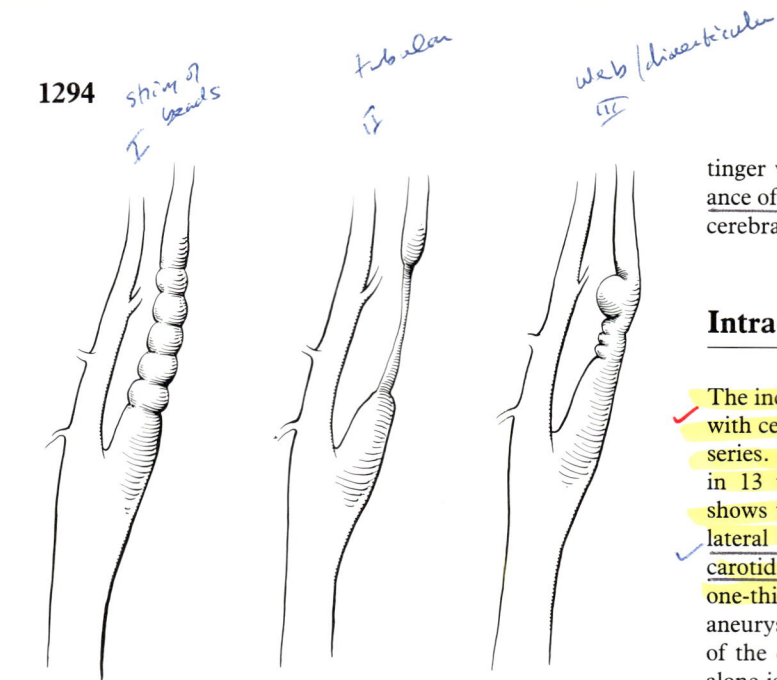

Figure 156-1 Angiographic appearance of carotid fibromuscular dysplasia. *Left.* Type 1, "string of beads." *Center.* Type 2, tubular stenosis. *Right.* Type 3, atypical fibromuscular dysplasia. (Modified from Osborn and Anderson.[8])

secondary to decreased distal blood flow, and vascular spasm. The characteristic location of the FMD lesion in the distal ICA helps to distinguish it from other disease entities.

Type 3 "Atypical FMD" (Fig. 156-1) usually affects only one wall of the involved segment with a diverticulum-like smooth or corrugated outpouching of the vessel wall. Type 3 lesions are quite rare and are sometimes associated with typical type 1 lesions. Most type 3 lesions probably represent complications of type 1 FMD. There are numerous case reports of other atypical types of FMD, including several examples of fibrous webs at the common carotid bifurcation area and tubular stenosis of the common carotid artery.[8,9,12]

The great majority of cerebral FMD is located in the high cervical ICA, and is bilateral in 60 to 86 percent of reported cases. The vertebral arteries are affected in 10 to 33 percent of patients. Most patients with vertebral involvement also have carotid lesions. Intracranial disease is found in 7 to 20 percent of cases.[3,6,7,10] Angiographic studies reported in the literature rarely included pancerebral and renal studies. Thus, the above percentages may be somewhat low.

Clinical Aspects

Renal artery FMD is usually diagnosed before the age of 45 in patients undergoing a workup for hypertension, whereas cerebral FMD is usually found about one decade later. The incidence of FMD in autopsy and angiographic series ranges from 0.5 to 1.5 percent.[1,6,7,9] FMD is primarily a disease of Caucasians, although 30 of 1100 patients reviewed by Mettinger were black. There was a marked female preponderance of greater than 3:1 in Mettinger's review of 321 cases of cerebral FMD.[6]

Intracranial Aneurysms

The incidence of intracranial berry aneurysms in association with cerebral FMD varies from 20 to 50 percent in reported series. Subarachnoid or intracerebral hemorrhage occurred in 13 to 51 percent of cases.[1,2,6,7,8,9] Mettinger's review shows that the aneurysms are most commonly located ipsilateral to the cervical carotid lesion on the supraclinoid carotid or middle cerebral artery. They are multiple in one-third of cases. Patients with FMD and intracranial aneurysm are noted to be hypertensive in less than one-half of the cases, which suggests that increased blood pressure alone is not the major etiologic factor. However, two-thirds of FMD patients with subarachnoid or intracerebral hemorrhage have a prior history of hypertension, implicating increased blood pressure as a cause of hemorrhage.[6] Aneurysms may occur with or without angiographic evidence of intracranial FMD. Usually the disease is limited to the cervical internal carotid artery (Fig. 156-2). Evidence that FMD is a widespread congenital mesenchymal disorder with multiple areas of defective media may help explain the development of intracranial aneurysms in FMD patients with otherwise normal intracranial vasculature.

Ischemic Symptoms

The relationship between cerebral FMD and ischemic symptoms is unclear. There is little doubt that FMD is responsible for symptoms of cerebral ischemia in selected cases. Patients presenting with symptoms and signs of cerebral ischemia are reported in 18 to 56 percent of cases. Often, there are no other associated lesions besides FMD to explain the symptoms; and in some cases, platelet and fibrin debris and even well-formed thrombi have been demonstrated on the fibrous webs, which suggest FMD as a source of emboli. Occasionally, the lesions are hemodynamically significant as well.[2,6,7,9,11] This may be especially significant in type 1 FMD. Each fibromuscular ring may represent a separate site of resistance to flow with the total resistance then being additive, and with blood flow beyond a diseased segment being decreased more than what might be expected from a relatively moderate stenosis. FMD is also known to be associated with spontaneous dissection of the carotid artery with all of its ischemic complications.[6]

The angiographic diagnosis of FMD must be interpreted with caution. Up to one-half of these patients have associated atherosclerotic lesions located appropriate to the symptoms.[1,9] Corrin et al. have pointed out that patients with a known diagnosis of FMD followed up to 5 years rarely experience further cerebral ischemic events.[1] Their review suggests that in many cases cerebral FMD is an incidental finding that does not require aggressive treatment.

Fibromuscular Dysplasia

The fact remains, however, that in most reported series, a significant percentage of patients present with cerebral ischemia.

Additional Clinical Observations

Although most reports suggest a variable clinical presentation, Mettinger has defined a clinical syndrome associated with cerebral FMD where headache, ECG abnormalities, hypertension, mental distress, tinnitus, vertigo, arrhythmia, cerebral ischemic events, syncope, and subarachnoid hemorrhage are frequent components. Headache is extremely common in both renal and cerebral FMD. It is quite commonly unilateral and occasionally presents as typical migraine. Atypical facial pain and pain in the cervical region are occasionally seen in patients with advanced disease. Horner's syndrome is occasionally seen and may relate to extension of the disease into the cervical sympathetic nerves. Involvement of the carotid sinus nerves may explain the occurrence of recurrent syncope in some patients. ECG abnormalities were seen in one-third of Mettinger's patients. They were usually confined to T-wave abnormalities and may be due to involvement of the coronary arteries. Carotid bruits are commonly seen in patients with FMD, although they are nonspecific and nondiagnostic. Hypertension is commonly seen in patients with cerebral FMD and is often associated with renal involvement. Noninvasive workup with Doppler imaging, etc., is unlikely to reveal the diagnosis because the dysplastic webs of tissue are thin and located high in the ICA. Good-quality digital subtraction angiography, however, can be diagnostic.[2,6,7,8,9,11]

Cerebral FMD is known to occasionally occur in children and to be progressive in one-third of cases where angiographic follow-up is available. The remainder of cases show no significant change, but there is no reported case of angiographic regression of the disease. Frens et al. revealed a 7 percent intracranial and a 10 percent vertebral artery incidence of FMD.[3] The true incidence is probably higher in view of the fact that many cases may have gone unrecognized.

Treatment

Various treatment modalities have been recommended—from medical therapy with anticoagulation and antiplatelet drugs to a multitude of surgical approaches. Early surgical procedures included endarterectomy of the affected segment or resection and interposition of vein grafts. These procedures were technically difficult and associated with relatively significant morbidity due to the usual location of cerebral FMD high in the cervical carotid artery near the base of the skull.[2,11] More recently, large numbers of patients have been effectively treated with transluminal dilatation procedures in which the fibromuscular rings are disrupted and normal flow restored. (Fig. 156-3). The most commonly employed technique involves operative exposure of the carotid bifurcation and internal carotid artery in the neck. A small arteriotomy is made near the bifurcation, and Bakes' gallbladder dilators are used to gradually dilate the arterial lumen from 2 mm up to 5 or 6 mm. The surgeon can feel the rings of tissue break loose as the dilators are passed up the vessel lumen.[2,11,12] Extreme caution must be exercised to prevent embolization of fragments or disruption of the arterial wall with the dilators. Carotid cavernous fistulas and perforations have been reported as complications. It is important that the patient be volume-expanded, and moderate induced hypertension can be employed to promote back bleeding during the procedure, which facilitates removal of potential embolic debris. Patients with significant atherosclerotic disease of the carotid bulb are subjected to endarterectomy as well.

Recent reports advocate the use of the Gruntzig percutaneous transluminal angioplasty technique for cervical carotid FMD.[5] Although preliminary reports are encouraging, potential embolic complications present a formidable risk. The use of a Gruntzig balloon or Fogarty catheter to progressively dilate the involved segment can easily and more safely be employed in an open technique where back bleeding can be allowed to occur and complications can be dealt with immediately and directly.[4] If possible, the technique

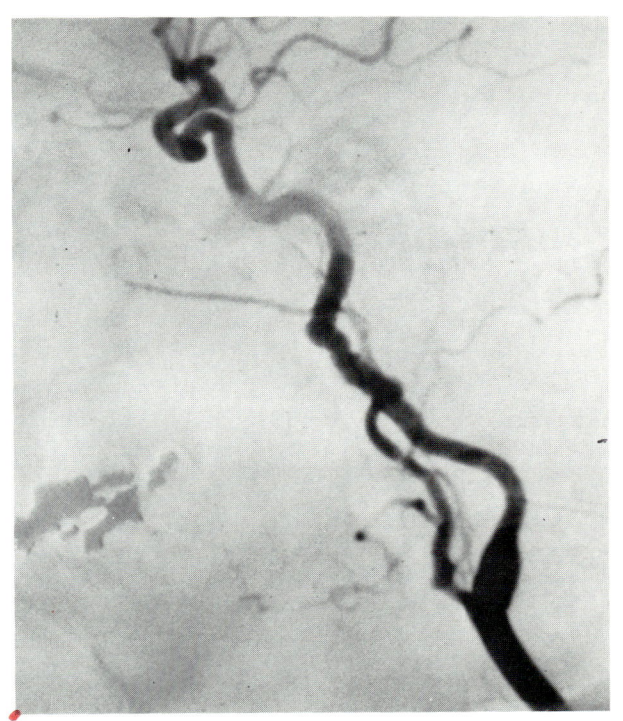

Figure 156-2 Angiogram of a 65-year-old woman who presented with a subarachnoid hemorrhage. The "string of beads," which was asymptomatic, is typical of cervical carotid FMD. Also note the small aneurysm of the carotid infundibulum intracranially. The opposite carotid angiogram showed a large aneurysm of the carotid artery, which was responsible for the subarachnoid hemorrhage.

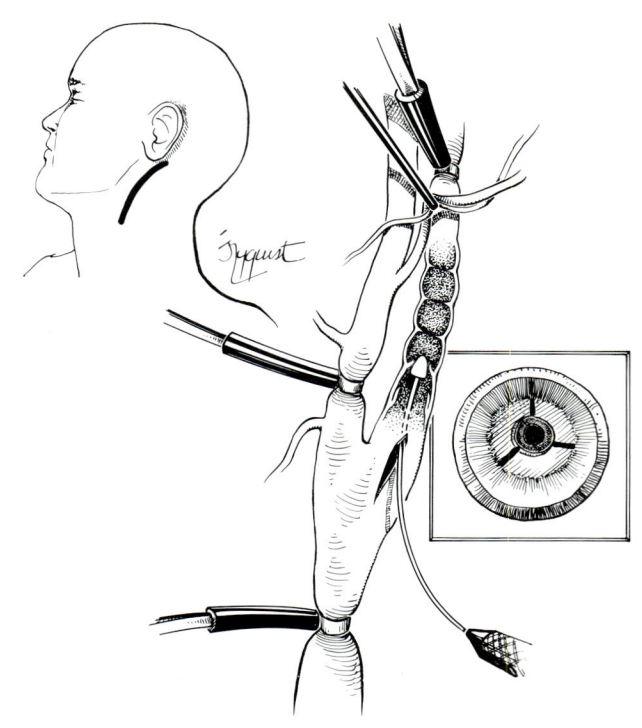

Figure 156-3 The open technique for either the balloon catheter or Bakes' method of progressive dilatation of the internal carotid artery. The inset shows a cross section of a FMD web inside the lumen. Back bleeding is encouraged at intervals throughout the procedure. Extreme caution is necessary to prevent rupture of the artery.

should be performed under direct fluoroscopic control. Intraoperative angiography may be of help in selected cases.

Most surgical series show good resolution of symptoms (including unilateral headache and facial pain) with minimal recurrence of ischemic symptoms.[2,11] However, the association between clinical symptoms and angiographic FMD must be interpreted carefully. There is considerable evidence to suggest that isolated cerebral FMD is a relatively benign disorder which rarely results in ischemic symptoms.[1] Surgical treatment should therefore be reserved for those patients with clear-cut clinical symptoms referable to their angiographic disease in whom no other obvious cause can be found. Patients shown to have cervical carotid FMD should certainly be subjected to four-vessel cerebral angiography to rule out associated aneurysms, particularly in the face of hypertension. Renal arteriograms should also be performed in hypertensive patients.

References

1. Corrin LS, Sandok BA, Houser OW: Cerebral ischemic events in patients with carotid artery fibromuscular dysplasia. Arch Neurol 38:616–618, 1981.
2. Effeney DJ, Ehrenfeld WK, Stoney RJ, Wylie EJ: Fibromuscular dysplasia of the internal carotid artery. World J Surg 3:179–186, 1979.
3. Frens DB, Petajan JH, Anderson R, Deblanc HJ Jr: Fibromuscular dysplasia of the posterior cerebral artery: Report of a case and review of the literature. Stroke 5:161–166, 1974.
4. Garrido E, Montoya J: Transluminal dilatation of internal carotid artery in fibromuscular dysplasia: A preliminary report. Surg Neurol 16:469–471, 1981.
5. Hasso AN, Bird CR, Zinke DE, Thompson JR: Fibromuscular dysplasia of the internal carotid artery: Percutaneous transluminal angioplasty. AJR 136:955–960, 1981.
6. Mettinger KL: Fibromuscular dysplasia and the brain: II. Current concept of the disease. Stroke 13:53–58, 1982.
7. Mettinger KL, Ericson K: Fibromuscular dysplasia and the brain: Observations on angiographic, clinical and genetic characteristics. Stroke 13:46–52, 1982.
8. Osborn AG, Anderson RE: Angiographic spectrum of cervical and intracranial fibromuscular dysplasia. Stroke 8:617–626, 1977.
9. So EL, Toole JF, Dalal P, Moody DM: Cephalic fibromuscular dysplasia in 32 patients: Clinical findings and radiologic features. Arch Neurol 38:619–622, 1981.
10. Stanley JC, Gewertz BL, Bove EL, Sottiurai V, Fry WJ: Arterial fibrodysplasia: Histopathologic character and current etiologic concepts. Arch Surg 110:561–566, 1975.
11. Starr DS, Lawrie GM, Morris GC Jr: Fibromuscular disease of carotid arteries: Long term results of graduated internal dilatation. Stroke 12:196–199, 1981.
12. Wirth FP, Miller WA, Russell AP: Atypical fibromuscular hyperplasia: Report of two cases. J Neurosurg 54:685–689, 1981.

157
Arterial Dissections

Allan H. Friedman

Although dissecting aneurysms of the head and neck were once thought to be extremely rare lesions, they are now recognized with increasing frequency as a cause of stroke. Arterial dissection occurs when blood is forced between the tissue planes of a vessel wall, and although trauma or some disease states may predispose a vessel to dissection, a dissecting hemorrhage may also occur spontaneously in a seemingly normal artery. The diagnosis of arterial dissection always must be considered in the young patient who presents with cerebral ischemia, as well as in the trauma patient who has a focal neurological deficit and a normal CT scan.

Fortunately, the neurological deficit associated with a dissection is frequently delayed in onset. A patient with a dissecting aneurysm may present with a transient ischemic attack or with only mild neurological dysfunction prior to developing a completed stroke. The diagnosis must therefore be made early so that appropriate therapeutic intervention can halt the evolution of the disease.

Internal Carotid Artery

A number of recent reports have dispelled the misconception that idiopathic carotid dissections are rare.[7] Dissection of the internal carotid artery may occur spontaneously in a seemingly healthy patient. Alternatively, dissection may result from vessel damage caused by cystic medial necrosis, fibromuscular dysplasia, Marfan's disease, or syphilitic arteritis. A rare cause of internal carotid dissection is the propagation of a dissection originating in the aortic arch.

Dissecting aneurysms may also result from direct arterial trauma. The most common type of injury is a stretch injury to the internal carotid as it passes over the upper vertebral bodies during hyperextension of the neck.[10] Longitudinal basilar skull fractures, however, have also been implicated as a cause of arterial contusion and subsequent dissection, as has the rarer case of direct intraoral trauma to the carotid at the level of the tonsillar pillar.

The site of origin of the arterial dissection generally lies distal to the carotid bifurcation and proximal to the vertical petrous segment of the carotid artery.[2] Once the media is broached, blood dissects upward within the media or between the media and adventitia of the vessel, narrowing the true lumen of the carotid artery and producing an abnormal dark blue or purple discoloration of the involved arterial segment. A false aneurysm may result when the dissection tracks between the media and adventitia (Fig. 157-1). Dissections of traumatic origin and rarely "spontaneous" dissections of the internal carotid artery may occur bilaterally.

The initial complaint of two-thirds of patients with carotid dissection is neck pain that frequently radiates into the mastoid or suboccipital area. A Horner's syndrome, resulting from injury to the pericarotid sympathetic plexus, is present in one-half of cases. A high cervical lesion may be associated with a bruit, and a lower cervical lesion may sometimes present as a pulsatile mass in the neck. Difficulty with taste or tongue movements can also occur as a result of injury to adjacent cranial nerves.

Unfortunately, however, the diagnosis of carotid dissection is not made in 90 percent of cases until the patient has suffered a neurological deficit in the form of a transient ischemic attack, a reversible ischemic neurological deficit, or a stroke.[10] In the majority of patients, these neurological symptoms are delayed, and only 10 percent of patients develop symptomatic cerebral ischemia coincident with the onset of dissection. In the case of dissecting aneurysms precipitated by trauma, the injury precedes the onset of neurological symptoms by an average of 10 h. A few reported cases describe latent periods of 1 to 2 years, although none of these reports documented an arterial dissection prior to the onset of symptoms. Although carotid stenosis or complete

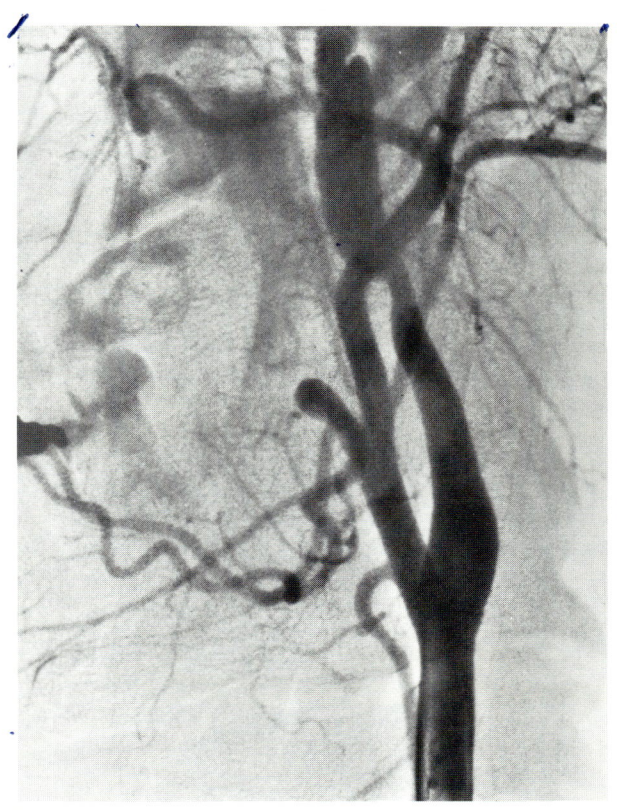

Figure 157-1 Carotid angiogram demonstrating a dissection of the internal carotid artery with a pseudoaneurysm.

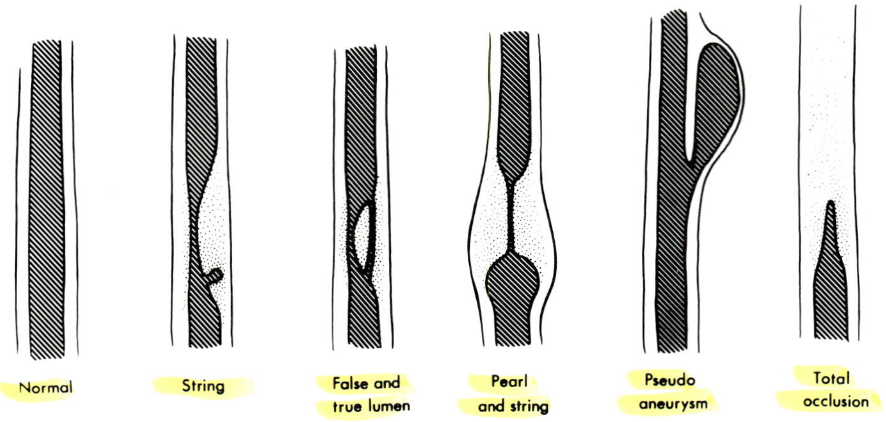

Figure 157-2 Types of dissections of cranial arteries. The patent lumen as it would appear on an arteriogram is represented by cross-hatching. Hematoma within the vessel is represented by stippling. Note the small diverticulum accompanying the string sign. This diverticulum is commonly seen when the dissection involves the internal carotid artery.

occlusion of the arterial lumen is responsible for the development of neurological deficit in some cases, embolization to the intracranial vessels has been documented angiographically in several cases.

The diagnosis of carotid dissection is made angiographically, and depends upon the recognition of the relationship between the true carotid lumen and the dissection cavity (Fig. 157-2).[3b] Occasionally the false channel caused by the dissecting blood will rupture back into the true lumen, and both channels will be patent to blood flow. On a carotid angiogram, the double lumen will appear as a double density of contrast material. More commonly, the true lumen is compressed by clotted blood lying within its arterial wall, and is therefore markedly thinned over the involved arterial segment. This segmental luminal constriction is known as the angiographic "string sign." As the dissection normally involves only a portion of the arterial wall, the true lumen will not be concentrically narrowed, but rather will be asymmetrically compressed off to one side. This asymmetrical focal constriction helps differentiate the luminal narrowing of carotid dissection from that of fibromuscular dysplasia, which concentrically narrows the vessel lumen (and more commonly involves multiple arteries). Carotid dissection must also be distinguished from atherosclerotic arterial disease. Atherosclerosis usually involves the carotid bifurcation and carotid siphon, whereas dissecting aneurysms generally do not. It should also be noted that both fibromuscular dysplasia and atherosclerosis are slowly progressive diseases, and so sequential angiograms will show stable or slowly progressive lesions. With carotid dissection, however, sequential angiograms will generally show either rapid progression of the disease with arterial occlusion or, more commonly, restoration of normal arterial caliber 1 to 3 months later.[3]

Pseudoaneurysm formation may also occur, generally in association with dissection of traumatic origin (Fig. 157-1). These false aneurysms may not become radiographically apparent until several days following trauma.[9]

The natural history of carotid dissection is not fully known, as the diagnosis may easily be missed in patients with neurologically asymptomatic lesions. In general, dissecting aneurysms that cause luminal stenosis without a concomitant pseudoaneurysm will frequently resolve in 1 to 3 months with restoration of the carotid lumen to a normal caliber. Distal embolization to branches of the middle cerebral artery has been demonstrated, however, prior to the resolution of the stenosis. In a small number of patients, stenosed vessels will progress to complete occlusion, and this group of patients tends to suffer more severe neurological deficits than do those patients whose carotid arteries remain patent.

If pseudoaneurysm formation occurs, the lesion may not resolve spontaneously. Serial angiography has demonstrated that some pseudoaneurysms have a propensity to enlarge or to remain stable.

A large number of patients may have spontaneous partial or complete resolution of their initial neurological deficits. As is the case with all forms of cerebrovascular disease, there is no known effective therapy for a completed stroke. Treatment of carotid dissection is therefore aimed at the prevention of a completed stroke. In order to prevent carotid occlusion or distal embolization, several authors have advocated treating these patients with anticoagulants. This mode of therapy appears to be successful, and although the number of cases reported is too small to establish firmly the benefits of any particular therapeutic modality, anticoagulation seems to be the treatment of choice in most lesions.

Because most of these lesions extend to the base of the skull, they are usually inaccessible to the surgeon. However, a small number of localized dissections have been treated with endarterectomy or vascular grafts. Carotid ligation with or without a superficial temporal to middle cerebral artery anastomosis should be considered in patients who have persistent emboli despite adequate anticoagulation.

Vertebral Artery

Dissection of the vertebral artery, like carotid artery dissection, may present with neck pain or a stroke. As complete occlusion of a vertebral artery can often be tolerated without adverse effect, dissection of the vertebral artery may frequently pass unnoticed.

Vertebral dissection is most commonly associated with cervical hyperextension and rotation, such as may occur with trauma or with chiropractic manipulation of the neck.[7] Vertebral dissections may occur spontaneously or in association with fibromuscular dysplasia and other systemic diseases that affect the arterial wall.[4]

The dissection is heralded by neck pain that radiates into the suboccipital region and is exacerbated by head turning. Neurological symptoms may include vertigo, ataxia, blurred vision, slurring of speech, memory loss, and drowsiness. Physical examination may reveal a miotic pupil, cranial nerve abnormalities, nystagmus, homonymous visual defects, or ataxia.

Although a neurological deficit may result solely from vessel occlusion, distal emboli have also been documented, with lodging of emboli in the posterior cerebral artery.[1] Symptoms are delayed in 30 percent of cases from minutes to days, and in an additional one-third of patients the symptoms are gradually progressive. An early diagnosis should be made so that prophylactic treatment can be instituted.

Angiographic studies have shown that although the dissection may occur anywhere along the cervical portion of the vertebral artery, the most common site of involvement lies between the second cervical vertebra and the occiput. The most common angiographic finding is irregular vessel narrowing at C1-2. Pseudoaneurysm formation occurs at the site of dissection in 75 percent of cases. As with carotid dissection, the lesion generally heals spontaneously, although in some cases the vertebral artery may thrombose entirely.

In a small series of patients, anticoagulants have been shown to lower the morbidity associated with vertebral dissection.

Intracranial Arterial Dissection

The dissection of an intracranial artery is a rare event that most frequently involves the middle cerebral or basilar arteries. Unlike dissection of extracranial vessels, the hemorrhage spreads between the intima and the media of the intracranial vessel. Although many intracranial dissections have occurred in healthy patients with apparently normal intracranial arteries, the disease has also been reported in association with syphilitic arteritis, polyarteritis nodosa, fibromuscular dysplasia, and mucoid degeneration of the media. Other cases have been reported in connection with head trauma and surgical manipulation of the intracranial vessels.[6] Although migraine headache has been identified as a possible risk factor in intracranial dissection, the number of reported cases is small. A curious theory that has been put forth is that a dissection represents the rupture of a small aneurysm into the media of a blood vessel.

In 95 percent of reported cases, the dissection causes severe headache. Neurological deficits may be delayed up to 4 weeks from the onset of headache, and the resulting stroke is one which frequently evolves over time. Middle-aged patients are most commonly affected, although intracranial arterial dissection may cause a juvenile stroke or infantile hemiplegia. A rare patient may present with a subarachnoid hemorrhage.[3] This last group of patients most frequently have dissections involving the arteries of the posterior fossa.

The angiographic findings are most often those of focal narrowing of the vessel lumen (string sign), preceded by a small aneurysmal dilatation of the vessel (pearl sign) (Fig. 157-3). This combination is frequently misdiagnosed as a congenital aneurysm with adjacent vasospasm. Occasionally the contrast medium will fill both the true and the false vessel lumens, creating a double density on the angiogram film.[11]

Because of the paucity of cases, the optimum therapy of these lesions is unclear. Patients who present with a completed stroke are beyond primary therapy. This group should be treated for brain swelling if it occurs, and then rehabilitated. Patients presenting with subarachnoid hemorrhage have been treated most frequently by ligation of the involved vessel just proximal to the area of dissection. The treatment of patients undergoing a stroke in evolution is speculative. Although it is possible that this group would benefit from revascularization of the ischemic area, the effect of this mode of therapy is unknown.

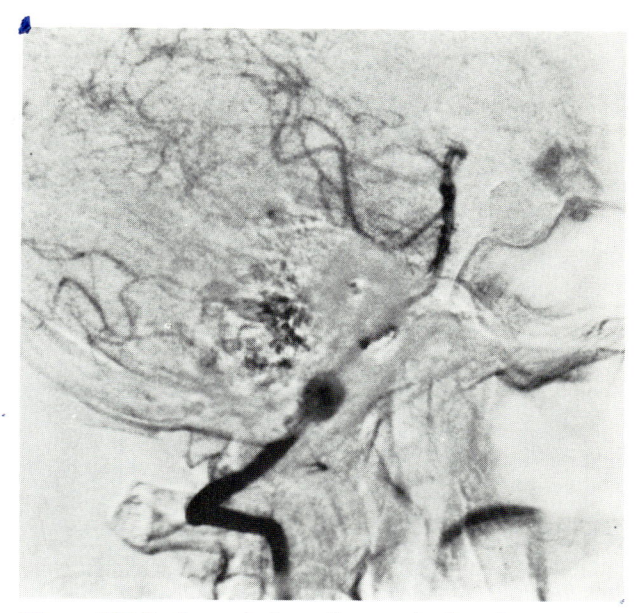

Figure 157-3 Lateral view of a vertebral angiogram demonstrating a dissection of the vertebral artery. Note the pearl and string sign. (Courtesy of Charles G. Drake, M.D.)

References

1. Bladin PF: Dissecting aneurysm of the carotid and vertebral arteries: A clinical and angiographic study of early diagnosis, natural history, and pathophysiology of cerebral lesions. Vasc Surg 8:203–223, 1974.
2. Fisher CM, Ojemann RG, Roberson GH: Spontaneous dissection of cervico-cerebral arteries. Can J Neurol Sci 5:9–19, 1978.
3. Friedman AH, Drake CG: Subarachnoid hemorrhage from intracranial dissecting aneurysms. J Neurosurg 60:325–334, 1984.
3a. Friedman WA, Day AL, Quisling RG, Sypert GW, Rhoton AL Jr: Cervical carotid dissecting aneurysms. Neurosurgery 7:207–214, 1980.
3b. Houser OW, Mokri B, Sundt TM Jr, Baker HL Jr, Reese DF: Spontaneous cervical cephalic arterial dissection and its residuum: Angiographic spectrum. AJNR 5:27–34, 1984.

4. Hugenholtz H, Pokrupa R, Montpetit VJA, Nelson R, Richard MT: Spontaneous dissecting aneurysm of the extracranial vertebral artery. Neurosurgery 10:96–100, 1982.
5. Luken MG III, Ascherl GF Jr, Correll JW, Hilal SK: Spontaneous dissecting aneurysms of the extracranial internal carotid artery. Clin Neurosurg 26:353–375, 1979.
6. Pilz P, Hartjes HJ: Fibromuscular dysplasia and multiple dissecting aneurysms of intracranial arteries: A further cause of moyamoya syndrome. Stroke 7:393–398, 1976.
7. Sherman DG, Hart RG, Easton JD: Abrupt changes in head position and cerebral infarction. Stroke 12:2–6, 1981.
8. Stringer WL, Kelley DL Jr: Traumatic dissection of the extracranial internal carotid artery. Neurosurgery 6:123–130, 1980.
9. Sullivan HG, Vines FS, Becker DP: Sequelae of indirect internal carotid injury. Radiology 109:91–98, 1973.
10. Yamada S, Kindt, GW, Youmans JR: Carotid artery occlusion due to nonpenetrating injury. J Trauma 7:333–342, 1967.
11. Yonas H, Agamanolis D, Takaoka Y, White RJ: Dissecting intracranial aneurysms. Surg Neurol 8:407–415, 1977.

158
Nonseptic Venous Occlusive Disease

John P. Kapp

Of all the organ systems in human beings, the cerebral veins are perhaps the most resistant to disease processes. Their common disorders are related to infectious processes, especially involving the face, cranial air sinuses, and meninges. If inflammatory thrombosis of cerebral veins and dural sinuses is removed from consideration, trauma is probably the most common etiologic factor in cerebral venous disease, followed by involvement of cerebral venous structures by neoplasms, metabolic or endocrinologically related venous thrombosis, and thrombosis of intracranial structures secondary to propagation of thrombus from the neck veins.

Anatomically, one may speculate that the design of the cerebral venous system functions to keep the vascular channels from collapsing in the face of negative intracranial venous pressure. The veins bridging from the brain to the venous sinuses usually enter the sinus in a direction opposite the flow of blood within the sinus. The Venturi effect, which would collapse the veins, is therefore minimized. The major sinuses are formed by splits in the dura of the cerebral convexity and the major intracranial partitions, the falx cerebri and tentorium cerebelli. They are thus triangular structures rigidly anchored at three points and are noncollapsible. Anatomical features that are present in the cerebral venous system and not in the peripheral venous system are the lateral lacunae, which accept arachnoid granulations and bridging veins, and the cords of Willis, or septations within the sinuses (Fig. 158-1). These features must be accommodated in planning surgical operations on the sinuses.

The superficial location of the major dural sinuses makes them susceptible to injury. Dural venous sinus injury occurs in about 10 percent of combat wounds involving the brain. The exact incidence of dural sinus injury in blunt trauma of the head is not known. Injury to a dural sinus may be immediate and obvious or may become apparent only when delayed thrombosis has occurred.[13,21,43,58] In neonates, compressions of the superior sagittal sinus by calvarial molding had been documented angiographically and has been proposed as a cause of intracerebral hemorrhage in infants.[54]

Meningiomas commonly involve the dural sinuses. Since progression to total occlusion is gradual and allows time for development of collateral circulation, symptoms of sinus obstruction are rarely important clinically. Malignant tumors of the scalp and skull may involve the adjacent sinus, and metastasis of lesions to a sinus wall is not uncommon.[53] Sinus thrombosis secondary to leukemic infiltration of the walls has been reported.[17,68]

The importance of the intraluminal tumors of arachnoid granulations that have been described by Browder et al. remains to be determined.[8] The suggestion that these lesions may obstruct the venous outflow of the brain and cause a syndrome comparable to pseudotumor cerebri is appealing, and the possibility that they may arise from a tissue that proliferates in response to endocrine changes cannot be dismissed.

Thrombosis of a jugular vein may be associated with retrograde propagation of thrombus into the lateral sinus, torcular, and sagittal sinus. This complication has been reported to follow radical neck dissection[25] and transvenous pacemaker implantation.[27]

Spontaneous thrombosis of cerebral veins and dural sinuses is seen during pregnancy and delivery and is most common during the first 2 postpartum weeks. Spontaneous cerebral venous thrombosis has been reported on numerous occasions in young women receiving oral contraceptives, and a causal relationship has been suggested. The event commonly occurs within a few weeks after the patient starts

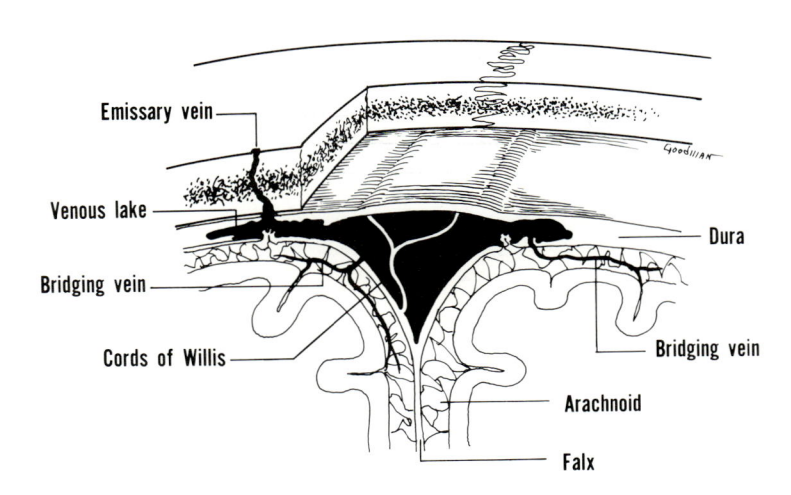

Figure 158-1 Drawing of a cross section of a dural sinus showing triangulation, lateral lacunae, and cords of Willis. (From Kapp JP: Surgical management of dural sinus lacerations, in Schmidek HH, Sweet WH (eds): *Operative Neurosurgical Techniques: Indications, Methods, and Results.* New York, Grune & Stratton, 1982, pp 205–213.)

taking the medication. The diverse disease states in which cerebral venous thrombosis have been reported, with relevant references, are listed in Table 158-1.

Clinical Features

In patients who have sustained trauma, venous sinus injury will be suspected when the wound or impact site lies over a dural venous sinus, when a fracture line crosses a venous sinus, or when the path of a missile crosses a venous sinus. Except for these criteria, clinical determination of venous sinus involvement based on examination is often unreliable. Sinus thrombosis following trauma may occur in the absence of a skull fracture.[13,43] There is no clinical syndrome associated with occlusion of the anterior portion of the sagittal sinus. When the midportion of the sagittal sinus is occluded, increase in muscle tone in the extremities innervated by the involved cortex is usually seen, and it may range from spastic hemiparesis or quadriparesis to decerebrate rigidity. In lesions involving the posterior portion of the sagittal sinus, visual field defects or cortical blindness are common, and coma is frequently seen. Occlusion of the transverse sinus produces no neurological deficit unless its mate on the opposite side is hypoplastic or does not drain the torcular. If this is the case, the clinical syndrome associated with transverse sinus occlusion may be identical to the clinical syndrome produced by occlusion of the posterior portion of the sagittal sinus.

Spontaneous cerebral venous thrombosis may be heralded by convulsions and by focal neurological deficit if the process is localized to a single cortical vein. Often the thrombotic process is more diffuse, involving multiple cortical veins and dural sinuses. In these cases, the clinical presentation may closely resemble spontaneous subarachnoid hemorrhage. The ictal event may be immediately catastrophic, with headache, collapse, seizures, and coma with stiff neck and blood-tinged cerebrospinal fluid. More often, the patient has the onset of an unusual type of headache several days prior to the development of a neurological deficit. Nausea, vomiting, drowsiness, focal neurological deficit, and seizures may develop as the disease progresses. The most consistent hematologic abnormality is moderate to extreme elevation of the erythrocyte sedimentation rate.[44] Lumbar puncture usually demonstrates increased cerebrospinal fluid pressure with bloody and xanthochromic cerebrospinal fluid in some cases. A syndrome of benign increased intracranial pressure indistinguishable clinically from pseudotumor cerebri and characterized by headaches, papilledema, absence of localizing neurological signs, a normal or smaller than normal ventricular system, and normal cerebrospinal fluid except for the increase in pressure has been associated with angiographically proven occlusion of the posterior sagittal sinus or a transverse sinus.[30,58]

TABLE 158-1 Diseases Associated with Thrombosis of Cerebral Veins and Dural Sinuses

Dehydration and cachexia[5,59,69]
Ulcerative colitis[6,34]
Cardiac disease[5,44,47,69]
Behçet's syndrome[7,36,55]
Use of oral contraceptives[3,9,18,22,24,48,51,56,62,63,72]
Nonmetastatic cancer[64]
Pregnancy and puerperium[1,14,16,26,38,44,49,50]
Periarteritis nodosa[45]
Polythemia rubra vera[5]
Regional enteritis[65]
Wegener's granulomatosis[52]
Sickle cell trait[61]
Thrombocytopenia[32]
Paroxysmal nocturnal hemoglobinuria[37]
Budd-Chiari syndrome[38]
Cryofibrinogenemia[20]
Trichinosis[23]
Diabetes mellitus[2]
Nephrotic syndrome[46]
Cerebral arterial occlusion[5,38]
Hypertensive intracerebral hemorrhage[5]
Following fever therapy[5]
Following intrauterine instillation of hypertonic saline[31]

Radiographic Features

Computed tomography (CT) may suggest the diagnosis of cerebral venous or dural sinus thrombosis. A normal CT scan has been noted in about 10 percent of cases and does not exclude this diagnosis. Both noncontrasted and contrast-enhanced scans are necessary, and the findings on CT depend on the timing of the scan in relation to the onset of symptoms. Early changes include small ventricles (33 percent), although as time passes the ventricles may become larger than normal. Fresh clot within the venous structures or cortical veins may be visualized on a noncontrasted scan, or low-density filling defects may be visualized within the venous structures on a contrast-enhanced scan. When the CT slice is perpendicular to a sinus, the high-density triangle with the low-density center creates the so-called empty delta sign, which has been noted in about 35 percent of reported cases.[10,12,57] High splitting of the sagittal sinus may mimic the empty delta sign but can be excluded if the sign is seen on adjacent sections at different levels. Epidural abscess may appear on the CT scan as a triangular low density with the contrast-enhanced sinus forming one of its margins, and may thus be confused with the delta sign.

Parenchymal hemorrhages are noted in about 20 percent of the reported cases, and, although nonspecific, if these are in an unusual location for hypertensive or aneurysmal hemorrhage, venous thrombosis should be suspected. A solitary intracerebral hematoma may occur, but has been extremely rare. Gyral enhancement following contrast infusion has been noted in 32 percent of patients, and when seen in combination with an empty delta sign is highly suggestive of sinus thrombosis. Intense tentorial enhancement, presumably representing tentorial collateral pathways, has been reported in straight sinus thrombosis. The "cord sign," representing high-density clot in a cerebral cortical vein seen on an unenhanced scan, is a pathognomonic sign of cortical vein thrombosis, but has been reported in only 2 of 30 cases.[57]

Radionuclide scans may show uptake in areas of venous infarction. Dynamic radionuclide brain scanning is noninvasive and may provide useful information regarding the posterior sagittal and transverse sinuses.[11,39] Resolution may be enhanced by photographic or computerized summation of counts during the sinus phase of the isotope angiogram. Resolution is not adequate for visualization of cortical veins, the deep venous system, or intraluminal filling defects in patent sinuses. Because the absence of a lateral sinus may be a normal anatomical variant, nonvisualization of a sinus must be taken in context. Radiographic criteria for sinus occlusion are:

1. Nonvisualization of the sinus on an isotope angiogram with a normal sinus groove for the sinus demonstrated by x-ray films of the skull
2. Nonvisualization of the sinus on an isotope angiogram with normal or increased visualization of the sinus on static images
3. Abrupt termination of radionuclide activity within the sinus, leaving a stump proximal to the point of termination (stump sign)

The extreme posterior aspect of the sagittal sinus and transverse sinuses are well visualized on the posteroanterior view (Fig. 158-2). For more extensive visualization of the sagittal sinus, we have found a vertex view to be helpful.

With the advent of rapid sequence filming and radiographic subtraction, direct sinography and retrograde jugular venography are rarely necessary for the diagnosis of cerebral venous disease, since adequate visualization of the major cerebral veins and dural sinuses can be achieved in virtually every case by angiography. In patients who have thrombosis of major venous channels, the cerebral circulation time may be prolonged, and delayed filming may be required in order to adequately visualize the venous system. For visualization of the superior sagittal sinus in two planes, an oblique projection is necessary, since superimposition of the anterior and posterior portions of the sinus may obscure filling defects. In the interpretation of intraluminal filling defects, one must remember that blood entering the sinus from a vessel that had not been injected with the contrast agent may appear as an intraluminal defect in the contrast pool. Finally, total absence of venous channels, especially the transverse sinus, may be due to normal anatomical variation. Visualization of stumps or of abnormal collateral pathways supports the diagnosis of an occlusive process.

Although specific reports concerning the use of digital intravenous subtraction angiography are not available at this

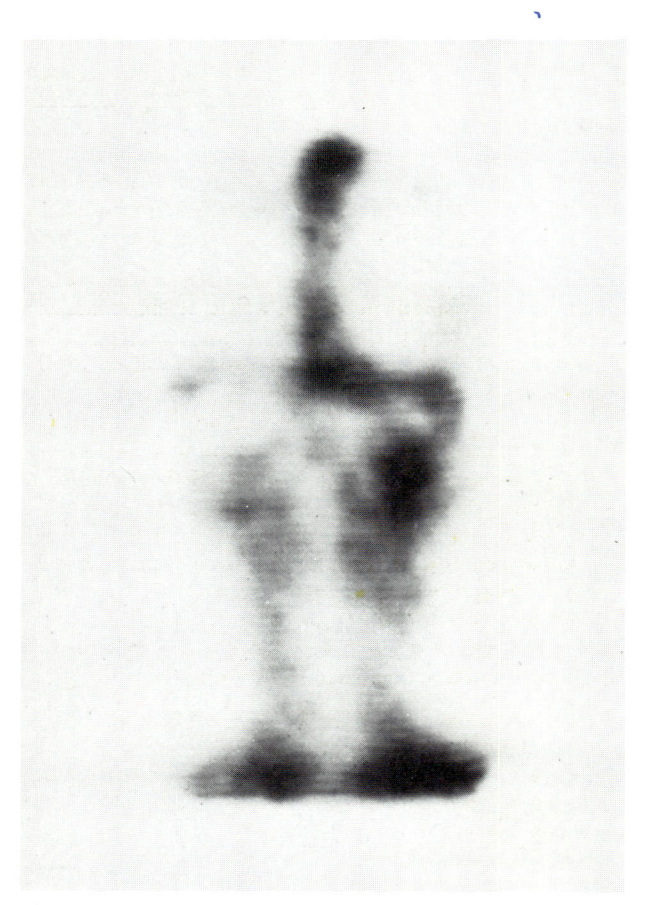

Figure 158-2 Isotope sinogram, posterior view, with computer assisted enhancement.

time, it seems clear that this radiographic technique will revolutionize the diagnosis of cerebral venous disease. Limited studies to date in our institution confirm that excellent visualization, not only of the major venous sinuses but also of the deep venous system, is possible with the equipment that is currently available (Fig. 158-3). Larger receiving tubes, biplane imaging, and the development of special projections will undoubtedly permit accurate and noninvasive diagnosis of lesions involving all areas of the cerebral venous system, including the sinuses on the floor of the skull and the jugular bulb.

Therapy

When one reviews the recorded clinical experience with the fatal cases of cerebral venous thrombosis, it becomes apparent that the thrombotic process is usually not well localized but involves multiple dural sinuses and cerebral veins. If one considers therapy of venous thrombosis in the brain, overall objectives must be threefold: (1) to correct the basic pathological process that caused the problem, (2) to prevent extension of thrombus into patent vessels after treatment is instituted, and (3) to control increased intracranial pressure until the involved vessels are recanalized or until collateral channels develop.

Theoretical or practical problems have arisen with virtually every approach to therapy, and most often an attempt to respond to one objective creates a problem in another area. Corticosteroids have been shown to interfere with reactive fibrinolysis.[28] Administration of corticosteroids to control increased intracranial pressure may interfere with clearance of intravascular thrombi, and thereby augment an abnormal coagulation state. Dehydration of the patient through fluid restriction or by the administration of diuretics or hyperosmolar agents may increase blood viscosity and sludging and result in extension of thrombus or may increase an already high risk of thromboembolic complications elsewhere in the body.

The tendency for venous infarcts to be hemorrhagic is well known, and administration of heparin or other anticoagulants to prevent extension of thrombus may result in additional intracranial hemorrhage. Objective data on which to base decisions are not available. Krayenbühl had no complications related to the use of heparin in the 17 patients in his series who received the drug.[44] Fairburn[24] and Castaigne et al.[15] each reported three additional patients who received heparin and recovered without complication, although these patients had bloody cerebrospinal fluid. Kalbag and Woolf advocated early diagnosis by angiography and supported the use of anticoagulant therapy early in the disease.[38] However, they thought that the onset of seizures signaled the development of hemorrhagic infarction and that after hemorrhagic infarction had occurred, the use of anticoagulants was contraindicated. Gettelfinger and Kokmen reported that two of the three patients in their series who received heparin died, and recommended that anticoagulants not be used in the treatment of cerebral venous thrombosis.[29] One must note, however, that both of these patients who developed fatal complications were receiving heparin at the time they developed intracranial venous thrombosis, and are thus unusual. Comparison of various isolated case reports from the literature are not valid because of the variety of associated predisposing disease processes and differences in anticoagulant regimens. It appears, however, that a strong argument can be made for the use of heparin anticoagulation since the intracranial process may progressively extend to noninvolved veins and since there is a high incidence of concurrent thromboembolic disease in other organ systems.[5,69]

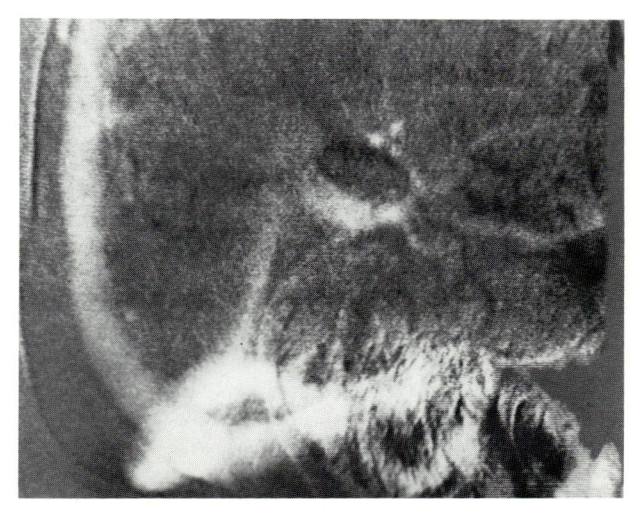

Figure 158-3 Digital subtraction angiogram showing the posterior sagittal and transverse sinuses, as well as the deep venous system.

The heparin dosage and schedule of administration may be crucial, and certainly a schedule that minimizes peaks and valleys in the level of anticoagulation is preferable. A rational schedule for medical management of sinus or cortical venous thrombosis would include:

1. Intravenous heparin infused at a rate of approximately 750 to 1000 units per hour
2. Elevation of the patient's head to promote venous drainage
3. Use of hyperosmolar agents and/or diuretics as necessary to control life-threatening increased intracranial pressure
4. Avoidance of corticosteroids because of their inhibition of fibrinolysis and increased risk of gastrointestinal hemorrhage in heparinized patients
5. Careful medical control of hypertension to minimize the risk of intracranial bleeding
6. Control of seizures with anticonvulsants
7. If possible, correction of the primary problem responsible for the intracranial venous thrombosis.

The successful intravenous use of the fibrinolytic agents urokinase and streptokinase has been reported.[3,19,24,70] In the five cases reported by Di Rocco et al., recovery was complete in all patients, improvement was evident within 1 week, and post-treatment sinus patency was proven by angiography in four of the cases.[19] Gettelfinger et al.[29] and Rousseaux et al.[60] each reported one death involving patients with extensive intracranial venous thrombosis who received heparin and urokinase.

Surgical thrombectomy of the superior sagittal and transverse sinuses is technically possible but has not as yet received a place in the therapeutic armamentarium because of the extension of clot into tributary veins and lateral lacunae and because of the problem of rethrombosis.

The need for operative treatment of lesions involving the venous system of the brain, especially the dural sinuses, arises most often in the management of head injuries, and less frequently in the management of neoplasms. At this time, involvement of a dural venous sinus by a localized malignant neoplasm involving scalp, skull, or dura would constitute a strong indication for resection of the involved sinus and, if necessary, its replacement with a graft. Indications for resection of dural sinuses involved by the meningioma are less definite. Conventional management dictates that if the sinus cannot be sacrificed, gradually occlusion will occur as tumor left attached to the sinus wall grows, and the sinus can be resected at less risk at a subsequent operation. Resection of sinuses that have been totally occluded by meningiomas is not without risk, however, probably because of interference with collateral venous channels in the scalp, in the skull, or in the brain itself.[71] It appears likely that as surgeons become more comfortable with the techniques of dural sinus reconstruction, more aggressive attempts will be made to totally remove meningiomas involving the venous sinuses at the first operation.

The techniques for surgical reconstruction of dural venous sinuses are based on the established principles of peripheral vascular surgery, i.e., adequate exposure of all sides of the involved vascular structure, proximal and distal control of hemorrhage, and accurate approximation of endothelial surfaces with fine sutures.[40] Certain accommodations must be made because of the unique anatomical features of the dural venous sinuses. Extensive mobilization of a dural sinus is hampered by rigid triangulation, by veins entering at frequent intervals along the course of the sinus, and by the lateral lacunae that may be opened when the dura is incised parallel to the lumen of the sinus. Therefore, intraluminal occlusion of a sinus by inflation of a balloon is usually utilized to control bleeding. Likewise, shunts for use in dural sinus reconstruction are held in place by balloon cuffs on each end of the shunt rather than by tourniquets around the vessel. Passage of tubes and shunts within a sinus may be obstructed by the cords of Willis, unless a rigid tube is first inserted with sufficient force to break them. A shunt tube inserted into the lumen of a sinus may enter a lateral lacuna and fail to function.

For sinus grafting, autogenous vein has proved to be a very satisfactory material. Arterial grafts in the dural venous sinuses have been reported to progressively fibrose and constrict, giving rise to a high incidence of late thrombosis.[66] There has been virtually no experience with the use of synthetic materials in the cerebral venous system.

When one anticipates the need to resect or to graft a venous sinus, the operation should be planned to provide wide exposure of the injured sinus, means for rapid, massive blood replacement, and tissue for use in sinus reconstruction.

A segment approximately 20 cm in length should be removed from the greater saphenous vein. The segment is flushed with heparinized saline and hydrostatically dilated to overcome spasm. It is then placed in the heparinized saline for later use. A large intravenous tube is inserted into the proximal stump of the vein and threaded centrally. This provides the best possible route for rapid transfusion or infusion of fluid. If the condition of the patient is not urgent, the proximal portion of the greater saphenous vein should be removed before the craniotomy is started. This procedure usually requires 20 to 30 min. If a delay of this magnitude is deemed unwise and the prone position is required for the cranial surgery, a segment of greater saphenous vein below the knee can be removed by a second surgical team after the craniotomy has started.

In trauma cases the injured area of the sinus should be left undisturbed until adequate exposure has been completed. Prior to the introduction of the balloon catheter or shunt into the sinus, thrombi and foreign material must be removed from the lumen of the sinus. In the resection of tumors, the sinus wall involved with the tumor is usually removed after the bulk of the tumor has been excised.

Control of hemorrhage is achieved by digital pressure in the case of small lacerations, or by inserting a balloon-tipped catheter, such as a large Fogarty catheter, into the lumen of the sinus and inflating the balloon. If occlusion of the involved sinus would not be tolerated, a shunt, which can be fashioned from a pediatric anode endotracheal tube with a short pediatric tracheostomy tube cuff on each end, will afford control of hemorrhage as well as diversion of blood (Fig. 158-4). The shunt must be prepared preoperatively, siliconized by the application of a thin layer of Dow-Corning (Midland, Mich.) high-vacuum silicone stopcock grease to both the lumen and the exterior surface, and gas-sterilized prior to use.[41]

Small lacerations in the venous sinuses can often be closed with small interrupted sutures. Relaxing incisions in the dura on each side of the involved sinus may reduce tension on the closure. Some stenosis of the sinus at the suture

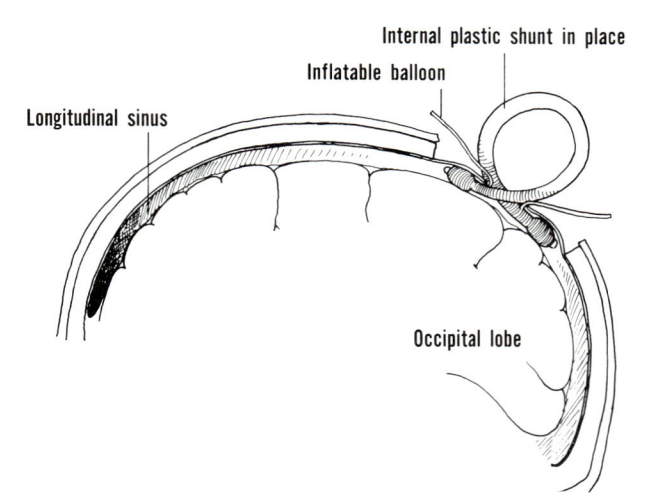

Figure 158-4 Shunt illustrating the balloon tips inflated within the sinus. (From Kapp JP: Surgical management of dural sinus lacerations, in Schmidek HH, Sweet WH (eds): *Operative Neurosurgical Techniques: Indications, Methods, and Results*. New York, Grune & Stratton, 1982, pp 205–213.)

line is acceptable, and we have found that stenosis of a venous sinus of 50 percent causes no problem. It is also possible to tie the sutures over a small roll of pericranium or dura if the closure is particularly tight.

Consideration for ligation should be given when the lesion is in a noncritical area and primary suture repair would result in stenosis of such magnitude that postoperative thrombosis would be expected. It should also be considered when the proximal venous flow is insignificant because of involvement of multiple bridging cortical veins. The areas that have been considered noncritical are the portions of the superior sagittal sinus anterior to the entrance of the rolandic vein, the nondominant transverse sinus or sigmoid sinus, the inferior sagittal and straight sinus, and the minor sinuses on the floor of the skull.

In the areas of the superior sagittal sinus posterior to the rolandic vein, the torcular, and the dominant transverse sinus, where one or more walls of the sinus have been destroyed by injury or are invaded by neoplasm, the sinus walls can be replaced with an autogenous vein graft.

Circulation through the operative area is controlled by the use of digital pressure, Fogarty catheters, or immediate insertion of the shunt. The lumen of the sinus is irrigated with heparinized saline, the anatomy of the lesion is defined, and if the shunt is not already in place, it is inserted at this time.

If profuse hemorrhage from the sinus wound makes it impossible to define the lumen of the sinus, a small sinotomy that is barely large enough to admit a no. 7 Fogarty catheter can be made proximal to the injury, and the Fogarty catheter inflated within the sinus. Digital pressure is usually sufficient to control bleeding from the distal sinus and to prevent air embolism.

The previously prepared vein graft is opened. A no. 5-0 nonabsorbable synthetic vascular suture is placed to approximate the end of the defect and the end of the graft. Because of the possible presence of valves, the graft must be properly oriented. One side of the graft is sutured into the defect with a continuous suture. The remainder of the graft is tailored to fit the defect, and the suture line is partially completed with a continuous suture to the point where the opening will allow easy removal of the shunt (1 to 2 cm). Interrupted sutures are placed but not tied to close the remaining defect that has admitted the shunt. The shunt is removed, a large-bore sucker is passed in each direction within the sinus to remove clots, and the preplaced sutures are tied down to complete the suture line (Fig. 158-5).

Efforts should be made to triangulate the grafted segment of the sinus by attaching it to dura or dural grafts at multiple points with fine vascular sutures placed through the adventitia. Compression of the grafted sinus by tight scalp flaps or by extradural fluid collections may lead to thrombosis. A soft-suction drain should be placed in the epidural space and brought out through a stab wound in the scalp. Systemic anticoagulants and low molecular weight dextran are not recommended.

Outcome

The results of treatment of lesions involving cerebral veins and dural sinuses is strongly influenced by the underlying disease process and by associated lesions. Surgical problems are most clear-cut, although both medical and surgical series are small and randomized studies are not available.

Nonseptic thrombosis of a cerebral venous sinus carries a variable mortality rate. In 1942, Stansfield reported a mortality of 56 percent in cases collected from the literature.[67] The figures in other reports have ranged from 5 percent to 71 percent.[4,22,29,35,44,73] Kendall estimated that 30 percent of recorded cases were fatal.[42] This appears to remain a reasonably correct approximation.

While the mortality associated with the surgical manage-

Figure 158-5 *Left.* The shunt has been placed, and the saphenous vein graft has been sutured into the defect on the right side with a continuous suture. *Right.* Interrupted sutures have been placed on the left side to be tied down when the shunt is removed. (From Kapp JP: Surgical management of dural sinus lacerations, in Schmidek HH, Sweet WH (eds): *Operative Neurosurgical Techniques: Indications, Methods, and Results.* New York, Grune & Stratton, 1982, pp 205–213.)

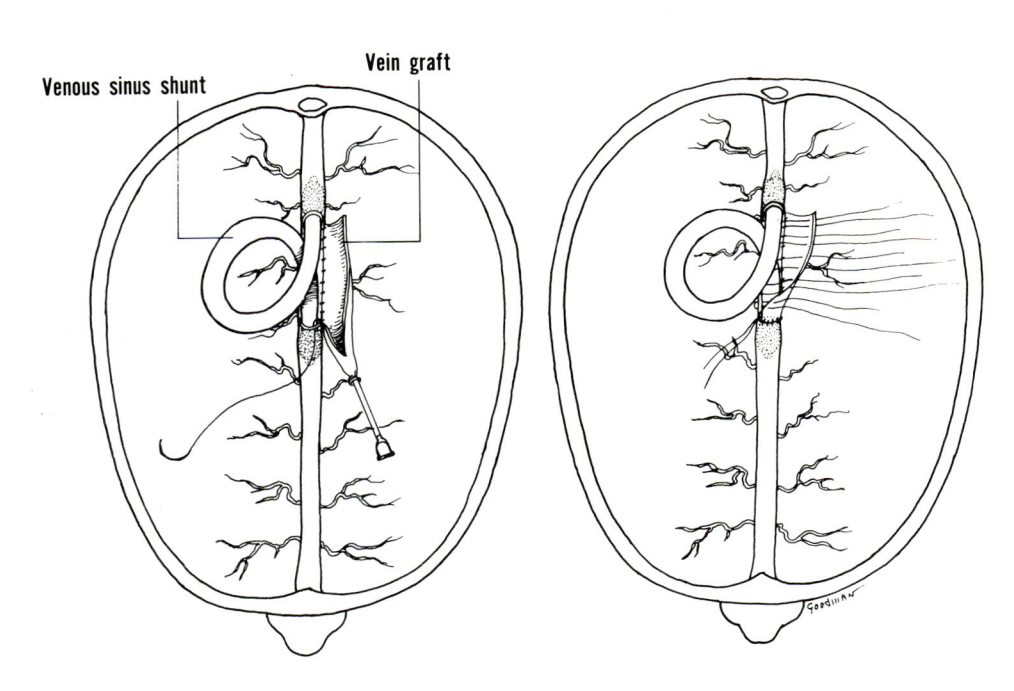

ment of lesions of the anterior portion of the sagittal sinus has not been influenced by changes in technique, the mortality associated with management of penetrating injuries of the posterior sagittal sinus was reduced from 42 percent to 0 percent, and the overall mortality in patients with dural sinus injury was reduced from 27 percent to 6 percent by the application of the surgical techniques described in this chapter.[40] Successful application of these techniques to the resection and replacement of segments of the cerebral venous system has been reported,[33] although too few cases have been described to permit any conclusions regarding mortality to be drawn.

References

1. Amias AG: Cerebral vascular disease in pregnancy. Br J Obstet Gynaecol 77:312–325, 1970.
2. Askenasy HM, Kosary IZ, Braham J: Thrombosis of the longitudinal sinus: Diagnosis by carotid arteriography. Neurology (Minneap) 12:288–292, 1962.
3. Atkinson EA, Fairburn B, Heathfield KWG: Intracranial venous thrombosis as a complication of oral contraceptives. Lancet 1:914–918, 1970.
4. Averback P: Primary cerebral venous thrombosis in young adults: The diverse manifestations of an underrecognized disease. Ann Neurol 3:81–86, 1978.
5. Barnett HJM, Hyland HH: Non-infective intracranial venous thrombosis. Brain 76:36–49, 1953.
6. Borda IT, Southern RF, Brown WF: Cerebral venous thrombosis in ulcerative colitis. Gastroenterology 64:116–119, 1973.
7. Bousser MG: Cerebral vein thrombosis in Behcet's syndrome. Arch Neurol 39:322, 1982.
8. Browder J, Kaplan HA, Howard EM: Hyperplasia of pacchionian granulations. Arch Pathol Lab Clin Med 95:315–316, 1973.
9. Buchanan DS, Brazinsky JH: Dural sinus and cerebral venous thrombosis: Incidence in young women receiving oral contraceptives. Arch Neurol 22:440–444, 1970.
10. Buonanno FS, Moody DM, Ball MR: CT scan findings in cerebral sinovenous occlusion. Neurology (NY) 29:1433–1434, 1979.
11. Buonanno FS, Moody DM, Ball MR, Cowan RJ, Laster DW, Ball JD: Radionuclide sinography: Diagnosis of lateral sinus thrombosis by dynamic and static brain imaging. Radiology 130:207–213, 1979.
12. Buonanno FS, Moody DM, Ball MR, Laster DW: Computed cranial tomographic findings in cerebral sinovenous occlusion. J Comput Assist Tomogr 2:281–290, 1978.
13. Carrie AW, Jaffé FA: Thrombosis of superior sagittal sinus caused by trauma without penetrating injury. J Neurosurg 11:173–182, 1954.
14. Carroll JD, Leak D, Lee HA: Cerebral thrombophlebitis in pregnancy and the puerperium. Q J Med 35:347–368, 1966.
15. Castaigne P, Laplane D, Bousser MG: Superior sagittal sinus thrombosis. Arch Neurol 34:788–789, 1977.
16. Cross JN, Castro PO, Jennett WB: Cerebral strokes associated with pregnancy and the puerperium. Br Med J 3:214, 1968.
17. David RB, Hadfield MG, Vines FS, Maurer MD: Dural sinus occlusion in leukemia. Pediatrics 56:793–796, 1975.
18. Dinder F, Platts ME: Intracranial venous thrombosis complicating oral contraception. Can Med Assoc J 111:545–548, 1974.
19. Di Rocco C, Iannelli A, Leone G, Moschini M, Valori VM: Heparin-urokinase treatment in aseptic dural sinus thrombosis. Arch Neurol 38:431–435, 1981.
20. Dunsker SB, Torres-Reyes E, Peden JC Jr: Pseudotumor cerebri associated with idiopathic cryofibrinogenemia: Report of a case. Arch Neurol 23:120–127, 1970.
21. Ecker AD: Linear fracture of the skull across the venous sinuses. NY State J Med 46:1120–1121, 1946.
22. Estanol B, Rodriquez A, Conte G, Aleman JM, Loyo M, Pizzuto J: Intracranial venous thrombosis in young women. Stroke 10:680–684, 1979.
23. Evans RW, Patten BM: Trichinosis associated with superior sagittal sinus thrombosis. Ann Neurol 11:216–217, 1982.
24. Fairburn B: Intracranial venous sinus thrombosis complicating oral contraception: Treatment by anticoagulant drugs. Br Med J 2:647, 1973.
25. Fielding IR, Grant JMF, Selby G: Lateral sinus thrombosis following radical neck dissection for malignant melanoma. Aust NZ J Surg 43:228–231, 1973.
26. Fishman RA, Cowen D, Silberman M: Intracranial venous thrombosis during the first trimester of pregnancy. Neurology (Minneap) 7:217–220, 1957.
27. Floyd WL, Mahaley MS: Cerebral dural venous sinus thrombosis following cardiac pacemaker implantation. Arch Intern Med 124:368–372, 1969.
28. Gerrits WBJ, Prakke EM, Van der Meer J, Feltkamp-Vroom TM, Vreeken J: Corticosteroids and experimental intravascular coagulation. Scand J Haematol 13:5–10, 1974.
29. Gettelfinger DM, Kokmen E: Superior sagittal sinus thrombosis. Arch Neurol 34:2–6, 1977.
30. Gills JP Jr, Kapp JP, Odom GL: Benign intracranial hypertension: Pseudotumor cerebri from obstruction of dural sinuses. Arch Ophthalmol 78:592–595, 1967.
31. Goldman JA, Eckerling B: Intracranial dural sinus thrombosis following intrauterine instillation of hypertonic saline. Am J Obstet Gynecol 112:1132–1133, 1972.
32. Greitz T, Link H: Aseptic thrombosis of intracranial sinuses. Radiol Clin Biol 35:111–123, 1966.
33. Hakuba A, Huh CW, Tsujikawa S, Nishimura S: Total removal of parasagittal meningioma of the posterior third of the sagittal sinus and its repair by autogenous vein graft: Case report. J Neurosurg 51:379–382, 1979.
34. Harrison MJG, Truelove SC: Cerebral venous thrombosis as a complication of ulcerative colitis. Am J Dig Dis 12:1025–1028, 1967.
35. Huhn A: Die Differentialdiagnose der Hirnvenen- und Sinusthrombose. Acta Neurochir (Wien) [Suppl] 7:355–361, 1961.
36. Imaizumi M, Nukada T, Yoneda S, Abe H: Behçet's disease with sinus thrombosis and arteriovenous malformation in brain. J Neurol 222:215–218, 1980.
37. Johnson RV, Kaplan SR, Blailock ZR: Cerebral venous thrombosis in paroxysmal nocturnal hemoglobinuria. Neurology (Minneap) 20:681–686, 1970.
38. Kalbag RM, Woolf AL: *Cerebral Venous Thrombosis*. London, Oxford University Press, 1967, pp 247–248.
39. Kapp JP, Alfred HC, Jones T: Isotope sinograms: Technical note. J Neurosurg 44:393–394, 1976.
40. Kapp JP, Gielchinsky I, Deardourff SL: Operative techniques for management of lesions involving the dural venous sinuses. Surg Neurol 7:339–342, 1977.
41. Kapp JP, Gielchinsky I, Petty C, McClure C: An internal shunt for use in the reconstruction of dural venous sinuses: Technical note. J Neurosurg 35:351–354, 1971.
42. Kendall D: Thrombosis of intracranial veins. Brain 71:386–402, 1948.
43. Kinal ME: Traumatic thrombosis of dural venous sinuses in closed head injuries. J Neurosurg 27:142–145, 1967.
44. Krayenbühl HA: Cerebral venous and sinus thrombosis. Clin Neurosurg 14:1–24, 1966.
45. Kulawik H, Hoppe W: Thrombose der intrakraniellen Venen

and Sinus bei Periarteriitis nodosa. Schweiz Arch Neurol Neurochir Psychiatr 109:237–244, 1971.
46. Lau SO, Bock GH, Edson JR, Michael AF: Sagittal sinus thrombosis in the nephrotic syndrome. J Pediatr 97:948–950, 1980.
47. Lhermitte J, Lereboullet J, Kaplan B: Ramollissement hémorragipare d'origine nerveuse chez un enfant, atteint de malformation cardiaques. Rev Neurol (Paris) 65:305–312, 1936.
48. Lorentz IT: Parietal lesion and "enavid." Br Med J 2:1191, 1962.
49. Lorincz AB, Moore RY: Puerperal cerebral venous thrombosis. Am J Obstet Gynecol 83:311–319, 1962.
50. Martin JP, Sheehan HL: Primary thrombosis of the cerebral veins (following childbirth). Br Med J 1:349–353, 1941.
51. McFarland HR: Regression of cerebral lesions after cessation of oral contraceptives. South Med J 63:145–151, 1970.
52. Mickle JP, McLennan JE, Chi JG, Lidden CW: Cortical vein thrombosis in Wegener's granulomatosis: Case report. J Neurosurg 46:248–251, 1977.
53. Mones RJ: Increased intracranial pressure due to metastatic disease of venous sinuses: A report of six cases. Neurology (Minneap) 15:1000–1007, 1965.
54. Newton TH, Goodling CA: Compression of superior sagittal sinus by neonatal calvarial molding. Radiology 115:635–639, 1975.
55. Pamir MN, Kansu T, Erbengi A, Zileli T: Papilledema in Behçet's syndrome. Arch Neurol 38:643–645, 1981.
56. Poltera AA: The pathology of intracranial venous thrombosis in oral contraception. J Pathol 106:209–219, 1972.
57. Rao KCVG, Knipp HC, Wagner EJ: Computed tomographic findings in cerebral sinus and venous thrombosis. Radiology 140:391–398, 1981.
58. Ray BS, Dunbar HS: Thrombosis of the dural venous sinuses as a cause of "pseudotumor cerebri." Ann Surg 134:376–386, 1951.
59. Reddy CR, Rao MS: Cerebral infarction due to intracranial venous sinus thrombosis. J Indian Med Assoc 50:98–102, 1968.
60. Rousseaux P, Bernard MH, Scherpereel B, Guyot JF: Thrombose des sinus veineux intra-craniens (à propos de 22 cas). Neurochirurgie 24:197–203, 1978.
61. Schenk EA: Sickle cell trait and superior longitudinal sinus thrombosis. Ann Intern Med 60:465–470, 1964.
62. Shafey S, Scheinberg P: Neurological syndromes occurring in patients receiving synthetic steroids (oral contraceptives). Neurology 16:205, 1966.
63. Shende MC, Lourie H: Sagittal sinus thrombosis related to oral contraceptives: Case report. J Neurosurg 33:714–717, 1970.
64. Sigsbee B, Deck MDF, Posner JB: Nonmetastatic superior sagittal sinus thrombosis complicating systemic cancer. Neurology 29:139–146, 1979.
65. Sigsbee B, Rottenberg DA: Sagittal sinus thrombosis as a complication of regional enteritis. Ann Neurol 3:450–452, 1978.
66. Sindou M, Mazoyer JF, Fischer G, Pialat J, Fourcade C: Eperimental bypass for sagittal sinus repair: Preliminary report. J Neurosurg 44:325–330, 1976.
67. Stansfield FR: Puerperal cerebral thrombophlebitis treated by heparin. Br Med J 1:436–438, 1942.
68. Steinherz PG, Miller LP, Ghavimi F, Allen JC, Miller DR: Dural sinus thrombosis in children with acute lymphoblastic leukemia. JAMA 246:2837–2839, 1981.
69. Towbin A: The syndrome of latent cerebral venous thrombosis: Its frequency and relation to age and congestive heart failure. Stroke 4:419–430, 1973.
70. Vines FS, Davis DO: Clinical-radiological correlation in cerebral venous occlusive disease. Radiology 98:9–22, 1971.
71. Waga S, Handa H: Scalp veins as collateral pathway with parasagittal meningiomas occluding the superior sagittal sinus. Neuroradiology 11:199–204, 1976.
72. Walsh FB, Clark DB, Thompson RS, Nicholson DH: Oral contraceptives and neuro-ophthalmologic interest. Arch Ophthalmol 74:628–640, 1965.
73. Weber G: Treatment of cerebral venous and sinus thrombosis, in *Pathogenesis and Treatment of Thromboembolic Diseases (International Symposium, Basel, 1965)*. Stuttgart, Schattauer-Verlag, 1966 (Thromb Haemost [Suppl] 21:435–448, 1966).

SECTION B

Intracranial Aneurysms

159

Intracranial Aneurysms and Subarachnoid Hemorrhage: An Overview

Bryce Weir

The dawn of modern aneurysm surgery came in 1933 when Egas Moniz demonstrated an aneurysm by the technique of cerebral angiography, which he had discovered.[66] The first malleable hemostatic clips in neurosurgery had been introduced by Cushing in 1911, but they were not appropriate for aneurysms. Schwartz developed a spring clip with cross legs, which was modified by Mayfield by making a smaller, tweezer-like applicator for it.[59] This paved the way for the introduction of a host of different spring clips in a variety of strengths and configurations. Other brilliant technical progress included the demonstration by Lundberg in 1960 of the feasibility of intraventricular catheters to continuously record and control ventricular fluid pressure.[56] Two years after that the first report appeared of an intracranial vascular procedure carried out with the aid of the operating microscope, which brought the twin blessings of magnification and illumination.[47] By 1971 the first computed tomographic (CT) head scanner was operational, having been developed by a group that included Godfrey Hounsfield.[12] The first planned intracranial operation for a saccular aneurysm was conducted by Dott in 1933.[21] He stuffed a muscle fragment against an aneurysm that had ruptured intraoperatively and succeeded in stopping the bleeding and obtaining a good long-term result. Credit for the first definitive treatment of a preoperatively diagnosed intracranial aneurysm (by virtue of a third nerve palsy) goes to Dandy, who in 1937 clipped the neck of an aneurysm with a metal clip and shriveled the sac with electrocautery[19] (Fig. 159-1). Aided by technical advances and general progress in radiology, anesthesia, and intensive care, many neurosurgeons achieved progressively lower postoperative mortality rates after operations for intracranial aneurysms in the 1960s and 1970s. Preeminent among these workers are Yaşargil of Zürich[123] and Drake of London, Ontario,[23] who have established benchmarks of excellence in huge series of aneurysms in the anterior and posterior circulations, respectively. Their careful anatomical observations and technical advice will be of immense help to the generations of surgeons that follow them.

A step forward in understanding the course of this disease came with the introduction by Botterell, Lougheed, and others of a neurological grading system in 1956.[9] In May

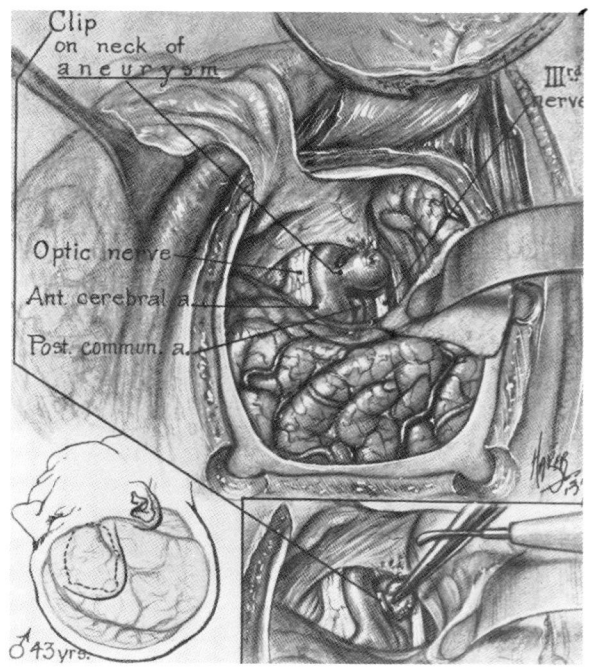

Figure 159-1 Operation of March 23, 1937: "The present effort is but a beginning or a suggestion that an aneurysm at the circle of Willis is not entirely hopeless . . . So far as I know this is the first attempt to cure an aneurysm at the circle of Willis by direct attack upon the aneurysm." (From Dandy[19].)

of the following year a central registry for aneurysm cases was begun at the University of Iowa, and a Cooperative Study was initiated. This has been a continual source of accurate data and an increasingly sophisticated guide to the efficacy of different therapeutic approaches.[80] The definitive study of the natural history of aneurysms was published by Pakarinen in 1967.[73] Lougheed later introduced the concept of management mortality rather than simple postoperative mortality in the assessment of surgical treatment.[55]

Classification, Characteristics, and Occurrence of Intracranial Aneurysms

A surgical classification of intracranial arterial aneurysms is proposed in Table 159-1. Such lesions can also be classified with respect to their presumed etiology. Some causative factors in intracranial arterial saccular and fusiform aneurysms are given in Table 159-2.

Bacterial aneurysms make up under 5 percent of all cases of intracranial aneurysms. The commonest cause is a streptococcal infection in a patient with bacterial endocarditis. Mortality is relatively low in patients treated with appropriate high-dose antibiotics and surgery. The majority of these aneurysms are on the distal middle cerebral circulation.[32] Fungal aneurysms are considerably rarer, are usually associated with arteritis and thrombosis, and have so far been uniformly fatal.[62] Traumatic aneurysms are uncommon and can result from either blunt or penetrating head trauma. The majority of patients have associated skull fractures. Penetrating injuries result from a variety of missiles and surgical instruments. These aneurysms are usually located on the supratentorial circulation at sites other than branching points and are most commonly single. Their presence should be considered when there is a syndrome of delayed deterioration following head injury. The sac may have an irregular contour and a neck may be absent. The outlook is poor without direct surgical treatment.[53]

Some aneurysms can be caused by tumor embolization, particularly choriocarcinoma. The possibility that some tumors stimulate the growth of aneurysms in nearby blood vessels has also been raised, but it is not clear whether the incidence exceeds what would normally be expected from the fact that brain tumors and aneurysms are both relatively common so that instances of both conditions in the same patient are inevitable. However, there is considerable surgical relevance to the finding of an aneurysm in the intracavernous or supraclinoid portion of the carotid artery in 5.4 percent of 183 pituitary adenomas or craniopharyngiomas[48] and 7.4 percent of 95 pituitary adenomas.[107]

TABLE 159-1 Surgical Classification of Intracranial Arterial Aneurysms

I. Morphology
  A. Saccular
  B. Fusiform
  C. Dissecting
II. Size
  A. < 3 mm
  B. 3–6 mm
  C. 7–10 mm
  D. 11–25 mm
  E. > 25 mm (giant)
III. Location
  A. Anterior circulation arteries
    1. Internal carotid
      a. Carotid canal
      b. Intracavernous
      c. Paraclinoid (ophthalmic)
      d. Posterior communicating region
      e. Anterior choroidal region
      f. Carotid bifurcation
    2. Anterior cerebral
      a. A_1 (main branch)
      b. Anterior communicating region
      c. A_2 (distal): callosomarginal region or distal pericallosal
    3. Middle cerebral
      a. M_1 (main branch) lenticulostriate or temporal branch regions
      b. Bifurcation
      c. Peripheral
  B. Posterior circulation arteries
    1. Vertebral
      a. Main trunk
      b. Posterior inferior cerebellar artery region
    2. Basilar
      a. Bifurcation
      b. Superior cerebellar artery region
      c. Anterior inferior cerebellar artery region
      d. Basilar trunk
      e. Vertebrobasilar junction region
    3. Posterior cerebral
      a. P_1 (first branches of basilar-distal to apex)
      b. P_2 (distal posterior cerebral)

Anatomical Sites of Aneurysms

The relative frequency of aneurysms at different anatomical sites is illustrated in Fig. 159-2. Ninety-five percent of aneurysms occur close to the circle of Willis in relation to the anterior and posterior communicating arteries and the bifurcations of the internal carotid, middle cerebral, and basilar arteries. Aneurysms usually arise from the distal carina of a bifurcation. They are usually on the convexity of a curve and point in the direction that the proximal axial bloodstream would have taken if the curve were not there.[76]

Size of Aneurysms

The frequency distribution of aneurysm size is illustrated in Fig. 159-3. It can be seen that ruptured aneurysms tend to be larger than unruptured aneurysms and that symptomatic aneurysms are larger than asymptomatic aneurysms. The size at which aneurysms usually begin to rupture is about 3 mm in maximum diameter and the size at which they begin to produce symptoms by means other than rupture is around 7 mm. In a planned autopsy study, the mean size of ruptured aneurysms was 8.6 mm, almost twice the mean size of the nonruptured aneurysms, which was 4.7 mm.[16] In an-

TABLE 159-2 Etiology of Intracranial Arterial Aneurysms

Saccular Aneurysms

A. Hemodynamic
 1. Uneven pulsatile pressure head distribution at apex of bifurcations, branchings, or outer aspect of curves, causing local degeneration of internal elastica
 2. Increased flow from:
    a. Distal arteriovenous malformation
    b. Aplasia, hypoplasia, or ligation of contralateral vessel normally present
    c. Persistent carotid-basilar anastomosis (trigeminal, otic, hypoglossal, proatlantal) and basilar-middle meningeal anastomosis
 3. Increased blood pressure (and possibly associated vessel defect in)
    a. Coarctation of aorta
    b. Polycystic kidney disease
    c. Fibromuscular dysplasia, renal arteries
B. Structural
 1. Combined media and elastica defects
 2. Preaneurysmal lesions: infundibulae, thin areas, microaneurysms
C. Genetic
 1. Familial intracranial aneurysms—dominant inheritance
 2. Genetic or possibly genetic syndromes associated with blood vessel abnormalities and reported with intracranial aneurysms: Ehlers-Danlos syndrome, Marfan's syndrome, pseudoxanthoma elasticum, Rendu-Osler-Weber syndrome, Klippel-Trenaunay-Weber syndrome
D. Traumatic
 1. Skull fracture
 2. Penetrating foreign body
 3. Surgical injury
E. Infectious
 1. Bacterial
 2. Fungal
F. Neoplastic embolization
 1. Choriocarcinoma
 2. Atrial myxoma
 3. Undifferentiated carcinoma
G. Other disorders affecting blood vessels
 1. Granulomatous (giant cell) angiitis
 2. Systemic lupus erythematosus
 3. Moyamoya disease

Fusiform Aneurysms

A. Atherosclerosis
 • Commonest cause of elongated, distended (dolichoectatic) cerebral vessels
 • Posterior circulation most affected
B. Structural
 1. Long areas of loss of normal elastica and media
 2. Diffuse arterial fibromuscular dysplasia
C. Genetic
 Possibly genetic conditions associated with fusiform aneurysms include Marfan's syndrome, pseudoxanthoma elasticum
D. Infectious
 Syphilis
E. Other disorders of blood vessels
 Giant cell arteritis
F. Hemodynamic
 Coarctation of aorta

---

other pathological series,[60] 16 percent of aneurysms 10 mm or less in size were ruptured, whereas 91 percent of aneurysms 11 mm or greater were ruptured. In 2329 cases, the size distribution was as follows: under 12 mm, 79 percent; 12 to 24 mm, 19 percent; over 24 mm, 2 percent.[50]

Multiple Aneurysms

In Suzuki's personal series of 1080 cases, single aneurysms comprised 85 percent of the series and multiple aneurysms 15 percent.[94] He reviewed seven other clinical series, totaling 10,795 cases, in which the incidence of multiple aneurysms was 14.1 percent overall, with a range of 7.7 to 29.8 percent. He similarly reviewed six autopsy series in which 1404 cases were studied to reveal multiple aneurysm cases in 23.5 percent (range 18.9 to 50 percent).[94] In Sahs et al.'s cooperative study of 3321 aneurysm cases, the rate of multiple aneurysms at autopsy was 22 percent, compared with the angiographically demonstrated rate of 18.5 percent.[80] This is probably a reflection of the fact that four-vessel angiography was not routinely carried out in 1969. In the multiple aneurysm cases of the conservatively managed patients in the cooperative study and in Suzuki's personal series, patients having two aneurysms comprised 71 and 77 percent; three aneurysms, 23 and 15 percent; and four or more aneurysms, 7 and 6 percent of multiple aneurysm cases, respectively. Multiple aneurysms are relatively more common in females (74 percent) than males.[80] The same study showed that 47 percent of multiple aneurysms are on opposite sides, 21 percent are on the same side, 29 percent have one in the midline and one on the side, and 3 percent are both midline. When two internal carotid aneurysms coexist, the chance of them being "mirror" aneurysms is three times greater than that of them both being on the same side. Similarly, with two middle cerebral aneurysms the chance is four times greater. When an aneurysm on the anterior circulation is found, the chance of a second aneurysm existing on the posterior circulation is between 3 and 5 percent. With internal carotid and middle cerebral aneurysms, there is a tendency toward either symmetrical aneurysms or a second aneurysm on the same vessel.

How is it possible to tell which aneurysm has ruptured? In 87 percent of 105 cases of multiple aneurysms studied by Wood,[121] the largest of the aneurysms had ruptured. Other angiographic signs of rupture were a local mass or vasospasm, irregular aneurysm shape, or intra-aneurysmal clot. When two aneurysms are on the same vessel, unless the proximal aneurysm is thrombosed, it is the proximal aneurysm which has ruptured.[17] The contribution of CT scanning to the accurate delineation of the offending lesion is now considerably higher with better-resolution scanners. Focal neurological signs and symptoms may also point to the offending lesion.

Occurrence of Aneurysms

Age

Aneurysmal rupture is extremely uncommon in the first decade of life. The incidence gradually increases for each decade and peaks in the sixth decade. In Pakarinen's review of the literature, the prevalence in each decade was as follows: first, less than 1 percent; second, 2 percent; third, 6

Intracranial Aneurysms and Subarachnoid Hemorrhage: An Overview

SINGLE ANEURYSMS PRODUCING SAH
(After Cooperative Study)

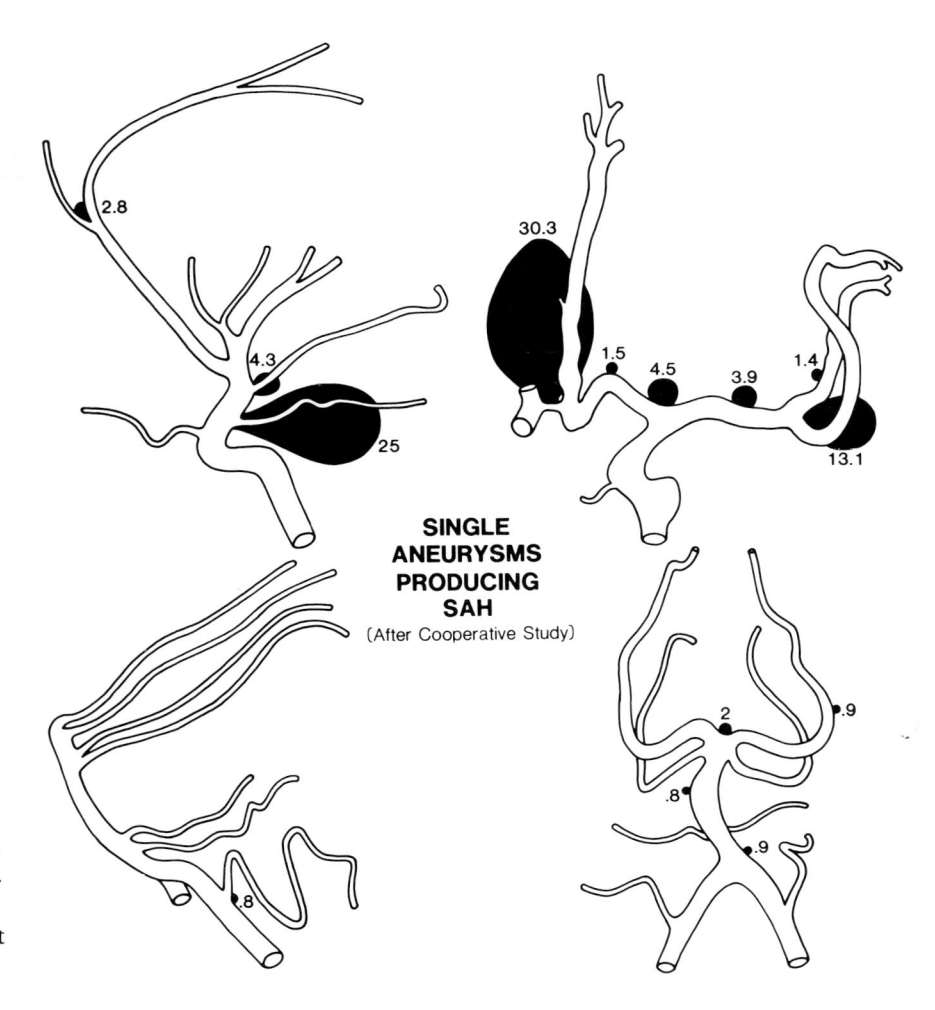

Figure 159-2 Schematic representation of the frequency (in percent) of single aneurysms producing subarachnoid hemorrhage, based on cooperative study data from Sahs et al.[80]

percent; fourth, 15 percent; fifth, 26 percent; sixth, 28 percent; seventh, 16 percent; and eighth, 6 percent.[73] These data were from 15 series comprising 5679 cases. Phillips et al. showed a steadily increasing incidence of aneurysms with increasing age level when correction was made for the smaller numbers of old persons in the population.[75]

SIZE OF ANEURYSMS (mm)				
Ruptured Symptomatic	<3 2%	3-10 60%	10-25 35%	>25 3%
Unruptured Symptomatic	<3 0%	3-10 70%	11-25 17%	>25 13%
Unruptured Asymptomatic	<3 19%	3-10 75%	11-25 6%	NIL
Sudden Fatal Ruptures	<5 12%	6-9 50%	±10 12%	>10 20%

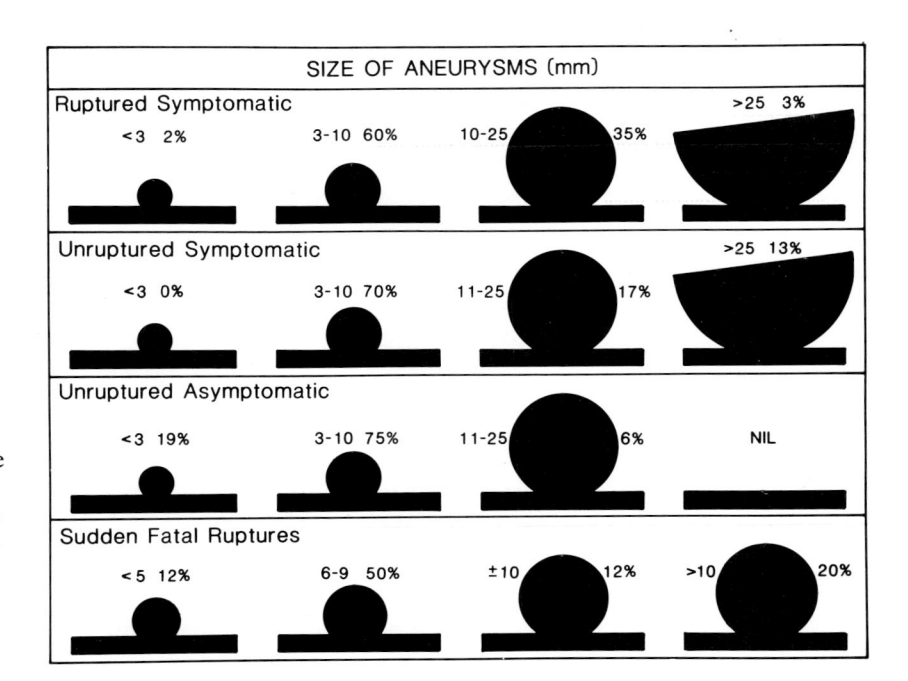

Figure 159-3 Size of aneurysms. The frequencies for ruptured aneurysms are those of 350 cases from the University of Alberta. The frequencies for unruptured aneurysms are from the cooperative study (Sahs et al.[80]) and those for sudden fatal ruptures are from Freytag.[33] Six percent of aneurysms could not be measured.

Sex

Figure 159-4 shows the sex and age distribution of cases. There is no doubt that there is a clear female predominance overall. Pakarinen analyzed 7010 cases in 21 series and found that 56.1 percent involved females.[73] There was a tendency for males to predominate until about the fifth decade, and thereafter females predominated. This late-life predominance of females may be partly, but is probably not entirely, due to the increasing proportion of females in the population.

Geographic Factors

All races share a propensity to develop intracranial aneurysms. The gross disparities in the availability and quality of neurosurgical care make it impossible to state at present whether there is a true racial or national difference in the occurrence of aneurysmal rupture.

Incidence of Aneurysm Rupture

The percentage of autopsied cases showing aneurysms will obviously be a function of the enthusiasm with which they are sought, as well as the age and sex mix of any particular institution's cases. Jellinger reviewed 12 series totaling 87,772 postmortem examinations, which revealed aneurysms in 1.6 percent of cases (range, 0.2 percent to 9 percent).[49] Bannerman et al. reviewed eight autopsy series comprising 51,360 cases[5] in which the total prevalence of aneurysms was 1.43 percent, 0.34 percent being unruptured and 1.09 percent ruptured. The occurrence of aneurysms is higher in forensic pathological series since aneurysms are a relatively more important cause of unexpected sudden death. In four such series, Pakarinen found the percentage of aneurysms to be 2, 2.4, 4, and 4.7 percent.[73] He also quoted the incidence as 5 percent in a military series of autopsies.

There are few studies of subarachnoid hemorrhage as the cause of death in whole populations. Brule (1958), in more than half a million deaths, found aneurysmal rupture to be the reported cause in 0.59 percent. Falconer (1950), in more than 50,000 deaths, found the corresponding figure to be 0.46 percent (both quoted by Pakarinen[73]).

The incidence of subarachnoid hemorrhage (new cases in a year) was reported to be between 6 and 10.9 per 100,000 population in the six series reviewed by Pakarinen.[73] They had been reported between 1950 and 1966. In those series, aneurysms comprised 77.2 percent of cases of subarachnoid hemorrhage. Of two reliable studies of incidence, one was that of Pakarinen himself in his Helsinki study, in which the incidence of aneurysmal rupture as a cause of subarachnoid hemorrhage was 10.3 per 100,000 per year. The 10.5 per 100,000 per year figure of Phillips et al. was based on a population study in Rochester, Minnesota.[75]

In the pathological study of McCormick and Acosta-Rua of 136 patients with aneurysms, 40 percent had ruptured aneurysms at autopsy.[60] In a similar pathological study of Chason and Hindman of 137 autopsies in which aneurysms were found, 42 percent of the patients had ruptured aneurysms.[16]

Based on the above data, it is probably a reasonable first-order approximation to say that less than 2 percent of the entire population will have an aneurysm; such an intracranial aneurysm will rupture in less than 1 percent of the population and will be the cause of death in 0.5 percent.

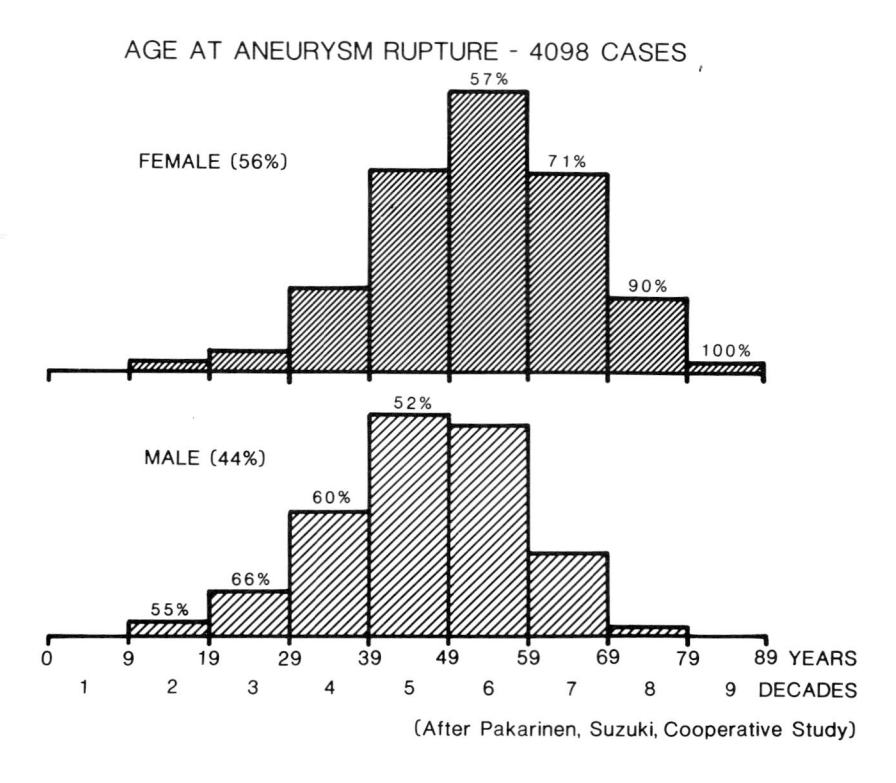

Figure 159-4 Age distributions of patients with ruptured aneurysms showing male predominance to the fifth decade and female predominance thereafter. Combined data of Sahs et al.[80] (cooperative study), Suzuki and Yoshimoto,[98] and Pakarinen.[73]

Familial Occurrence of Aneurysms

A minority of patients with aneurysms have such a high rate of saccular aneurysms occurring in their close relatives that a genetic mechanism may be assumed. The percentage of these patients in the total aneurysm population is unknown. In three of 39 such families, aneurysms occurred in identical twins.[81] Aneurysms occurred in siblings in 25 of 39 families. There were 34 affected males with 44 aneurysms and 38 affected females with 54 aneurysms. The incidence of multiplicity is therefore higher than in the general aneurysm population. The peak incidence occurred at 30 to 39 years and patients younger than 29 years made up 26.9 percent of the total, which compares with only 5.9 percent in all aneurysm cases studied in the cooperative study. It is therefore likely that a single autosomal dominant mechanism is involved. Since aneurysms are relatively common in the population at large, some familial aggregations are bound to occur on the basis of pure chance. However, if two or more siblings or a parent and child have aneurysms, it is reasonable to investigate the apparently uninvolved siblings. A family has been reported in which four members had aneurysms and one additional member was suspect. Elective angiography on five asymptomatic members of the family disclosed asymptomatic aneurysms in two.[40] In a fatal case involving two intracranial aneurysms the victim, who had previously refused elective angiography, was one of 13 siblings, 7 of whom were known to have had aneurysms.[30]

In an even smaller percentage of cases, there are familial aggregations with aneurysms due to the effects of known hereditary syndromes or suspected hereditary syndromes (Table 159-2). The Ehlers-Danlos syndrome is characterized by fragmentation or absence of elastic tissue in small arteries and probably also by collagen defects. There is hyperelasticity of the skin, subcutaneous nodules, and increased joint mobility, as well as easy bruisability. Angiography and surgery are extremely hazardous. Patients with coarctation of the aorta also have a greatly increased chance of having intracranial aneurysms, which tend to rupture when the patients are in their twenties. There is a high incidence of multiplicity of aneurysms. Early diagnosis and treatment is imperative. It is not certain whether or not there is an associated vascular intracranial anomaly with the aortic vascular lesion or whether the aneurysms result from the arterial hypertension secondary to the coarctation. A similar problem exists in determining the relationship of polycystic kidney disease to intracranial aneurysms. Aneurysms have been reported in 7.3 and 16.6 percent of cases of polycystic kidney disease in two series.[10]

Aneurysms of Infancy and Childhood

The Cooperative Aneurysm Study included one case of an aneurysm in a child under 4 years of age.[80] Pakarinen found no cases involving children among 511 patients.[73] Patel and Richardson found that among 3000 cases of aneurysms, only 58 patients were under 20 years of age and none were under 2 years of age.[74]

Among 27 reported cases of aneurysm in early childhood, 10 were found at autopsy and 14 were confirmed by angiography.[72] Sixty-three percent of the patients were males, and half of the patients had clinical symptoms in the first 6 months of life. Symptoms included seizures and evidence suggestive of a tumor. Of 11 patients treated surgically, nine survived.[72] In another review of saccular aneurysms in infancy and early childhood, only one of the 11 patients who were operated upon died.[7]

Thirty-nine patients with intracranial saccular aneurysms who were under 30 years of age were studied from the 1000-patient series of Suzuki.[125] One-third of them had arterial hypertension (greater than 150/100 mmHg) although no coarctation of the aorta or polycystic kidney disease was present. Eighty-six percent of the patients had excellent or good surgical results and only 2.6 percent died postoperatively. Multiple aneurysms were more common in the juvenile patients than in the series as a whole. None of the juvenile patients had middle cerebral aneurysms, as opposed to 17.4 percent for all cases.

Stehbens critically assessed the histology of published cases of aneurysms in infants.[89] He stated that inadequate pathological examination or atypical histological features in many of the cases gave little support to the theory of a congenital origin of these aneurysms. He thought that the existence of even a few authentic cases of saccular aneurysms at birth does not warrant the conclusion that all such aneurysms are due to a developmental defect.

Hemodynamics of Aneurysms

It is now generally considered that the impingement of an axial bloodstream on a distal carina can generate forces that cause local destruction of the internal elastic membrane. The resultant saclike outpouching increases the turbulence of flow in the area. This in turn can cause the wall to vibrate and accelerate the degenerative process.[26] Studies of static pressure-volume curves obtained on aneurysm and arterial material from human autopsies have shown that aneurysms are much less distensible than arteries.[84] At a given pressure therefore, the intracranial aneurysm must withstand a greater wall tension than the artery because of its different size and elasticity. The stress in the aneurysm wall is greater than in the arterial wall because it is stiffer and larger and also because it is thinner. It has been postulated that large fluctuations in stress in the aneurysm wall result from the pulsating blood pressure, which produces structural fatigue in the wall and further degeneration of the elastica. In an animal model of aneurysms involving a tail artery, at all flow rates no flow occurred beyond 2.5 tube diameters downstream from the mouth of the aneurysm. This is the probable explanation of why large aneurysms thrombose.[77]

In morphological studies of the internal elastic lamina at the bifurcation of human cerebral arteries, the mean diameter of the fenestrations in the elastica was found to increase in the vicinity of the apex, and the proportion of the area of internal elastic lamina composed of fenestrations also increased significantly.[15] On the basis of a comparison of stress concentration factors, it was proposed that the presence of enlarged fenestrations weakens the lamina and contributes to the initiation of microaneurysms.

Pathological observations relative to the hemodynamics of aneurysms have been made in 289 cases of fatal aneurysm rupture.[17] The actual site of aneurysmal rupture was most commonly the distal apex. Thin surface bubbles or multiloculations were present in 57 percent of ruptured aneurysms but only in 16 percent of unruptured aneurysms. Multiloculations were more common as aneurysms increased in size. In 88 percent of 90 cases with multiple aneurysms, the aneurysm with the greatest maximum external diameter had ruptured. The critical size beyond which aneurysms suddenly became unstable and likely to rupture was 4 mm. When combinations of middle cerebral and internal carotid aneurysms were present on the same side, the proximal aneurysm was the one which ruptured first in 70 percent of cases. Aneurysmal rupture is determined by an equation of enormous complexity, which reflects factors such as the number of water hammer pulses delivered, the pressure configurations, the brittleness of the wall, and the relative sizes and geometry of the aneurysm, its orifice, and the feeding artery.

Pathology and Pathogenesis of Aneurysms

Current concepts on the pathology of aneurysms are summarized in Table 159-3[18,38,42,49,60,80,87,88,95] and are illustrated in Figure 159-5. In 1934 it was suggested that elastica could herniate through areas of medial defects and then undergo degeneration secondary to the strain produced by overdistension.[28] However, a decade later Glynn[38] was unable to produce bulging of the unsupported elastic elements of arterial vessel walls even when these were subjected to pressures of 600 mmHg. Since probably everyone has medial defects in the cerebral arteries and since probably fewer than 5 percent (more likely 2 percent) of all persons have aneurysms, some pathological factor other than a medial defect must be at play. It is now widely accepted that damage to the internal elastic lamina by hemodynamic factors is the critical pathological change. However, it should not be forgotten that in addition to absence of the elastica, all aneurysms show absence of the media as well.

Crompton examined 149 cases at autopsy.[18] He found medial defects, intimal hyperplasia, and even changes in the internal elastica in cerebral arterial forks at birth, although he did note an increasing number in size with aging. Elastic degeneration appeared first in the intimal pads around the bifurcation, then in the elastica over medial defects. He found that large medial defects were unusual in the first decade but thereafter became progressively more common. Arterial hypertension and renal polycystic disease were associated with increased numbers of large medial defects. Atheromas were found in 52 percent of aneurysm cases—76 percent of such cases when there was evidence of hypertension and only 22 percent when there was not.

The consensus now is that atherosclerosis does not lead directly to the formation of aneurysms. When arteries feeding aneurysms were studied in 100 patients, in all but 12 there was evident atherosclerosis of the parent vessel.[87] Intimal proliferations occurred at the mouths of all aneurysms and to some extent at the sites of early aneurysmal change.

Elastic tissue alterations and loss in early aneurysmal changes were similar to, although greater than, the changes at forks without aneurysms. Apical regions were affected much more frequently than could be explained by chance alone. The absence of a distinct media in the sac wall was emphasized. The sac wall was still capable of organization

TABLE 159-3 Pathology of Intracranial Arterial Saccular Aneurysms

A. Light microscopy: The aneurysmal sac lacks normal layers.
 1. Intima: Normal or shows subendothelial proliferations consisting of several layers of smooth muscle cells and connective tissue enveloped by internal elastic membrane usually situated at the mouth of the sac; there may be foam cells.
 2. Internal elastic lamina: Usually absent or reduced to fragments; may be hypertrophied and duplicated at margin of aneurysm.
 3. Muscularis layer of media: Ends abruptly at neck of aneurysm.
 4. Aneurysm wall: May vary greatly in thickness. Larger aneurysms with thick walls may have a laminated appearance, with fibrous tissue layers having hemosiderin deposits and cholesterol and foam cells interposed between them. Thin areas may consist of only endothelium and adventitial fibrous tissue but usually some fibrohyaline tissue is interposed.
 5. Rupture site: Usually the thinnest area of the dome of the sac. Fibrin plug or layer is present at break in the wall. Thrombus is associated within the sac. In remote ruptures the fibrin is infiltrated by capillaries from the arachnoid. These can traverse the wall to regions of intimal proliferation. Microhemorrhages can occur in the wall from these capillaries.
 6. Lumen: May contain thrombus of varying degrees of organization; dense hyaline acellular tissue may occur in an organized thrombus.
 7. Adventitia: The loose fibrous tissue may be infiltrated by leukocytes, lymphocytes, and hemosiderin-laden phagocytes if there has been previous hemorrhage.
 8. Parent artery: Usually shows atherosclerotic changes, most marked in intimal pads at entrance to sac; foam cells, lipophages, and cholesterol clefts are seen.

B. Electron microscopy
 1. Scanning microscopy shows:
  a. Regressive changes in endothelium, such as ballooning, craters, and cytoplasmic bridges. At gaps between endothelial cell junctions, platelets and leukocytes adhere. Endothelium may be missing altogether.
  b. Adventitia may look normal.
 2. Transmission microscopy shows:
  a. Endothelial cells containing intracytoplasmic vacuoles, empty or full of lipid material.
  b. Beneath the endothelium there is often a grossly thickened basement membrane, which is multilaminar or reticulated.
  c. Fragments of elastica still present have lost their fibrillar structure.
  d. Scanty and sclerotic smooth muscle cells exist in the wall. Some contain hyaline patches, others autophagic vacuoles. Connective tissue contains some well-preserved fibroblasts. Extracellular lipid is common. Collagen fibers of variable length are arranged haphazardly. There is an abundant intercellular space containing lipofuscin granules.

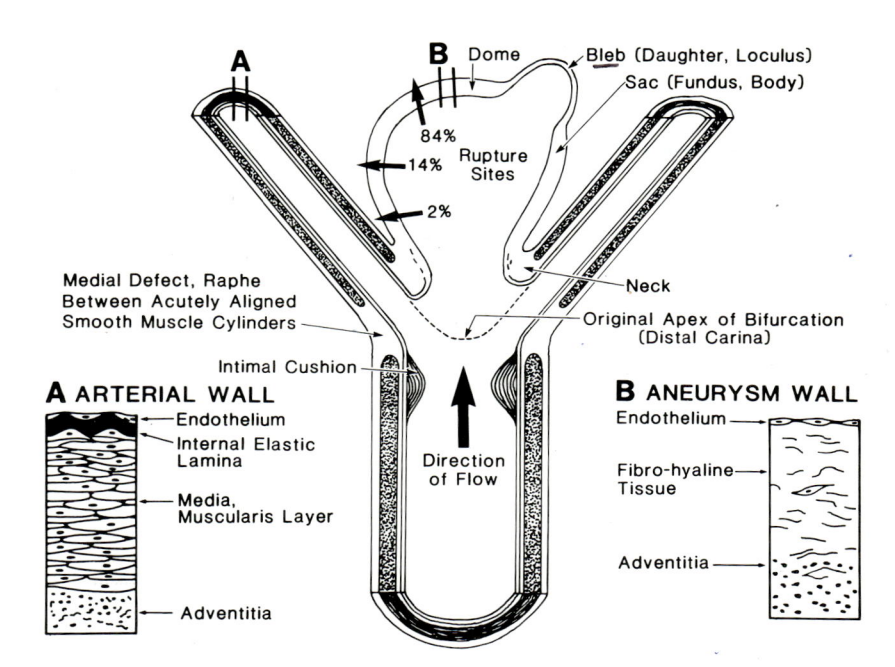

Figure 159-5 Diagram of aneurysmal pathology based on various authors. The data on frequency of rupture at different aneurysmal sites are from Crompton.[17]

and repair. Rather than a medial defect being the earliest change, funnel-shaped dilatations, areas of thinning, and small evaginations were thought to be the essential preaneurysmal lesions since they were associated with severe degenerative changes in the internal elastic lamina that had areas of thinning or evagination. Stehbens denied that small vessels arising from the apex of forks, vestiges of primitive capillary plexuses, or inflammatory processes are important in the pathogenesis of aneurysms.[88]

The pathological sequelae of aneurysmal rupture are listed in Table 159-4. The most feared by neurosurgeons are rebleeding and focal ischemic infarction due to severe vasospasm. In the cooperative study of Sahs et al.[80] 13 percent of initial survivors who were unoperated rebled in the first week, 12 percent in the second, 6 percent in the third, and 6 percent in the fourth. The mortality rate for the second bleeding episode was 43 percent. In 502 patients, the proven rebleeding rate for the first 2 weeks when patients received antifibrinolytic therapy was 12.7 percent.[68] A focal ischemic deficit occurred in 11 percent of 2265 cases.[50] In a control group of 63 grade 1 and 2 cases, 26 percent suffered a delayed ischemic neurological deficit due to vasospasm, which resulted in a severe neurological deficit in 8 percent and death in 5 percent.[2] In 98 cases, including patients in poorer grades, 10 percent died from vasospasm.[109]

Association of Aneurysms with Other Vascular Lesions

Anatomical Variants

Figure 159-6 illustrates some of the structural anomalies that have been reported in association with intracranial aneurysms. It may be that such anomalies cause altered flow patterns, which generate aneurysms through hemodynamic mechanisms. An alternative explanation is that there are common embryonic processes that predispose to both the anatomical variants and the arterial wall defects that result in the aneurysm.

Of 232 patients with primitive trigeminal artery, 14 percent had associated aneurysms, and of these aneurysms, 13 percent were on the primitive trigeminal artery itself.[36] All the primitive caroticobasilar anastomoses have been reported in association with intracranial aneurysms, including the rare otic artery.[120]

TABLE 159-4 Pathological Sequelae of Aneurysmal Rupture

A. Immediate
1. Hemorrhage
   a. Subarachnoid
   b. Intracerebral
   c. Intraventricular
   d. Subdural
   e. Intra-aneurysmal
2. Acute brain swelling
3. Acute ventricular dilatation
4. Brain shifts
   a. Tentorial herniation
   b. Foraminal impaction of cerebellar tonsils

B. Delayed
1. Hemorrhage
   a. Repeat aneurysmal rupture
   b. Secondary midbrain hemorrhages
2. Chronic hydrocephalus
3. Arterial vasospasm
4. Brain infarction
   a. Direct pressure from space-occupying lesion
   b. Vessel compression from brain shift
   c. Severe diffuse vasospasm
   d. Systemic hypotension, decreased cardiac output, decreased red cell mass and blood volume, hypoxia, acidosis, other fluid and electrolyte abnormalities

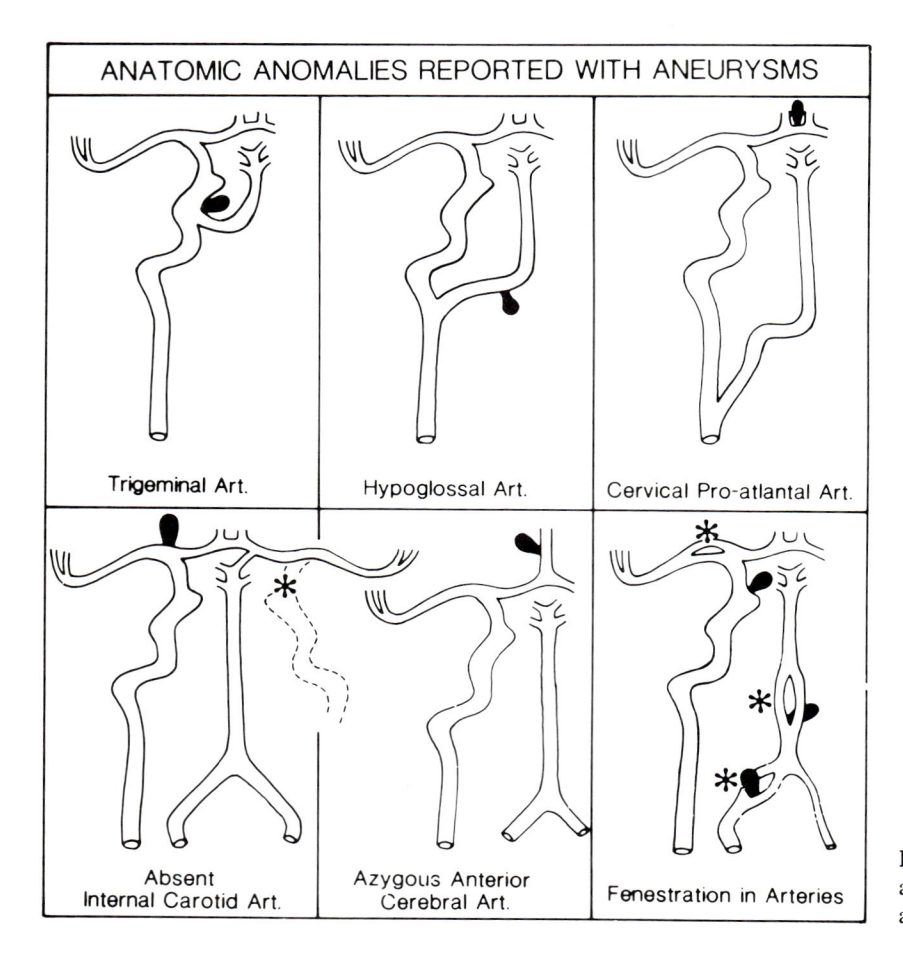

Figure 159-6 Synopsis of some of the anomalies that have been reported in association with intracranial aneurysms.

Figure 159-7 is based on an analysis of 143 ruptured and 39 unruptured aneurysms in 143 autopsy cases.[117] It is evident that hyperplasia of one anterior cerebral artery is associated with a relatively high incidence of aneurysms in the region of the anterior communicating artery. However, relative hyperplasia of one posterior communicating artery was not associated with a relative increase of aneurysms in that region. The meticulous operative findings of Yaşargil in anterior communicating artery region aneurysms substantiate the increased frequency of aneurysms when there is one hyperplastic or dominant A1 segment (75 percent of 203 cases).[122] The aneurysm in 97 percent of his 145 cases of unilateral hyperplasia was on the wall opposite the incoming dominant axial flow.

Arteriovenous Malformations

Of 3265 patients with intracranial aneurysms in the cooperative study, 1 percent also had intracranial arteriovenous malformations (AVMs).[80] In these patients, 34 percent of the aneurysms were on a major feeding artery to the malformation and 25 percent were on the same feeding system more proximally. Of 29 patients with both lesions reported, 14 were treated surgically and 15 conservatively; the mortality rate in the latter group was 60 percent. Nine cases of aneurysm and AVM from a total of 140 AVM cases (6.4 percent) have been reported.[96] Both lesions were treated definitively in eight of the nine cases. There were no deaths and seven of the nine patients were capable of working. This study reviewed five series of AVMs comprising 890 cases and found the incidence of associated aneurysm to be 7 percent. Hemodynamic stress is the factor most likely to be responsible for the formation of aneurysms in patients who have AVMs.[43] The principal evidence is that 77 percent of the aneurysms reviewed were on a proximal artery hemodynamically related to the AVM. Additional evidence of a flow-related origin for these aneurysms was that two aneurysms not surgically treated disappeared almost completely several months after excision of the AVM.

Infundibular Widenings of the Posterior Communicating Artery

Infundibula are pyramidal in shape, under 3 mm in maximum diameter, and located at arterial origins with small arteries coming from the apex. Miyasaka et al. studied 132 patients with AVMs, of whom 16.7 percent had associated aneurysms;[64] 10 patients had aneurysms and infundibula and 20 had infundibula alone. Miyasaka et al. found that infundibula were more likely to occur in older patients and in patients with larger AVMs. Of the infundibula, 65 percent occurred at the junction of the internal carotid and posterior communicating arteries and 82 percent were located on arteries supplying the AVM or on the internal carotid artery ipsilateral to the AVM. In four patients the infundibulum decreased in size following successful treatment of the

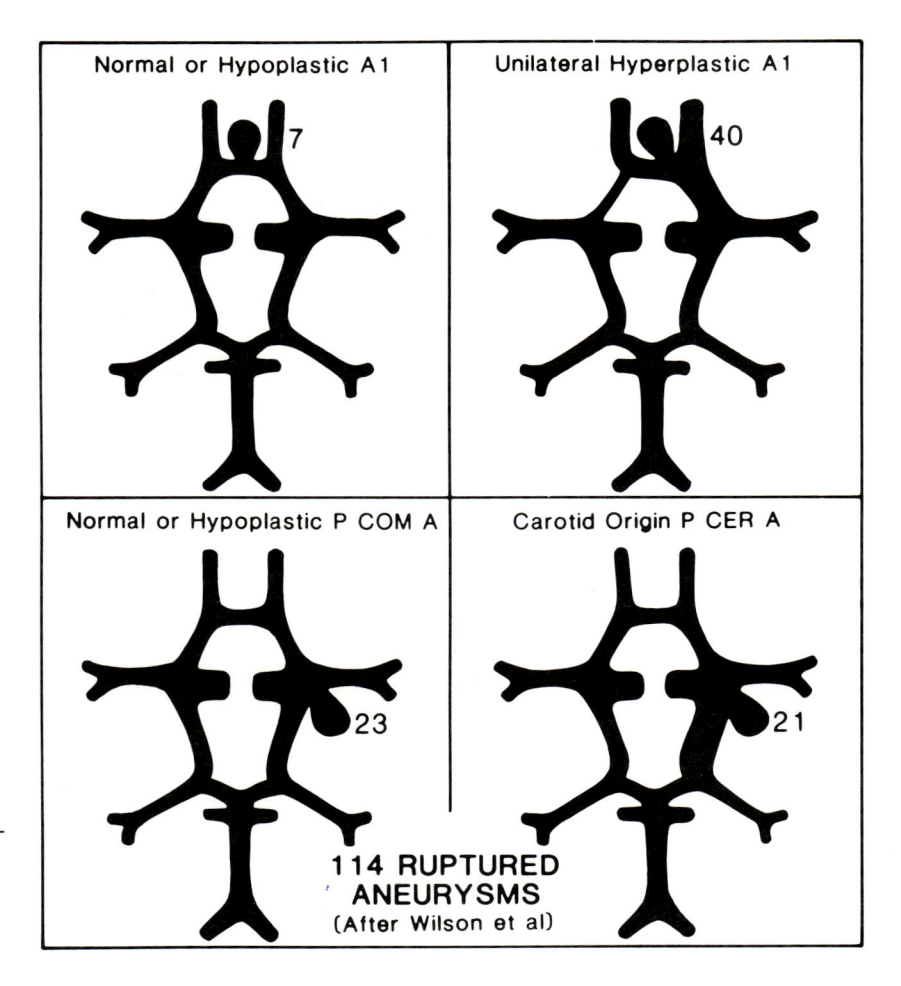

Figure 159-7 Pictorial depiction of data of Wilson et al.[117] showing the increased frequency of unilateral hyperplasia of the A1 segment of the anterior cerebral artery with anterior communicating aneurysms but no such association in the posterior circle.

AVM. In the same study, 3 of 43 aneurysms decreased in size after removal of the AVM. It has been suggested that infundibula occur in about 7 percent of normal angiograms and that the frequency increases with age.[104] A case of infundibular enlargement over a period of 9 years with evolution into an aneurysm that was unruptured has been documented. There are five similar case reports in the literature. Others have assessed the gross and histological findings in seven junctional dilatations discovered at autopsy.[24] No significant histological abnormalities were found in any case and it was concluded that a junctional dilatation was neither aneurysmal nor preaneurysmal. If an infundibulum does evolve into an aneurysm, it must be an unusual event. A rupture is even rarer.

Hypertension

The relationship between blood pressure and aneurysmal rupture was investigated in 212 cases seen between 1964 and 1976.[3] Blood pressures were determined by the patient's medical record preceding admission for aneurysmal rupture and/or by the stable blood pressure off medication as long as possible after the initial bleeding. The series was compared with Department of Health and Human Services data for approximately 10,000 patients in each matched age group. Mean systolic and diastolic blood pressures were not elevated to a statistically significant extent in patients with aneurysms as compared with the general population, except for a minor elevation in systolic blood pressure in a few subsets of younger male and female patients. A hypertensive patient under 55 years of age of either sex was found to be twice as likely to have multiple aneurysms as a normotensive patient.

McCormick and Schmalstieg used both blood pressure records and myocardial hypertrophy found at autopsy to assess hypertension and reported no increase in hypertension in aneurysm patients as compared with controls.[61] In their 250 aneurysm patients, there was also no evident association of hypertension with multiplicity of aneurysms, age at which aneurysms presented clinically, or age at rupture. These results cast serious doubt on hypertension as a major cause of intracranial aneurysms.[61]

A comparison was made of 319 cases of subarachnoid hemorrhage with an equal number of controls and almost half a million discharges from the Veterans Administration hospitals of the United States.[51] Among the 173 patients in whom angiograms were performed, aneurysms were found in 74 percent of the 109 normotensive but only 58 percent of the 64 hypertensive patients. Conversely, hypertension existed in 49 percent of 55 patients without aneurysms but only 31 percent of 118 with aneurysms. The coexistence of aneurysms and hypertension was therefore uncommon. In addition, the marked excess of hypertension among blacks was not associated with a corresponding excess of aneurysms. It can reasonably be concluded that hypertension is not a major factor in the etiology of saccular aneurysms. This finding should not be confused with the fact that immediately following the ictus of aneurysmal rupture, the occurrence of hypertension has been universally found to be a very important negative prognostic factor (Table 159-8). In these circumstances, however, it is probably partly a reflection of the Cushing response to intracranial hypertension.

Processes Affecting Carotid Blood Flow

Two patients with aneurysms who underwent cervical carotid artery ligation after several years developed aneurysms on the contralateral intracranial internal carotid artery that had not been present on the original angiograms.[82] Follow-up angiography of 25 aneurysms of the intracranial carotid artery following carotid ligation in the neck showed disappearance or diminution in size of aneurysms in 17 cases and no change in 5.[37]

Stern et al. reviewed 20 patients with anterior circulation aneurysms coexisting with carotid stenosis that was ipsilateral to the aneurysm in 13 cases and contralateral in 7.[90] The stenosis was greater than 70 percent in all cases. One-third of the patients had intracavernous carotid aneurysms. Two patients in all were known to have died from rupture of their aneurysms following carotid reconstruction; the mean follow-up time was not stated. These data suggested that there was little additional risk in performing carotid endarterectomy in patients with asymptomatic aneurysms, but this risk was considerably increased if the endarterectomy was being performed in the feeding vessel of a symptomatic or previously ruptured aneurysm.

Fields and Weibel reported a 67-year-old patient who presented with an aneurysmal rupture and third nerve palsy.[27] A left carotid endarterectomy was performed and 10 months later the patient had a recurrent hemorrhage, which ultimately proved fatal. A reasonable conclusion is that in the presence of a symptomatic internal carotid artery stenosis and asymptomatic aneurysm(s), the endarterectomy should be performed if clinically indicated, and subsequently the aneurysm should be operated upon if the patient is a good risk or there is evidence of growth of the aneurysm on follow-up angiography.

A case of anterior communicating artery aneurysm associated with absence of a left cervical carotid artery was reviewed and 15 previously published cases were analyzed.[106] Of these aneurysms 63 percent were on the anterior communicating artery and 19 percent on the basilar bifurcation. In these cases two vessels would be subjected to increased flow to compensate for the unilateral carotid absence. The occurrence of an intracranial aneurysm in 9 of 36 patients with an absent internal carotid artery has been described.[85]

Two cases of pulseless disease (Takayasu's disease) associated with aneurysmal rupture have been presented.[58] In one patient both carotid arteries were occluded and in the other one carotid was. The aneurysms and cerebral arteries did not show the panarteritis with giant cell granulomas typical of the occlusive lesions in the aortic arch and pulmonary artery with this entity. The patient with absent carotid arteries bilaterally had a basilar tip aneurysm and the one with a unilaterally absent carotid artery had a carotid–posterior communicating artery aneurysm on the contralateral side.

Experimental Aneurysms

Cerebral aneurysms have been induced in rats by feeding them β-aminoproprionitrile, which causes a connective tissue abnormality due to defects in cross-linkage between elastin and collagen. The rats were also rendered hypertensive by a variety of means. Flow was increased through one carotid system by ligation of the other common carotid.[41] Ligation of the carotid artery in rabbits induced exceptionally large defects in the media, especially at the distal end of the basilar artery.[42] Very rare reports have also appeared in the literature of post-traumatic intracranial aneurysms in animals. There is not yet a naturally occurring model of aneurysms in animals.

Predisposing Factors to Aneurysm Rupture

Activities at Time of Rupture

Among 2228 cases in the cooperative study, the onset of subarachnoid hemorrhage was associated with lifting or bending in 12 percent, emotional strain in 4 percent, defecation in 4 percent, coitus in 4 percent, trauma in 3 percent, coughing in 2 percent, urination in 2 percent, and parturition in 0.35 percent.[80] In about one-third of cases, rupture was said to have occurred during sleep or in unspecified circumstances. In the absence of data on the time spent by age- and sex-matched nonaneurysmal cases in these strenuous activities, it is not possible to prove that they in fact precipitate aneurysmal rupture. Notwithstanding this, it is very likely that peaks of arterial hypertension, rapid oscillations in venous and cerebrospinal fluid pressure, and possibly movement of brain structures in relation to one another can all precipitate aneurysmal rupture.

Smoking

A retrospective study of 208 patients with ruptured cerebral aneurysms found a highly significant excess of cigarette smokers compared with the expected incidence. It was suggested that continued smoking increases the risk of suffering a subarachnoid hemorrhage by a factor of 3.9 for men and 3.7 for women.[8]

Alcohol Consumption

In 25 percent of 75 aneurysmal ruptures in a Finnish study, the bleeding was preceded within 24 h by a bout of alcohol consumption.[46] This intoxication preceding the ictus was two to four times as common in male patients and three to five times as common in female patients as alcohol intoxication in the general Finnish population of the same age and sex.

Pregnancy and Puerperium

During a 24-year period from 1950 to 1973 a Minnesota maternal mortality study found that 4.4 percent of maternal deaths were due to spontaneous subarachnoid hemorrhage[6] and 51 percent of the cerebral hemorrhages were due to rupture of an aneurysm or AVM. Toxemia was the next most common cause. In 29 autopsies, a ruptured aneurysm was found in 52 percent of cases, and AVM in 34 percent, and no definite cause of massive hemorrhage in 35 percent. Other large studies also indicate that rupture of an aneurysm and AVM are about as common as hemorrhage from toxemia. In the Minnesota study, 68 percent of the patients died within the first 24 h from the hemorrhage and 86 percent died within 4 days. Rapid irreversible coma occurred in 76 percent of cases, and 42 percent of the fetuses died. An important observation from their data was that the aneurysmal rupture rate was 0.4 per week during pregnancy (undelivered), 35 per week during labor or the immediate few hours postpartum, and 1.4 per week in the first 3 months postpartum. The ratio of aneurysms to AVMs in pregnancy in Robinson's review of the literature was 1.75:1.[78] The frequency of aneurysmal rupture increases as pregnancy progresses. In 77 cases, 4 percent ruptured in the first 10 weeks, 19 percent in the second 10 weeks, 30 percent in the third 10, 44 percent in the fourth 10, and 3 percent in labor or the early puerperium.[78] A patient with aneurysmal subarachnoid hemorrhage is six times more likely than her counterpart with an AVM to have had a previous normal pregnancy.

In a review of five surgical series including 36 patients, 44 percent had conservative management, 56 percent had surgical treatment,[63] 24 percent of the deliveries were by cesarean section, and 61 percent of the mothers and 78 percent of the infants were alive and well.

From the point of view of the aneurysmal rupture, the mother should be treated the same as if she were not pregnant. The aneurysm should be clipped as soon as possible. There is no evidence that the fetus is more susceptible to induced hypotension than the mother but discretion would clearly indicate that as little hypotension as necessary should be used. In the presence of an unsecured aneurysm, it is usually recommended that Valsalva maneuvers be avoided as much as possible and that the second stage of labor be shortened with forceps and lumbar epidural anesthesia. Cesarean section should be for primarily obstetrical indications.

Aneurysmal Rupture During Angiography

It has been stated that a dangerous rise in blood pressure precipitating aneurysmal rupture could result from the quick injection of a large volume of contrast medium, particularly if there is spasm at the tip of the catheter, increased blood pressure, raised intracranial pressure, or spasm of intracranial arteries.[54] Conditions leading to excessive spontaneous cross-circulation should be avoided. A review of 10 new cases of aneurysmal rupture during angiography and 20 other well-documented cases from the literature[52] indicated that internal carotid injections were not more dangerous than common carotid injections. Overall, these patients tended to be in poor condition, with 18 percent being grade 4 and 32 percent grade 5 at the time of angiography, which was performed in 53 percent within 12 h of admission to the hospital; 45 percent had common carotid injections and 42 percent had internal carotid injections. Of these patients 84 percent died following the extravasation. The authors suggested that a mixture of blood and hyperosmolar contrast agent must be more toxic than blood alone. They found no correlation between the volume of contrast material and the number of injections prior to the one associated with rupture. Unfortunately, detailed data on arterial blood pressure, injection pressures, and flow rates were not obtainable.

Thirty-two cases of aneurysmal rupture during angiography provided no definite proof that an acute phase of intracranial arterial spasm occurs.[116] Where vasospasm was present, it was assumed in most cases to have been related to a prior episode of bleeding. It is possible, of course, that the hyperosmolar contrast material has a vasodilating effect that counteracts the acute vasoconstricting effect of blood.

Diagnosis of Aneurysmal Rupture

Warning Symptoms and Signs

In 2621 aneurysm cases from the cooperative study of Sahs et al.,[80] symptoms antedating the first subarachnoid hemorrhage occurred as follows: headache, 48 percent; dizziness, 10 percent; orbital pain, 7 percent; diplopia, 4 percent; and loss of vision, 4 percent. Signs antedating the first hemorrhage were motor or sensory disturbances, 6 percent; seizures, 4 percent; ptosis, 3 percent; bruits, 3 percent; and dysphasia, 2 percent. Of the total number of patients with unruptured symptomatic aneurysms, 68 percent had third cranial nerve involvement. It was suggested that only 10 to 15 percent of all aneurysm cases presented the opportunity for diagnosis before rupture.

In an analysis of 112 single aneurysm cases, the most frequent warning symptoms and signs prior to rupture were generalized headache 25 percent, localized head pain 18 percent, lethargy 8 percent, impairment of extraocular movements 7 percent, face and eye pain 6 percent, and neck and back pain 6 percent. Internal carotid–posterior communicating artery region aneurysms were associated with impairment or extraocular movements in 23 percent of cases and visual field defects, eye pain, and face pain in 8 percent each. The average interval between the warning signs and major hemorrhage in these patients was 3 weeks. Patients with warning signs tended to be younger.[71]

Another study of 192 patients found that warning signs occurred in 59 percent.[105] The latent interval to major hemorrhage was about 1 week for middle cerebral and internal carotid aneurysms and over 2 weeks for anterior communicating aneurysms. The incidence was much higher for internal carotid aneurysms (69 percent) and for multiple aneurysms (67 percent) than for other situations. It was not possible to decide whether warning signs occurred from a minor hemorrhage or from expansion of the aneurysm. Twenty-nine percent of patients were operated upon on the basis of warning signs prior to the development of a major hemorrhage. It is clear from the very nonspecific nature and ubiquitousness of such symptoms in the general population that it will require a considerable amount of professional and public education to improve the proportion of cases coming to a definitive diagnosis prior to a major hemorrhage.

Clinical Presentation of Aneurysmal Rupture

Sarner and Rose studied 962 patients with ruptured aneurysms.[83] Symptoms and signs occurred with decreasing frequency as follows: meningism, 64 percent; coma, 52 percent; nausea and vomiting, 45 percent; generalized headache, 32 percent; classical occipital headaches, 21 percent; reflex changes, 19 percent; motor deficit, 17 percent; dysphasia, 13 percent; confusion, 12 percent; intraocular hemorrhage, 12 percent; anisocoria, 11 percent; papilledema, 9 percent; homonymous hemianopia, 9 percent; lateralized headache, 8 percent; third nerve palsy, 7 percent; and sensory disturbances, 5 percent. No localizing signs occurred in 39 percent. The cardinal diagnostic points remain a headache of unusual severity for a particular patient with very sudden onset.

Symptoms and Signs Not Due to Rupture

Distal Embolization from Partially Thrombosed Aneurysms

Sixteen cases are known.[34] Transient ischemic attacks can be considered secondary to an aneurysm if no other lesion or predisposing risk factor is present, if there is no recent evidence of subarachnoid hemorrhage or vasospasm, if the aneurysm is located proximal to the territory involved in the symptomatology, if there is evidence of thrombus in the sac, and if the attacks cease when the aneurysm is excluded from the circulation. Of these cases 75 percent had no recurrence of symptoms following definitive treatment of the aneurysm, 13 percent had continued or recurrent symptoms when the aneurysm was not excluded from the circulation, and 6 percent (one case) had no recurrence despite the fact that the aneurysm was only wrapped.

Neurological Signs from Giant Aneurysms

Aneurysms larger than 2.5 cm in maximum diameter are called *giant*. Figure 159-3 illustrates the frequency with which such aneurysms are found in ruptured and unruptured groups as well as in symptomatic and asymptomatic groups. Of Drake's series of 174 giant aneurysms, 38 percent involved the anterior circulation and 62 percent involved the posterior circulation.[22] The high incidence of vertebrobasilar giant aneurysms probably was at least partly a reflection of his expertise in dealing with such aneurysms. Of his cases 36 percent presented with subarachnoid hemorrhage.

In another series of 28 giant aneurysms, 39 percent occurred in the cavernous sinus.[67] This indicates that the surrounding dural structures permitted some external support to the aneurysmal wall, preventing rupture and permitting enlargement to the giant size. The rate of subarachnoid hemorrhage was 47 percent for extracavernous giant aneurysms. The only cavernous one to rupture had enlarged out of the confines of the cavernous sinus. The frequency of signs referable to a given cranial nerve was as follows: third, 32 percent; second, 25 percent; sixth, 25 percent; fourth, 14 percent; fifth, 11 percent; eighth, ninth, and tenth, 4 percent; and eleventh and twelfth, 7 percent. The most common site was the internal carotid artery, followed by the middle cerebral artery. In another series of 22 extracavernous giant aneurysms, 23 percent occurred at the apex of the basilar artery, 18 percent on the vertebral and basilar arteries, 14 percent on the middle cerebral artery, and 9 percent on both the internal carotid and anterior communicating arteries.[11] There was a 2.7:1 female predominance.

Cranial Nerve Signs from Nongiant Aneurysms

In the cooperative study, there were 86 patients with unruptured, symptomatic posterior communicating–internal carotid artery aneurysms.[80] Of these patients 87 percent had signs of third cranial nerve involvement. Only 2 and 1 percent had evidence of sixth and fourth cranial nerve palsies, respectively. The same study included 37 patients with ophthalmic–internal carotid artery aneurysms. Of these cases 29 percent presented with loss of vision and 19 percent had symptoms referable to the third cranial nerve, 13 percent to the fifth, 10 percent to the fourth, and 6 percent to the sixth. For unruptured symptomatic aneurysms of the internal carotid artery, the maximum frequency occurred with aneurysms 7 to 10 mm in size.

Natural History of Aneurysms

Table 159-5 summarizes some of the major contributions to our understanding of the prognosis when an aneurysm is present. The major observation to emerge is that the principal mortality occurs immediately following the hemorrhage and that the death rate diminishes rapidly thereafter. A fact of paramount importance from the cooperative study was that the mortality rate over the entire first week was 27 percent for single aneurysms after subarachnoid hemorrhage.[80] Figure 159-8 is a graphic estimate as to what might happen to the total population of aneurysmal rupture cases in North America. The 1980–1981 census figures give a total population of about 251 million. The incidence of ruptured aneurysms in two careful studies in the United States and Europe was 10.5 and 10.3 per 100,000 population per year. In the cooperative study, 37 percent of patients were admitted more than 3 days after their subarachnoid hemorrhage and 16 percent had minimal symptoms.[80] Of 5831 patients with subarachnoid hemorrhage, 17 percent were admitted after

TABLE 159-5 Prognosis for Surgically Untreated Saccular Intracranial Aneurysms

A. Ruptured
  1. *Unselected*, entire city, minimal surgical withdrawals, all sudden deaths autopsied. Helsinki 1954–1961, 363 cases. Mortality: 1 day 32%; 1 week 43%; 1 month 56%; 6 months 60%.[73]
  2. *Selected* by virtue of surgical withdrawals, admissions to many hospitals. Cooperative study, 1958–1965, 830 single aneurysm cases. Mortality: 1 day 10%; 1 week 27%; 1 month 49%; 6 months 61%.[80]
  3. *Unselected* since surgical withdrawals were randomized, admissions to two hospitals. London 1958–1967, 364 cases, anterior communicating aneurysms. Mortality: 6 months 41%; 5 years 48%; 10 years 51%.[119]
  4. *Partly selected*, entire city, 27 surgical withdrawals at a mean time of 9 days postrupture. Rochester 1945–1974, 119 cases (estimated from an illustration). Mortality: 1 day 8%; 1 week 40%; 1 month 60%.[75]

B. Unruptured
  1. *Asymptomatic* multiple aneurysms associated with other previously ruptured and clipped aneurysms. Helsinki, 1956–1970, 61 cases, follow-up 10 to 24 years. Mortality from rupture of different aneurysms at 10 years after original aneurysm rupture 6.6%. Mortality at last available follow-up 11.5%.[45]
  2. *Asymptomatic* multiple aneurysms associated with other previously ruptured and clipped aneurysms. London, 46 cases, follow-up mean 7 years. Mortality from rupture of different aneurysms at mean follow-up 7 years 6.5%.[118]
  3. Combined *asymptomatic* (71%) and *symptomatic* (29%), no surgical withdrawals. Rochester, 1955–1975, 65 cases, follow-up mean 8 years. Mortality from aneurysm rupture 11%.[115]
  4. *Asymptomatic*, no surgical withdrawals. Cooperative study, 1958–1965, 50 cases, follow-up not stated, said to be "less satisfactory" than for other groups. Mortality at 5 years 2%.[80]
  5. *Asymptomatic*, estimates using prevalence averages and decremental life table analysis methods. 1982. Estimated mortality for a 20-year-old by age 75 years 16.6%. Estimated mortality for a 60-year-old by age 75 years 4.68%.[20]
  6. *Symptomatic*, no surgical withdrawals. Cooperative study, 1958–1965, 32 cases. Mortality at mean follow-up 41 months 28%.[80]

hemorrhage or would have died from the hemorrhage, again without a diagnosis. Drake reported that neurosurgeons were operating upon 1.6 per 100,000 per year in Japan and 3.6 per 100,000 per year in Ontario.[23] We are therefore not operating on the majority of aneurysm rupture cases and, for the most part, are probably simply treating the "survivors." Even in Rochester, Minnesota, 8 percent of patients with ruptured aneurysms died before reaching medical attention.[75] Pakarinen found that 15 percent of patients died before they reached a hospital.[73] The natural history of a patient admitted to the hospital is still bleak. From the data presented in Table 159-6, it can be seen that for those patients admitted to neurosurgeons very early, the postoperative mortality can be reduced by delaying operation, but this is a spurious gain because overall management mortality usually increases. A recent study of 249 patients with aneurysmal rupture between 1974 and 1977, admitted within 3 days to American hospitals and treated with antifibrinolytic therapy, has been reported.[1] Operation was not carried out before 11 days after rupture. There was a 36.2 percent mortality; 17.9 percent survived with serious neurological sequelae; and only 46 percent had a favorable outcome at 90 days. Outcome would, of course, have been worse if all admissions had been on the day of hemorrhage. How can we reconcile these bleak figures with the reports of others who are obtaining very low postoperative mortality figures overall in very large series? The explanation in part lies in the delay in transfer to, and natural selection that occurs prior to arrival at, major tertiary referral centers. This can be seen in Table 159-7, in which the lower overall postoperative mortality rate in three large series was due to the delay in operation compared with a smaller series in which the patients were more commonly admitted to the neurosurgeon immediately following their aneurysmal rupture.

It is obviously of vital importance to a neurosurgeon to be able to advise a patient and the patient's relatives as to the possible outcome with different courses of action. In the past decade, more sophisticated methods of analysis using multiple regression (or multivariant) techniques have permitted the simultaneous analysis of potentially important preoperative prognostic factors. Table 159-8 lists some of these studies. It is clear that we are still a long way from predicting with 100 percent accuracy what is likely to happen to an individual patient, but neurological grade, blood pressure, the presence of intraventricular or intracerebral hemorrhage, and advanced age are obviously important clinical factors.

more than one hemorrhage. The number of cases initially misdiagnosed must have been greater than this figure since some patients would not have had a second subarachnoid

TABLE 159-6 Proportion of Early Operations and Occurrence of Intraventricular Hemorrhage as Determinants of Management Mortality. Admissions to Hospital Day 0–1 after Aneurysm Rupture

Reference	Types of Aneurysms	Number of Cases	Postoperative Mortality, % ≤7 days	Postoperative Mortality, % >7 days	Management Mortality, % ≤7 days	Management Mortality, % >7 days
Weir and Aronyk[110]	All	224	30	7	53	64
Wheelock et al.[114]	With intracerebral hematoma	103	40	18	46	47
Mohr et al.[65]	With intraventricular hemorrhage	74	22	40	71	89

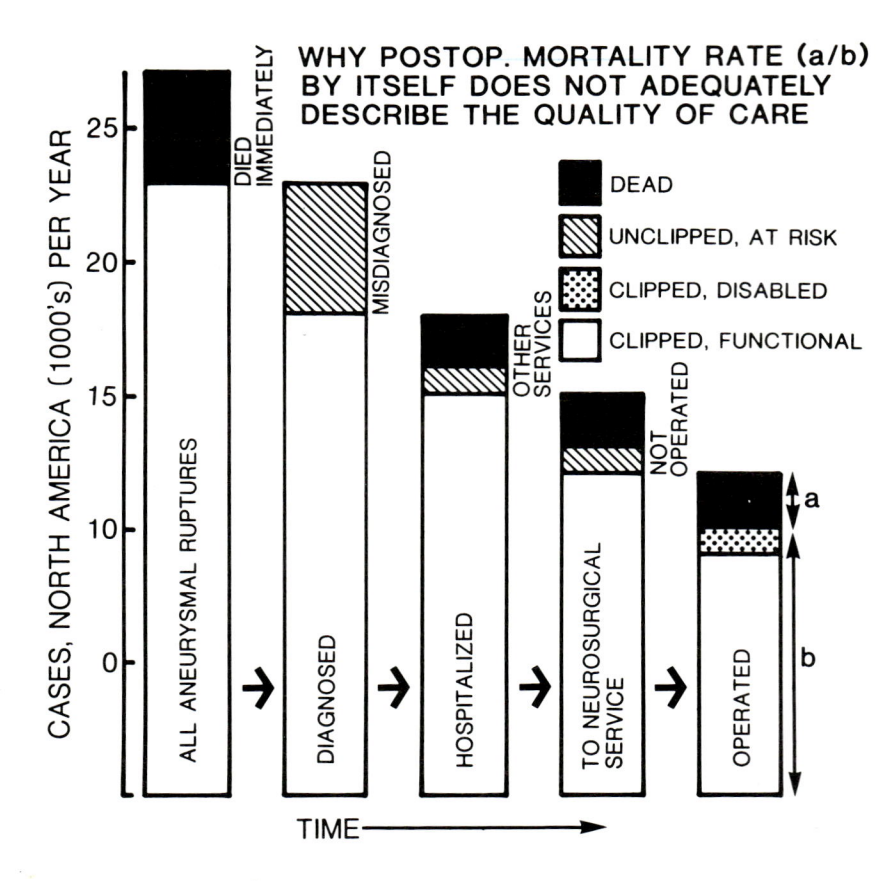

Figure 159-8 Schematic representation of patient flow following aneurysm rupture. The actual numbers can best be described as an educated guess in the absence of any hard epidemiologic data.

The results that any given neurosurgeon can achieve in the treatment of aneurysmal rupture are as individual as his fingerprints. Although most of us would wish otherwise, individual technical skill is probably of lesser importance than geographic, sociological, and organizational factors in our area of practice, which ultimately determine the nature of the patient group referred to us and the time at which this is done. In analyzing the reports of neurosurgical series, the reader should note whether it is stated when the patients were admitted to the neurosurgeons in relation to the time of their aneurysmal rupture, what grade they were, whether or not there were any arbitrary exclusions of cases on the basis of age or neurological status, and whether all aneurysmal ruptures in that geographic area were likely to have been included.

Medical Complications of Aneurysm Rupture

General

Table 159-9 lists the preliminary experience from the latest cooperative study on the timing of aneurysm surgery, directed by Kassell and Torner.[50] The most frequently encountered medical complications are hypertension, cardiac arrhythmias and hypotension, pneumonia and atelectasis, inappropriate secretion of antidiuretic hormone, gastrointestinal hemorrhage, and anemia.

Infections can also be a major source of danger to a patient with an aneurysm. Weir, in a study of 100 consecutive

TABLE 159-7 Proportion of Early Operations as a Determinant of Total Postoperative Mortality Rate

Reference	Yaşargil[123]	Suzuki[97]	Sundt[93]	Weir[111]
Number of cases	638	625	271	67
Postoperative mortality < 7 days, %	15	16	18	10
Postoperative mortality 7–14 days, %	2	5	8*	0
Postoperative mortality > 14 days, %	2	3	2†	0
Total postoperative mortality, %	4	5	6	7
Percent of cases operated < 7 days	18	17	17‡	73

*7–9 days.
† ≥ 10 days.
‡ ≤ 6 days.

Intracranial Aneurysms and Subarachnoid Hemorrhage: An Overview

TABLE 159-8 Relative Strength of Preoperative Factors as Predictors of Mortality after Aneurysmal Rupture (Multiple Regression Analyses)*

A. All Aneurysmal Ruptures
  1114 cases, 1970–1977, 14-day mortality[100]
  1. Neurological status   17.74
  2. Diastolic blood pressure   11.66
  3. Interval to treatment   9.44
  4. Vasospasm   8.51
  5. Medical condition   5.51

  265 cases, 1972–1977, 5-year postoperative mortality, excluding preoperative deaths and postoperative deaths from unrelated causes[4]
  1. Botterell grade   0.65
  2. Age   0.47
  3. Blood pressure   0.31
  4. Interval to operation   0.20
  5. Aneurysm side   0.19

  135 cases, 1968–1973, mortality 2 months after aneurysmal rupture[112]
  1. Neurological grade   0.36
  2. Grade at operation   0.34
  3. Preoperative vasospasm   0.28
  4. Mass lesion   0.23
  5. Blood pressure   0.20
  6. Interval to surgery   0.00
  7. Age   0.06

B. Aneurysmal Rupture Producing Intracerebral Hematoma
  132 cases, 1982, mortality during initial admission[114]
  1. Systolic blood pressure   0.37
  2. Preoperative herniation   0.35
  3. Grade at clipping   0.33
  4. Grade at evacuation of clot 0.27
  5. Diastolic blood pressure   0.16
  6. Grade at initial CT scan   0.14
  7. Size of hematoma   0.14
  8. Vasospasm   0.13

C. Aneurysmal Rupture Producing Intraventricular Hemorrhage
  91 cases, 1982, mortality during initial admission[65]
  1. Size of ventricles   0.56
  2. Systolic blood pressure   0.38
  3. Age   0.37
  4. Diastolic blood pressure   0.32
  5. Grade on admission   0.31
  6. Associated intracerebral clot 0.17
  7. Location of aneurysm   0.15
  8. Location of clot   0.11

*Numbers in each series are only relative within the series.

patients, found that 16 percent developed cystitis and 9 percent developed vaginitis.[109] Three percent showed evidence of gram-negative septicemia or fungal superinfection.

Pulmonary Edema

Among the most dramatic and dangerous acute complications of aneurysm rupture is pulmonary edema. Of 141 patients with fatal aneurysm rupture 13 percent showed clinical evidence of this entity.[108] All patients had shown sudden onset of coma and virtually instantaneous onset of breathing difficulties. Respirations were irregular and pink foam issued from the airways. Skin was cyanotic, moist, and cool. These patients tended to be young. The treatment of the pulmonary problem is intubation, artificial ventilation with positive end-expiratory pressure, and massive doses of furosemide (Lasix; Hoechst, Willowdale, Ontario).[109]

Fluid and Electrolyte Disturbances

In a review of Suzuki's 1000 surgically treated aneurysms, hyponatremia (<130 meq Na per liter) occurred in 4 percent of cases, hypernatremia (>155 meq Na per liter) in 2.1 percent, both disorders in 1 percent, and polyuria in 0.7 percent.[99] These abnormalities occurred with aneurysms of the anterior communicating artery more commonly than with aneurysms at all other sites combined. The death rate associated with hypernatremia was 43 percent; with diabetes insipidus 25 percent; and with hyponatremia 15 percent. The abnormalities reached a peak (20 percent) between the third and seventh day after the last hemorrhage. Patients coming to autopsy showed hypothalamic hemorrhage.

The syndrome of inappropriate antidiuretic hormone secretion is of great importance following aneurysmal rupture because its time course and symptomatology are very similar to those of the delayed ischemic deficit from vaso-

TABLE 159-9 Medical Complications of Aneurysm Rupture*

	Preoperative, % of 2265 cases	Postoperative, % of 1892 cases
Cardiovascular		
Hypertension	16.4	12.4
Arrhythmia	2.4	2.4
Hypotension	1.4	2.3
Cardiac failure	1.2	1.6
Angina	0.7	0.4
Myocardial infarct	0.6	0.4
Thrombophlebitis	0.6	1.7
Respiratory		
Pneumonia	2.9	5.7
Atelectasis	1.2	2.3
Adult respiratory distress syndrome	0.9	1.8
Asthma	0.8	1.0
Pulmonary edema	0.7	1.2
Pulmonary embolism	0.2	0.6
Endocrine		
Inappropriate ADH secretion	1.9	2.7
Metabolic		
Diabetes mellitus	1.6	1.8
Gastrointestinal		
Hemorrhage	1.3	3.2
Hepatic failure	0.4	1.6
Hepatitis	0.1	1.0
Renal		
Failure	0.9	1.2
Hematologic		
Anemia	1.9	5.5
Bleeding disorder	0.4	0.9

*Preliminary data, Kassell and Torner.[50]

spasm. The classical features of the syndrome are serum sodium < 135 meq per liter, serum osmolality < 280 mosmol per kilogram, urinary sodium > 25 meq per liter, and a urine osmolality greater than plasma osmolality. The urinary sodium wasting must not be due to renal or adrenal disease and there should be absent peripheral edema and dehydration and a poor response to hypertonic saline infusion.[31]

Diabetes insipidus is a rarer condition. When urinary output exceeds fluid intake or when absolute urine volume is in excess of 3 liters per day, diabetes insipidus should be suspected.[86] The urinary specific gravity is < 1.005, urine osmolality is between 50 and 150 mosmol/kg, and serum sodium levels are usually normal or increased. Treatment consists of maintaining accurate fluid balance. Fluid intake should be almost solely dextrose and water solutions. Aqueous vasopressin is the preferred treatment in the early stages. Frequent accurate monitoring of body weight and electrolyte levels are essential.

Maroon and Nelson drew attention to the fact that red blood cell mass and total blood volume can be significantly decreased in patients following subarachnoid hemorrhage.[57] They listed possible causes of a contracted blood volume as bed rest, supine diuresis, pooling in the peripheral vascular beds, negative nitrogen balance, decreased erythropoiesis, and iatrogenic blood loss. Their data supported the use of intravascular volume expansion with red blood cells and colloid to prevent delayed ischemic infarction due to vasospasm.

Intracranial Pressure Elevations

Nornes and Magnaes recorded extradural pressure from nine patients during a subarachnoid hemorrhage.[70] In massive hemorrhage, there was an instantaneous rise in intracranial pressure with a leveling off at levels approaching the systemic blood pressure, which was associated with death. A second type was characterized by an instantaneous rise followed by a rapid fall to a level higher than the initial level, frequently followed by a lower secondary rise. Subsequently, it was noted that 77 percent of the hemorrhages started when the intracranial pressure was below 29 mmHg. Most hemorrhages arrested at or below the diastolic blood pressure. At the height of the hemorrhage, the forward flow in the carotid artery was arrested at the end of diastole but continued during systole; 1 or 2 min following the peak of the hemorrhage, diastolic blood pressure averaged 111 mmHg and intracranial pressure 128 mmHg.[69]

Intraventricular pressure in 52 cases of aneurysmal rupture was measured for a mean of 8 days each.[102] The ventricles were drained if pressure was greater than 25 mmHg for more than 30 min. Clinical grades I and II had a mean intraventricular pressure of 10; II and III 18; and III and IV 29 mmHg. All patients who improved clinically had progressive reductions in their intraventricular pressure. Of 16 who deteriorated, 44 percent showed a progressive increase in intraventricular pressure. Patients with no vasospasm had a mean intraventricular pressure at angiography of 16 mmHg whereas those with severe vasospasm had a mean level of 27 mmHg. Eighteen patients with a mean intraventricular pressure greater than 25 mmHg had a 77 percent mortality rate; of 34 patients with a mean intraventricular pressure below 25 mmHg only 26 percent died. B waves were recorded persistently at all intraventricular pressure levels. These are 1-per-second waves (range 0.5 to 2 per second) with an amplitude of under 50 mmHg. A waves (plateau waves) were extremely rare or absent in patients with aneurysmal rupture. In five cases cerebrospinal fluid was drained during the rebleeding episode.[103] The steady-state intraventricular pressure level after the repeat rupture was significantly increased in comparison with that of patients in whom cerebrospinal fluid was not drained during the rupture. Four of five such patients died with large intracerebral hemorrhages. The usual profile for intracranial pressure changes based on their seven cases of observed ruptures without drainage was as follows: initial intracranial pressure, 18 mmHg, peaked at 2½ min to 95 mmHg; in another 3 min it fell to 40 mmHg and in another 5 min to 22 mmHg. At peak, the intracranial pressure was 10 to 15 mmHg greater than diastolic blood pressure.

Many authors have now noted clinical improvement coincident with ventricular drainage and reduction of elevated intracranial pressure. Continuous ventricular drainage to a level of 15 mmHg in 88 patients produced marked clinical improvement.[92] A reduction in intracranial pressure in acute subarachnoid hemorrhage cases resulted in an increase in cerebral blood flow if the intracranial pressure was initially elevated.[39]

It is usually assumed that the corpuscular elements of the blood block the arachnoidal villi and thereby cause acute elevations in intracranial pressure. It has also been observed that a sudden release of large amounts of blood into the subarachnoid space of rats can cause an acute alteration of vesicular cerebrospinal fluid transport through the arachnoid villi, leading to increased pressure.[13] The increase in outflow resistance could be simulated by macromolecular substances associated with the clotting cascade in the absence of foreign blood cells. Late hydrocephalus is probably due to fibrotic obliteration of cerebrospinal fluid pathways at many points.

Hydrocephalus

Table 159-10 reviews some of the major series that have added to our understanding of hydrocephalus as it complicates aneurysm rupture. Acute ventricular dilatation should be treated with external ventricular drainage as an emergency. The more insidious chronic hydrocephalus, if it is delaying full recovery or is associated with regression and neurological signs, should be treated with a ventriculoperitoneal shunt.

The Neurological Complications of Aneurysm Rupture

The neurological complications of aneurysmal rupture represent an infinite spectrum of brain dysfunction. Epilepsy is obviously a significant problem. This is reviewed in Table 159-11. It seems reasonable that most young patients with middle cerebral aneurysms should be treated with anticon-

TABLE 159-10 Hydrocephalus Complicating Aneurysm Rupture

1. Of 100 patients studied by angiography, 19 percent of total developed neurological deficit secondary to hydrocephalus (HC) although 33.4 percent developed ventricular enlargement diagnosed by angiography. Of patients with HC, the 26 percent with most severe involvement showed dementia, arterial hypertension, gait impairment, headache, epilepsy, incontinence, akinetic mutism, and slowed circulation time. Dilatation began in the month following aneurysm rupture but could proceed over several months.[35]
2. Of 280 cases diagnosed by echograms, cisternography, and pneumography, HC developed in 9 percent of operated and 15 percent of unoperated cases. Most shunts were carried out between 2 and 6 weeks following the last subarachnoid hemorrhage (SAH). The larger the ventricles before shunting, the greater was the clinical improvement.[124]
3. All of 167 patients studied by CT scans were below 65 years in age and either never lost consciousness or regained it following SAH; only 15 percent were grade 3, 4, or 5. Acute ventricular dilatation was associated with intraventricular clots in 35 percent of cases. Of the 26 cases with early (< 14 days post-SAH) ventricular dilatation, 35 percent showed progression and surgery was carried out in 31 percent. HC developed in 10.5 percent of 210 cases in all types of SAH after 2 weeks and was clinically significant in 7 percent. Indications for shunting were lack of improvement from a neurological plateau or deterioration with marked ventricular dilatation, periventricular lucencies, rounding of frontal horns, and obliteration of cerebral sulci.[101]
4. CT scans were used to study 91 patients with intraventricular hemorrhage. Of 54 having CT scan on same day as rupture, 85 percent had ventricular dilatation. The degree of dilatation was the most powerful preoperative indicator of mortality. Progressive chronic enlargement was more common in survivors than a spontaneous relapse to normal size ventricles.[65]

vulsants for at least 2 years following their aneurysm rupture. Decisions regarding other patients should probably be individualized.

The most common psychiatric problems after aneurysmal rupture (Table 159-8) are intellectual impairment and depression. The psychiatric disability and the neurological deficits tend to go *pari passu*; however, the occasional patient can have a reactive depression out of proportion to the neurological dysfunction. Surgeons should be aware of this in order to obtain appropriate consultation.

The syndrome of disorientation and lethargy associated with damage to the small hypothalamic arteries leaving the posterior aspect of the anterior communicating artery has been described by Yaşargil et al.[122] Their insistence on the careful preservation of these fine vessels will tend to reduce this complication.

Nonaneurysmal Subarachnoid Hemorrhage

Subarachnoid hemorrhage can be due to the rupture of any vascular structure that communicates in some fashion with the intracranial or intraspinal subarachnoid space. The ruptured vessel can be normal or pathological. Numerous traumatic, infectious, neoplastic, toxic, inflammatory, and degenerative factors can induce the hemorrhage. Trauma is the most common cause of subarachnoid hemorrhage but, excluding this, the relative frequencies in the cooperative study were as follows: aneurysm 51 percent; AVM 6 percent; aneurysm and arteriovenous malformation 0.7 percent; and "other" causes 43 percent.[80] This latter group comprises hypertension and/or arteriosclerotic disease 64 percent, brain tumors 7 percent, endocarditis 3 percent, anticoagulants 3 percent, infections 1 percent, and unknown 22 percent. The latter category existed despite both angiographic and autopsy studies. The most important cause of fatal subarachnoid hemorrhage in cases not due to aneurysm or AVM is intracerebral hemorrhage associated with hypertension and arteriosclerotic disease in older persons. No particular tumor type in either primary or metastatic cases dominates the neoplasms with associated subarachnoid hemorrhage. Similarly, no specific infectious agents ac-

TABLE 159-11 Other Neurological Complications of Aneurysm Rupture

Epilepsy
1. Of 1009 cases, 1958–1962, with average follow-up less than 5 years, 10.4 percent of patients developed epilepsy according to clinic notes. A follow-up detailing examination and history of 61 cases showed a rate of 14.8 percent. Rate by decade: 3rd to 5th—15.8 percent; 6th to 7th—6.4 percent. Rate by location of aneurysm: middle cerebral artery—25 percent; posterior communicating artery—9 percent; anterior communicating artery—2.5 percent. For cases with hematoma—20 percent. The rate was not increased if a fit occurred at the time of aneurysm rupture. After aneurysm rupture, 72 percent of seizures began within 1 year, 94 percent within 2 years. No patients were on adequate dosage of anticonvulsants at the time of first seizure.[79]
2. Of 152 patients operated upon, 1945–1973, with mean follow-up of 7 years, 22 percent developed epilepsy (28 percent rate for intracranial surgery, 5 percent for carotid ligation). If severe postoperative deficit, 50 percent developed epilepsy, if mild or negligible, 20 percent became epileptic. Of middle cerebral aneurysm cases with moderate and severe neurological sequelae, 56 percent became epileptic. This was the highest risk group.[14]
3. In 109 patients from neurological series, grade 1 to 3 only, with a follow-up time of 1½ to 5½ years, the only significant risk factor was younger age. Seizures developed 10 to 54 months postoperatively; 4.5 percent developed seizures. In 4 patients having seizures in less than 24 h, none developed late epilepsy. No patient was on anticonvulsants at the time of first seizure.[25]

Psychiatric Illness
1. A study of 209 patients from 1958 to 1964, with a follow-up time less than 3 years in 56 percent, revealed that 45 percent were normal, 24 percent had mild intellectual impairment, and 18 percent had moderate disability (could not do skilled work, had deteriorated personal relationships, showed severe depression); 10 percent showed severe disability (unemployed, markedly deteriorated family relationships, personality damage, severe depression); 3 percent suffered from very severe disability (demented, inaccessible, bedfast, grossly dysphasic).[91]
2. Of 203 patients with anterior cerebral artery aneurysms operated upon, 20 percent developed confusion, disorientation, dementia, and lethargy lasting days and, rarely, weeks; this was permanent in 4 percent of cases.[122]

count for the majority of subarachnoid hemorrhages in this class.

Of "other" subarachnoid hemorrhage patients, 79 percent survived 1 year from the day of hemorrhage. The prognosis is therefore much better than for aneurysms or AVMs. Among 465 cases studied by angiography, the rebleeding rate was only 5 percent in the time of follow-up; this was considerably lower than for aneurysms. Good functional recovery and survival both fell sharply over the age of 60 for these patients.[80]

The Negative Workup for Aneurysms as a Cause of Subarachnoid Hemorrhage

The proportion of patients who have a negative workup has fallen steadily over the past few decades with the advent of higher-resolution diagnostic techniques. Heidrich reviewed 15 series, published between 1952 and 1966 and comprising 4111 cases, and found that in 43 percent no origin for the subarachnoid hemorrhage was evident.[44] Pakarinen reviewed nine series as well as his own data on the prognosis in subarachnoid hemorrhage with normal angiograms.[73] Excluding missed aneurysms shown at autopsy, the mortality rate was 3 percent for 1513 cases followed for several years on the average. He concluded that the mortality rate was approximately one-tenth that for aneurysms.

In six series, autopsies on patients who had died following subarachnoid hemorrhage with normal angiograms revealed that an aneurysm was present in 47 percent of the cases. This had presumably been the cause of the original subarachnoid hemorrhage and was the cause of the final fatal subarachnoid hemorrhage. Most investigators feel therefore that a missed aneurysm is the commonest cause of the normal angiogram in the presence of subarachnoid hemorrhage. West et al.[113] evaluated four major series of subarachnoid hemorrhage totaling almost 7000 patients and found a reported normal angiographic incidence of 18 to 27 percent. Those studies had been carried out between 1962 and 1967. In their own series of 220 patients using femoral catheterization, magnification angiography, oblique and basal projections, and subtraction, only 7 percent of patients had normal angiograms. Forster et al[29] carried out repeat four-vessel angiography in 56 patients with confirmed subarachnoid hemorrhage in whom the first investigation failed to reveal an aneurysm. Only one aneurysm was demonstrated in the second group of studies. They suggested that with good technique, a complete study, and careful interpretation, a false-negative rate of less than 2 percent would seldom justify repeat panangiography.

The best estimate of the prognosis for patients who have a subarachnoid hemorrhage without a known cause probably comes from Pakarinen's own series of 55 cases, followed up for a mean of 4.9 (1 to 9) years[73]; 7.3 percent of patients had recurrent subarachnoid hemorrhage and 3.6 percent died of this. One patient was autopsied and no aneurysm was demonstrated. The risk of a fatal recurrent hemorrhage where good four-vessel studies have been carried out initially can therefore be placed at well under 1 percent per year.

Workup of Patients Suspected of Having Recent Aneurysmal Rupture

Patients suspected of recent aneurysmal rupture should be rapidly admitted to a neurosurgical service experienced in their care. Intensive care measures should be instituted for those who are in very poor neurological condition with respiratory distress, and CT scans should then be carried out immediately. Lumbar puncture is performed if the CT scan does not show unequivocal evidence of abnormal blood collections. Complete angiographic workup should be performed as soon as possible if the CT scan or lumbar puncture shows evidence of hemorrhage. There is no advantage in delaying the definitive investigation.

References

1. Adams HP Jr, Kassell NF, Torner JC, Nibbelink DW, Sahs AL: Early management of aneurysmal subarachnoid hemorrhage: A report of the Cooperative Aneurysm Study. J Neurosurg 54:141–145, 1981.
2. Allen GS, Ahn HS, Preziosi TJ, Battye R, Boone SC, Chou SN, Kelly DL, Weir BK, Crabbe RA, Lavik PJ, Rosenbloom SB, Dorsey FC, Ingram CR, Mellits DE, Bertsch LA, Boisvert DPJ, Hundley MB, Johnson RK, Stron JA, Transou CR: Cerebral arterial spasm: A controlled trial of nimodipine in patients with subarachnoid hemorrhage. N Engl J Med 308:619–624, 1983.
3. Andrews RJ, Spiegel PK: Intracranial aneurysms: Age, sex, blood pressure, and multiplicity in an unselected series of patients. J Neurosurg 51:27–32, 1979.
4. Artiola-Fortuny L, Prieto-Valiente L: Long-term prognosis in surgically treated intracranial aneurysms: Part 1. Mortality. J Neurosurg 54:26–34, 1981.
5. Bannerman RM, Ingall GB, Graf CJ: The familial occurrence of intracranial aneurysms. Neurology 20:283–292, 1970.
6. Barno A, Freeman DW: Maternal deaths due to spontaneous subarachnoid hemorrhage. Am J Obstet Gynecol 125:384–392, 1976.
7. Becker DH, Silverberg GD, Nelson DH, Hanbery JW: Saccular aneurysm of infancy and early childhood. Neurosurgery 2:1–7, 1978.
8. Bell BA, Symon L: Smoking and subarachnoid haemorrhage. Br Med J 1:577–578, 1979.
9. Botterell EH, Lougheed WM, Scott JW, Vandewater SL: Hypothermia, and interruption of carotid, or carotid and vertebral circulation, in the surgical management of intracranial aneurysms. J Neurosurg 13:1–42, 1956.
10. Brackett CE, Morantz RA: Special problems associated with subarachnoid hemorrhage, in Youmans JR (ed): *Neurological Surgery: A Comprehensive Reference Guide to the Diagnosis and Management of Neurosurgical Problems*, 2d ed. Philadelphia, Saunders, 1982, pp 1807–1820.
11. Bull J: Massive aneurysms at the base of the brain. Brain 92:535–570, 1969.
12. Bull J: History of computed tomography, in Newton TH, Potts DG (eds): *Radiology of the Skull and Brain, vol 5: Technical Aspects of Computed Tomography*. St. Louis, Mosby, 1981, pp 3835–3849.
13. Butler AB, Maffeo CJ, Johnson RN, Bass NH: Impaired absorption of CSF during experimental subarachnoid hemorrhage: Effects of blood components on vesicular transport in

arachnoidal villi, in Shulman K, Marmarou A, Miller JD, Becker DP, Hochwald GM, Brock M (eds): *Intracranial Pressure IV*. Berlin, Springer, 1980, pp 245–248.
14. Cabral RJ, King TT, Scott DF: Epilepsy after two different neurosurgical approaches to the treatment of ruptured intracranial aneurysm. J Neurol Neurosurg Psychiatry 39:1052–1056, 1976.
15. Campbell GJ, Roach MR: Fenestrations in the internal elastic lamina at bifurcations of human cerebral arteries. Stroke 12:489–496, 1981.
16. Chason JL, Hindman WM: Berry aneurysms of the circle of Willis: Results of a planned autopsy study. Neurology 8:41–44, 1958.
17. Crompton MR: Mechanism of growth and rupture in cerebral berry aneurysms. Br Med J 1:1138–1142, 1966.
18. Crompton MR: The pathogenesis of cerebral aneurysms. Brain 89:797–814, 1966.
19. Dandy WE: Intracranial aneurysm of the internal carotid artery: Cured by operation. Ann Surg 107:654–659, 1938.
20. Dell S: Asymptomatic cerebral aneurysm: Assessment of its risk of rupture. Neurosurgery 10:162–166, 1982.
21. Dott NM: Intracranial aneurysms: Cerebral arterio-radiography: Surgical treatment. Edinburgh Med J 40:219–240, 1933.
22. Drake CG: Giant intracranial aneurysms: Experience with surgical treatment in 174 patients. Clin Neurosurg 26:12–95, 1979.
23. Drake CG: Management of cerebral aneurysm. Stroke 12:273–283, 1981.
24. Epstein, F, Ransohoff J, Budzilovich GN: The clinical significance of junctional dilatation of the posterior communicating artery. J Neurosurg 33:529–531, 1970.
25. Fabinyi GCA, Artiola-Fortuny L: Epilepsy after craniotomy for intracranial aneurysm. Lancet 1:1299–1300, 1980.
26. Ferguson GG: Physical factors in the initiation, growth, and rupture of human intracranial saccular aneurysms. J Neurosurg 37:666–667, 1972.
27. Fields WS, Weibel J: Coincidental internal carotid stenosis and intracranial saccular aneurysm. Trans Am Neurol Assoc 95:237–238, 1970.
28. Forbus WD: On the origin of miliary aneurysms of the superficial cerebral arteries. Bull Johns Hopkins Hosp 47:237–284, 1930.
29. Forster DMC, Steiner L, Hakanson S, Bergvall U: The value of repeat pan-angiography in cases of unexplained subarachnoid hemorrhage. J Neurosurg 48: 712–716, 1978.
30. Fox JL: Familial intracranial aneurysms: Case report. J Neurosurg 57:416–417, 1982.
31. Fox JL, Falik JL, Shalhoub RJ: Neurosurgical hyponatremia: The role of inappropriate antidiuresis. J Neurosurg 34:506–514, 1971.
32. Frazee JG, Cahan LD, Winter J: Bacterial intracranial aneurysms. J Neurosurg 53:633–641, 1980.
33. Freytag E: Fatal rupture of intracranial aneurysms: Survey of 250 medicolegal cases. Arch Pathol 81:418–424, 1966.
34. Fukuoka S, Suematsu K, Nakamura J, Matsuzaki T, Satoh S, Hashimoto I: Transient ischemic attacks caused by unruptured intracranial aneurysm. Surg Neurol 17:464–467, 1982.
35. Galera R, Greitz T: Hydrocephalus in the adult secondary to the rupture of intracranial arterial aneurysms. J Neurosurg 32:634–641, 1970.
36. George AE, Lin JP, Morantz RA: Intracranial aneurysm on a persistent primitive trigeminal artery: Case report. J Neurosurg 35:601–604, 1971.
37. Gibbs JR: Effects of carotid ligation on the size of internal carotid aneurysms. J Neurol Neurosurg Psychiatry 28:383–394, 1965.
38. Glynn LE: Medical defects in the circle of Willis and their relation to aneurysm formation. J Pathol 51:213–222, 1940.
39. Hartmann A, Alberti E, Lange D: Effects of CSF-drainage on CBF and CBV in subarachnoid hemorrhage and communicating hydrocephalus. Acta Neurol Scand [Suppl] 64:336–337, 1977.
40. Hashimoto I: Familial intracranial aneurysms and cerebral vascular anomalies. J Neurosurg 46:419–427, 1977.
41. Hashimoto N, Handa H, Nagata I, Hazama F: Experimentally induced cerebral aneurysms in rats. V. Relation of hemodynamics in the circle of Willis to formation of aneurysms. Surg Neurol 13:41–45, 1980.
42. Hassler O: Experimental carotid ligation followed by aneurysmal formation and other morphological changes in the circle of Willis. J Neurosurg 20:1–7, 1963.
43. Hayashi S, Arimoto T, Itakura T, Fujii T, Nishiguchi T, Komai N: The association of intracranial aneurysms and arteriovenous malformations of the brain: Case report. J Neurosurg 55:971–975, 1981.
44. Heidrich R: Subarachnoid haemorrhage, in Vinken PJ, Bruyn GW (eds): *Handbook of Clinical Neurology, vol 12: Vascular Diseases of the Nervous System, Part II.* Amsterdam, North-Holland, 1972, pp. 68–204.
45. Heiskanen O: Risk of bleeding from unruptured aneurysms in cases with multiple intracranial aneurysms. J Neurosurg 55:524–526, 1981.
46. Hillbom M, Kaste M: Does alcohol intoxication precipitate aneurysmal subarachnoid haemorrhage? J Neurol Neurosurg Psychiatry 44:523–526, 1981.
47. Jacobson JH II, Wallman LJ, Schumacher GA, Flanagan M, Suarez EL, Donaghy RMP: Microsurgery as an aid to middle cerebral endarterectomy. J Neurosurg 19:108–114, 1962.
48. Jakubowski J, Kendall B: Coincidental aneurysms with tumours of pituitary origin. J Neurol Neurosurg Psychiatry 41:972–979, 1978.
49. Jellinger K: Pathology and aetiology of intracranial aneurysms, in Pia HW, Langmaid C, Zierski J (eds): *Cerebral Aneurysms. Advances in Diagnosis and Therapy.* New York, Springer, 1979, pp 5–19.
50. Kassell NF, Torner JC: Unpublished observations. International Cooperative Study on the Timing of Aneurysm Surgery. US Public Health Service Grant No. IRION1590, 1982.
51. Keller AZ: Hypertension, age and residence in the survival with subarachnoid hemorrhage. Am J Epidemiol 91:139–147, 1970.
52. Koenig GH, Marshall WH Jr, Poole GJ, Kramer RA: Rupture of intracranial aneurysms during cerebral angiography: Report of ten cases and review of the literature. Neurosurgery 5:314–324, 1979.
53. Laun A: Traumatic aneurysms: Survey, in Pia HW, Langmaid C, Zierski J (eds): *Cerebral Aneurysms. Advances in Diagnosis and Therapy.* New York, Springer, 1979, pp 364–375.
54. Liliequist B, Lindqvist M, Probst F: Rupture of intracranial aneurysm during carotid angiography. Neuroradiology 11:185–190, 1976.
55. Lougheed WM: Selection, timing, and technique of aneurysm surgery of the anterior circle of Willis. Clin Neurosurg 16:95–113, 1968.
56. Lundberg N: Continuous recording and control of ventricular fluid pressure in neurosurgical practice. Acta Psychiatr Scand [Suppl] 149:1–193, 1960.
57. Maroon JC, Nelson PB: Hypovolemia in patients with subarachnoid hemorrhage: Therapeutic implications. Neurosurgery 4:223–226, 1979.
58. Masuzawa T, Shimabukuro H, Sato F, Furuse M, Fukushima

K: The development of intracranial aneurysms associated with pulseless disease. Surg Neurol 17:132–136, 1982.
59. Mayfield FH, Kees G Jr: A brief history of the development of the Mayfield clip: Technical note. J Neurosurg 35:97–100, 1971.
60. McCormick WF, Acosta-Rua GJ: The size of intracranial saccular aneurysms: An autopsy study. J Neurosurg 33:422–427, 1970.
61. McCormick WF, Schmalstieg EJ: The relationship of arterial hypertension to intracranial aneurysms. Arch Neurol 34:285–287, 1977.
62. Mielke B, Weir B, Oldring D, von Westarp C: Fungal aneurysm: Case report and review of the literature. Neurosurgery 9:578–582, 1981.
63. Minielly R, Yuzpe AA, Drake CG: Subarachnoid hemorrhage secondary to ruptured cerebral aneurysm in pregnancy. Obstet Gynecol 53:64–70, 1979.
64. Miyasaka K, Wolpert SM, Prager RJ: The association of cerebral aneurysms, infundibula, and intracranial arteriovenous malformations. Stroke 13:196–203, 1982.
65. Mohr G, Ferguson G, Khan M, Malloy D, Watts R, Benoit B, Weir B: Intraventricular hemorrhage from ruptured aneurysm: Retrospective analysis of 91 cases. J Neurosurg 58:482–487, 1983.
66. Moniz E: Anévrysme intra-cranien de la carotide interne droite rendu visible par l'artériographie cérébrale. Rev Otoneuroophthalmol 11:746–748, 1933.
67. Morley TP, Barr HWK: Giant intracranial aneurysms: Diagnosis, course, and management. Clin Neurosurg 16:73–94, 1969.
68. Nibbelink DW, Torner JC, Henderson WG: Antifibrinolytic therapy in recent onset subarachnoid hemorrhage, in Sahs AL, Nibbelink DW, Torner JC (eds): *Aneurysmal Subarachnoid Hemorrhage: Report of the Cooperative Study*. Baltimore, Urban & Schwarzenberg, 1981, pp 297–306.
69. Nornes H: The role of intracranial pressure in the arrest of hemorrhage in patients with ruptured intracranial aneurysm. J Neurosurg 39:226–234, 1973.
70. Nornes H, Magnaes B: Intracranial pressure in patients with ruptured saccular aneurysm. J Neurosurg 36:537–547, 1972.
71. Okawara S: Warning signs prior to rupture of an intracranial aneurysm. J Neurosurg 38:575–580, 1973.
72. Orozco M, Trigueros F, Quintana F, Dierssen G: Intracranial aneurysms in early childhood. Surg Neurol 9:247–252, 1978.
73. Pakarinen S: Incidence, aetiology, and prognosis of primary subarachnoid haemorrhage: A study based on 589 cases diagnosed in a defined urban population during a defined period. Acta Neurol Scand [Suppl] 29:1–128, 1967.
74. Patel AN, Richardson AE: Ruptured intracranial aneurysms in the first two decades of life: A study of 68 patients. J Neurosurg 35:571–576, 1971.
75. Phillips LH II, Whisnant JP, O'Fallon WM, Sundt TM Jr: The unchanging pattern of subarachnoid hemorrhage in a community. Neurology (NY) 30:1034–1040, 1980.
76. Rhoton AL Jr: Anatomy of saccular aneurysms. Surg Neurol 14:59–66, 1980.
77. Roach MR: A model study of why some intracranial aneurysms thrombose but others rupture. Stroke 9:583–587, 1978.
78. Robinson JL, Hall CJ, Sedzimir CB: Subarachnoid hemorrhage in pregnancy. J Neurosurg 36:27–33, 1972.
79. Rose FC, Sarner M: Epilepsy after ruptured intracranial aneurysm. Br Med J 1:18–21, 1965.
80. Sahs AL, Perret GE, Locksley HB, Nishioka H (eds): *Intracranial Aneurysms and Subarachnoid Hemorrhage: A Cooperative Study*. Philadelphia, Lippincott, 1969.
81. Sakai N, Sakata K, Yamada H, Yamamoto M, Aiba T, Takeda F: Familial occurrence of intracranial aneurysms. Surg Neurol 2:25–29, 1974.
82. Salar G, Mingrino S: Development of intracranial saccular aneurysms: Report of two cases. Neurosurgery 8:462–465, 1981.
83. Sarner M, Rose FC: Clinical presentation of ruptured intracranial aneurysm. J Neurol Neurosurg Psychiatry 30:67–70, 1967.
84. Scott S, Ferguson GG, Roach MR: Comparison of the elastic properties of human intracranial arteries in aneurysms. Can J Physiol Pharmacol 50:328–332, 1972.
85. Servo A: Agenesis of the left internal carotid artery associated with an aneurysm on the right carotid syphon: Case report. J Neurosurg 46:677–680, 1977.
86. Shucart WA, Jackson I: Management of diabetes insipidus in neurosurgical patients. J Neurosurg 44:65–71, 1976.
87. Stehbens WE: Histopathology of cerebral aneurysms. Arch Neurol 8:272–285, 1963.
88. Stehbens WE: Ultrastructure of aneurysms. Arch Neurol 32:798–807, 1975.
89. Stehbens WE: Intracranial berry aneurysms in infancy. Surg Neurol 18:58–60, 1982.
90. Stern J, Whelan M, Brisman R, Correll JW: Management of extracranial carotid stenosis and intracranial aneurysms. J Neurosurg 51:147–150, 1979.
91. Storey PB: Psychiatric sequelae of subarachnoid haemorrhage. Br Med J 3:261–266, 1967.
92. Sundbärg G, Pontén U: ICP and CSF absorption impairment after subarachnoid hemorrhage, in Beks JWF, Bosch DA, Brock M (eds): *Intracranial Pressure III*. Berlin, Springer, 1976, pp 139–146.
93. Sundt TM Jr: Cerebral vasospasm following subarachnoid hemorrhage: Evolution, management, and relationship to timing of surgery. Clin Neurosurg 24:228–247, 1977.
94. Suzuki J: Multiple aneurysms: Treatment, in Pia HW, Langmaid C, Zierski J (eds): *Cerebral Aneurysms: Advances in Diagnosis and Therapy*. Berlin, Springer, 1979, pp 352–363.
95. Suzuki J, Ohara H: Clinicopathological study of cerebral aneurysms: Origin, rupture, repair, and growth. J Neurosurg 48:505–514, 1978.
96. Suzuki J, Onuma T: Intracranial aneurysms associated with arteriovenous malformations. J Neurosurg 50:742–746, 1979.
97. Suzuki J, Onuma T, Yoshimoto T: Results of early operations on cerebral aneurysms. Surg Neurol 11:407–412, 1979.
98. Suzuki J, Yoshimoto T: Distribution of cerebral aneurysms, in Pia HW, Langmaid C, Zierski J (eds): *Cerebral Aneurysms: Advances in Diagnosis and Therapy*. Berlin, Springer, 1979, pp 127–133.
99. Takaku A, Shindo K, Tanaka S, Mori T, Suzuki J: Fluid and electrolyte disturbances in patients with intracranial aneurysms. Surg Neurol 11:349–356, 1979.
100. Torner JC, Kassell NF, Wallace RB, Adams HP Jr: Preoperative prognostic factors for rebleeding and survival in aneurysm patients receiving antifibrinolytic therapy: Report of the Cooperative Aneurysm Study. Neurosurgery 9:506–513, 1981.
101. Vassilouthis J, Richardson AE: Ventricular dilatation and communicating hydrocephalus following spontaneous subarachnoid hemorrhage. J Neurosurg 51:341–351, 1979.
102. Voldby B, Enevoldsen EM: Intracranial pressure changes following aneurysm rupture: 1. Clinical and angiographic correlations. J Neurosurg 56:186–196, 1982.
103. Voldby B, Enevoldsen EM: Intracranial pressure changes following aneurysm rupture: 3. Recurrent hemorrhage. J Neurosurg 56:784–789, 1982.
104. Waga S, Morikawa A: Aneurysm developing on the infundibular widening of the posterior communicating artery. Surg Neurol 11:125–127, 1979.

105. Waga S, Ohtsubo K, Handa H: Warning signs in intracranial aneurysms. Surg Neurol 3:15–20, 1975.
106. Waga S, Okada M, Kojima T: Saccular aneurysm associated with absence of the left cervical carotid arteries. Neurosurgery 3:208–212, 1978.
107. Wakai S, Fukushima T, Furihata T, Sano K: Association of cerebral aneurysm with pituitary adenoma. Surg Neurol 12:503–507, 1979.
108. Weir BKA: Pulmonary edema following fatal aneurysm rupture. J Neurosurg 49:502–507, 1978.
109. Weir B: Medical aspects of the preoperative management of aneurysms: A review. Can J Neurol Sci 6:441–450, 1979.
110. Weir B, Aronyk K: Management mortality and the timing of surgery for supratentorial aneurysms. J Neurosurg 54:146–150, 1981.
111. Weir B, Aronyk K: Management and postoperative mortality related to time of clipping for supratentorial aneurysms: A personal series. Acta Neurochir (Wien) 63:135–139, 1982.
112. Weir B, Rothberg C, Grace M, Davis F: Relative prognostic significance of vasospasm after subarachnoid hemorrhage. Can J Neurol Sci 2:109–114, 1975.
113. West HH, Mani RL, Eisenberg RL, Tuerk K, Stucker TB: Normal cerebral arteriography in patients with spontaneous subarachnoid hemorrhage. Neurology 27:592–594, 1977.
114. Wheelock B, Weir B, Watts R, Mohr G, Khan M, Hunter M, Fewer D, Ferguson G, Durity F, Cochrane D, Benoit B: Timing of surgery for intracerebral hematomas due to aneurysm rupture. J Neurosurg 58:476–481, 1983.
115. Wiebers DO, Whisnant JP, O'Fallon WM: The natural history of unruptured intracranial aneurysms. N Engl J Med 304:696–698, 1981.
116. Wilkins RH: Aneurysm rupture during angiography: Does acute vasospasm occur? Surg Neurol 5:299–303, 1976.
117. Wilson G, Riggs HE, Rupp C: Pathological anatomy of ruptured cerebral aneurysms. J Neurosurg 11:128–142, 1954.
118. Winn HR, Berga SL, Richardson AE, Waldman MTG, O'Brien WM, Jane JA: Long-term evaluation of patients with multiple cerebral aneurysms. Ann Neurol 10:106, 1981. (Abstr.)
119. Winn HR, Richardson AE, Jane JA: The assessment of the natural history of single cerebral aneurysms that have ruptured, in Hopkins LN, Long DM (eds): *Clinical Management of Intracranial Aneurysms.* New York, Raven Press, 1982, pp 1–10.
120. Wollschlaeger G, Wollschlaeger PB: The circle of Willis, in Newton TH, Potts DG (eds): *Radiology of the Skull and Brain: Angiography,* vol 2, book 2. St. Louis, Mosby, 1974, pp 1171–1201.
121. Wood EH: Angiographic identification of the ruptured lesion in patients with multiple cerebral aneurysms. J Neurosurg 21:182–198, 1964.
122. Yaşargil MG, Fox JL, Ray MW: The operative approach to aneurysms of the anterior communicating artery. Adv Tech Stds Neurosurg 2:113–170, 1975.
123. Yaşargil MG, Smith RD: Management of aneurysms of anterior circulation by intracranial procedures, in Youmans JR (ed): *Neurological Surgery: A Comprehensive Reference Guide to the Diagnosis and Management of Neurosurgical Problems,* 2d ed. Philadelphia, Saunders, 1982, pp 1663–1696.
124. Yaşargil MG, Yonekawa Y, Zumstein B, Stahl HJ: Hydrocephalus following spontaneous subarachnoid hemorrhage: Clinical features and treatment. J Neurosurg 39:474–479, 1973.
125. Yoshimoto T, Uchida K, Suzuki J: Intracranial saccular aneurysms in the first three decades. Surg Neurol 9:287–291, 1978.

160

Microsurgical Anatomy of Saccular Aneurysms

Albert L. Rhoton, Jr.

Basic Anatomical Principles

Three aspects of the anatomy of saccular aneurysms should be considered when planning the operative approach to these lesions.[9] These three aspects will be reviewed in relation to each of the common aneurysm sites.

First, these aneurysms arise at a branching site on the parent artery. This site may be formed either by the origin of a side branch from the parent artery, such as the origin of the posterior communicating artery from the internal carotid artery, or by subdivision of a main arterial trunk into two trunks, as occurs at the bifurcation of the middle cerebral artery. The operative approach should be planned so as to protect the flow through these branching sites, which seem to be a part of the basic substrate essential to the formation of a saccular aneurysm (Fig. 160-1).

Second, saccular aneurysms arise at a turn or curve in the artery. These curves, by producing local alterations in intravascular hemodynamics, exert unusual stresses on apical regions, which receive the greatest force of the pulse wave. The sites of the curves associated with the common intracranial aneurysms are reviewed in the discussion that follows.

Third, saccular aneurysms point in the direction that the blood would have gone if the curve at the aneurysm site were not present. The aneurysm dome or fundus points in the direction of the maximal hemodynamic thrust in the preaneurysmal segment of the parent artery. The operation to obliterate an aneurysm should be designed to allow the surgeon to control and reduce the hemodynamic thrust in the parent artery until after the aneurysm is obliterated. As a saccular aneurysm enlarges, it may encounter obstacles that change the direction of growth from that based solely on the direction of the maximal hemodynamic thrust.

Aneurysms are infrequently encountered on a straight, nonbranching segment of an intracranial artery. The aneurysms occurring on straight, nonbranching segments are more often found to have sacs that point longitudinally along the wall of the artery in the direction of blood flow and project only minimally above the adventitial surface. Aneurysms having these characteristics are of a dissecting type rather than of the congenital saccular type, and their development is heralded more frequently by the onset of ischemic neurological deficits than by the subarachnoid hemorrhage associated with congenital saccular aneurysms. It is rare to find an aneurysm on the concave side of an arterial curve or to find one that points in a direction opposite to that of the flow in the parent artery.

Internal Carotid Artery Aneurysms

These three facets of anatomy as they apply to aneurysm sites on the supraclinoid portion of the internal carotid artery are considered first.[2,10] These aneurysms arise at four sites (Figs. 160-2 and 160-3): the upper surface of the inter-

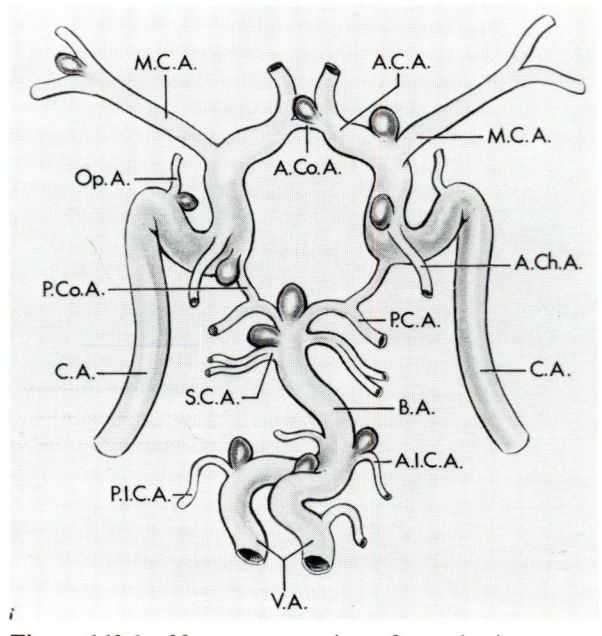

Figure 160-1 Most common sites of saccular intracranial aneurysms. Each aneurysm arises from the branching site of a large artery. Most are located on or near the circle of Willis. Over 90 percent are located at one of the following five sites: (1) the internal carotid artery (C.A.) at the level of the posterior communicating artery (P.Co.A.); (2) the junction of the anterior cerebral (A.C.A.) and anterior communicating (A.Co.A) arteries; (3) the proximal bifurcation of the middle cerebral artery (M.C.A.); (4) the junction of the posterior cerebral (P.C.A.) and basilar (B.A.) arteries; and (5) the bifurcation of the carotid artery into the anterior cerebral and middle cerebral arteries. Other aneurysm sites on the carotid artery are at the origins of the ophthalmic (Op.A.) and anterior choroidal (A.Ch.A.) arteries. Other sites on the vertebral (V.A.) and basilar arteries include the sites of origin of the posterior inferior cerebellar (P.I.C.A.), the anterior inferior cerebellar (A.I.C.A.), and the superior cerebellar (S.C.A.) arteries and the junction of the basilar and vertebral arteries. (From Rhoton.[7])

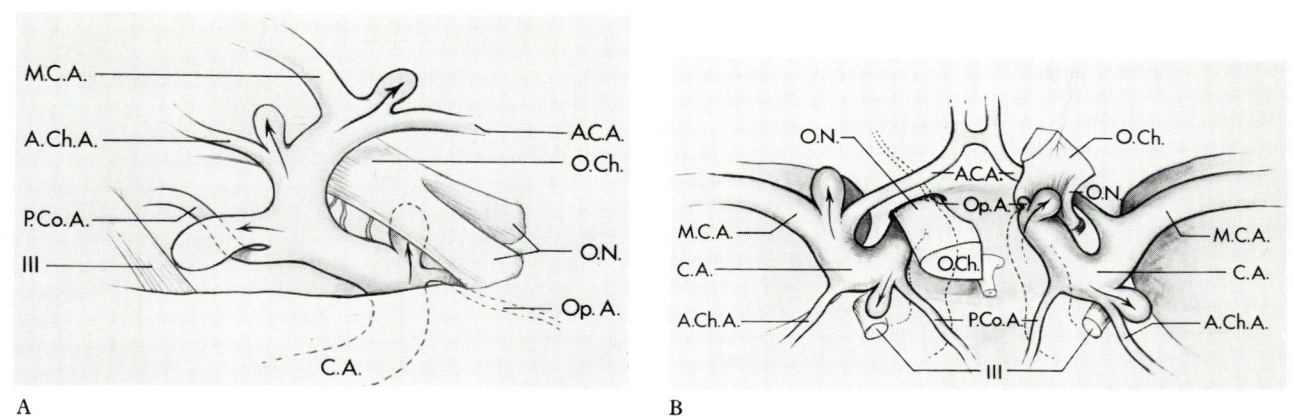

Figure 160-2 Lateral (A) and superior (B) views of common aneurysm sites on the supraclinoid portion of the internal carotid artery. A. Lateral view of the right internal carotid artery. B. Superior view of the internal carotid arteries, with the right optic nerve and right half of the optic chiasm reflected forward to expose the origin of the ophthalmic artery. The intracavernous portion of both carotid arteries and the course of the left ophthalmic artery are shown by dotted lines. The aneurysms arise on curves in the artery at the site of origin of its branches. The aneurysms point in the direction (*arrows*) of the maximal hemodynamic force immediately proximal to the aneurysm site and in the direction the blood would have gone if there were no curve at the aneurysm site. The aneurysm sites on the internal carotid artery (C.A.) are usually located immediately distal to the origins of its branches. Aneurysms arising at the origin of the ophthalmic artery (Op.A.) point upward into the optic nerve (O.N.). Aneurysms arising near the origin of the posterior communicating artery (P.Co.A) point posteriorly toward the oculomotor nerve (III) and are usually located superolateral to the posterior communicating artery. Aneurysms arising near the origin of the anterior choroidal artery (A.Ch.A) point posterolaterally and are usually located immediately superior to the origin of the anterior choroidal artery. Aneurysms arising at the carotid bifurcation into the anterior (A.C.A.) and middle (M.C.A.) cerebral arteries point upward laterally to the optic chiasm (O.Ch.) toward the anterior perforated substance. (From Rhoton.[7])

nal carotid artery at the origin of the ophthalmic artery, the posterior wall near the origin of the posterior communicating artery, the posterior wall at the origin of the anterior choroidal artery, and the apex of the carotid artery bifurcation into the anterior and middle cerebral arteries.

An aneurysm at the carotid-ophthalmic artery junction arises from the superior wall of the carotid artery distal to the origin of the ophthalmic artery immediately above the roof of the cavernous sinus where the superiorly directed intracavernous segment turns posteriorly. At this turn, the maximal hemodynamic thrust is directed toward the superior wall of the carotid artery just distal to the ophthalmic artery, and the aneurysm projects upward toward and eventually against the optic nerve (Figs. 160-2, 160-3).

The initial segment of the supraclinoid portion of the carotid artery is directed posterolaterally, but distally the portion giving rise to the posterior communicating or anterior choroidal artery curves upward toward its bifurcation (Figs. 160-2 and 160-3). An aneurysm at the carotid–posterior communicating artery junction usually arises from the posterior wall of the carotid artery near the apex of this turn immediately above the level of the origin of the posterior communicating artery. The aneurysm points posteriorly toward the oculomotor nerve. The posterior communicating artery is usually found on the inferomedial side of the aneurysm. The anterior choroidal artery is located superior or superolateral to the aneurysm arising at the level of the posterior communicating artery. The apex of the posteriorly convex curve may also be located at the level of origin of the anterior choroidal artery, which shifts the hemodynamic force distally from the level of origin of the posterior communicating artery to that of the anterior choroidal artery. An aneurysm arising at the level of the anterior choroidal artery is usually located superior or superolateral to the origin of the anterior choroidal artery (Figs. 160-2, 160-3).

The aneurysm arising at the terminal bifurcation of the internal carotid artery most easily fits these principles (Figs. 160-2, 160-3). It arises at the level of the T-shaped bifurcation formed by the origin of the anterior and middle cerebral arteries and points upward in the direction of the long axis of the prebifurcation segment of the internal carotid artery.

Middle Cerebral Artery Aneurysms

Aneurysms arising on the middle cerebral artery also conform to these three anatomical precepts (Fig. 160-4).[1] They arise at the level of the bifurcation or trifurcation of the ar-

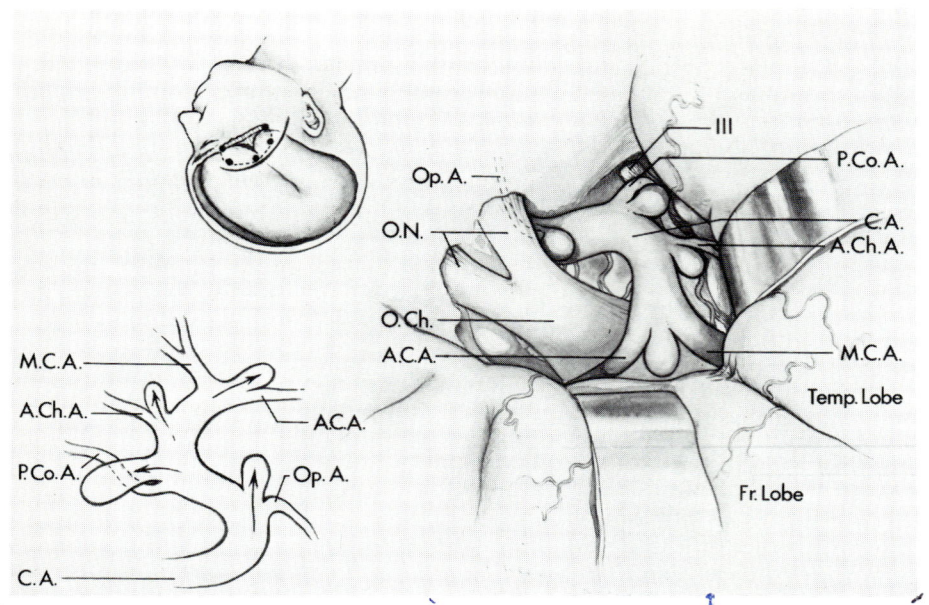

Figure 160-3 Operative view of common aneurysm sites on the supraclinoid portion of the internal carotid artery. *Upper left:* Head position, scalp incision (*solid line*), bone flap (*dotted line*), and craniectomy (*oblique lines*) used to approach internal carotid artery aneurysms. *Right:* Operative view provided by a right frontotemporal craniotomy with retractors on the frontal and temporal lobes. *Lower left:* Lateral view of the right internal carotid artery showing aneurysm sites. These aneurysms point in the direction (*arrows*) of the maximal hemodynamic force proximal to the aneurysm site and in the direction the bood would have gone if there were no curve in the parent artery at the aneurysm site. The aneurysm sites on the internal carotid artery (C.A.) are usually located immediately distal to the origins of its branches. Aneurysms arising at the origin of the ophthalmic artery (Op.A.) point upward into the optic nerve (O.N.). Aneurysms arising near the origin of the posterior communicating artery (P.Co.A.) point posteriorly toward the oculomotor nerve (III) and are usually located superolateral to the posterior communicating artery. Aneurysms arising near the origin of the anterior choroidal artery (A.Ch.A.) point posterolaterally and are usually located immediately superior to the origin of the anterior choroidal artery. Aneurysms arising at the carotid bifurcation into the anterior (A.C.A.) and middle (M.C.A.) cerebral arteries point upward lateral to the optic chiasm (O.Ch.) toward the anterior perforated substance. Each of the aneurysms can be approached through a frontotemporal craniotomy. (From Rhoton.[7])

tery. The angulation with which the bifurcating trunks arise from the main trunk forms the turn or curve. These aneurysms usually point laterally in the direction of the long axis of the prebifurcation segment of the main trunk.

Anterior Cerebral Artery Aneurysms

The most common aneurysm site on the anterior cerebral artery is at the level of the anterior communicating artery (Fig. 160-5).[6] The aneurysm usually arises at the point where the dominant proximal or precommunicating segment bifurcates at the level of the anterior communicating artery to give rise to both distal segments. These aneurysms usually point away from the dominant proximal segment toward the opposite side. They may also project in other directions. The direction in which the fundus points is determined by the course of the anterior cerebral arteries proximal to their junction with the anterior communicating artery. Tortuosity of the arteries may create a situation in which the hemodynamic thrust varies so that these aneurysms may project not only to the opposite side but also in the anterior, posterior, superior, or inferior direction.

The next most common aneurysm site on the anterior cerebral artery is at the level of origin of the callosomarginal artery from the pericallosal artery (Fig. 160-6). The curve is formed by the angulation of branching and the artery's passage around the rostrum of the corpus callosum. The aneurysm points distally into the interval between the junction of the pericallosal and callosomarginal arteries.

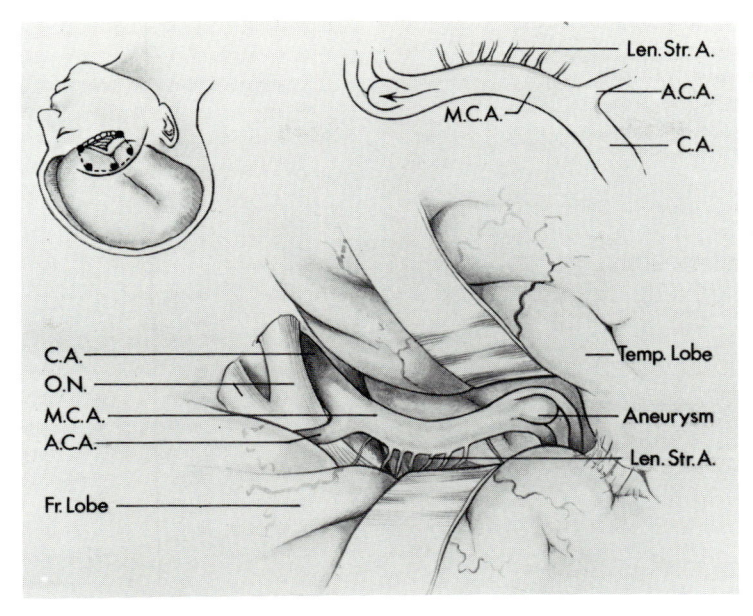

Figure 160-4 Middle cerebral artery aneurysm. *Upper right:* Anterior view of an aneurysm at the bifurcation of the right middle cerebral artery (M.C.A.). Aneurysms arising on the M.C.A. are usually located at the proximal bifurcation near the genu of the artery. The arrow shows the direction of hemodynamic force at the aneurysm site. *Upper left:* Head position, scalp incision (*solid line*), bone flap (*dotted line*), and craniectomy (*oblique lines*) for the approach to these aneurysms. *Lower center:* Operative view provided by a right frontotemporal craniotomy. The right sylvian fissure has been split to provide this view of the optic nerves (O.N.) and the carotid (C.A.) and anterior cerebral (A.C.A.) arteries. Retractors are on the temporal and frontal lobes. The lenticulostriate arteries (Len.Str.A.) arise proximal to the bifurcation of the M.C.A. and the aneurysm. (From Rhoton.[7])

Vertebral and Basilar Artery Aneurysms

Aneurysms arising on the branches of the vertebral and basilar arteries also share the same three facets of anatomy: they arise at a branching site on a curve and point in the direction the blood would have followed if the curve were not present (Fig. 160-7). The basilar apex aneurysm arises at the branching of the posterior cerebral arteries from the basilar artery. The curve at the aneurysm site is related to the change from the vertical direction of the basilar artery to a lateral direction of the posterior cerebral arteries. These aneurysms project upward in the direction of the long axis of the basilar artery (Fig. 160-8*A,B*).

Aneurysms arising from the basilar artery at the level of origin of the superior cerebellar or anterior inferior cerebellar artery or from the vertebral artery at the level of origin of the posterior inferior cerebellar artery initially appear to conform poorly to the three facets of anatomy applicable to the other aneurysms because the basilar and vertebral arteries are often pictured as straight arteries, with the cerebellar arteries arising at right angles from them (Fig. 160-7).[9] However, most of the arteries harboring aneurysms are tortuous, and the change in direction of flow associated with the curves creates hemodynamic stress on the wall of the basilar or vertebral arteries near the origins of the cerebellar arteries. These aneurysms point in the direction the blood would have gone had there not been a curve at the level of origin of the involved branch. For example, a basilar aneurysm at the level of the superior cerebellar artery often arises where there is a curvature and tilt of the upper basilar artery, so that the hemodynamic thrust created by flow along the basilar artery is just above the origin of the superior cerebellar artery rather than at the basilar apex (Fig. 160-8*C*).[3]

The aneurysm located at the origin of the anterior inferior cerebellar artery commonly arises from the convex side of the curve in the basilar artery and points in the direction of the long axis of the basilar segment immediately proximal to the aneurysm (Figs. 160-7 and 160-8*D*).[5]

The most common aneurysm site on the vertebral artery is at the level of origin of the posterior inferior cerebellar artery. The vertebral artery is often depicted as being straight; however, if an aneurysm is present, the vertebral artery is often found to have a convex upward curve from the apex, where the posterior inferior cerebellar artery arises (Figs. 160-7 and 160-8*F*).[4] The aneurysm arises from the apex of this curve at the origin of the posterior inferior cerebellar artery and points upward.

Aneurysms arising infrequently at the junction of the two vertebral arteries with the basilar artery may initially seem difficult to fit into these precepts. When examined in multiple angiographic projections, however, they are often found to conform to these same anatomical principles applied in predicting the site and direction of projection of the more common saccular aneurysms. These aneurysms often arise on the convex side of a tortuous curve formed at the vertebrobasilar junction (Figs. 160-7 and 160-8*E*), and the junction of the two vertebral arteries with the basilar artery creates a configuration similar to the branching at other aneurysm sites.

Anatomical Principles Directing Surgery

The following basic anatomical principles are helpful in directing the surgical attack on intracranial aneurysms.

1. The parent artery should be exposed proximal to the aneurysm. This allows control of flow to the aneurysm if it ruptures during dissection. Exposure of the internal carotid artery above the cavernous sinus will give proximal control for aneurysms arising at the level of the posterior communicating or anterior choroidal artery. The internal carotid ar-

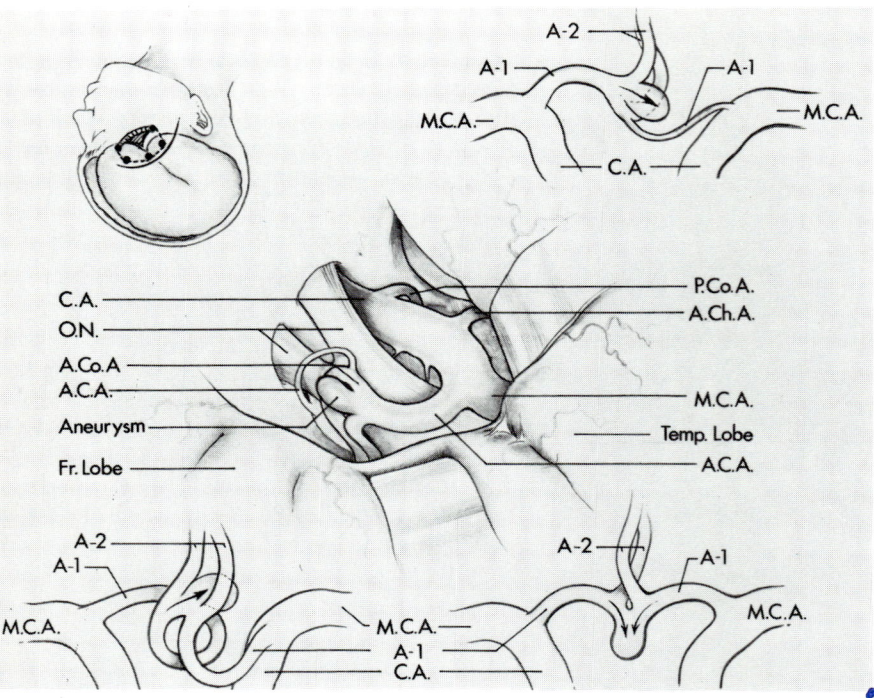

Figure 160-5 Anterior and operative views of anterior communicating artery aneurysms. *Upper right, lower right,* and *lower left:* Anterior views show three different aneurysm configurations created by the different hemodynamic forces (*arrows*) associated with the various sizes and shapes of proximal (A-1) and distal (A-2) segments of the anterior cerebral arteries. The most common configuration (*upper right*) is associated with a hypoplastic A-1 segment. Less common projections of these aneurysms are straight forward (*lower right*) or posterior (*lower left*). The direction in which the fundus points is determined by the course of the artery proximal to its junction with the anterior communicating artery. *Upper left and center:* Operative view of an anterior communicating artery aneurysm: scalp incision (*solid line*), bone flap (*dotted line*), and craniectomy (*oblique lines*). The aneurysm points downward and forward away from the dominant anterior cerebral artery. The anterior cerebral (A.C.A.) and anterior communicating (A.Co.A.) arteries are located above the optic nerves (O.N.) and chiasm. The carotid arteries (C.A.) also give rise to the middle cerebral (M.C.A.), posterior communicating (P.Co.A.), and anterior choroidal (A.Ch.A.) arteries. The retractors are on the frontal and temporal lobes. (From Rhoton.[7])

tery should also be exposed initially to obtain proximal control of middle cerebral and anterior cerebral artery aneurysms. The exposure can be directed laterally from the internal carotid artery for middle cerebral aneurysms and medially over the optic nerves and chiasm for anterior communicating aneurysms. For basilar apex aneurysms, control of the basilar artery proximal to the aneurysm can be obtained by following the inferior surface of the posterior cerebral artery or the superior surface of the superior cerebellar artery to the basilar artery and then working up the side of the basilar artery to the neck of the aneurysm.

2. If possible, the side of the parent vessel opposite the side on which the aneurysm arises should be exposed before dissecting the neck of the aneurysm. The dissection can then be carried around the side of the parent vessel to the origin of the aneurysm.

3. The aneurysmal neck should be dissected before the fundus. The neck is the area that can tolerate the greatest manipulation, has the least tendency to rupture, and is to be clipped. Unfortunately, it is the portion of the aneurysm that is most likely to incorporate the origin of a vessel. Therefore, dissection of the neck and proximal part of the fundus should be done carefully with full visualization to prevent passage of a clip around the arterial branches, described previously, which arise near the neck of the aneurysm. The dissection should not be started at the dome because this is the area most likely to rupture before or during surgery.

4. All perforating arterial branches should be separated from the aneurysmal neck prior to passing the clip around the aneurysm. A detailed review of the important perforating arteries at each common aneurysm site has been presented elsewhere.[8] Prior to the use of magnification there was a tendency to keep dissection of aneurysms to a minimum because of the hazard of rupture. The use of magnification has permitted increased accuracy of dissection of the

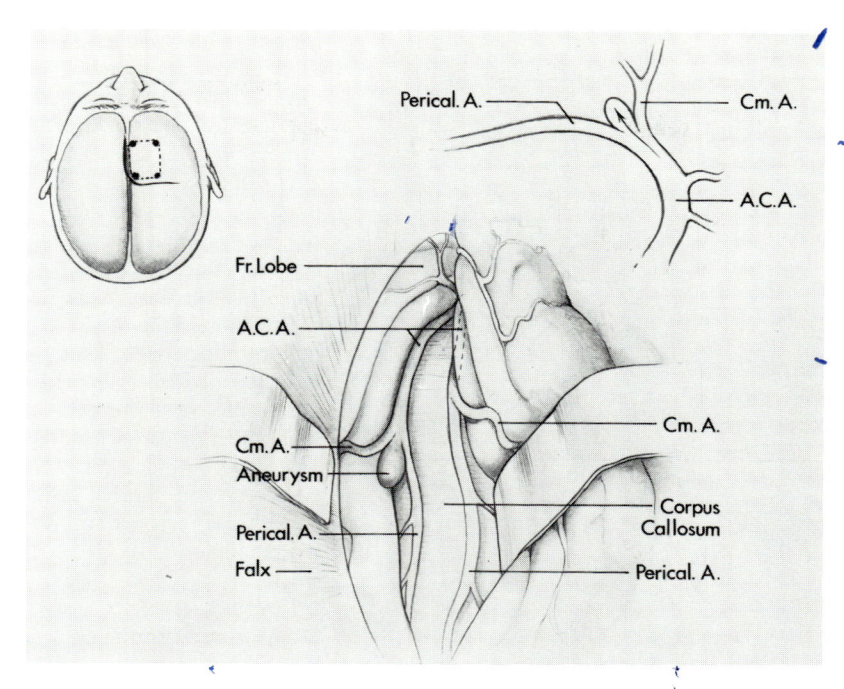

Figure 160-6 Lateral and operative views of the most common aneurysm site on the distal part of the anterior cerebral artery. *Upper right:* Medial surface of the right anterior cerebral artery. The aneurysm arises on the medial surface of the frontal lobe at the anterior margin of the corpus callosum. The hemodynamic thrust (*arrow*) and the aneurysm are directed distally in the interval between the pericallosal (Perical.A.) and callosomarginal (Cm.A.) arteries. *Upper left:* Scalp incision (*solid line*) and bone flap (*dotted line*). *Lower:* The right frontal lobe (Fr. Lobe) is retracted to expose the anterior cerebral arteries (A.C.A.), the falx, and the aneurysm arising above the corpus callosum at the origin of the callosomarginal and pericallosal arteries. (From Rhoton.[7])

aneurysmal neck and more frequent preservation of the recurrent and other perforating arteries.[2,6,8,11] The risk of occlusion of perianeurysmal perforating arterioles that results from placement of a clip on an inadequately exposed aneurysm is greater than the hazard of rupture with microsurgical dissection.

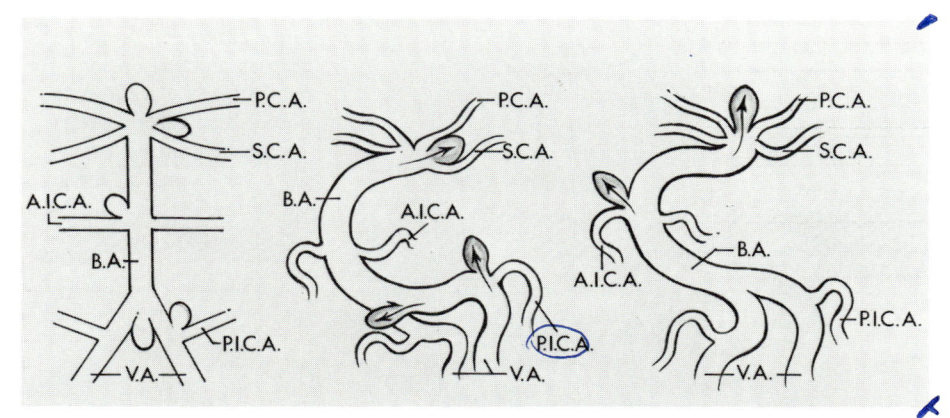

Figure 160-7 Aneurysm sites on the vertebral and basilar arteries. *Left:* Frequently used diagrammatic representation of the vertebral and basilar arteries and aneurysm sites. The vertebral (V.A.) and basilar (B.A.) arteries are shown as straight vessels, and the posterior cerebral (P.C.A.), superior cerebellar (S.C.A.), anterior inferior cerebellar (A.I.C.A.), and posterior inferior cerebellar (P.I.C.A.) arteries are shown as arising at right angles from the parent arteries, with the aneurysm projecting at nearly right angles to the direction of flow in the parent arteries. *Center and right:* Frequent configurations associated with aneurysms in which the tortuosity of the basilar and vertebral arteries creates a hemodynamic force directed at the wall near a branching site, with the aneurysms pointing in the direction of hemodynamic thrust in the segment proximal to the aneurysm site. The aneurysms of the vertebral artery arise at its junctions with the posterior inferior cerebellar and basilar arteries (*center*). The aneurysms of the basilar artery arise between the posterior cerebral and superior cerebellar arteries (*center*), at the basilar apex (*right*), and at the origin of the anteror inferior cerebellar artery (*right*). All point in the direction of the long axis of the preaneurysmal segment of the artery and in the direction of maximal hemodynamic thrust (*arrows*) at the aneurysm site. (From Rhoton.[7])

Figure 160-8 (*Continued*)
A. A basilar apex aneurysm is shown arising at the origin of the posterior cerebral arteries as exposed by a right subtemporal craniotomy. Note scalp incision (*dotted line*) and bone flap or craniectomy (*solid line*). The retractor is on the temporal lobe, and the tentorium cerebelli (Tent.) has been divided to expose the basilar, posterior cerebral, superior cerebellar, posterior communicating (P.Co.A.) and internal carotid (C.A.) arteries and the oculomotor (III), trochlear (IV), and trigeminal (V) nerves. *B.* A basilar apex aneurysm is exposed by a frontotemporal approach. The sylvian fissure has been split and the frontal and temporal lobes are retracted to expose the aneurysm. The middle cerebral (M.C.A.), anterior cerebral (A.C.A.), and anterior choroidal (A.Ch.A.) arteries and the optic nerves (O.N.) are also exposed. The carotid artery is retracted with a blunt dissector to expose the aneurysm.

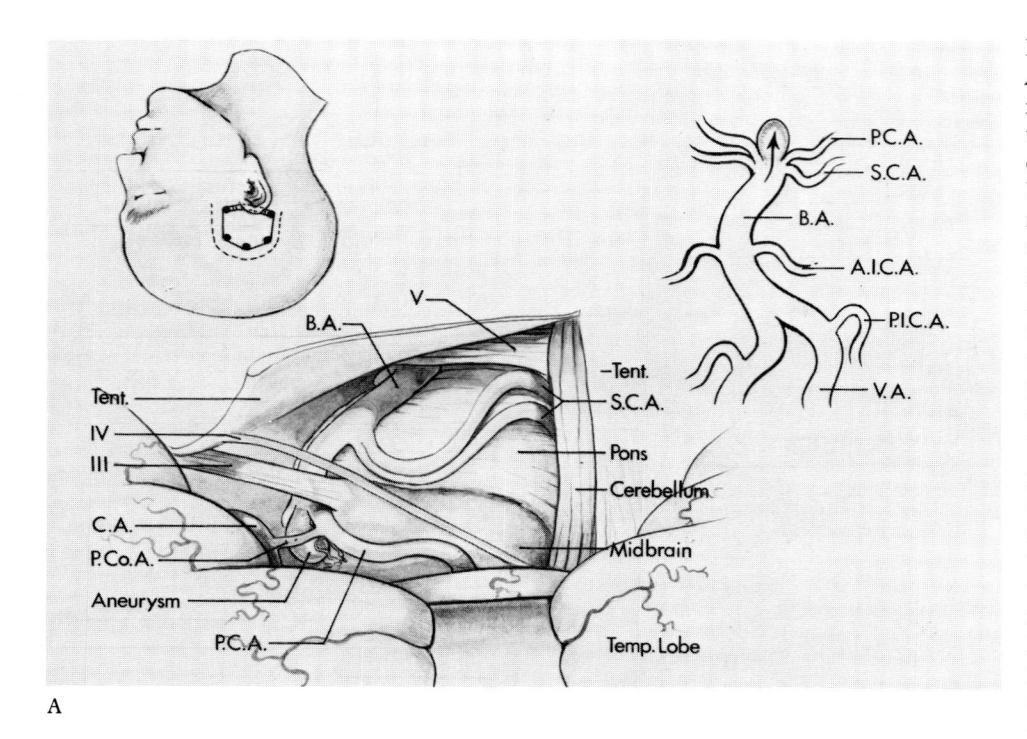

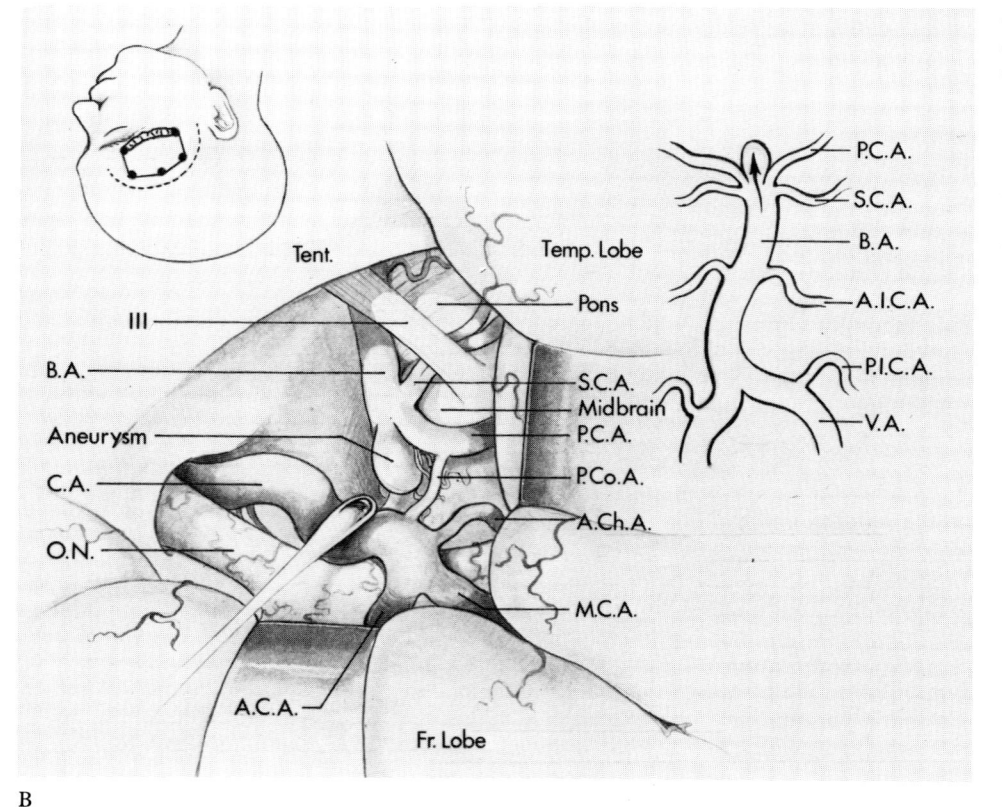

Figure 160-8 *A* to *E*. Common aneurysm sites in the posterior cranial fossa. Diagrams on the upper right show the basilar (B.A.), vertebral (V.A.), posterior cerebral (P.C.A.), superior cerebellar (S.C.A.), posterior inferior cerebellar (P.I.C.A.), and anterior inferior cerebellar (A.I.C.A.) arteries; the site of the aneurysm; and the direction of hemodynamic force (*arrow*) at the aneurysm site. Diagrams on the upper left show the scalp incision and bone flap or craniectomy used to expose the aneurysm.

Figure 160-8 (*Continued*) *C.* Subtemporal exposure of a basilar aneurysm arising between the origin of the superior cerebellar and posterior cerebral arteries. The basilar artery curvature creates a hemodynamic thrust (*arrow*) against the wall of the artery at the junction of the upper two branches of the basilar artery. The aneurysm projects laterally below or into the oculomotor nerve. *D.* Subtemporal exposure of a basilar aneurysm arising at the origin of the anterior inferior cerebellar artery. The abducens nerve (VI) is below the anterior inferior cerebellar artery. The tentorium is split laterally above the trigeminal nerve to expose the facial (VII) and vestibulocochlear (VIII) nerves. The curvature of the basilar artery creates a hemodynamic thrust (*arrow*) against the wall of the artery at the junction of the basilar and anterior inferior cerebellar arteries.

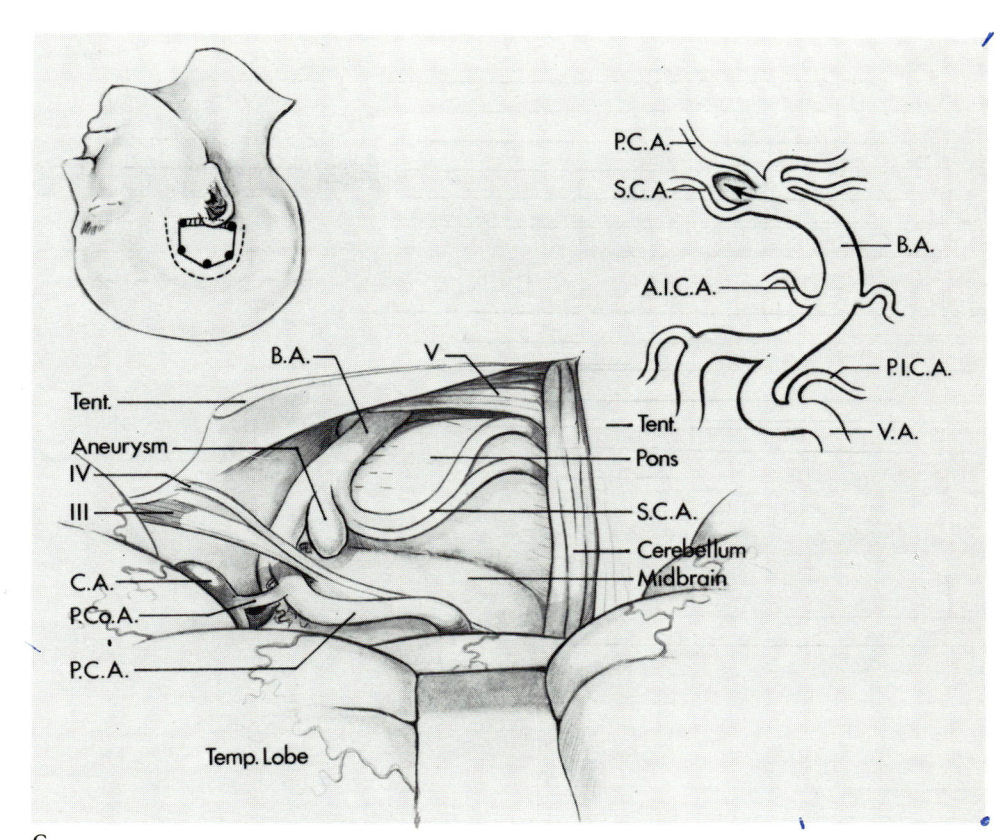

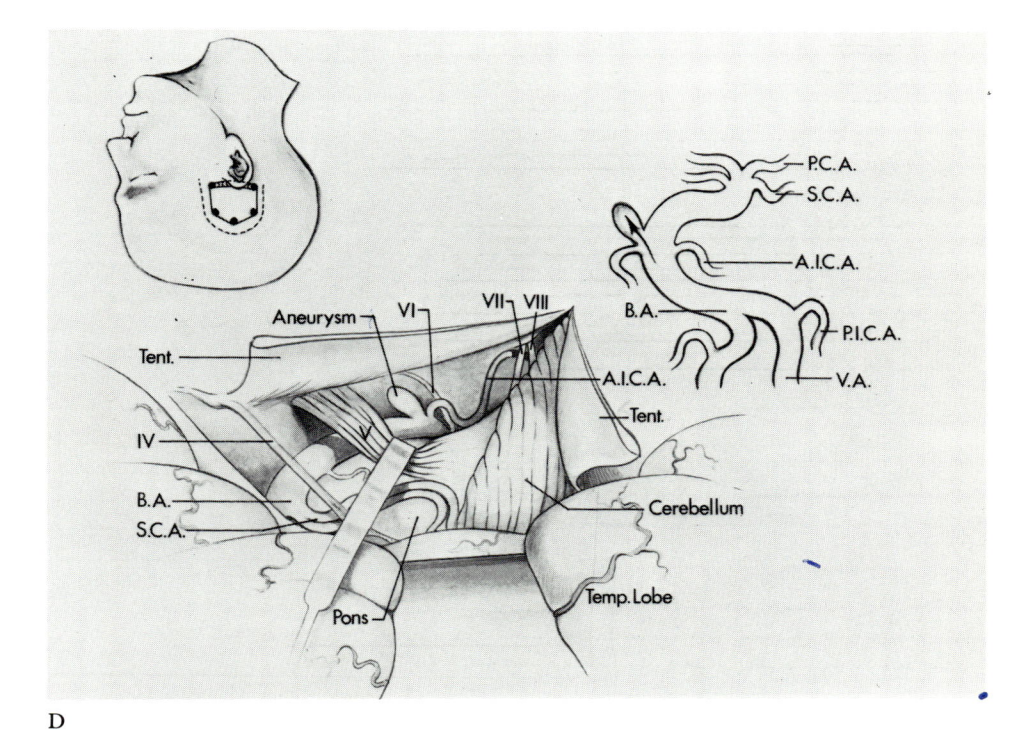

5. If rupture occurs during microdissection, bleeding should be controlled by applying a small cotton pledget to the bleeding point and concomitantly reducing mean arterial pressure. If this technique does not stop the hemorrhage, a temporary clip can be applied to the proximal blood supply, but only for the briefest possible time.

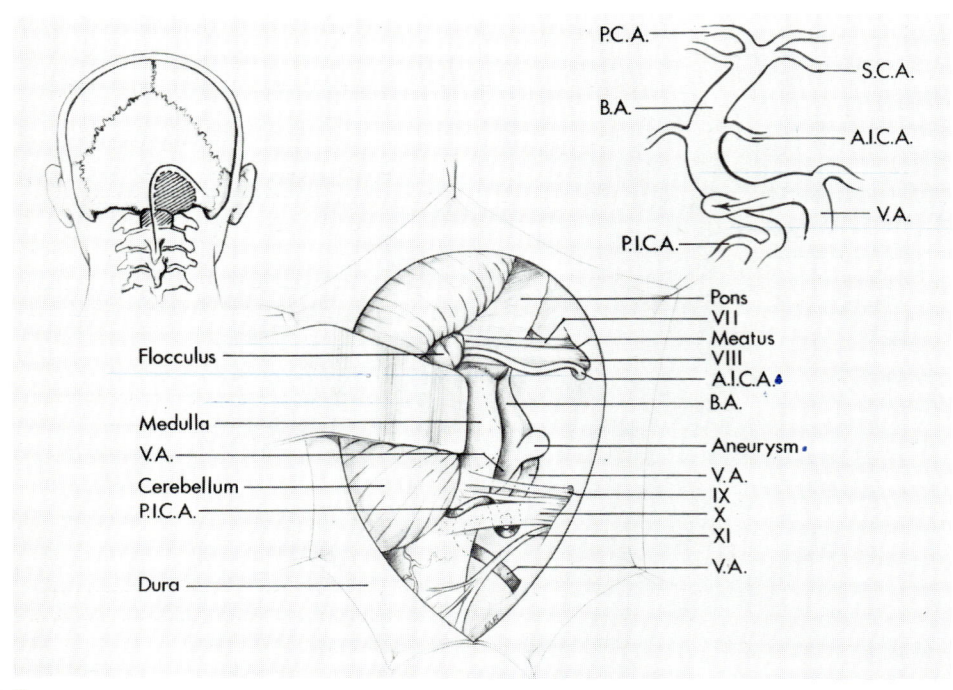

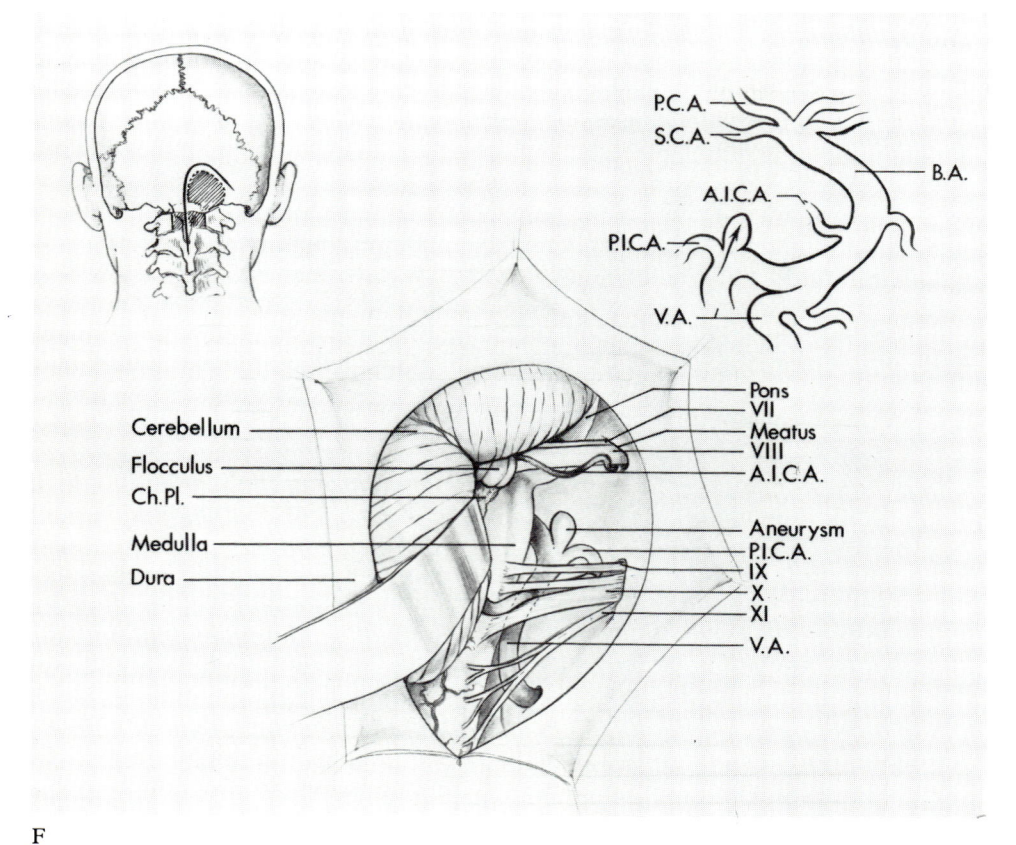

Figure 160-8 (*Continued*) *E.* Suboccipital exposure of an aneurysm arising at the junction of the vertebral and basilar arteries. The patient is in the sitting position. The right half of the cerebellum is retracted to expose the facial, vestibulocochlear, glossopharyngeal (IX), vagus (X), and spinal accessory (XI) nerves and the internal acoustic meatus. One of the vertebral arteries often joins the other in a configuration resembling the branching seen at other aneurysm sites. Angiographic views in multiple projections reveal the aneurysm pointing in the direction of flow in the preaneurysmal segment of the larger vertebral artery. *F.* Suboccipital exposure of an aneurysm arising at the origin of the right vertebral and posterior inferior cerebellar arteries. The angulation of the vertebral artery creates a hemodynamic thrust (*arrow*) in the direction in which the aneurysm points. The flocculus and choroid plexus (Ch.Pl.) protrude into the cerebellopontine angle. (From Rhoton.[7])

6. The bone flap should be placed as low as possible to minimize the need for retraction of the brain. Most aneurysms are located on or near the circle of Willis under the central portion of the brain. A low flap minimizes the amount of brain retraction needed to reach these areas.

7. A clip with a spring mechanism that allows it to be removed, repositioned, and reapplied should be used.

8. After the clip is applied, the area should be inspected to make certain the clip does not kink or obstruct a major vessel and that no perforating branches are included in it.

Microsurgical Anatomy of Saccular Aneurysms

9. If an aneurysm has a broad-based neck that will not accept the clip easily, the neck may be reduced by bipolar coagulation. Nearby perforating arteries are protected with a cottonoid sponge during coagulation. The tips of the bipolar coagulation forceps are inserted between adjacent vessels and the neck of the aneurysm and are gently squeezed during coagulation. Short bursts of low current are used, and the tips of the forceps are relaxed and opened between applications of current to prevent them from adhering to the aneurysm and to evaluate the degree of shrinkage.

10. If a clip or ligature cannot be applied to obliterate the neck of the aneurysm, the sac should be encased in surgical gauze or plastic. Wrapping with muscle is probably ineffective.

Operative Approaches

Ninety-five percent of aneurysms are found at one of five sites, all of which are located in close proximity to the circle of Willis (Fig. 160-1). These sites are: (1) the internal carotid artery between the posterior communicating and the anterior choroidal arteries; (2) the anterior communicating artery area; (3) the proximal bifurcation of the middle cerebral artery; (4) the internal carotid bifurcation; and (5) the basilar bifurcation. The frontotemporal craniotomy with slight modifications is suitable for approaching all these aneurysms arising from the anterior circle of Willis and for some originating from the upper basilar artery (Figs. 160-2 to 160-5, 160-8, 160-9).

A small frontotemporal flap centered at the pterion may be used for internal carotid artery aneurysms (Fig. 160-3). It may be enlarged posterosuperiorly for reaching aneurysms of the middle cerebral artery and of the internal carotid artery bifurcation (Fig. 160-4), forward for approaches to the anterior communicating area (Fig. 160-5), and posteriorly to provide a pterion–anterior subtemporal approach for an aneurysm of the basilar apex (Fig. 160-8B).

The scalp incision for this flap begins above the zygoma and extends across the temporal region and forward to the frontal region behind the hairline (Fig. 160-9). The scalp, galea, pericranium, and temporalis muscle and fascia are reflected as a single layer. A small bone flap having the center of its base at the pterion is elevated. The opening in the skull is extended inferiorly and medially by removing the lateral two-thirds of the sphenoid ridge. The time required to prepare this flap, in which all the soft tissue layers are reflected together, is less than that required to separate and reflect each layer individually. The incidence of weakness of the frontalis muscle is reduced because the layers superficial to the temporalis fascia are not disturbed. Decreased dissection around the temporalis muscle diminishes the incidence of contractions that limit opening of the mouth and reduces cosmetic deformities caused by scarring and atrophy of the temporalis muscle. Any burr holes or craniectomy site that would heal with a cosmetic deformity are closed with acrylic, mixed at the time the flap is replaced. The soft acrylic is molded into position and allowed to harden under direct vision to ensure that it fits the natural contour of the area (Fig. 160-9).

After the bone flap is elevated, the dura mater is opened

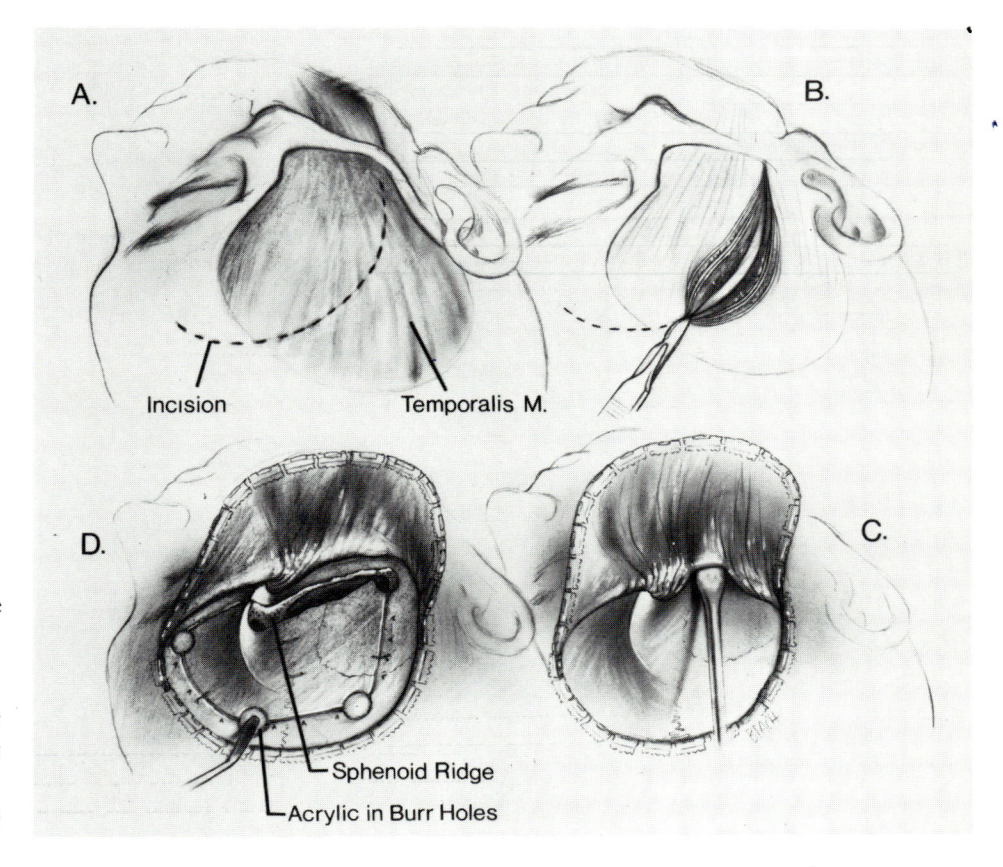

Figure 160-9 Frontotemporal craniotomy used to expose aneurysms on the anterior part of the circle of Willis. A to C. The scalp and temporalis muscle and fascia are elevated as a single layer. D. As the craniotomy flap is closed, soft acrylic is molded into the burr holes and allowed to harden under direct vision to minimize the cosmetic deformity associated with this bone removal. (From Rhoton.[7])

and the posterior inferior frontal lobe is elevated with the use of a self-retaining brain retractor to expose the sphenoid ridge to the depth of the anterior clinoid process. The cistern over the optic nerve and carotid artery is opened, and a suction drain protected with a cottonoid pledget is inserted to remove cerebrospinal fluid to relax the brain and increase exposure. One is at the desired location if the aneurysm arises from the internal carotid artery (Figs. 160-2 and 160-3). For anterior communicating artery aneurysms, the dissection is directed superiorly to the bifurcation of the internal carotid artery and over the optic nerve and chiasm along the anterior cerebral artery to the neck of the aneurysm (Fig. 160-5). Middle cerebral artery aneurysms are exposed by splitting the Sylvian fissure beginning at the internal carotid artery (Fig. 160-4). Some basilar artery aneurysms may be exposed through this approach by working through the space between the optic nerve and internal carotid artery if the interval between those two structures is sufficiently wide and the aneurysm projects superiorly or anteriorly.[10] If this approach is used, care should be taken to preserve the vital perforating branches that arise on the internal carotid artery and cross this space to supply the optic nerve and tract and diencephalon.[2] More commonly, the aneurysm must be approached through the space between the internal carotid artery and the oculomotor nerve. This exposure is facilitated by elevating the internal carotid artery with a dissector (Fig. 160-8B). If a basilar aneurysm arises from the posterior aspect of the upper basilar artery, it is best to elevate the temporal lobe and approach the area along the floor of the middle fossa (Fig. 160-8A).

Most basilar artery aneurysms are approached through a subtemporal craniotomy (Fig. 160-8A). This approach under the temporal lobe gives better exposure of the perforating arteries that commonly arise from the posterior aspect of the basilar artery than does the frontotemporal approach along the sphenoid ridge. These perforating branches are especially important because they supply diencephalic areas controlling consciousness. The subtemporal approach, when combined with section of the tentorium cerebelli posterior to the trochlear nerve, can be used to reach basilar aneurysms arising from the junction of the basilar artery and the superior cerebellar or anterior inferior cerebellar arteries (Figs. 160-8C,D).

Aneurysms arising at the vertebrobasilar junction may be reached through a subtemporal-transtentorial exposure if this junction is high. Otherwise, aneurysms arising at the vertebrobasilar junction are approached through a suboccipital craniectomy (Fig. 160-8E). Vertebral artery aneurysms arising at the origin of the posterior inferior cerebellar artery are approached through a suboccipital craniectomy (Fig. 160-8F). The arch of the C1 vertebra is removed to provide adequate exposure of the segment of the vertebral artery proximal to the aneurysm. The side for the suboccipital approach should be selected only after careful review of the angiogram because aneurysms of one vertebral artery may lie on the opposite side of the brain stem because of the extreme tortuosity of these arteries.

References

1. Gibo H, Carver CC, Rhoton AL Jr, Lenkey C, Mitchell RJ: Microsurgical anatomy of the middle cerebral artery. J Neurosurg 54:151–169, 1981.
2. Gibo H, Lenkey C, Rhoton AL Jr: Microsurgical anatomy of the supraclinoid portion of the internal carotid artery. J Neurosurg 55:560–574, 1981.
3. Hardy DG, Peace DA, Rhoton AL Jr: Microsurgical anatomy of the superior cerebellar artery. Neurosurgery 6:10–28, 1980.
4. Lister JR, Rhoton AL Jr, Matsushima T, Peace DA: Microsurgical anatomy of the posterior inferior cerebellar artery. Neurosurgery 10:170–199, 1982.
5. Martin RG, Grant JL, Peace D, Theiss C, Rhoton AL Jr: Microsurgical relationships of the anterior inferior cerebellar artery and the facial-vestibulocochlear nerve complex. Neurosurgery 6:483–507, 1980.
6. Perlmutter D, Rhoton AL Jr: Microsurgical anatomy of the anterior cerebral–anterior communicating–recurrent artery complex. J Neurosurg 45:259–272, 1976.
7. Rhoton AL Jr: Anatomy of saccular aneurysms. Surg Neurol 14:59–66, 1980.
8. Rhoton AL Jr, Saeki N, Perlmutter D, Zeal A: Microsurgical anatomy of common aneurysm sites. Clin Neurosurg 26:248–306, 1979.
9. Saeki N, Rhoton, AL Jr: Microsurgical anatomy of the upper basilar artery and the posterior circle of Willis. J Neurosurg 46:563–578, 1977.
10. Yaşargil MG, Fox JL: The microsurgical approach to intracranial aneurysms. Surg Neurol 3:7–14, 1975.
11. Zeal AA, Rhoton AL Jr: Microsurgical anatomy of the posterior cerebral artery. J Neurosurg 48:534–559, 1978.

161
Radiology of Intracranial Aneurysms

Eugene F. Binet
Edgardo J. C. Angtuaco

Aneurysms are the most common nontraumatic cause of subarachnoid hemorrhage in adults but they may also present as mass lesions or cause neurological symptoms and signs not secondary to hemorrhage.

Classically, the first radiological procedure undertaken in a patient suspected of having an intracranial aneurysm is plain skull radiography. These roentgenograms are reviewed for displacement of the pineal body or choroid plexus that occurs secondary to an intracerebral or subdural hematoma. Very rarely, calcification is seen in the walls of a giant aneurysm. In a small percentage of patients, bony erosion of the clivus, pituitary fossa, or sphenoid wing will indicate a giant aneurysm.

High-Resolution Computed Tomography

More recently, high-resolution computed tomography (CT) has become the procedure of choice for the detection of subarachnoid hemorrhage and the localization of intracranial aneurysms.[7,14,15] It may obviate lumbar puncture in a patient at risk for transtentorial herniation. The CT scan should be performed within the first 24 h of the ictus. Sections should be obtained both before and after intravenous injection of a contrast medium. Ultra-thin sections encompassing the circle of Willis should be obtained following a second bolus injection to detect small aneurysms arising from the arteries at the base of the skull (Fig. 161-1).

Unenhanced CT Scans

On the unenhanced CT scan subarachnoid hemorrhage will be identified as areas of increased density in the subarachnoid spaces along the base of the skull, within the sylvian fissures, within the sulci over the periphery of the brain, along the falx and tentorium, and even in the interhemispheric fissure (Figs. 161-1A, 161-8A, 161-11A). The development of a full-fledged appearance, with Hounsfield units ranging from 60 HU to 80 HU, may take several hours following the hemorrhage. The detection of subarachnoid hemorrhage on unenhanced CT scans depends on the cooperation of the patient, the time since the subarachnoid hemorrhage, and the employment of a high-resolution CT scanner.[9]

In patients with severe anemia, subarachnoid, intracerebral, and intraventricular hemorrhages may be only slightly more dense than the surrounding brain tissue. Subarachnoid hemorrhage in the presence of a bleeding aneurysm will be detected in more than 90 percent of the patients in the first 24 h and in over 50 percent within the first week.[5] Following the seventh day, these percentages drop off dramatically. Significant subarachnoid hemorrhage seen 10 or more days following an episode of bleeding is suspicious for the occurrence of rebleeding. If the unenhanced CT scan does not demonstrate subarachnoid hemorrhage, a lumbar puncture should be done in the absence of an intracranial mass lesion.

In addition to subarachnoid hemorrhage, the unenhanced study should be evaluated for intraventricular or intracerebral hemorrhage (Figs. 161-2A and B, 161-3A). Extensive intraventricular hemorrhage may completely fill both lateral ventricles as well as the third and fourth ventricles. More commonly, however, the CT scan shows a thin layer of blood confined to the occipital horns. Intracerebral hemorrhage may be identified as a large area of increased density within the substance of the temporal or frontal lobes associated with edema and mass effect. Subdural hematomas occur in 1 to 8 percent of patients with subarachnoid hemorrhage due to bleeding aneurysms and these may be identified on CT scans as areas of increased density paralleling the inner table of the skull.[4]

The location of the subarachnoid blood may frequently suggest the site of the bleeding aneurysm. It is very common for anterior communicating artery aneurysms to bleed into the interhemispheric fissure. Hemorrhage into the septum pellucidum and adjacent frontal lobe alone is almost pathognomonic for an anterior communicating artery aneurysm (Fig. 161-2B). Unenhanced scans showing hemorrhage into the temporal lobe and sylvian fissure alone are frequently obtained with a middle cerebral artery aneurysm (Fig. 161-3A). Aneurysms at the internal carotid artery bifurcation may bleed into the basal ganglia, the frontal and medial temporal lobes, and the adjacent subarachnoid space. The location of the subarachnoid hemorrhage associated with bleeding posterior communicating artery aneurysms varies depending upon the direction to which the aneurysm points. Hemorrhages into the sylvian fissure and temporal lobe are often present where the tip of the aneurysm points laterally. On the other hand, a tip pointing posteriorly may be associated with hemorrhage into the interpeduncular cistern. Hemorrhage into the brain stem as well as the interpeduncular cistern may be the presenting findings for distal basilar artery aneurysms, although hemorrhage into the third ventricle has also been recorded with these lesions. Posterior inferior cerebellar artery aneurysms often bleed into the medullary cistern, with blood also appearing in the fourth ventricle. In general, posterior fossa aneurysms do not frequently bleed into the supratentorial subarachnoid space or into the lateral ventricles. More blood is present in the

1341

A   B

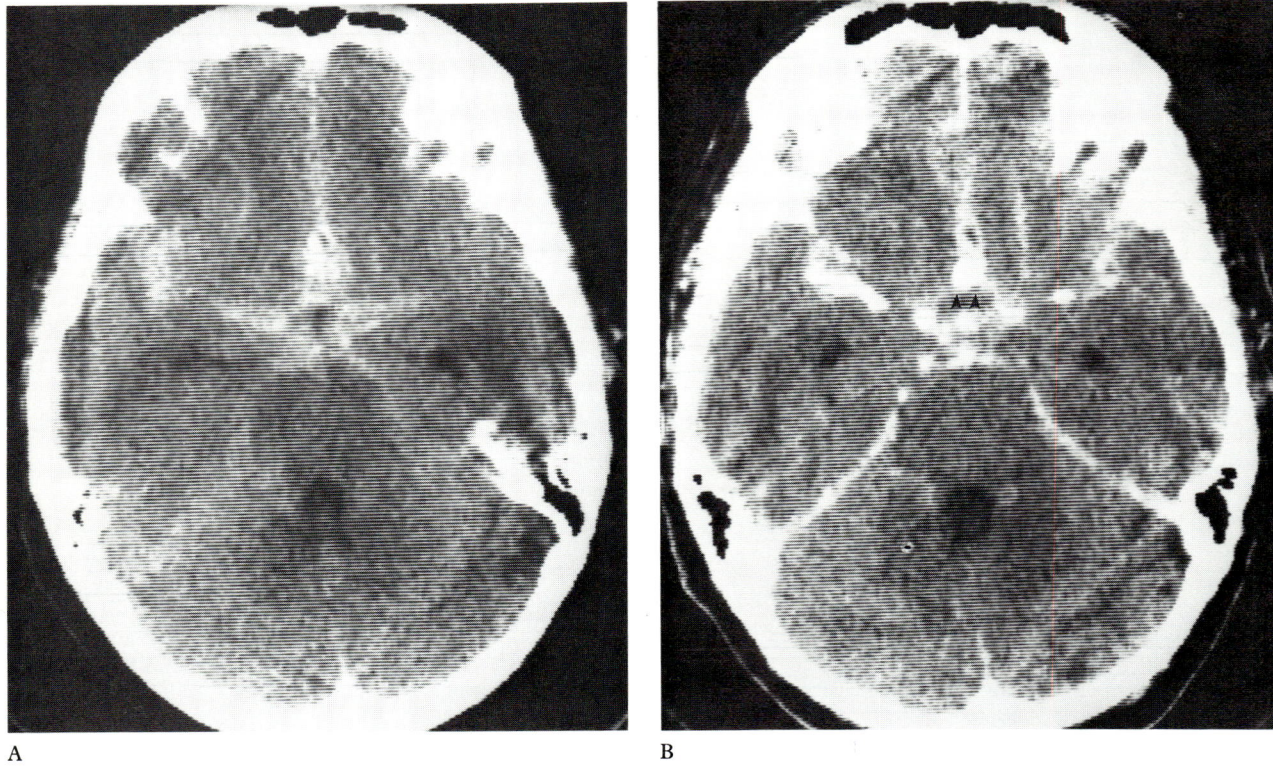

Figure 161-1 *A.* Unenhanced 10 mm-thick CT scan at the level of the basilar cisterns shows subarachnoid hemorrhage in the interhemispheric fissure, the suprasellar cistern, and the interpeduncular cistern and along the tentorium. *B.* A 1.5 mm-thick enhanced high-resolution CT scan shows an anterior communicating artery aneurysm 5 mm in diameter (*arrowheads*).

fourth ventricle than the third ventricle with posterior fossa aneurysms.

Enhanced CT Scans

Following analysis of the unenhanced CT scans, all patients (unless contraindicated) should receive a large bolus of intravenous contrast medium and the routine intracranial sections should be repeated. This should be followed by thin sections encompassing the base of the skull and circle of Willis after a second contrast bolus. The contraindications to enhanced scans include absolute sensitivity to intravenous contrast agents, complete renal shutdown, and severe patient jeopardy. The use of contrast-enhanced scans for detection of the cause of subarachnoid hemorrhage is so important that dialysis following the CT scan should be considered for patients with impaired renal function. The final decision as to whether a given patient should have a postcontrast study lies with the referring physician after consultation with the supervising neuroradiologist. That decision should take into account the great amount of information that is provided on thin-section high-resolution CT scans.

Enhanced studies have several purposes. First and foremost, they will identify the cause of subarachnoid hemorrhage in most patients (Figs. 161-1 and 161-3*A* to *C*). Although the localization of subarachnoid hemorrhage on unenhanced studies frequently points to the site of an aneurysm, enhanced CT scans confirm this location and may show the presence of a second aneurysm as well (Fig. 161-4*A* and *B*). The size, shape and relationship of an aneurysm to its parent vessel can easily be determined with high-resolution techniques (Figs. 161-3*B* and *C*, 161-7). Aneurysms greater than 5 mm can be seen (Fig. 161-1*B*). The magnification mode is also helpful to delineate fine detail (Fig. 161-4*A* and *B*). The use of sagittal coronal reformatting or direct coronal scanning will provide additional information concerning the aneurysm's relationship to other vital structures at the base of the brain (Figs. 161-3*B* and *C*, 161-12*A* and *B*). The enhanced CT scan provides a road map for angiography when preoperative fine detail analysis of the aneurysm becomes necessary. In the great majority of patients, the localization of subarachnoid hemorrhage and its cause can therefore be made on a relatively noninvasive, low-morbidity study, and angiography can be deferred until such time as the patient is more stable, the angiography team better prepared, and the angiographer better informed.

Enhanced studies will occasionally show that an aneurysm is not the cause of subarachnoid hemorrhage. An arteriovenous malformation may be identified on enhanced CT scans as a serpiginous tangle of enlarged feeding arteries and draining veins. Cavernous hemangioma and venous angioma may present with subarachnoid hemorrhage; they also have distinctive CT appearances on enhanced studies. Even rarer

Radiology of Intracranial Aneurysms

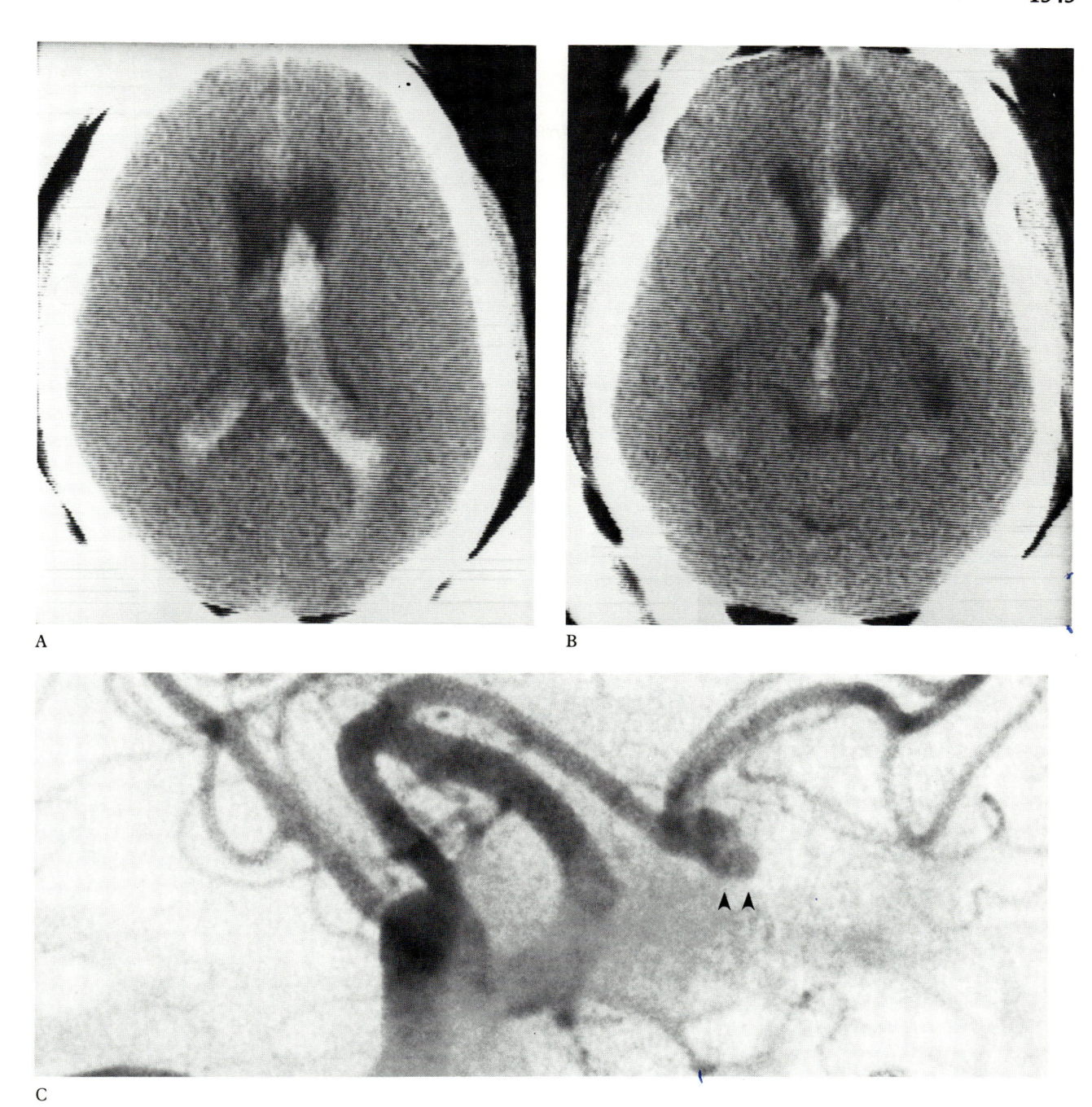

Figure 161-2 *A.* Unenhanced CT scan shows massive hemorrhage within both lateral ventricles. *B.* Unenhanced CT scan shows hemorrhage into the septum pellucidum and the third ventricle. *C.* Right common carotid angiogram, oblique projection, subtraction print, shows anterior communicating artery aneurysm (*arrowheads*).

lesions such as metastatic melanoma to the brain, which occasionally causes subarachnoid hemorrhage, can be detected on enhanced studies.

With present techniques, high-resolution CT scanning with and without contrast enhancement will detect the cause of nontraumatic subarachnoid hemorrhage in most patients. Utilizing this first radiological step, the neurosurgeon and neuroradiologist will be better able to evaluate the patient's status and plan the remainder of the patient's diagnostic workup. If immediate surgery is required to remove a subdural or intracerebral hematoma or to place an intraventricular catheter, the precise localization of the aneurysm on the enhanced CT scan will allow the surgeon to determine the approach to the problem without waiting for the corroborative angiogram or approaching the aneurysm unknowingly (Fig. 161-3*B*, *C*).

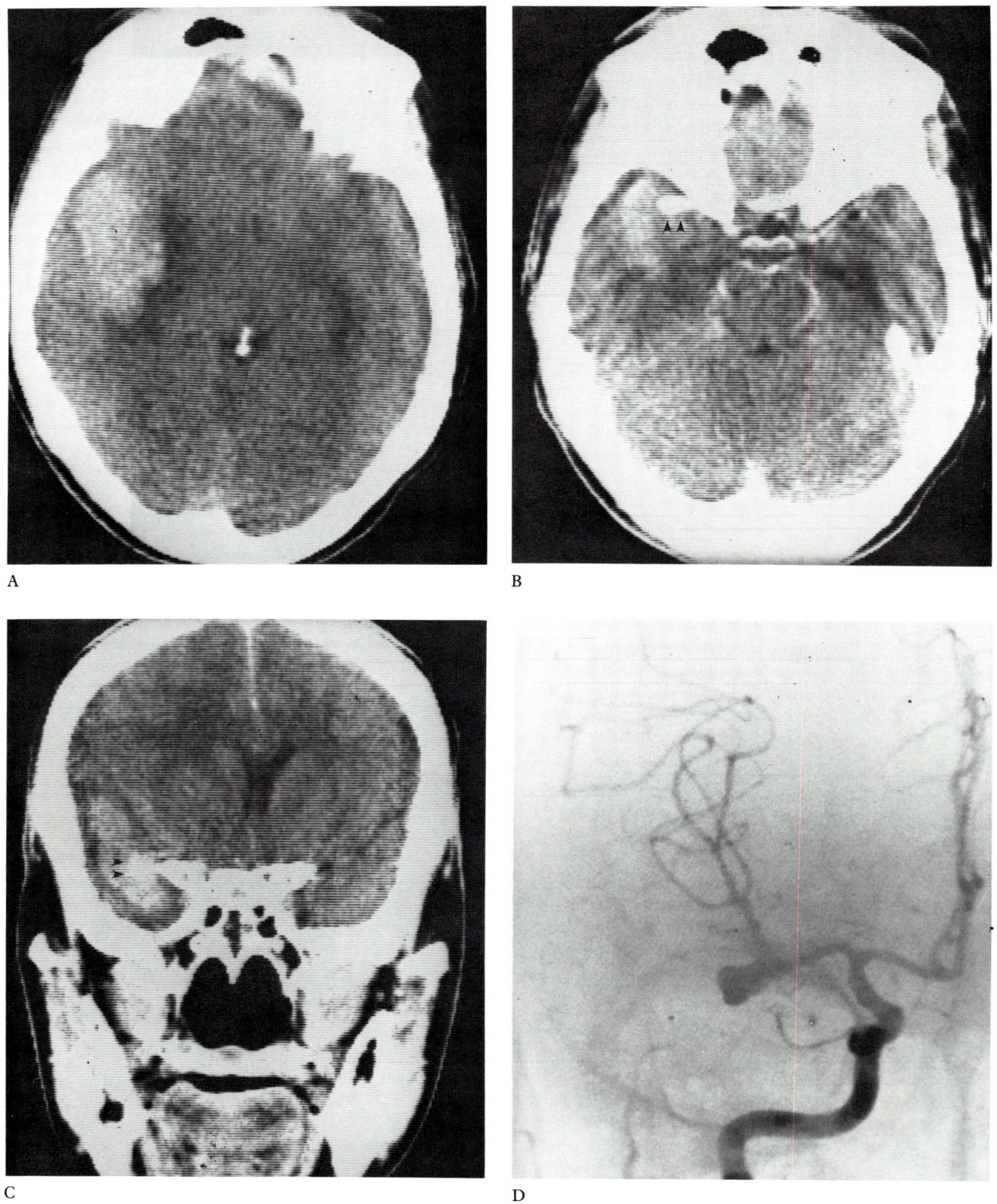

Figure 161-3 *A.* Unenhanced CT scan shows intracerebral hematoma in the right temporal lobe. *B.* Thin-section high-resolution enhanced CT scan shows a right middle cerebral artery aneurysm projecting to the edge of the right temporal lobe hematoma (*arrowheads*). *C.* Direct coronal, thin-section high-resolution enhanced CT scan shows the right middle cerebral artery aneurysm projecting into the right temporal lobe hematoma (*arrowheads*). *D.* Right common carotid angiogram, transorbital projection, subtraction print, shows the large right middle cerebral artery aneurysm. The large right temporal lobe hematoma causes medial displacement of the middle cerebral artery and contralateral displacement of the anterior cerebral artery.

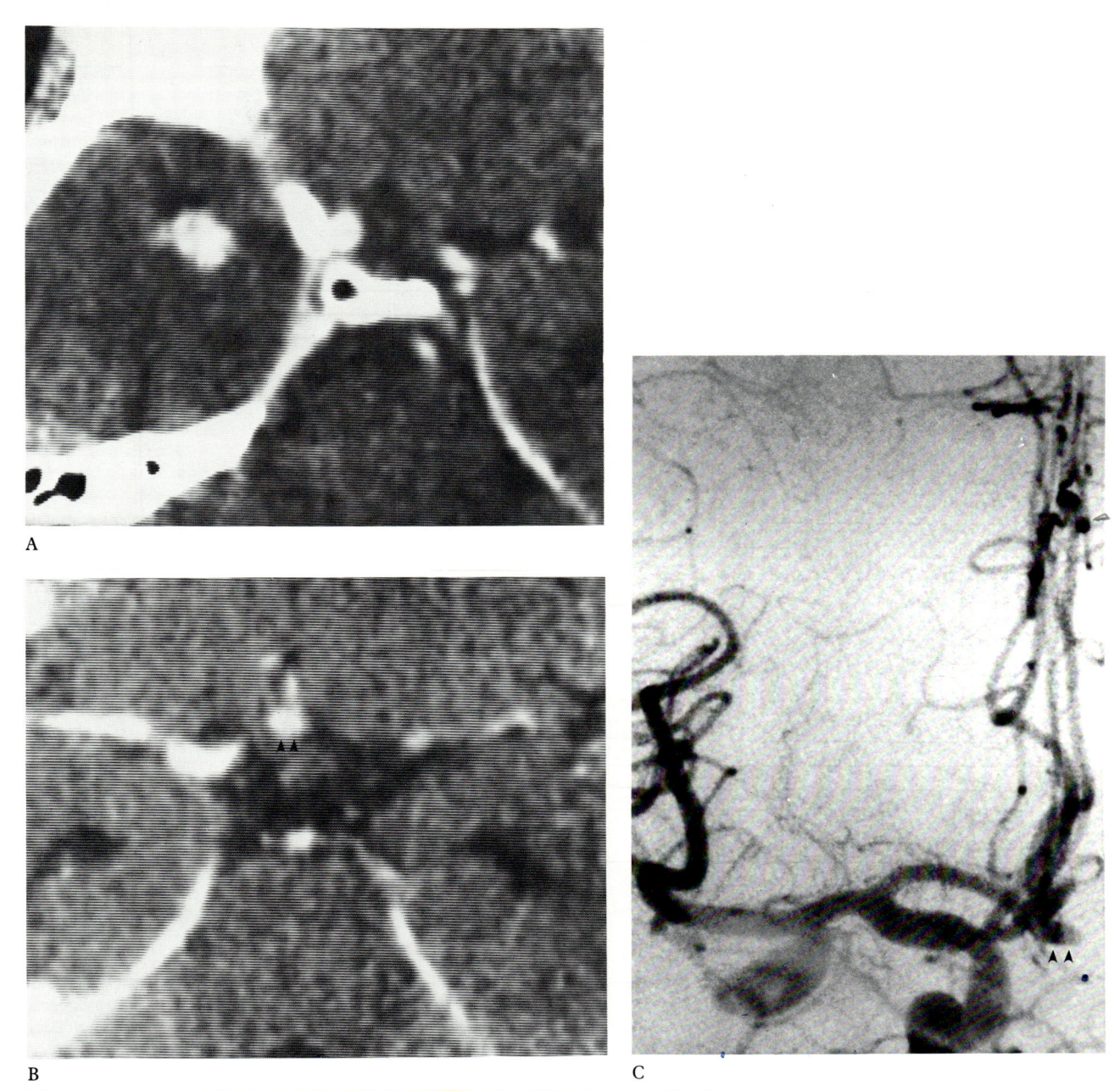

Figure 161-4 *A.* Enhanced high-resolution thin-section CT scan, magnification mode, shows a right middle cerebral artery aneurysm with irregular margins. A small clot is seen within the lumen of the aneurysm. *B.* Enhanced high-resolution CT scan, magnification mode, shows a second smaller anterior communicating artery aneurysm (*arrowheads*). *C.* Right common carotid angiogram shows the right middle cerebral artery aneurysm with clot within its lumen. Also observed is the small anterior communicating artery aneurysm (*arrowheads*).

Transfemoral Cerebral Angiography

The second step in the radiological evaluation of patients with suspected subarachnoid hemorrhage due to a ruptured aneurysm is a complete transfemoral cerebral angiogram. This can be performed immediately preceding surgery. A catheter study is indicated as this is the only method whereby complete evaluation of the vasculature to both cerebral hemispheres and the posterior fossa can be accomplished with one vessel puncture. In patients with aortofemoral grafts, axillary puncture with selective catheterization of the brachiocephalic vessels is easily accomplished. In older patients it may be necessary to evaluate the aortic arch and carotid bifurcations in the neck to exclude the presence of significant vascular disease. Patients

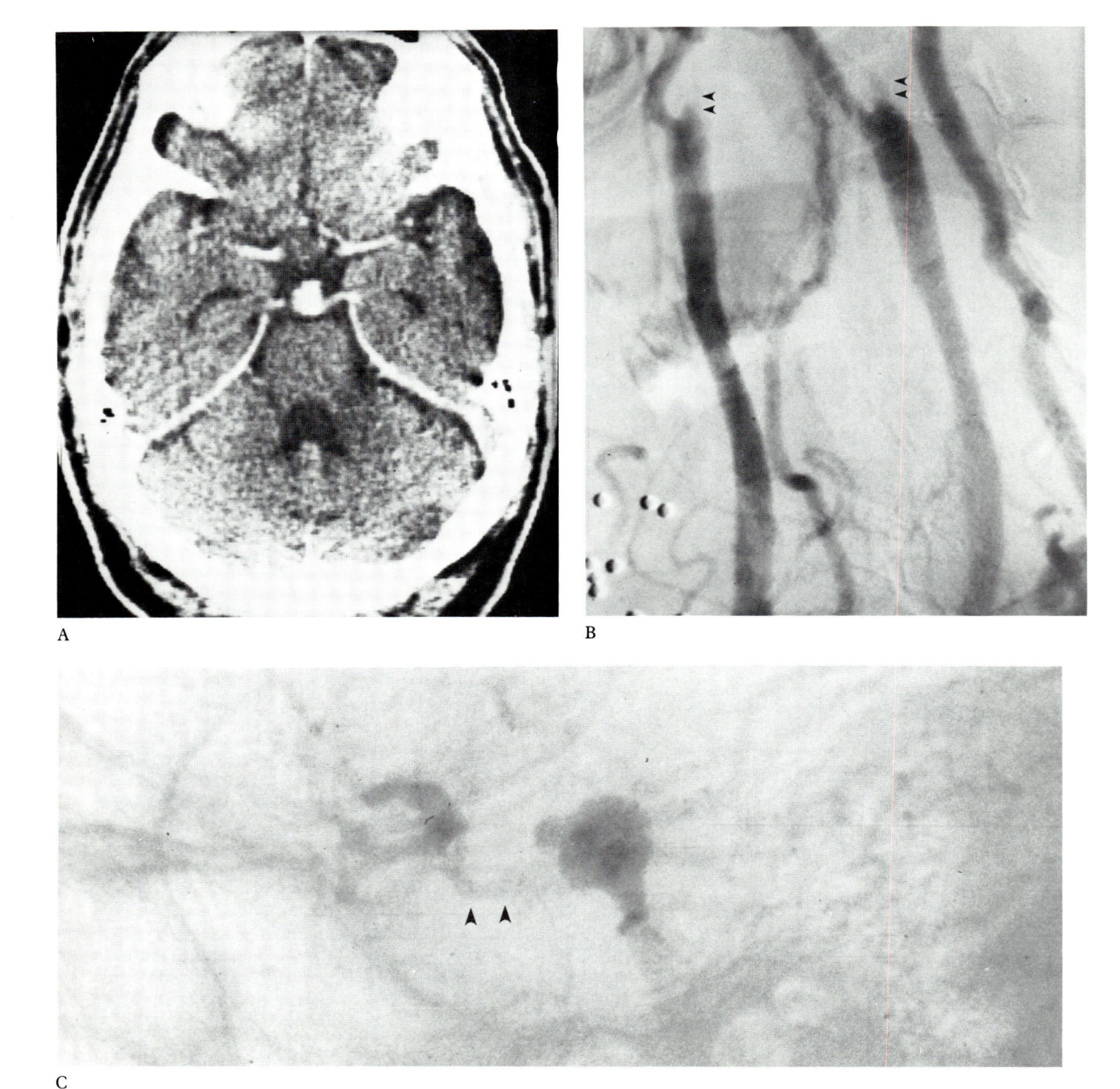

Figure 161-5 *A.* Enhanced thin-section CT scan shows a large basilar artery aneurysm. *B.* An arch aortogram, subtraction print, demonstrates complete occlusion of both internal carotid arteries at their origins (*arrowheads*). *C.* Vertebral angiogram, lateral projection, subtraction print, shows the basilar artery aneurysm. The supraclinoid portion of both the right and the left internal carotid arteries are filled via the posterior communicating arteries (*arrowheads*).

with an antecedent history of transient ischemic attacks or previous strokes should have an arch aortogram prior to selective catheterization of the neck vessels. It is not uncommon to find significant cervical lesions in older patients with a bleeding aneurysm (Fig. 161-5).

Selective injection of small amounts of contrast medium (6 to 10 ml) into the common carotid and vertebral arteries will usually suffice to demonstrate the circle of Willis in great detail. Selective injections into the internal carotid artery or high in the vertebral artery are usually not necessary and are contraindicated, as they may cause intra-angiographic rupture of an aneurysm. Steps should be taken to correct any bleeding diathesis prior to angiography. Replacement blood transfusions should be considered for patients with sickle cell anemia.

The initial angiogram should be performed by utilizing the standard anteroposterior and lateral projections. Biplanar magnification techniques should be used if available, and subtraction films should always be obtained in all projections, not only to clarify details about observed aneurysms but also to exclude additional aneurysms obscured by overlying bone. It is best to perform the angiogram on the "side closer to the aneurysm" first. The side of the bleeding aneurysm can usually be discerned from the CT if the neurological findings are nonlocalizing. If the blood supply to the aneurysm is in the distribution of one carotid circulation, that vessel should be examined first. Then the contralateral common carotid artery and the larger or more accessible vertebral artery should be injected. If the aneurysm is in the posterior fossa, then the larger, more accessible vertebral artery should be cannulated first and this should be followed by selective injections into both common carotid arteries. There are several advantages to performing the angiogram first in the artery "closest to the aneurysm." If there is severe spasm of the cerebral vasculature on the first angiographic run, at least a "peek" at the aneurysm will have been obtained prior to terminating the study. In addition, if there is a technical malfunction of the equipment during or after the first angiographic run, again a peek will have been obtained. The same is true if the patient has an allergic reaction or a cardiorespiratory failure during the procedure. If all goes well, the films from the first run will be developed first and be available for detailed scrutiny while the other vessels are being examined. The angiographer can then plan and carry out special views of the aneurysm while the additional routine runs are being processed. This plan of sequencing ensures a greater likelihood of a successful angiogram and reduces the length of time that the catheter is in the bloodstream, an important consideration in the prevention of complications.

Special views are often necessary to identify the neck of an aneurysm.[8] For suspected anterior communicating artery aneurysms, the patient's head should be turned away from the side of injection (Fig. 161-2C). Middle cerebral artery aneurysms are often best identified by placing the area of suspicion within the bony orbit (Fig. 161-3D). This is accomplished by utilizing the transorbital oblique view with the head in moderate extension. Basilar artery aneurysms are often best identified in the base view (Fig. 161-6B). The submentovertical view is also helpful in anterior communicating artery and middle cerebral artery aneurysms (Fig. 161-7B). The special view technique chart described by Lin and Kricheff should be utilized as a guide to the proper projection for any given aneurysm.[8]

If no aneurysm is identified on the routine studies, the other vertebral artery should be injected if it has not been already visualized adequately. If this is not helpful and the enhanced CT scan is not diagnostic, consideration should be given to obtaining additional special views of those areas demonstrating subarachnoid or intracerebral hemorrhage on

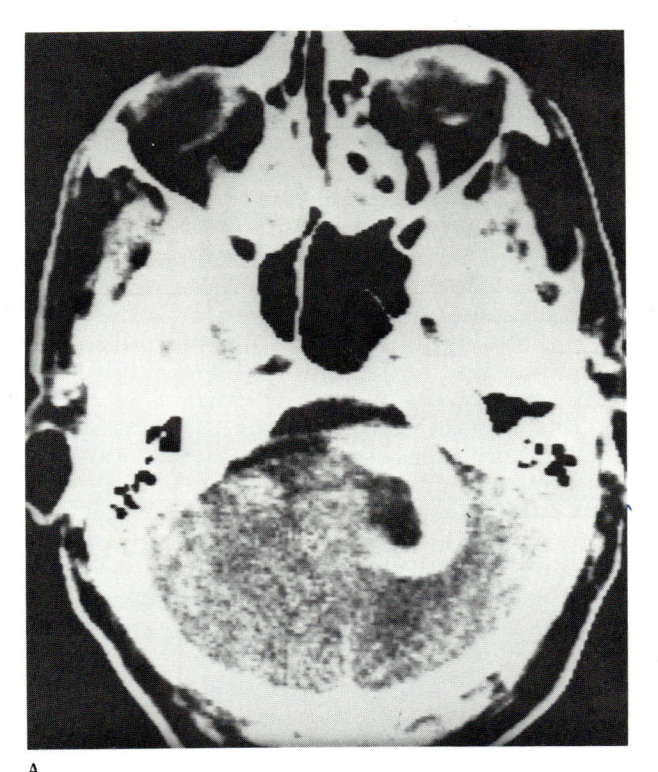

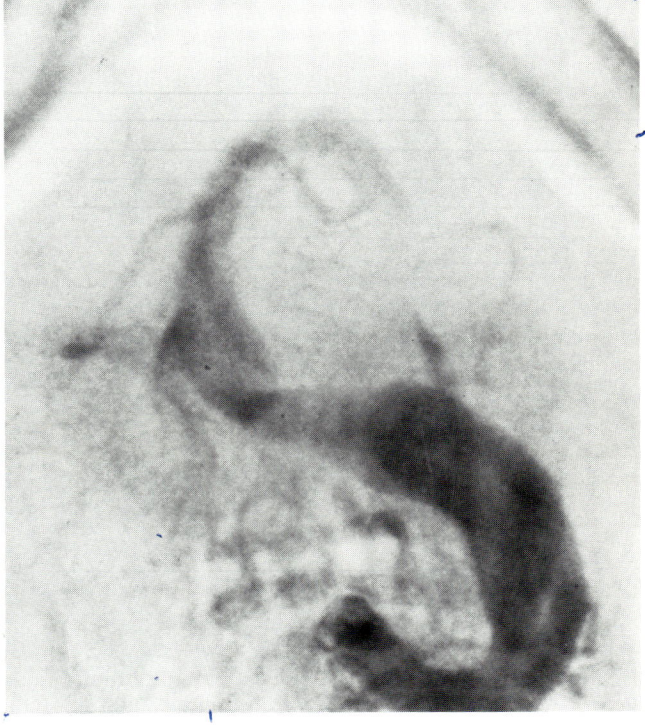

Figure 161-6 *A.* Enhanced CT scan shows a large atherosclerotic aneurysm of the basilar artery. *B.* Left vertebral angiogram, submentovertical projection, subtraction print, shows the large atherosclerotic aneurysm of the basilar artery.

A   B

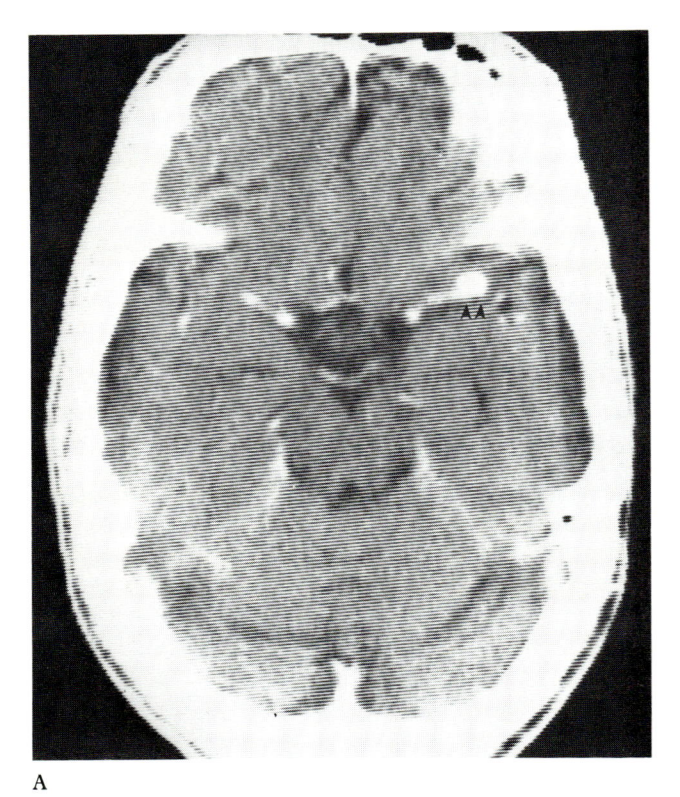

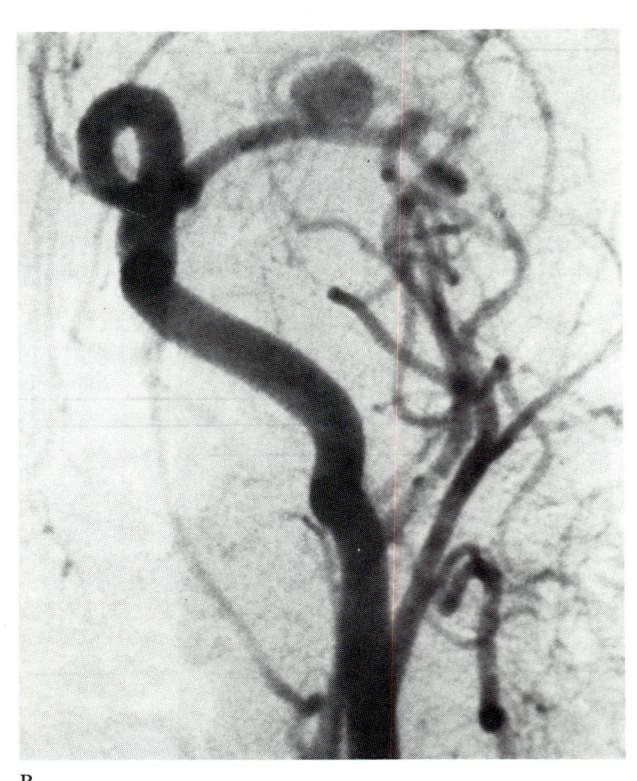

Figure 161-7 *A.* Enhanced thin-section high-resolution CT scan shows a left middle cerebral artery trifurcation aneurysm (*arrowheads*). *B.* Left common carotid angiogram, submentovertical projection, subtraction print, shows an irregularly marginated aneurysm projecting anteriorly from the left middle cerebral artery.

the CT scan. For example, if the standard views do not demonstrate an aneurysm of the anterior communicating artery and the CT scan shows interhemispheric hemorrhage or hemorrhage into the septum pellucidum, either an oblique or base angiogram of the anterior communicating artery should be obtained, as most surely the aneurysm will be found in this location.

The standard angiographic runs should be carried out well into the venous phase of the cerebral circulation and analyzed for the presence of other lesions. If no aneurysm has been seen on the routine and special views, a careful analysis of the arterial, capillary, and venous phases of the angiogram may reveal a small, cryptic arteriovenous malformation that has not only bled but has defied detection by CT scanning. This important analysis is often overlooked in the flurry of activity to find the more dramatic saccular aneurysm.

Cross-compression techniques are seldom performed as they are not physiological, do not accurately predict the change in flow patterns that will occur as a result of surgery, and are technically difficult to perform correctly.

The accuracy of the initial angiogram in detecting a bleeding aneurysm varies from investigator to investigator, depending on observer error, the use of magnification and subtraction techniques, and whether or not all four vessels are examined.[3] With modern techniques, one should expect to identify more than 75 percent of the aneurysms on the first study. Causes for nonvisualization of an aneurysm on the first study may be due to its being totally thrombosed or completely "blown out" at the time of the first hemorrhage. The cryptic arteriovenous malformation that has destroyed itself at the time of first hemorrhage also falls into this category. A second high-quality angiogram will usually discover 5 to 10 percent more aneurysms. Two high-quality cerebral angiograms should have been interpreted as normal before searching for a spinal arteriovenous malformation or spinal cord tumor. How soon a high-quality but completely negative angiogram should be repeated depends on several factors, not the least of which is the condition of the patient. It is said that the maximal spasm of the cerebral vasculature occurs between the fourth and fourteenth day after bleeding.[2] Certainly an angiogram should not be performed during this period of time unless absolutely necessary. The use of intra-arterial digital angiography as a screening procedure to rule out spasm before proceeding to a full-fledged second angiogram is helpful.

Follow-Up Studies

Follow-up CT studies are also promising. They may determine the cause of the neurological deficits that may occur during this waiting period. These include rehemorrhage,

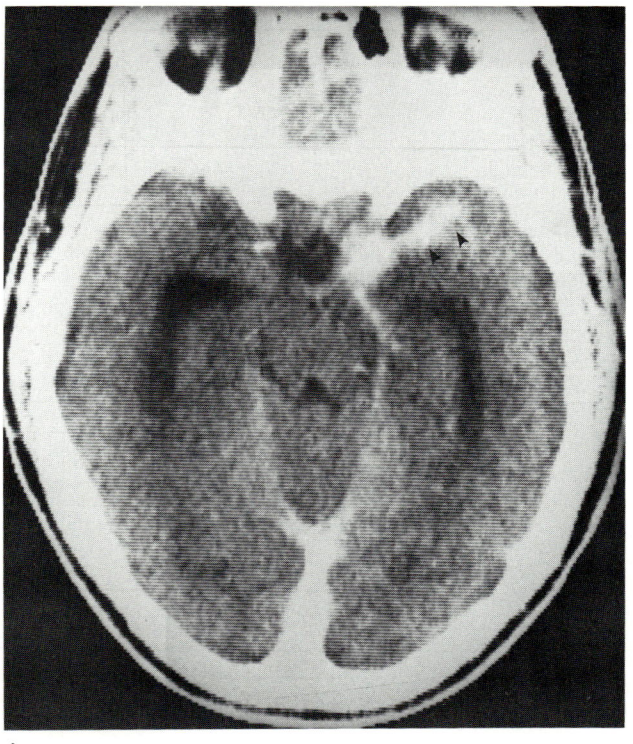

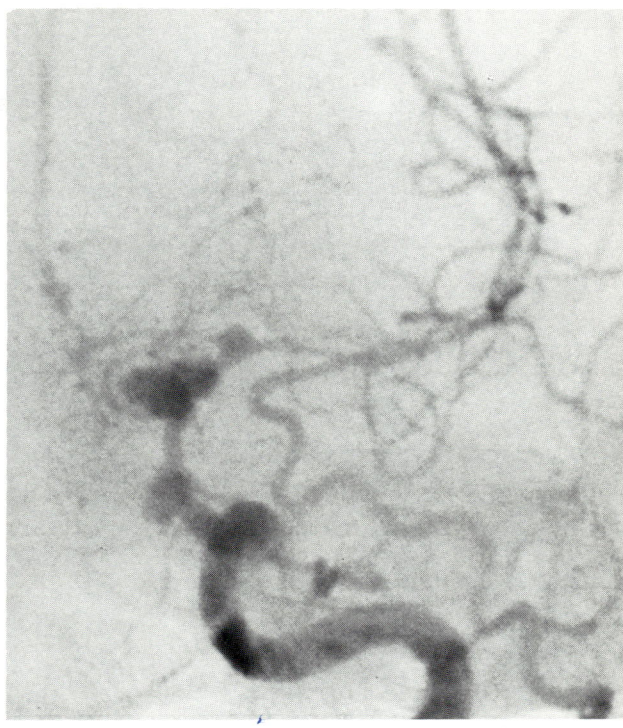

A   B

Figure 161-8 *A.* Enhanced thin-section high-resolution CT scan shows a left posterior communicating artery aneurysm with hemorrhage into the adjacent subarachnoid space (*arrowheads*). *B.* Left common carotid angiogram, subtraction print, demonstrates marked spasm of the supraclinoid portion of the left internal carotid artery and the horizontal rami of the left anterior and middle cerebral arteries. A large left posterior communicating artery aneurysm is seen.

hydrocephalus, and vasospasm. A rebleed is identified as an area of increased density in the subarachnoid cisterns. It may also extend into the ventricles or into the brain parenchyma. Hydrocephalus can be easily recognized by comparing the ventricular size with that shown by the initial scan. Frequently the hydrocephalus is accompanied by periventricular edema, occurring most prominently adjacent to the frontal horns. Hydrocephalus is caused by the blockage of the pacchionian granulations by erythrocytes, which prevent absorption of cerebrospinal fluid. The possibility of a rebleed or the development of hydrocephalus cannot be predicted either clinically or from the initial CT scan.

Vasospasm is related directly to the presence of blood in the subarachnoid space. It occurs when blood comes into direct contact with the adventitia of an artery. On the initial CT scan, the thickness of blood clot in the subarachnoid cisterns correlates highly with the severity of vasospasm seen at angiography (Fig. 161-8). The angiographic finding of severe vasospasm, judged as greater than 75 percent compromise of the vascular lumen with poor cephalad flow of contrast medium, directly correlates with the development of permanent neurological deficits. On CT scans, the effects of vasospasm are manifested as low-density changes within the brain parenchyma. These low-density appearances, however, do not represent permanent brain damage and may disappear with improvement in the neurological status.

Delayed enhancement of the low-density areas on CT scans has been associated with permanent brain damage. In effect then, the severity of angiographic vasospasm is directly proportional to the thickness of the blood clot found on the initial scan following aneurysm rupture.[1] The development of cerebral infarcts following vasospasm directly correlates with the severity of angiographic vasospasm.

Postoperative CT has been useful in the detection of residual lesions such as encephalomalacia or cerebral infarction (Fig. 161-9). In some instances faulty placement of the aneurysm clip may even be detected (Fig. 161-10). The development of postoperative hydrocephalus, whether due to the original bleeding insult or the operation itself, is best analyzed by serial CT scans. The ease of performance of postoperative CT has reduced the need for postoperative angiography.

Types of Intracranial Aneurysms

Congenital

The incidence of congenital aneurysms will vary from investigator to investigator depending on whether statistics were derived from a study of partial or complete angiograms, au-

A   B

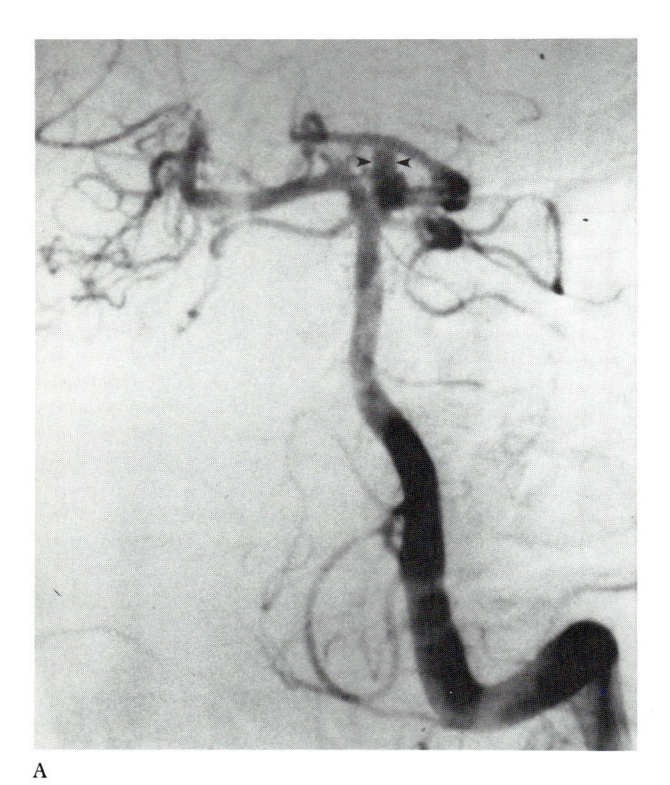

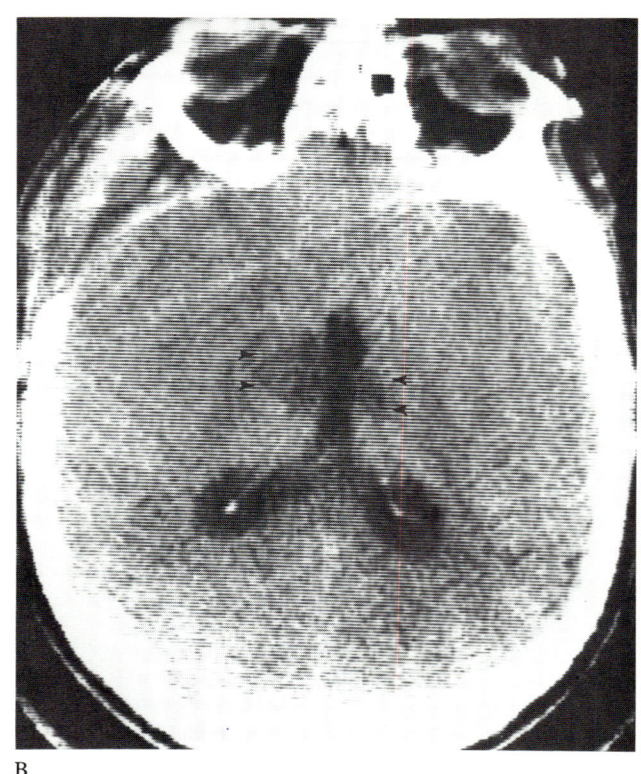

Figure 161-9 *A.* Selective left vertebral angiogram, subtraction print, shows an irregularly marginated basilar artery aneurysm (*arrowheads*). *B.* Computed tomogram following successful aneurysm surgery shows areas of decreased density in the right and left thalami, representing thalamic infarctions (*arrowheads*).

topsy series, or autopsy series with selective injection of the arteries at the base of the skull with x-ray analysis and microdissection.[10] Estimates as low as 8 percent and as high as 20 percent have been recorded based on these differing analyses. It is not unreasonable to expect the incidence of congenital aneurysms to approach 15 percent. Etiologically, there is a definite relationship between atherosclerosis and aneurysm formation. Aneurysms are also seen in the presence of developmental anomalies such as polycystic kidneys, aortic coarctation, fibromuscular dysplasia, and lupus erythematosus. The precise statistic as to which is the most common location of an intracerebral aneurysm also depends on the investigator being quoted. In the opinion of Taveras and Wood, middle cerebral artery aneurysms are most common, with posterior communicating artery aneurysms second in frequency and anterior communicating artery aneurysms third.[18] Up to 20 percent of aneurysms are multiple. Bilateral middle cerebral artery bifurcation and posterior communicating artery aneurysms are often symmetrical.

Atherosclerotic

Atherosclerotic aneurysms also occur at the base of the brain and are most common on the basilar artery, where they may block the outlet of the third ventricle and produce hydro-cephalus. They can occur on the internal carotid artery as well. The vessel involved with the atherosclerotic aneurysm is usually uniformly enlarged, somewhat irregular, tortuous, and elongated.[11] Atherosclerotic aneurysms seldom produce subarachnoid hemorrhage but more often present as masses, producing cranial nerve deficits and in some instances even mimicking extra-axial brain tumors.

Infectious

Infectious (mycotic) aneurysms represent approximately 6 percent of all intracranial aneurysms. They usually involve peripheral branches. They may produce an infected hematoma by bleeding into either the brain or the subdural space.[16]

Traumatic

Traumatic aneurysms are usually secondary to blunt trauma to the skull and result when a spicule of bone in a depressed skull fracture lacerates an adjacent cortical branch of the middle cerebral artery. They may occur on the pericallosal artery where it lies adjacent to the rigid falx (Fig. 161-11).[17] Rarely, penetrating skull trauma may result in laceration of

Radiology of Intracranial Aneurysms

1351

A

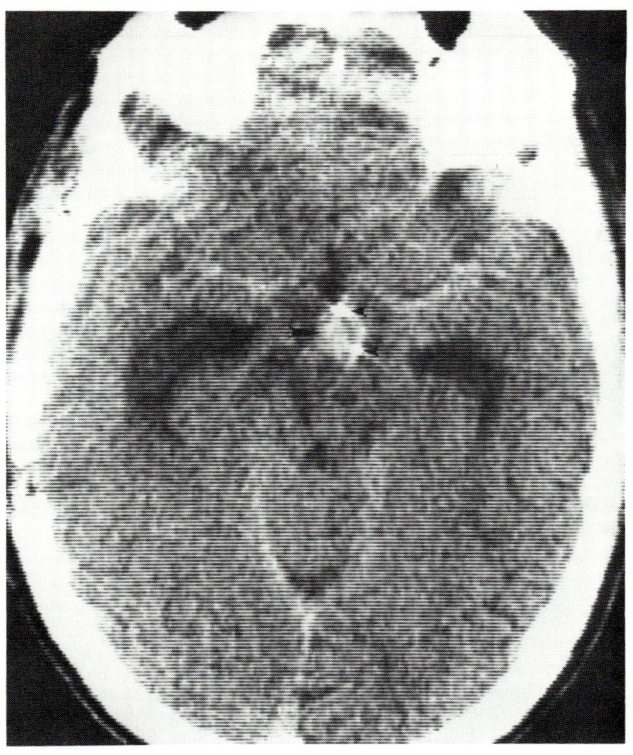

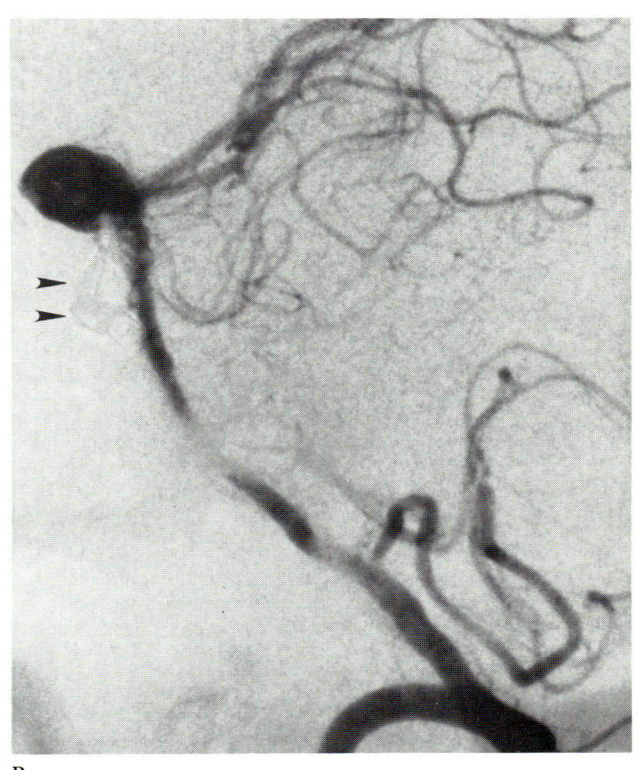

B

Figure 161-10 *A.* Enhanced thin-section high-resolution CT scan performed following basilar artery aneurysm surgery shows persistent filling of a basilar artery aneurysm (*large arrowhead*). Two small metallic densities adjacent to the aneurysm are tips of the aneurysm clip (*small arrowheads*). *B.* Selective left vertebral angiogram, lateral view, subtraction print, shows persistence of the basilar artery aneurysm. The misplaced aneurysm clip is seen adjacent to the aneurysm (*arrowheads*).

a cerebral vessel, producing a false aneurysm. Many of these lesions are associated with an adjacent intracerebral hematoma or cerebral edema.

Neoplastic

Neoplastic aneurysms have been reported in patients with metastatic atrial myxoma and choriocarcinoma. Infectious, traumatic, and neoplastic aneurysms are rare and may be suspected on the basis of clinical information. While they may rarely be centrally located, more often than not they lie peripherally in the distribution of the middle cerebral artery and can be easily identified on magnified subtracted cerebral angiograms. If the lesions are large, they may be seen on contrast-enhanced CT scans.[16]

Giant

Giant aneurysms by definition must be greater than 2.5 cm in greatest diameter. They represent 5 percent of all verified aneurysms. They most often present clinically as intracranial masses with focal neurological signs. Lower cranial nerve deficits occur with posterior fossa giant aneurysms

(Fig. 161-12). There are two types of giant aneurysms, *globoid* and *serpentine*. The globoid are thought to be large examples of the more commonly seen small saccular aneurysms. They are congenital lesions with a defective internal elastic membrane and may contain either a central or an eccentric thrombus within their lumen with circumferential flow about the thrombus. By distinction, the serpentine subgroup, also called *fusiform*, shows a snakelike vascular channel surrounded by a large thrombus. This variety should not be confused with diffuse arterial ectasia, in which a tortuous vessel with an enlarged lumen is present but without mass effect or thrombus (Fig. 161-6). The serpentine variety does not necessarily occur at arterial bifurcations and is not associated with atherosclerosis. It is most common on the middle cerebral artery. An arteriovenous malformation should not be confused with the serpentine aneurysm as there are no early filling veins present. The etiology of serpentine giant aneurysms is not certain. They may be expansions of smaller saccular aneurysms or may arise by a different pathological process and represent a congenitally different subgroup.

The characteristic plain radiographic findings in giant aneurysms include calcification and bony erosion. The calcification seen in approximately 18 percent of proven giant aneurysms may be either curvilinear, ringlike, or even shell-

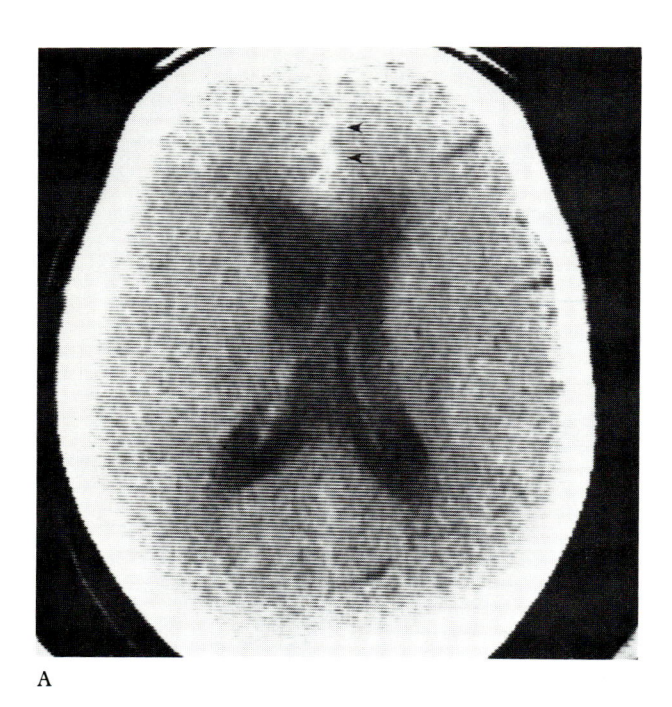

Figure 161-11 *A.* Unenhanced CT scan shows subarachnoid hemorrhage in the interhemispheric fissure (*arrowheads*). *B.* Left carotid angiogram, lateral view, subtraction print, shows a small pericallosal artery aneurysm (*arrowheads*) with marked spasm of the adjacent pericallosal and callosomarginal arteries.

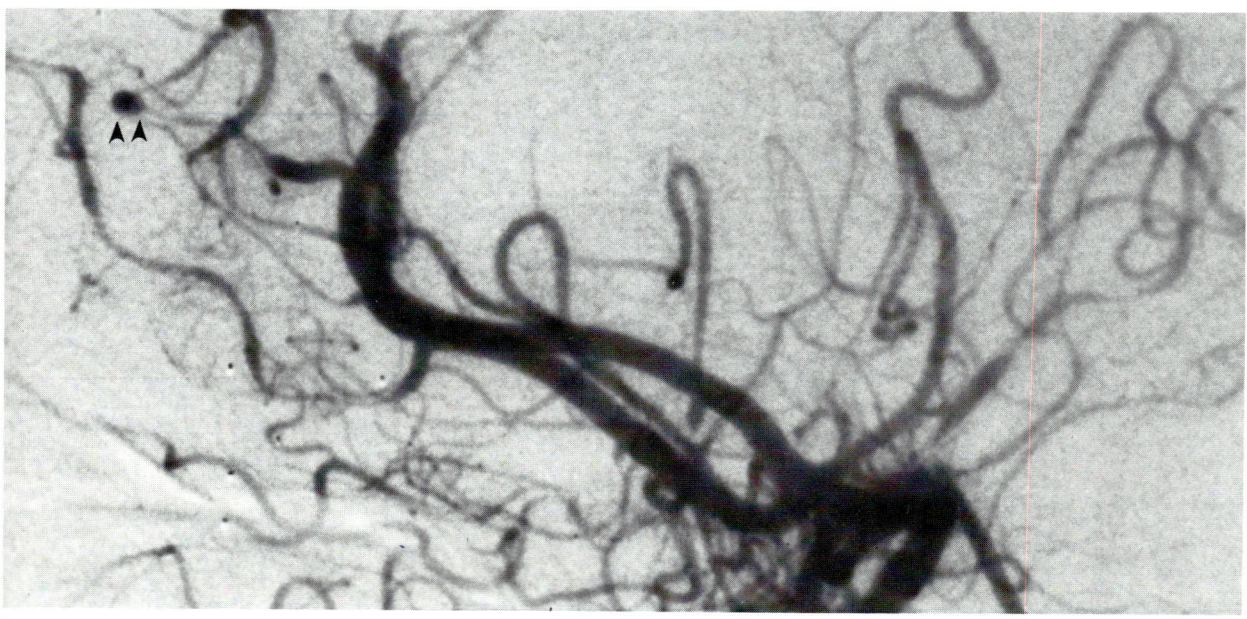

like but is usually thinner than that seen with intracranial tumors. In an additional 18 percent of cases the plain films will show bone erosion. This erosion may involve the petrous bone, the floor of the middle cranial fossa, the sella turcica, the anterior clinoid, or even the superior orbital fissure. Although bone erosion is not a specific finding for giant intracranial aneurysms, it should be carefully looked for and properly documented.

The CT findings of giant aneurysms will vary depending whether the lumen of the aneurysm is totally patent, partially thrombosed, or completely thrombosed. In the completely patent giant aneurysm the nonenhanced CT scan will show a round or oval mass of slightly increased density (as compared with the adjacent brain), with varying amounts of calcification at its circumference. Following intravenous contrast infusion, intense enhancement of the lumen occurs. While there is intense enhancement of the aneurysm wall as well as the lumen, it usually cannot be identified separately. This rim enhancement is due to the presence of increasing numbers of adventitial vessels in the rim of the giant aneurysm. In a completely thrombosed giant aneurysm, the unenhanced CT scan usually shows an area of increased density greater than the adjacent brain, with a somewhat mottled appearance again accompanied by varying amounts of calcification at its periphery. This area of significantly increased density represents the completely clotted lumen. Following

Radiology of Intracranial Aneurysms

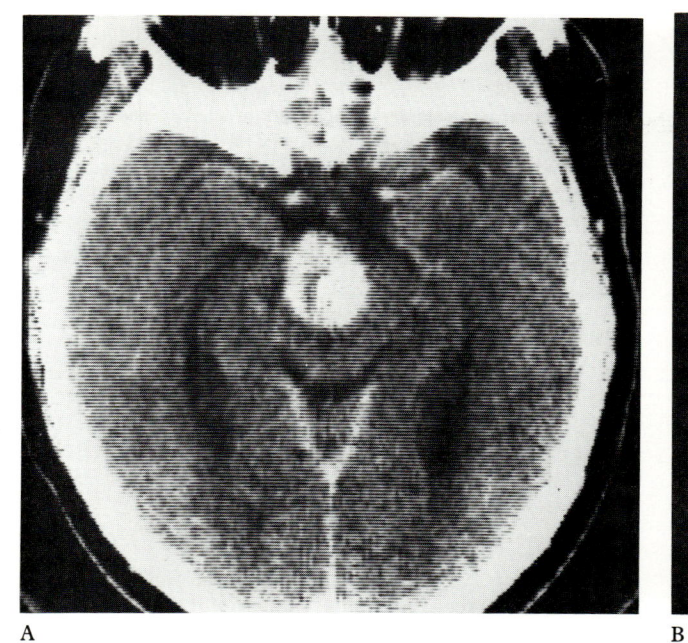

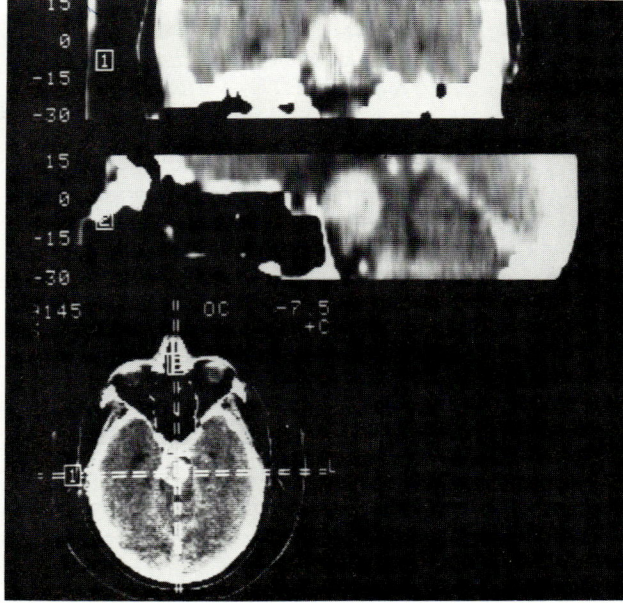

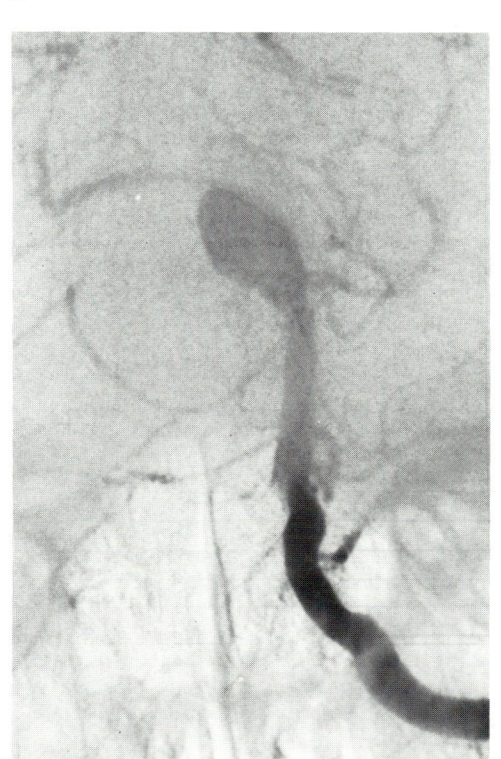

Figure 161-12 *A.* Enhanced high-resolution thin-section CT scan shows a giant basilar artery aneurysm. The area of marked enhancement is the residual lumen. The area of lesser density represents intraluminal thrombus. The markedly thickened wall of the aneurysm also enhances. *B.* Enhanced high-resolution thin-section CT scan with sagittal and coronal reformatting shows the partially thrombosed giant basilar artery aneurysm compressing the upper brain stem. *C.* Selective left vertebral angiogram, anteroposterior view, subtraction print, shows the giant basilar artery aneurysm. The mass of the aneurysm causes upward bowing of the right posterior cerebral artery and downward displacement of the right superior cerebellar artery. Only the residual lumen of the aneurysm is identified on the angiogram.

the intravenous infusion of a contrast agent, the clotted lumen is not enhanced but the richly supplied vascular wall of the giant aneurysm is well luminated. In those cases in which a partial thrombosis of a giant aneurysm has occurred, the CT appearance is more complex. The unenhanced CT study will usually show a round or oval lesion with mixed densities. There will be a central or eccentric area of significantly increased density, which is the thrombosed portion of the aneurysm surrounded or capped by a slightly less dense area (but denser than the adjacent brain), which represents the remaining patent lumen of the aneurysm. This in turn is surrounded by a peripheral zone of increased density containing variable amounts of calcification, which represents the aneurysm wall. Following intravenous contrast enhancement, the residual patent lumen intensely enhances, as does the vascular rim of the aneurysm. This has been referred to as the *target sign* and is quite specific for a partially thrombosed aneurysm on CT (Fig. 161-12).[12] As by definition giant aneurysms of the serpentine subcategory are partially thrombosed, their appearance fits into this last category.

The differential diagnosis of a giant aneurysm seen on computed tomography includes pituitary adenoma, craniopharyngioma, chordoma, germinoma, epidermoid tumor, chemodectoma, glioma, colloid cyst, choroid plexus papilloma, pinealoma, and metastasis. While angiography is usually required to make a definitive differential diagnosis, certain CT features of giant aneurysms may allow a differentiation. Little or no surrounding edema is seen on the CT scan in patients with giant intracranial aneurysms. Giant aneurysms are found almost exclusively on the circle of Willis or occur only as far distally as the proximal middle cerebral artery bifurcation. Transit time analysis of patent giant aneurysms demonstrates washin and washout phases with timing similar to that of the larger adjacent cerebral vessels. This will allow distinction from vascular tumors which do not show this washin and washout phenomenon.[12]

Bleeding Aneurysms

The criteria for determining which of multiple aneurysms has bled were established in the neuroradiological literature prior to CT scanning[19]; CT scanning has affected these criteria only minimally.[13] The most significant single criterion for concluding that a given aneurysm among several has bled is to see the aneurysm actually bleed during angiography (a rare event) or during the enhanced CT study (an even rarer event).[6] More often, the presence of a mass near or adjacent to an aneurysm indicts that aneurysm as the one having most recently bled. While classically this mass has been first detected at angiography, more recently CT scanning has disclosed the presence of even small hemorrhages adjacent to aneurysms, thereby affirming the bleeding lesion (Fig. 161-8). Much less localizing is the presence of spasm adjacent to a particular aneurysm. While it has been said that spasm localized to the vicinity of but one aneurysm strongly suggests that that aneurysm is the bleeding site, in most instances the spasm may involve several vessels having aneurysms. It is usually wise not to attempt to determine which is the offending aneurysm in the presence of severe spasm but to wait for a more complete angiographic study of all intracranial vessels after the spasm has subsided. The more irregularly shaped, larger aneurysm is usually the offender (Fig. 161-4A, B). Bleeding aneurysms are often associated with a small hematoma within their lumen (Fig. 161-4A, B). Proximity to the circle of Willis is also a consideration. Regardless of the above criteria, if an anterior communicating artery aneurysm is present, it is often the offender.

References

1. Davis JM, Davis KR, Crowell RM: Subarachnoid hemorrhage secondary to ruptured intracranial aneurysm: Prognostic significance of cranial CT. AJR 134:711–715, 1980.
2. Davis KR, Kistler JP, Heros RC, Davis JM: A neuroradiologic approach to the patient with a diagnosis of subarachnoid hemorrhage. Radiol Clin North Am 20:87–94, 1982.
3. Forster DMC, Steiner L, Hakanson S, Bergvall U: The value of repeat pan-angiography in cases of unexplained subarachnoid hemorrhage. J Neurosurg 48:712–716, 1978.
4. Handel SF, Perpetuo FOL, Handel CH: Subdural hematomas due to ruptured cerebral aneurysms: Angiographic diagnosis and potential pitfall for CT. AJR 130:507–509, 1978.
5. Inoue Y, Saiwai S, Miyamoto T, Ban S, Yamamoto T, Takemoto K, Taniguchi S, Sato S, Namba K, Ogata M: Postcontrast computed tomography in subarachnoid hemorrhage from ruptured aneurysms. J Comput Assist Tomogr 5:341–344, 1981.
6. Jordan K, Lefkowitch J, Hays A, Sane P: Rupture of intracranial aneurysm during computerized tomography. Arch Neurol 37:465–466, 1980.
7. Liliequist B, Lindqvist M: Computer tomography in the evaluation of subarachnoid hemorrhage. Acta Radiol [Diagn] (Stockh) 21:327–331, 1980.
8. Lin JP, Kricheff II: Angiographic investigation of cerebral aneurysms. Radiology 105:69–76, 1972.
9. Modesti LM, Binet EF: Value of computed tomography in the diagnosis and management of subarachnoid hemorrhage. Neurosurgery 3:151–156, 1978.
10. Newton TH, Potts DG: *Radiology of the Skull and Brain*. St Louis, CV Mosby, 1974.
11. Peterson NT, Duchesneau PM, Westbrook EL, Weinstein MA: Basilar artery ectasia demonstrated by computed tomography. Radiology 122:713–715, 1977.
12. Pinto RS, Cohen WA, Kricheff II, Redington RW, Berninger WH: Giant intracranial aneurysms: Rapid sequential computed tomography. AJNR 3:495–499, 1982.
13. Schnapf DJ: Multiple aneurysms of the intracranial arteries: Computed tomography in detecting the site of bleeding. JAOA 81:208–211, 1981.
14. Scotti G, Ethier R, Melançon D, Terbrugge K, Tchang S: Computed tomography in the evaluation of intracranial aneurysms and subarachnoid hemorrhage. Radiology 123:85–90, 1977.
15. Silver AJ, Pederson ME Jr, Ganti SR, Hilal SK, Michelson WJ: CT of subarachnoid hemorrhage due to ruptured aneurysm. AJNR 2:13–22, 1981.
16. Simmons KC, Sage MR, Reilly PL: CT of intracerebral haemorrhage due to mycotic aneurysms—case report. Neuroradiology 19:215–217, 1980.
17. Smith KR Jr, Bardenheier JA, III: Aneurysm of the pericallosal artery caused by closed cranial trauma: Case report. J Neurosurg 29:551–554, 1968.
18. Taveras JM, Wood EH: *Diagnostic Neuroradiology*, 2d ed. Baltimore, Williams & Wilkins, 1976.
19. Wood EH: Angiographic identification of the ruptured lesion in patients with multiple cerebral aneurysms. J Neurosurg 21:182–198, 1964.

162

Intracranial Arterial Spasm

Robert R. Smith
Junji Yoshioka

The Nature of Intracranial Arterial Spasm

The terms *intracranial arterial spasm* and *cerebral vasospasm* have been used to describe a radiological and clinical phenomenon that occurs after the rupture of an intracranial aneurysm and less frequently in a few other clinical settings (for example, following head trauma, after surgery in the hypothalamic-pituitary area, and following subarachnoid hemorrhage due to a cause other than a ruptured aneurysm). Intracranial arterial spasm was first described as an arteriographic finding.[11] After the rupture of an intracranial aneurysm, narrowing of short (focal vasospasm) or long segments (diffuse vasospasm) of one or more intracranial arteries may be seen by arteriography. It is rare to see such changes within the first 48 h after a patient's first subarachnoid hemorrhage. The radiographic changes are ordinarily delayed in onset and are most frequent and most striking during the second week after the hemorrhage. More than 35 percent of patients with a ruptured intracranial aneurysm will exhibit such intracranial arterial narrowing, especially during the second week. A patient who has a significant amount of blood in the basal subarachnoid cisterns as shown by a CT scan performed within a few days after the aneurysm rupture usually will then develop arterial narrowing as shown arteriographically. In contrast, the patient without this finding on the initial CT scan is unlikely to subsequently develop arterial narrowing.

Such narrowing is an intradural phenomenon and affects the intradural portions of the internal carotid arteries (and less frequently the intradural portions of the vertebral arteries) while ordinarily sparing the extradural portions of these vessels. Intracranial arterial spasm affects the anterior intracranial circulation [especially the distal internal carotid and proximal anterior and middle cerebral arteries (Fig. 162-1)] more than the posterior circulation, which is usually not involved to a noticeable degree unless the ruptured aneurysm is on the posterior circulation. Once radiographic evidence of intracranial arterial spasm has developed, it ordinarily resolves gradually over one to a few weeks.

It has been known for many years that patients who experience the rupture of an intracranial aneurysm may subsequently develop clinical and pathological evidence of one or more cerebral infarcts. Such delayed neurological deficits have been presumed to be due to the delayed development of intracranial arterial spasm (symptomatic vasospasm). The basic concept therefore arose that the initial deposition of blood in the subarachnoid spaces around the circle of Willis caused by the rupture of an aneurysm induces the delayed constriction of these arteries, perhaps owing to a factor or factors liberated from the clotted blood, and that the arterial constriction then leads to cerebral ischemia and infarction.

This basic idea still is pertinent today, but there have been many confusing discrepancies discovered. For example, the mere presence of blood in the subarachnoid spaces at the base of the human brain may not provoke the radiological and/or clinical syndrome of intracranial arterial spasm. Furthermore, there is no animal model that accurately mimics what happens in the human patient who develops the syndrome. The introduction of blood into the basal cisterns of animals, even with concomitant arterial injury, ordinarily causes immediate arterial constriction (which has not been shown to occur in humans) and only a minor delayed arterial constriction with no cerebral infarction or delayed neurological deficits.

At the extremes of the spectrum (i.e., severe aneurysm rupture, resulting in a large amount of subarachnoid blood and leading to severe diffuse cerebral vasospasm and delayed neurological deficits, or a mild rupture with little subarachnoid blood and no delayed deficits) correlations can be made among the degree of subarachnoid hemorrhage, degree and distribution of arteriographic vasospasm, cerebral blood flow values, clinical status and outcome, and pathological evidence of cerebral infarction. Yet when patients are considered in groups or when individual patients have a subarachnoid hemorrhage of moderate severity, such correlations may not exist. This indicates that the entry of blood into the subarachnoid cisterns may be only one of several events that must occur simultaneously or in sequence to cause cerebral vasospasm and that such vasospasm is only one of several factors (such as cardiac output, rate, and rhythm; blood viscosity and pressure; collateral routes of circulation; intracranial pressure) that together determine the actual regional cerebral blood flow and hence whether the patient will develop symptoms and signs of cerebral ischemia and infarction.

There is even more confusion when one further considers the nature, etiology, and pathogenesis of the intracranial arterial narrowing seen angiographically and called vasospasm. According to definition, a spasm is a sudden but transitory contraction of a muscle or group of muscles that occurs involuntarily. Such a reaction can be produced in cerebral arterial smooth muscle by both chemical and mechanical stimulation. There is, however, little evidence to link the brief transitory constriction of the cerebral artery that can be produced in the laboratory with the complex series of clinical and radiographic events that occur in humans following rupture of an intracranial aneurysm. It is unfortunate that the observed constriction of surface pial arteries in response to mechanical and electrical stimulation elegantly shown by Florey[15] and Echlin[8] would be linked to the cerebral infarction that develops as late as 3 weeks after

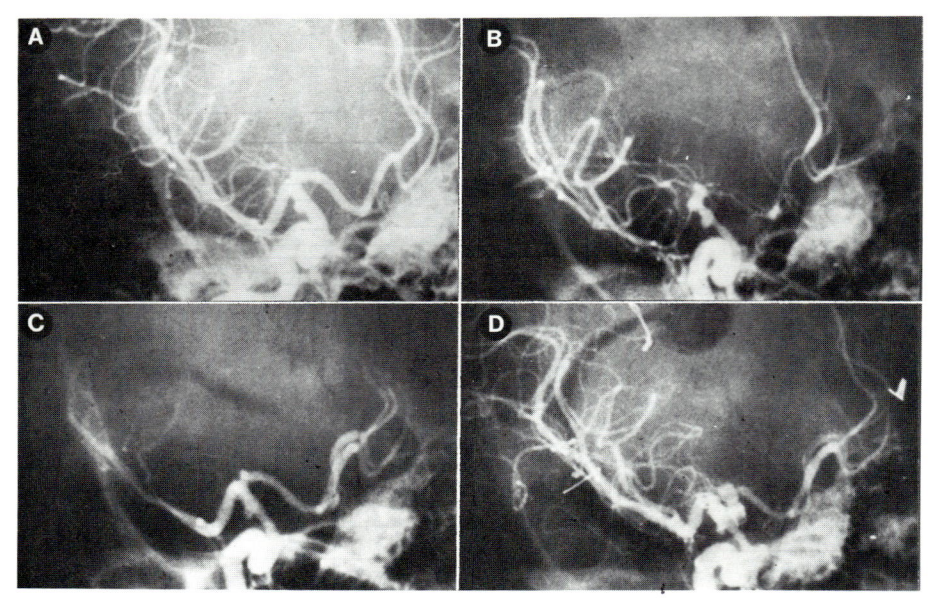

Figure 162-1 Comparable oblique view from four sets of right carotid arteriograms of a 27-year-old woman with three aneurysms of the internal carotid artery, one of which had ruptured: *A.* One day after subarachnoid hemorrhage (SAH), the patient was alert with headache. *B.* Seven days later the patient was drowsy and hemiplegic; diffuse vasospasm is present (primarily affecting the intradural portion of the internal carotid artery and the proximal portions of the anterior and middle cerebral arteries); the aneurysms, which have no smooth muscle layer, are not constricted and are more apparent. *C.* At 30 days after SAH, the patient was alert and hemiparetic; the vasospasm is resolving. *D.* At 45 days after SAH and 1 day after aneurysm clipping, the patient was alert and hemiparetic; some residual vasospasm is still present. (From Weir BKA: The effect of vasospasm on morbidity and mortality after subarachnoid hemorrhage from ruptured aneurysm, in Wilkins RH (ed): *Cerebral Arterial Spasm.* Baltimore, Williams & Wilkins, 1980, pp 385–393.)

aneurysm rupture. Convincing evidence has never been presented that long-lasting or propagated spasm due to involuntary constriction of cerebral arterial smooth muscles actually occurs.

Ecker and Riemenschneider first called attention to angiographic narrowing of cerebral arteries after aneurysm rupture and concluded that traction on the wall was probably the responsible mechanism.[11] Later, Echlin showed that if fresh blood was applied directly to the adventitia of the exposed basilar artery, marked vasospasm resulted.[9] Serotonin and a number of blood-related products produce a similar reaction although perhaps not as forceful as that caused by blood. The constriction is usually of short duration and a delayed phase associated with neurological deficit has not been shown following direct application of blood to cerebral vessels.

Clinical studies applied to large groups of patients suggest that the "vasospasm complex" may be delayed. Although angiographic constriction may be seen as early as 1 day after aneurysm rupture, in the majority of cases it tends to appear at the beginning of the second week and to last for days or weeks. A number of hypotheses have been offered to explain the onset latency. The concept that a substance might be released by the lysis of blood has been proposed. Initial evidence seemed confirmatory. Blood left in a test tube for 1 week to 12 days has been shown to cause marked spasm when applied to the basilar artery.[10] Kapp et al. isolated a fraction from feline blood serum that could cause marked constriction when applied to the outer wall of the artery.[20] Most surgeons, however, readily affirm that blood or blood clot in contact with a major cerebral artery does not invoke the vasospasm complex and that the condition, although perhaps encountered rarely in cases of intracranial hemorrhage of other causes, is essentially one associated with aneurysm rupture.

The denervation hypersensitivity concept was brought forward by Fraser et al.[17] and Peerless and Yasargil[30]. These investigators showed that experimental subarachnoid hemorrhage was followed by depletion of catecholamines in perivascular nerves and vesicles. Further, the application of phenoxybenzamine, a long-acting alpha-receptor blocking agent, reversed the constriction produced by the topical application of blood. In essence, the empty receptors lie unprotected and sensitized to catecholamines, which are known to be elevated in the circulating blood of patients with ruptured aneurysms. Unfortunately, while acute vasoconstriction may be favorably influenced by alpha blocking agents, the recurrent phase (of clinical importance) is unaffected by these agents.

The possibility that prostaglandin $F2_{\alpha}$, a potent vasoconstrictor, may be involved in vasospasm was first proposed by Robertson[32] and co-workers. It appears that extremely high

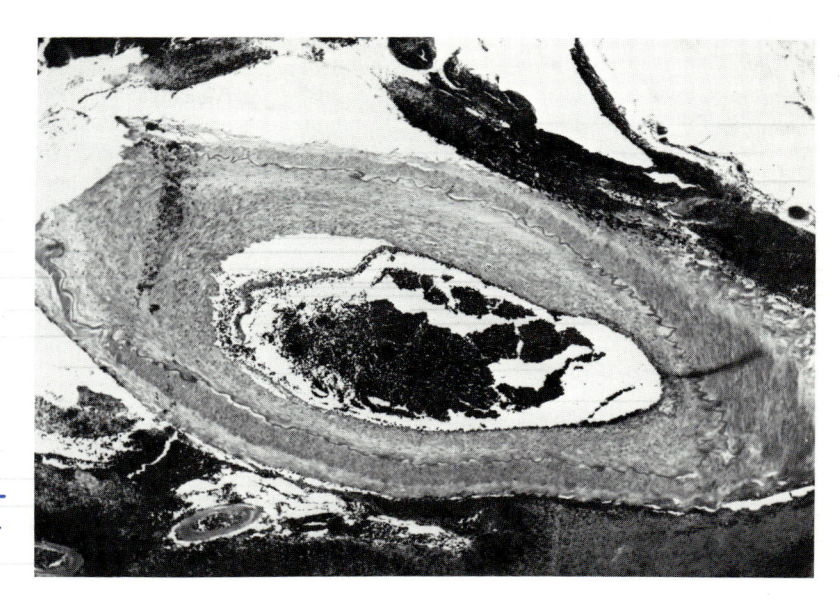

Figure 162-2 Cross section of an intracranial artery. There is thickening of the layer between the internal elastic membrane and the endothelium due to smooth muscle cell migration and proliferation.

concentrations would be required to produce intense constriction, and such levels seem out of the question.

A number of workers have recently emphasized the morphological aspects of the vasospasm complex. Thickening and subintimal proliferation associated with myonecrosis of arteries can be seen in many individuals after aneurysm rupture (Fig. 162-2). Similar findings have been associated with severe head injury and the inference can be made that the changes are due to vessel injury. The primary difference in the pathology of vessels associated with subarachnoid hemorrhage and that seen after injury due to other causes is the diffuse nature and apparent propagation of the arterial wall damage. The lesion has been compared histologically with that seen with peripheral vasospastic disorders such as Buerger's disease. The principal fact that detracts from the morphological hypothesis is that until recently the changes have been described quite late in the course of subarachnoid hemorrhage, weeks and months after its occurrence. Also, the magnitude of vascular thickening has not been sufficient to explain the radiographic appearance seen in premortem angiography. Protagonists of the morphological hypothesis, however, emphasize that the vessel wall becomes rigid and loses compliance to elastic expansion much earlier, before the florid changes can be observed with a light microscope.[7] Apparently, smooth muscle cells penetrate into the subintimal layer and may be in a functional state in this site to promote the vasoconstriction. The cause of the diffuse vascular injury associated with subarachnoid hemorrhage has been the subject of several studies but no definitive answers have yet appeared. Intramural hemorrhage has been a feature of the more pronounced cases. In addition, the possibility that norepinephrine or serotonin released by platelets may be the factor promoting structural changes has been raised by Kapp et al.[21] In a few cases, at least, the constrictive endarteriopathy that develops after aneurysm rupture may be responsible for the radiographic appearance seen late, in the second and third weeks after aneurysm rupture, and may be related to the cerebral infarction observed.[38]

Zervas et al. have questioned the metabolic pathways of cerebral vascular smooth muscle.[46] Apparently there are no vasa vasorum along intracranial arteries to nourish the multiple layers of smooth muscle cells found in the media. The source of nutrients for this layer has not been identified but Zervas and co-workers, using the horseradish peroxidase method, have demonstrated crypts connecting the subarachnoid space to the muscular layer. The effect of subarachnoid hemorrhage on these delicate communicating channels and the relationship to diffuse vascular injury has been questioned.

Innervation of Intracranial Vessels

Brain vessels are unique in that innervation plays little role in the control and regulation of blood flow. The minimal effect of sympathetic stimulation was first demonstrated in Forbes' laboratory in 1938.[16] The conclusive evidence for a well-developed sympathetic nerve supply was developed by use of fluorescent methods in humans in 1976.[13] A rich adrenergic plexus of nerves is placed delicately upon the arteries and arterioles of the brain but does not seem to penetrate into the medial layer. A plexus of nerves follows the arteries into the parenchyma along the penetrating arterioles. Nelson and Rennels noted that vessels containing only two layers of muscle cells were also supplied by nerves containing adrenergic vesicles.[28]

The origin of the perivascular neural plexus has been a subject of much concern. It appears that the larger basal vessels, including the carotid artery, the middle cerebral artery, and the basilar artery, are supplied, in part at least, by the superior cervical ganglion. However, most of the brain arterioles and capillaries are innervated by central axon terminals, perhaps associated with cranial nerves.

A rich cholinergic innervation of the cerebrovascular bed has also been demonstrated[12]; these nerve fibers do not accompany intracerebral vessels. In addition, a third type of fiber containing a vasoactive intestinal polypeptide was recently found among the perivascular nerves of the brain by immunochemical techniques.[25] This peptide is known to be vasodilatory in intestinal vessels. Cervical ganglionectomy causes no change in these sparse structures, and thus their origin is still unknown. There may also be histamine receptors, 5-HIAA receptors, and dopamine receptors on cerebral vessels. In physiological concentrations, histamine causes vasodilatation, serotonin causes marked vasoconstriction, and dopamine produces a dilatory response. In addition to alpha receptors, both β_1- and β_2-adrenergic receptors have been demonstrated on the cerebral vessels. There may be species variability, however.

The Pharmacology of Smooth Muscle Contraction

The numerous factors involved in smooth muscle activity have come to light recently. Neurotransmitters, transmembrane mechanisms, and calcium flux all play important parts in smooth muscle contraction. The cyclic nucleotides also are vital in the relaxation of vascular smooth muscle as an energy substrate. Adenyl cyclase, an enzyme bound to the cell membrane, is activated by beta-adrenergic stimulation. Upon stimulation, cyclic adenosine monophosphate (cAMP) is converted into two fractions within the cell, each of which has a distinct role (Fig. 162-3). A cytoplasmic fraction activates protein kinase, which in turn activates the phosphorylase system, leading to the conversion of glycogen to glucose-1-phosphate. Energy-rich adenosine triphosphate and creatine phosphate are thus produced. The microsomal fraction ultimately binds calcium to protein. This binding of the ionic calcium causes relaxation of the actin and myosin filaments of vascular smooth muscle cells.

Guanyl cyclase, which is also a membrane-bound enzyme, is activated by the alpha receptor agent and catalyzes reaction of guanosine triphosphate. Its product, cyclic guanosine monophosphate (cGMP), leads to increased permeability of the cell membrane to ionic calcium and initiates contraction of the actin and myosin filaments. Thus, these two enzymes have opposite roles, effected through calcium binding to relax or constrict the smooth muscle cell. Activation of the cAMP system and inhibition of the cGMP system causes smooth muscle cells to relax. The opposite reaction causes them to constrict. Stimulation of cAMP can be achieved with salbutamol, a β_2-adrenergic drug. The phosphodiesterase system can be effectively inhibited with aminophylline. Unfortunately, neither of these agents has proved consistently effective in relieving vasospasm, and their use has been largely abandoned.

Ultimately, it is the calcium influx through the cell membrane and the binding of the actin and myosin compound that results in active constriction. Through Bohr's work it is now clear that this calcium influx into the cell is closely regulated by norepinephrine and the adrenergic receptor[5] (Fig. 162-3). There is, however, great variability among arteries of different vascular beds. Calcium antagonism reduces constriction of the coronary arteries, for instance, but has little effect upon the aorta. Likewise, in Prinzmetal's angina, caused by sympathetic stimulation, the pain is effectively relieved by nifedipine, a calcium blocker.

Clinical Events

The appearance of vasospasm after aneurysm rupture may exert a crucial influence on morbidity and mortality. There are a number of ways that the diagnosis may be established but angiographic demonstration is critical. Various studies using radiographic criteria have indicated that between 35 and 60 percent of patients with ruptured aneurysms show

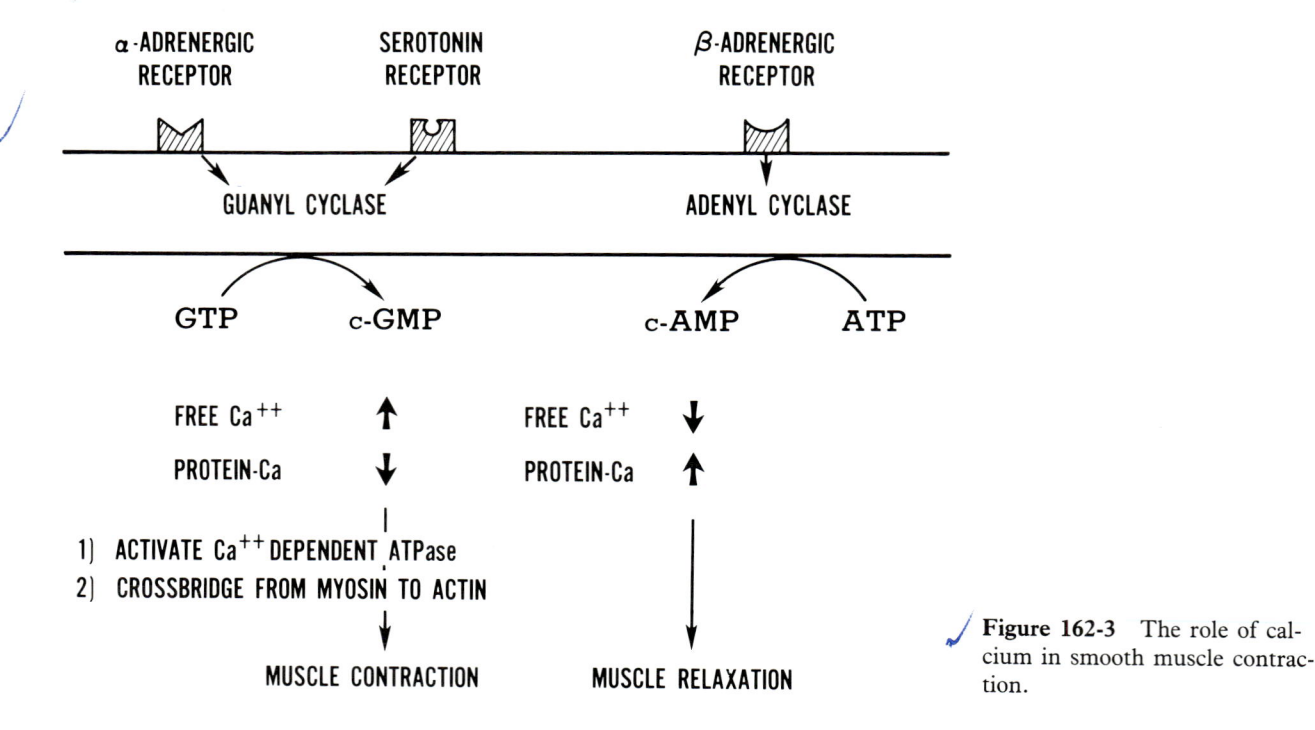

Figure 162-3 The role of calcium in smooth muscle contraction.

constriction at some time in their course and probably more frequently postoperatively. Early angiography may fail to demonstrate the process, which usually begins in the second posthemorrhage week. In the Saito and Sano series, in no case was vasospasm identified before the fifth day and the latest appearance was on the sixteenth day.[35] The exact location of a supratentorial aneurysm seems to have little influence on the development of vasospasm, although it is perhaps more often recognized in patients who are in better neurological condition at the outset. Contraction reaches its greatest intensity from 4 to 6 days after onset or 10 to 12 days after subarachnoid hemorrhage. It often migrates from the proximal to the distal segments. Weir found no cases of vasospasm in 106 patients studied within 24 h of their subarachnoid hemorrhage.[43] Thus, there is little radiographic evidence to support a biphasic component of the vasospasm complex.

The clinical manifestations are: (1) increasing headaches, (2) increasing nuchal rigidity, (3) increasing lethargy, (4) deteriorating neurological status, (5) low-grade fever, and (6) anhydrosis. The fever has been attributed to blood in the cerebrospinal fluid, defective hypothalamic heat loss mechanisms, and failure of peripheral sweat glands.[18,33] Often there are focal changes in the electroencephalogram, and characteristically these consist of slowing in the wave pattern, which correlates well anatomically with the radiographic picture. Focal hematomas, however, may produce an identical pattern.[34] Cerebral blood flow (CBF) has been measured in both clinical and experimental subarachnoid hemorrhage. While there is nothing specifically diagnostic about CBF, in some cases flow is diminished considerably and in others there is apparent autoregulatory failure. The reduction in CBF to about half the normal value is usually accompanied by an unsatisfactory outcome.[31]

Cerebral infarction is not an invariable accompaniment of cerebral vasospasm, although immediately after rupture increased intracranial pressure reduces perfusion pressure. Cerebral infarction can thus occur in the absence of demonstrated arteriographic vasoconstriction. There may be systemic manifestations of cerebral vasospasm.[24] In a small series of patients studied at our center, there was evidence of loss of peripheral sympathetic function concomitant with a tremendous decrease in serum dopamine beta-hydroxylase activity.[18] The disorders were manifested clinically by depressed levels of consciousness and supersensitivity to catecholamines peripherally. This can be best demonstrated by placing one drop of 0.5% epinephrine into the conjunctival sac. Normally, 0.5% epinephrine causes no reaction. In the sympathetic depleted state after subarachnoid hemorrhage, the pupils dilate maximally, apparently because the alpha receptors of the iris are not saturated.

The significance of angiographic vasospasm has been rightfully questioned. Millikan found essentially no difference in the clinical condition of those patients who showed angiographic vasospasm and those who did not.[26] Likewise, there was no influence of vasospasm on mortality. Many others do not share this view. In the series of Fisher et al., virtually all patients who showed severe vasospasm on angiography also developed severe ischemic deficits.[14] The latter view probably more adequately expresses neurosurgical opinion.

Ancillary diagnostic tests may be helpful in predicting vasospasm. Although the actual measurement of subarachnoid blood from the CT scan is limited, estimations can be quite valuable. For patients who show no blood in the subarachnoid space on the CT scan, almost 70 percent never develop vasospasm. On the other hand, localized blood clots in the subarachnoid space or layers of blood 1 mm or more in thickness are almost universally associated with cerebral vasospasm.[14] In cases in which there is intracerebral or intraventricular blood there may or may not be vasospasm. Symon et al. also reported increasingly poor results based on the density of the blood within the subarachnoid space.[39] When high-density material filled the subarachnoid space, almost one-fourth of the patients died or were disabled. An elevated lactate value in the ventricular fluid is an excellent indicator of cerebral hypoxia and vasospasm. Levels greater than 2 mmol per liter are usually associated with severe vasospasm and a poor outcome.

Postoperative vasospasm is a subject about which even less can be certain. The clinical onset occurs within 10 h after operation and angiographic changes are usually apparent. In some cases, however, there is little narrowing of the major vessels. Usually the syndrome is associated with high intracranial pressure, greater than 25 mmHg. Presumably, this is due to ischemia and edema.[1] Basically, the patient fails to awaken from anesthesia quickly, the vessels show narrowing on the first angiogram, and the intracranial pressure is greater than 15 mmHg. Whether surgery activates this type of vasospasm is not yet clear. It is, however, difficult to ignore the time relationship of the phenomenon itself to the operation.

Prevention and Treatment

Zervas et al.[45] first observed that vasospasm could be prevented in monkeys and dogs by drugs designed to lower the levels of active monamines such as serotonin and norepinephrine in the brain and circulating blood. Reserpine and kanamycin were initially used, and on the basis of success a randomized study was carried out on a small number of patients at the Massachusetts General Hospital. Ischemic deficits developed in 12 percent of the treated, as opposed to 39 percent of the untreated patients. However, Blumenkopf et al. were unable to show any benefit of the method.[4] Though not infallible, perhaps it does no harm. From our own laboratory experience, reserpine appears to inhibit the exuberance of the reaction caused by vascular injury, and the constrictive endarteriopathy is lessened in magnitude. Apparently the agent functions by inhibiting the migration of smooth muscle cells into the subintimal layer via its effect on platelet serotonin.

The possibility that calcium blocking agents, such as nifedipine and nimodipine, might be effective in causing vascular smooth muscle relaxation is currently being tested. Both these drugs inhibit the influx of extracellular calcium into the smooth muscle cell. In vitro both are effective in preventing the contraction of isolated arteries. Unfortunately, the water content of the brain in treated animals increases significantly, perhaps owing to increased blood flow.[40] Auer et al. administered nimodipine topically through a plastic cannula into the basal cisterns and by continuous infusion.[3] Dilatation was found in all observed vessel treated intraoperatively. It is of significance that one patient treated with nimodipine developed vasoconstriction and neurological deterioration postoperatively, which was not influenced by intracisternal nimodipine. Although the latter agent has been shown to preferentially affect cerebral vascular beds, systemic reactions such as bradycardia and hypotension are regularly described.[40]

The recently discovered vasodilator prostacyclin may have a role in the treatment of symptomatic vasospasm.[6] Prostacyclin synthetase has been demonstrated in human isolated cerebral arteries. Prostacyclin dilates cerebral arteries predictably but its life cycle is short, in the order of seconds (Fig. 162-4). Recently, it has been used in vitro to dilate vasospastic arteries. The major actions of prostacyclin, which is synthesized in the vessel wall, is inhibition of platelet aggregation and promotion of dilatation. This effect may be augmented by drugs such as dipyridamole, which blocks phosphodiesterase and mimics the effect of prostacyclin.

On the other hand, thromboxane A_2 (TXA2) released from platelets counteracts prostacyclin, promoting platelet aggregation and vascular constriction. Both prostacyclin and TXA2 are synthesized from cyclic endoperoxides (prostaglandin G2 and H2), mainly in endothelial cells of the vessel wall and platelet, respectively, and have been suggested to be important for maintaining peripheral blood flow. Prostacyclin synthesis may diminish in the cerebral artery after experimental subarachnoid hemorrhage, causing a disproportionate increased synthesis of TXA2 (mainly a platelet factor). In order to correct this disproportionate synthesis of TXA2, TXA2 inhibitor(s) might be useful. Imidazole[27] and pyridine[41] have been reported to inhibit synthesis of TXA2. Recently, a pyridine derivative, OKY-1581 [sodium-(E)-3-(4(3-pyridylmethyl)phenyl)-2-methyl-2-propenoate], was found effective in experimental vasospasm[36] and a cooperative study of this agent is currently being planned for aneurysm patients in Japan.

Wilkins has reviewed all agents that have been used to prevent the development of or to relieve intracranial arterial spasm.[44] Over 80 agents have been employed and none has produced consistently uniform success. Indeed, it may be questioned whether any are useful in dilating the constricted arterial muscle at which they are aimed. Investigators who use certain drug combinations have had other goals in mind. Phenylephrine constricts the peripheral beds, while sodium nitroprusside is used to release cerebrovascular contraction.[2] This combination has produced mixed results. The combination of alpha-blocking (phentolamine) and beta-blocking (propranolol) agents is an interesting combination that has been employed in 100 patients in a continuing clinical trial. At present, the results have been more favorable in females, whereas in males untreated patients have fared somewhat better.[42] At present, no conclusions can be drawn about this regimen.

Hydrocortisone in high doses apparently suppresses the activity of vasoconstrictive nerves, but again in human cases the effect has been inconsistent.[19] Kassell et al. have presented preliminary studies on the use of barbiturates in reducing intracranial pressure associated with ischemia and vasospasm. Overall, 10 of the 11 patients included in these studies died, which does not generate a great deal of enthusiasm for the method.[23] Barbiturate coma, in general, has been associated with a high complication rate in our hands, largely attributable to the loss of clinical markers so necessary to good neurosurgical care.

Hypervolemia and induced arterial hypertension have been recently advocated as a therapy for patients with vasospasm.[23] Needless to say, the method is best suited to patients whose aneurysms have been successfully clipped. It is

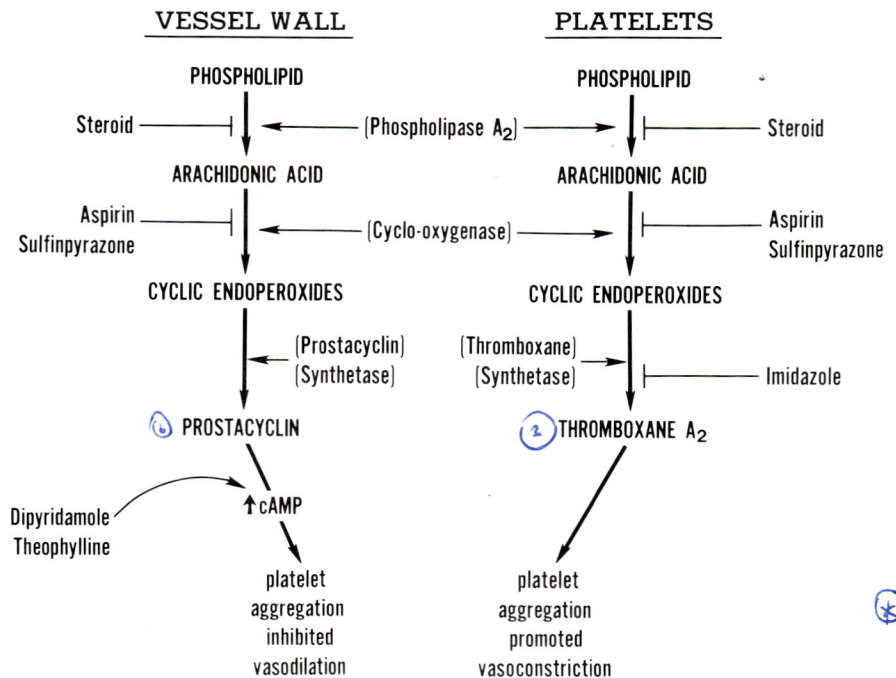

Figure 162-4 Factors influencing constriction and relaxation of vascular smooth muscle.

also necessary to monitor continuously systemic arterial pressure, central venous pressure (CVP), pulmonary wedge pressure, intracranial pressure, hemoglobin and hematocrit, electrolytes, osmolarities, blood gases, fluid balance, and cardiac function. Crystalloid solutions must be infused to maintain serum electrolytes at a normal level. Arterial pressure may be elevated by using dopamine. Arterial lines must be used for continuous monitoring and recording of blood pressure. The intravascular volume may be expanded by use of whole blood, packed cells, plasma fractionate, albumin, or low-molecular-weight dextran. The latter agent may be associated with coagulation abnormalities. Fludrocortisone and vasopressin may be used to assist in maintaining the hypervolemia/hypertension, and atropine may be used to counteract the vagal depressor effect caused by the hypervolemia and hypertension. The CVP should be elevated to 10 to 17 mmH$_2$O while cardiac function is monitored carefully with continuous ECG recordings. Among 58 patients so treated, 43 were said to be permanently improved. On the other hand, the regimen was started at the first sign of any neurological regression and the natural history of this group of minimally affected individuals is not known. There are theoretical limitations to hypervolemia and hypertension. In the presence of defective autoregulation or infarction, cerebral edema might be considerably affected. Kassell et al. recorded that pulmonary edema and aneurysmal rebleeding complicated hypervolemia-hypertensive treatment in 17 and 19 percent, respectively, in their series.[23]

It is unlikely that hypervolemic therapy would be of any lasting benefit in a patient with constrictive endarteropathy. Ultimately, infarcts in the territory of the affected vessel are likely if blood flow is reduced significantly. The treatment, however, may have merit in the early case, especially if the aneurysm has been clipped and if there is no evidence of infarction clinically or on the basis of CT scanning.

Proponents of the "something in the blood" theory contend that bleeding within the subarachnoid space precipitates vasospasm and that the volume of blood present determines the course of the disorder and predicts clinical outcome. Removal of this clot from the subarachnoid space early should, logically, be the most effective preventative of the disorder.[37] Preliminary surveys indicated that it is not always possible to remove the greatest portion of the clot. Early operation, on the other hand, does not seem to aggravate spasm and in some cases seems to prevent its development. Ohta et al. observed that extensive clot evacuation within 48 h after the onset of subarachnoid hemorrhage did not prevent the development of vasospasm but may have reduced the severity of it.[29] There is little question, however, that excessive clot evacuation seems to worsen brain swelling and sometimes leads to the development of hematomas.

References

1. Adams CBT: Postoperative vasospasm after aneurysm surgery, in Wilkins RH (ed): *Cerebral Arterial Spasm*. Baltimore, Williams and Wilkins, 1980, pp 433–434.
2. Allen GS: Cerebral arterial spasm: Update on treatment of delayed ischemic neurological deficits with sodium nitroprusside and phenylephrine, in Wilkins RH (ed): *Cerebral Arterial Spasm*. Baltimore, Williams & Wilkins, 1980, pp 589–590.
3. Auer LM, Ito Z, Suzuki A, Ohta H: Prevention of symptomatic vasospasm by topically applied nimodipine. Acta Neurochir (Wien) 63:297–302, 1982.
4. Blumenkopf B, Wilkins RH, Feldman JM: Cerebral vasospasm and delayed neurological deficit after aneurysm rupture despite administration of reserpine and kanamycin, in Wilkins RH (ed): *Cerebral Arterial Spasm*. Baltimore, Williams & Wilkins, 1980, pp 518–524.
5. Bohr DF: Electrolytes and smooth muscle contraction. Pharmacol Rev 16:85–111, 1964.
6. Boullin DJ: Potential use of prostacyclin in the treatment of vasospasm, in Wilkins RH (ed): *Cerebral Arterial Spasm*. Baltimore, Williams & Wilkins, 1980, pp 533–539.
7. Clower BR, Haining JL, Smith RR: Pathophysiological changes in the cerebral artery after subarachnoid hemorrhage, in Wilkins RH (ed): *Cerebral Arterial Spasm*. Baltimore, Williams & Wilkins, 1980, pp 124–131.
8. Echlin FA: "Cerebral Ischemia and Its Relation to Epilepsy," thesis, McGill University, Montreal, 1939.
9. Echlin FA: Spasm of basilar and vertebral arteries caused by experimental subarachnoid hemorrhage. J Neurosurg 23:1–11, 1965.
10. Echlin FA: Current concepts in the etiology and treatment of vasospasm. Clin Neurosurg 15:133–159, 1968.
11. Ecker A, Riemenschneider PA: Arteriographic demonstration of spasm of the intracranial arteries: With special reference to saccular arterial aneurysms. J Neurosurg 8:660–667, 1951.
12. Edvinsson L, Nielsen KC, Owman C, Sporrong B: Cholinergic mechanism in pial vessels: Histochemistry, electron microscopy and pharmacology. Z Zellforsch Mikrosk Anat 134:311–325, 1972.
13. Edvinsson L, Owman C, Sjöberg NO: utonomic nerves, mast cells, and amine receptors in human brain vessels. A histochemical and pharmacological study. Brain Res 115:377–393, 1976.
14. Fisher CM, Kistler JP, Davis JM: The correlation of cerebral vasospasm and the amount of subarachnoid blood detected by computerized cranial tomography after aneurysm rupture, in Wilkins RH (ed): *Cerebral Arterial Spasm*. Baltimore, Williams & Wilkins, 1980, pp 397–408.
15. Florey H: Microscopical observations on the circulation of the blood in the cerebral cortex. Brain 48:43–64, 1925.
16. Forbes HS, Cobb S: Vasomotor control of cerebral vessels. Res Publ Assoc Res Nerv Ment Dis 18:201–217, 1938.
17. Fraser RAR, Stein BM, Barret RE, Pool JL: Noradrenergic mediation of experimental cerebrovascular spasm. Stroke 1:356–362, 1970.
18. Harden TK, Klein RL, Smith RR, Thureson-Klein ÅK, Lowry MW: Serum dopamine B-hydroxylase activity following subarachnoid hemorrhage in man. Med Biol 53:100–106, 1975.
19. Hashi K, Matsuoka Y, Tanaka K, Ohkawa N: Treatment of cerebral vasospasm with large doses of hydrocortisone, in Wilkins RH (ed): *Cerebral Arterial Spasm*. Baltimore, Williams & Wilkins, 1980, pp 611–618.
20. Kapp J, Mahaley MS Jr, Odom GL: Cerebral arterial spasm: Part 3. Partial purification and characterization of a spasmogenic substance in feline platelets. J Neurosurg 29:350–356, 1968.
21. Kapp JP, Neill WR, Neill CL, Hodges LR, Smith RR: The three phases of vasospasm. Surg Neurol 18:40–45, 1982.
22. Kassell NF, Peerless SJ, Drake CG, Adams HP: High dose barbiturate therapy of cerebral vasospasm: Preliminary results, in Wilkins RH (ed): *Cerebral Arterial Spasm*. Baltimore, Williams & Wilkins, 1980, pp 628–633.
23. Kassell NF, Peerless SJ, Durward QJ, Beck DW, Drake CG,

Adams HP: Treatment of ischemic deficits from vasospasm with intravascular volume expansion and induced arterial hypertension. Neurosurgery 11:337–343, 1982.
24. Kelly PJ, Gorten RJ, Rose JE, Grossman RG: Cerebral infarction and ruptured intracranial aneurysms, in Wilkins RH (ed): *Cerebral Arterial Spasm*. Baltimore, Williams & Wilkins, 1980, pp 366–371.
25. Larsson LI, Edvinsson L, Fahrenkrug J, Håkanson R, Owman C, Schaffalitzsky de Muckadell O, Sundler F: Immunohistochemical localization of vasodilatory polypeptide (VIP) in cerebrovascular nerves. Brain Res 113:400–404, 1976.
26. Millikan CH: Cerebral vasospasm and ruptured intracranial aneurysm. Arch Neurol 32:433–449, 1975.
27. Moncada S, Bunting S, Mullane K, Thorogood P, Vane JR, Raz A, Needleman P: Imidazole: A selective inhibitor of thromboxane synthetase. Prostaglandins 13:611–618, 1977.
28. Nelson E, Rennels M: Neuromuscular contacts in intracranial arteries of the cat. Science 167:301–302, 1970.
29. Ohta H, Ito Z, Yasui N, Suzuki A: Extensive evacuation of subarachnoid clot for prevention of vasospasm—effective or not? Acta Neurochir (Wien) 63:111–116, 1982.
30. Peerless SJ, Yasargil MG: Adrenergic innervation of the cerebral blood vessels in the rabbit. J Neurosurg 35:148–154, 1971.
31. Pickard JD, Matheson M, Paterson J, Wyper DJ: Autoregulation of cerebral blood flow and the prediction of late morbidity and mortality after cerebral aneurysm surgery, in Wilkins RH (ed): *Cerebral Arterial Spasm*. Baltimore, Williams & Wilkins, 1980, pp 350–355.
32. Robertson JT: Cerebral arterial spasm: Current concepts. Clin Neurosurg 21:100–106, 1974.
33. Rousseaux P, Scherpereel B, Bernard MH, Graftieaux JP, Guyot JF: Fever and cerebral vasospasm in ruptured intracranial aneurysms. Surg Neurol 14:459–465, 1980.
34. Rumpl E, Bauer G, Gerstenbrand F, Stampfel G: Focal electroencephalographic changes associated with vasospasm after subarachnoid hemorrhage, in Wilkins RH (ed): *Cerebral Arterial Spasm*. Baltimore, Williams & Wilkins, 1980, pp 356–360.
35. Saito I, Sano K: Vasospasm after aneurysm rupture: Incidence, onset, and course, in Wilkins RH (ed): *Cerebral Arterial Spasm*. Baltimore, Williams & Wilkins, 1980, pp 294–301.
36. Sasaki T, Wakai S, Asano T, Takakura K, Sano K: Prevention of cerebral vasospasm after SAH with thromboxane synthetase inhibitor, OKY-1581. J Neurosurg 57:74–82, 1982.
37. Shigeno T, Saito I, Sano K, Takakura K, Brock M: Roles of subarachnoid blood clots and norepinephrine in cerebral vasospasm. Acta Neurochir (Wien) 63:277–280, 1982.
38. Smith RR, Clower BR, Peeler DF Jr, and Yoshioka J: The angiopathy of subarachnoid hemorrhage: Angiographic and morphologic correlates. Stroke 14:240–245, 1983.
39. Symon L, Bell Ba, Kendall B: Relationship between effused blood and clinical course and prognosis in aneurysmal subarachnoid hemorrhage: A preliminary computerized tomography scan study, in Wilkins RH (ed): *Cerebral Arterial Spasm*. Baltimore, Williams & Wilkins, 1980, pp 409–411.
40. Symon L, Harris RJ, Branston NM: Calcium and calcium antagonists in ischaemia. Acta Neurochir (Wien) 63:267–275, 1982.
41. Tai HH, Tai CL, Lee N: Selective inhibition of thromboxane synthetase by pyridine and its derivatives. Arch Biochem Biophys 203:758–763, 1980.
42. Walter P, Neil-Dwyer G, Parsons V: The effect of phentolamine and propranolol in subarachnoid hemorrhage, in Wilkins RH (ed): *Cerebral Arterial Spasm*. Baltimore, Williams & Wilkins, 1980, pp 584–588.
43. Weir BKA: The incidence and onset of a vasospasm after subarachnoid hemorrhage from ruptured aneurysm, in Wilkins RH (ed): *Cerebral Arterial Spasm*. Baltimore, Williams & Wilkins, 1980, pp 302–305.
44. Wilkins RH: Attempted prevention or treatment of intracranial arterial spasm: A survey, in Wilkins RH (ed): *Cerebral Arterial Spasm*. Baltimore, Williams & Wilkins, 1980, pp 542–555.
45. Zervas NT, Kistler JP, Ploetz J: Effect of reserpine and kanamycin on postoperative delayed ischemic deficits in patients with subarachnoid hemorrhage after aneurysm rupture, in Wilkins RH (ed): *Cerebral Arterial Spasm*. Baltimore, Williams & Wilkins, 1980, pp 514–517.
46. Zervas NT, Liszczak TM, Mayberg MR, Black PM: Cerebrospinal fluid may nourish cerebral vessels through pathways in the adventitia that may be analogous to systemic vasa vasorum. J Neurosurg 56:475–481, 1982.

163
Timing of Aneurysm Surgery

Neal F. Kassell
David J. Boarini

The primary purpose of surgery for ruptured aneurysms of the circle of Willis is to prevent rebleeding, and the secondary purpose is to facilitate the management of vasospasm. Rebleeding occurs with the greatest frequency in those days immediately after the initial bleeding.[2] Vasospasm peaks between the fifth and ninth day after the ictus (Fig. 163-1). Accordingly, it would appear logical that in order to minimize the chances of rebleeding and to favorably affect the course of vasospasm, surgery should be performed as soon as possible after the subarachnoid hemorrhage. However, experience over the past three decades suggests that this approach cannot be applied in many instances without unacceptable operative morbidity and mortality rates.

At this time most neurosurgeons in North America prefer to treat patients medically for at least 1 to 2 weeks after aneurysm bleeding and operate after this delay only if the patients are neurologically and medically stable. This approach has resulted in good surgical results in most centers over the past decade. However, in the past 5 to 10 years there has been an increasing awareness of the distressing number of patients who succumb to rebleeding or vasospasm during the waiting interval and who thus never survive to have surgery. While the surgical results have continued to improve, overall management results, which take into account those patients who die or are disabled prior to surgery, have remained at unacceptable levels.[1] This has given impetus to a reevaluation of early surgery as a means for decreasing the overall mortality and morbidity.

History of the Delayed Surgery Approach

In the early days of aneurysm surgery, circa 1950, operations were generally performed as soon as possible after admission in an attempt to prevent the cataclysmic event—rebleeding. However, the pioneering aneurysm surgeons were often confronted with a swollen brain and an aneurysm that ruptured before the dissection was complete, eliminating any hope of visualizing the neck of the sac, the parent vessels, or contiguous vital structures. There were many surgical catastrophes, and even when the operative procedure was accomplished uneventfully, patients not infrequently were left with disabling deficits from occlusion of perforating arteries not visualized at operation or from vasospasm that would develop at a later date. An operative mortality rate of 80 percent was not unheard of for surgery performed in the acute period during that era. Within several years, however, it became apparent that if surgery was intentionally delayed for 1 or 2 weeks after the most recent hemorrhage and was reserved for patients in good neurological condition, the operative conditions were much more favorable and excellent surgical results could be achieved. In 1953, Norlén and Olivecrona published their remarkable results on 100 consecutive anterior communicating artery aneurysms operated upon with a 3 percent mortality rate.[3] This landmark paper, as much as anything, defined the strategy to be employed by most neurosurgeons over the next three decades. During this interval many reports of excellent results of delayed surgery appeared to strengthen support for this approach.

However, since 1973 there has been a growing awareness of the plight of those patients who succumb while awaiting surgery, mostly from rebleeding and vasospasm. Thus, while the operative results have evolved to a point of excellence, the overall management results remain distressingly poor, with only perhaps one in three victims of aneurysmal subarachnoid hemorrhage returning to the premorbid state.[1]

In an attempt to improve the situation, a number of surgeons have re-examined early operation. In contrast to the disastrous results reported in the early 1950s, the recently reported results of early surgery are much more optimistic, with good operative conditions and mortality rates in the vicinity of 10 percent noted in certain communications.[1]

There are a variety of factors that may account for the differences in the results of early operation practiced in the early 1950s and that practiced now. The definition of early surgery has changed. Originally *early surgery* meant as soon as possible after admission whether that was Day 0 or Day 5 or 6. Now early surgery is generally (although not universally) understood as that which takes place within 48 to 96 h after subarachnoid hemorrhage. Vasospasm increases by the end of the first week after bleeding and there may be differences between the results of surgery performed in the first few days compared with the results obtained in subsequent days. This is most likely to be true in the case of patients who have serious neurological impairments. Patients who are in poor condition in the first day or two after subarachnoid hemorrhage have a reasonable chance of recovering, whereas those noted at the end of 1 week do not.

In the past three decades there has been a marked improvement in neuroanesthesia. In most circumstances the anesthetists are able to provide the surgeon with a slack brain requiring minimal retraction. Also, controlled hypotension is available to provide safer manipulation and dissection of the aneurysm and to make the hemorrhage easier to control should the sac rupture.

Also, tremendous advances in neurosurgical technique have been achieved with the advent of the microsurgical

1363

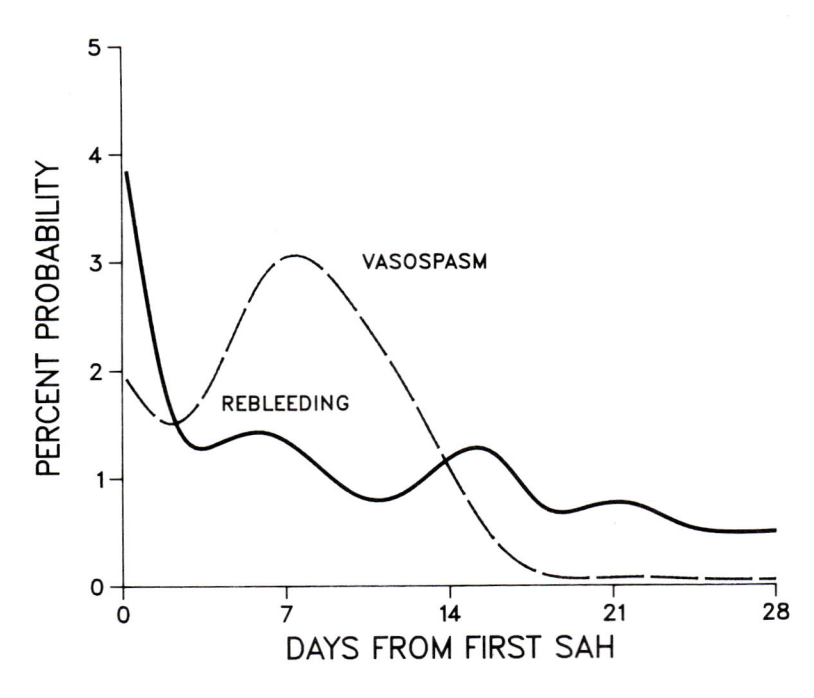

Figure 163-1 Time course of rebleeding and vasospasm. (Kassell NF, Torner JC: Unpublished observations from the Cooperative Aneurysm Study, 1982.)

approach to aneurysms. The operating microscope provides vastly improved illumination and visualization of the aneurysm and nearby vital structures. This is complemented by the fine microsurgical instruments. Removable clips in a large variety of configurations have been of great assistance in accurate obliteration of aneurysms.

Early Versus Delayed Surgery

Theoretical Considerations

There are a number of theoretical factors favoring surgery in the acute period following subarachnoid hemorrhage.

1. *Rebleeding* Surgical correction of the aneurysm essentially eliminates the possibility of subsequent subarachnoid hemorrhage.

2. *Management of Vasospasm* Craniotomy in the first days after aneurysm rupture affords the opportunity to open the major cisterns and fissures and remove much of the subarachnoid clot and thereby perhaps decrease the incidence and severity of subsequent vasospasm. To be effective, this must be accomplished as soon as possible after the hemorrhage. Clearly, this represents a rather gross approach. The morbidity from bruising of pial banks and injury to small vessels remains to be documented. Furthermore, once the sac is protected from the arterial circulation, reversal of ischemic deficits can be pursued more vigorously by increasing the arterial pressure.

3. *Prevention of Medical Complications* Securing the aneurysm early eliminates the need for prolonged treatment with antifibrinolytics, antihypertensives, sedatives, and bed rest and thus the frequency of atelectasis, pneumonia, deep vein thrombosis, and pulmonary embolus should decrease.

4. *Psychological Factors* Being removed from the precipice of sudden death has a positive influence on the patient's mood. This attitude is shared to some extent by the patient's family members and physicians and nurses.

5. *Length of Hospitalization* Early operation should theoretically decrease the average stay in the hospital by at least several days.

While the factors in favor of early operation are appealing theoretically, there are a variety of considerations strongly in support of delayed surgery.

1. *Brain Slackness* Brain edema and swelling result from subarachnoid hemorrhage. Less forceful brain retraction should be required if surgery is performed after the edema has resolved.

2. *Autoregulation* Autoregulation of the cerebral circulation is transiently disturbed after subarachnoid hemorrhage.[4] Patients should tolerate reduction in arterial pressure from brain retraction more satisfactorily after autoregulation has been restored.

3. *Ease of Aneurysm Dissection* By 1 week after subarachnoid hemorrhage, much of the blood in the subarachnoid space obscuring anatomical detail will have lysed and been washed away by the cerebrospinal fluid, which allows better visualization and makes dissection of the aneurysm easier and safer. Furthermore, that clot which remains sealing the hole in the aneurysm should be firmer than in the acute stage, which results in a decreased tendency for premature rupture during exposure and dissection of the sac.

4) Logistics With delayed surgery, there is more opportunity to observe and study the patient. Scheduling the various diagnostic examinations and surgery is simpler. Also, there is a better chance to assemble the best team, including neuroanesthetist and nurses, to approach the difficult and challenging cases.

5) Results The most compelling argument for delayed surgery is still the fact that good results are obtained from this modality in a variety of settings, including large and smaller neurosurgical services in university and community hospitals. While the overall management results of early surgery reported from certain series are superior to those generally achieved with delayed operation, it is yet to be determined whether these optimistic results are as reproducible and generally applicable as those of delayed surgery.

The Timing of Surgery Controversy

From the above, it can be surmised that the fundamental issues in the controversy about the timing of aneurysm surgery are those relating to the theoretical advantages of preventing rebleeding and facilitating the management of vasospasm versus the disadvantages involved in the hasty evaluation and operation on a sick patient with a recently injured, swollen brain with disturbed autoregulation. In an attempt to resolve this controversy, the Cooperative Aneurysm Study has undertaken a major project on the timing of aneurysm surgery. This project is funded by the National Institute of Neurological and Communicative Disorders and Stroke and is an epidemiological survey on the influence of the timing of surgery on overall outcome following aneurysmal subarachnoid hemorrhage. It covers 3000 patients admitted to more than 70 neurosurgical units throughout the world within 3 days of their first aneurysmal subarachnoid hemorrhage. The results will be available in late 1984 or early 1985.

Timing of Aneurysm Surgery: Practical Considerations

Currently, the optimal timing of operation for patients with a ruptured aneurysm has not been established. Accordingly, no dogmatic approach can be recommended. Rather, it is essential to consider each case individually and assess the prognosis and its likely modification and develop a plan based on the factors discussed below.

Neurological Status

Patients in poor condition neurologically have a reasonable chance to recover if seen within a day or two after their hemorrhage and may be considered as candidates for early surgery. However, if profound deficits have persisted for more than several days since the time of the ictus, the outcome will generally be poor and no surgery should be planned until such time as significant improvement occurs.

Age

Older patients have more difficulty with surgery of any sort. In particular, the brains of older individuals recover more slowly and less completely than those of younger persons and should be less likely to tolerate the additional stresses imposed by early operation. Accordingly, it may be prudent to delay surgery in the elderly until they have fully recovered from the effects of the hemorrhage—usually at least 10 to 14 days.

Medical Condition

Patients with serious medical problems should have surgery deferred until such time as their condition has stabilized. However, solution of the problems causing a delay in surgery should be sought with the utmost expediency.

Vasospasm

The presence of a significant degree of angiographic arterial narrowing should be considered to be a relative contraindication to surgery—even in patients with a good neurological status. This is rarely an issue in patients in whom surgery is planned within 4 days of the bleeding episode, unless they have had more than one hemorrhage. If angiography reveals vasospasm, operation is deferred an additional 5 to 7 days and the study repeated if the patient's status is stable. If the narrowing has diminished, surgery is scheduled for the following day; otherwise the cycle is repeated. Generally, however, it is relatively safe to operate on patients with a moderate degree of vasospasm who are in good condition after the beginning of the third week since the last hemorrhage. It is hoped that cerebral blood flow studies, perhaps performed with a trial of hypotension, will facilitate the selection of those patients with vasospasm in whom surgery can be performed safely.

Brain Swelling

An intraparenchymal mass effect from infarction with edema and a shift of the midline structures on a CT scan is an absolute contraindication to surgery, unless there is an accompanying large hematoma that can be removed at time of craniotomy. Increased intracranial pressure per se is not a contraindication, since in many instances hydrocephalus is a major component contributing to the intracranial hypertension, and this can be dealt with readily at the time of operation. A CT scan is critical in these circumstances.

Change in Aneurysm Size

An increase in the size of an aneurysm, either angiographically or as evidenced by the development of a third nerve palsy in the case of the posterior communicating artery aneurysm, is often ominous for rebleeding. In this event, serious consideration should be given to advancing the planned interval of surgery.

Aneurysm Configuration

In those instances in which the aneurysm is particularly large or complicated or located in a difficult site, it is probably judicious to delay surgery until all circumstances are optimal.

Rebleeding

In situations in which the aneurysm rebleeds and the patient survives in reasonable condition, serious consideration must be given to proceeding with surgery on an urgent basis. This is particularly true in cases in which rebleeding has occurred more than once.

Size of Hemorrhage

The size of the hemorrhage and the corresponding likelihood for the patient to develop vasospasm can be estimated from the CT scan. Patients who are least likely to have difficulty from vasospasm, as predicted by only a small amount of blood on the CT scan, are least likely to accrue the benefits from those aspects of early surgery concerned with the management of vasospasm. On the other hand, those patients with a large amount of blood on the CT scan are most likely to develop ischemic neurological deficits and therefore theoretically should benefit most from early operation.

Experience of the Surgeon

Indications are that surgery in the acute stage may be more difficult for a variety of reasons. The brain may be fuller, somewhat softer, and more prone to bruising. The aneurysm may be more likely to rupture prematurely, and the subarachnoid clot makes identification of neural and vascular structures more difficult. A surgeon who performs relatively few aneurysm operations but achieves excellent results with delayed surgery may have considerably more difficulty in the acute situation.

References

1. Kassell NF, Boarini DJ, Adams HP Jr, Sahs AL, Graf CJ, Torner JC, Gerk MK: Overall management of ruptured aneurysm; Comparison of early and late operation. Neurosurgery 9:120–128, 1981.
2. Kassell NF, Torner JC: Time of rebleeding after aneurysmal subarachnoid hemorrhage. Presented at the 32d Annual Meeting of the Congress of Neurological Surgeons, Toronto, October 7, 1982.
3. Norlén G, Olivecrona H: The treatment of aneurysms of the circle of Willis. J Neurosurg 10:404–415, 1953.
4. Symon L: Disordered cerebro-vascular physiology in aneurysmal subarachnoid hemorrhage. Acta Neurochir (Wien) 41:7–22, 1978.

164
Patients with Ruptured Aneurysm: Pre- and Postoperative Management

Neal F. Kassell
David J. Boarini

The effective pre- and postoperative management of patients who undergo surgery to correct ruptured intracranial aneurysms has its foundation in the prevention or the early detection and correction of complications. The most important neurological and general medical complications that occur in these patients are listed in Table 164-1.

At the University of Iowa, patients with aneurysms are housed in specialized units. An eight-bed acute care stroke unit is used for uncomplicated pre- and postoperative patients. This unit has full monitoring capability and specially trained neurological nurses in a nurse-patient ratio of approximately 1:2. More complicated cases, particularly those requiring ventilatory support, and all patients in the first 12 to 24 h after operation are kept in the neurosurgical intensive care unit, where the nurse-patient ratio is 1:1.

Ischemia from Vasospasm

Vasospasm is the leading cause of morbidity following aneurysmal subarachnoid hemorrhage and is second only to the destructive effects of the initial hemorrhage as a cause of mortality.[10] Arterial narrowing that can be demonstrated angiographically probably occurs in nearly 80 percent of patients following aneurysm rupture.[23] Ischemic neurological deficits attributable to vasospasm and increased cerebrovascular resistance occur in approximately 30 percent of patients either pre- or postoperatively.[10]

At present there is no clearly proven method for preventing the arterial narrowing. However, removal of the subarachnoid clot by early craniotomy and opening of the basal cisterns may be beneficial in certain circumstances.[15] Furthermore, calcium channel blocking agents have recently been demonstrated to favorably affect the outcome of those patients who develop deficits from vasospasm.[2] The use of calcium antagonists in the management of vasospasm appears most promising and warrants careful attention.

Once vasospasm develops, there is no effective agent for dilating the narrowed segments.[24] The other possibilities for the management of vasospasm include reversal of the ischemic deficits once they occur and if this cannot be accomplished, decreasing the cerebral metabolic rate so that the brain can survive on the compromised level of substrates provided by the reduced blood flow.[6]

Reversal of ischemic deficits can be achieved by improving the rheological characteristics of the blood, increasing cardiac output, or improving perfusion pressure.[6] Avoidance of a high hematocrit,[13] continuous mannitol in a dose of 1 to 2 g/kg per day by continuous infusion,[12,19] and administration of albumin and plasma fractionate[21] all favorably affect the rheology of the blood.

Barbiturate Therapy

High-dose barbiturate therapy decreases the cerebral metabolic rate and would appear to have significant theoretical advantages in protecting the brain from infarction when adequate levels of perfusion cannot be obtained.[3,4,11,14] However, empiric evidence to date with this modality for treatment of patients with profound neurological deficits from vasospasm has been disappointing.[8] Whether this is a manifestation of the severity of the disease or an inherent inadequacy of this form of treatment remains to be determined.

TABLE 164-1 Frequent Complications of Aneurysmal Subarachnoid Hemorrhage[10]

Complication	Approximate Occurrence, percent
Ischemic focal deficits	27
Hypertension	19
Brain swelling	12
Hydrocephalus	12
Recurrent subarachnoid hemorrhage	11
Intraparenchymal hemorrhage	8
Pneumonia	8
Anemia	6
Seizures	5
Gastrointestinal hemorrhage	4
Inappropriate antidiuretic hormone secretion	4
Thrombophlebitis, pulmonary emboli	3
Cardiac arrhythmias	3
Atelectasis	3
Hypotension	3
Iatrogenic arterial occlusion	2

Hypervolemic-Hypertensive Therapy

The cornerstone of our current theoretical basis for this therapeutic approach is as follows. The neurological deficits that are related to vasospasm are secondary to the increased cerebrovascular resistance due to the arterial narrowing. As previously mentioned, measures to decrease cerebrovascular resistance by producing vasodilatation have been unrewarding. The alternatives that remain for enhancing cerebral perfusion in these circumstances are (1) to improve the rheological characteristics of the blood (as noted above) or (2) to increase the cerebral perfusion pressure. Increased perfusion pressure increases cerebral blood flow in the ischemic regions because autoregulation is impaired.[22] Also, through mechanisms poorly understood at present, hypervolemia increases cerebral blood flow in ischemic zones.[18]

Patients who require this form of therapy must be monitored intensively. Systemic arterial pressure is measured continuously through an indwelling arterial line. The Swan-Ganz catheter is most useful for measuring both pulmonary artery wedge pressure and diastolic pressure as well as for making intermittent determinations of cardiac output, although a central venous pressure line is a good second choice since most aneurysm patients have healthy hearts and lungs. When intracranial hypertension appears to be a major problem, intracranial pressure is monitored. The electrocardiogram is monitored continuously and arterial blood gases, hemoglobin, hematocrit, serum electrolytes, and osmolarity are measured at least twice daily, and usually more frequently in the first 1 to 2 days of this treatment. Fluid balance is assessed carefully on an hourly basis and chest x-ray filming is performed daily to look for early signs of congestive heart failure or pulmonary edema.

The patient is kept flat in bed, elastic stockings are applied, and oxygen is administered to maintain arterial P_{O_2} greater than 70 torr. If intracranial hypertension is a problem, measures for reducing intracranial pressure are employed.

Therapy commences with volume expansion, initially with plasma fractionate followed by blood and electrolyte solutions to maintain a hematocrit of approximately 40 and normal serum electrolytes. The initial goal is to create a positive fluid balance of between 1 and 2 liters. When the hypervolemic state is reached, two things occur. First, the patient begins to diurese. This can result in a situation in which intravenous fluids are being used to "chase" urine losses in excess of 500 to 1000 ml per hour. To minimize this response and simplify the patient's management, aqueous vasopressin is administered in a dose of 5 units intramuscularly every 3 to 4 h if the urine output exceeds 100 ml per hour. The second response that occurs to the hypervolemia is a vagal depressor reflex, which results in decreased cardiac output. Atropine, 1 mg intramuscularly every 2 to 4 h, is used to block this and maintain the heart rate in excess of 80 but less than 120 to assure adequate filling volumes for the heart. When further increases in cardiac output are required, isoproterenol may be used. If arterial blood gases deteriorate, signs of congestive heart failure are noted on the chest film, or the cardiac output decreases, suggesting incipient congestive heart failure, digitalis is administered.

In over half of the patients these measures alone will result in an increase in cardiac output as well as an increase in arterial blood pressure. If further increases in arterial pressure are required, dopamine is administered. Conversely, if the arterial pressure reaches excessive levels, especially in patients whose aneurysms are not corrected, hydralazine is used to lower the arterial pressure without decreasing cardiac output.

In patients with uncorrected aneurysms, hypervolemia is initially induced and arterial blood pressure is allowed to rise to 160 mmHg systolic. Occasionally situations are encountered in which this level of hypertension is not sufficient to reverse the ischemic neurological deficits. At that time, a decision must be reached as to whether it is preferable to allow the patient to develop an infarction and a permanent neurological deficit or whether to accept the chance that the aneurysm will rebleed in the face of arterial pressures in excess of 160 mmHg. For those patients whose aneurysms have been corrected, hypertension is induced by using dopamine simultaneously with the infusion of large amounts of fluids. An attempt is made to titrate the blood pressure against neurological status. The objective is to achieve an acceptable although perhaps not entirely normal level of neurological function at the lowest level of arterial pressure. Blood pressure elevations are limited to 240 systolic and 120 mean to avoid breakthrough of autoregulation.[5,20] There is a hysteresis effect: on occasion as the blood pressure is raised, neurological impairments resolve rapidly; as the blood pressure is lowered in an attempt to find the threshold level, 2 to 3 h must elapse before the neurological deficits reappear; when the blood pressure is raised again, the impairments resolve rapidly. No explanation is available for this phenomenon.

In our experience, length of treatment has varied between 12 h and 8 days.[9] However, if an acceptable level of neurological function can be maintained for 3 days, the outcome will generally be favorable.

Using this hypervolemic-hypertensive therapy, permanent improvement can be obtained in approximately two-thirds to three-quarters of the patients who develop ischemic neurological deficits from vasospasm.[9] The results are more favorable in patients whose aneurysms have been already corrected and who can be treated more aggressively. Causes of failure have mostly been related to unrelenting progression of vasospasm. The therapy must be initiated promptly because once infarction has occurred, no improvement can be expected. Furthermore, in this situation the risks of vasogenic edema and hemorrhagic infarction are probably greater, although we have not found this to be a problem. Most complications have been related to fluid overload and include pulmonary edema and dilutional hyponatremia. These can be minimized by judicious monitoring of central pressures, cardiac output, arterial blood gases, fluid balance, and chest x-ray films.

Rebleeding

Rebleeding is the most dramatic and second most important complication of aneurysmal rupture in terms of death and disability.[10] There are two strategies currently employed to decrease the incidence of rebleeding in the acute period following subarachnoid hemorrhage. The first is to minimize the *transmural* or *bursting pressure* of the aneurysm, which is defined as the difference between the mean systemic arterial pressure and the intracranial pressure. The second is to decrease the lysis of the clot that seals the rent in the aneurysm.

Transmural Pressure

The transmural pressure can be decreased by reducing the arterial pressure. Also, reductions in transmural pressure can be minimized by avoiding abrupt or uncontrolled decreases in intracranial pressure, since intracranial pressure exerts a tamponade effect on the aneurysm. When possible, the use of lumbar puncture, ventriculostomy, or CSF shunts should be avoided in the preoperative period.

Arterial pressure in excess of that required for brain perfusion, especially hypertension associated with pain, anxiety, excitement, straining, or hypoxia, must be eliminated. The patient should be kept at strict bed rest in a private room, with no television or radio. Only decaffeinated coffee should be permitted and the use of flurazepam for sleep should be avoided owing to the high levels of REM (rapid eye movement) sleep associated with this drug. Likewise, the use of sympathomimetic drugs such as phenylephrine nose drops should be discouraged. Stool softeners are administered and analgesics are given to keep the patient pain-free. If headache and stiff neck are particularly severe, intravenous or intramuscular morphine is used initially, followed by oral codeine when the pain has decreased. Sufficient sedatives and tranquilizers are given to make the patient drowsy enough to sleep most of the day. For these purposes, we prefer to use phenobarbital since it is also a good anticonvulsant. Occasionally it is supplemented with diazepam.

If the blood pressure is elevated owing to essential hypertension, antihypertensive agents should be administered. Long-acting or cardiac depressant drugs should be avoided. Also, fluid restriction must not be used as an adjunct for the control of arterial pressure. Antihypertensive drugs should be used with extreme caution during the period when vasospasm is at its maximum, roughly the fifth through the ninth day following the last subarachnoid hemorrhage. The drug of choice for control of essential hypertension is hydralazine administered either orally or intravenously. Occasionally, propranolol is used, particularly if the patient shows evidence of sympathetic hyperactivity associated with subarachnoid hemorrhage. This drug also facilitates the use of intraoperative hypotension with sodium nitroprusside.[17]

Recent data suggest that the peak incidence of rebleeding is in the first 24 to 48 h following subarachnoid hemorrhage rather than at the end of the first or the beginning of the second week, as traditionally believed.[10] In the first day or two after the hemorrhage, patients will generally not have vasospasm. Accordingly, drugs to induce hypotension (blood pressures lower than normal) should in theory be used safely during this interval. However, for this purpose only intravenous, rapidly reversible drugs should be used.

The most reasonable choice at this time for a hypotensive drug is sodium nitroprusside, although significant problems with tachyphylaxis and toxicity are associated with its use. These problems may be minimized through the adjunctive use of propranolol and saralasin.[17] Still, sodium nitroprusside is not an ideal agent, and other drugs such as adenosine are under current investigation.[7]

Clot Lysis

Although the use of antifibrinolytic agents to minimize clot lysis is controversial, the bulk of the evidence still favors the use of these drugs.[1] Epsilon-aminocaproic acid (EACA) is administered to patients admitted within the first 10 to 14 days after their most recent subarachnoid hemorrhage in whom the plan is to delay surgery at least for several days. An initial dose of 48 g per day by continuous intravenous infusion for the first 2 days is given, followed by 36 g per day for 14 days. The medication is then switched from the intravenous to the oral route and tapered over 1 week if the patient does not have surgery. The drug is discontinued 6 h prior to any planned operation or angiography. The rational use of EACA suggests monitoring of streptokinase clot level times or EACA levels, although this is rarely done.

A word of caution regarding rebleeding: The clinical picture of rebleeding is not infrequently masked or confused with that of vasospasm. Accordingly, the cause of neurological deterioration must always be documented with a CT scan (or lumbar puncture if the CT scan is not helpful). The treatment of rebleeding is usually the same as that of the initial hemorrhage, although at times a patient who rebleeds more than once and/or shows significant enlargement of the aneurysm may become a candidate for an early operation. A patient who has a coma-producing rebleed while in the hospital and does not regain consciousness within 10 to 15 min after the ictus should be intubated, hyperventilated, and given 1 to 2 g/kg of mannitol. Such a patient should be taken immediately for a CT scan and if an intracerebral hematoma is noted, should be taken immediately to the operating room for evacuation of the clot as a salvage procedure. These heroic efforts can at times yield quite gratifying results.

Brain Swelling and Edema

Patients with subarachnoid hemorrhage have many reasons for developing brain swelling and edema, including irritation of the parenchyma by the subarachnoid clot, ischemia from vasospasm or iatrogenic vascular compromise, operative retraction of the brain, abrupt increase in intracranial pressure secondary to the subarachnoid hemorrhage, and edema around an intracerebral hematoma. Accordingly, in the preoperative period patients receive dexamethasone, between 12 and 24 mg per day in four divided doses. Postoperatively, the steroids are usually tapered over 1 week. In addition, normal plasma osmotic and oncotic pressure should be maintained by careful attention to electrolyte balance and appropriate selection of fluid replacement.

Ischemia from Operative Vascular Compromise

Postoperatively patients may develop cerebral ischemia from intentional or unintentional compromise of arterial or venous structures. Management of this complication is based on the same principles as the treatment for ischemic deficits from postoperative vasospasm.

Seizures

Not counting the epileptiform activity that occurs during a hemorrhage, approximately 3 percent of patients with ruptured aneurysms will have seizures during their acute illness, either pre- or postoperatively.[10] In patients who have a normal level of consciousness, phenobarbital is used both as an anticonvulsant and a sedative. However, in a patient with an impaired level of consciousness, hydantoin is the preferred agent.

Hydrocephalus

The incidence of hydrocephalus noted on CT scans performed shortly after subarachnoid hemorrhage is between 15 and 20 percent. Clinically, between 10 and 15 percent of patients with aneurysmal subarachnoid hemorrhage will evidence hydrocephalus. Between 5 and 10 percent of patients with ruptured aneurysms will ultimately require a cerebrospinal fluid (CSF) shunt.[10]

Some investigators have speculated that early operation with the removal of clot from the subarachnoid space and ventriculocisternal drainage can decrease the incidence of hydrocephalus.[25] Others have hypothesized that steroids decrease the incidence of hydrocephalus while some observers think that antifibrinolytics increase the incidence of hydrocephalus.[16] There is little evidence to support any of these views.

Preoperatively, it has been our general policy to avoid shunting or ventricular drainage whenever possible because of our concerns regarding the loss of tamponade effect. Also, we think that a moderate degree of hydrocephalus provides a greater volume of CSF to be drained at operation and will thus afford the opportunity to produce a slacker brain. Also, we are still concerned about the problems of infection with ventriculostomy. We avoid shunting patients at the time of craniotomy for fear of increasing the incidence of postoperative subdural hematoma or hygroma formation, although this practice is not based on sound evidence. Generally, when a CSF diversion is required, we prefer a lumboperitoneal shunt performed 1 or more weeks postoperatively.

Other Complications

Fluid and Electrolyte Abnormalities

Patients with subarachnoid hemorrhage are particularly prone to develop fluid and electrolyte abnormalities. Essentially all patients will have some degree of inappropriate antidiuretic hormone secretion. Furthermore, hyponatremia in patients with subarachnoid hemorrhage can also be attributable to a decrease in total body sodium. Meticulous attention must be paid to fluid balance and serum electrolyte concentrations in these patients. Fluid restriction is no longer employed because hypovolemia is a factor in cerebral ischemia. Hypotonic fluids are generally not administered. Sodium and potassium replacement is essential.

Hematoma Formation

Epidural, subdural, and intracerebral hematomas can all occur in patients with ruptured aneurysms, the latter two preoperatively. A large subdural or intracerebral hematoma is an indication for early operation if the patient's neurological condition is unstable, deteriorates, or is initially unacceptable. Repeated CT scans to monitor the degree of brain edema around the hematoma and any midline shift are required both pre- and postoperatively.

Wound Infection, Meningitis, Septicemia

Prophylactic methicillin and gentamicin starting 12 h preoperatively and continuing for 48 h postoperatively are employed with all our patients. This is used not only as prophylaxis against wound infection and meningitis from the craniotomy but also to prevent infectious complications from the extensive invasive monitoring employed during the perioperative period.

Deep Vein Thrombosis and Pulmonary Embolus

Sometime during their hospital course approximately 2 percent of patients with ruptured aneurysms will develop deep vein thrombosis and 1 percent will have a pulmonary embolus.[10] Postoperatively patients with these disorders are treated with systemic heparinization. Preoperatively there are only three choices: (1) systemic heparinization followed by surgery at the previously planned interval; (2) immediate surgery followed by heparinization postoperatively; (3) insertion of an antiembolism umbrella into the inferior vena cava. The choice must be based on the individual patient since there is not sufficient experience to make a general statement. The prevention of these complications includes active and passive leg exercises in patients who are at bed rest, elastic stockings, intermittent pressure stockings, and early postoperative mobilization.

Atelectasis and Pneumonia

Atelectasis will occur in 3 percent of patients and pneumonia in 8 percent.[10] Pre- and postoperative management consists of frequent turning and chest physiotherapy, chest x-ray films and arterial blood gases at the early suspicion of pulmonary congestion, and early postoperative mobilization.

Gastrointestinal Bleeding

Gastrointestinal bleeding is noted in approximately 4 percent of patients following aneurysm rupture.[10] Most often it occurs in those individuals who have an impaired level of consciousness and disturbed vegetative functions. Hypovolemia from gastrointestinal hemorrhage can be disastrous in the presence of vasospasm.

Prevention of gastrointestinal bleeding is based on the routine use of cimetidine and antacid preparations. Treatment of gastrointestinal bleeding after subarachnoid hemorrhage is similar to that employed in patients with other underlying disorders, with the exception that more attention must be paid to maintaining normal circulating blood volume and levels of hemoglobin.

References

1. Adams HP Jr: Current status of antifibrinolytic therapy for treatment of patients with subarachnoid hemorrhage. Stroke 13:256–259, 1982.
2. Allen GS, Battye R, Boone S, Chou S, Kelly D, Weir B: Preliminary results of multicenter double blind prospective study of nimodipine in the prevention of delayed neurological deficits from cerebral arterial spasm. Presented at the 32nd Annual Meeting of the Congress of Neurological Surgeons, Toronto, October 7, 1982.
3. Demopoulos HB, Flamm ES, Seligman ML, Jorgensen E, Ransohoff J: Antioxidant effects of barbiturates in model membranes undergoing free radical damage. Acta Neurol Scand [Suppl] 64:152–153, 1977.
4. Flamm ES, Demopoulos HB, Seligman ML, Ransohoff J: Possible molecular mechanisms of barbiturate-mediated protection in regional cerebral ischemia. Acta Neurol Scand [Suppl] 64:150–151, 1977.
5. Häggendal E, Johansson B: Effect of increased intravascular pressure on the blood-brain barrier to protein in dogs. Acta Neurol Scand 48:271–275, 1972.
6. Kassell NF, Boarini DJ: Cerebral ischemia in the aneurysm patient. Clin Neurosurg 29:657–665, 1982.
7. Kassell NF, Boarini DJ, Olin JJ, Sprowell JA: Cerebral and systemic circulatory effects of arterial hypotension induced by adenosine. In press.
8. Kassell NF, Peerless SJ, Drake CG, Boarini DJ, Adams HP: Treatment of ischemic deficits from cerebral vasospasm with high dose barbiturate therapy. Neurosurgery 7:593–597, 1980.
9. Kassell NF, Peerless SJ, Durward QJ, Beck DW, Drake CG, Adams HP: Treatment of ischemic deficits from vasospasm with intravascular volume expansion and induced arterial hypertension. Neurosurgery 11:337–343, 1982.
10. Kassell NF, Torner JC: Unpublished observations from the Cooperative Aneurysm Study, 1982.
11. Lafferty JJ, Keykhah MM, Shapiro HM, Van Horn K, Behar MG: Cerebral hypometabolism obtained with deep pentobarbital anesthesia and hypothermia (30°C). Anesthesiology 49:159–164, 1978.
12. Little JR: Modification of acute focal ischemia by treatment with mannitol. Stroke 9:4–9, 1978.
13. Merrill EW: Rheology of blood. Physiol Rev 49:863–888, 1969.
14. Michenfelder JD: The interdependency of cerebral functional and metabolic effects following massive doses of thiopental in the dog. Anesthesiology 41:231–236, 1974.
15. Mizukami M, Kawase T, Usami T, Tazawa T: Prevention of vasospasm by early operation with removal of subarachnoid blood. Neurosurgery 10:301–307, 1982.
16. Park BE: Spontaneous subarachnoid hemorrhage complicated by communicating hydrocephalus: Epsilon aminocaproic acid as a possible predisposing factor. Surg Neurol 11:73–80, 1979.
17. Pertuiset B, Ancri D, Lienhart A: Profound arterial hypotension (MAP ≤ 50 mmHg) induced with neuroleptanalgesia and sodium nitroprusside (series of 531 cases): Reference to vascular autoregulation mechanism and surgery of vascular malformations of the brain. Adv Tech Stds Neurosurg 8:75–122, 1981.
18. Pritz MB, Giannotta SL, Kindt GW, McGillicuddy JE, Prager RL: Treatment of patients with neurological deficits associated with cerebral vasospasm by intravascular volume expansion. Neurosurgery 3:364–368, 1978.
19. Quest DO, Burke AM, Chien S: The effect of mannitol on blood viscosity. Presented at the 30th Annual Meeting, Congress of Neurological Surgeons, Houston, October 9, 1980.
20. Strandgaard S, Mackenzie ET, Sengupta D, Rowan JO, Lassen NA, Harper AM: Upper limit of autoregulation of cerebral blood flow in the baboon. Circ Res 34:435–440, 1974.
21. Sundt TM Jr, Waltz AG, Sayre GP: Experimental cerebral infarction: Modification by treatment with hemodiluting, hemoconcentrating, and dehydrating agents. J Neurosurg 26:46–56, 1967.
22. Symon L: Disordered cerebro-vascular physiology in aneurysmal subarachnoid haemorrhage. Acta Neurochir (Wien) 41:7–22, 1978.
23. Weir B, Grace M, Hansen J, Rothberg C: Time course of vasospasm in man. J Neurosurg 48:173–178, 1978.
24. Wilkins RH: Attempted prevention or treatment of intracranial arterial spasm: A survey. Neurosurgery 6:198–210, 1980.
25. Yamamoto I: Early operation for ruptured intracranial aneurysms: Comparative study with computerized tomography. Presented at the 32d Annual Meeting, Congress of Neurological Surgeons, Toronto, October 7, 1982.

165

Aneurysm Clips

John M. Tew, Jr.
Hans Jacob Steiger

Cushing described the use of a malleable silver vascular clip in 1911. Malleable tantalum or gold clips were commonly used for obliteration of most intracranial aneurysms until the first spring clips were developed by Schwartz and Mayfield in the 1950s. Despite early problems with these designs, such as slippage and a tendency to cut the aneurysm in the crotch of the blades, the advantage of the easily removable clip was obvious, since it did not commit the surgeon to a perfect clip application on the first attempt. The Mayfield clip was required for aneurysm surgery during the 1950s and 1960s. Subsequently, a variety of spring clips have been developed (Fig. 165-1). New aneurysm clips have a more consistent occlusive force, corrosion resistance has been improved, and versatility has been increased by a variety of different blade configurations. The recently developed clip appliers that permit flexible positioning of the clip between the jaws at various angles also facilitate proper application and adjustment of a clip.[7]

Most neurosurgeons use only few of the more than 50 available aneurysm clips. The cost of the different sets of clips and appliers limits the number of different types stocked in the operating room. Comparison of objective performance data enables the neurosurgeon to make an optimal choice. The prime requirements for aneurysm clips are easy handling, acceptable mechanical properties, and inertness. Comparative studies concerned with closing forces, metallic fatigue, and corrosion of clips have been published by many authors.[1-5] It is more difficult to be objective about the handling qualities of a clip and applier combination, and the choice remains partially a matter of personal preference.

Classification of Aneurysm Clips

Dujovny classifies spring clips according to their mechanical principle. He and his associates distinguish among alpha, pivot, and mobile fulcrum type clips.[2] The Mayfield clip is the prototype of the alpha class. This type is an integral crossed-leg design, which resembles the Greek letter alpha (α). This class includes the Yasargil (Fig. 165-2), McFadden (Fig. 165-3), Drake and Sugita (Fig. 165-4), and Rhoton (Fig. 165-5) aneurysm clips,[6] as well as the Biemer clip (Aesculap Instruments) for temporary microvascular occlusion.

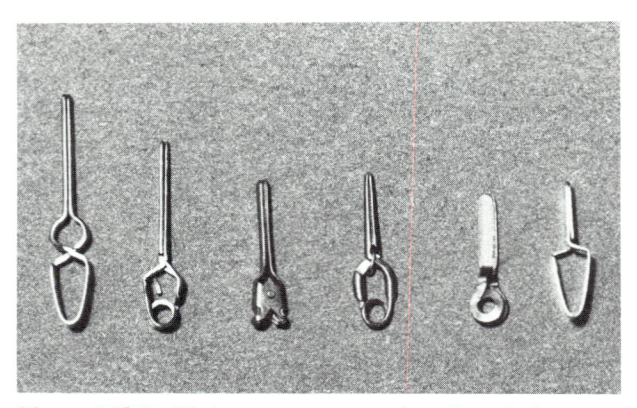

Figure 165-1 Various aneurysm spring clips. *Left to right:* Drake, McFadden, Heifetz, Yasargil, Scoville, and Mayfield designs. The distributors of these clips are: Drake clips, Codman & Shurtleff, Inc., Randolph, Mass.; McFadden and Mayfield clips, V. Mueller & Co., Chicago, and Codman & Shurtleff; Heifetz clips, Edward Weck & Co., Inc., Research Triangle Park, N. C.; Yasargil clips, Aesculap Instruments, New York; and Scoville clips, Downs Surgical, Inc., Decatur, Ga.

Mayfield, Drake, McFadden, and Biemer clips consist of only one part, whereas Yasargil, Rhoton, and Sugita clips have an additional small ringlet or strut as an alignment guide. Pivot clips, in contrast, consist of several parts. The blades rotate or rock around a central pivot, and a separate coil spring provides the closing force.[8] The Heifetz clip is the prototype of the pivot class. Pivot (V. Mueller & Co) Kleinert-Kutz (Edward Weck & Co., Inc.) clips for temporary use are other popular members of this family. In the Scoville clip, an example of the mobile fulcrum clip, part of the integral spring coil acts as a fulcrum around which the blades rotate and the position of the fulcrum depends on the gap between the blades. The Acland clip, which is designed for temporary microvascular occlusion, is another example of this class.

Aside from the mechanical principle, spring clips are classified as permanent or temporary according to their closing force. Yasargil, Sugita, and Pivot clips are offered with a

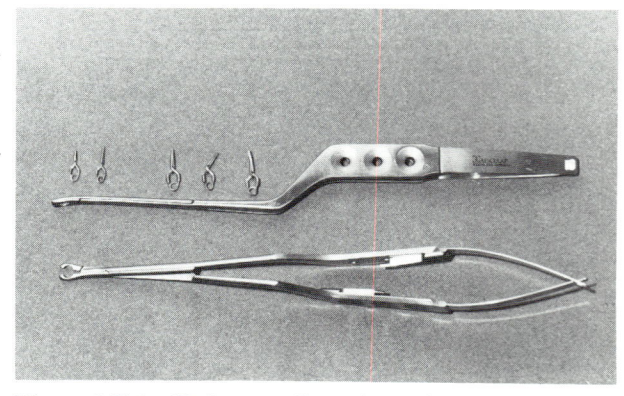

Figure 165-2 Various configurations of Yasargil clips and the bayonet applier.

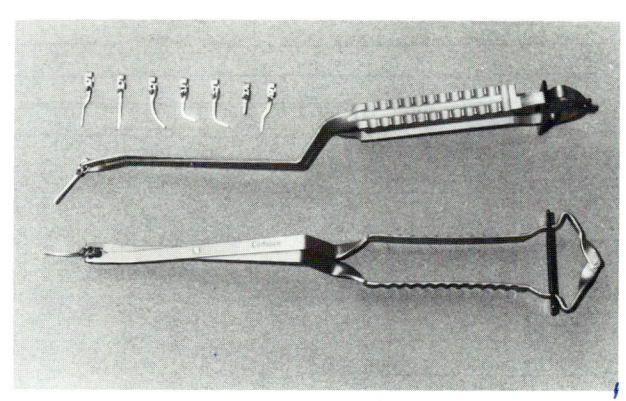

Figure 165-3 McFadden clips and applier. The clip can be locked at various angles.

reduced closing force for temporary vessel occlusion. The temporary Yasargil clip was originally designed as a pilot clip for preliminary clipping of an aneurysm, since the blades open wider than in most other clips and permit easier application of the clip. Biemer, Acland, and Kleinert-Kutz clips are strictly designed for temporary occlusion and not for permanent implantation.

Despite the predominant use of spring clips, there is occasionally a place for malleable clips, especially when dealing with broad-based or fusiform aneurysms that require aneurysmorrhaphy. The Weck Hemoclip (Edward Weck & Co, Inc.) and the Ethicon Ligaclip (Ethicon, Inc., Somerville, N.J.), which are made of tantalum, are used primarily.

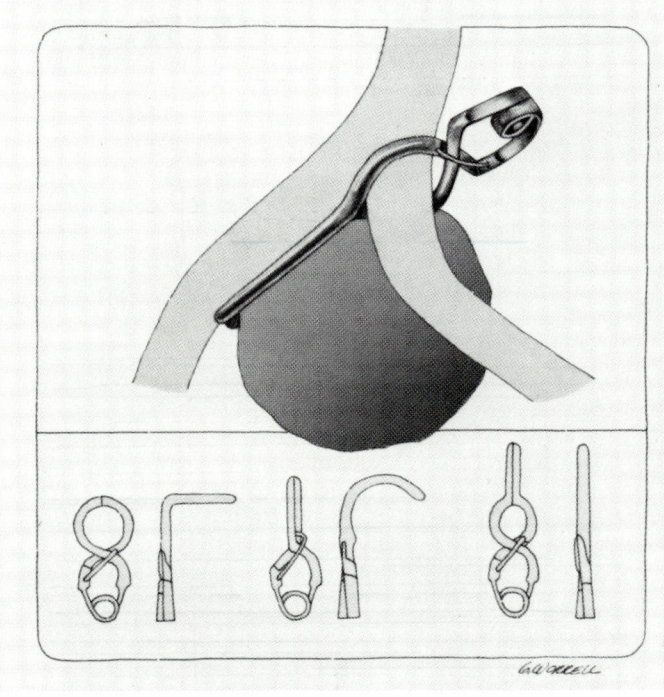

Figure 165-4 Sugita aneurysm clips (Downs Surgical, Inc.). A variety of different configurations, including fenestrated types, increases the versatility of this system.

The original silver clips have been abandoned because they induce an inflammatory tissue reaction and have poor functional properties.

Principles of Aneurysm Obliteration

In the past only relatively small aneurysms not hidden behind vital structures could be eliminated directly by ligation or with the available simple clips. Large aneurysms were often dealt with indirectly by ligation of the parent vessel or by coating the aneurysm with muscle, gauze, or adhesives. The modern sophisticated clips permit direct ablation of almost all intracranial aneurysms, even large fusiform aneurysms hidden behind vital structures. A variety of different clip configurations must be available in the operating room to permit selection of the proper method for clipping.

The size and the geometrical configuration of aneurysm, parent artery, and surrounding structures determine the proper clipping technique. If the size of the aneurysmal neck is large compared with the diameter of the parent artery, the clip blade must be applied parallel to the parent artery to avoid constriction of the arterial wall. If the parent vessel, or vascular or neural structures obstruct direct access to the aneurysm, a fenestrated clip should be chosen. Fenestrated clips were originally designed by Drake for clipping basilar-tip aneurysms hidden behind the posterior cerebral artery. More recently, Sugita has developed angled fenestrated clips for fusiform aneurysms of the carotid and vertebral arteries. Large broad-based aneurysms can also be dealt with effectively by aneurysmorrhaphy if they are accessible. After temporary occlusion of the proximal and distal parent artery, the aneurysmal sac is excised and the vessel is reconstructed with a series of malleable clips (Fig. 165-6) or sutures. Temporary clips are useful not only for isolation of an aneurysm during the ablation but also to serve as a test occlusion of the aneurysm. The blades of the temporary clips open wider than the blades of permanent aneurysm clips, and the blades slide more easily around a large aneurysm. Temporary Pivot clips are often necessary when angled clips are chosen as final clips because angled blades cannot be opened widely. Intraoperative systemic hypotension greatly facilitates application of the clip. A mean arterial pressure of 45 to 55 mmHg is recommended for normotensive patients.

Difficulty may arise when operating in a deep surgical cavity. Because of the limited freedom of motion, it is often difficult to align the clip blades in the desired line of action. Careful selection of the optimal clip and applier combination is necessary. The new variable angle appliers used for Pivot, McFadden, and Rhoton clips and the Sano all-angle applier for Sugita, Yasargil, and Heifetz clips facilitate proper setting of the clip. The clip often changes its position after release from the applier. Sugita, Yasargil, and Heifetz clips are then often very difficult to recapture with the applier if adjustment of the clip position becomes necessary. This task is much easier with the Pivot, McFadden, and Rhoton clips since the jaws of the corresponding appliers can be locked into the two sides of the clip body in a sequential fashion and can be slid into the locking position not only straight over the top of the clip but also from any side of the clip.

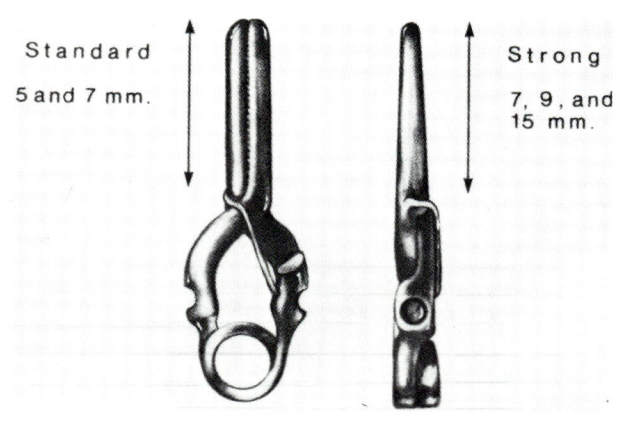

Figure 165-5 The Rhoton aneurysm clip is a revised construction and a further development of the popular Yasargil clip. It is distributed by V. Mueller & Co. in a normal version and a strong version suitable also for large aneurysms. A varied angle applier has been designed for this system. (From Rhoton and Merz.[6])

Closing Force

The closing force of an aneurysm clip is one of the most important factors when choosing a clip for a particular aneurysm. In practice a clip may be too weak to occlude a large aneurysm, and the trial-and-error method for selection of a sufficient clip is dangerous because manipulation of an aneurysm can lead to premature rupture. The neurosurgeon should know from performance data which clip will provide sufficient force to close a given aneurysm but will not damage the vessel by applying excessive force.

The force necessary to occlude an aneurysm or artery is impossible to assess without a method for precise measurement. Additional factors such as blood pressure, clip blade width, diameter of the aneurysm, stiffness of the aneurysm wall, and geometrical configuration of the aneurysm must be considered. If the blades of the clip are parallel to the parent artery, more force is transmitted from the arterial wall. Requisite occlusive forces for arteries are less complicated to establish. Dujovny et al. have published tables of minimal occlusive forces for various vessel diameters, blood pressures, and clip blade widths.[2,3] These data were generated by a computer program and were verified by measurements in vivo. A study by the same group also indicates that small arteries do not tolerate excessive compression loads because endothelial disruption and clot formation may occur.

On the other hand, performance data for the various clips need consideration. Only two clip distributors in the United States print the closing force of a clip with package labeling. Several independent studies have provided comparative data of clip performance. However, the conditions of force measurements vary and make deductions and comparison difficult. The occlusive force of a spring clip depends on the gap between the blades and the position of the vessel or aneurysm in the clip. According to the "spring law," closing force increases in a linear fashion with increasing gap between the blades, and according to the "lever law," the force exerted on a vessel increases hyperbolically with decreasing distance from the fulcrum of the clip. Finally, when a clip closes, the spring may exert a force at a given gap between the blades that is lower than the opening resistance at the same gap. This phenomenon is known as *hysteresis* and is a sign of internal friction. All popular clip designs are mechanically reliable today. However, significant differences of closing forces and hysteresis may be present between various production lots. Knowledge of this fact places the responsibility for proper clip performance on the surgeon. Various clip closure force meters are commercially available. These devices can be used to examine all clips prior to implantation and also permit periodic examination of clips that have been used but not permanently implanted.

Matching the proper clip to a particular aneurysm must remain a matter of surgical experience, to be fortified with knowledge of aneurysm configuration and clip performance. The McFadden clip is the strongest commercially available clip and the only design able to occlude an aneurysm with a neck diameter greater than 8 to 10 mm. If a single clip turns out to be insufficient, a parallel second clip may help (Fig. 165-7). Some surgeons favor the use of "booster clips" placed on the blades of the initial clip. The new Rhoton clip promises to be extremely strong; clinical testing is pending.

Metallurgical Considerations

Freedom from corrosion is the prime requirement for a metal suitable for biological implantation. Corrosion may lead to mechanical failure of the implanted device and cause unwanted inflammatory tissue reaction. Slippage and fracture of aneurysm clips due to corrosion has been reported by several authors.[4]

Corrosion is an electrochemical reaction consisting of oxidation of an anodic metal (negative pole) and simultaneous reduction of a cathodic metal (positive pole). An alloy composed of different metallic elements may have a heterogeneous surface, which can form anodic and cathodic poles. Electrolysis may also be induced by scratches on the surface or by enclosure of the surface by foreign materials. Clips composed of several parts are more prone to corrosion than integral devices.

Stainless steel and cobalt-based alloys form a passivated chromium oxide surface layer, which inhibits corrosion. This film depends on homogeneous availability of oxygen. Partial encasement of a clip with synthetic material interferes with oxygen contact. Corrosion of aneurysm clips can be a consequence of partial oxygen deprivation.

Stainless steel is classified into ferritic, martensitic, and austenitic steels according to the metallic composition and crystalline structure. The modern steel aneurysm clips such as Yasargil, Rhoton, and Scoville clips are constructed of austenitic steel. They resist corrosion and are nonmagnetic. Absence of ferromagnetism deserves attention because of the new nuclear magnetic resonance (NMR) scanners. A strong magnetic field exerts considerable forces on magnetic aneurysm clips and implanted clips are currently considered a contraindication for NMR examinations. Mayfield, Heifetz, and other clips consist partially of martensitic steel. Corrosion resistance is relatively minor and these materials are ferromagnetic. Cobalt-based superalloys are a viable al-

Aneurysm Clips 1375

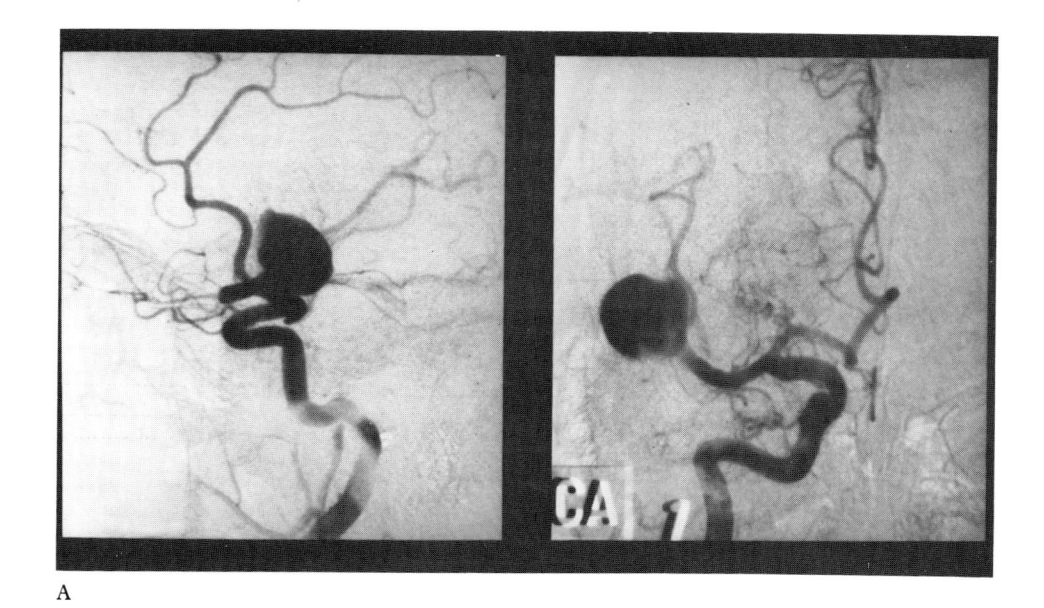

Figure 165-6 A giant right middle cerebral artery aneurysm and the technique of aneurysmorrhapy applied to this case. *A.* Preoperative arteriographic views in the lateral (*left*) and anteroposterior (*right*) projections. *B.* Similar postoperative arteriographic views. The aneurysm was treated by aneurysmorrhapy with temporary clipping of the proximal and distal middle cerebral artery, excision of the fundus of the aneurysm, and arterial reconstruction with a series of malleable tantalum clips.

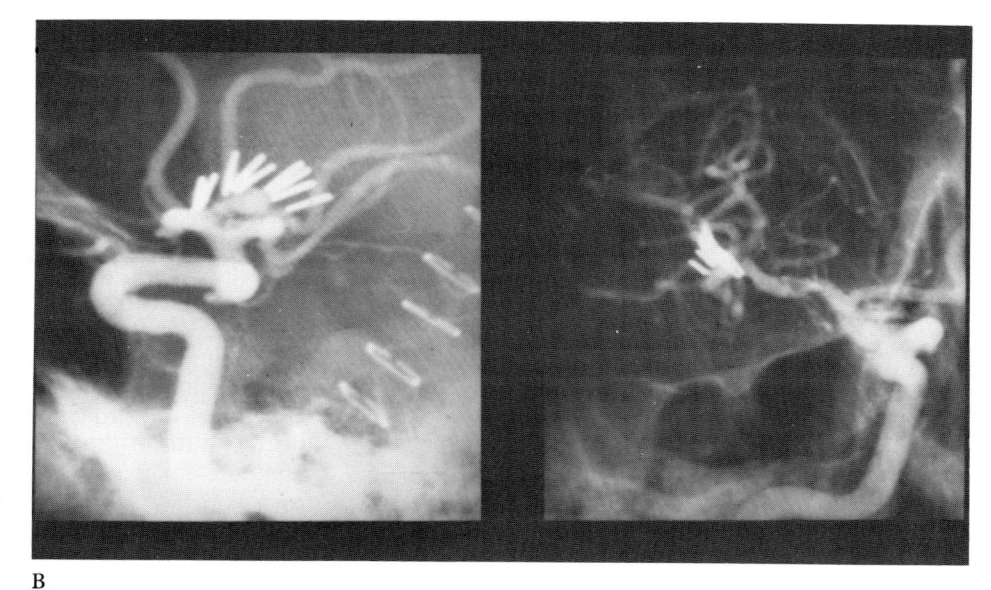

Figure 165-7 Arteriograms of a large basilar tip aneurysm. Preoperative views, lateral (*left*) and anteposterior (*middle*). A Drake clip was chosen for initial application since it would encircle the third nerve, which blocked direct access to the aneurysm. The closing force was insufficient, but parallel application of a McFadden clip led to complete occlusion of the aneurysm, as seen in the postoperative view (*right*).

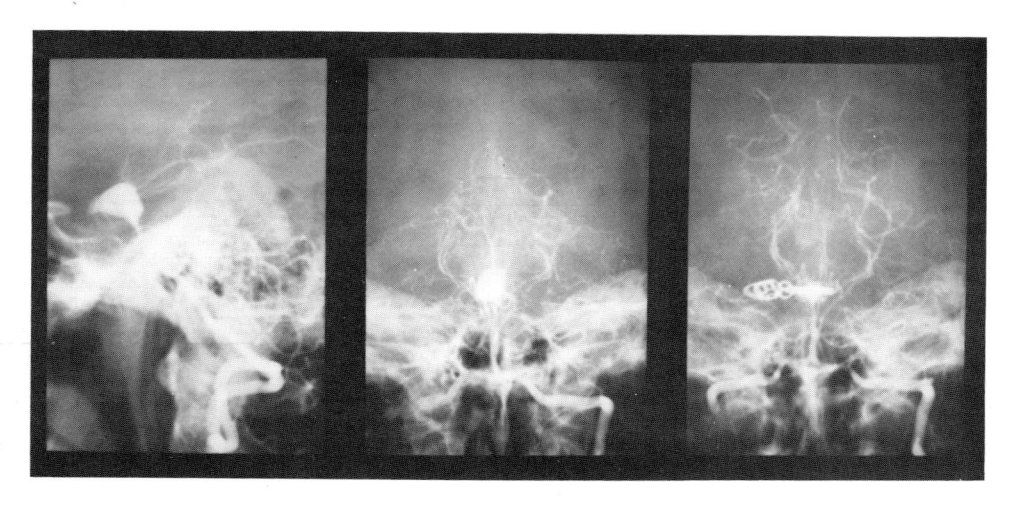

ternative to stainless steel for integral spring clips. These materials are very resistant to corrosion and are nonmagnetic. The Sugita and McFadden clips are both made of cobalt alloys.

Tantalum is another metal suitable for biological implantation. It does not corrode and leads to minimal tissue reaction. However, tantalum is too soft for spring clips and can be used only for malleable clips.

References

1. DeLong WB, Ray RL: Metallurgical analysis of aneurysm and microvascular clips. J Neurosurg 48:614–621, 1978.
2. Dujovny M, Ressler EO, Kossovsky N, Tucker JB, Wackenhut N, Leff L: Vascular clip closure force meter. Surg Neurol 14:107–109, 1980.
3. Dujovny M, Wakenhut N, Kossovsky N, Gomes CW, Laha RK, Leff L, Nelson D: Minimum vascular occlusive force. J Neurosurg 51:662–668, 1979.
4. Kossowsky R, Dujovny M, Kossovsky N, Keravel Y: Failure of a Heifetz aneurysm clip. J Neurosurg 57:233–239, 1982.
5. McFadden JT: Metallurgical principles in neurosurgery. J Neurosurg 31:373–385, 1969.
6. Rhoton A, Merz W: Spring clip for aneurysm surgery. Surg Neurol 19:14–16, 1983.
7. Sano K: A multipurpose all-angle clip applier for aneurysm surgery: Technical note. J Neurosurg 53:260–261, 1980.
8. Sugita K, Kobayashi S, Kyoshima K, Nakagawa F: Fenestrated clips for unusual aneurysms of the carotid artery. J Neurosurg 57:240–246, 1982.

166
Middle Cerebral Artery Aneurysms
Roberto C. Heros

Clinical Aspects

Middle cerebral artery (MCA) aneurysms account for approximately 20 percent of all intracranial aneurysms.[9,12] The majority are located at the first major bifurcation of the MCA. A few arise more proximally on the main trunk, at the origin of an early frontotemporal or anterior temporal branch or in relation to the perforating lenticulostriate vessels. Another small proportion arise at a more distal bifurcation of one of the main divisions. A review of the literature and personal experience suggest that giant MCA aneurysms are more common than giant aneurysms in other locations, with the possible exception of the paraclinoid region of the internal carotid artery. This observation might relate to the fact that MCA aneurysms can reach massive proportions without producing symptoms from encroachment on vital structures.

When large enough, unruptured MCA aneurysms can produce clinical symptoms from mass effect. Headaches associated with signs of increased intracranial pressure, including papilledema, occur rarely with the larger aneurysms. Temporal lobe epilepsy is another symptom that occurs rarely as a result of MCA aneurysms but only exceptionally as a result of aneurysms in other locations. Ischemic symptoms such as transient ischemic attacks and small strokes, although rarely due to aneurysms, occur more frequently with aneurysms of the MCA than with aneurysms in other locations. These symptoms are thought to result from intra-aneurysmal thrombosis with subsequent embolism. Only exceptionally has a major stroke occurred as a consequence of spontaneous thrombosis of the MCA or one of its major divisions as a result of aneurysmal expansion.

Rupture of an MCA aneurysm usually results in a syndrome indistinguishable from that associated with subarachnoid hemorrhage from rupture of an aneurysm in any other location. Certain clinical characteristics, however, favor the diagnosis of a ruptured MCA aneurysm. These characteristics were first described in detail by Höök and Norlén.[4] About 60 percent of patients with an MCA aneurysm lose consciousness at the onset of rupture, a higher proportion than with aneurysms at other locations. Diffuse headache is, of course, of no localizing significance, but about one-third of patients with a ruptured MCA aneurysm have primarily unilateral headache, which is much less commonly seen after rupture of aneurysms elsewhere. When such unilateral headache is present, it is almost always on the side of the aneurysm. About 80 percent of the patients in Höök and Norlén's series had focal neurological deficits when first seen. Such deficits were severe in half of the patients and usually consisted of hemiparesis, aphasia, visual field deficits, and central facial weakness. Only 34 percent of patients with ruptured aneurysms in other locations had such findings when first seen and only 7 percent had severe deficits.[4] When a patient with a ruptured aneurysm is first seen awake but with a severe hemiparesis, the most likely location of the aneurysm by far is the MCA. These aneurysms are also slightly more likely to result in seizures after rupture than aneurysms in other locations. In all likelihood, the propensity of MCA aneurysms to cause focal signs and symptoms is due to their tendency to bleed at least partially into the brain parenchyma as well as into the subarachnoid space. Thus, the incidence of intracerebral hematomas in patients with ruptured MCA aneurysms is between 30 and 50 percent, which is considerably higher than with aneurysms in other locations.[1,5] These intracerebral hematomas are frequently of great diagnostic value when identified by computed tomography (CT). A hematoma extending into both the frontal and the temporal opercula, bridging the sphenoid ridge, is virtually pathognomonic of a ruptured MCA aneurysm.

In terms of radiological diagnosis, little can be said specifically for MCA aneurysms. An early CT scan is mandatory to establish the diagnosis of SAH, to localize and quantitate the amount of blood in the cisterns in order to predict the likelihood and location of vasospasm, and to determine whether an intracerebral hematoma is present. The timing of angiography is related to each surgeon's particular bias about the timing of surgery. My personal policy is to perform early angiography in patients with a large intratemporal hematoma whether or not early surgery is contemplated. These patients can deteriorate abruptly, and surgical evacuation of the clot may suddenly become mandatory. Under such circumstances, it is comforting to have in hand an angiogram delineating the anatomy of the lesion, which is usually dealt with when the clot is evacuated. Angiography is, of course, essential in demonstrating the presence and location of the aneurysm and in providing a rough guide to the relation of the aneurysm to the major branches of the MCA. My experience indicates that it is not necessary to obtain multiple views to ascertain the presence or absence of a neck or the relationship of the MCA branches to the neck. Whether demonstrated or not, a neck is almost invariably present in all but the largest aneurysms. The anatomical details must be worked out at surgery by thorough exposure of the aneurysmal complex and cannot be predicted accurately even with the best angiographic technique.

The question of early versus late surgery remains as unsettled for MCA aneurysms as for aneurysms in other locations. Some comments, however, are pertinent in a discussion of MCA aneurysms. As discussed earlier, these aneurysms are frequently associated with temporal lobe hematomas, which may require emergency drainage. It is possible, of course, to gently evacuate a portion of the clot, enough to effect adequate decompression, and to leave the clot around the aneurysm until the aneurysm is clipped at a later date. I prefer, however, always to clip the aneurysm at the time of evacuation of the clot. There is usually a large space to work through without brain retraction after the hematoma is evacuated and, in my opinion this facilitates dissection and clipping of the aneurysm. Also, I worry about rebleeding from the unclipped aneurysm once the clot has been evacuated. Additionally, in many of these patients the bleeding has been primarily into the brain parenchyma rather than into the subarachnoid space, and therefore vasospasm is not a significant problem. It is in this group of patients with large temporal lobe hematomas that we have seen our only successful outcomes after operation on grade 4 patients and even on one occasion on a moribund patient. These comments, of course, do not apply to patients with deep hematomas in the frontal lobe or basal ganglia, since evacuation of these clots does not necessarily facilitate exposure.

Patients with MCA aneurysms, even without a temporal hematoma, may still be good candidates for early surgery. These aneurysms are located peripherally, and therefore deep retraction is not necessary, since they can be exposed by opening the fissure peripherally or by suctioning some of the superior temporal gyrus without much retraction at all, as will be discussed below. In addition, the subarachnoid clots in these patients are frequently localized in the sylvian fissure, and removal of the clot can be accomplished more thoroughly through a unilateral exposure than with centrally located aneurysms. This more thorough clot removal may be a factor in decreasing the incidence of vasospasm. Even when vasospasm supervenes, it has been our clinical impression that its consequences are less devastating when the subarachnoid clot, and hence the resultant vasospasm, is limited to one major arterial territory.

Because of the preceding considerations, it seems that patients with peripherally located MCA aneurysms who are in good neurological condition or whose poor neurological condition can be attributed to an intratemporal hematoma may represent an ideal group to be considered for early surgery even by surgeons who, like myself, remain skeptical about the advantages of early surgery.

Surgical Approaches

There are three basic approaches to MCA aneurysms. They involve (1) opening the sylvian fissure medially and following the MCA trunk distally or following the major division proximally either (2) by opening the fissure peripherally or (3) by subpial dissection after resection of a portion of the superior temporal gyrus. At times a surgeon can use a combination of these approaches or change from one approach to another when difficulties are encountered. It is important that the surgeon be familiar with each of these approaches because although he may use one preferentially, there are specific instances in which an alternative approach may be necessary.

Medial Trans-Sylvian Approach

When the aneurysm is approached by initially opening the sylvian fissure, the scalp incision and bone flap are the same as used for other aneurysms of the anterior circle of Willis. I use the basic pterional approach elaborated by Yasargil[12] and described in detail elsewhere in this book. The importance of a thorough removal of the pterion and of the lateral wing of the sphenoid to achieve a low approach at the expense of bone removal rather than of brain retraction cannot be overemphasized. Just as important is the vigorous downward retraction of the muscle toward the temporal fossa, since nothing is gained by a thorough bone removal if overhanging muscle obstructs the view. I prefer to use a free bone flap and turn the flap of skin and muscle together by opening the fascia and the muscle along the same line of the skin incision posteriorly and then detaching the muscle from the bone by subperiosteal dissection and leaving it attached to the skin flap. I have found that cutting the anterior (frontal) attachments of the muscle fibers from within facilitates retraction of the muscle backwards and downwards toward the temporal fossa with barbless fishhooks or sutures attached to strong rubber bands. If this is done, it is important to resuture the muscle anteriorly during closure to avoid a cosmetically unpleasant depression over the pterional region. If the anterior incision of the muscle attachment is made only through the muscle fibers down to the plane of areolar and fatty tissue between the muscle and the temporalis fascia, the frontal branch of the facial nerve, which runs in this plane, will not be injured. Another step I have found useful in preventing injury to the frontalis nerve is to start the incision at the level of the zygoma just in front of the tragus, as opposed to 1 or 1.5 cm in front of the tragus as is frequently illustrated. By starting the incision just in front of the tragus, one spares not only the frontalis nerve, but also the superficial temporal artery, or at least its frontal branch, which may, on occasion, be used later for a bypass graft.

After the dura is opened and tented inferiorly to allow a flat subfrontal approach along the sphenoid ridge, cerebrospinal fluid (CSF) can be suctioned from the medial cisterns to facilitate exposure. I have not found it necessary to insert a lumbar CSF drain routinely, but this is a matter of preference. After adequate relaxation is obtained, the surgeon decides whether the exposure will proceed from medial to lateral or vice versa. In the former case, the carotid cistern is opened by sharp arachnoidal dissection, and then the medial aspect of the sylvian fissure is opened, preferably on the frontal side of the sylvian veins.[6] I have never hesitated to coagulate any vein that bridged the medial aspect of the fissure, regardless of its size. It must be pointed out that the exact location of the fissure medially is not always apparent and that the fissure does not always "open" in a clean arachnoidal plane, as is frequently illustrated. It has been my experience, particularly in cases of recent hemorrhage, that more frequently than not a small amount of brain must be suctioned in order to follow the carotid artery as it continues to curve laterally to become the MCA. The placement of the self-retaining retractors at this stage is critical. The frontal and temporal opercula must be gently retracted to put the medial aspect of the fissure under some stretch. This is best accomplished by gradually opening the tips of the retractors as the dissection proceeds. It is preferable to retract more on the temporal side, since excessive retraction of the frontal operculum can be harmful, particularly on the dominant side, where it can result in expressive aphasia.[7]

The MCA is followed along its anterior-inferior aspect, away from the perforating vessels. Usually one or two temporal or frontotemporal branches will be seen before the aneurysm is reached. I do not hesitate to resect a small amount of brain tissue from the temporal lobe to facilitate exposure. When the aneurysm arises from the M_1 segment in relation to a perforating branch, all that is necessary is to carefully separate the perforators from the neck enough to pass a clip. These aneurysms usually are not too large and point straight upward into the frontal lobe; it is not necessary to dissect the dome completely. In aneurysms of the bifurcation (or, rarely, trifurcation) of the MCA, however, complete dissection of the aneurysmal complex is usually preferable. This can be done with relative safety after a small portion of the MCA just proximal to the aneurysm has been prepared for temporary clipping in case of rupture. After preparing the neck as well as possible for clipping, the surgeon can advance the dissection distally, frequently in a subpial plane, leaving a small amount of adherent clot and brain with the dome. The relationship of the divisions to the dome is then worked out and, more frequently than not, at least one division must be carefully separated from the base of the aneurysm by sharp dissection to define the true neck. Particular care must be taken in sparing the important recurrent perforators that so frequently come from the origin of the major divisions.[2,6] Except in the case of small aneurysms, it is frequently necessary to replace the clip several times because of kinking of one division or "slipping" of the clip proximally onto the MCA. This frequently is an indication for further dissection to separate the divisions more proximally down to a narrower neck. With large aneurysms, I have found it helpful to use a small self-retaining retractor on the aneurysm itself. A small Rhoton-type dissector fits nicely into the arm of the Greenberg self-retaining retractor and can be used for this purpose, freeing both the surgeon's hands. With the aneurysm retracted in one direction, the surgeon can retract the vessel gently away from the aneurysm to stretch the arachnoid bands that must be sharply divided to separate the vessel from the aneurysm.[3]

Lateral Trans-Sylvian Approach

Some surgeons prefer to open the sylvian fissure peripherally, find the distal divisions, and dissect proximally toward the aneurysm. This approach has the advantage of facilitating exposure of the distal anatomy of the aneurysmal complex, which is usually the difficult aspect of the case. The major disadvantage is that the surgeon reaches the aneurysm before achieving proximal control. To correct this situation, Yasargil recommends starting the dissection medially on the fissure to expose the MCA and to achieve proximal control, and then moving laterally, starting the dissection distally in the fissure, and from there proceeding proximally.[12] As mentioned previously, the exact location of the sylvian fissure may not always be obvious. A helpful maneuver is to pick a relatively large cortical vessel and follow it medially toward the fissure.[7,12]

Superior Temporal Gyrus Approach

My preferred approach for the majority of MCA aneurysms has been transtemporal through a small incision, with subpial resection in the anterior portion of the superior temporal gyrus.[3] When this approach is planned, the patient is placed in the supine position with the head turned about 60 degrees to the contralateral side, which is a slightly greater angle than for the usual pterional approach. A roll placed under the ipsilateral shoulder sometimes facilitates turning of the neck.

The incision is started at the level of the zygoma, just in front of the tragus, as discussed for the medial trans-sylvian approach. The only difference here is that the incision curves slightly backward above the ear before starting to swing forward to a point just about 1 cm in front of the hairline at about the level of the pupil (Fig. 166-1). As already discussed, this type of incision will preserve the frontalis branch of the facial nerve and the frontal branch of the superficial temporal artery. The muscle is turned down with the skin flap, as already discussed, and the anterior attachments of the muscles are cut so that the muscle can be retracted backward and downward into the temporal fossa. The bone flap is then cut in the same manner as for the standard pterional approach, but the cut is extended farther back into the temporal bone to expose more of the temporal lobe (Fig. 166-1). The pterion and the lateral aspect of the sphenoid ridge are totally removed. This step is important because it exposes the anterior aspect of the sylvian fissure, which allows dissection of the aneurysm and clip application from an anterolateral direction as well as from a posterior direction. If the pterion is not removed completely, the surgeon is forced to work only from behind, underneath the overhanging bone, which may be a significant handicap.

The dura is opened inferiorly in a crescentic fashion with a perpendicular posterior cut along the sylvian fissure, as illustrated in Fig. 166-2. When I use this approach, I do not open the medial cisterns, since brain relaxation is less critical with this approach than with the others because the exposure is obtained by suction of nonessential brain tissue. As soon as the dura is opened, the microscope is brought into the field, and a 2- to 3-cm incision is made in the superior temporal gyrus beginning about 1 cm behind the front of the sylvian fissure and continuing posteriorly in a direction parallel to the fissure (Fig. 166-2). With suction and bipolar coagulation, the incision is extended medially into the vertical segment of the sylvian fissure over the insula. The sylvian veins are not disturbed. By microsurgical technique the branches of the MCA are followed proximally toward the aneurysm (Fig. 166-3). It is usually possible to follow one of the two major divisions toward the base of the aneurysm without disturbing the dome. This is done by following the division on the side away from the aneurysm until the distal portion of the MCA can be seen. Only enough of the distal trunk of the MCA is exposed to allow the application of a

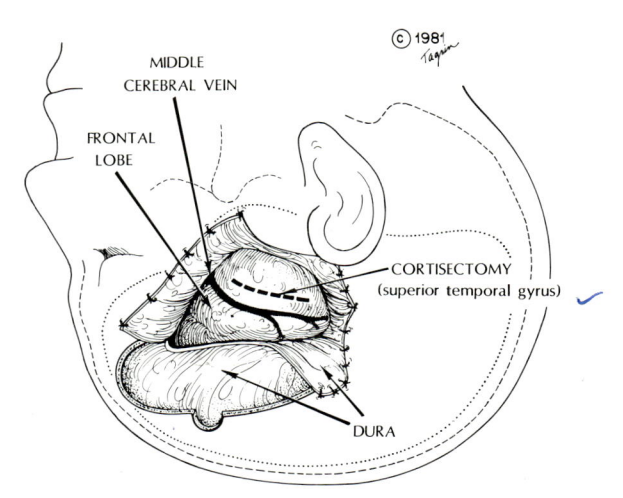

Figure 166-2 A diagram showing the dural opening and line of cortisectomy in the superior temporal gyrus (*dashed line*). (From Heros et al.[3])

temporary clip, should such become necessary. By this time the second division is usually in view and can also be followed to the aneurysm. Once the distal part of the trunk of the MCA and the origins of the main divisions have been identified, we usually proceed with a dissection of the entire aneurysmal complex, taking the precaution of leaving adherent brain and clot on the dome in the area of likely rupture (Fig. 166-4).

For this final step of aneurysmal dissection, we use some hypotension. Until recently we were using rather significant hypotension, such that mean systemic pressure was 50 to 60 torr. More recently, I have not found it necessary to lower the blood pressure this much and am usually content with a mean systemic pressure of about 75 torr. In patients who have significant angiographic vasospasm or who have been clinically symptomatic from vasospasm, I prefer not to lower the blood pressure at all. If the aneurysm ruptures, the first instinct is usually to lower the blood pressure further. I have had problems in the past by doing just that and then finding it necessary to place a temporary clip in the efferent vessel. The combination of temporary vessel occlusion plus deep systemic hypotension is a particularly deadly one. Therefore, my most recent inclination is to raise the blood pressure when there is a rupture, rather than to lower it. The amount of bleeding does not seem to change very much, and having a better mean perfusion pressure will allow for safer application of a temporary clip on the efferent vessel should such become necessary.

Even though most of these aneurysms come from a true bifurcation, there is usually a third branch from the MCA just before the origin of the aneurysm or from one of the major divisions just after the origin of the aneurysm. Of course, every effort should be made to preserve each of these branches. In addition, it is very important to keep in mind the recurrent perforating vessels that can arise from the divisions, as discussed earlier. The approach through the superior temporal gyrus is particularly well suited to large aneurysms, since the surgeon has better circumferential access to the aneurysm and is able to retract it in any direction in

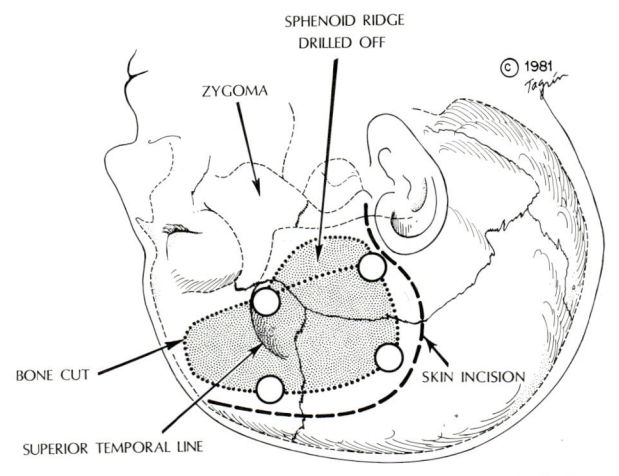

Figure 166-1 A diagram of the skin incision (*dashed line*) and bony opening (*stippled area*) for the superior temporal gyrus approach. (From Heros et al.[3])

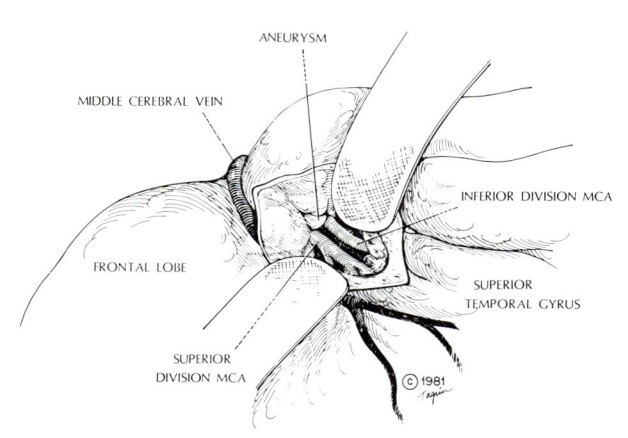

Figure 166-3 A diagram of the exposure of the main divisions of the middle cerebral artery through the superior temporal gyrus. (From Heros et al.[3])

order to expose the anatomy at the base and neck of the aneurysm.

The choice of approach to MCA aneurysms is largely determined by the individual surgeon's preference. Most MCA bifurcation aneurysms project laterally as a direct continuation of the MCA; less commonly they project caudally or rostrally.[3,8] In these cases, the superior temporal gyrus approach allows the surgeon to expose the main trunk of the MCA without disturbing the dome of the aneurysm by following the branches proximally to the base of the aneurysm. In the rare cases in which the aneurysm projects mostly backwards over the insula, the dome of the aneurysm is in the way when the aneurysm is approached from a distal position. Therefore, we prefer to approach these aneurysms from a medial position by splitting the sylvian fissure. It must be emphasized that this latter type of projection is unusual, and we have found it only once.

The superior temporal gyrus approach is not suited to aneurysms of the main trunk of the MCA proximal to the bifurcation or to those aneurysms that arise from the MCA at the point of origin of an early temporal branch. This approach is also not suitable for patients in whom the main trunk of the MCA is short and the aneurysm arises from an early bifurcation that occurs before the genu, that is, from the point at which the MCA starts to turn upward around the limen of the insula. In these instances, the aneurysm arises from the horizontal segment of the MCA beneath the insula, and nothing is gained by a temporal lobe resection since the surgeon must work from an anterior position to avoid damage to the insular region.

Table 166-1 is a summary of the advantages and disadvantages of the superior temporal gyrus approach to MCA aneurysms. With this approach, significant retraction of the frontal operculum is avoided, and the exposure is achieved by suctioning nonessential brain tissue rather than by retraction. This advantage would seem to be particularly important in acute operations when the brain is swollen and hyperemic. There is also no doubt about the advantage of this approach in cases of a large anterior temporal hematoma, and even surgeons who routinely prefer to use the medial approach would ordinarily approach these aneurysms through the clot under such circumstances. Another relative advantage of working through the temporal lobe is that the sylvian veins are left undisturbed. Although we are not convinced that occlusion of these veins definitely leads to any difficulty, there is, of course, the theoretical possibility of venous congestion if the sylvian veins are occluded, as they may need to be occasionally with the approach through the fissure. The transtemporal approach also avoids manipulation of the medial circle of Willis and of the proximal portion of the MCA with its important dorsal perforators. Whether such manipulation has any relationship to postoperative vasospasm is a question that remains unsettled.

The most important advantage of this approach is that the distal, dorsal aspect of the aneurysmal complex is more thoroughly exposed. This is the most difficult portion of the aneurysmal anatomy to visualize, and it should be defined as well as possible before clipping is attempted, especially in the case of larger aneurysms. The transtemporal approach combined with a thorough removal of the pterion allows, as discussed above, circumferential access to the aneurysm and placement of the clip from any direction. The main disadvantage of the approach through the superior temporal gyrus is that the base of the aneurysm is encountered before

TABLE 166-1 Superior Temporal Gyrus Approach to MCA Aneurysms

Advantages
1. Minimal brain retraction
2. Preservation of sylvian veins
3. Minimal manipulation of main trunk and perforators of the MCA
4. Better visualization of posterior aspect of the aneurysmal complex
5. Easier manipulation of the aneurysm and definition of the distal branches

Disadvantages
1. Lack of "proximal control" until the base of the aneurysm is reached
2. Increased potential risk of epilepsy
3. Slightly larger bone flap is required
4. Unsuitable for "proximal" MCA aneurysms

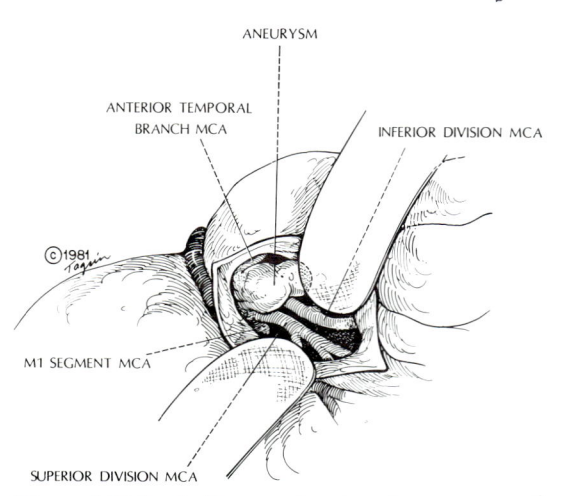

Figure 166-4 A diagram showing the exposure of the middle cerebral artery aneurysm through the superior temporal gyrus. (From Heros et al.[3])

proximal control of the efferent vessel is assured. However, it is almost always possible to expose enough of the distal MCA to allow for the application of a temporary clip, should such become necessary, before exposing the dome of the aneurysm. A minor disadvantage of this approach is the need for a slightly larger skin and bone flap than is required for the usual pterional approach. A theoretical disadvantage of this approach is the possibility of increasing the risk of epilepsy by the cortical resection. The length of follow-up in our patients does not allow us to reach any conclusions in this respect.

In conclusion, I have found the superior temporal gyrus approach most satisfactory for the majority (about 85 percent) of MCA aneurysms. I cannot state that the transtemporal approach is superior to more conventional approaches to these aneurysms; however, it may be the preferred approach in patients with a temporal lobe hematoma, in patients operated upon early when considerable brain swelling is still present, and in patients with large aneurysms that project laterally, anteriorly, or inferiorly.

Results

Table 166-2 summarizes the surgical results of 68 consecutive operations for MCA aneurysm performed on 65 patients (3 patients had bilateral MCA aneurysms). These operations were performed personally or under the supervision of Robert Crowell, Robert Ojemann, or myself during the last 6 years. Table 166-2 includes data from 49 patients operated upon through the superior temporal gyrus and described in a recent report.[3] The grade immediately before operation is compared with the result at the time of the last follow-up available, usually 6 months to a year after operation. A good result means a normal patient or a patient who had a minor neurological deficit that resolved completely within 3 months. A fair result indicates a patient who is ambulatory and independent but with a persistent mild to moderate neurological deficit. A poor result implies a patient incapacitated with a permanent moderate to severe neurological deficit.

Table 166-3 compares the size of the aneurysm as estimated from the preoperative angiograms (and CT scan in cases of partially thrombosed aneurysms). In this series, no patient in good condition preoperatively (grade 0, I, II, or III by Hunt's classification) has died. The series contains 12 patients with asymptomatic unruptured aneurysms and 1 patient (to be described) with a massive unruptured but severely symptomatic aneurysm who presented with signs of herniation from the mass effect. When analyzing these results, it must be kept in mind that these are surgical results and not "management" results. Unfortunately, we are unable to retrospectively analyze our total case management morbidity and mortality, since many patients with aneurysms did not come onto our service until the time of operation. In addition, it is important to point out that day 14 was the median day of operation, and thus, in general, "late" surgery was favored in this series. With rare exceptions (Hunt grade I patients seen within the first 48 h), the only patients operated upon early in this series were patients with severely symptomatic temporal lobe hematomas. For the rest, we planned the operation generally between the tenth and twelfth day but deferred it further if the patient developed symptomatic vasospasm or showed severe diffuse angiographic vasospasm.

In this series, four aneurysms were wrapped with gauze and coated with plastic adhesives. Another aneurysm was excised, and an aneurysmorrhaphy of the base was carried out. The rest were clipped. Of the latter group, postoperative angiography was carried out in 36 patients. In two patients (to be described), the MCA was found to be occluded. In another patient (to be described), a third, previously unrecognized branch was occluded, and in another patient there was partial kinking of one division. The rest of the postoperative angiograms were unremarkable except for filling in a minor portion of the neck in two patients and varying degrees of vasospasm in a few other patients. Except for the patients whose aneurysms were only wrapped, the patients who did not have postoperative angiography had their aneurysm opened and collapsed or excised at surgery.

These results are similar to other recent reports of MCA aneurysm surgery by experienced surgeons.[10-12]

Complications

With the exception of herniation from the mass effect of a temporal hematoma, no preoperative complication is peculiar to MCA aneurysms. The incidences of rebleeding, vasospasm, and hydrocephalus are probably not significantly different from those associated with aneurysms in other locations.[1] It has been our experience that the incidence of electrolyte disturbances and other evidence of hypothalamic dysfunction is a bit lower with MCA aneurysms than with aneurysms located more proximally in the circle of Willis, such as aneurysms of the anterior communicating complex.

Our operative complications are summarized in Table 166-4. They will be discussed in some detail since they are

TABLE 166-2 Middle Cerebral Artery Aneurysms

Preoperative Grade (Hunt)	Number of Cases	Surgical Result			
		Good	Fair	Poor	Dead
0, I, II	47	45	2	0	0
III	12	4	6	2	0
IV	5	1	2	1	1
V	4	0	1	0	3
Total	68	50	11	3	4

TABLE 166-3 Middle Cerebral Artery Aneurysms

Size	Number of Cases	Surgical Result			
		Good	Fair	Poor	Dead
<7 mm	6	6	0	0	0
7–15 mm	29	21	5	1	2
15–25 mm	21	15	5	1	0
>25 mm	12	8	1	1	2
Total	68	50	11	3	4

TABLE 166-4 Middle Cerebral Artery Aneurysms: Operative Complications

Intracerebral hemorrhage after artificially induced hypertension
Death as a result of massive brain swelling after excision of a giant aneurysm
Hemiplegia as a result of occlusion of the MCA after attempted repair of an intraoperative rupture of a giant aneurysm
Broca's aphasia from excessive frontal retraction
Mild hemiparesis from occlusion of an unrecognized large branch
Moderate hemiparesis from postoperative vasospasm after "early" surgery
Thrombophlebitis (eight patients)
Pulmonary embolism, nonfatal (two patients)
Subdural empyema
Subdural hematoma

---

representative of those frequently encountered when dealing with aneurysms in this location.

A few years ago it was our policy to check for hemostasis by increasing the blood pressure artificially to hypertensive levels before closing. In one patient an intracerebral hemorrhage developed during this period of induced hypertension after the aneurysm had been clipped. We believe that this complication may have been related to an impairment in autoregulation caused by the period of hypotension induced during clipping of the aneurysm. We have since discontinued this practice.

Another unfortunate patient had what we consider to be a rare, but interesting and poorly understood, problem. She had been followed by us for 3 years with a known giant aneurysm of the left MCA that occupied most of the temporal fossa. Initially the aneurysm was treated by carotid ligation and extracranial tointracranial bypass grafting. The aneurysm continued to enlarge, however, and the graft, which was initially patent, was later found to be occluded. We believed that this was related to the fact that there was excellent collateral supply through a very large posterior communicating artery that filled the entire middle cerebral territory in an anterograde fashion. This was also probably the cause of continuing enlargement of the aneurysm. Eventually, the patient presented with a syndrome of headaches for a few days, then nausea and vomiting, and finally unconsciousness. When first seen, she had a large left pupil and a dense right hemiparesis. The CT scan showed a tremendous mass effect on the left side with considerable evidence of brain edema around the partially thrombosed aneurysmal mass. She was treated successfully with vigorous medical management of her brain edema and intracranial hypertension. Nevertheless, a week later she developed, again rather abruptly, signs of herniation with marked drowsiness, enlargement of the left pupil, worsening right hemiparesis, and aphasia. Since this syndrome progressed in spite of maximal medical therapy, we decided to proceed with surgical excision of the aneurysm. We planned to temporarily occlude the MCA and its branches under hypothermic anesthesia with barbiturate coverage. Owing to technical difficulty in exposing and excising the aneurysm, we required a period of clamping of approximately 45 min for the MCA and its branches. During this time the temperature was kept at about 30 to 31°C.

The patient never awoke from the operation. A CT scan revealed massive swelling of the left hemisphere with severe downward herniation of the brain stem. An angiogram showed that the basilar artery was pushed downward and the posterior communicating artery, which previously supplied the middle cerebral territory, was occluded at the petroclinoid ligament, where it had to take a sharp turn to come upward from its markedly displaced downward position. The entire trunk of the MCA was occluded. The patient died shortly after the angiogram. The MCA may have occluded after aneurysmorrhaphy, even though at surgery the flow appeared to be excellent through the trunk and all of the branches. If the artery occluded postoperatively, this could have produced massive cerebral infarction with subsequent herniation. Alternatively, the brain could have become tremendously swollen as a result of ischemia suffered during the period of occlusion at operation, and the resulting herniation with downward displacement of the basilar artery could have led to occlusion of the posterior communicating artery and hence the middle cerebral trunk, which was being fed by the former vessel.

If faced with a similar case again, we would consider performing the operation under profound hypothermia with cardiac arrest and the patient under cardiopulmonary bypass. Whether this would make a difference in a patient such as the one described above, who was in an extremely serious neurological state prior to surgery, remains to be seen, but certainly our approach to the problem was not successful. The aspect of this case that we find interesting and puzzling is the intractable brain edema encountered preoperatively in relation to the partially thrombosed giant aneurysm. Even though the aneurysm had enlarged only slightly since the last CT scan, the amount of surrounding edema found when the patient presented was much more impressive.

Another patient became hemiplegic because of MCA occlusion resulting from the tearing of a giant aneurysm at surgical exposure during an attempted operative repair. In another case, severe expressive aphasia developed, which fortunately improved significantly. This patient was perfectly normal before operation, and we believe that the aphasia was related to excessive retraction on the frontal operculum. This particular small aneurysm was approached medially by splitting the sylvian fissure, since the aneurysm was located fairly proximally beneath the insula. Another patient suffered a mild postoperative hemiparesis, and on postoperative angiography we found occlusion of a branch that we had failed to recognize either in the preoperative angiogram or intraoperatively. One of the very few patients in this series who underwent early operation suffered significant postoperative vasospasm that resulted in a serious neurological deficit. A subdural hematoma developed in one patient, and a subdural empyema was found in another; neither of these patients suffered serious permanent neurological disability.

When we initially reviewed this series, we were surprised at the frequency with which thrombophlebitis was encountered. There were eight patients with this complication. Two had a pulmonary embolus, which fortunately was of no lasting significance. We cannot help speculating that aminocaproic acid, which most of these patients received, played a role in this high incidence of phlebitis.

References

1. Graf CJ, Nibbelink DW: Cooperative Study of Intracranial Aneurysms and Subarachnoid Hemorrhage: Report on a randomized treatment study. III. Intracranial surgery. Stroke 5:559–601, 1974.
2. Grand W: Microsurgical anatomy of the proximal middle cerebral artery and the internal carotid artery bifurcation. Neurosurgery 7:215–218, 1980.
3. Heros RC, Ojemann RG, Crowell RM: Superior temporal gyrus approach to middle cerebral artery aneurysms: Technique and results. Neurosurgery 10:308–313, 1982.
4. Höök O, Norlén G: Aneurysms of the middle cerebral artery. Acta Chir Scand [Suppl] 235:1–39, 1958.
5. Lougheed WM, Marshall BM: Management of aneurysms of the anterior circulation by intracranial procedures, in Youmans JR (ed): *Neurological Surgery: A Comprehensive Reference Guide to the Diagnosis and Management of Neurosurgical Problems*, 1st ed. Philadelphia, Saunders, 1973, pp 731–767.
6. Peerless SJ: The surgical approach to middle cerebral and posterior communicating aneurysms. Clin Neurosurg 21:151–165, 1974.
7. Rand RW: Microneurosurgery in cerebral aneurysms, in Rand RW (ed): *Microneurosurgery*, 2d ed. St Louis, CV Mosby, 1978, pp 311–324.
8. Rhoton AL Jr, Saeki N, Perlmutter D, Zeal A: Microsurgical anatomy of common aneurysm sites. Clin Neurosurg 26:248–306, 1979.
9. Robinson RG: Ruptured aneurysms of the middle cerebral artery. J Neurosurg 35:25–33, 1971.
10. Sundt TM Jr, Kobayashi S, Fode NC, Whisnant JP: Results and complications of surgical management of 809 intracranial aneurysms in 722 cases: Related and unrelated to grade of patient, type of aneurysm, and timing of surgery. J Neurosurg 56:753–765, 1982.
11. Suzuki J, Kodama N, Fujiwara S, Ebina T: Surgical treatment of middle cerebral artery aneurysms: From the experience of 174 cases, in Suzuki J (ed): *Cerebral Aneurysms: Experience with 1000 Directly Operated Cases*. Tokyo, Tokyo Press Co Ltd, 1979, pp 278–283.
12. Yasargil MG, Smith RD: Middle cerebral artery aneurysms, in Youmans JR (ed): *Neurological Surgery: A Comprehensive Reference Guide to the Diagnosis and Management of Neurosurgical Problems*, 2d ed. Philadelphia, Saunders, 1982, pp 1663–1696.

167
Distal Anterior Cerebral Artery Aneurysms

Alan S. Fleischer
Daniel L. Barrow

Incidence, Etiology, and Anatomy

Aneurysms of the distal anterior cerebral artery (DACA) comprise between 2 and 4.5 percent of all intracranial aneurysms. In the largest reported series there was a nearly equal incidence in males and females.[1–3,5,9,10] There have been a variety of diseases and anomalies associated with DACA aneurysms, including other intracranial aneurysms,[5,10] arteriovenous malformations,[5] polycystic kidney disease,[3] coarctation of the aorta,[5] hypertension, craniosynostosis,[5] and agenesis of the corpus callosum.

DACA aneurysms, like other intracranial aneurysms, can be categorized as saccular (berry, "congenital"), mycotic, atherosclerotic, or traumatic. The large majority of DACA aneurysms are of a saccular type, presumably of congenital etiology. The location of the aneurysm on the anterior cerebral artery (ACA) is related to the etiology.

The DACA includes the ACA and its branches distal to the anterior communicating artery. The ACA courses anteriorly and superiorly from the anterior communicating artery to the genu of the corpus callosum, where it bifurcates into the more superior callosomarginal and inferior pericallosal arteries. A few centimeters distal to the anterior communicating artery, the prefrontal and frontopolar arteries arise from the anterior cerebral artery. The two DACAs run parallel to each other a few millimeters apart on the medial surface of the olfactory area in the interhemispheric fissure. Beyond the origin of the callosomarginal artery, the anterior, middle, and posterior inferior frontal arteries arise as branches of the DACA. At about the midportion of the corpus callosum, the paracentral artery and, more distally, the precuneal and parieto-occipital arteries arise. About 25 percent of human brains will have an anomalous pattern of the DACA, including an unpaired ACA, an artery feeding the opposite hemisphere, a triplicate vestigial vessel, and intercommunicating vessels between the DACAs beyond the anterior communicating artery.

The overwhelming majority of DACA aneurysms are located near the genu of the corpus callosum at the bifurcation of the pericallosal and callosomarginal arteries, where the pericallosal artery frequently makes an abrupt bend posteriorly. The etiology of most of these aneurysms is believed to be similar to that of the more common berry aneurysms located on the circle of Willis, which occur at the bifurcations of vessels and are characterized pathologically by fragmentation and loss of the internal elastica and thinning of the media.[7] The description by Laitinen and Snellman[5] of the occurrence of a communication between the pericallosal arteries at the genu of the corpus callosum in conjunction with DACA aneurysms has been cited as evidence for a congenital etiology. These authors have termed this anomalous communicating vessel the *supreme anterior communicating artery*. Yasargil and Carter have likewise noted similar arterial connections and suggest that although a developmental etiology is possible, it is just as likely that an anatomical variation may create a flow disturbance leading to aneurysm formation.[10] In support of this view, only five DACA aneurysms have been reported in children under 5 years of age.

Most of the DACA aneurysms located beyond the genu of the corpus callosum are secondary to trauma, infection (mycotic), or tumor embolus or are idiopathic.[7] A larger percentage of DACA aneurysms than of aneurysms at other intracranial locations occur as a result of infection or trauma. Traumatic aneurysms, of which DACA aneurysms are second in incidence only to those of cortical branches of the middle cerebral artery, are the result of either direct or indirect trauma. Direct trauma results in aneurysm formation when a penetrating object, surgical manipulation, or overlying skull fracture damages the wall of an artery in the pathway of the trauma. Indirect vascular injury is usually associated with a significant closed head injury and is probably secondary to the deformity, shearing and compression occurring with the traumatic acceleration and deceleration of the brain. The arterial injury producing DACA aneurysms may be secondary to compression of the vessel on the adjacent free edge of the falx during a transient shift of the brain beneath this rigid structure. If the injury to the arterial wall is incomplete, the damaged internal elastic lamina and media of the artery allow dilatation in a manner similar to a congenital (true) berry aneurysm. False aneurysms occur when all layers of the arterial wall are lacerated, with resultant hemorrhage. The hematoma is contained by surrounding brain and the periphery becomes organized over the next few days.[4]

Mycotic aneurysms occur as a result of infected emboli (usually from bacterial endocarditis) that infect the arterial wall by direct extension from the lumen.[8] The DACA aneurysms of embolic infectious origin are usually located on the most distal branches. A DACA aneurysm in a location not near the genu of the corpus callosum should raise the suspicion of either a mycotic or traumatic origin.

Clinical Presentation

The most common presentation of DACA aneurysms is subarachnoid hemorrhage, with or without residual neurological deficit. It is often difficult to clinically differentiate the subarachnoid hemorrhage caused by a DACA aneurysm from that resulting from other intracranial aneurysms, especially those of the anterior communicating artery. There is, however, a high incidence of pyramidal signs, especially a crural predominant hemiparesis[1] or contralateral lower extremity monoparesis.[5] This signature may be transient and should be looked for early. DACA aneurysms may also present with mental deterioration and urinary incontinence, simulating a frontal lobe tumor or normal pressure hydrocephalus. Laitinen and Snellman reported mental confusion in one-half and papilledema in about one-third of their 14 patients, 13 of whom presented with a subarachnoid hemorrhage.[5] Other manifestations have included intraventricular hemorrhage and compression of the optic nerves by an inferiorly directed frontopolar aneurysm, as well as the incidental finding of a DACA aneurysm during arteriography for unrelated symptoms.[1]

Management

The overall management of DACA aneurysms except for the surgical approach is the same as for other intracranial aneurysms. The results of a cooperative study would indicate, however, that DACA aneurysms "appear to carry a worse prognosis for survival than [aneurysms at] any other site."[6]

The etiology of the aneurysm will dictate the form of therapy in some instances. Berry or traumatic aneurysms that have ruptured should be surgically repaired in our opinion. Mycotic aneurysms occurring on the DACA should be treated with appropriate antibiotic therapy. If the aneurysm is nonvisualized or smaller on a repeat angiogram performed 2 weeks after the start of therapy, antibiotics should be continued for a full course. Should the aneurysm enlarge over this period, surgical intervention should be considered.

Incidental DACA aneurysms are managed as are other incidental aneurysms.

Surgical Approaches

Aneurysms that arise immediately distal to the anterior communicating artery or at any point proximal to the middle of the genu of the corpus callosum are within the operating field of the anterior communicating artery and are approached subfrontally or pterionally. Laitinen and Snellman operated on 10 of their patients with DACA aneurysm through a subfrontal approach by locating the internal carotid artery and following the ACA to the pericallosal bifurcation.[5] These authors and others have pointed out the difficulty of the approach. All other series have utilized an interhemispheric approach to DACA aneurysms as described by Yasargil and Carter[10] and Wilson et al.[9] This is the surgical approach we recommend for any DACA aneurysm distal to the mid-genu of the corpus callosum. Preoperative treatment is identical to that for any other intracranial aneurysm.

The patient is placed in the supine position with the head slightly flexed in a brow-up manner. We do not use spinal drainage routinely. A coronal skin incision is made and reflected anteriorly. A rectangular bone flap is elevated on the right side of midline. The dural flap is based on the superior sagittal sinus. A self-retaining brain retractor is used to maintain gentle lateral retraction on the right frontal lobe, exposing the interhemispheric fissure. At this point the operating microscope is utilized and the ACA is located anterior to the aneurysm for proximal control should an untimely rupture occur. The aneurysm is then dissected from surrounding vessels and brain until the neck is well delineated. The ACA and the pericallosal and callosomarginal arteries should be well visualized before clip application to avoid the potential significant morbidity associated with interruption of these vessels. If possible, a clip is applied across the base of the aneurysm to isolate it from the normal cerebral circulation. If the anatomy of the aneurysm precludes clip ligation, acrylic coating is indicated. If the aneurysm sac collapses after clipping, no further manipulation is necessary. Should it remain tense, a 27-gauge needle is used to aspirate the sac to be sure it is adequately clipped. Postoperative angiography is not performed routinely.

The results of surgical treatment of DACA aneurysms has been generally good. Operative mortality ranges in the literature from 0 to 25 percent, with a morbidity of approximately 15 percent.

References

1. Becker DH, Newton TH: Distal anterior cerebral artery aneurysm. Neurosurgery 4: 495–503, 1979.
2. Dechaume JP, Aimard G, Michel D, Bret P, Desgeorges M, Lapras C, Lecuire J: Les anévrysmes de l' artère péri-calleuse: A propos d'une série de 12 observations. Neurochirugie 19: 135–150, 1973.
3. Fisher RG, Ciminello V: Pericallosal aneurysms. J Neurosurg 25: 512–515, 1966.
4. Fleischer AS, Patton JM, Tindall GT: Cerebral aneurysms of traumatic origin. Surg Neurol 4: 233–239, 1975.
5. Laitinen L, Snellman A: Aneurysms of the pericallosal artery: A study of 14 cases verified angiographically and treated mainly by direct surgical attack. J Neurosurg 17: 447–458, 1960.
6. Nishioka H: Report on the Cooperative Study of Intracranial Aneurysms and Subarachnoid Hemorrhage. Section VII, Part 1. Evaluation of the conservative management of ruptured intracranial aneurysms. J Neurosurg 25: 574–592, 1966.
7. Olmsted WW, McGee TP: The pathogenesis of peripheral aneurysms of the central nervous system: A subject review from the AFIP. Radiology 123: 661–666, 1977.
8. Roach MR, Drake CG: Ruptured cerebral aneurysms caused by microorganisms. N Engl J Med 273: 240–244, 1965.
9. Wilson CB, Christensen FK, Subrahmanian MV: Intracranial aneurysms at the pericallosal artery bifurcation. Am Surg 31: 386–393, 1965.
10. Yasargil MG, Carter LP: Saccular aneurysms of the distal anterior cerebral artery. J Neurosurg 40: 218–223, 1974.

168

Carotid-Ophthalmic Artery Aneurysms

Gary G. Ferguson

Carotid-ophthalmic aneurysms may be defined as those aneurysms taking origin from the carotid artery at the level of the ophthalmic artery. They were first reported as a unique class of carotid aneurysm by Drake et al. in 1968.[5] Although these lesions are relatively uncommon, accounting for about 5 percent of all intracranial saccular aneurysms, they have attracted considerable interest because of their distinctive clinical features and the surgical challenge they provide.[1,5,7,8,10–12,15,19,22] The details of the clinical presentation and the treatment of carotid-ophthalmic aneurysms outlined in this chapter are based on experience with 100 cases seen at our institution.

Presentation

General Clinical Features

The clinical characteristics of the 100 patients and their aneurysms are summarized in Table 168-1, together with a comparison of these features in patients presenting with and without visual signs.

TABLE 168-1 General Clinical Features in 100 Patients with Carotid-Ophthalmic Aneurysms

Feature	All Cases ($N = 100$)	Cases with Visual Signs ($N = 32$)	Other Cases ($N = 68$)
Age, years			
Mean	48	48	48
Range	10–71	10–66	12–71
Sex			
Female, %	84	91	81
Male, %	16	9	19
Aneurysm			
Ruptured, %	39	22	47
Intact, %	61	78	53
Giant size, %	32	88	6
Multiple, %	56	44	68

Age

The age of presentation is not distinctive and is in keeping with that for intracranial aneurysms at other sites. The majority of patients are in their fifth to seventh decades of life, although on occasion a patient below the age of 20 is seen.

Sex

These aneurysms usually occur in women. The female preponderance is greater than that for other intracranial aneurysms. Intact aneurysms presenting with visual signs are almost exclusively a female phenomenon.

Mode of Presentation

Carotid-ophthalmic aneurysms come to attention most frequently because of subarachnoid hemorrhage. In our series, 39 of the patients had sustained aneurysmal rupture. Of 61 patients with intact aneurysms, 36 aneurysms were discovered in the course of investigation of other cerebral symptoms or of subarachnoid hemorrhage that proved to be from another aneurysm; 25 presented solely because of visual symptoms. In 3 of these 25 patients, there was a history of subarachnoid hemorrhage in the distant past. Most patients with giant, visually symptomatic aneurysms do not have headache, although ipsilateral periorbital pain may be a feature. In spite of their strategic location, giant carotid-ophthalmic aneurysms rarely produce hypothalamic-pituitary axis dysfunction.

Aneurysm Size

A characteristic feature of carotid-ophthalmic aneurysms is their remarkable and unexplained tendency to grow to giant size without hemorrhage. Sacs greater than 2.5 cm in diameter were found in 32 patients in our series (in 28 of the cases with visual signs and in 4 of the other cases). Of the 25 patients with intact, visually symptomatic aneurysms, 24 harbored giant aneurysms.

Multiple Aneurysms

More than half of the patients with a carotid-ophthalmic aneurysm will have at least one other intracranial aneurysm. Most commonly this will be on the contralateral carotid artery, the most frequent site being the opposite carotid-ophthalmic junction.

Radiological Features

Curvilinear suprasellar or parasellar calcification indicative of a giant aneurysm will be seen occasionally on the plain x-ray films of the skull. CT scanning will reveal all giant aneurysms and most large aneurysms. A uniformly enhancing mass is the usual finding, although irregular enhancement because of intraluminal thrombosis may occur.[18] As the CT scan will not reliably distinguish an aneurysm from other suprasellar or parasellar mass lesions, angiography is required in every case.

Carotid-ophthalmic aneurysms may be classified into two types according to their projection in relation to the carotid artery: *superomedial aneurysms*, projecting in an anterior and superomedial direction (Fig. 168-1), and *posteromedial aneurysms*, projecting in an inferior and posteromedial direction (Fig. 168-2). The posteromedial aneurysms have been classified by some authors as *paraophthalmic aneurysms*.[17] The variation in the projection of these aneurysms probably relates to variation in the exact point of origin of the ophthalmic artery from the circumference of the parent carotid artery. The superomedial aneurysms are more common (4:1) and are more likely to have associated visual signs, and their surgical treatment is generally more straightforward.

Visual Symptoms and Signs

Sir Geoffrey Jefferson gave the first detailed accounts of compression of the optic nerves and chiasm by saccular aneurysms.[13,14] He failed to recognize that some of his patients had aneurysms arising at the origin of the ophthalmic artery. More recent reports have described symptomatic optic apparatus compression in association with aneurysms at many intracranial sites without recognizing the particular significance of those aneurysms arising at the level of the ophthalmic artery.[2,3,16,20] The earlier reports on carotid-ophthalmic aneurysms suggested that associated visual symptoms were uncommon.[1,5,19,22] More recent experience indicates that aneurysms arising at the carotid-ophthalmic junction are the most frequent cause of aneurysmal compression of the optic nerves and chiasm.[4,7,8] This is not surprising in view of their location, large size, and usual projection.

Table 168-2 summarizes the visual signs in 32 patients in our series, 25 with intact aneurysms and 7 with ruptured aneurysms. A detailed account of the visual presentation and the results of treatment in this group of patients is given in the reports of Ferguson and Drake.[7,8] Visual acuity is almost always impaired. This impairment usually involves both eyes, although as a rule the loss of vision begins on the side of a single aneurysm or on the side of the larger of bilateral aneurysms and is most advanced on that side. In the majority of patients with intact aneurysms, the visual loss is slowly progressive over many months or a few years, the cause being unrecognized. However, the progression may be rapid, with blindness occurring in a few weeks. In patients with ruptured aneurysms, the visual symptoms are most commonly coincident with the hemorrhage, although there may be an antecedent history of visual disturbance, unrecognized as to its significance. Optic pallor is a common sign, as is the Marcus Gunn pupillary sign, both reflecting major impairment of optic nerve function.

Some abnormality of the visual fields is the rule. Involvement may be restricted to the side of the aneurysm, but bilateral defects are common. The visual field abnormalities that occur with carotid-ophthalmic aneurysms are remarkably diverse, reflecting the various ways in which such aneurysms may displace the optic nerves and chiasm. The most common abnormalities are unilateral or bilateral temporal defects or hemianopsias, but nasal defects, altitudinal hemianopsias, and central scotomas are seen. Homonymous defects reflecting a tract lesion are rare. It has been sug-

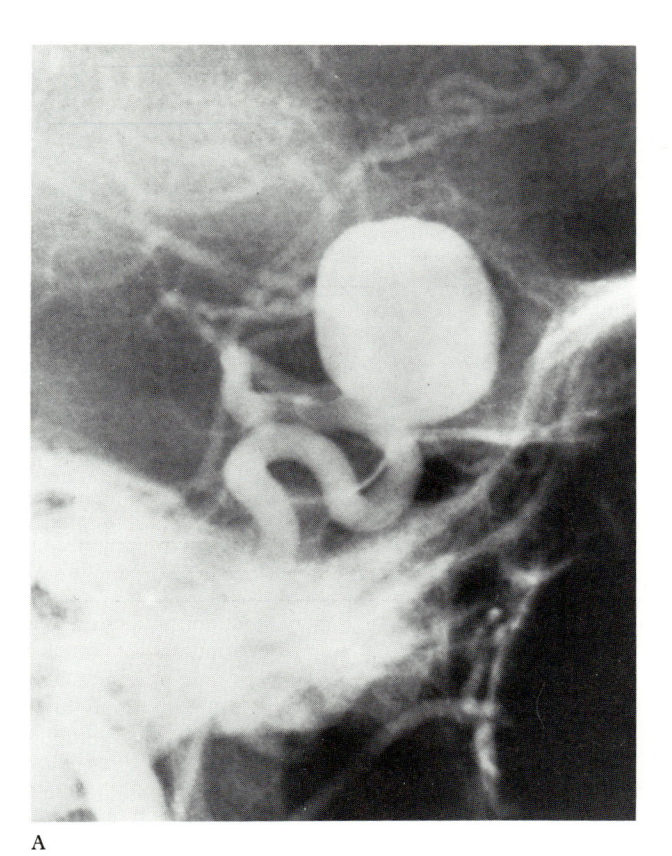

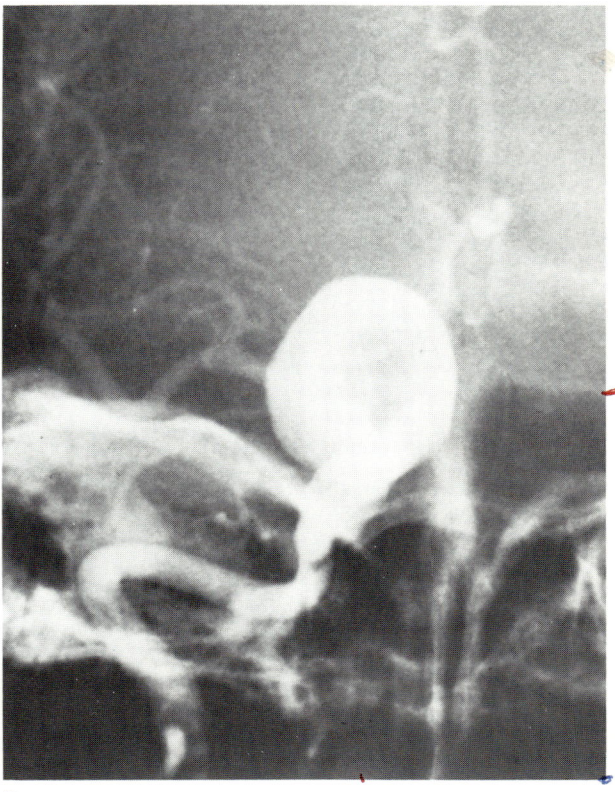

A   B

Figure 168-1 Giant right carotid-ophthalmic aneurysm demonstrating the usual superomedial projection of such an aneurysm in relation to the internal carotid artery. This type of aneurysm is certain to present with visual signs. *A.* Lateral view. *B.* Anteroposterior view.

gested that the pattern of visual field loss with supraclinoid carotid aneurysms is distinctive, allowing clinical differentiation from sellar and other parasellar mass lesions. This is not the case. Carotid-ophthalmic aneurysms may simulate pituitary and like tumors exactly in their visual presentation, and failure to recognize this fact may result in serious errors in diagnosis.[7,8,21]

Methods of Surgical Treatment

Carotid-ophthalmic aneurysms present particular difficulties for the surgeon that relate to their proximal location on the carotid artery and the fact that they are often of giant size and intimately involved with the optic apparatus, which is likely to be already seriously compromised in function and intolerant of anything but the most gentle manipulation. In contemplating the correct course of action with such aneurysms, each of the surgical techniques available for the management of aneurysms in general will need to be considered in turn. This is reflected in the wide variety of techniques employed to treat these aneurysms in our series, as summarized in Table 168-3.

The need for treatment of a ruptured aneurysm is self-evident. The decision to treat a patient with an intact aneu-

rysm is not as straightforward, as the risk can be considerable. In the case of a visually symptomatic aneurysm (which is almost certain to be of giant size) some attempt is usually justified, for the history is invariably one of progressive visual loss ending in blindness. There is also a serious risk of future hemorrhage and death from giant aneurysms.[4] In the case of an asymptomatic or incidentally discovered carotid-ophthalmic aneurysm, the decision regarding treatment relates to the size of the aneurysm, as with aneurysms at other sites.[6] In our center, a recommendation in favor of surgery is usually made when the aneurysm is greater than 5 mm in diameter and capable of treatment by a direct approach.[9]

TABLE 168-2 Visual Signs in 32 Patients with Carotid-Ophthalmic Aneurysms

Visual Sign	Intact Aneurysm (N = 25)	Ruptured Aneurysm (N = 7)	All Cases (N = 32)
Impairment of visual acuity	24	7	31
Optic pallor	20	3	23
Marcus Gunn pupil	12	2	14
Visual field abnormality	25	7	32

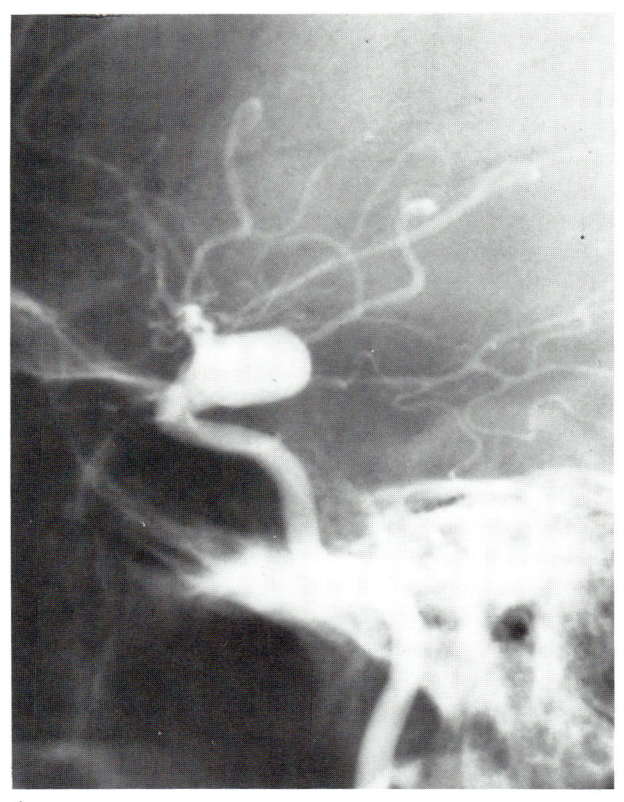

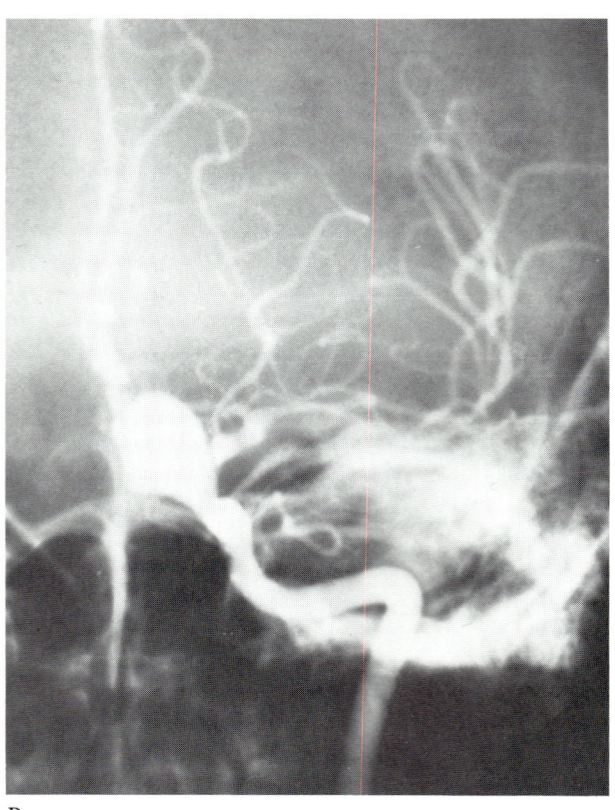

Figure 168-2 Large left carotid-ophthalmic aneurysm with a posteromedial projection in relation to the carotid artery. These are also known as *paraophthalmic aneurysms*. Carotid-ophthalmic aneurysms of this type are less common than those projecting superomedially and are often more difficult to treat. *A.* Lateral view. *B.* Anteroposterior view.

Direct Approach

A direct intracranial approach is the preferred method of treatment, as it allows immediate obliteration of the neck and collapse of the sac with decompression of the visual apparatus in those patients presenting with visual signs and with preservation of the carotid and ophthalmic arteries. A direct approach is generally possible in smaller aneurysms, and is often successful in surprisingly large aneurysms.[7] A direct approach is contraindicated in those patients with aneurysms that are partly intracavernous and in those in whom the extraordinary size of the aneurysm obviously precludes successful obliteration of the neck.

These aneurysms are usually approached through an anterolateral (pterional) craniotomy, with the head turned 45 degrees away from the side of the aneurysm. Lumbar drainage of cerebrospinal fluid and the administration of diuretics are used to produce a slack brain, as considerable frontal retraction may be required. In the case of giant aneurysms projecting to the midline with major bilateral visual involvement, the craniotomy should be extended medially to allow a more subfrontal approach. Although bilateral aneurysms may be clipped successfully from a unilateral approach, a bifrontal craniotomy is probably safer. With giant aneurysms, the superficial temporal artery should be carefully preserved, as an extracranial-intracranial (EC-IC) bypass may be required.

On elevation of the frontal lobe, the fundus of the aneurysm is usually encountered immediately (Fig. 168-3). In large or giant aneurysms, the aneurysm ordinarily projects beneath the ipsilateral optic nerve displacing it superiorly and medially. The optic nerve is often surprisingly splayed and thinned by these aneurysms, even in the absence of preoperative visual signs. A clear dissection plane between the lateral edge of the optic nerve and the sac of the aneurysm may not be obvious. Rarely, the sac projects above the optic nerve, which is then displaced posteriorly and medially. The internal carotid artery is swept laterally and posteriorly by giant sacs. The dissection of the aneurysm begins by opening the arachnoid over the distal portion of the internal carotid artery. The proximal sylvian fissure is split to allow easier retraction. Gentle retraction of the tip of the temporal lobe, with care to preserve bridging veins, is required. The arachnoid is further divided so as to reveal most of the sac, the optic apparatus, and most of the intracranial portion of the internal carotid artery. The identification and dissection of the distal side of the neck of the aneurysm is generally not difficult. It is usually clear of the optic nerve. The proximal

TABLE 168-3 Summary of the Surgical Treatment of 84 Carotid-Ophthalmic Aneurysms*

Treatment	Ruptured (N = 39)	Intact Symptomatic (N = 25)	Intact Asymptomatic (N = 20)	Total (N = 84)
Direct	32	18	20	70
Clip	16	14	18	48
Ligature and clip	3	2	2	7
Ligature	6			6
Packing	4			4
Cardiopulmonary bypass		1		1
Exploration only	3	1		4
Indirect	7	7		14
Carotid occlusion	5	3		8
EC-IC bypass	1	3		4
Trapping		1		1
Mullan clamp	1			1

*Excluded are 16 patients in whom carotid-ophthalmic aneurysms were discovered incidentally in the course of investigation for subarachnoid hemorrhage from another aneurysm.

side of the neck, however, is often obscured by the anterior clinoid process, the ipsilateral optic nerve, and the sac, as illustrated in Fig. 168-3. This may be true even with relatively small aneurysms.

The following techniques aid in exposure of the proximal neck: controlled hypotension, temporary occlusion of the internal carotid artery in the neck, removal of the anterior clinoid process, and unroofing of the optic canal. Hypotension reduces the tension in the wall of the aneurysm, allowing for safer and bolder manipulation of the sac.[9] The need for temporary occlusion of the internal carotid artery will depend on the size of the aneurysm and the experience of the operator. If the surgeon is confident that the situation is unlikely to be unduly difficult, intermittent digital compression by the anesthetist or an assistant will suffice. Otherwise, the artery should be exposed directly to allow certain short-term occlusion, as required during the dissection of the sac and the application of the clip. Removal of all or part of the anterior clinoid process is not necessary routinely but may be necessary if the carotid artery and the aneurysm are rather more laterally situated than is usually the case. A very useful and commonly required step is to unroof the optic canal.[12] To accomplish this, the sac of the aneurysm must first be freed from the overlying portion of the tuberculum sellae and anterior clinoid process. This step is necessary to expose the proximal neck, even if unroofing of the optic canal is not required. Although the aneurysm may appear to be densely adherent to the dura, sharp dissection with a knife under high magnification allows freeing of the sac. That part of the tuberculum and clinoid process covering the optic nerve is next denuded of dura and the overlying bone removed with a high-speed drill or fine laminectomy punch. The dura propria overlying the optic nerve is then incised longitudinally. In this way up to 1 cm of the optic nerve in its canal can be exposed. Careful retraction of the nerve medially brings the most proximal portion of the internal carotid artery and the neck of the aneurysm into view (Fig. 168-3). The ophthalmic artery, arising from the superomedial aspect of the internal carotid artery, can usually be identified.

Once exposure has been achieved, the application of a clip to the neck of a small or medium-sized sac is generally straightforward. Aneurysm clips with smooth, narrow blades, such as Drake clips (Codman and Shurtleff Inc., Randolph, Mass.) or Sugita clips (Downs Surgical Canada Ltd., Mississauga, Ont.), are best because of the narrow confines of the proximal neck in particular. A giant aneurysm with a very broad neck is much more of a problem. A single long clip may not completely close about a very broad neck and is likely to kink or occlude the internal carotid artery as it is pushed down by a bulbous sac. The imaginative use of clips alone or in combination is often necessary. The use of tandem clips can be very helpful (Fig. 168-3). A clip with an aperture is applied first with part of the neck of the aneurysm enclosed in the aperture. A second clip is then applied parallel to the first to occlude that part of the neck enclosed in the aperture. The two clips in tandem are of sufficient closing strength to completely occlude the neck. The internal carotid artery can also be enclosed in the aperture of a clip (Fig. 168-3), and this may be the only method of treating the neck of an aneurysm that is directed posteromedially. On occasion, the optic nerve has been enclosed in the clip aperture (Fig. 168-3).

A useful technique in applying the clips is to trap the aneurysm temporarily between an occlusion of the internal carotid artery in the neck and a clip applied to the intracranial portion of the internal carotid proximal to the posterior communicating artery. The aneurysm can then be punctured with a fine needle and partially collapsed with a sucker. The neck can then be more readily identified in relation to the internal carotid artery, which allows accurate application of the clips.

In the case of giant aneurysms with visual signs, it is important to collapse the aneurysm to decompress the visual apparatus. Extensive dissection of the optic nerves and chiasm is not necessary and may interfere with their blood supply. Failure to collapse the sac in the presence of visual signs may result in blindness because of swelling of the intra-aneurysmal clot. Delayed removal of this clot does not ensure recovery.

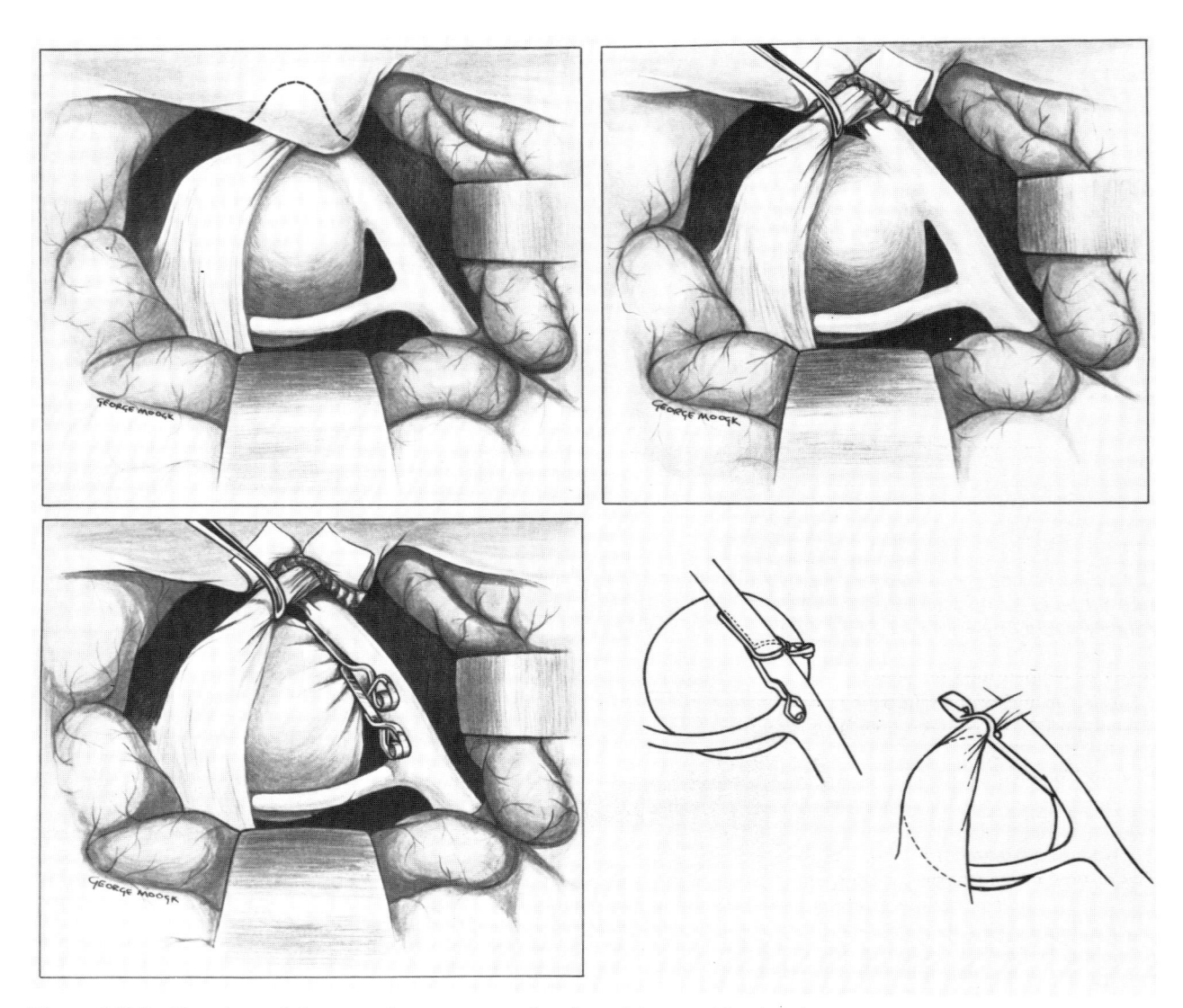

Figure 168-3 Drawings of the operative treatment of a giant right carotid-ophthalmic aneurysm similar to that shown in Fig. 168-1. *Upper left:* Initial exposure following the dissection of the arachnoid layer. The proximal neck of the aneurysm is obscured by the anterior clinoid process and right optic nerve and to a lesser extent by the sac of the aneurysm itself. *Upper right:* Exposure of the proximal neck by unroofing of the optic canal. To accomplish this the overlying clinoid process and tuberculum sellae have been denuded of dura and the bone removed with a high-speed drill. In aneurysms that are more medially located, it may not be necessary to remove any of the clinoid process. Gentle retraction of the optic nerve brings the proximal neck into view. The ophthalmic artery is not often seen as clearly as illustrated. *Lower left:* Obliteration of the neck by the use of tandem clips. The sac of the aneurysm is then collapsed to decompress the optic apparatus. *Lower right (left drawing):* Tandem clip application for a posteromedially projecting aneurysm in which the aperture of one Sugita clip has been used to encircle the internal carotid artery; *right drawing:* Drake clip application to a superomedially projecting aneurysm, with the aperture of the clip enclosing the optic nerve.

Early in our series, aneurysmal necks occasionally were either narrowed by means of a ligature and then clipped or were occluded with a ligature alone. These techniques have been superseded by the use of the multiple clip combinations described above. Occasionally an aneurysm is so proximal that the only feasible treatment is packing of the dome.

TABLE 168-4 Neurological Results of Surgical Treatment in 84 Patients with Carotid-Ophthalmic Aneurysms Based on Presentation*

Type of Aneurysm	Number of Cases	Excellent	Good	Poor	Dead
Intact					
Visually symptomatic	25	17 (68%)	4 (16%)	3 (12%)	1 (4%)
Asymptomatic	20	17 (85%)	2 (10%)		1 (5%)
Ruptured	39	28 (72%)	3 (8%)		8 (20%)
Total	84	62 (74%)	9 (10%)	3 (4%)	10 (12%)

*The 16 patients with incidentally discovered carotid-ophthalmic aneurysms are excluded, as the results of treatment are attributable to another aneurysm.

Indirect Approach

A direct approach may be judged impossible because of the extraordinary size of an aneurysm, the absence of a clearly defined neck (especially in posteromedially projecting aneurysms), or the location of part of the aneurysm within the cavernous sinus. In such cases, internal carotid artery occlusion in the neck with or without EC-IC bypass grafting can be an effective form of treatment, resulting in complete thrombosis of the aneurysm and visual recovery. The risk of stroke is real, however. Patients at risk of hemodynamic stroke can be identified by cerebral blood flow studies and trial occlusion and systematic angiographic study of the collateral potential.[7] If collateral flow is not adequate, a bypass procedure is indicated. A bypass is not necessary in all patients, and its use does not guarantee prevention of a stroke; a stroke in such cases is presumably the result of embolism from the thrombosing sac.[7] Common carotid artery occlusion does not guarantee thrombosis of the aneurysm, as reversal of flow in the external carotid artery may occur. Occlusion of the internal carotid artery is more reliable.

Results

In assessing the overall effectiveness of treatment of patients with carotid-ophthalmic aneurysms, both the neurological and visual results need to be assessed. In addition, the relative effectiveness of a direct versus an indirect approach should be considered. Tables 168-4 to 168-7 present the details of the experience in our series.

Neurological Results

Overall, three-quarters of the patients had excellent neurological results with no persisting neurological abnormalities besides those of the visual system (Table 168-4). Ten percent, with persisting neurological abnormalities that were not functionally significant, had good results; four percent developed new and disabling neurological deficits. Twelve percent of the patients died.

Intact visually symptomatic aneurysms are a particular challenge. In our series, three patients had a poor neurological outcome. In two patients, this was associated with indirect treatment by internal carotid occlusion. In one of these, hemiplegia followed the inadvertent avulsion of the internal carotid artery during an attempt to remove the stem of a Selverstone clamp. In the other, hemiplegia was not prevented in spite of prior treatment with an EC-IC bypass graft. Angiography demonstrated an embolic occlusion of the middle cerebral artery trunk, in all probability the result of an embolus from the thrombosing aneurysm. The third poor result was associated with direct clipping of an aneurysm. One patient with an intact visually symptomatic aneurysm died from anoxic encephalopathy, which complicated the use of cardiopulmonary bypass and circulatory arrest as an adjunct to the surgical procedure. With the development of temporary trapping procedures, the use of cardiopulmonary bypass is not necessary for the successful direct treatment of these aneurysms.

Results with asymptomatic aneurysms must be generally excellent to justify their treatment. The results in our series were satisfactory except with one patient, who died as a result of hemorrhage from a previously unruptured aneurysm associated with slippage of the clip postoperatively.

The outcome of treatment of ruptured carotid-ophthalmic aneurysms is related principally to the fact that hemorrhage has occurred and thus to the clinical grade of the patient at the time of operation (Table 168-5) and is in keeping with the experience for ruptured aneurysms at other intracranial sites. Although 80 percent of the patients in our series had a satisfactory outcome, 8 of 39 patients died. Most of these deaths occurred early in the series. One grade 3 patient died of massive postoperative infarction related to arterial vasospasm; the other grade 3 patient died from rebleeding before

TABLE 168-5 Neurological Results of Surgical Treatment in 39 Patients with Ruptured Carotid-Ophthalmic Aneurysms Based on Clinical Grade

Clinical Grade	Number of Cases	Excellent	Good	Dead
1	25	23 (92%)	2 (8%)	
2	7	5 (72%)	2 (28%)	
3	4		2 (50%)	2 (50%)
5	3		1 (33%)	2 (67%)
Total	39	28 (72%)	7 (18%)	4 (10%)

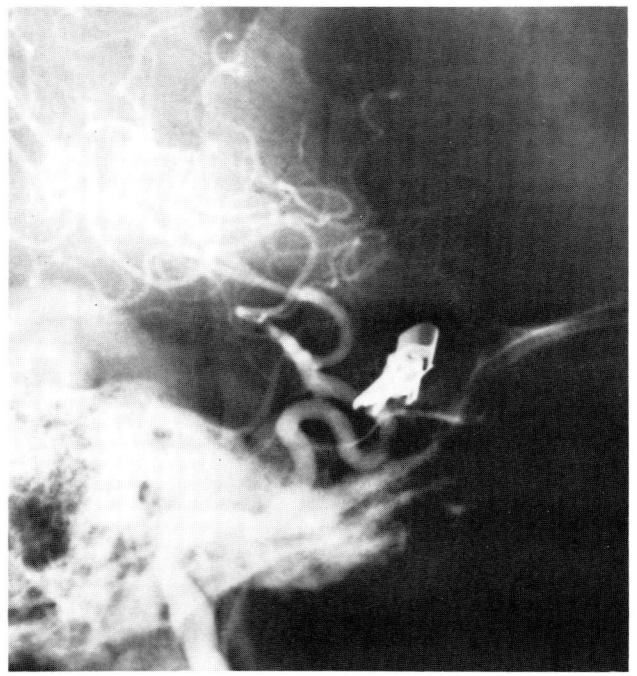

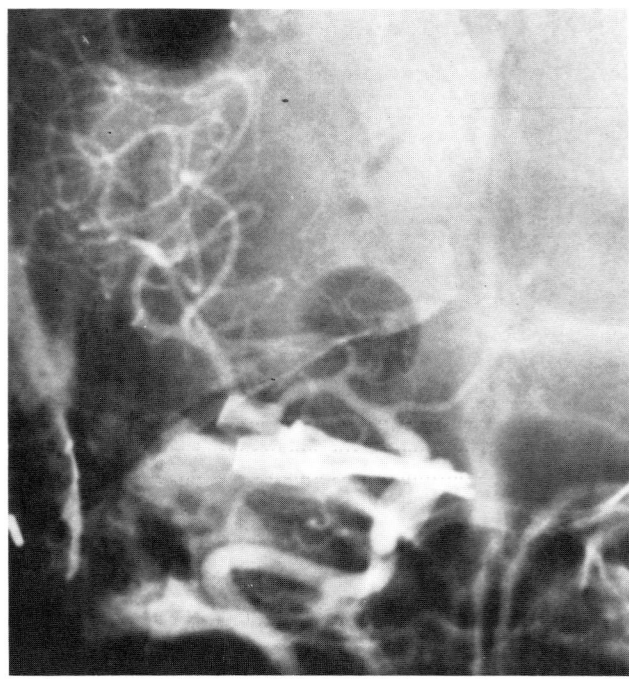

Figure 168-4 Postoperative angiogram of the aneurysm shown in Figure 168-1. A tandem clip technique has been used. Temporary trapping of the aneurysm and partial collapse of the sac were necessary before the clips could be applied without occluding the carotid artery. *A.* Lateral view. *B.* Anteroposterior view.

definitive treatment of the aneurysm, despite the use of a stenosing clamp on the internal carotid artery. The grade 5 patients would not be treated surgically today. Of the four good grade patients who died, one died from rupture of the aneurysm coincident with the skin incision, one from a pulmonary embolus, and two from arterial vasospasm.

The neurological results of indirect treatment of these aneurysms compares favorably with those of direct treatment (Table 168-6). The higher incidence of poor results with indirect treatment relates specifically to the major ischemic complications that may occur with proximal internal carotid artery occlusion.

With a direct approach, it is usually possible to completely obliterate the neck while sparing both the internal carotid and ophthalmic arteries (Fig. 168-4). Indirect treatment usually results in complete thrombosis of the aneurysm, if not immediately, then with time.

Visual Results

The visual results in the 29 survivors in our series who had had preoperative visual signs are given in Table 168-7. Two patients with ruptured aneurysms and one patient with an

TABLE 168-6 Neurological Results of Surgical Treatment in 84 Patients with Carotid-Ophthalmic Aneurysms Based on Method of Treatment

Method of Treatment	Type of Aneurysm	Number of Cases	Excellent	Good	Poor	Dead
Direct						
	Intact					
	Visually symptomatic	18	13 (72%)	3 (16%)	1 (6%)	1 (6%)
	Asymptomatic	20	17 (85%)	2 (10%)		1 (5%)
	Ruptured	32	22 (69%)	3 (9%)	—	7 (22%)
	Total	70	52 (75%)	8 (11%)	1 (1%)	9 (13%)
Indirect						
	Intact					
	Visually symptomatic	7	4 (57%)	1 (14%)	2 (29%)	
	Ruptured	7	6 (86%)	—	—	1 (14%)
	Total	14	10 (72%)	1 (7%)	2 (14%)	1 (7%)

TABLE 168-7 Visual Results in 29 Survivors

Visual Function	Improved	Unchanged	Worsened
Visual acuity	12	11	6
Visual fields	14	12	3
Overall visual function	15	9	5

intact aneurysm died. Overall visual function improved in just over half of the patients but worsened in 5 of the 29. In general, visual recovery is greatest in those in whom preoperative symptoms have been of the shortest duration.[8]

The pattern of visual recovery is unpredictable and variable. Recovery may begin immediately, particularly if it has been possible to collapse the aneurysm (Fig. 168-5). Such recovery may continue for as long as 2 years. Recovery may be delayed, even when the optic apparatus has been decompressed acutely. A delay in recovery is to be expected with indirect treatment, but the ultimate recovery in such cases can be very gratifying, and marked reduction in mass effect can usually be demonstrated on follow-up angiography.[7] It is also possible to have initial worsening with ultimate complete recovery. The risk of worsening of visual function is greatest in those patients whose vision is extremely compromised preoperatively. Postoperative blindness is usually not reversible, especially if the optic apparatus was decompressed at operation. If the aneurysm can not be collapsed at the first operation and blindness occurs, then immediate reoperation, clot evacuation, and decompression can result in recovery of vision.[7,9] In general, the postoperative changes in the visual fields parallel the changes in visual acuity. Although a considerable number of patients will have no improvement in visual function, the results can be regarded as satisfactory if vision has not worsened, as there is no longer a risk of further visual loss or of future hemorrhage. In general, the best visual results occur with direct treatment of the aneurysm.

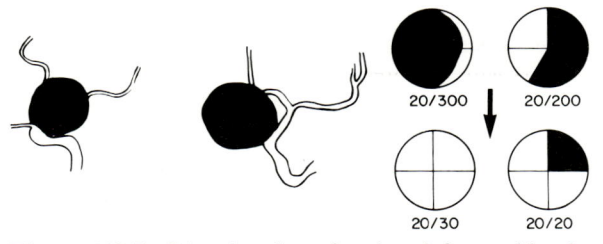

Figure 168-5 Line drawing of a giant left carotid-ophthalmic aneurysm in a patient presenting with a 1-month history of profound visual loss, greater in the left eye than the right eye. Visual field examination revealed a dense bitemporal hemianopsia with nasal encroachment. The aneurysm was successfully clipped, and the sac collapsed. Visual recovery began immediately, and continued for 2 years, at which time the only abnormality was a persisting right upper temporal quadrantanopsia.

References

1. Almeida GM, Shibata MK, Bianco E: Carotid-ophthalmic aneurysms. Surg Neurol 5:41–45, 1976.
2. Berson EL, Freeman MI, Gay AJ: Visual field defects in giant suprasellar aneurysms of the internal carotid artery: Report of three cases. Arch Ophthalmol 76:52–58, 1966.
3. Cullen JF, Haining WM, Crombie AL: Cerebral aneurysms presenting with visual field defects. Br J Ophthalmol 50:251–256, 1966.
4. Drake CG: Giant intracranial aneurysms: Experience with surgical treatment in 174 patients. Clin Neurosurg 26:12–95, 1979.
5. Drake CG, Vanderlinden RG, Amacher AL: Carotid-ophthalmic aneurysms. J Neurosurg 29:24–31, 1968.
6. Ferguson GG: Physical factors in the initiation, growth, and rupture of human intracranial saccular aneurysms. J Neurosurg 37:666–677, 1972.
7. Ferguson GG, Drake CG: Carotid-ophthalmic aneurysms: The surgical management of those cases presenting with compression of the optic nerves and chiasm alone. Clin Neurosurg 27:263–308, 1980.
8. Ferguson GG, Drake CG: Carotid-ophthalmic aneurysms: Visual abnormalities in 32 patients and the results of treatment. Surg Neurol 16:1–8, 1981.
9. Ferguson GG, Peerless SJ, Drake CG: Natural history of intracranial aneurysms. N Engl J Med 305:99, 1981.
10. Guidetti B, La Torre E: Management of carotid-ophthalmic aneurysms. J Neurosurg 42:438–442, 1975.
11. Heros RC, Nelson PB, Ojemann RG, Crowell RM, DeBrun G: Large and giant paraclinoid aneurysms: Surgical techniques, complications, and results. Neurosurgery 12:153–163, 1983.
12. Iwabuchi T, Suzuki S, Sobata E: Intracranial direct operation for carotid-ophthalmic aneurysm by unroofing of the optic canal. Acta Neurochir (Wien) 43:163–169, 1978.
13. Jefferson G: Compression of the chiasma, optic nerves, and optic tracts by intracranial aneurysms. Brain 60:444–497, 1937.
14. Jefferson G: Further concerning compression of the optic pathways by intracranial aneurysms. Clin Neurosurg 1:55–103, 1955.
15. Kothandaram P, Dawson BH, Kruyt RC: Carotid-ophthalmic aneurysms: A study of 19 patients. J Neurosurg 34:544–548, 1971.
16. Peiris JB, Russell RWR: Giant aneurysms of the carotid system presenting as visual field defect. J Neurol Neurosurg Psychiatry 43:1053–1064, 1980.
17. Pia HW: Classification of aneurysms of the internal carotid system. Acta Neurochir (Wien) 40:5–31, 1978.
18. Pinto RS, Kricheff II, Butler AR, Murali R: Correlation of computed tomographic, angiographic, and neuropathological changes in giant cerebral aneurysms. Radiology 132:85–92, 1979.
19. Sengupta RP, Gryspeerdt GL, Hankinson J: Carotid-ophthalmic aneurysms. J Neurol Neurosurg Psychiatry 39:837–853, 1976.
20. Walsh FB: Visual field defects due to aneurysms at the circle of Willis. Arch Ophthalmol 71:15–27, 1964.
21. White JC: Aneurysms mistaken for hypophyseal tumors. Clin Neurosurg 10:224–250, 1964.
22. Yasargil MG, Gasser JC, Hodosh RM, Rankin TV: Carotid-ophthalmic aneurysms: Direct microsurgical approach. Surg Neurol 8:155–165, 1977.

169

Aneurysms of Internal Carotid and Anterior Communicating Arteries

Eugene S. Flamm

This chapter will focus on the preoperative and operative management of patients with aneurysms located at the posterior communicating (PCA) and anterior choroidal (ACh) arteries, the internal carotid artery bifurcation (ICAB), and the anterior communicating artery (ACA). Aneurysms at other locations are dealt with elsewhere in this book. Although there are many similarities in managing all patients with subarachnoid hemorrhage (SAH) from aneurysms, specific details of these locations will be stressed. The aneurysms to be discussed in this chapter constitute approximately 60 percent of all intracranial aneurysms and thus are among the most frequently encountered causes of subarachnoid hemorrhage.

The diagnostic methods currently used to document the specific location of a cerebral aneurysm are discussed in another chapter. CT scanning, angiography, and digital intravenous angiography (DIVA) are highly effective tools for arriving at a correct diagnosis of SAH, but they are only useful once the diagnosis has been suspected clinically. Although this is not usually a problem for the neurological specialist, it is important to realize that the first physician called to see a patient with the sudden onset of headache may not have the same high index of suspicion.

Preoperative Preparation

The preoperative care of patients with SAH is as important to their overall outcome as is the actual surgical procedure.[5] The major steps, once the correct diagnosis is made, include determining the neurological status of the patient, localizing the site of the SAH, and embarking on a course that will prepare the patient for surgical obliteration of the aneurysm. Three major developments that must be looked for and dealt with should they occur during the preoperative period are rebleeding, vasospasm, and hydrocephalus. The regimen that is presented here is predicated on the hypothesis that surgery is better tolerated and that the outcome in terms of morbidity and mortality is improved if patients are operated upon after a suitable period of delay after the SAH. This is usually about 2 weeks.

Once the diagnosis has been made, the patient is placed at bed rest in the neurosurgical intensive care unit. Although this may not be the most quiet environment for these patients, it provides them with a team of skilled nursing personnel. Attention must be given to the patient's discomforts such as headache, bowel and bladder function, and the general apprehension associated with hospitalization.

Control of Rebleeding

Since the original Cooperative Study of aneurysms, it has been generally accepted that patients are at greatest risk for a second hemorrhage toward the end of the first week after the initial bleed.[19] Although recent data from the Cooperative Study suggest that the peak incidence of rebleeding may actually be during the first 24 h, management of these patients has focused on reducing the rebleeding while awaiting operation.[9] One approach that has been recently espoused is to operate as soon as possible after the SAH and thereby eliminate the source of any secondary hemorrhage.[9,20,21,26] The question of timing of surgery is dealt with in a previous chapter. Until this issue is resolved, we continue to allow patients to stabilize for about 2 weeks before surgery. This approach requires a regimen that addresses itself to such problems as control of blood pressure, sedation, and antifibrinolytic therapy.

Antifibrinolysis

Many papers have appeared that support or condemn the efficacy of antifibrinolytic therapy to prevent recurrent SAH.[1,3,6,22,23] Although antifibrinolytic agents are of major importance in reducing the incidence of rebleeding, it should be emphasized that the use of epsilon aminocaproic acid (EACA) or tranexamic acid is only part of a total regimen of management of these patients. To ignore the many other factors that must be controlled, such as blood pressure, temperature, seizures, and sedation, places an unrealistic burden on antifibrinolysis and makes it difficult to compare the conflicting reports in the literature.

We currently begin the intravenous administration of EACA in all patients with SAH as soon as the diagnosis is made, even before the angiogram has been performed. Patients receive EACA at 36 g/24 h as a continuous infusion until the time of operation or for 3 weeks if an operation is not performed. The use of a continuous infusion of 3 g/50 ml per hour reduces the incidence of local phlebitis and avoids the side effects encountered with oral administration of EACA.

Sedation

Sedation is determined by frequent evaluation of the patient. It is hard to apply any one drug or dose to all patients. The goal is to have the patient dozing but easily arousable when evaluated by physicians or nursing staff. To achieve this, 45 mg of phenobarbital every 6 h is used; this can be supplemented with diazepam as needed. It is also important to calm the patient's family and enlist their help in reassuring the patient.

Control of Blood Pressure

If the patient is known to be hypertensive, the blood pressure is lowered from his known level by about 30 percent. In normotensive patients the aim is to reduce the systolic pressure by 30 percent. It is important not to use the blood pressure obtained on admission as an indication of the patient's usual pressure since this is often elevated by the SAH itself. If signs of cerebral ischemia due to vasospasm develop, the blood pressure is allowed to normalize.

Anticonvulsants

All patients with SAH are placed on phenytoin as soon as the diagnosis has been made. This is continued postoperatively for 1 year even in patients who have never had a seizure. Richardson and Uttley reviewed the occurrence of seizures in 508 of 1009 patients who survived a SAH for at least 1 year.[18] The total epilepsy rate during a 5-year follow-up period was 10.5 percent. There was considerable variation according to the location of the aneurysm. Anterior cerebral region aneurysms had a 2.5 percent incidence, while PCA and middle cerebral artery aneurysms had rates of 9 and 20 percent, respectively. They recommend maintaining adequate doses of anticonvulsants for 6 to 12 months in cases of ACA aneurysms and 2 to 3 years in patients with other aneurysms or those who had an intracerebral hematoma.

With the use of diuretics and dehydrating agents such as mannitol during surgery, we have found that plasma levels of phenytoin may be well below the therapeutic level at the completion of the operation. To prevent this we now administer phenytoin 200 mg bid from the time of admission; an additional dose of 500 mg orally is given the night before operation. At the conclusion of the operation the patient is given an additional 200 mg of phenytoin intravenously. Following this regimen we have been able to maintain plasma levels within the therapeutic range of 10 to 20 μg/ml without seizures during the acute postoperative period.

Steroids

Corticosteroids are not used routinely during the preoperative period unless there is evidence of increased intracranial pressure. In preparation for surgery patients are started on methyl prednisolone on the day before the operation. An intravenous dose of 250 mg every 6 h is given; this is continued at this level during the first 3 postoperative days and then tapered over the next 4 to 5 days. While on steroids, patients receive antacids but not histamine blockers unless there is a history of peptic ulcer disease.

Fluids

No attempt is made to restrict fluid intake in patients with SAH. The usual daily intake is 2500 to 3000 ml per day either orally or intravenously. This is particularly important in patients who develop cerebral vasospasm either with or without clinical signs of ischemia.[13,14]

This regimen does not eliminate rebleeding; it controls it and allows us to gain time to carry out surgery safely at 2 weeks when the incidence of postoperative spasm is quite low and the brain has recovered from the effects of the hemorrhage. Utilizing this regimen our incidence of rebleeding has been maintained at a level of 6.3 percent (Table 169-1).

Timing of Angiography

If surgery is planned for 2 weeks after the SAH, angiography could be delayed until just before the operation. We prefer to carry out angiography soon after the patient is admitted. This is done when the full neuroradiological team is available and not on an emergency basis. Although a second study will be necessary, this permits an early diagnosis which is of obvious importance for managing the patient. To obviate the need for a second angiogram just before operation, we now perform a digital intravenous angiogram on the day before surgery. This is an effective method to determine the presence of spasm and also to follow patients during the preoperative period while they are being treated for spasm[16] (Fig. 169-1). Although the DIVA is not suitable for diagnosing small aneurysms, it is ideal for these follow-up studies. Cooper et al. suggested that the presence of vasospasm at the time of operation has an unfavorable effect on outcome even in patients who are clinically asymptomatic.[2] If spasm is present on the follow-up DIVA, surgery is delayed until repeat studies show the spasm beginning to resolve. It is not necessary to wait until the spasm has completely cleared.

Case Material

This chapter is based on the author's experience with 400 aneurysms; 289 aneurysms have been operated upon in the past 5 years. All patients were admitted to our center, usually in transfer from other hospitals. The mean time of admission was 12 days after subarachnoid hemorrhage. Seventy-five percent of the patients were in Grades I to III, eleven percent were in Grades IV and V, and fourteen percent had unruptured aneurysms (Grade 0 according to the Hunt classification). These data are summarized in Tables 169-1 and 169-2. The distribution of aneurysms is shown in Table 169-3. From this series, 60 percent form the basis of

TABLE 169-1 Case Material

	1978	1979	1980	1981	1982	Total
Numbers of patients	38	45	52	49	55	239
Patients with subarachnoid hemorrhage	29	40	44	44	48	205
Numbers of aneurysms	47	50	63	62	67	289
Multiple aneurysms, %	19	10	18	21	18	21
Patients receiving epsilon aminocaproic acid	27	39	39	40	45	190
Rebleeding from aneurysm	2	3	2	2	3	12
Rebleeding rate, %	7.4	7.7	5.1	5.0	6.7	6.3
Rebleeding mortality	2/2	2/3	2/2	1/2	2/3	9/12(75%)

this chapter, excluding ophthalmic, middle cerebral, and vertebrobasilar aneurysms, which are dealt with in other chapters.

Anesthesia

Preoperative Medication, Preparation, and Induction

Patients receive phenytoin, methyl prednisolone, and furosemide on call to the operating room. In addition to these medications, 0.4 mg of atropine sulfate is given. The patient arrives in the operating room with a radiographically confirmed central venous line. Electrocardiogram leads are placed, and the patient is ready for induction.

Anesthesia is induced with morphine sulfate (5 to 10 mg) and thiopental (4 mg/kg) intravenously. After consciousness is lost, the patient is ventilated with a 50:50 mixture of nitrous oxide and oxygen. In preparation for intubation, pancuronium bromide (0.1 mg/kg) is given to ensure complete paralysis during intubation. Laryngoscopy with topical spraying of the vocal cords with 4% lidocaine is performed only after the patient is fully anesthetized and relaxed. This ensures a smooth intubation without any bucking, hypertension, or increased intracranial pressure.

At this point additional lines are inserted. An arterial line is essential for monitoring blood pressure and following blood gases. In addition to the central venous line, two large-bore peripheral intravenous lines are placed. A Foley catheter is also inserted.

Maintenance of Anesthesia and Hypotension

Anesthesia is maintained with a 50:50 mixture of nitrous oxide and oxygen to which halothane (0.5 to 1.0%) is added. With this regimen, blood pressure can be maintained at 100 torr systolic without difficulty. Increasing the halothane concentration or giving additional morphine sulfate can be used to achieve the desired level of hypotension.

If lower levels of hypotension are desired, an infusion of nitroprusside can be used. An infusion pump is used for

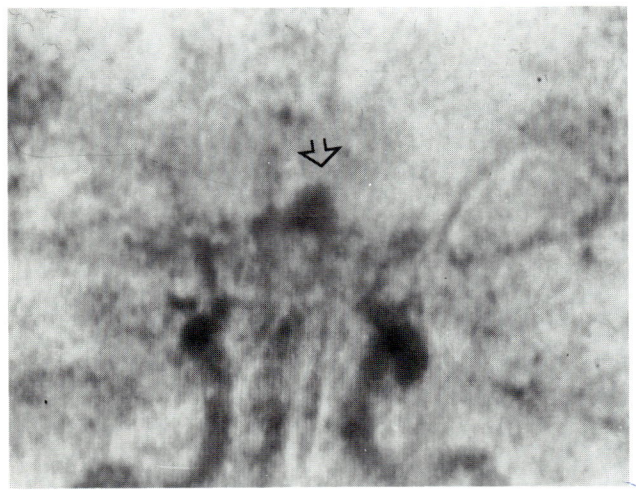

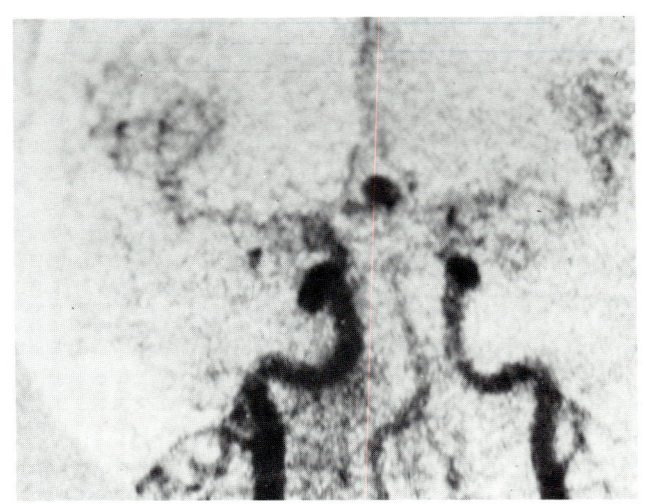

A   B

Figure 169-1 A. A digital intravenous angiogram performed 8 days after a subarachnoid hemorrhage when the patient was confused and drowsy. The arrow indicates an anterior communicating artery aneurysm. There is poor filling of the anterior and middle cerebral arteries as a result of cerebral vasospasm. B. A digital intravenous angiogram performed 5 days later. The aneurysm is seen, and there is good filling of the intracranial vessels.

TABLE 169-2 Grades of Patients Admitted 1978–1982

Grade	Number	Percent
0	34	14
I & II	140	60
III	40	15
IV	23	10
V	2	1
Total	239	100

administering this agent with a mixture of 25 mg/500 ml of 5% dextrose in water (0.005%). Although this was frequently used several years ago, it has not been routinely used in the past 2 years. At the present time most surgery around the aneurysm is carried out at a systolic pressure of 80 to 85 torr. This level of hypotension is easily achieved by controlling the anesthetic concentration and with the use of controlled respiration.

Aids to Exposure

To maximize the exposure of the circle of Willis and reduce the amount of retraction required, several adjuncts are utilized. An infusion of 20% mannitol (0.5 to 1.0 g/kg) is begun at the time of the skin incision. Patients also receive furosemide (40 mg) on the morning of the operation. This combination results in a slack brain even before the dura is opened.

The other important adjunct is spinal drainage. A catheter introduced through a Touhey needle is inserted into the lumbar subarachnoid space after the induction of anesthesia. The drainage is not opened at this time. When the dura has been exposed and tented, the spinal drainage is begun. This delay prevents stripping away of the dura, which may cause epidural bleeding that is difficult to control. Furthermore it is easier to open the leaves of the arachnoid in the sylvian fissure if there is some CSF present. In addition to the relaxation of the brain and reduction of the need for retraction, this method facilitates the microdissection since the surgeon can work in a drier field and does not constantly have to remove CSF while working on the aneurysm. The final step to achieve a slack brain is to maintain a P_{CO_2} in the range of 25 to 30 torr before the dura is opened; thereafter P_{CO_2} is kept between 30 and 35 torr.

TABLE 169-3 Location of Aneurysms Operated Upon

Parent Artery	Number	Percent
Ophthalmic	28	9.7
Posterior communicating	73	25.2
Anterior choroidal	16	5.5
Carotid bifurcation	15	5.2
Anterior communicating	62	21.5
Pericallosal	7	2.4
Middle cerebral	56	19.4
Vertebral or basilar	32	11.1
Total	289	100

Equipment

Operating Microscope

Our preferred objective lens for the operating microscope is 300 mm; this allows ample room to work between the lens and point of focus. A 20× ocular lens in an inclined f-160 eyepiece to achieve the maximum possible magnification with 300-mm objective lens is preferred. Although the overall field is smaller, this poses no problem for aneurysm surgery and is offset by the advantage of the increased magnification. It is essential to be able to focus the microscope without using one's hands; this allows the surgeon to keep both hands in the field at all times and make minor adjustments of the focus as the dissection proceeds. This is particularly important when the arachnoid is being dissected from the neck of the aneurysm. The surgeon should be seated, and both the surgeon and the microscope should be free to move and change positions with minimal effort.

Instrumentation

Fairly rigid, moderately heavy bipolar forceps with different tip sizes and angulations are used. By using heavier stainless steel, rather than titanium, instruments, it is possible to use them for both dissection and coagulation. The lighter instruments do not have sufficient spring to be used in a spreading fashion to divide the arachnoid and do not provide enough proprioceptive feedback to the surgeon.

A variety of sharp arachnoid knives are an important part of the equipment needed. These can be used effectively in places that scissors cannot; small disposable blades such as the Beaver blades (Rudolph Beaver, Inc., Waltham, Mass.) can be used to good advantage for this purpose. Less traction is transmitted to the aneurysm if the arachnoid is divided sharply rather than tearing it with forceps.

An adequate array of microsurgical instruments is necessary. In addition to the standard instruments, dissectors with varying curved and straight tips, on both bayonet and straight handles, are helpful for retracting vessels and the aneurysm itself. A no. 7 vented Frazier-type suction tip is used on the left side with a vacuum of 100 torr. A larger tip is kept on the right side for the first assistant in the event of rupture of the aneurysm.

Although aneurysm clips are discussed in another chapter, certain points should be stressed here. Several suitable clips should be selected and loaded by the surgeon before the dura is opened. My own preference is for larger clips that will fit the aneurysm. There is no advantage in stuffing a large aneurysm into a small clip. In addition to a large array of Yasargil clips, McFadden and Sundt clips are available. The former are particularly helpful for large broad-necked aneurysms. The Sundt clip is not often used but has been helpful in several dire emergencies. With the introduction of the Sugita clips an even greater variety of clip sizes and configurations are now available.

The use of a self-retaining system for brain retractors is essential for all microsurgery and particularly for surgery of aneurysms. Since the operative exposure is small, there is usually insufficient room for the hands of an assistant on a brain retractor. Furthermore the brain retraction must be gentle and precise; this can only be achieved with a mechanically secured retractor.

Surgical Technique

Preparation

The patient is positioned with the head secured in a three-pin head holder. This is necessary to reduce any movement of the head which will interfere with the microdissection that is carried out at 16× magnification. The head is turned to a full lateral position, and the vertex is dropped slightly toward the floor. This extension permits better direct visualization of the region of the optic nerve and carotid artery and reduces any obstruction to vision by the temporalis muscle or floor of the skull. The zygoma is almost parallel with the floor.

A curvilinear incision begins at the upper border of the zygoma, 1 cm in front of the tragus. It is extended upward following the hairline in a gentle curve. It should be placed as low as possible, and yet remain behind the hairline (Fig. 169-2). The medial extent of the incision is the midpupillary line. It is not necessary to bring the medial portion of the incision onto the forehead. If a larger flap is required, the incision can be extended toward the midline. As the incision is made in front of the ear, care should be exercised to avoid injuring the superficial temporal artery.

The scalp flap is reflected inferiorly in a single layer including the temporalis muscle. This eliminates any injury to branches of the facial nerve to the frontalis muscle; if the scalp is separated from the underlying muscle as would be necessary for an osteoplastic flap, such injury with a loss of frontalis movement usually ensues.

After the incision is made, scalp clips are applied. The temporalis fascia is incised with a scalpel so that a good closure can be achieved. The temporalis muscle is then incised with the cutting cautery and separated from the skull. The entire scalp flap is reflected in a single layer down to the level of the supraorbital ridge. The bony landmark for this step is the zygomatic process of the frontal bone; it is important to expose at least 2 cm of frontal bone along the supraorbital ridge in front of the zygomatic process. This is particularly important when the flap is on the left side. Failure to do this will limit the angle at which a right-handed surgeon can introduce instruments through this small craniotomy.

A single burr hole is placed in the temporal region. From this a free bone flap measuring 6 × 4 cm is created with the craniotome. An initial cut is made from the burr hole toward the sphenoid wing as far as is possible. The craniotome is then returned to the burr hole and the remainder of the flap created; it is usually necessary to crack the bone at the sphenoid wing by elevating the flap. It is essential that the bony opening be flush with the floor of the frontal fossa. The lateral aspect of the sphenoid wing is then rongeured away so that it will offer no obstruction to the line of vision. It is not necessary to drill this away, and 1.5 cm of the wing can

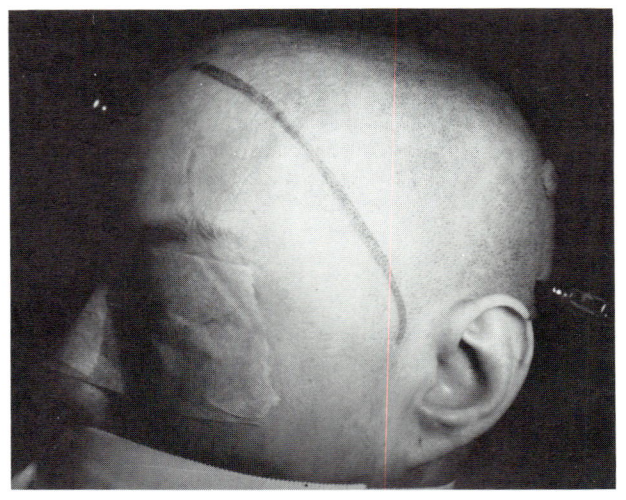

Figure 169-2 The scalp incision for the usual pterional approach. The incision is completely behind the hairline.

easily be removed with rongeurs (Fig. 169-3). After dural tenting sutures have been placed, the spinal drainage is opened.

It is difficult to describe all the nuances of the dissection techniques used in aneurysm surgery. For aneurysms of the carotid artery such as posterior communicating, anterior choroidal, and bifurcation locations, certain general maneuvers can be outlined. The first step is the identification of the optic nerve. Once this has been seen, the exposure is maintained with a self-retaining retractor. The landmarks for identifying the optic nerve are the olfactory tract and the sphenoid wing. The nerve is found at the point of intersection of these two structures.

The operating microscope is now brought into use, by increasing magnification from the 6× setting initially to 16× for dissection along the parent vessel and aneurysm. The first step of the microdissection is to divide various

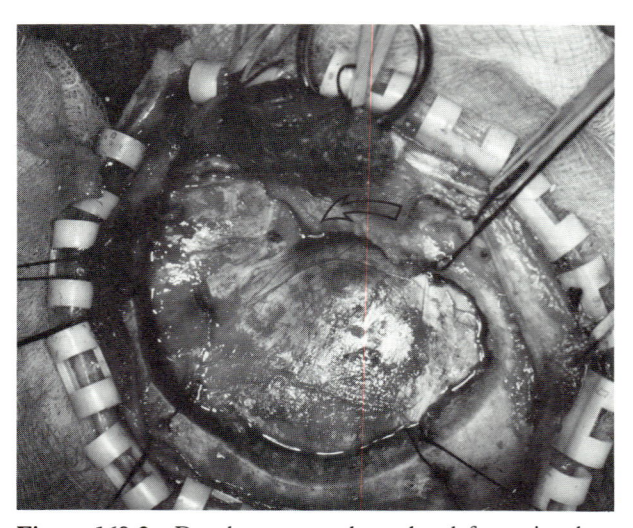

Figure 169-3 Dural exposure through a left pterional flap. The lateral aspect of the sphenoid wing (*arrow*) has been removed. The opening measures 4 × 5 cm.

arachnoid connections. This frees the aneurysm from any undue traction and increases the room in which to operate within the subarachnoid space. The arachnoid between the frontal lobe and optic nerve is first divided. This plane is extended laterally into the medial portion of the sylvian fissure. As the arachnoid is divided, additional retraction increases the exposure of the carotid artery. The next step is to obtain control of the carotid artery; this is particularly important for carotid artery aneurysms. The best place to begin this portion of the dissection is between the optic nerve and the artery. Once this arachnoid is opened, the dissection can proceed along the carotid to the point of origin of the aneurysm.

Techniques for Large Aneurysms

In addition to these general methods that apply to the specific aneurysm sites discussed below, some special techniques for dealing with large aneurysms at these locations are necessary. Although large aneurysms arising from the carotid artery are usually found at the origin of the ophthalmic artery, large and giant aneurysms may be found at the locations under discussion in this chapter. Several problems that occur with aneurysms of 2-cm diameter or larger must be recognized before the clip application is attempted. The method and principles of the dissection are the same, but special attention must be given to the selection and application of the clip. Although Yasargil has advocated the use of bipolar coagulation of the aneurysm neck to reduce its size and permit safer clipping,[11] I do not often use this method. I prefer a larger clip when possible. The large variety of aneurysm clips now available makes it easier to find an appropriate clip for most aneurysms. Another alternative is to apply more than one clip, usually from different directions, to obliterate some of the larger aneurysms.

Another problem encountered with large aneurysms is that the wall of the neck is quite thick. This together with the large aneurysm sac may cause the clip to slip proximally and compromise the parent vessel. To prevent this it is often helpful to enlarge the length of the neck by placing a ligature around the neck. This ligature is tightened enough to reduce the diameter of the neck but not to obliterate it completely. A heavy silk ligature will create a good area to which a clip can be applied. The ligature, in addition to fashioning a neck, provides a region of better purchase for the clip and prevents it from slipping into an undesired attitude (Fig. 169-4).

An additional problem encountered with carotid aneurysms, especially a large one, is the tension within the aneurysm. This often prevents the clip from closing completely; there is also an increased chance of rupture if the clip does not completely obliterate the aneurysm when it is applied. Several techniques are available to reduce the tension within the aneurysm. Temporary occlusion of the internal carotid artery in the neck dramatically reduces the pressure in the supraclinoid carotid artery and within the aneurysm. The use of this method must be anticipated so that the carotid can be exposed in the neck before craniotomy. Although temporary clips can be applied directly to the supraclinoid carotid artery, this often reduces the working space necessary to clip the aneurysm and carries the risk of endothelial damage.

Another technique that has been helpful with large thick-walled aneurysms is suction decompression.[4] A 21-gauge scalp vein needle with the flanges removed is connected to the operating room suction. By puncturing the dome of the aneurysm where it is thick, blood can be suctioned through the aneurysm and the intraluminal tension reduced. Although this may not cause the thick-walled aneurysm to collapse, the aneurysm will become softer and more pliable. The clip can then be closed down easily and more safely. Blood loss has not been more that 150 ml when this technique is employed.

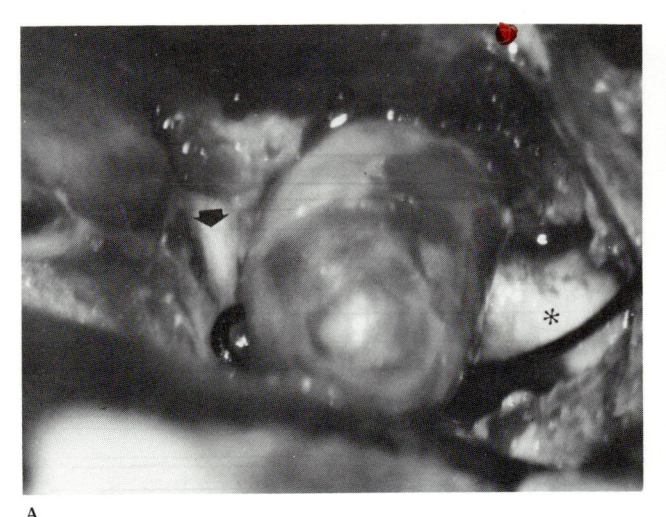

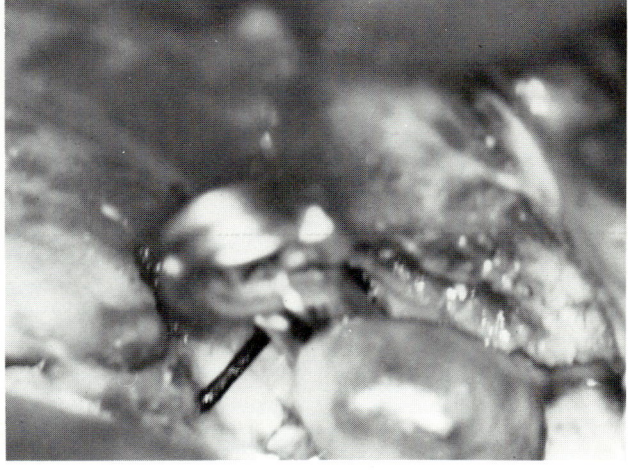

Figure 169-4 *A.* A ligature being passed around the base of a right carotid artery aneurysm before clip application. *Carotid artery; *arrow*, right optic nerve. ×16. *B.* A clip applied over the ligature which fashioned a discrete neck for the clip. ×7.5.

Posterior Communicating Artery Aneurysms

The most characteristic presentation of this aneurysm is the sudden appearance of a partial third nerve palsy at the time of the SAH. This almost always manifests itself with some pupillary abnormality. A recent report has described pupillary sparing with PCA aneurysms, but this is quite unusual.[10] In addition to anisocoria there may be ptosis and varying degrees of limitation of eye movements under the control of the third nerve. This is probably the only pathognomonic sign associated with SAH; with aneurysms in any other location it is usually not possible to be certain of the specific site.

Another common presentation of the PCA aneurysm is the development of a third nerve deficit in the absence of a SAH. The appearance of an enlarged pupil with or without involvement of other third nerve functions should be taken as diagnostic of a PCA aneurysm until proven otherwise. This usually requires angiography since neither CT scanning nor DIVA is sufficient to rule out a small aneurysm in this location. Although this will undoubtedly result in some negative studies being performed, it can be fully justified since the greatest risk that such a patient can have is to sustain a SAH. If the diagnosis can be made before rupture of the aneurysm, the surgical management and overall prognosis are much improved.

About 10 percent of PCA aneurysms will not produce any third nerve deficit. When this occurs, special attention should be given to the angiogram since this often indicates that the aneurysm is projecting laterally onto the medial edge of the temporal lobe rather than in the more common downward position. This is of great importance in planning the surgical approach since care must be taken not to retract the temporal lobe prematurely and thereby rupture the aneurysm before the dissection has begun (Fig. 169-5).

The dissection for exposure of this aneurysm proceeds along the carotid artery. The arachnoid between the optic nerve and the carotid artery is fully opened, as is the medial portion of the sylvian fissure. These steps are important to minimize brain retraction and the resultant forces applied to the aneurysm as well as to improve the visualization of the aneurysm and the pertinent branches of the carotid artery. The dissection should be carried out within the subarachnoid space. By elevating the arachnoid from the carotid artery, the region of the aneurysm can be easily identified. It is safer to enter this plane over the carotid artery than over the aneurysm itself.

The neck of the aneurysm is now freed of arachnoid both by sharp dissection and by the spreading of the dissecting forceps. The elevated arachnoid can be removed or coagulated to improve the exposure. Once a plane has been established on either side of the neck, attempts to identify the posterior communicating artery are made. Gentle lateral retraction of the carotid artery toward the aneurysm allows good visualization between the optic nerve and carotid artery. Usually the communicating artery can be identified and spared. If necessary, this vessel can be included within the clip, provided it is truly a communicating artery and not a posterior cerebral artery arising directly from the carotid artery (Fig. 169-6). If the PCA aneurysm is somewhat distal on the carotid artery, an additional precaution is to identify the anterior choroidal artery. This vessel, unlike the posterior communicating artery, must always be preserved. Once the aneurysm has been clipped, it should be punctured to ensure that it is completely obliterated and to achieve maximum decompression of the third nerve. Further dissection of the aneurysm from the third nerve is not necessary.

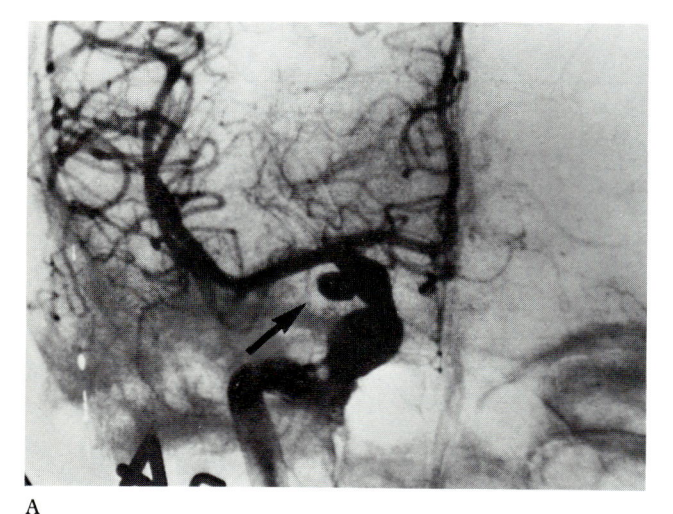

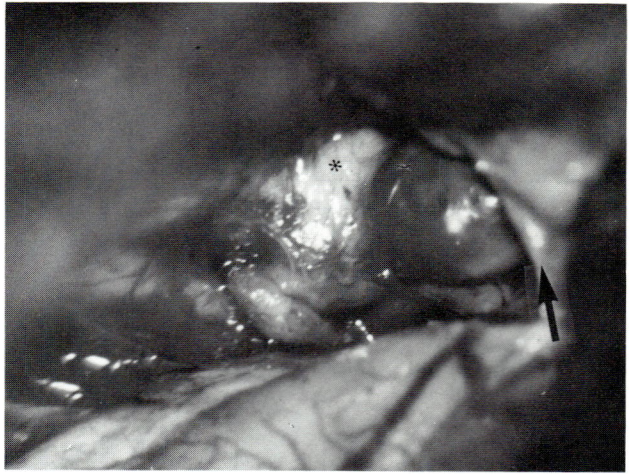

Figure 169-5 *A.* A right carotid angiogram which shows a posterior communicating artery aneurysm (*arrow*) pointing laterally toward the temporal lobe. The patient did not have a third nerve palsy. *B.* The same aneurysm exposed at operation. *Right carotid artery; *arrow*, arachnoid of the sylvian fissure. The dome of the aneurysm is adherent to the medial aspect of the temporal lobe. ×12.

Anterior Choroidal Artery Aneurysms

There is no specific clinical presentation of aneurysms that arise from the region of the anterior choroidal artery. They are relatively uncommon, composing only 5.5 percent of the present series. Such aneurysms presented with SAH in 14 of 16 cases, temporal lobe seizures in 1, and a partial third nerve palsy in 1. They were found in association with another aneurysm in 9 cases, the most common association being with an adjacent PCA aneurysm. Because of the important territory of the brain supplied by the anterior choroidal artery, every effort should be made preoperatively to identify the origin of this aneurysm and the artery itself.[8] At the time of the operation, great care must be taken to identify the anterior choroidal artery. Failure to do this will frequently cause the vessel to be included in the clip. This is poorly tolerated and results in an infarction in the internal capsule which produces a severe hemiparesis from which recovery is incomplete at best.

The dissection and clipping of aneurysms in this location are quite similar to the methods described for PCA aneurysms. The major difference is the need to identify with certainty the anterior choroidal artery. An important aid to visualizing the anterior choroidal artery is to obtain adequate room to work at the distal end of the carotid artery. This is facilitated by widely opening the sylvian fissure. Although this is generally done as part of the initial approach to carotid aneurysms and certainly for aneurysms of the carotid bifurcation, an extra effort should be made in cases of anterior choroidal aneurysms because there is often a tendency to regard them as PCA aneurysms which do not require the same amount of exposure. The anterior choroidal artery may course medial to the aneurysm; it becomes necessary to separate it from the aneurysm neck to prevent its inclusion in the clip. Often this can be done by working from the medial side of the carotid artery between the vessel and the optic nerve (Fig. 169-7).

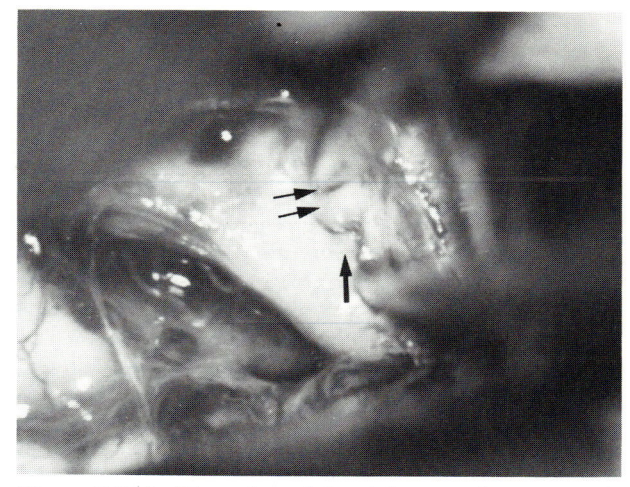

Figure 169-6 Dissection of the right posterior communicating artery from the aneurysm dome. The arrow indicates the origin of the right posterior communicating artery; the double arrow points to the wall of the aneurysm displaced by the forceps.

It is imperative that the leaves of the sylvian fissure be opened so that good visualization of the artery and control of the related vessels can be obtained. This requires the use of two self-retaining retractors, one on the frontal and one on the temporal lobe. Of particular importance is the exposure of the proximal anterior and middle cerebral arteries. To achieve this exposure, more retraction is needed than for other carotid artery aneurysms. These lesions often lie buried in the anterior perforated substance, a portion of the brain that should be carefully preserved.

The initial dissection is similar to that for other carotid aneurysms. The carotid artery is exposed in its proximal supraclinoid segment, and dissection is carried up the sylvian fissure. It is important to divide the arachnoid bridging

Internal Carotid Bifurcation Aneurysms

Aneurysms at the distal end of the internal carotid artery are among the less frequent aneurysms of the anterior circulation. Nevertheless they can be a most challenging problem because of the size that they may attain, the increased likelihood of intraoperative rupture, and the involvement of several major vessels (namely, the anterior and middle cerebral arteries, the anterior choroidal artery, and the internal carotid artery itself).

In most reported series and in my experience, aneurysms at the ICAB constitutes 5 percent of intracranial aneurysms (Table 169-3).[15,25] They may present as mass lesions or following SAH. There is no specific clinical presentation that increases the probability of finding an aneurysm in this location. The special considerations for this aneurysm revolve around the local anatomy, particularly the arrangement of the perforating arteries near the bifurcation of the carotid artery and the path of the anterior choroidal artery in relation to the aneurysm.[8,15]

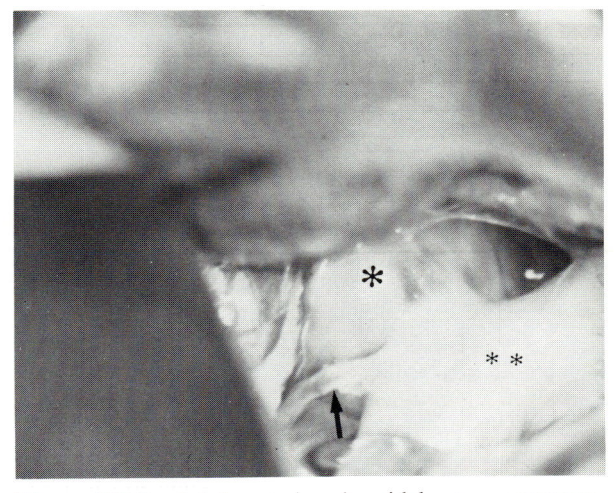

Figure 169-7 A left anterior choroidal artery aneurysm (*). The arrow indicates the anterior choroidal artery that has been separated from the neck of the aneurysm.
**Left internal carotid artery.

the lips of the sylvian fissure to gain adequate exposure. My own approach is not to proceed directly to the distal side of the bifurcation and the region of the aneurysm. When working up the carotid artery, one first encounters the anterior surfaces of the anterior and middle cerebral arteries. The dissection is then carried laterally along the middle cerebral artery and medially along the anterior cerebral artery to expose these segments before the aneurysm is confronted. By doing this, one can then return toward the aneurysm working along each of these vessels (Fig. 169-8). This allows one to identify and establish a cleavage plane between the dome of the aneurysm itself and the carotid bifurcation. The danger of proceeding directly to the bifurcation and dissecting the aneurysm is that one may enter the dome of the aneurysm while trying to establish the planes around the neck. By proceeding toward the aneurysm from the lateral and medial sides one can establish the cleavage plane and creep up on the neck of the aneurysm. It is important to bear in mind that the perforating arteries rarely arise in the immediate vicinity of the bifurcation.[8] While dissecting on these vessels, one should stay on the anterior and inferior surfaces of the vessels to avoid sacrificing any of the perforators. Once again, a path is established on either side of the neck. It is important that this be clearly visualized before attempts to pass a clip are made. Failure to do this may result in a tear of the aneurysm by one of the blades of the clip.

Even before these planes are well established, the surgeon should develop a mental picture of the location of the neck. Should rupture occur before the dissection has been completed, it is helpful to have a good idea of where the neck is so that a rapid and accurate dissection and application of the clip can be carried out while bleeding is controlled by the suction.

A point to remember is that the anterior choroidal artery passes behind the carotid artery as seen in this approach. This artery should be located before the clip is applied so that it is not included in the clip as it passes deep to the aneurysm. This is a small but important detail of this aneurysm's location.

Anterior Communicating Artery Aneurysms

The effectiveness of microsurgical approaches to cerebral aneurysms is best illustrated by the change in techniques that have developed for dealing with ACA aneurysms since the introduction and widely accepted use of the operating microscope. Perhaps the influence of microsurgery on the field of aneurysm surgery is not better emphasized than in the surgery of ACA aneurysms.[24] In the 1950s and early 1960s a variety of approaches to this aneurysm were advocated. Pool utilized a wide bifrontal exposure, Lougheed favored an interhemispheric approach, and French used resection of the medial portion of the hemisphere to gain exposure. With the widespread use of the pterional approach, these other methods are of only historical interest now.[7,12,17]

There has been some variation in the selection of the side of approach to these midline aneurysms. Almost all aneurysms are more safely managed by gaining control of the

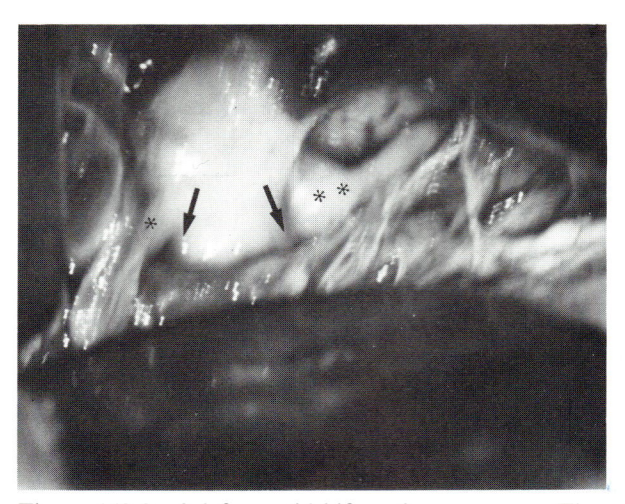

Figure 169-8 A left carotid bifurcation aneurysm. The arrows indicate both sides of the neck. *Middle cerebral artery; **anterior cerebral artery. Both vessels were separated before the neck was dissected.

parent vessel before dissecting the neck of the aneurysm. In cases of ACA aneurysms this means that all patients should not be operated from the right or nondominant side. If the aneurysm is truly midline, that is, arising from the communicating artery itself, a right-sided approach can be used. However, this situation is found in only about 30 percent of cases.[15,24] Most ACA aneurysms arise from the junction of the major anterior cerebral artery with the communicating artery. The experienced aneurysm surgeon has a better chance of controlling this aneurysm safely and effectively by approaching it from the side of its major blood supply, be it left or right. This advantage is significant enough to offset the possible risk to dominant hemisphere function. It should be emphasized that these considerations apply to the experienced aneurysm surgeon, who should be comfortable and confident with aneurysm surgery before dealing with ACA aneurysms and certainly before adopting a method of approach from the side of the dominant hemisphere.

The preliminary steps for the surgical approach to ACA aneurysms are similar to those for the other sites discussed above. It is usually unnecessary to proceed along the carotid artery to the bifurcation before the anterior cerebral artery is identified. By first dividing the arachnoid between the undersurface of the frontal lobe and the optic nerve, one can usually identify the anterior cerebral artery and the recurrent artery of Heubner. The anterior cerebral artery can then be followed medially to the region of the midline. By dividing the arachnoid of the interhemispheric fissure, additional exposure and relaxation can be achieved.

It is often helpful to resect about 1 cm^3 of brain of the gyrus rectus at this juncture to expose the curve of the anterior cerebral artery as it changes from the A_1 to the A_2 segment. This simple maneuver enables the surgeon to see both the proximal and distal anterior cerebral artery, the anterior communicating artery, the origin of the recurrent artery of Heubner, and some portion of the aneurysm. In cases in which the aneurysm points anteriorly and inferiorly above the chiasm this resection is usually not needed.

It is important to identify the contralateral anterior cerebral artery early in the course of the operation. Because of the angle of the approach, this vessel is sometimes seen before the ipsilateral one. As Yasargil has pointed out, it is essential to visualize the entire "H" complex of the anterior cerebral–anterior communicating artery region.[24] Only in this way can inadvertent clipping of one of these major vessels be avoided (Fig. 169-9).

The other vessels that must be recognized and spared are the lenticulostriate and other perforating arteries. If the dissection proceeds along the anterior half of the circumference of the anterior cerebral arteries, these small branches can be preserved; often they need not be visualized at all. Once again, the aneurysm should be punctured after it has been clipped to be certain that it has been completely obliterated.

Postoperative Management

The goals of postoperative care are to maintain adequate cerebral perfusion, reduce any postoperative cerebral swelling and increase in intracranial pressure, and prevent the occurrence of seizures. These aims can be accomplished by continuing the preoperative medical regimen of corticosteroids, anticonvulsants, and fluids.

Upon the patient's transfer to the recovery room, blood pressure is maintained at normal to slightly elevated levels. Central venous pressure is maintained at 4 to 6 cmH$_2$O by administering colloid and/or whole blood. Corticosteroids (in our practice, 250 mg of methyl prednisolone every 6 h) are maintained at this level for 3 days and then tapered over the next 5 days. Levels of anticonvulsants are determined initially after surgery and during the postoperative period.

Since most aneurysms have been opened intraoperatively, we do not routinely perform postoperative angiography. If there is any change in the patient's neurological condition or if the aneurysm was not opened at operation, angiography is carried out.

TABLE 169-4 Management Results, 1978–1982

Number of patients	239
Number with subarachnoid hemorrhage	205
Number operated upon	200
Mortality	
Surgical—Grades I to III	2.0%
Surgical—all grades	5.0%
Nonsurgical	15.0%
Case mortality	20.0%

Results

By following this regimen we have not experienced any postoperative cerebral vasospasm. The management of this vexing problem is discusssed in another chapter. During the preoperative period while awaiting surgery we manage the problem of vasospasm with volume expansion and continuous infusions of aminophylline and isoproterenol.[5] The overall results and surgical results are summarized in Table 169-4. In patients with these aneurysms who were better than Grade IV preoperatively, the surgical mortality has been 2.0 percent, and the morbidity 1.5 percent. Unfortunately, the overall case mortality has been 20 percent. The cause of death or morbidity in these patients has been ischemia in 15 percent and rebleeding in 5 percent. Until the efficacy of early surgery is established, we will continue to recommend a delay of 10 to 14 days between the onset of the SAH and surgery. This is particularly appropriate for aneurysms of the internal carotid artery bifurcation and the anterior communicating artery region. Both of these sites require considerably more dissection and brain retraction than do PCA aneurysms. This seems to be better accomplished and tolerated if the swelling and perturbation of the brain produced at the time of the hemorrhage have subsided.

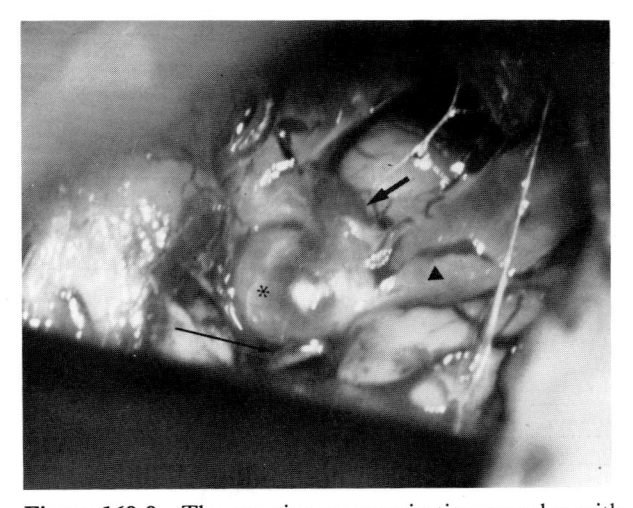

Figure 169-9 The anterior communicating complex with an aneurysm (*) arising from the junction of the right A$_1$ (*triangle*) and communicating (*short arrow*) arteries. The long arrow indicates the right artery of Heubner which overlies and obscures the right A$_2$.

References

1. Adams HP Jr, Nibbelink DW, Torner JC, Sahs AL: Antifibrinolytic therapy in patients with aneurysmal subarachnoid hemorrhage, in Sahs AL, Nibbelink DW, Torner JC (eds): *Aneurysmal Subarachnoid Hemorrhage: Report of the Cooperative Study*. Baltimore, Urban & Schwarzenberg, 1981, pp 331–339.
2. Cooper PR, Shucart WA, Tenner M, Hussain S: Preoperative arteriographic spasm and outcome from aneurysm operation. Neurosurgery 7:587–592, 1980.
3. Flamm ES: Parasurgical treatment of aneurysms. Clin Neurosurg 24:240–247, 1977.
4. Flamm ES: Suction decompression of aneurysms: Technical note. J Neurosurg 54:275–276, 1981.
5. Flamm ES: Antifibrinolysis and the preoperative management of subarachnoid hemorrhage, in Hopkins LN, Long DM (eds): *Clinical Management of Intracranial Aneurysms*. New York, Raven Press, 1982, pp 49–58.
6. Fodstad H, Liliequist B, Schannong M, Thulin CA:

Tranexamic acid in the preoperative management of ruptured intracranial aneurysms. Surg Neurol 10:9–15, 1978.
7. French LA, Ortiz-Suarez HJ: Anterior communicating artery aneurysms: Technique of operation and results. Clin Neurosurg 21:115–119, 1974.
8. Gibo H, Lenkey C, Rhoton AL Jr: Microsurgical anatomy of the supraclinoid portion of the internal carotid artery. J Neurosurg 55:560–574, 1981.
9. Kassell NF, Drake CG: Timing of aneurysm surgery. Neurosurgery 10:514–519, 1982.
10. Kissel JT, Burde RM, Klingele TG, Zeiger HE: Pupil-sparing oculomotor palsies with internal carotid-posterior communicating artery aneurysms. Ann Neurol 13:149–154, 1983.
11. Krayenbühl H, Yasargil MG, Flamm ES, Tew JM Jr: Microsurgical treatment of intracranial saccular aneurysms. J Neurosurg 37:678–686, 1972.
12. Lougheed WM, Marshall BM: Management of aneurysms of the anterior circulation by intracranial procedures, in Youmans JR (ed): *Neurological Surgery: A Comprehensive Reference Guide to the Diagnosis and Management of Neurosurgical Problems*. Philadelphia, WB Saunders, 1973, pp 731–767.
13. Maroon JC, Nelson PB: Hypovolemia in patients with subarachnoid hemorrhage: Therapeutic implications. Neurosurgery 4:223–225, 1979.
14. Nibbelink DW, Torner JC, Burmeister LF: Fluid restriction in combination with antifibrinolytic therapy, in Sahs AL, Nibbelink DW, Torner JC (eds): *Aneurysmal Subarachnoid Hemorrhage: Report of the Cooperative Study*. Baltimore, Urban & Schwarzenberg, 1981, pp 307–330.
15. Pia HW: Classification of aneurysms of the internal carotid system. Acta Neurochir (Wien) 40:5–31, 1978.
16. Pinto RS, Kricheff II, De Filipp G, Flamm ES, Lin JP: Digital intravenous angiography in the assessment of vasospasm secondary to ruptured intracranial aneurysms. In press.
17. Pool JL: Bifrontal craniotomy for anterior communicating artery aneurysms. J Neurosurg 36:212–220, 1972.
18. Richardson AE, Uttley D: Prevention of postoperative epilepsy. Lancet 1:650, 1980.
19. Sahs AL, Perret GE, Locksley HB, Nishioka H: *Intracranial Aneurysms and Subarachnoid Hemorrhage: A Cooperative Study*. Philadelphia, JB Lippincott, 1969.
20. Saito I, Ueda Y, Sano K: Significance of vasospasm in treatment of ruptured intracranial aneurysms. J Neurosurg 47:412–429, 1977.
21. Samson DS, Hodosh RM, Reid WR, Beyer CW, Clark WK: Risk of intracranial aneurysm surgery in the good grade patient: Early versus late operation. Neurosurgery 5:422–426, 1979.
22. Sengupta RP, So SC, Villarejo-Ortega FJ: Use of epsilon aminocaproic acid (EACA) in the preoperative management of ruptured intracranial aneurysms. J Neurosurg 44:479–484, 1976.
23. Shucart WA, Hussain SK, Cooper PR: Epsilon-aminocaproic acid and recurrent subarachnoid hemorrhage: A clinical trial. J Neurosurg 53:28–31, 1980.
24. Yasargil MG, Fox JL, Ray MW: The operative approach to aneurysms of the anterior communicating artery. Adv Tech Stds Neurosurg 2:113–170, 1975.
25. Yasargil MG, Smith RD, Gasser C: Microsurgery of the aneurysms of the internal carotid artery and its branches. Prog Neurol Surg 9:58–121, 1978.
26. Yoshimoto T, Uchida K, Kaneko U, Kayama T, Suzuki J: An analysis of follow-up results of 1000 intracranial saccular aneurysms with definitive surgical treatment. J Neurosurg 50:152–157, 1979.

170

Giant Intracranial Aneurysms

Yoshio Hosobuchi

Intracranial aneurysms that have a diameter greater than 2.5 cm are considered giant aneurysms.[24] In its most common form, the giant aneurysm is presumed to evolve from an initially smaller congenital saccular aneurysm that undergoes continued enlargement, during which time it may or may not rupture. In addition to this saccular form, fusiform giant aneurysms may arise in the posterior circulation, probably as a consequence of ectasia of the parent artery resulting from atherosclerotic degeneration of the vessel wall.

Black and German proposed that the size of any aneurysm is proportional to the size of its neck.[2] Certainly, one might expect that the greater the area of the aneurysmal neck, the greater will be the fluxional turbulence in the sac. Ferguson provided experimental evidence to this effect:[10] that turbulence within the sac of the aneurysm produces vibration of the wall, causing it to degenerate and thereby allowing the aneurysm to enlarge.[33,37,40] This finding may apply also to those giant aneurysms that are located at the terminations of the carotid and basilar arteries but it would not seem to apply to the more distally located giant aneurysms of the middle cerebral artery (MCA). There is no satisfactory explanation as to why many giant aneurysms of the MCA continue to enlarge without rupturing. These lesions are unusual also in that they often contain a large, laminated thrombus,[18,41] which when dissected by blood flow, may produce a peculiar angiographic appearance of serpentine channeling.[5,44]

From the few available reports, the prognosis in the natural course of unoperated giant aneurysms would appear to be grim. As many as 80 percent of patients die within a few years after the discovery of the aneurysm,[4,30,48] either from subarachnoid hemorrhage (SAH) or from cerebral ischemia presumably due to compression of major arteries by the progressive enlargement of the aneurysm. Conversely, however, there are some reports of spontaneous diminution or even disappearance of a giant aneurysm.[6,30,43]

Although the introduction of microsurgical technique has resulted in great improvements in the surgical management of intracranial aneurysms,[22] large aneurysms still present obstacles to direct surgical intervention because of a number of factors: their large size and often large neck; their proximity to the diencephalon and brain stem structures; the incorporation of perforating vessels into the wall of the aneurysmal neck; occasionally the incorporation of the parent artery into the sac; and the likelihood of atheromatous involvement at the neck of the aneurysm.[9] During the past 12 years, I have managed 84 cases of large intracranial aneurysm that were classified as giant on the basis of either radiological or direct intraoperative measurement. I will review the clinical features of these intracranial giant aneurysms, the surgical techniques used in treating them, and the outcome in these cases, and will discuss the pertinent literature.

Clinical Presentation

Giant intracranial aneurysms are found predominantly in females, the female-male ratio being 3 to 1, and they occur most commonly in patients 30 to 60 years of age (Table 170-1). The reported incidence of giant aneurysms varies, but they probably constitute no more than 5 percent of all intracranial aneurysms,[24,26,30,45] and 15 percent of giant aneurysms are associated with either multiple intracranial aneurysms or an arteriovenous malformation. No familial association has been reported. It is well known that most aneurysms of this type arise at the junction of the carotid and ophthalmic arteries, and there is a high incidence of cases in which vestigial vessels are found connecting two internal carotid arteries in the fetus.[12] Otherwise, the distribution of giant aneurysms in various branches of the cerebral arteries is similar to that found with smaller aneurysms (Table 170-2).

Most giant aneurysms present with signs of a mass lesion, such as chronic headache, visual disturbance, and oculomotor palsies—all of which are common symptoms and signs of carotid-ophthalmic artery giant aneurysm and cavernous carotid aneurysm.[9,16,20,30,48] Other cranial nerve palsies and signs of brain stem compression are common manifestations

TABLE 170-1 Sex and Age Distributions of 84 Patients with Intracranial Giant Aneurysm

Sex
  Male 26   Female 58

Age (yr)
  0–10   2   41–50   22
  11–20   1   51–60   25
  21–30   6   61–70   14
  31–40 13   71–80   1

TABLE 170-2 Anatomical Locations of Intracranial Giant Aneurysms

Anatomical Location	Number of Aneurysms
Cavernous carotid artery	18
Internal carotid–ophthalmic artery junction	28
Carotid termination	5
Posterior communicating artery	5
Anterior communicating artery	9
Middle cerebral artery	4
Basilar or vertebral artery	15
Total	84

of vertebrobasilar artery giant aneurysm.[8,9,17] The mass effect of the giant aneurysm arising in other areas may be more subtle.[34] Slowly progressive dementia may be a primary presenting symptom of a giant aneurysm of the anterior communicating artery,[9,17] whereas progressive hemiparesis may signify a giant aneurysm of the MCA causing not only direct mass effect on the brain but also compression of the sylvian vessels.[5,9,17,30] We have had one patient in whom an aneurysm located at the base of the skull presented with cerebrospinal fluid rhinorrhea as a primary symptom resulting from erosion of the planum sphenoidale.[17] Despite the frequent occurrence of giant aneurysms at the carotid-ophthalmic junction, hypopituitarism is a rare sequela of these lesions.[11,39]

Although the prevailing opinion is that giant aneurysms seldom rupture, there are only a few studies in the literature to support such a notion.[19] On the contrary, my experience and series reported by others show that a surprising proportion of them present with SAH in a frequency varying from 30 to 80 percent.[9,17,24,30,36,45,51] Often, giant aneurysms that do not present with recent SAH show evidence of a more remote history of bleeding that probably occurred when the aneurysm was small. The incidence of SAH for aneurysms of the anterior circulation does not differ significantly from that for aneurysms of the posterior circulation. Drake reported that massive mural thrombosis in a giant sac did not seem to provide protection from bleeding, as a thrombus was present in about one-third of the recently ruptured giant aneurysms in his series.[9]

Radiological Diagnosis

Since the advent of computed tomography (CT), plain x-ray films of the skull are used only rarely for the radiological diagnosis of neurosurgical problems except in cases of head injury. In the diagnosis of giant aneurysms, however, they may afford some useful information. Occasionally, curvilinear calcification can be seen along the perimeter of a giant aneurysm on the plain films. Erosion of the base of the skull resulting from the chronic mass effect has also been reported.[4,17,30]

CT provides a tentative diagnosis of this lesion.[17,23,51] A telltale radiological sign of a giant aneurysm is a large, spherical mass in the basal area showing contrast filling to varying degrees and a partially contrast-enhancing intramural thrombus. A coronal reformation may be necessary to appreciate the true size of the lesion and its relationship to the diencephalon and brain stem. An ectatic fusiform aneurysm in the posterior fossa may be slightly more difficult to delineate clearly by CT.

Cerebral angiography may fail to show the actual size of the aneurysm because of the intramural thrombus; however, angiography is essential to demonstrate the artery from which the aneurysm arises, the size of the neck, and its relationship to adjacent perforating vessels.[4,9,17,30,36,42,48,51] It is crucial to include the external carotid circulation in the angiographic study, as the size of the superficial temporal artery (STA), of the occipital artery, or of both may become important in deciding whether it may be possible to manage the lesion with an extracranial-intracranial (EC-IC) vascular bypass.[50]

Methods of Treatment

Until recently, Hunterian occlusion of the parent artery has been the technique used most frequently to treat these formidable lesions.[8,9,13,34,38,52,53] The artery can be ligated at a distance from the aneurysm, as in the ligation of the internal carotid or vertebral artery in the neck; or as described by Drake, it can be ligated near the aneurysm by intracranial occlusion of the carotid, middle cerebral, anterior cerebral, vertebral, upper and lower basilar, superior cerebellar, or posterior cerebral artery.[9]

Mere occlusion of the common carotid artery probably is not adequate for the treatment of a giant carotid aneurysm, however.[7,17] In my series, six patients with a giant aneurysm of the carotid artery had been treated previously with common carotid ligation but the aneurysm had continued to enlarge, as was manifested by a progressive visual deficit and the angiographic demonstration of an enlarging lesion.[17]

Internal carotid artery ligation for the treatment of a giant aneurysm presents significant problems because of the unpredictable possibility of delayed and devastating ischemia and cerebral infarction, even in cases in which preoperative angiography has demonstrated good cross-circulation. It appears that 80 percent of patients can tolerate acute occlusion of one carotid artery but 20 percent will not[28]; and opening the carotid artery immediately after the first sign of ischemia does not reverse all neurological deficits. There also appears to be a long-term risk of ischemia associated with occlusion of the carotid artery.[1,21,25,35] In a long-term follow-up study of 35 cases reported by German and Black, 10 of the 33 patients who left the hospital (30 percent) died during the follow-up period of 13 years.[13] One other patient developed hemiparesis and aphasia 25 months after internal carotid artery ligation, and at least two patients (6 percent) developed late cerebral ischemic episodes. Similarly, Oldershaw and Voris reported two cases of late stroke occurring 1 and 13 years, respectively, after carotid artery occlusion.[35]

Based on such observations, some surgeons have advocated the use of an EC-IC vascular bypass in conjunction with carotid occlusion for the treatment of the giant carotid aneurysm.[9,50,54] The STA-MCA bypass is the most commonly used; however, a reasonably good collateral circulation is still required for the patient to be able to withstand acute occlusion of the carotid flow.[49] In my series, two patients who were treated with internal carotid artery ligation (entrapment) and an STA-MCA bypass died from massive cerebral infarction despite having had a patent vascular bypass (Table 170-3). In any patient it is difficult to estimate precisely the state of collateral blood flow to the hemisphere, although as shown by Miller et al., it can be predicted with reasonable confidence through a combination of studies of blood flow at the carotid bifurcation and measurements of stump pressure.[28] Any patient with an internal carotid artery stump pressure of less than 30 mmHg will not tolerate acute internal carotid artery occlusion, even with an optimally patent STA-MCA anastomosis. In such a case, a vein graft rather than an STA-MCA bypass is needed to substitute for the carotid circulation because it affords more blood delivery to the brain (Fig. 170-1).

A low internal carotid artery stump pressure may be merely a reflection of the compression of collateral circulation caused by the mass effect of the giant aneurysm. If the surgeon temporarily entraps the aneurysm and aspirates its contents to reduce its mass effect, the distal intracranial arterial pressure may rise suddenly to within a high range of stump pressure without an immediate need for an EC-IC bypass.[17] This observation and the technical approach of evaluation in such a situation are illustrated by one case in my series. The patient, who presented with a chronic right frontal headache and progressive visual difficulty in 1972, was found to have a giant right carotid–ophthalmic aneurysm (Fig. 170-2). She underwent a ligation of the right

TABLE 170-3 Results in 56 Patients with Intracranial Giant Aneurysm of the Internal Carotid Artery*

Result	Neck Occlusion	Proximal Occlusion	Trapping	Intramural Thrombosis
Excellent	10	14†	8	9
Good	—	—	3‡	3
Poor	—	2	—	2
Died	1	—	2†	2
Total	11	16	13	16

*Cavernous carotid, internal carotid-ophthalmic artery junction, carotid termination, posterior communicating artery.
†With STA-MCA bypass.
‡With vein graft EC-IC vascular bypass.

Giant Intracranial Aneurysms

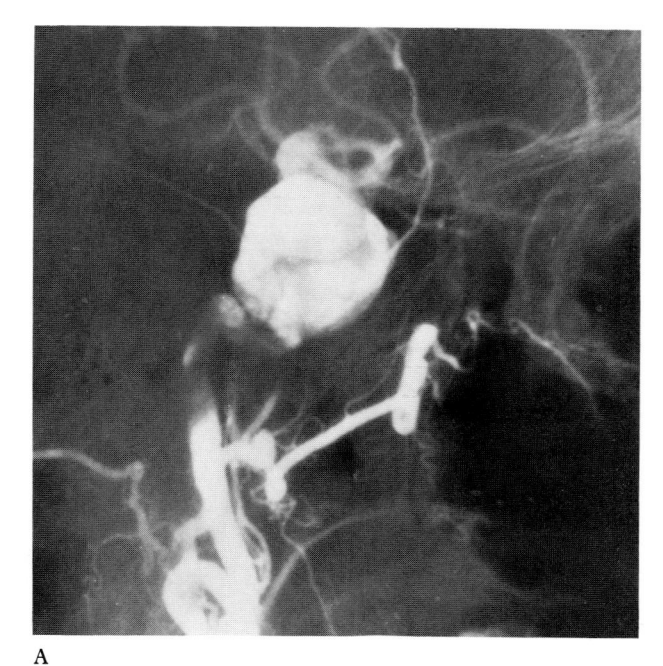

Figure 170-1 A 68-year-old female with chronic right retro-orbital pain and a 2-year history of a progressive decrease in visual acuity in the right eye presented with the sudden onset of a right abducens nerve palsy. *A.* The preoperative arteriogram demonstrates a giant right cavernous carotid aneurysm. *B.* The postoperative arteriogram demonstrates the entrapped aneurysm and the EC-IC vascular bypass made by using a saphenous vein graft.

common carotid artery. For a short time, her symptoms diminished somewhat, but they recurred within a year and progressively became worse. When she was evaluated again in March 1974, the vision in her right eye had diminished markedly and she reported paroxysmal attacks of paresthesia in her left hand. An angiogram showed that the aneurysm was definitely larger than it had been in 1972. It filled from the right carotid artery, which received substantial flow from the right vertebral artery through anastomosis of the muscular branches. There was little collateral flow to the right hemisphere (Fig. 170-3).

A right frontotemporal craniotomy was performed, and the cervical carotid bifurcation was also exposed. The systemic arterial pressure was 130/70 mmHg. The intra-arterial pressure was measured at 110/60 mmHg by a technique similar to that described by Bloor et al.[3] A 27-gauge needle connected by plastic tubing to a strain gauge was inserted into the intracranial carotid artery distal to the aneurysm. When a vascular clamp was placed temporarily on the cervical internal carotid artery, the arterial pressure distally fell to 50/30 mmHg with minimal pulsatile excursion (Fig. 170-4A). The contents of the aneurysm were then aspirated by clipping the intracranial carotid artery just distal to the aneurysm and inserting a large-bore suction needle obliquely through the wall. When the sac was collapsed (Fig. 170-4B), the distal arterial pressure rose suddenly to 90/50 mmHg, clearly indicating that the collateral circulation to the right cerebral hemisphere was increased by decompression of the mass.

On the basis of this observation, I decided to trap the aneurysm by ligating the cervical internal carotid artery and clipping it intracranially just distal to the aneurysm. A large clip was placed across the neck of the aneurysm to prevent refilling of the sac by flow through the ophthalmic artery and the intracavernous anastomosing branches of the carotid artery. The sac was then opened and the thrombosed content evacuated. The postoperative angiogram (Fig. 170-5) showed improved collateral circulation. The patient's chronic headache disappeared after the operation and her vision rapidly improved. At follow-up examination in November 1977, her visual fields were normal and the acuity in her right eye was 20/30.

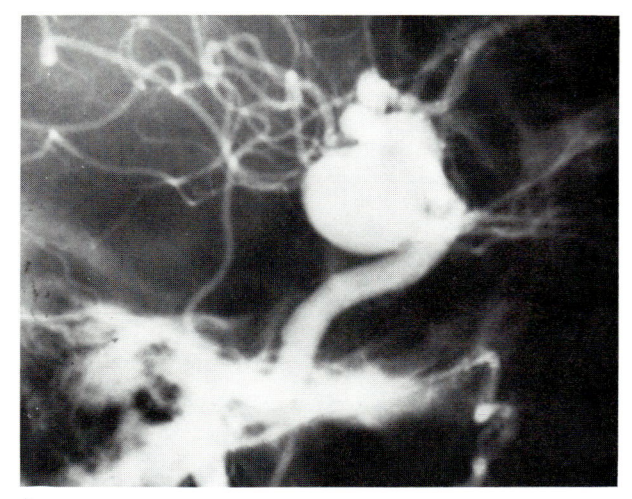

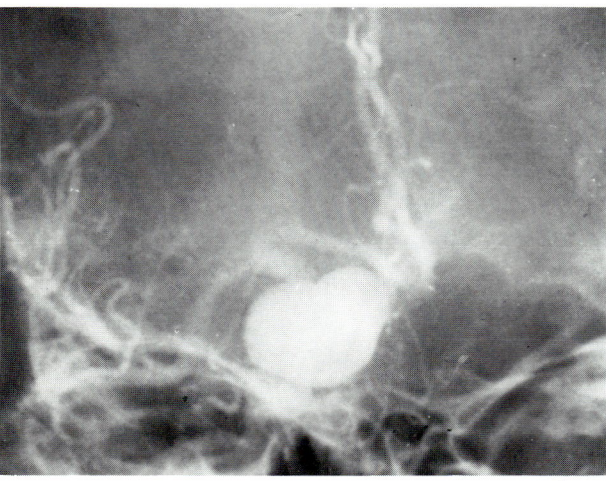

Figure 170-2 This patient presented with a chronic right frontal headache and progressive visual difficulty in 1972. These angiograms were obtained in 1974. The lateral (A) and anteroposterior (B) projections of the right carotid artery show a giant carotid-ophthalmic aneurysm. (From Hosobuchi.[17])

Without doubt, the most effective approach to giant aneurysms is occlusion of the aneurysmal neck, although in most of the major series of giant aneurysms that were managed surgically, fewer than 70 percent of the lesions could be treated in this manner.[9,51] The main difficulty is that the neck of a giant aneurysm is often bulbous and firm because of its thickness or because of atheroma, mural thrombus, or the pressure within it; thus the clip applied to the neck easily slides off or occludes the parent artery. In many cases, pharmacologically induced hypotension or acute proximal occlusion of the parent artery reduces the intramural tension, allowing a clip to be applied reliably. It is usually more effective to apply the clip perpendicular to the course of the artery and to either place the cross-clip from the opposite direction (Fig. 170-6) or piggyback another clip to reinforce the closing tension of the first clip. When the round, thick neck of a carotid aneurysm will not hold a clip, I have found a curved Potts clamp to be very useful. The clamp is placed across the neck and held gently but firmly closed during temporary cervical carotid artery occlusion. This gentle crushing of the neck of the aneurysm creates an indentation that helps to hold the blades of a strong clip.

Many large aneurysmal necks are rigid with mural thrombus that has to be removed to make them soft enough for clipping. This can be accomplished by a temporary entrapment of the aneurysm. I keep the patient normotensive, fully heparinized, and under mild hypothermia (30 to 32°C). Pentobarbital (3 to 4 mg/kg) is given in a single intravenous bolus injection before the initiation of entrapment.[14,15,27,29,46,47,55] Under this condition, the surgeon has the benefit of about 10 min in which to perform the thrombectomy and to clip the aneurysm in the manner described earlier. Thrombectomy is not performed easily, however. The thrombus is thick, tough, stringy, and adherent to the aneurysm wall, and the neck is fragile. It is best to find the plane at which the thrombus cleaves from the wall of the sac and to separate as much of the mass of thrombus as possible by a piecemeal removal with end-biting forceps. The duration of the patient's tolerance to the temporary entrapment depends on the availability of collateral circulation, although a rising mean arterial pressure during entrapment is a certain warning sign of cerebral intolerance to the ischemia, and reperfusion should be established without delay. Because of this brief interval in which to work during temporary entrapment, some surgeons advocate approaching the problem by performing a cardiopulmonary bypass while the patient is under hypothermia. Silverberg et al. have reported favorable results with this approach,[45] although Drake has been discouraged by instances of silent hematoma caused by the intraoperative use of heparin.[9] The Sundt-Kee circumferential clip is rarely usable for clipping giant aneurysms because of its feeble closure tension; either it is spit off by the re-expanding aneurysm or it pinches the parent artery, resulting in occlusion of the vessel.

Some giant aneurysms are simply not amenable to Hunterian ligation, entrapment, or clipping. In such situations, intramural thrombosis induced with metallic material, such as stainless steel or beryllium-copper wire, may better protect the patient from further enlargement or rupture of the aneurysm than will simple exploration.[16,17,31,32] The fine (25-μm) wires are inserted into the sac of the aneurysm under direct visualization. Only a part of the sac needs to be exposed. The wall of the aneurysm is punctured with a 30-gauge needle, and the fine wire, which is guided into the needle by 22-gauge steel tubing to prevent it from kinking (Fig. 170-7), is inserted through the needle into the sac of the aneurysm. As these wires do have some memory property, they can be coiled before they are inserted. The wire should be packed into the aneurysm as much as possible, and the degree of induced intramural thrombosis must be checked occasionally by intraoperative angiography. To thrombose a giant aneurysm of 3 to 4 cm in diameter requires at least 30 to 50 ft of wire (Fig. 170-8). In my series, 33 aneurysms were treated by means of this technique; complete thrombosis was induced in 27 cases. A follow-up review of 2 years' duration with angiographic data shows continued thrombosis in 21 cases. Among patients with 2 to 10

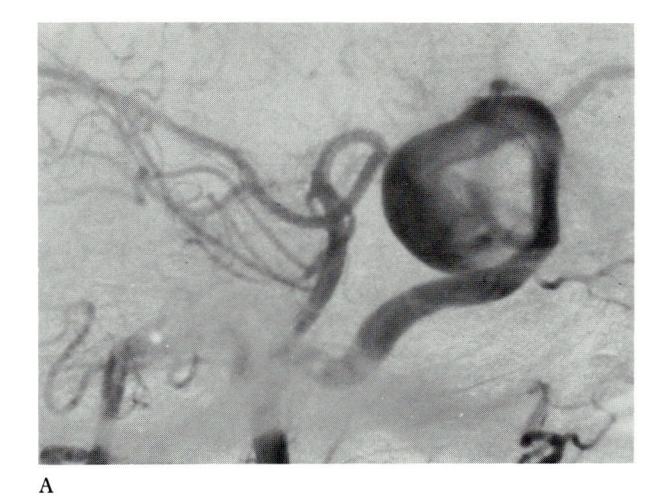

Giant Intracranial Aneurysms

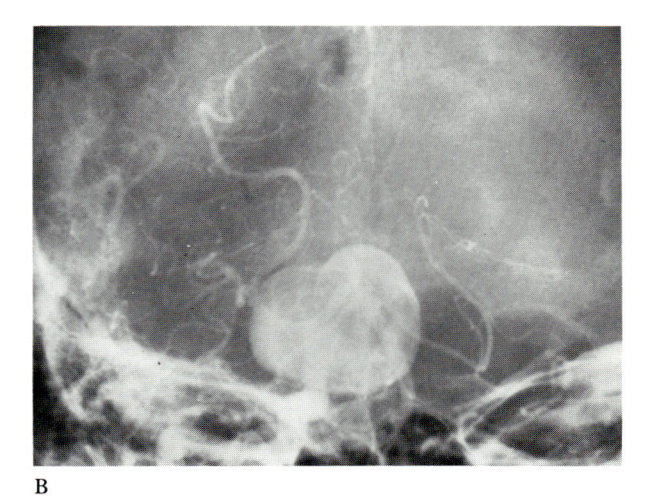

Figure 170-3 Same patient as shown in Fig. 170-2. Right vertebral angiograms in the lateral (*A*) and anteroposterior (*B*) projections show further enlargement of the giant carotid-ophthalmic aneurysm. A left carotid angiogram (*C*) shows minimal collateral circulation to the right cerebral hemisphere. (From Hosobuchi.[17])

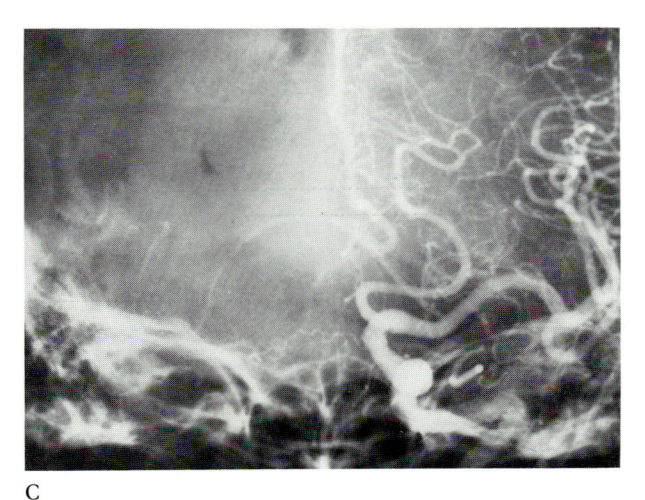

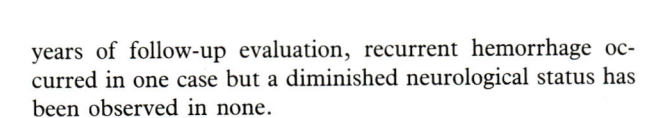

years of follow-up evaluation, recurrent hemorrhage occurred in one case but a diminished neurological status has been observed in none.

Surgical Results

How a giant aneurysm is managed surgically depends on many factors. Its size and location and the incorporation of important perforating arterial branches into the lesion may determine the approach, but the skill and experience of the surgeon undoubtedly constitute the critical element.

Drake recently reviewed his entire series of giant aneurysms.[9] Of the 174 lesions, 66 were on the carotid system and 108 were vertebrobasilar. SAH had occurred in 36 percent of his patients; one-third of these had mural thrombi, sometimes massive, within the aneurysmal sac. He classified his results as good to excellent in 71.5 percent of the series, 13 percent of the patients had a poor outcome, and 15.5 percent died. Occlusion of the aneurysmal neck could be accomplished in only 38.5 percent of cases, however. Thirteen patients had exploration only, and the remainder underwent a number of procedures, including

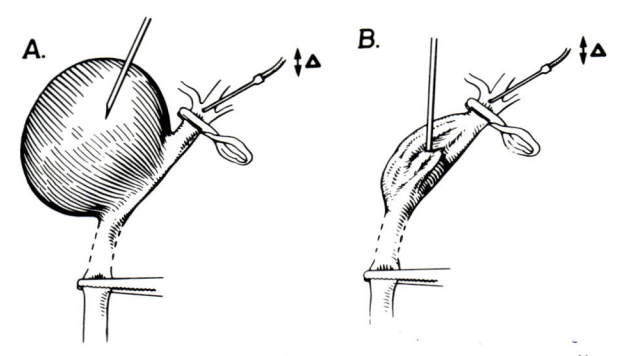

Figure 170-4 Diagram of an entrapment maneuver, illustrated by the case of a giant aneurysm of the left carotid artery. The distal branches shown are, from left to right, the posterior communicating, middle cerebral, and anterior cerebral arteries; the ophthalmic and anterior choroidal arteries are not shown. *A.* The pressure is measured with a 27-gauge needle connected by plastic tubing to a strain gauge. When the distal pressure (Δ) is less than 50 mmHg, the pulsatory excursion of the blood pressure is minimal and only systolic pressure is recorded. *B.* The contents of the aneurysm are aspirated with a 20- or 18-gauge needle (connected to suction tubing) inserted obliquely through the wall of the aneurysm. (From Hosobuchi.[17])

A   B

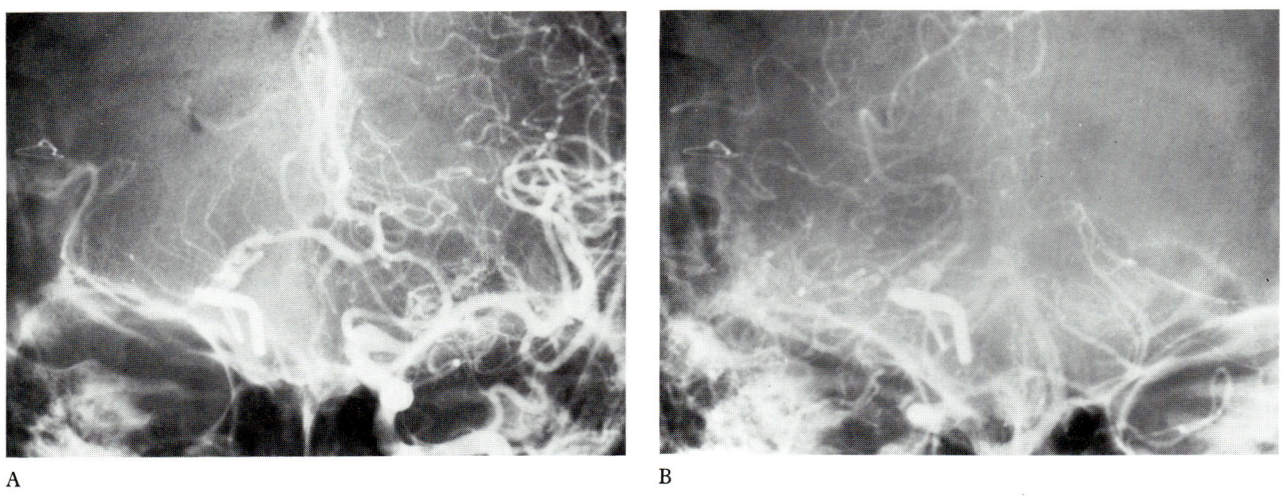

Figure 170-5 Postoperative angiograms of the patient shown in Figs. 170-2 and 170-3 show anteroposterior projections of the left carotid (A) and right vertebral (B) arteries. (From Hosobuchi.[17])

wrapping, intraluminal thrombosis with hair or wire, and proximal occlusion or trapping. An EC-IC bypass was performed before proximal occlusion in some cases, and it was thought to provide a measure of protection to the patient. An ingenious delayed proximal arterial occlusion was performed in a number of patients with the patient awake, after an arterial snare had been applied to the parent artery during surgical exploration when it was clear that the aneurysm could not be ligated at its neck.

Other surgeons have reported giant aneurysms on the MCA that were treated by STA-MCA anastomosis followed by proximal occlusion of the MCA. One must gamble in such a case that the fresh anastomosis can supply sufficient blood to the middle cerebral arterial tree to prevent ischemia. Still other surgeons have simply excised the giant aneurysm, sacrificing the parent artery; sometimes this approach yields an acceptable result. Sundt and Piepgrass, reviewing 80 cases of giant aneurysm among 594 operations for aneurysm (13.5 percent), reported commendable rates of mortality (4 percent) and morbidity (14 percent).[51] Direct clipping

A   B

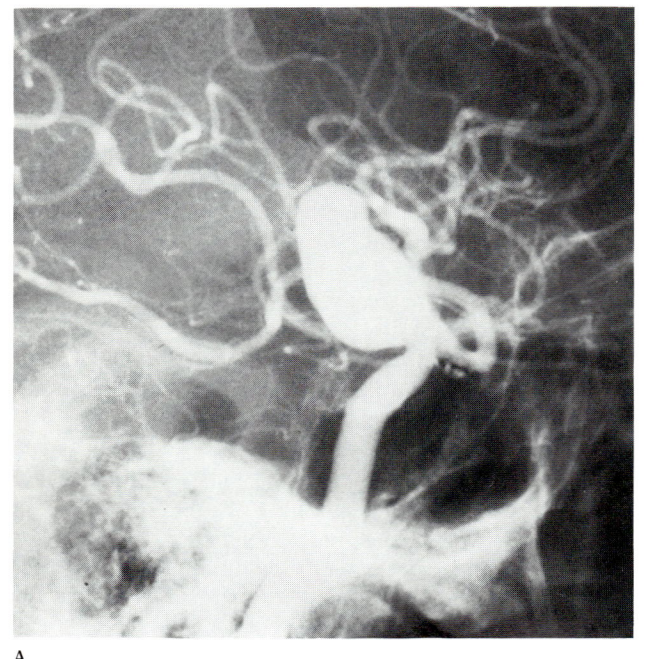

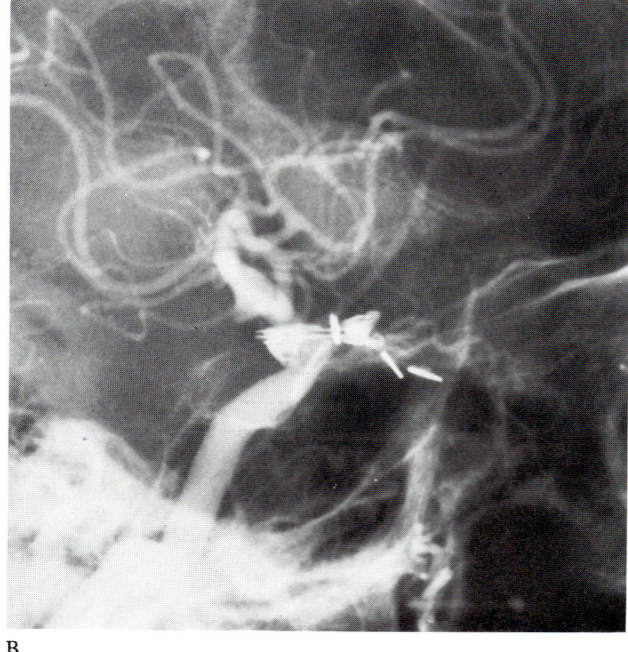

Figure 170-6 Angiograms of a giant aneurysm of the right carotid-ophthalmic artery junction (lateral projection) before (A) and after (B) successful obliteration with use of two opposed aneurysm clips. (From Hosobuchi.[17])

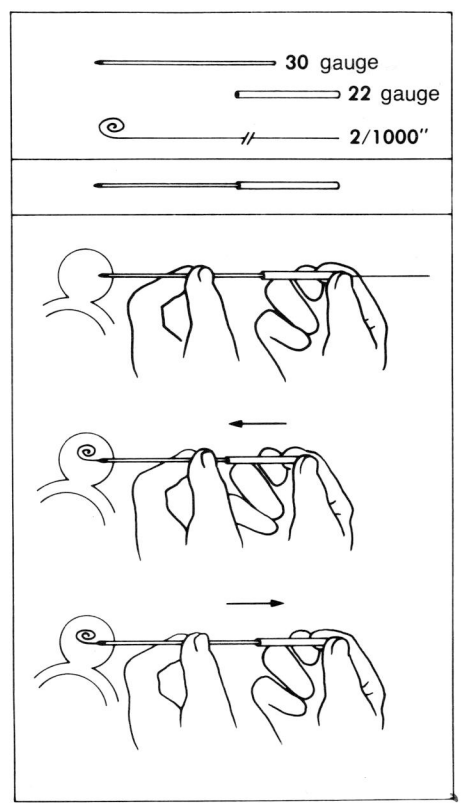

Figure 170-7 Diagram of insertion of a 30-gauge needle into the sac of a giant aneurysm and the pumping action of a segment of 22-gauge tubing to feed the metallic wire. This is essential to prevent kinking of the wire during insertion.

or excision was accomplished in 55 patients (69 percent), and the remainder had either proximal ligation (with or without an EC-IC bypass) or a trapping procedure. Their results with aneurysms of the carotid circulation were good, but those with aneurysms of the posterior circulation were less so: there was a 30 percent morbidity and a 7 percent mortality among patients with these latter lesions. The rate of morbidity among their patients with basilar head aneurysm was 50 percent.

Onuma and Suzuki reviewed 32 giant aneurysms, of which seven were infraclinoid in location.[36] In their series, 72 percent of patients presented with SAH. Twenty-four patients underwent a direct approach to the aneurysm and four had a carotid ligation. Some patients were operated upon under mild hypothermia (without cardiac arrest). In 10 cases the lesions could be extirpated after the neck had been ligated; in 12 the surgeon had to settle for partial ligation plus reinforcement of the aneurysm by wrapping with muscle. Neither two patients in whom a trapping procedure was necessary survived. Overall, the mortality in cases approached by direct surgery was 20.8 percent and the morbidity was 37.5 percent.

The surgical results in my series of 84 giant intracranial aneurysms are summarized in Tables 170-3, 170-4, and 170-5. The cavernous carotid giant aneurysms generally responded well to proximal ligation of the carotid artery. When the stump pressure of the carotid artery was low (less than 50 mmHg), a bypass procedure to anastamose the common carotid artery with the MCA was performed, which involved a saphenous vein graft before proximal occlusion of the carotid artery, entrapment of the aneurysm, or both (Fig. 170-1). Symptoms of involvement of the oculomotor and trigeminal nerves dissipated rapidly after the surgical treatment of the aneurysms, but abducens nerve palsy did not resolve in any case.

Of the 38 intradural carotid giant aneurysms, it was possible to occlude the neck of the aneurysm with clips in 11 cases. One patient died because of severe hyponatremia 5 days after the operation. Of 13 patients who underwent an entrapment procedure, 2 died of massive cerebral ischemia despite a patent STA-MCA bypass. These cases indicate that the STA-MCA bypass is unlikely to afford acute replacement of the carotid blood flow.

Of 14 patients treated by the intramural thrombosis technique, 2 died postoperatively, one because of a massive extension of the thrombus from the aneurysm sac to the lumen of the carotid artery that caused total occlusion of carotid blood flow. The other death was caused by a massive pulmonary embolism that occurred during the sixth postoperative day. Unlike the basilar-tip giant aneurysms, the carotid-ophthalmic aneurysms have a relatively large orifice in relation to the parent artery and therefore involve a higher risk of distal embolization after induced intramural thrombosis. Such a complication occurred in two patients treated by intramural thrombosis and in each case this resulted in major hemispheric deficits; these cases are listed among the poor results.

Giant aneurysms of the anterior communicating artery are the most difficult to treat among all the intracranial giant aneurysms because if one attempts to clip the neck, it is often impossible to see the vessels on the other side, or the sac may be quite adherent to the hypothalamus. On the other hand, if one induces intramural thrombosis, the mass effect may not be totally eliminated, even after satisfactory obliteration of the lumen. This frustrating quandary is reflected well in my results (Table 170-4).

Of the two giant aneurysms of the MCA in my series, one was totally excised after I failed to find recipient MCA branches large enough to permit an STA-MCA anastomosis. The other MCA giant aneurysm was treated by aneurysmorrhaphy.

In my experience the intramural thrombosis technique has been the most effective method for treating the basilar

TABLE 170-4 Results in 9 Patients with Intracranial Giant Aneurysm of the Anterior Communicating Artery

| Result | Type of Treatment ||
	Neck Occlusion	Intramural Thrombosis
Excellent	1	3
Good	1	1
Poor	1	1
Died	—	1
Total	3	6

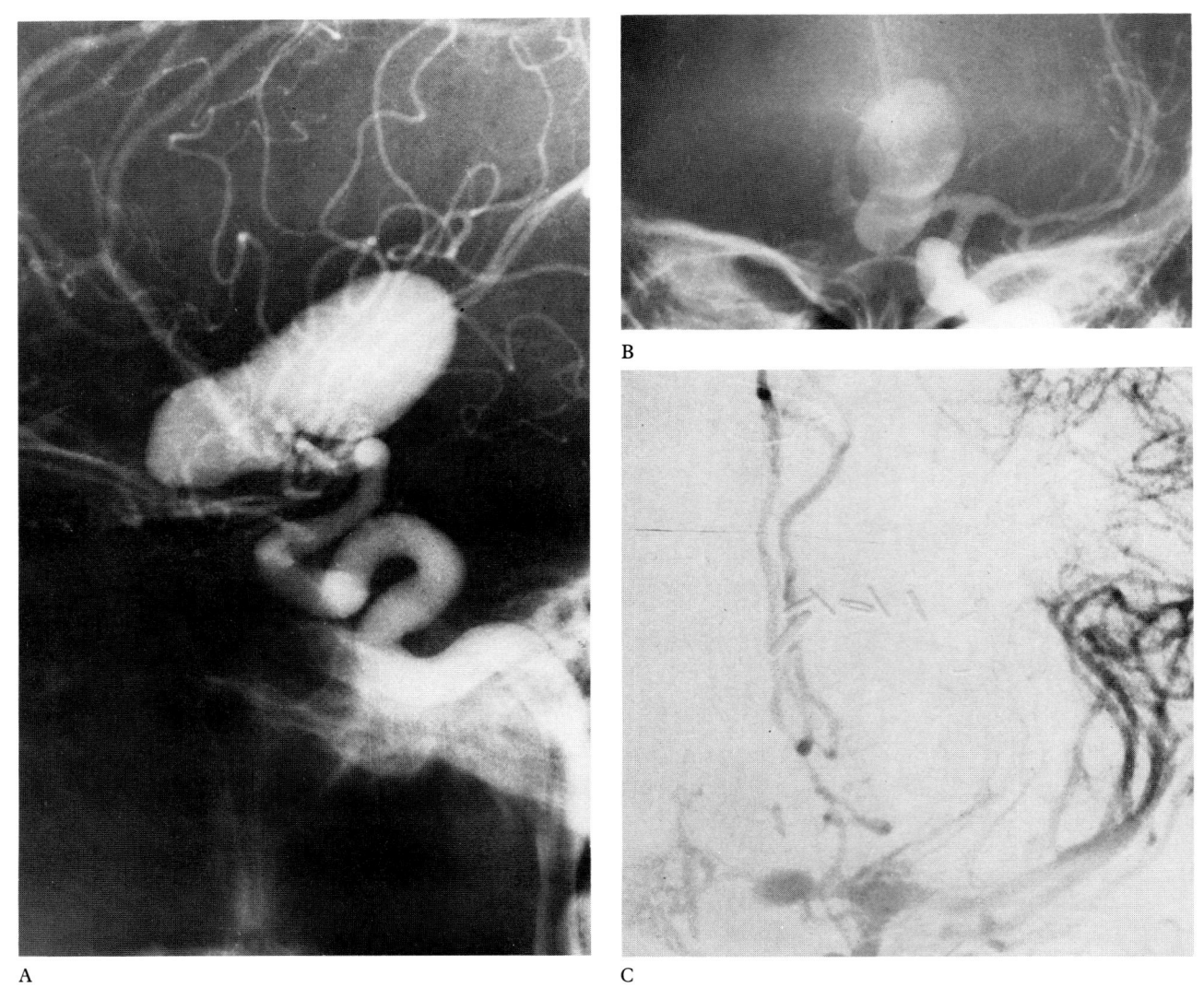

Figure 170-8 Angiograms of a giant aneurysm of the anterior communicating artery, lateral (*A*) and anteroposterior (*B*) projections. *C*. The postoperative angiogram shows the intact anterior communicating artery, which was preserved by controlled progressive intramural thrombosis with use of intraoperative arteriograms. The residual dilatation of the base was reinforced with muslin. (From Hosobuchi.[17])

giant aneurysms (Table 170-5). Over a 10-year period of follow-up review for the earliest cases, there has been no recurrent SAH or increasing mass effect. These results exceed those obtained in other series.[9,51]

Silverberg et al. have reported no mortality and low morbidity rates with the use of hypothermia and cardiac arrest in the treatment of giant aneurysms.[45] The aneurysm was excluded from the cerebral circulation in all but one case. They proposed that the success of their procedure is attributable to collapse of the aneurysm so that the vascular anatomy at the base of the aneurysm can be more easily appreciated without being inundated by a swirling pool of blood. In contrast to Drake's experience, their series included only one case of a small intracerebral hematoma postoperatively.

Despite there still being considerable operative morbidity and mortality among cases of giant intracranial aneurysm, patients harboring these lesions do better when treated surgically than when managed conservatively. The exceptions are those patients with a giant aneurysm arising from the cavernous carotid artery. These lesions rarely cause more than cranial nerve palsy and facial pain, and unless the surgeon can assure the lowest possible incidence of morbidity and no mortality, a surgical procedure should not be ventured.

There is no single best surgical approach to the intracranial giant aneurysm. The neurosurgeon must be prepared to apply all possible means to reduce the risk of hemorrhage and the mass effect from these devastating lesions. Hypothermia with cardiac arrest, as reported by Silverberg's group, may provide the surgeon with additional working time and a clear operative field. With regard to the use of induced intraluminal thrombosis, my experience clearly

TABLE 170-5 Results in 15 Patients with Intracranial Giant Aneurysm of the Posterior Circulation

Result	Type of Treatment		
	Neck Occlusion	Trapping	Intramural Thrombosis
Excellent	—	1	10
Good	1	1	1
Poor	1	—	—
Died	—	—	—
Total	2	2	11

indicates that, although the results do not match those obtained with clipping of the aneurysmal neck, the technique provides an exceedingly high percentage of satisfactory results in the surgical treatment of giant aneurysms of the posterior circulation. This experience is at variance with that of Drake and Sundt. Drake has rejected this technique, although he has reported as a good result a case in which spontaneous thrombosis occurred postoperatively in an aneurysm that he had found untreatable during the surgical exploration.[9] Considering that instances of spontaneous thrombosis are relatively rare and in view of the grim prognosis that can be expected when a giant aneurysm remains untreated, it would seem preferable to induce thrombosis intentionally rather than to leave the aneurysm untreated. My experience indicates also that further trials with the use of metallic wire to induce luminal thrombosis are warranted.

References

1. Barnett HJM: Delayed cerebral ischemic episodes distal to occlusion of major cerebral arteries. Neurology 28:769–774, 1978.
2. Black SPW, German WJ: Observations on the relationship between the volume and the size of the orifice of experimental aneurysms. J Neurosurg 17:984–990, 1960.
3. Bloor BM, Odom GL, Woodhall B: Direct measurement of intravascular pressure in components of the circle of Willis. Arch Surg 63:821–823, 1951.
4. Bull J: Massive aneurysms at the base of the brain. Brain 92:535–570, 1969.
5. Cantu RC, LeMay M: A large middle cerebral aneurysm presenting as a bizarre vascular malformation. Br J Radiol 39:317–319, 1966.
6. Carlson DH, Thomson D: Spontaneous thrombosis of a giant cerebral aneurysm in five days: Report of a case. Neurology 26:334–336, 1976.
7. Cuatico W, Cook AV, Tyshchenko V, Khatib R: Massive enlargement of intracranial aneurysms following carotid ligation. Arch Neurol 17:609–613, 1967.
8. Drake CG: Ligation of the vertebral (unilateral or bilateral) or basilar artery in the treatment of large intracranial aneurysms. J Neurosurg 43:255–274, 1975.
9. Drake CG: Giant intracranial aneurysms: Experience with surgical treatment in 174 patients. Clin Neurosurg 26:12–95, 1979.
10. Ferguson GG: Physical factors in the initiation, growth, and rupture of human intracranial saccular aneurysms. J Neurosurg 37:666–677, 1972.
11. Gallagher PG, Dorsey JF, Stefanini M, Looney JM: Large intracranial aneurysm producing panhypopituitarism and frontal lobe syndrome. Neurology 6:829–837, 1956.
12. Garcia-Bengochea F, Deland FH: Bilateral giant carotid-ophthalmic aneurysms: Case report. J Neurosurg 42:589–592, 1975.
13. German WJ, Black SPW: Cervical ligation for internal carotid aneurysms: An extended follow-up. J Neurosurg 23:572–577, 1965.
14. Hoff JT, Pitts LH, Spetzler R, Wilson CB: Barbiturates for protection from cerebral ischemia in aneurysm surgery. Acta Neurol Scand [Suppl] 64:158–159, 1977.
15. Hoff JT, Smith AL, Hankinson HL, Nielsen SL: Barbiturate protection from cerebral infarction in primates. Stroke 6:28–33, 1975.
16. Hosobuchi Y: Electrothrombosis of carotid-cavernous fistula. J Neurosurg 42:76–85, 1975.
17. Hosobuchi Y: Direct surgical treatment of giant intracranial aneurysms. J Neurosurg 51:743–756, 1979.
18. Howe JF, Harris AB, Sypert GW: Giant aneurysm of the middle cerebral artery. Surg Neurol 6:231–233, 1976.
19. Jain KK: Surgery of intracranial berry aneurysms: A review. Can J Surg 8:172–187, 1965.
20. Jefferson G: Compression of the chiasma, optic nerves, and optic tracts by intracranial aneurysms. Brain 60:444–497, 1937.
21. Kak VK, Taylor AR, Gordon DS: Proximal carotid ligation for internal carotid aneurysms: A long-term follow-up study. J Neurosurg 39:503–513, 1973.
22. Krayenbühl HA, Yasargil MG, Flamm ES, Tew JM, Jr: Microsurgical treatment of intracranial saccular aneurysms. J Neurosurg 37:678–686, 1972.
23. Lavyne MH, Kleefield J, Davis KR, Ojemann RG, Crowell RM: Giant intracranial aneurysms of the anterior circulation: Clinical characteristics and diagnosis by computed tomography. Neurosurgery 3:356–363, 1978.
24. Locksley HB: Report on the cooperative study of intracranial aneurysms and subarachnoid hemorrhage, Sect. V, Part II. Natural history of subarachnoid hemorrhage, intracranial aneurysms and arteriovenous malformations: Based on 6368 cases in the cooperative study. J Neurosurg 25:321–368, 1966.
25. Love JG, Dart LH: Results of carotid ligation with particular reference to intracranial aneurysms. J Neurosurg 27:89–93, 1967.
26. Matson DD: Intracranial arterial aneurysms in childhood. J Neurosurg 23:578–583, 1965.
27. Michenfelder JD, Milde JH, Sundt TM Jr: Cerebral protection by barbiturate anesthesia: Use after middle cerebral artery occlusion in Java monkeys. Arch Neurol 33:345–350, 1976.
28. Miller JD, Jawad K, Jennett B: Safety of carotid ligation and its role in the management of intracranial aneurysms. J Neurol Neurosurg Psychiatry 40:64–72, 1977.
29. Molinari GF, Oakley JC, Laurent JP: The pathophysiology of barbiturate protection in focal ischemia. Stroke 7:3–4, 1976. (Abstr.)
30. Morley TP, Barr HWK: Giant intracranial aneurysms: Diagnosis, course, and management. Clin Neurosurg 16:73–94, 1969.
31. Mullan S: Experiences with surgical thrombosis of intracranial berry aneurysms and carotid cavernous fistulas. J Neurosurg 41:657–670, 1974.
32. Mullan S, Reyes C, Dawley J, Dobben G: Stereotactic copper electric thrombosis of intracranial aneurysms. Prog Neurol Surg 3:193–211, 1969.
33. Nyström SHM: Development of intracranial aneurysms as revealed by electron microscopy. J Neurosurg 20:329–337, 1963.
34. Obrador S, Dierssen G, Hernandez JR: Giant aneurysm of the posterior cerebral artery: Case report. J Neurosurg 26:413–416, 1967.

35. Oldershaw JB, Voris HC: Internal carotid artery ligation: A follow-up study. Neurology (NY) 16:937–938, 1966.
36. Onuma T, Suzuki J: Surgical treatment of giant intracranial aneurysms. J Neurosurg 51:33–36, 1979.
37. Polis Z, Brzeziński J, Chodak-Gajewicz M: Giant intracranial aneurysm: Case report. J Neurosurg 39:408–411, 1973.
38. Poppen JL, Fager CA: Intracranial aneurysms: Results of surgical treatment. J Neurosurg 17:283–296, 1960.
39. Raymond LA, Tew J: Large suprasellar aneurysms imitating pituitary tumour. J Neurol Neurosurg Psychiatry 41:83–87, 1978.
40. Roach MR: Changes in arterial distensibility as a cause of poststenotic dilatation. Am J Cardiol 12:802–815, 1963.
41. Sadik AR, Budzilovich GN, Shulman K: Giant aneurysm of middle cerebral artery: A case report. J Neurosurg 22:177–181, 1965.
42. Sarwar M, Batnitzky S, Schechter MM: Tumorous aneurysms. Neuroradiology 12:79–97, 1976.
43. Scott RM, Ballantine HT Jr.: Spontaneous thrombosis in a giant middle cerebral artery aneurysm: Case report. J Neurosurg 37:361–363, 1972.
44. Segal HD, McLaurin RL: Giant serpentine aneurysm: Report of two cases. J Neurosurg 46:115–120, 1977.
45. Silverberg GD, Reitz BA, Ream AK: Hypothermia and cardiac arrest in the treatment of giant aneurysms of the cerebral circulation and hemangioblastoma of the medulla. J Neurosurg 55:337–346, 1981.
46. Smith AL, Hoff JT, Nielson SL, Larson CP: Barbiturate protection in acute focal cerebral ischemia. Stroke 5:1–7, 1974.
47. Smith RW, Alksne JF: Stereotaxic thrombosis of inaccessible intracranial aneurysms. J Neurosurg 47:833–839, 1977.
48. Sonntag VKH, Yuan RH, Stein BM: Giant intracranial aneurysms: A review of 13 cases. Surg Neurol 8:81–84, 1977.
49. Spetzler R, Chater N: Microvascular bypass surgery. Part 2: Physiological studies. J Neurosurg 45:508–513, 1976.
50. Spetzler RF, Schuster H, Roski RA: Elective extracranial-intracranial arterial bypass in the treatment of inoperable giant aneurysms of the internal carotid artery. J Neurosurg 53:22–27, 1980.
51. Sundt TM Jr, Piepgrass DG: Surgical approach to giant intracranial aneurysms: Operative experience with 80 cases. J Neurosurg 51:731–742, 1979.
52. Tindall GT, Odom GL: Treatment of intracranial aneurysms by proximal carotid ligation. Prog Neurol Surg 3:66–114, 1969.
53. Tytus JS, Ward AA Jr.: The effect of cervical carotid ligation on giant aneurysms. J Neurosurg 33:184–190, 1970.
54. Yasargil MG: *Microsurgery Applied to Neurosurgery*. New York, Academic Press, 1969, pp 105–117.
55. Yatsu FM, Diamond I, Graziano C, Lindquist P: Experimental brain ischemia: Protection from irreversible damage with a rapid-acting barbiturate (methohexital). Stroke 3:726–732, 1972.

171

Carotid Ligation

Richard A. Roski
Robert F. Spetzler

Carotid artery ligation has been used for many years as an alternative method for treating intracranial aneurysms. Its place in the armamentarium of modern neurosurgery, however, constantly needs to be reassessed. As with many neurosurgical procedures, its role has been dramatically affected by the evolving changes in microneurosurgery. Improved techniques for intracranial aneurysm surgery have eliminated the necessity of carotid ligation in the treatment of many types of aneurysms. In contrast, the development of extracranial to intracranial (EC-IC) arterial bypass surgery has helped to augment the usefulness of carotid ligation in the treatment of difficult giant intracranial aneurysms. The present role of carotid ligation in the treatment of intracranial aneurysms will be reviewed, as well as the history, physiological effects, and complications of the procedure.

History

The first reports of carotid ligation described its use in controlling severe hemorrhage from the neck.[34] This was most often encountered as a complication of a penetrating injury to the carotid artery, the rupture of an aneurysm of the extracranial portion of the internal carotid artery, or erosion into the carotid artery by a tumor of the head and neck region. One of the earliest such reports was by Paré in 1585, who reported the emergent use of carotid ligation to control life-threatening hemorrhage in a patient who had sustained a stab wound of the neck. Lynn in 1792 reported the use of common carotid ligation to control hemorrhage encountered during the removal of a tumor from the neck. Similar reports by Abernathy, Fleming, and Twitchell followed in the late 1700s and early 1800s. In 1805, Sir Astley Cooper performed the first "elective" ligation of the internal carotid artery in a patient with an extracranial internal carotid artery aneurysm. Although Cooper's first patient died, he subsequently reported a successful result in 1808. Carotid ligation continued to gain considerable popularity during the early 1800s. It was used not only for the treatment of hemorrhage but also for a variety of other problems, including trigeminal neuralgia, epilepsy, and psychosis. Pilz in 1868 published a series of over 600 common carotid artery ligations with an operative mortality rate of 43 percent.[32] He stressed that the use of carotid ligation should be limited to controlling severe hemorrhage and to treating aneurysms of the carotid artery. Those two problems have subsequently remained its primary clinical indications.

The role of carotid ligation in treating intracranial aneurysms was questioned because of the high mortality that had been reported in many series. In 1938 Jefferson stated that this poor reputation and high mortality resulted from its use in cases in which infection, secondary hemorrhage, and malignant disease of the neck were present. He suggested re-evaluating its use in the treatment of intracranial aneurysms. In 1940 Schorstein, following Jefferson's suggestion, reviewed 60 cases of intracranial aneurysm treated by carotid ligation.[37] That initial report included 27 cases from the literature as well as 33 previously unreported cases. The operative mortality and morbidity were each 13.3 percent. Schorstein's detailed analysis helped to highlight several important clinical factors regarding the use of carotid ligation. He noted that complications from internal carotid artery ligation were more common in patients with severe anemia from previous hemorrhage. He postulated that severe anemia, the mass effect of a giant aneurysm, or increased intracranial pressure produced poor cerebral perfusion. He observed better results in patients with infraclinoid as opposed to supraclinoid aneurysms and he noted a higher mortality rate in patients who had had a recent subarachnoid hemorrhage as compared with patients with a more remote hemorrhage. Although we are now better able to explain the operative risk factors in physiological terms, very little has been added to the clinical observations of the complications of carotid ligation since Schorstein's excellent description. The low operative morbidity and mortality rates have helped to establish carotid ligation as a major method of treatment for intracranial aneurysms.

Physiological Significance of Carotid Ligation

The rationale for using carotid ligation is based on the concept that ligating the carotid artery will produce a drop in blood pressure distal to the ligation and therefore help to potentiate thrombosis of the aneurysm. The effects of carotid ligation on the immediate and late changes in internal carotid artery pressure, the angiographic appearance of the aneurysm, and the blood flow changes in the carotid artery have all been studied extensively.

To document the change in the distal arterial pressure following carotid occlusion, Sweet et al. carried out pressure measurements in 26 patients who were undergoing cerebral arteriography.[42] When the internal carotid artery was occluded, the distal systolic pressure measured in the internal carotid artery dropped 49 percent, the pulse pressure dropped 69 percent, and the mean blood pressure dropped 43 percent. Extreme variability was seen. There were seven cases in which the systolic pressure drop was less than 30 percent and three cases in which the systolic pressure drop was greater than 70 percent. When the internal carotid artery pressure following common and external carotid artery ligation was measured, a minimal change in the distal internal carotid artery pressure was noted when the external carotid artery was opened. The minimal difference in distal internal carotid artery pressure observed in patients with a common carotid occlusion as contrasted with an internal carotid artery occlusion became an important point in later debates over whether to use common carotid or internal carotid artery ligation.

In subsequent work, Bakay and Sweet measured blood pressure in the intracranial vessels following carotid occlusion.[1] Mean pressures in the temporal branches of the middle cerebral artery averaged 86 percent of those measured in the common carotid artery. In five frontal branches and in three parietal branches, the pressures averaged 82 percent of the values measured in the common carotid artery. Bakay and Sweet demonstrated that carotid ligation could produce a reduction in the internal carotid artery pressure distal to the point of occlusion, as well as intracranially in blood vessels down to at least 0.4 mm in diameter. We have also reported that in patients with internal carotid artery occlusion secondary to atherosclerotic disease, the pressure measured in the middle cerebral artery showed a 42 percent reduction from normal.[35]

Bakay and Sweet assessed the prolonged effect of common carotid ligation by measuring internal carotid artery pressures in nine patients 6 days to 24 weeks following their initial ligation.[2] In the majority of patients, the repeat distal carotid pressure demonstrated a slight increase as contrasted with the immediate postocclusion pressure, except for two patients in whom there was a pronounced recovery of pressure almost to the preoperative level. Tindall et al. also recorded immediate and late pressure changes in the internal carotid artery following common carotid ligation.[43] The immediate pressure reductions ranged from 31 to 66 percent of the preocclusion values. The late pressure reductions, however, ranged from 25.5 to 30.8 percent. Retinal artery pressures, measured in the same group of patients, demonstrated an immediate drop in systolic and diastolic pressure of 40 and 33 percent, respectively, following ligation and 30 and 23 percent, respectively, on late follow-up examination. Others have found late pressure reductions in the internal carotid artery ranging from 16 to 44 percent.[16,48]

It is clearly established that ligation of either the common or internal carotid artery will produce a significant drop in the distal internal carotid artery pressure and that this drop in pressure is maintained well into the intracranial vasculature. With time, however, there appears to be an equilibration of the distal internal carotid artery pressure with a prolonged pressure reduction, which usually ranges from 20 to 30 percent of the mean systemic blood pressure.

The distal internal carotid artery pressure has also been correlated with the incidence of recurrent subarachnoid hemorrhage.[47] Among eight patients whose distal carotid pressure following ligation was greater than 100 mmHg, 80 percent had a recurrent hemorrhage. Of eight patients whose residual pressure ranged from 85 to 90 mmHg, two (25 percent) had a recurrent hemorrhage. Among 29 patients whose residual pressures ranged from 80 to 84 mmHg, two (7 percent) had a recurrent hemorrhage, and of 56 patients whose residual pressure was less than 70 mmHg, six (11 percent) had a recurrent hemorrhage.

Following common carotid ligation, blood flow in the internal carotid artery may be maintained in a forward direction or it may reverse, with flow coming down the internal carotid artery and proceeding up the external carotid artery.[45] With time, the reversed internal carotid artery flow will revert to a normal forward flow. The forward flow ranges from 24 to 50 percent of the preocclusion flow rate and it is usually stabilized by 9 h following ligation.[48]

Several authors have analyzed the angiographic change in intracranial aneurysms following carotid ligation. Table 171-1 summarizes 348 reported cases with follow-up arteriography.[10,13,23-25,30,39,43] Of the 348 patients, 30 percent were found on follow-up arteriography to have nonvisualization of their aneurysms and in 86 percent the aneurysms were found to be either nonvisualized or smaller than those seen preoperatively. Thirteen patients demonstrated nonocclusion of the carotid artery on follow-up arteriography. Interestingly, of these 13 patients only one was found on follow-up arteriography to have an aneurysm that was larger than that seen on the initial arteriogram. Despite the infrequent observation of an enlarging aneurysm in the series shown in Table 171-1, case reports have described late arteriographic enlargement of aneurysms following successful carotid ligation.[5]

Indications for Carotid Ligation

In the past, carotid ligation was considered an important alternative for the treatment of all types of intracranial aneurysms, excluding those of the posterior circulation. With present microsurgical techniques, however, most aneurysms of the internal carotid artery distal to the cavernous sinus and those of the middle cerebral, anterior cerebral, and anterior communicating arteries can be treated by direct intracranial clipping or wrapping procedures. The direct approach, we think, offers better operative morbidity and mortality than does carotid ligation and it avoids some of the long-term complications of carotid ligation that are discussed later in this chapter.

For aneurysms of the intracavernous segment of the internal carotid artery and for giant internal carotid artery aneurysms, which on intracranial exposure are found to be unclippable, carotid ligation remains the treatment of choice.

One of the major problems encountered with the use of carotid ligation is the selection of patients who will safely tolerate permanent occlusion. The Matas test was one of the earliest tests employed to select patients who could tolerate carotid occlusion. This technique involved manual compression of the carotid artery in the neck for a period of 10 to 15 min to determine if ischemic symptoms would develop. The test was helpful in predicting those patients who could not tolerate occlusion; however, it had very little predictive value in selecting patients who could tolerate occlusion. This is not surprising since many patients do not develop ischemic symptoms for 48 to 72 h following complete occlusion of the carotid artery.

The most comprehensive assessment to determine tolerance to carotid occlusion has been reported by Miller et al.[22] They established criteria for xenon cerebral blood flow (CBF) measurements, EEG changes, and distal internal carotid artery pressure measurements that allowed them to select patients who could safely tolerate carotid occlusion. According to Miller et al., ligation is safe if: (1) CBF is greater than 40 ml/min per 100 g during carotid clamping; (2) CBF during carotid clamping ranges from 20 to 40 ml/min per 100 g, providing the reduction from the control flow is less than 25 percent, (3) CBF ranges from 20 to 40 ml/min per 100 g with up to a 35 percent reduction in flow from the control level, provided that the distal internal carotid artery pressure is greater than 60 mmHg in normoten-

TABLE 171-1 Arteriographic Changes Following Carotid Ligation

Authors	Year	Number Patients	Aneurysm Location	Artery Ligated	Nonvisualized	Much Smaller	Smaller	Unchanged	Larger
Mount,	1956	10	ICA	ICA	8	—	0	2	0
Taveras		4	MCA	ICA	1	—	3	0	0
		8	ICA	Nonocc.	2	—	4	1	1
Harris, Udvarhelyi	1957	66	ICA-P. Com. A.	Various	7	8	51	0	0
Mount	1959	30	Various	Various	12	—	10	6	2
Morris	1963	13	ICA-P. Com. A.	ICA	0	10	2	1	0
		9	ICA-P. Com. A.	CCA	0	7	2	0	0
		5	ICA-P. Com. A.	Nonocc.	0	1	3	1	0
Gibbs	1965	24	ICA	Various	4	3	13	4	0
Somach, Shenkin	1966	4	ICA	ICA	1	—	3	0	0
		7	ICA	CCA-ECA	4	—	2	1	0
		9	ICA	CCA	5	—	3	1	0
Tindall et al.	1966	58	ICA	CCA	17	—	26	14	1
Odom, Tindall	1968	67	ICA	CCA	25	—	27	14	1
		19	ACA	CCA	13	—	3	1	2
		5	ACA	CCA + ACA	3	—	0	2	0
		10	MCA	CCA	4	—	3	3	0
Total		348			106	29	155	51	7

ACA: anterior cerebral artery
MCA: middle cerebral artery
ICA: internal carotid artery
CCA: common carotid artery
ECA: external carotid artery
P. Com. A.: posterior communicating artery
Nonocc.: vessel not occluded

sive patients. Ligation is always considered unsafe if the CBF during clamping is less than 20 ml/min per 100 g. If adequate flow rates cannot be obtained during ligation of the internal carotid artery, then common carotid ligation with flow rate measurements performed can be used as an alternative. By criteria of Miller et al. approximately 20 percent of the patients will be unable to tolerate carotid occlusion. Miller et al. noted from the use of the above criteria and their surgical results that there was no correlation between tolerance of carotid ligation and preoperative arteriographic findings, including cerebral filling on cross-compression arteriography, jugular venous blood sampling, or EEG measurements, all of which have been used previously for determining the safety of carotid ligation. Unfortunately, patient selection does remain a very difficult problem despite all attempts to find a foolproof method.

Contraindications to the use of carotid ligation include:

1. Severe hypovolemia
2. A poor rating on the Botterell or Hunt classification
3. Presence of a recent subarachnoid hemorrhage
4. Cerebral vasospasm noted on arteriogram
5. Presence of an intracerebral hematoma
6. Inability to tolerate carotid occlusion (positive Matas test)

The six listed contraindications reflect situations in which collateral blood flow to the cerebral hemisphere may be severely impaired and therefore may increase the risk from carotid ligation. Cerebral vasospasm may already be limiting CBF, and a further decrease of CBF by occluding a carotid artery may cause marked cerebral ischemia or infarction. There is frequently a marked decrease in cerebral perfusion pressure noted in patients who have increased intracranial pressure from a recent hemorrhage or intracerebral hematoma, which may increase the patient's susceptibility to cerebral ischemic complications from carotid occlusion. A poor rating on the Botterell or Hunt classification often reflects a combination of the above situations. Severe hypovolemia is not as common in patients with intracranial aneurysms as in patients who have suffered severe neck hemorrhages. It can develop, however, when a patient has been maintained on severe fluid restriction for several days to reduce cerebral edema. Preoperatively, such patients need volume expansion to help prevent the potential ischemic problems of carotid ligation. It is apparent that the listed contraindications are similar in part to currently held contraindications for intracranial aneurysm surgery. Therefore, the choice of operative intervention, whether it be carotid ligation or intracranial surgery, should be based on the acute and late morbidity and mortality of the operative procedure and not upon the patient's immediate clinical condition.

Relative contraindications to carotid ligation include (1) the presence of a contralateral internal carotid artery aneurysm and (2) the presence of contralateral atherosclerotic carotid disease. Following ligation of a carotid artery, increased blood flow develops through the contralateral internal carotid artery. If a contralateral internal carotid artery aneurysm exists, increased flow through that artery may increase the likelihood of subsequent aneurysm rupture. Furthermore, the presence of severe contralateral atherosclerotic carotid artery stenosis may make carotid artery ligation a more dangerous procedure by diminishing the potential for increased flow on the contralateral side.

Selection of Artery

Over the years numerous types of carotid ligation have been performed to treat intracranial aneurysms. These include ligation of the common carotid artery, ligation of the internal carotid artery, ligation of the common carotid artery in conjunction with the external carotid artery, and ligation of the common carotid artery with subsequent ligation of the internal carotid artery. Since the pressure changes in the distal internal carotid artery are similar if either the internal carotid or the common carotid artery is ligated, many authors have recommended the preferential use of common carotid ligation. The incidence of complications from various types of carotid ligation vary considerably from series to series. When Brackett analyzed the complications of internal carotid versus common carotid ligation in patients with supraclinoid aneurysms, there was a considerably lower incidence of complications with internal carotid ligation.[4] When he compared the two types of ligation in patients with infraclinoid aneurysms, however, there was essentially no change in the complication rate. Scott and Skwarok's review of 909 patients revealed that the operative mortality for internal carotid artery ligation was 6 percent as opposed to 11 percent for common carotid artery ligation.[38] The overall morbidity from internal carotid artery ligation, however, was 22 percent as compared with 11 percent for common carotid artery ligation. It is difficult to conclude from the literature whether internal carotid or common carotid ligation is the safer procedure. The data in Table 171-2 as well as the incidence of late rebleeding shown in Table 171-3 demonstrate the marked variability between the two procedures. We prefer to use internal carotid ligation in those patients with intracavernous internal carotid artery aneurysms or giant internal carotid artery aneurysms. This will often allow for an intracranial trapping procedure if the aneurysm is not completely obliterated following carotid ligation. In most cases we also prefer to carry out carotid ligation in conjunction with a superficial temporal artery–middle cerebral artery bypass, as will be discussed in the last section.

Although many authors advocate gradual occlusion of the carotid artery with the use of either the Selverstone, Crutchfield, or Kindt clamp, Landholt and Millikan[20] as well as Nishioka[29] have reported that there was no difference in morbidity from acute versus gradual occlusion of the carotid artery. We still prefer to use gradual occlusion with the Selverstone clamp since this permits quick reversal of the occlusion if ischemic symptoms do occur.

Procedure for Carotid Ligation

A patient who is considered ready for carotid ligation is first tested by percutaneous compression of the carotid artery prior to the open surgical placement of a Selverstone clamp. This procedure is carried out with EEG monitoring. If the patient develops a hemiparesis or major focal EEG changes

TABLE 171-2 Morbidity and Mortality of Carotid Ligation

Authors	Date	Number Patients	Artery Ligated	Aneurysm Location	Morbidity, % Temporary	Morbidity, % Permanent	Mortality, %
Poppen, Fager	1960	101	ICA	ICA	6.9		3.9
German, Black	1965	35	Various	ICA	–0–		6.0
Somach, Shenkin	1966	20	CCA	ICA	5.0		5.0
Nishioka	1966	785	Various	Various	31.9		—
		814	Various	Various	—		23.9
Love, Dart	1967	20	Various	Various	5.0		5.0
Neill	1968	146	CCA	ICA	—		13.0
Odom, Tindall	1968	220	CCA	Various	11.4	2.3	6.8
		143	CCA	ICA			16.7
Tindall et al.	1970	31	CCA + contralateral ACA	A. Com. A.	–0–		29.0
Kak et al.	1973	126	Various	ICA	27.0		4.7
Galbraith, Clark	1974	37	CCA	Various	5.4		2.7
Gurdjian et al.	1975	27	CCA	ICA	11.1		11.1
Miller et al.	1977	72	Various	ICA	21.0	5.0	–0–
		28	Nonocc.	ICA	32.0	11.0	–0–
Giannotta et al.	1979	21	Various	ICA	9.5		–0–
Roski et al.	1981	57	Various	Various	16.0		13.0

ICA: internal carotid artery
CCA: common carotid artery
ACA: anterior cerebral artery
A. Com. A.: anterior communicating artery
Nonocc.: vessel not occluded

within 3 min of carotid compression, plans for further carotid occlusion are delayed. If the patient is able to tolerate percutaneous compression, a Selverstone clamp is placed on the internal carotid artery. Giannotta et al. have stressed the importance of having a well-hydrated patient prior to performing the carotid ligation and the use of volume expansion whenever ischemic symptoms occur.[9] If there is concern that a patient, because of age or previous cardiac symptoms, may not tolerate a rapid infusion of intravenous fluids, then a flow-directed catheter should be used to monitor cardiac output, and prophylactic preoperative digitalization may be necessary.

Surgery can be carried out under local or light general anesthesia. The incision is made along the anterior border of the sternocleidomastoid muscle and dissection is taken down to the common carotid artery. The carotid bifurcation is identified and the carotid bulb is injected with 1% lidocaine. The hypoglossal nerve is identified and isolated from the field. The Selverstone clamp is placed around the internal carotid artery and the stem of the clamp is brought out through a separate stab wound in the skin. The clamp is partially closed to reduce the distal internal carotid artery pressure by 50 percent. This usually will require an 80 percent stenosis of the carotid artery. Postoperatively the clamp is further closed by increments over the next 3 days. If the patient develops focal cerebral ischemia, the clamp is immediately reopened and intravenous volume expansion with either low-molecular-weight dextran or Plasmanate (Cutter Laboratories, Inc., Berkeley, Calif.) is started. Vasopressors can be used along with volume expansion to increase cerebral perfusion should hypotension develop. When treating previously unruptured aneurysms, systemic heparinization can be used until the carotid artery is finally ligated.

Operative Complications

The operative morbidity and mortality for carotid ligation from previously reported series were reviewed by Scott and Skwarok in 1961.[38] The operative mortality in their review of 909 patients ranged from 0 to 18 percent. Table 171-2 summarizes the operative complications in the major series of carotid ligations reported since 1961.[6,8,9,11,18,21,22,28–30,33,36,39,44] Operative mortality still varies widely, from 0 to 29 percent. Significant variation in operative morbidity also exists.

Numerous factors have been shown to be significant in producing complications of carotid ligation. Some authors have suggested that older patients are at a higher risk; however, Schorstein, Brackett, and others believe that age is probably not a significant factor in the ability to tolerate carotid occlusion.[4,37] Higher morbidity and mortality rates have been reported when ligation is carried out within 10 days of an acute subarachnoid hemorrhage whereas delaying ligation beyond 10 days appears to decrease the risks.

The two major causes of complications immediately following carotid ligation are aneurysmal rebleeding and cerebral ischemia. Kak et al. reviewed the incidence of early aneurysmal rebleeding after carotid ligation in the major series reported in the literature from 1953 to 1973.[18] Their review included a total of 1298 patients, 57 of whom had early rebleeding for an overall incidence of 4.4 percent. Several factors have been found to aggravate cerebral ischemia following carotid occlusion. These include systemic hypotension, anemia, and hypovolemia. Correction of anemia and the use of volume expansion have been shown to be beneficial in preventing the ischemic complications from carotid ligation and in treating such complications when they do occur. Although severe bradycardia has been noted following carotid ligation, there has been little documentation to implicate the carotid sinus reflex as a significant cause of early ischemic complications.[20] Another potential cause of ischemia is propagation of a thrombus up the occluded artery; however, Brackett suggests that there is very little evidence to implicate thrombus propagation as a major cause of ischemic complications.[4] Miller et al., using xenon cerebral blood flow measurements, have demonstrated that regional cerebral hypoperfusion can occur following carotid occlusion.[22] This may very well be the most significant factor in the development of early ischemic complications.

Late Complications

Late complications from carotid ligation following discharge from the hospital have included aneurysmal rebleeding and ischemic complications on the side of the carotid ligation.[34] Table 171-3 outlines the incidence of late aneurysmal rebleeding. Wright and Sweet reviewed 112 patients who were followed for up to 16 years, 65 of them for over 3 years.[47] During the time of follow-up, there were 19 subarachnoid hemorrhages from the treated aneurysms, 12 of those within a 4-year period, and 2 others from a contralateral aneurysm. German and Black followed 18 patients with common carotid artery ligation and 15 with internal carotid artery ligation.[8] Three patients in each group died from aneurysm-related causes, for an incidence of 17 percent in cases of common carotid artery ligation and 20 percent in cases of internal carotid artery ligation. There were also two fatal subarachnoid hemorrhages from other aneurysms in their series. In the report by Miller et al. of 72 patients with carotid ligation, there were 4 subarachnoid hemorrhages, 3 of which were related to a previously undiagnosed aneurysm.[22] Winn et al. compared the late follow-up results of patients with internal carotid–posterior communicating artery aneurysms that were treated either conservatively or with common carotid artery ligation.[46] Of the 41 conservatively treated patients, 8 had late rebleeding from their aneurysms, 3 of which were fatal. Of the 37 patients with common carotid ligation, 4 had a fatal rebleed and 1 had a nonfatal rebleed. There was also one late hemorrhage from a contralateral aneurysm that was teated with intracranial clipping. Winn et al. concluded that although the long-term morbid-

TABLE 171-3 Late Rebleeding Following Carotid Ligation

Authors	Date	Number Patients	Artery Ligated	Subarachnoid Hemorrhage
Hardy et al.	1958	54	CCA	3 Fatal (5.5%)
Poppen, Fager	1960	96	ICA	4 Fatal (4.2%)
Scott, Skwarok	1961	21	CCA	4 Fatal (19.0%)
German, Black	1965	18	CCA	2 Fatal (11.1%)
		15	ICA	3 Fatal (20.0%)
Somach, Shenkin	1966	19	Various	1 Fatal (5.3%)
Nishioka	1966	462	Various	16 Fatal (3.4%)
Love, Dart	1967	3	ICA	–0–
		13	CCA	2 Fatal (15.4%)
Neill	1968	127	CCA	6 Fatal (4.7%)
Kak et al.	1973	84	Various	5 Fatal (5.9%)
Miller et al.	1977	72	Various	4 Fatal (5.5%)
Roski et al.	1981	39	Various	3 Fatal (7.5%)

ICA: internal carotid artery
CCA: common carotid artery

ity was somewhat better in the patients with common carotid ligation, the prevention of aneurysmal rebleeding after 6 months was no different for the operated patients than for those patients who were treated conservatively.

Development of a delayed hemiparesis following carotid ligation has also been reported by several authors. Black and German have recorded a 6 percent incidence of late ischemic problems following carotid ligation.[3] Roski et al. reported a late occurrence of transient ischemic attacks in 12.5 percent of their patients and a late occurrence of stroke in 7.5 percent.[36] Oldershaw and Voris reported hemiparesis developing in 2 of their 21 patients at 1 and 13 years following internal carotid artery ligation.[31] Love and Dart also reported two instances of delayed hemiparesis among the 40 patients in their series.[21]

Several other potential long-term effects of carotid ligation have been questioned.[46] Winn and Christiansson have noted an increased incidence of hypertension following common carotid ligation.[46] Subarachnoid hemorrhage occurring from previously unrecognized contralateral aneurysms has also been reported.[8,46,47] Hassler[15] and Hashimoto et al.[14] have demonstrated in an experimental model that ligation of the carotid artery can lead to contralateral aneurysm formation. All these data, however, need better statistical assessment to be confirmed.

Partial Carotid Ligation

The rationale behind the use of carotid ligation is to decrease the distal intraluminal pressure in an attempt to produce intra-aneurysmal thrombosis. These pressure changes occur following complete carotid occlusion. Other techniques have also been used to produce a similar change in the distal internal carotid artery. Early attempts were made to decrease the distal intraluminal pressure by inducing systemic hypotension. This proved to be difficult to control and did not provide significant protection against rebleeding. Two factors are known to affect a pressure and flow change across an area of stenosis. They are the cross-sectional diameter of the vessel and the length of the stenosis.[19] Very little alteration in the blood pressure across an area of stenosis is obtained until the stenosis reduces the cross-sectional diameter of the artery by at least 70 percent. The drop in pressure can be accomplished by increasing the degree of stenosis or by extending the stenosis over a longer area of the artery. Stenosis of the carotid artery that decreases the arterial diameter by 70 to 80 percent should produce a significant drop in the distal internal carotid artery pressure and potentially provide some protection from rebleeding.

Mullan et al. have reported using the Selverstone clamp to partially occlude the common carotid artery as a temporary means of preventing aneurysmal rebleeding in the time period prior to craniotomy.[26,27] In Mullan's first series, all 16 patients were treated with partial ligation of the common carotid artery by using the Selverstone clamp, 24 g per day of epsilon-aminocaproic acid, and a hypotensive regimen of reserpine, chlorothiazide, and chlorpromazine.[26] None of the 16 patients suffered a subsequent aneurysmal rebleed prior to surgery; however, one patient ruptured a contralateral intracavernous internal carotid artery aneurysm prior to operation and one patient ruptured her treated aneurysm as the dura was being opened during her craniotomy. One additional patient developed hemiplegia following the occlusion. It was unclear whether the partial occlusion or cerebral vasospasm caused the hemiplegia. Mullan et al. subsequently reported a series of 13 patients treated by subtotal carotid occlusion alone and 26 patients in whom partial occlusion was used in conjunction with other agents.[27] The average pressure reduction was 44 percent and the clamp was used for an average of 11 days. In five patients the clamp had to be reopened because of clinical deterioration. In two of those patients, symptoms progressed to hemiplegia despite the opening of the clamp. There were also two instances of embolization and three cases of infection. In patients in whom partial occlusion was used along with antifibrinolytic therapy and good control of blood pressure was obtained, there was no incident of rebleeding or death. Five of the six patients who did go on to rebleed from their aneurysm were patients who could not tolerate the hypotensive therapy. A definitive conclusion regarding the use of partial carotid ligation is currently unavailable. In selected cases of intracranial aneurysms, this therapy may prove to be beneficial.

EC-IC Bypass Surgery in Conjunction with Carotid Ligation

The advent of EC-IC arterial bypass surgery has added a new dimension to the use of carotid ligation. Two major concerns regarding the use of carotid ligation have included: (1) the development of a hemiplegia hours to days following complete occlusion of the carotid artery and (2) the significant incidence of late ischemic complications. It has been proposed that providing collateral blood flow to the cerebral hemisphere with EC-IC bypass surgery may decrease the complications. Hopkins and Grand reported a series of 11 patients who were treated by a combination of both internal carotid artery ligation and superficial temporal to middle cerebral artery (STA-MCA) bypass.[17] Three patients developed a cerebral infarct following the EC-IC bypass but prior to ligation of the internal carotid artery. One of their patients died from a ruptured aneurysm. Gelber and Sundt reported excellent results in a series of 10 patients with the same combination of internal carotid ligation and STA-MCA bypass.[7]

Spetzler et al. described a series of 21 patients who had an STA-MCA bypass in conjunction with staged occlusion of the internal carotid artery.[40,41] No ischemic complications developed in the perioperative period or in a 6- to 41-month follow-up. They recommended that the STA-MCA bypass be performed at the same time as the placement of a Selverstone clamp on the internal carotid artery. The Selverstone clamp is partially closed at the time of operation, producing

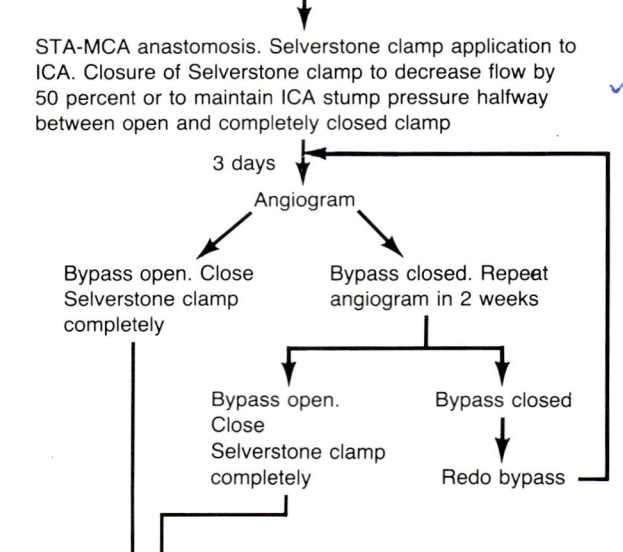

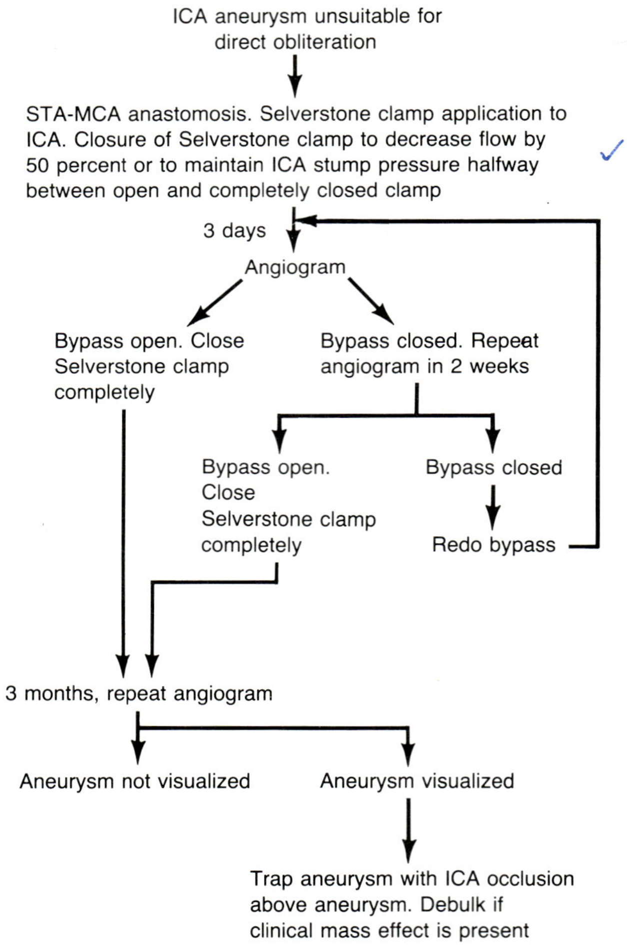

Figure 171-1 Summary of plan for treating internal carotid artery (ICA) aneurysms that are unsuitable for direct clipping. STA, superficial temporal artery; MCA, middle cerebral artery. (Modified from Spetzler et al.[41])

a 50 percent decrease in the distal internal carotid artery pressure. An arteriogram is performed on the third postoperative day to document bypass patency. The clamp is then completely closed. The staged occlusion of the internal carotid artery allows time for maturation of the bypass to occur. The clamp is not closed unless a patent bypass has been well demonstrated arteriographically. Three days later the clamp is removed and triple ligation of the internal carotid artery is performed. A follow-up arteriogram is obtained 1 month later to be sure that the aneurysm does not visualize. If it does visualize, then an intracranial trapping procedure is performed. Figure 171-1 outlines our protocol for managing patients with an internal carotid artery aneurysm.

References

1. Bakay L, Sweet WH: Cervical and intracranial intra-arterial pressures with and without vascular occlusion. Surg Gynecol Obstet 95:67–75, 1952.
2. Bakay L, Sweet WH: Intra-arterial pressures in the neck and brain: Late changes after carotid closure, acute measurements after vertebral closure. J Neurosurg 10:353–359, 1953.
3. Black SPW, German WJ: The treatment of internal carotid artery aneurysms by proximal arterial ligation. J Neurosurg 10:590–601, 1953.
4. Brackett CE Jr: The complications of carotid artery ligation in the neck. J Neurosurg 10:91–106, 1953.
5. Cuatico W, Cook AW, Tyshchenko V, Khatib R: Massive enlargement of intracranial aneurysms following carotid ligation. Arch Neurol 17:609–613, 1967.
6. Galbraith JG, Clark RM: Role of carotid ligation in the management of intracranial carotid aneurysms. Clin Neurosurg 21:171–181, 1974.
7. Gelber BR, Sundt TM Jr: Treatment of intracavernous and giant carotid aneurysms by combined internal carotid ligation and extra- to intracranial bypass. J Neurosurg 52:1–10, 1980.
8. German WJ, Black SPW: Cervical ligation for internal carotid aneurysms: An extended follow-up. J Neurosurg 23:572–577, 1965.
9. Giannotta SL, McGillicuddy JE, Kindt GW: Gradual carotid artery occlusion in the treatment of inaccessible internal carotid artery aneurysms. Neurosurgery 5:417–421, 1979.
10. Gibbs JR: Effects of carotid ligation on the size of internal carotid aneurysms. J Neurol Neurosurg Psychiatry 28:383–394, 1965.
11. Gurdjian ES, Lindner DW, Thomas LM: Experiences with ligation of the common carotid artery for treatment of aneurysms of the internal carotid artery. J Neurosurg 23:311–318, 1975.
12. Hardy WG, Thomas LM, Webster JE Gurdjian ES: Carotid ligaton for intracranial aneurysm: A follow-up study of 54 patients. J Neurosurg 15:281–289, 1958.
13. Harris P, Udvarhelyi GB: Aneurysms arising at the internal carotid–posterior communicating artery junction. J Neurosurg 14:180–191, 1957.
14. Hashimoto N, Handa H, Hazama F: Experimentally induced cerebral aneurysms in rats. Surg Neurol 10:3–8, 1978.
15. Hassler O: Experimental carotid ligation followed by aneurysmal formation and other morphological changes in the circle of Willis. J Neurosurg 20:1–7, 1963.
16. Heyman A, Tindall GT, Finney WHM, Woodhall B: Measurement of retinal artery and intracarotid pressures following carotid artery occlusion with the Crutchfield clamp. J Neurosurg 17:297–305, 1960.
17. Hopkins LN, Grand W: Extracranial-intracranial arterial bypass in the treatment of aneurysms of the carotid and middle cerebral arteries. Neurosurgery 5:21–31, 1979.
18. Kak VK, Taylor AR, Gordon DS: Proximal carotid ligation for internal carotid aneurysms: A long-term follow-up study. J Neurosurg 39:503–513, 1973.
19. Kindt GW, Youmans JR: The effect of stricture length on critical arterial stenosis. Surg Gynecol Obstet 128:729–734, 1969.
20. Landolt AM, Millikan CH: Pathogenesis of cerebral infarction secondary to mechanical carotid artery occlusion. Stroke 1:52–62, 1970.
21. Love JG, Dart LH: Results of carotid ligation with particular reference to intracranial aneurysms. J Neurosurg 27:89–93, 1967.
22. Miller JD, Jawad K, Jennett B: Safety of carotid ligation and its role in the management of intracranial aneurysms. J Neurol Neurosurg Psychiatry 40:64–72, 1977.
23. Morris L: Arteriographic studies in aneurysm of the internal carotid artery treated by carotid occlusion. Acta Radiol [Diagn] (Stockh) 1:367–372, 1963.
24. Mount LA: Results of treatment of intracranial aneurysms using Selverstone clamp. J Neurosurg 16:611–618, 1959.
25. Mount LA, Taveras JM: The results of surgical treatment of intracranial aneurysms as demonstrated by progress arteriography. J Neurosurg 13:618–626, 1956.
26. Mullan S: Conservative management of the recently ruptured aneurysm. Surg Neurol 3:27–32, 1975.
27. Mullan S, Hanlon K, Brown F: Management of 136 consecutive supratentorial berry aneurysms. J Neurosurg 49:794–804, 1978.
28. Neill CL, Hodges LR, Neill WR: Cerebral aneurysms treated by common carotid ligation. J Neurol Neurosurg Psychiatry 31:87, 1968. (Abstr.)
29. Nishioka H: Results of the treatment of intracranial aneurysms by occlusion of the carotid artery in the neck. J Neurosurg 25:660–682, 1966.
30. Odom GL, Tindall GT: Carotid ligation in the treatment of certain intracranial aneurysms. Clin Neurosurg 15:101–116, 1968.
31. Oldershaw JB, Voris HC: Internal carotid artery ligation. A follow-up study. Neurology 16:937–938, 1966.
32. Pilz C: Zur Ligatur der Arteria carotis communis, nebst einer Statistik dieser Operation. Arch Klin Chir 9:257–445, 1868.
33. Poppen JL, Fager CA: Intracranial aneurysms: Results of surgical treatment. J Neurosurg 17:283–296, 1960.
34. Roski RA, Spetzler RF: Carotid ligation in the treatment of cerebral aneurysms, in Hopkins LN, Long DM (eds): *Clinical Management of Intracranial Aneurysms*. New York, Raven Press, 1982, pp 11–19.
35. Roski RA, Spetzler RF: Middle cerebral artery perfusion pressure in occlusive cerebrovascular disease. Presented at the 51st Annual Meeting of the American Association of Neurological Surgeons, Honolulu, April 26, 1982.
36. Roski RA, Spetzler RF, Nulsen FE: Late complications of carotid ligation in the treatment of intracranial aneurysms. J Neurosurg 54:583–587, 1981.
37. Schorstein J: Carotid ligation in saccular intracranial aneurysms. Br J Surg 28:50–70, 1940.
38. Scott M, Skwarok E: The treatment of cerebral aneurysms by ligation of the common carotid artery. Surg Gynecol Obstet 113:54–61, 1961.
39. Somach FM, Shenkin HA: Angiographic end-results of carotid ligation in the treatment of carotid aneurysm. J Neurosurg 24:966–974, 1966.
40. Spetzler RF, Roski RA, Schuster H, Takaoka Y: The role of EC-IC in the treatment of giant intracranial aneurysms. Neurol Res 2:345–359, 1980.

41. Spetzler RF, Schuster H, Roski RA: Elective extracranial-intracranial arterial bypass in the treatment of inoperable giant aneurysms of the internal carotid artery. J Neurosurg 53:22–27, 1980.
42. Sweet WH, Sarnoff SJ, Bakay L: A clinical method for recording internal carotid pressure: Significance of changes during carotid occlusion. Surg Gynecol Obstet 90:327–334, 1950.
43. Tindall GT, Goree JA, Lee JF, Odom GL: Effect of common carotid ligation on size of internal carotid aneurysms and distal intracarotid and retinal artery pressures. J Neurosurg 25:503–511, 1966.
44. Tindall GT, Kapp J, Odom GL, Robinson SC: A combined technique for treating certain aneurysms of the anterior communicating artery. J Neurosurg 33:41–47, 1970.
45. Tindall GT, Odom GL, Dillon ML, Cupp HB Jr, Mahaley MS Jr, Greenfield JC Jr: Direction of blood flow in the internal and external carotid arteries following occlusion of the ipsilateral common carotid artery. J Neurosurg 20:985–994, 1963.
46. Winn HR, Richardson AE, Jane JA: Late morbidity and mortality of common carotid ligation for posterior communicating aneurysms. J Neurosurg 47:727–736, 1977.
47. Wright RL, Sweet WH: Carotid or vertebral occlusion in the treatment of intracranial aneurysms: Value of early and late readings of carotid and retinal pressures. Clin Neurosurg 9:163–192, 1962.
48. Youmans JR, Kindt GW, Mitchell OC: Extended studies of direction of flow and pressure in the internal carotid artery following common carotid artery ligation. J Neurosurg 27:250–254, 1967.

172

Posterior Circulation Aneurysms

S. J. Peerless
Charles G. Drake

Historical Review

Aneurysms arising from the posterior circulation are relatively uncommon, accounting for less than 15 percent of all intracranial aneurysms. Because of their infrequency, few surgeons have had the opportunity to become familiar with their treatment, which requires manipulation in the confined space in front of the brain stem and cerebellum. Prior to 1950, a few tumor-like masses in the posterior fossa were explored and, when shelled out, were found to be thrombosed aneurysms.[1,10,13] The true nature of these lesions always came as a surprise to the pioneer surgeons of this era, and required hurried trapping and occlusion of the parent vessels with ligatures and crude clips to control the hemorrhage.[4,5] Schwartz is credited with the first direct attack on an aneurysm in the posterior fossa. Using simple silver clips, he trapped a large sac buried in the pons without the use of magnification and with a successful outcome for the patient.[11] Drake first reported his own experience with four patients with aneurysms at the basilar bifurcation in 1961.[2] In reviewing the literature to that time, we find that 47 cases had been reported: 14 had been treated with vertebral artery ligation, and almost half of the remaining cases were unusual aneurysms arising peripherally off branches of the vertebral or basilar artery. Of the 10 aneurysms arising at the basilar bifurcation, only 4 were clipped; the remainder were packed with gauze.[7] In 1964, Jamieson published a gloomy report of the direct surgical treatment of 19 aneurysms of the vertebrobasilar system.[6] Postoperatively, only 4 of the patients were employable, 5 had significant neurological morbidity, and 10 died. In 1965, Drake expressed a note of optimism in the surgical treatment of aneurysms of the basilar trunk but emphasized the high morbidity and mortality of the direct surgical attack on aneurysms of the basilar bifurcation.[3] In his first seven patients with terminal basilar artery aneurysms, four had died, one was severely disabled, and only two had returned to normal life. It was in this communication that Drake pointed out the absolute importance of identifying and protecting the perforating vessels arising from the proximal posterior cerebral arteries in dealing with aneurysms at the basilar bifurcation.

With the advent of the operating microscope, fine instruments, and precise clips combined with modern techniques of neuroanesthesia and neuroradiology, there has been a remarkable improvement in the surgery of intracranial aneurysms. In the past 15 years, our experience has grown to more than 1100 surgically treated cases of vertebrobasilar aneurysms, and current results are comparable to the results of surgical treatment of aneurysms of the anterior circulation. Mortality and morbidity today are almost always limited to patients with giant aneurysms and those who are in a poor clinical state as a result of their initial subarachnoid hemorrhage.

Incidence

Aneurysms of the posterior circulation amount to approximately 15 percent of all intracranial aneurysms. Until the advent of routine bilateral vertebral angiography, their rec-

Posterior Circulation Aneurysms

ognition in life was infrequent, the larger masses being identified by pneumoencephalography and ventriculography. With modern imaging techniques, aneurysms of 1 cm in diameter are commonly imaged with computed tomography (CT) scanning. Bilateral injection of contrast substance into the vertebral arteries with anteroposterior (AP), Towne's, and lateral views, and occasionally basal views or angiotomography, are necessary for precise localization of these lesions.

The most common aneurysms of the posterior circulation are those arising at the basilar bifurcation, with those arising from the basilar-superior cerebellar artery (SCA) junction and from the vertebral artery at the posterior inferior cerebellar artery (PICA) origin being the next most common. Those sacs arising off the posterior cerebral artery, at the vertebrobasilar junction, and off the midportion of the basilar artery in the region of the anterior inferior cerebellar artery (AICA) have been, in our experience, the least common aneurysms arising from this circulation (Fig. 172-1).

Clinical Features

Subarachnoid hemorrhage, caused by rupture of an aneurysm arising in the posterior circulation, can only occasionally be distinguished clinically from rupture of an anterior cerebral circulation aneurysm. Sudden onset of headache, neck pain, nausea, and vomiting is shared commonly by both groups. Abrupt loss of consciousness is perhaps somewhat more common following rupture of a posterior circulation aneurysm, and respiratory and, less often, cardiac arrest may be seen in rupture of an aneurysm nestled close to the medulla, such as the vertebral-PICA aneurysm.

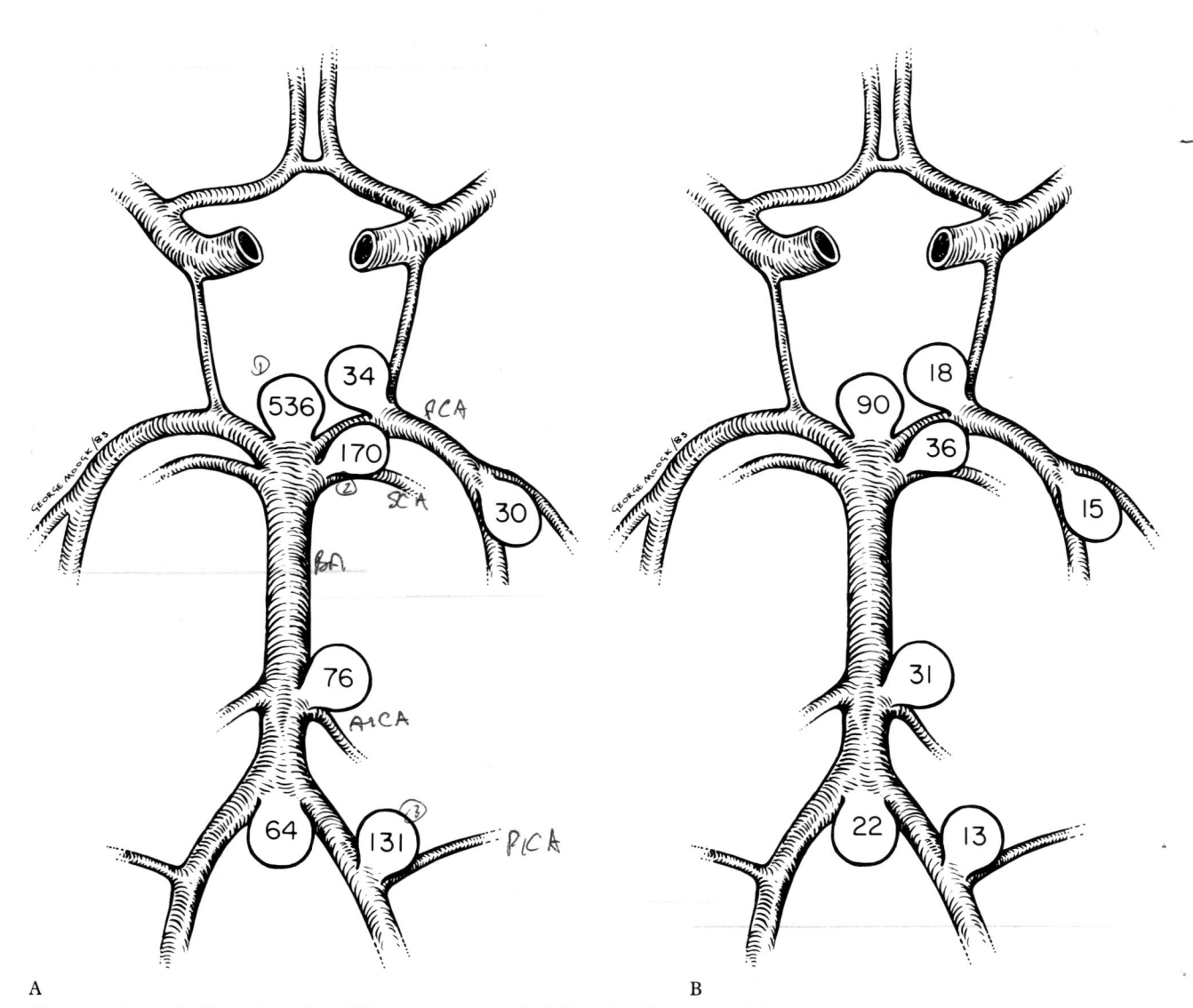

Figure 172-1 *A.* Site of small and large aneurysms (<2.5 cm in diameter) arising from the posterior circulation. Numbers in circles indicate patients operated upon in our series. *B.* Site of giant aneurysms (>2.5 cm in diameter) arising from the posterior circulation. Numbers in circles indicate patients operated upon in our series.

There is a close proximity of some of the cranial nerves to the common sites of aneurysms in the posterior circulation. Aneurysms of the basilar bifurcation, or more commonly the basilar-SCA junction, are in close proximity to the oculomotor nerve as it exits from the interpeduncular fossa. The abducens nerve bears a close relationship to basilar-AICA aneurysms, and the hypoglossal nerve to vertebral-PICA aneurysms. Occasionally, sudden enlargement of the aneurysmal sac may compress and deform one of these nerves, producing a specific nerve palsy. More often, large or giant aneurysms of the terminal basilar artery or those arising at the origin of the superior cerebellar artery will deform and compress the peduncle as well as the third nerve, producing a Weber's syndrome. It is remarkable, though, how often even with a large sac and major deformities of the pons and medulla the patient is asymptomatic and has no signs of neurological dysfunction. We have seen deafness, facial palsy, hemifacial spasm, and glossopharyngeal neuralgia only rarely. Of course, with giant sacs and severe compression of the medulla and pyramids, one can see quadriparesis and severe respiratory dysfunction and even obstruction of CSF pathways.

In our experience, vasospasm is as common after subarachnoid hemorrhage from aneurysms of the posterior circulation as it is following rupture of anterior circulation aneurysms. The same relationship exists between the amount of blood spilled into the subarachnoid space and the development of spasm. Rupture of a posterior circulation aneurysm can produce spasm of vessels in the anterior circulation. Vasospasm involving vessels of the vertebrobasilar system results in ischemia in the brain stem, cerebellum, temporal lobe, and occipital pole.

Operative Approaches to Posterior Circulation Aneurysms

Anesthesia and Monitoring Techniques

Much of the success of modern aneurysm surgery is directly related to the development of precise scientific neuroanesthesia. We have been fortunate in our unit to work with dedicated neuroanesthetists who have been responsible for the development of many of our current techniques.

The patient is brought to the operating room, lightly sedated and with an accurate assessment of fluid balance. Infused antifibrinolytic agents are continued into the operating room. A flexible needle is inserted into the radial or dorsalis pedis artery to provide a port for continuous monitoring of the systemic arterial pressure. In patients in whom cardiac function or fluid balance is in doubt, a Swan-Ganz catheter is installed. The patient is gently induced with Pentothal, paralyzed, and then intubated with an armored tube. The anesthetic techniques have varied over the years but basically consist of assisted ventilation using nitrous oxide or a narcotic technique. In the past few years, we have used isoflurane rather than halothane. Isoflurane has proved to be an excellent anesthetic, as well as a convenient way to induce hypotension. The anesthetic is kept reasonably light, with meticulous monitoring of blood gases to maintain the P_{CO_2} in the range of 35 to 45 torr and the P_{O_2} in excess of 100 torr.

After the patient is positioned, the anesthetist inserts a lumbar subarachnoid catheter through a Tuohy needle into the lumbar subarachnoid space and attaches this to an enclosed collection bag. Lumbar subarachnoid drainage is begun only after the dura is opened to aid intracranial relaxation. Adequate intracranial relaxation is essential for the success of surgical procedures at the base of the brain. To ensure a slack brain, we routinely administer 1 gm/kg of 20% mannitol and double this dose if we contemplate temporary occlusion of a major intracranial vessel. If necessary, we will administer furosemide (1 mg/kg) intravenously shortly after induction, also to enhance the intracranial relaxation process. Because of this vigorous application of both an osmotic agent and a loop diuretic, meticulous monitoring of the fluid balance is essential and complete replacement of the fluid loss by the end of the procedure is mandatory.

Drug-induced hypotension for some period of the procedure is almost routine in our theater. The arterial line is connected to a transducer positioned at the level of the brain and connected to a monitor to provide readings of systolic, diastolic, and mean pressures. In the past, hypotension was induced by intravenous infusion of trimethaphan camsylate or sodium nitroprusside. Because of the great variability of the response to these drugs in some individuals and untoward toxic effects, we have, in recent years, abandoned these intravenous medications in favor of simply deepening the isoflurane anesthesia. This technique of isoflurane hypotension has proved to be safe, reliable, and, most importantly, precise. By increasing the concentration of the inspired isoflurane, the anesthetist can bring about an exact decrease in blood pressure and hold it precisely at the predetermined level. When higher pressures are required, the isoflurane concentration is simply reduced without the fear of overshoot or long delays before the pressure returns to normal. Normally, mean systemic arterial pressures of 50 to 60 torr are used during the initial dissection around the aneurysm. With manipulation of the sac, or application of the clip, the pressure is lowered to 40 to 45 torr. These low pressures have been well tolerated for 30 to 40 min and, even in the elderly, are unlikely to be responsible for neurological or cardiac dysfunction when used for as long as 60 to 90 min. Of course, to maximize collateral flow we do not use systemic hypotension if we contemplate temporary proximal clipping of the vertebral or basilar artery.

After the patient is positioned, the anesthetist monitors fluid balance, ECG, mean systemic arterial blood pressure, and blood gases. Recently, we have been evaluating the utility of monitoring brain stem evoked potentials in the surgery of this region. This technique would appear to be promising in monitoring brain stem function, although, as yet, not entirely validated. Occasionally, we will employ brain retractor pressure monitoring, EEG, and intraoperative cerebral blood flow measures when we anticipate prolonged interruption of focal or general cerebral blood flow.[8]

Positioning

Most aneurysms of the basilar artery and its branches above the anterior inferior cerebellar arteries can be approached from the supratentorial compartment through the incisura.

Posterior Circulation Aneurysms 1425

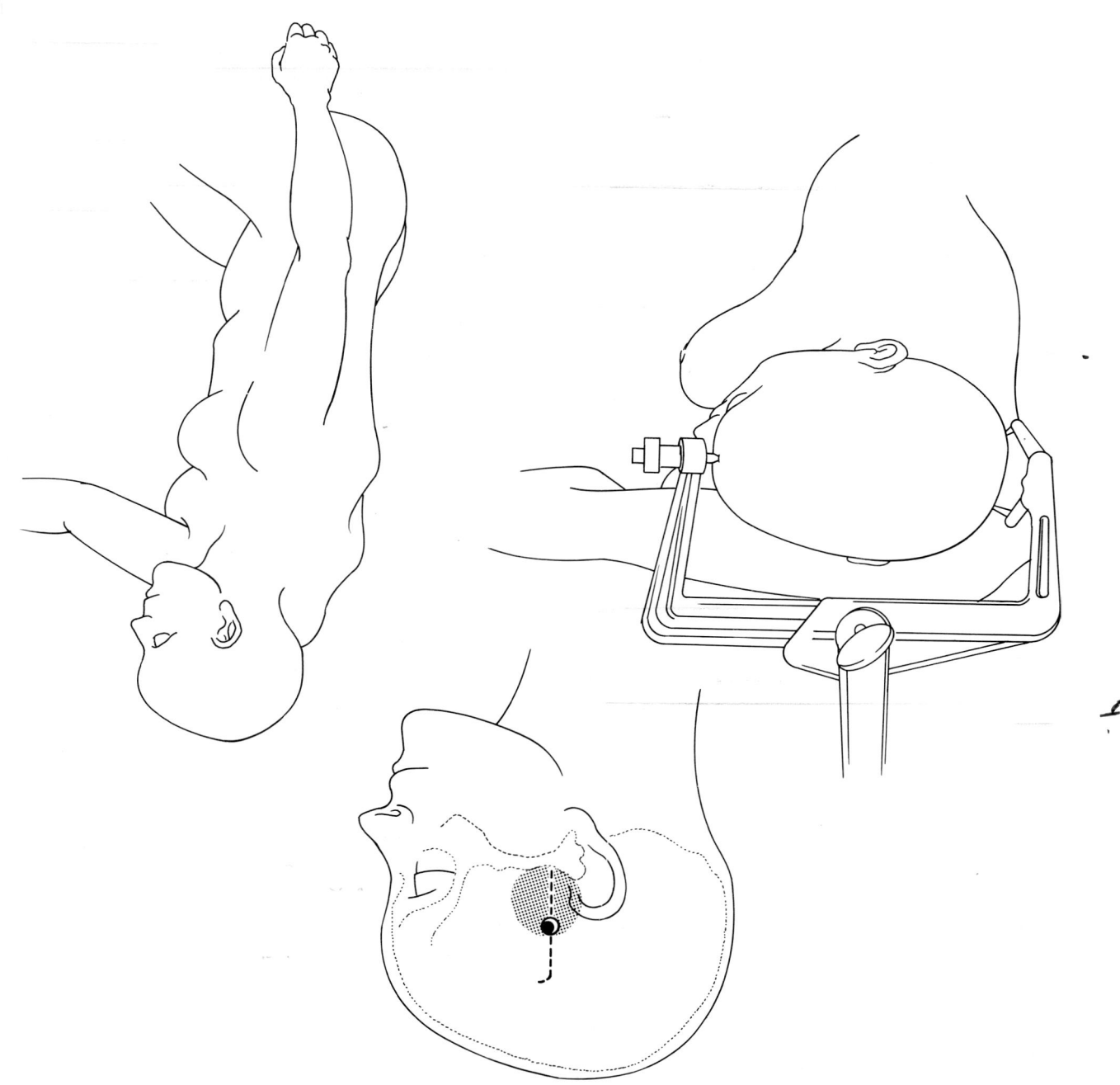

Figure 172-2 Lateral decubitus position for subtemporal approach to upper basilar artery. Note: Anteroposterior axis of head is parallel to floor. Dotted line and stippled area in the lower drawing show scalp incision and craniectomy site, respectively.

Normally, we use a subtemporal approach and, therefore, place the patient in the lateral decubitus or "park bench" position (Fig. 172-2). The patient is placed on the left side since we normally aim to retract the nondominant temporal lobe. The left axilla is supported on a sand bag, the chest is free, and the back is supported by a firm rest attached to the operating table. The head is attached to a pin headrest in a line so that the anteroposterior axis is precisely parallel to the floor and the sagittal plane angled 15 degrees toward the floor. Normally, we do not move the head again during the procedure, relative to the position of the body, but not infrequently we will tip the table head up or head down, or rotate it from side to side to enhance visualization of the upper basilar artery. The head clamp is positioned, and the head is clipped and prepared so as to permit extension of the normal tic craniectomy either forward or backward to fashion a frontotemporal or posterior temporal flap. As outlined below, most often a tic craniectomy has proved adequate to deal with most of the aneurysms of the upper basilar artery. In some circumstances, it will be necessary to convert the approach to the pterional trans-sylvian exposure, a combination of the subtemporal and trans-sylvian exposure, or the posterior temporal exposure. This flexibility must be planned for at the time of positioning.[9]

Subtemporal Approach to the Upper Basilar Artery

There exists a small controversy regarding the optimum method of approaching aneurysms of the upper basilar artery. We have favored the subtemporal approach; others have suggested that the ideal is the pterional approach. In reality, a true controversy does not exist. There are clear advantages and disadvantages to each method and to combinations of these methods, with certain configurations and positions of aneurysms clearly favoring one or another method. Most important is the surgeon's familiarity with the method, the anatomy, the configuration of the aneurysm, the depths of the wound, and, in particular, certain fundamental hazards that must be recognized and guarded against with each of the methods.

In our early experience, we routinely turned sizable temporal bone flaps in the subtemporal approach to aneurysms of the upper basilar artery. However, in our more recent 600 cases, this has proved unnecessary. With the routine use of the operating microscope, one needs a much smaller bony opening, large enough only to admit the light beam of the microscope, to manipulate the microinstruments, and to achieve sufficient retraction of the temporal lobe. The key to the exposure is to gain access to the base of the skull, at about the junction of the anterior and middle third of the temporal lobe where the temporal lobe has begun to turn upward to follow the convex floor of the middle cranial fossa. The surgeon gains nothing by exposing a large area of the lateral surface of the temporal lobe, either anteriorly or posteriorly, unless the exposure is to be converted to the frontotemporal approach or the posterior temporal approach. Certainly bony removal over the lateral surface of the temporal lobe is to no avail.

A linear incision extending vertically upward from the zygomatic process of the temporal bone, just in front of the main stem of the superficial temporal artery, for a distance of approximately 10 cm is sufficient. After the skin, subcutaneous tissue, and galea are divided, the temporalis fascia and muscle are incised using the monopolar cutting current, with the muscle fibers being cut at right angle to the vertical incision for about 5 mm on either side at the level of the zygomatic process. The scalp and soft tissue are then retracted, and a single burr hole is made in the squamous portion of the temporal bone. The burr hole is enlarged with rongeurs to form a pear-shaped opening approximately 4 cm wide at the base, with bone removed down behind the origin of the zygomatic process (Fig. 172-3A). The anterior branch of the superficial temporal artery will be divided, but the posterior branch is left intact because occasionally it may be necessary to use this scalp vessel to form a surgical collateral.

The triangular opening of the dura, based inferiorly, is fastened. The lumbar subarachnoid drain is normally opened at this point in the procedure, and drainage of cerebrospinal fluid is commenced. The undersurface of the temporal lobe is then gently inspected with a hand-held retractor to identify the position of any bridging veins anteriorly, and to identify and protect the vein of Labbé (Fig. 172-3B). We normally cover the vein of Labbé with several strips of Gelfoam to protect it. This critical vein and those at the tip

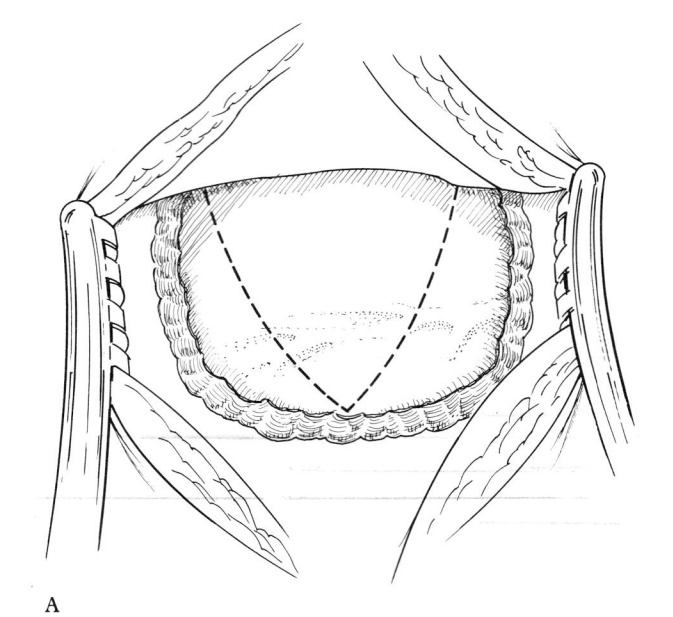

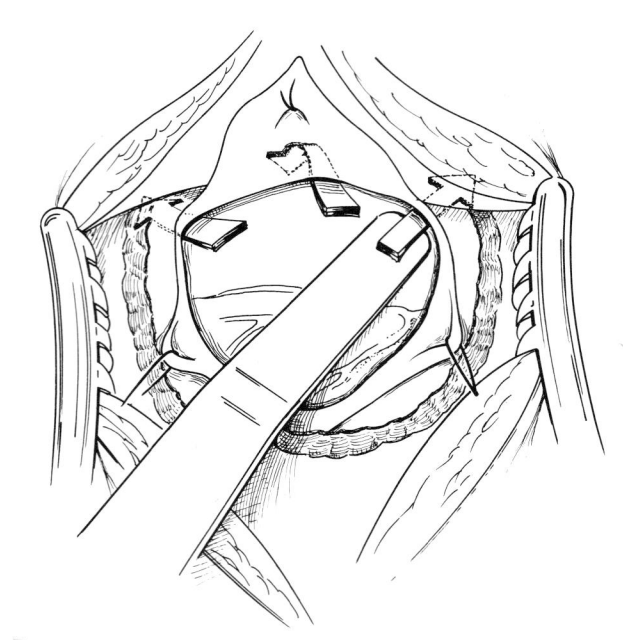

Figure 172-3 Subtemporal approach. *A.* Craniectomy to base of zygomatic process. *B.* After dura has been opened, initial inspection of surface of temporal lobe for position of bridging veins.

of the temporal lobe should be spared; tiny bridging veins on the undersurface of the temporal lobe, and particularly a commonly seen vein that runs between the uncus and the tentorial edge, may be coagulated and divided. The surface of the temporal lobe should then be covered with a compressed sheet of Gelfoam, and the temporal lobe gently retracted.

The key to this approach is to have sufficient intracranial relaxation. A slack brain is essential. The combination of mannitol and CSF drainage is usually sufficient to bring about relaxation, but if not, it is important to check the respiratory parameters, elevate the head, and wait until a little more CSF has been withdrawn, or give a second dose of mannitol. If retraction remains heavy, it is wise to abandon the procedure in favor of returning another day or make the attempt through another approach. Occasionally, a swollen brain that cannot be adequately retracted will be encountered. Heavy retraction and damage to surface veins, combined with hypotension, will set the stage for disastrous brain swelling, infarction, or hemorrhage into the temporal lobe.

After a self-retaining retractor is inserted, the edge of the tentorium will come into view. Retractor pressure is deepened and increased slightly so that the uncus, seen through the layer of overlying arachnoid, is displaced away from the free edge of the tentorium by 2 or 3 mm. The free edge of the tentorium is now sutured back into the floor of the middle cranial fossa. By tensioning this suture, the free edge is rolled laterally, giving another 3 to 5 mm of exposure and obviating the need for division of the tentorium for most aneurysms of the upper basilar artery.

The operating microscope is now brought into position and, under 10 to 16 times magnification, the surgeon should focus on the layer of arachnoid covering the uncus and cerebral peduncle. The trochlear nerve will be seen shining through the outer layer of arachnoid as it runs around the peduncle to pass to the underside of the tentorium. The arachnoid should be picked up just superior to this nerve and sharply incised with a fine knife and the incision extended anteriorly, opening the double layer of arachnoid as it crosses to form the lateral boundary of the interpeduncular cistern. Following subarachnoid hemorrhage, the cistern is typically filled with clotted blood. This blood can be removed with suction and dissection, taking care to avoid the likely site of rupture of the aneurysm. We normally identify the superior cerebellar artery as it courses around the peduncle, and dissecting the old clot off its surface, we follow it down to the lateral aspect of the basilar artery. Then, after identifying the basilar artery, it is a simple matter to move superiorly to expose the origins of the posterior cerebral artery on the near (right) side, on the left side, and on the anterior aspect of the neck of the aneurysm. By looking across the anterior aspect of the basilar artery, the origins of both proximal posterior cerebral (P1) arteries can be seen by gently compressing the neck and the ectatic basilar artery backward toward the pons. Similarly, with a small dissector, the terminal basilar artery can be gently lifted out of the interpeduncular fossa, bringing into view the posterior aspect of the neck and, more importantly, the fine perforating vessels that arise off the origins of P1 (Fig. 172-4A).

The third cranial nerve frequently need not be manipulated at all during this exposure. It is left attached to the uncus by the double layer of arachnoid, and because the retractor has lifted the uncus, the third nerve is displaced out of the operative field. The site at which the posterior cerebral artery courses over the nerve is a useful reference point, as it is between this point and the origin of the P1 segment that all of the terminal perforating vessels will be found. It cannot be overemphasized that these perforating vessels must be identified and protected at all cost. They are frequently adherent to the posterior and lateral aspects of the aneurysm, and should be dissected free and clearly preserved during clip placement. Working from the lateral aspect in this approach, it is necessary to displace the terminal basilar artery for several millimeters out of the interpeduncular fossa so as to look behind the aneurysm and see the perforators from the opposite (left) P1, and ensure that they are also protected and free. Again from the lateral approach, we have found the aperture clip, designed originally by Drake, to be most useful. The clip blades are measured to be precisely long enough to obliterate the neck of the sac. We would normally place the P1 segment into the aperture, often with one or two perforators (Fig. 172-4B). Occasionally, the third cranial nerve is included in the clip aperture so as to get an anatomical position of the blades across the neck of the aneurysm.

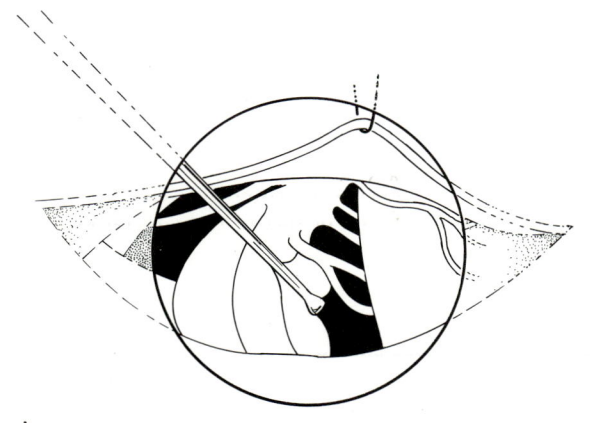

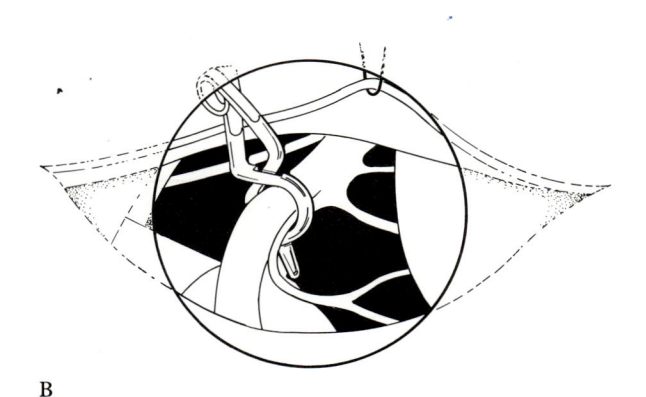

Figure 172-4 Subtemporal approach. *A.* Exposure of basilar bifurcation aneurysm. Dissector displacing aneurysm and terminal basilar artery away from interpeduncular fossa. Note perforating vessels arising from P1 segment. Edge of tentorium has been sutured back into middle fossa. *B.* Placement of aperture Sugita clip across neck of basilar bifurcation aneurysm. P1 segment and one perforator are patent in the aperture.

Several points need to be emphasized in dealing with basilar bifurcation aneurysms. Firstly, the neck of such an aneurysm is almost always wider in the coronal plane than in the anteroposterior dimension. This is another cogent reason for clipping from the subtemporal approach; one can compress the neck in its narrowest dimension without kinking or deforming the origins of the posterior cerebral arteries. It is critical always to review and identify the visible anatomy before applying the clip. It is easy to mistake the opposite superior cerebellar artery for the left P1, but by identifying the opposite oculomotor nerve, and recalling that this structure always runs between the superior cerebellar and posterior cerebral arteries, one should find that positive identification of the origin of P1 is not a problem. The precise length of the clip blade is essential. When too short, it will of course leave a portion of the neck open and the aneurysm still filling. A more troublesome error, however, is to place too long a clip blade, narrowing or occluding the origin of the opposite P1. We avoid this by actually measuring the width of the neck on its anterior and posterior surfaces with a slim dissector and choosing or, if necessary, cutting and filing the blades to exactly the required dimension (Fig. 172-5).[9]

Typically, we place, remove, and replace the clip many times before we are satisfied. After the clip placement and careful inspection on the posterior and anterior surfaces to ensure that the major vessels and their perforators are free, the dome of the aneurysm is punctured and its contents aspirated. With the extra room afforded by the collapsed sac, the anatomy is carefully inspected again. If precision has not been achieved with the clip in position, it should be immediately removed and repositioned.

The length of the basilar artery varies considerably. As such, the height of the bifurcation typically is just at or slightly above the level of the dorsum sellae. Occasionally, it may be much higher, reaching well above the mammillary bodies and indeed, at times, indenting the third ventricle. With a very high bifurcation aneurysm, the subtemporal approach may not be advantageous in that more temporal lobe retraction is necessary, requiring dissection between the uncus and oculomotor nerve. With a very high bifurcation, it is occasionally prudent to choose the pterional trans-sylvian approach (Fig. 172-6). If, on the other hand, the bifurcation is low (i.e., a centimeter or more below the level of the dorsum sellae), the pterional trans-sylvian approach may well be impossible as the bony barrier of the dorsum

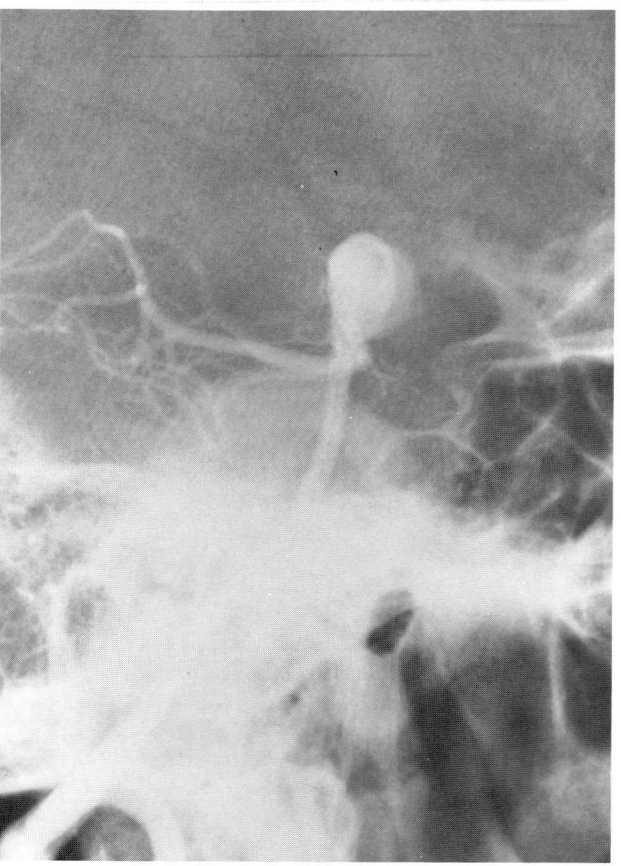

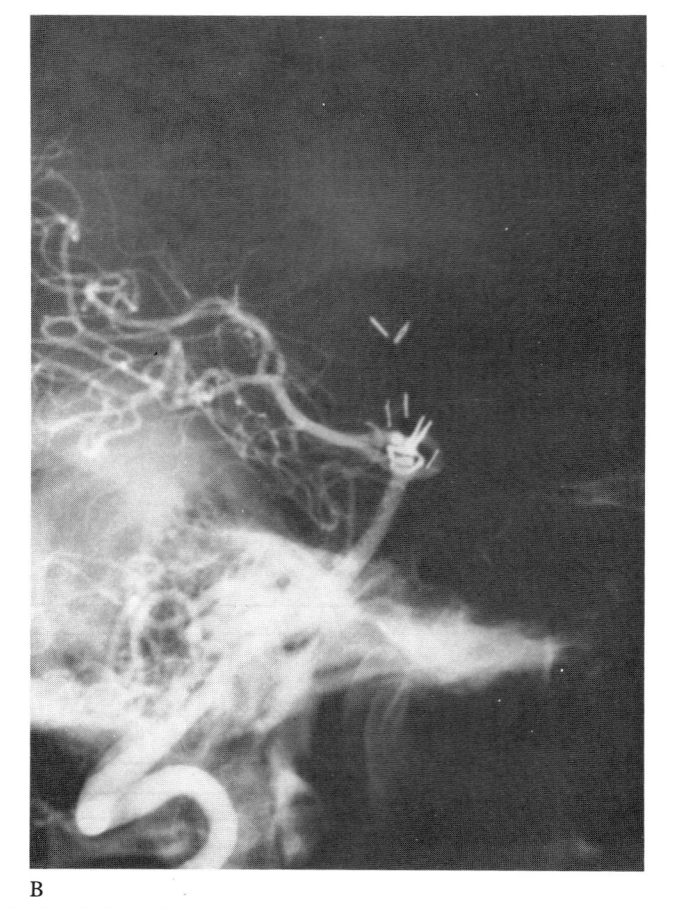

Figure 172-5 *A.* Lateral vertebral angiogram showing large basilar bifurcation aneurysm pointing upward. *B.* Postoperative angiogram after a subtemporal approach, showing small craniectomy and lateral orientation of clip obliterating neck of aneurysm.

sellae will prevent exposure and visualization of the neck of the aneurysm.

With the low-lying bifurcation aneurysms, the dissection and exposure is considerably more difficult, and indeed at times hazardous. The dome of the aneurysm and its original rupture site are often fused to the clivus or posterior aspect of the dorsum, making manipulation of the sac hazardous with an increased likelihood of intraoperative rupture. The space that contains these low-lying aneurysms is a narrow, truncated cone with the apex pointing downward. This forces the surgeon to gain visual access to the neck from the subtemporal approach, over the bulging belly of the pons in the depths of the wound. This approach is enhanced by retracting the temporal lobe somewhat more posteriorly to view the anterior aspect of the pons. Division of the tentorium is occasionally necessary to gain a better access to this region, and angled aperture clips are often essential to secure these low-placed aneurysms.

Another conceptual hazard in dealing with basilar bifurcation aneurysms is the appearance given by angiograms taken in the Towne's projection, which tend to show the P1 segments entirely separate from the neck of the aneurysm and coming straight laterally from the side of the basilar artery. In reality, and in particular when viewed from the surgical exposure of the subtemporal approach, the posterior cerebral arteries course forward, upward, and laterally before they turn out to cross above the oculomotor nerve and before swinging laterally around the peduncle under cover of the hippocampal gyrus. With the angiographic picture in mind, the surgeon will be surprised when faced with a large or bulbous bifurcation aneurysm to see from the lateral exposure what appear to be the P1 segments coming out of the side of the aneurysmal sac. As mentioned above, in the course of the development of the aneurysms, and particularly the larger ones, the terminal basilar artery becomes widened and ectatic. It is critical then for the surgeon to define the neck precisely, even though it may appear to be much wider than in the angiogram, and to spare the origins of both P1's and, of course, any adjacent perforators.

Superior Cerebellar Artery Aneurysms

Superior cerebellar artery aneurysms arise at the origin of the superior cerebellar artery off the basilar artery. This aneurysm almost always projects laterally and somewhat posteriorly, with the fundus imbedded in the peduncle. As the sac and neck enlarge, the aneurysm will occupy the whole length of the basilar artery between the distal carina of the superior cerebellar artery and the proximal origin of the posterior cerebral artery. The fundus of the aneurysm almost always has an intimate association with the oculomotor nerve and will stretch this nerve over or below the dome of the sac. With large superior cerebellar artery aneurysms, deformity and dysfunction of the third nerve, as well as compression of the peduncle, produces the common Weber's syndrome.

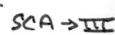

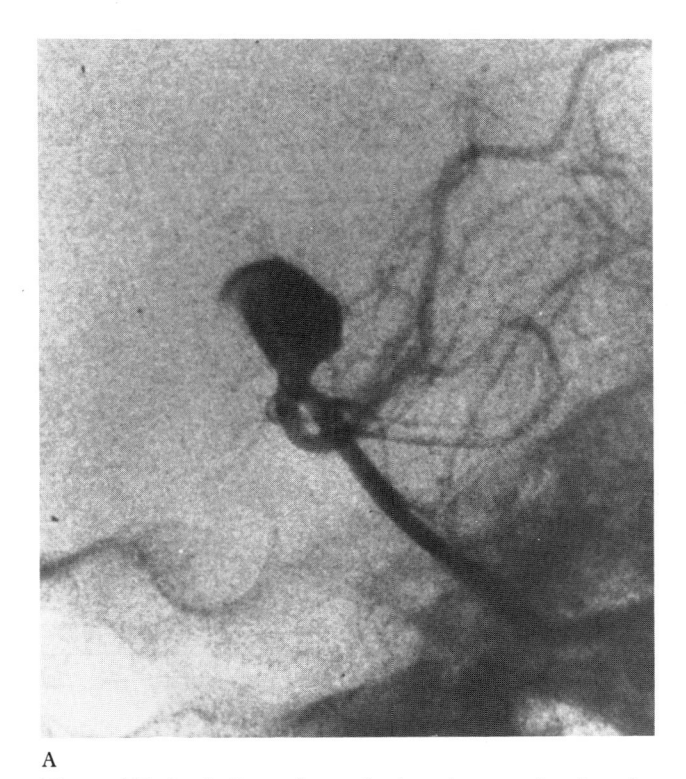

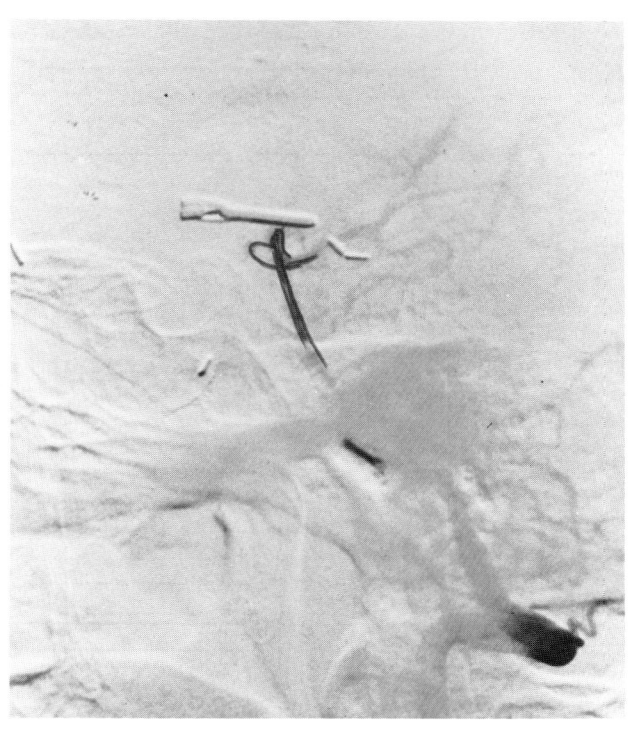

Figure 172-6 *A*. Lateral vertebral angiogram showing elongated basilar artery and neck of bifurcation aneurysm situated more than 1 cm above dorsum sellae. *B*. This bifurcation aneurysm was clipped via the pterional trans-sylvian approach.

Small and moderate-sized aneurysms of the basilar–superior cerebellar artery junction are usually quite straightforward to deal with. There are no perforators arising from the superior surface of the superior cerebellar artery, and the perforators arising from the inferior posterior surface of the posterior cerebral artery are usually displaced away from the sac and neck as the fundus enlarges. The subtemporal exposure gives an excellent exposure of this aneurysm. After defining the neck and being quite certain of the presence and position of the posterior cerebral perforators, the surgeon, following the natural line of the basilar artery as it turns to form the origin of the posterior cerebral artery, can usually work a clip across the neck of the aneurysm (Fig. 172-7).

Small aneurysms of the left superior cerebellar artery will require a left subtemporal approach. There is a slight but additional hazard to the patient with retraction of the dominant temporal lobe, but, in our experience, this has not been significant. Very large aneurysms arising from the left side of the basilar artery at this site may be approached from the right side because the basilar artery is usually displaced toward the right as the aneurysm enlarges. One then carries out the dissection over the front of the basilar artery, taking advantage of the shorter distances involved. The two major hazards of clipping these aneurysms are kinking or narrowing the basilar artery, and narrowing or occluding the origin of the superior cerebellar artery. These hazards may be avoided if, after the neck is secured with a clip, the sac is punctured and collapsed and careful inspection is made to ensure that both the basilar artery and the superior cerebellar artery are normally patent. The superior cerebellar artery normally has poor collateral circulation; narrowing or occlusion of this vessel with the tip of the clip blade will usually result in unwanted consequences for the patient.

Posterior Cerebral Artery Aneurysms

There are four typical sites of origin of aneurysms from the posterior cerebral artery: (1) at the origin of the large perforating branches on P1; (2) at the junction of the posterior communicating artery and P1 segment; (3) at the origin of the anterior and posterior occipital-temporal arteries along the side of the brain stem; and (4) at the terminal branching of the vessel into its parietal and calcarine branches. The most common sites are at the origin of the posterior communicating artery and where the first major branching occurs along the side of the brain stem.

The more proximal of these aneurysms can be dealt with

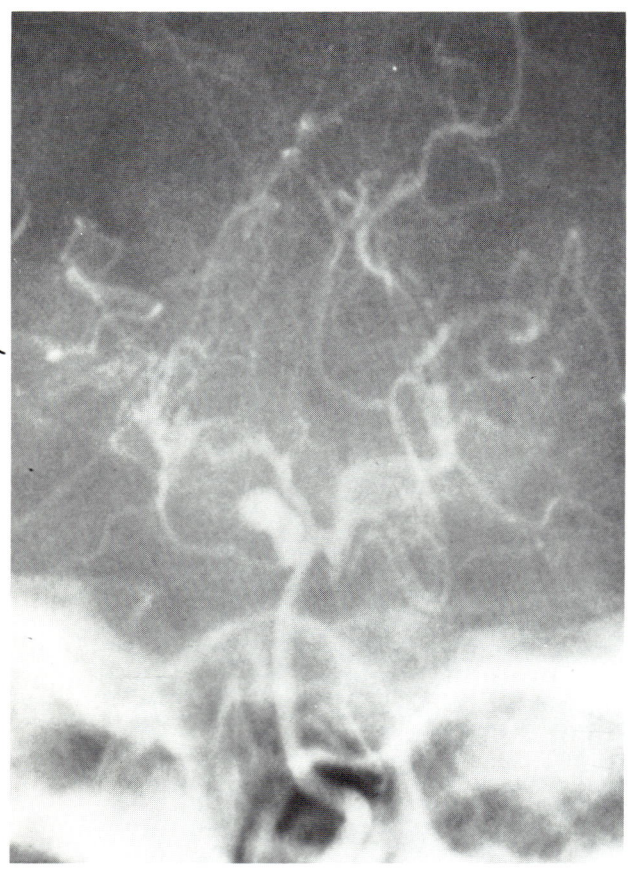

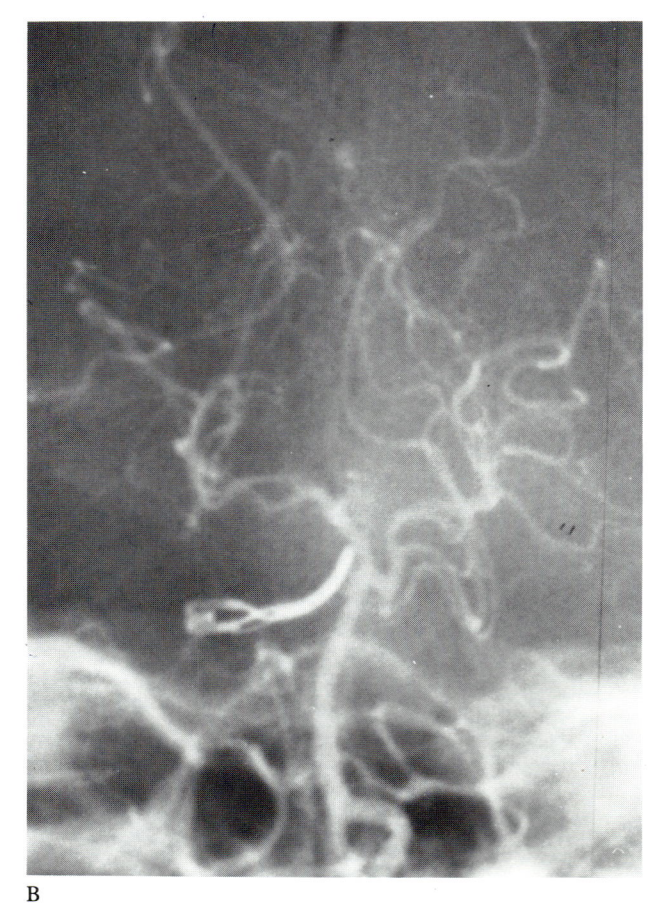

Figure 172-7 *A.* Anteroposterior angiogram showing a partially thrombosed giant aneurysm arising from the right basilar-SCA junction. *B.* It was clipped with a curved Sugita clip.

conveniently via the subtemporal approach. These aneurysms are relatively easy to dissect, being somewhat distal to the main perforators going to the perforated substance and peduncle, but the surgeon must always take care to spare these vessels without exception. The more distal of these aneurysms are typically hidden under the hippocampal gyrus, requiring more retraction of this gyrus or occasionally resection of a small portion of the gyrus to gain exposure. Resection of a portion of the hippocampal gyrus is almost always necessary with those aneurysms lying in the origin of the choroidal fissure. With giant aneurysms arising off the posterior cerebral artery, we have found that it is usually safe to proximally occlude the posterior cerebral artery distal to the perforators arising from the first and second segments and beyond the emergence of the major temporal branch of the posterior cerebral artery. The posterior cerebral artery has normally a rich collateral supply. In 22 cases where we have deliberately occluded the posterior cerebral artery, we have had only one incidence of a persistent visual field defect as the result of occipital infarction. Nevertheless, it is important to state that one must not occlude the posterior cerebral artery proximal to the origin of the posterior choroidal arteries or to trap any of the proximal perforators off the posterior cerebral artery in that ischemia or infarction in the territory of these vessels will be devastating.

Trans-sylvian Pterional Approach to Aneurysms of the Terminal Basilar Artery

The pterional approach has many proponents and some distinct advantages (Fig. 172-8). The approach also has some hazards and disadvantages, which should be known and appreciated. As described by Yasargil et al., this approach emphasizes a small frontotemporal craniotomy with removal of the lesser wing of the sphenoid at the pterion so as to give a greater exposure of the base of the brain by removing some of the base of the skull.[14] Although bony removal has been emphasized in this approach, the key to success is not only bony removal but a lengthy and careful splitting of the sylvian fissure. We think it would be more accurate to describe this as the trans-sylvian pterional approach to the basilar bifurcation, with the greater emphasis on opening the fissure. The fissure needs to be separated to the point where the carotid bifurcation and origin of the middle cerebral artery can easily be seen. Then with retraction of both the frontal and temporal lobes, and through the widely opened sylvian fissure, the dissection is carried deeply, usually on the lateral side of the carotid artery, following the posterior communicating artery backward to the posterior cerebral and thence to the bifurcation. Occasionally it will be necessary to clip and divide the posterior communicating artery (always between and sparing its vital perforators) to remove the curtain of vessels that will be between the operator and the operator's ultimate goal. With this exposure, the basilar artery and the bifurcation will appear obliquely oriented to the operator with the near (usually right side) P1 origin being clearly seen, with somewhat less visualization of the left P1. The neck of the aneurysm, in the case of the usual basilar bifurcation sac, will be nicely in view and easily dissected from this position. This immediate accessibility of the neck may prove a trap for the unwary. The hazard is that the P1 perforators are not immediately visible, arising as they do from the posterior aspect of the P1 segments, often wrapping around and behind the neck of the sac and often crossing the midline. A clip worked across the neck of the sac and closed, therefore, runs a considerable hazard of occluding one of these perforators without the vital vessel ever being seen.

In general, it is preferable to make this approach on the

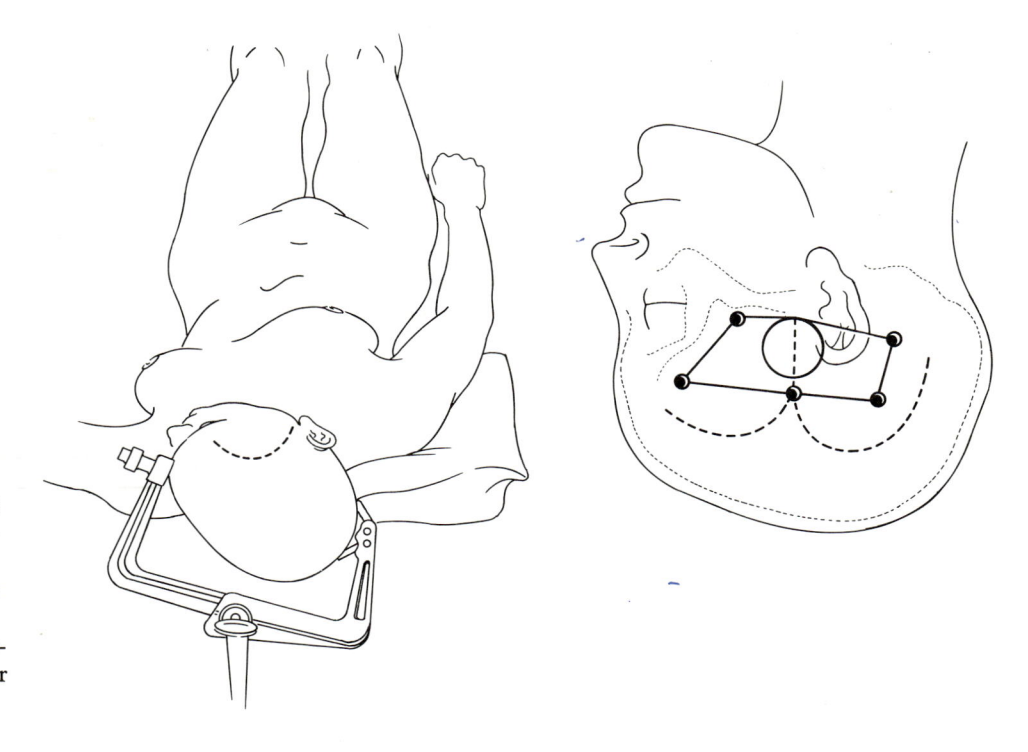

Figure 172-8 Position of patient for pterional trans-sylvian approach. Drawing on right depicts scalp incisions (*dotted lines*) and approximate craniotomy sites for the pterional, subtemporal, and posterior temporal approaches to the upper basilar artery.

lateral side of the carotid artery. It has been suggested that the approach can also be made on the medial side of the carotid artery. We believe this is hazardous and rarely necessary. It requires retraction on the carotid artery, which can be troublesome, particularly if the vessel is atherosclerotic. Moreover, the space between the carotid artery and the optic nerve presents yet another shutter of vital structures between the surgeon and the ultimate goal, increasing the difficulty of visualization and instrument manipulation.[12]

Certain disadvantages of the trans-sylvian pterional approach need be emphasized. The basilar bifurcation is at least 1 cm deeper via the trans-sylvian approach as compared with the subtemporal approach. This greater distance, coupled with a curtain of vital structures (optic nerve, carotid artery, posterior communicating and anterior choroidal arteries and their perforators) in the path, will frequently make the exposure more technically demanding. The orientation of the basilar artery is oblique, and is addressed from the anterolateral aspect when using the trans-sylvian approach, increasing the possibility of anatomical confusion and always making it difficult to see the P1 perforators with certainly. Low-lying bifurcation aneurysms and those aneurysms arising off the basilar artery at the superior cerebellar origin may have their necks largely obscured by the dorsum sellae. Bilobed aneurysms of the bifurcation, or those that project entirely backward into the interpeduncular fossa, cannot be approached by the trans-sylvian route (Figs. 172-9 and 172-10). Finally, a short, wide, or ectatic carotid artery may entirely block the operator's exposure of the terminal basilar artery.

On the other hand, an elongated basilar artery with a high-lying bifurcation can most often be conveniently approached by splitting the sylvian fissure. Certainly, the most common bifurcation aneurysm, pointing directly upward at or above the dorsum sellae, can be dealt with quite satisfactorily if the surgeon has familiarity with the trans-sylvian approach. In the final analysis, experience with the approach and familiarity with the anatomy, with careful attention to the many small details, will be the major factors that determine the success of the surgeon's choice of approach to this remote site of aneurysms.

Aneurysms of the Basilar Trunk

Basilar-Anterior Inferior Cerebellar Artery Aneurysms

The anterior inferior cerebellar artery (AICA) aneurysms usually arise at the distal carina of the origin of the anterior inferior cerebellar artery from the basilar artery. Occasion-

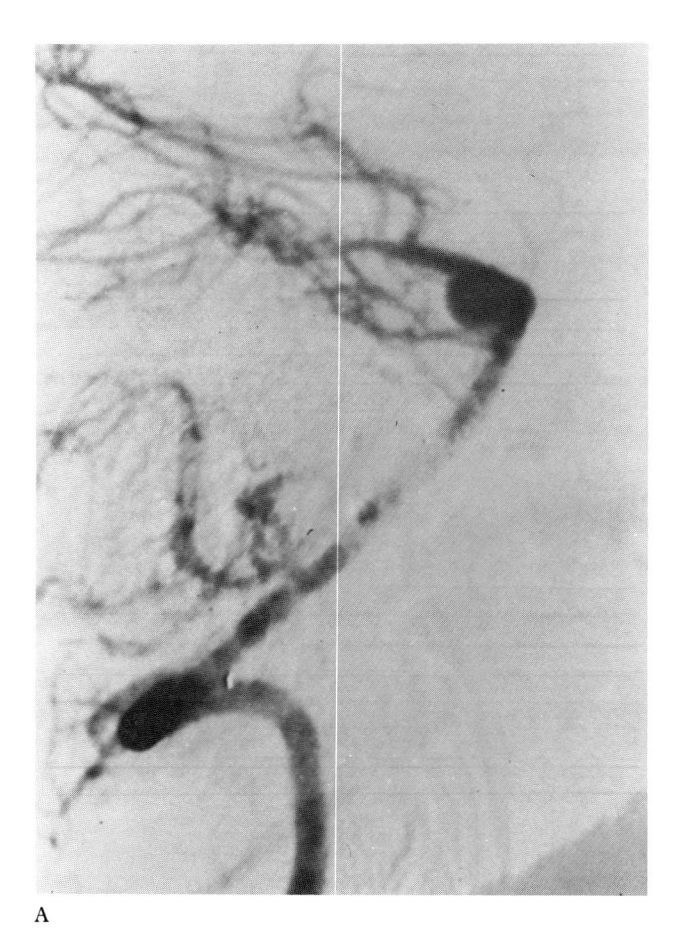

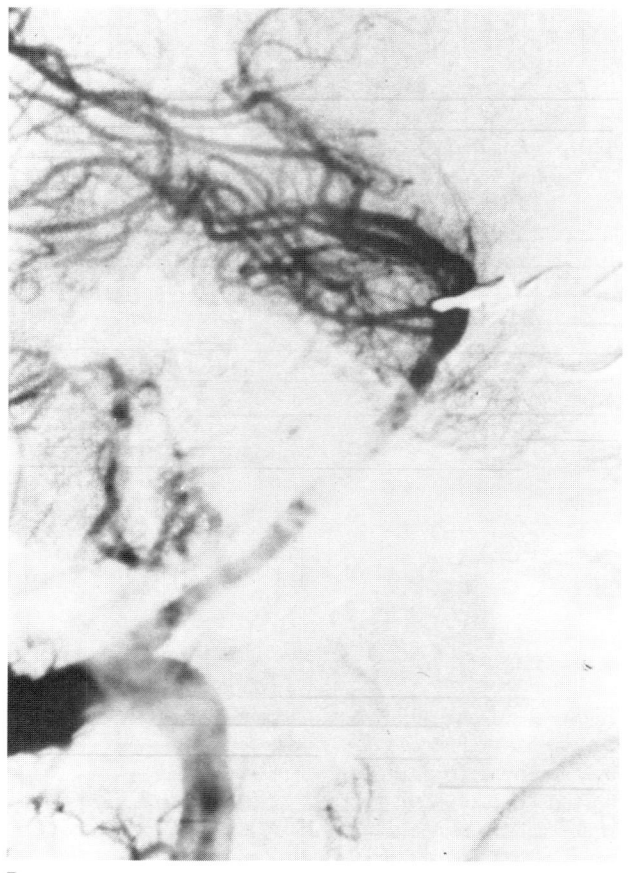

Figure 172-9 *A.* Posterior projecting basilar bifurcation aneurysm. This aneurysm is difficult to secure from pterional trans-sylvian approach. *B.* This posterior projecting bifurcation aneurysm was clipped from a lateral subtemporal approach.

Posterior Circulation Aneurysms

ally, however, these aneurysms will arise on the proximal side of this junction. This variation can usually be predicted on the preoperative angiogram. These aneurysms usually project laterally but may project anteriorly and be fused to the clivus, and occasionally may point backward and be buried in the pons or pontomedullary junction. Basilar-AICA aneurysms usually bear a close relationship to the abducens nerve.

These aneurysms may be approached subtemporally and transtentorially or, because of the variable site of origin of the AICA, suboccipitally, or occasionally by a combined subtemporal-suboccipital approach by dividing both the tentorium and the petrosal sinus. Rules regarding the choice of approach cannot be easily stated. It depends on the size, site of origin, and configuration of the aneurysm. Basilar trunk aneurysms bulging forward and originating well along the trunk of the basilar artery are usually best approached subtemporally. Those originating more proximally on the basilar artery may be exposed more easily and directly through the suboccipital approach. Generally it is best to approach the aneurysm from an exposure closest to the neck and where the operator will have the best opportunity to visualize and spare with certainty the major branch vessels in the region. Whatever the approach, these aneurysms lie in a narrow and confined space at some distance from either a supra- or infratentorial exposure. It is always best, therefore, to plan the approach that will most readily bring the neck into view.

With the subtemporal approach, it is necessary to turn a moderate-sized temporal bone flap, which is centered to permit a direct line of sight down the posterior slope of the petrous bone and clivus. With this exposure, the vein of Labbé will be in the anterior third and must be protected. The tentorium is then divided sharply behind the attachment of the trochlear nerve, with the division carried almost to the junction of the petrosal and lateral sinuses. The anterior leaf of the tentorium is then sutured forward into the middle fossa, and the posterior leaflet coagulated to shrink it back out of view. After the tentorium is divided, the arachnoid that forms the roof of the posterior fossa cisterns will be exposed, and under it the trochlear and trigeminal nerves will be seen. The petrosal vein piercing this arachnoid layer should be coagulated and divided. After the arachnoid lateral to the trigeminal nerve has been opened, a narrow retractor blade can be used to gently displace the anterosuperior aspect of the cerebellum to expose the pons and the abducens, facial, and auditory nerves. With the anterior and superior aspects of the cerebellopontine angle now open, the basilar artery, partially obscured by the bulge of the pontine hemisphere, can be seen, and if this vessel is followed inferi-

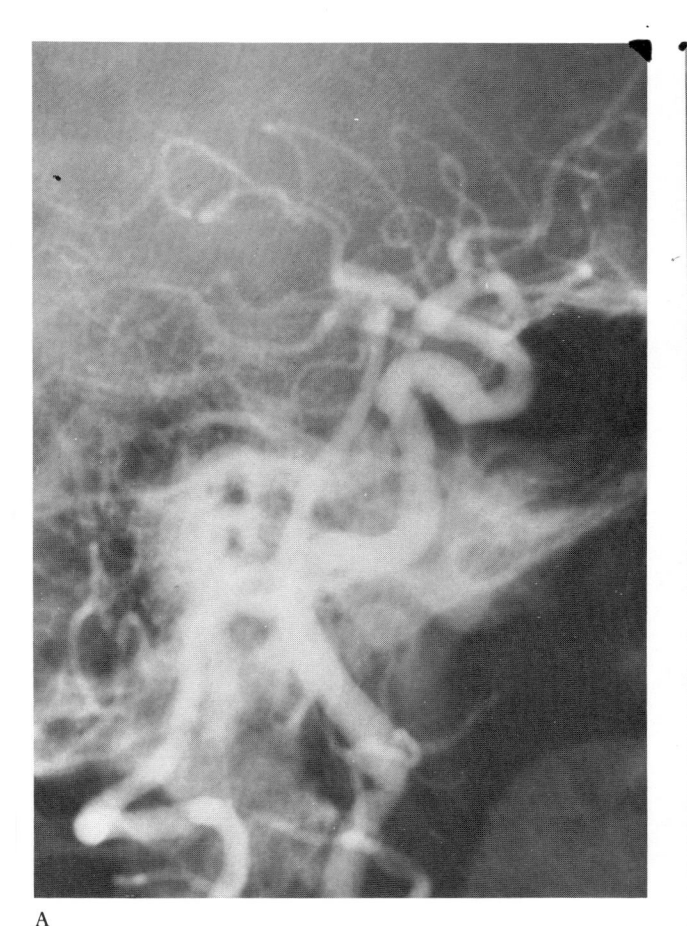

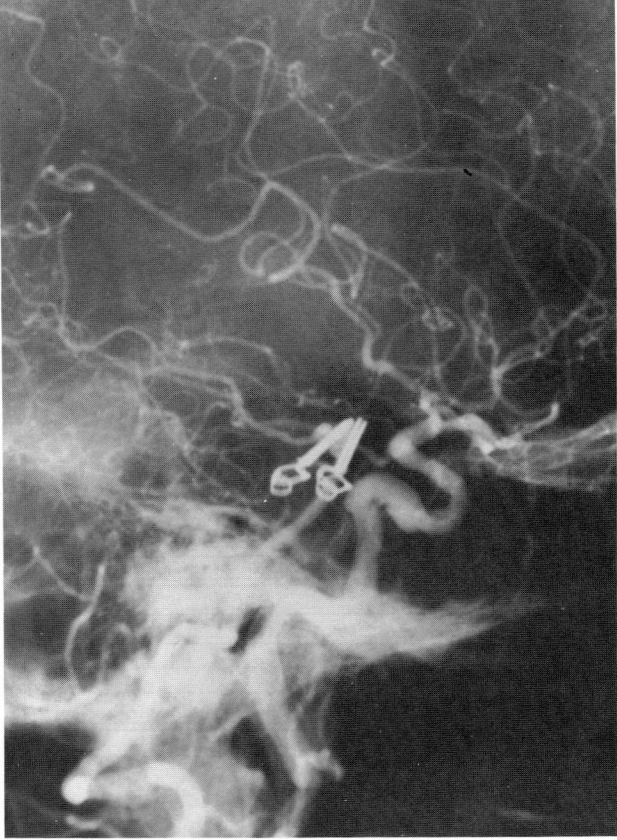

Figure 172-10 *A.* Lateral vertebral angiogram depicting a bilobed basilar bifurcation aneurysm. *B.* This bilobed aneurysm was secured with two clips from a lateral, subtemporal approach. This aneurysm configuration is extremely difficult to attack via the pterional trans-sylvian approach.

orly, the aneurysm can be exposed. After removing clot and CSF, this narrow space will gradually open to expose the pertinent anatomy. It is usually necessary to separate the sixth nerve from the aneurysm, but as this structure is usually slack as it courses upward to gain the cavernous sinus, it can be easily displaced to clear the neck of the aneurysm. From the subtemporal transtentorial approach, the origin of the AICA will not usually be seen since it will be on the inferior aspect of the sac. We have found it useful to expose this vessel by gently grasping the neck of the aneurysm with bipolar forceps and tipping the sac away from the pons so as to expose the AICA, and then sharply dissecting this vessel free from the neck. Obviously the AICA must be spared with the clip placement. In that these aneurysms normally point anteriorly, the definition of the AICA, the basilar artery, and those perforating branches coming from the basilar artery to irrigate the pons is quite straightforward. With aneurysms that are buried into the pons, visualization of these vessels will be much more difficult. This exposure is always confining because at the critical moment of clip application the essential anatomy is usually obscured by the clip applier and the handle of the clip. It is essential, once the clip is applied, that the surgeon quickly inspect the position of the blade to ensure absolute accuracy of clip placement. To narrow or occlude the basilar artery, trap perforators, or obstruct the origin of the AICA will have catastrophic consequences for the patient.[9]

Rarely we have encountered aneurysms arising from the trunk of the basilar artery, distal to the origin of the AICA, presumably at the site of origin of long or short pontine perforators or, even more rarely, at the origin of a primitive trigeminal artery. These aneurysms again are approached through the transtentorial route, but medial to the trigeminal nerve. It is necessary to gently retract the trigeminal nerve laterally while intermittently retracting on the belly of the pons with a narrow-bladed retractor. It is important to look for and spare the perforators arising from the basilar artery that will almost always be associated with these aneurysms.

Vertebral Junction Aneurysms

Even in our series, vertebral junction aneurysms are uncommon, which is fortunate because they are difficult to expose and clip placement is awkward. They have almost always been associated with anomalous development of the vertebral arteries, such as congenital absence of a vertebral artery, vertebral artery ending in the PICA, and fenestration of the basilar artery. Associated with these anomalies, the junction of the vertebral arteries may be higher or lower than the normal position, which is just at or slightly below the junction of the middle and inferior thirds of the clivus. The aneurysm may be displaced well off the midline.

Again, these aneurysms may be approached either subtemporally or suboccipitally depending primarily on the height of the aneurysm and, therefore, the distance the operator must trespass to reach the neck, and secondarily on the size and configuration of the aneurysm. The major difficulty with this aneurysm is its remoteness from the surface and the fact that it is buttressed by pons above and medulla below, which cannot easily be retracted. It is also difficult to visualize both the proximal vertebral and distal basilar vessels and to ensure their patency when the clip is applied. It is essential to take great care when approaching them from below to avoid injuring the lower cranial nerves. Inadvertent injury to the ninth, tenth, and eleventh cranial nerves will certainly cause significant morbidity and, not infrequently, mortality secondary to pharyngeal dysfunction, aspiration, and pneumonia.

For large aneurysms in this region, we have, on occasion, used a combined subtemporal-suboccipital approach, turning a generous temporal bone flap and joining this to a suboccipital craniectomy. After the tentorium is divided, the petrosal sinus is divided between clips as it enters the lateral sinus, and the dura incision is then continued into the posterior fossa. With the operating microscope placed halfway between the suboccipital and subtemporal approach, and retractors placed over the lateral aspect of the cerebellum, a very generous lateral exposure of the whole side of the brain stem is afforded, providing an excellent view. The major hazard is to the exposed cranial nerves and, in particular, an overstretching of the cochlear branch of the auditory nerve. In attacking a large, thrombosed, aneurysmal mass, this approach can be quite advantageous.

Vertebral Artery Aneurysms

Aneurysms that arise from the vertebral artery usually arise just beyond the origin of the posterior inferior cerebellar artery (PICA). Only rarely do these aneurysms arise from the vertebral artery more distal to the origin of the PICA, at the origin of unnamed branches, or at the origin of the anterior spinal artery. As a rule, the anatomy of the PICA is extremely variable, and, as a result, we have seen vertebral-PICA aneurysms lying in or below the foramen magnum and as high as the middle of the clivus. Although these aneurysms are usually found on the lateral aspect of the medulla, we have seen a left vertebral-PICA aneurysm lying largely in the right cerebellopontine angle. The aneurysms are typically nestled along the side of the medulla, with the twelfth cranial nerve intimately associated with the neck and, occasionally, even split by the sac as it enlarges. Frequently these aneurysms take origin from a significant portion of the proximal part of the PICA and, therefore, have a V-shaped neck, which presents a challenge to the surgeon in clip selection and placement so as to preserve the continuity of both the vertebral artery and the PICA.

Aneurysms arising from the vertebral artery are normally approached through the suboccipital exposure, with the patient in the lateral or "park bench" position, with the face turned slightly toward the floor. A lateral, curvilinear paramedian incision is made, and after the muscle is reflected, with care to preserve the occipital nerves, a small craniectomy is made well lateral to expose the mastoid air cells. The rim of the foramen magnum is usually removed (Fig. 172-11). In that these aneurysms usually lie relatively close to the midline, extreme lateral or medial exposures are unnecessary; it is desirable only to have a moderate lateral exposure

Posterior Circulation Aneurysms

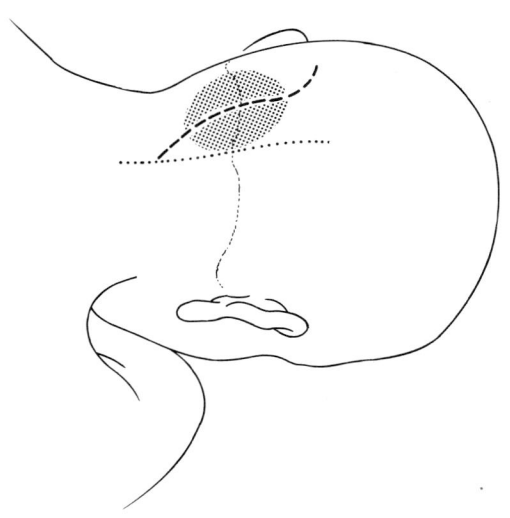

Figure 172-11 Suboccipital approach. Lateral decubitus position. Head positioned with face turned toward floor. Dotted line depicts scalp incision. Stippled area shows the bony removal.

of the medulla so as to see the vertebral artery as it enters the subarachnoid space (after the cisterna magna is opened). With removal of CSF and gentle upward and medial retraction of the cerebellar tonsil, the ninth, tenth, and eleventh cranial nerves come into view. The caudal loop of the PICA is immediately apparent, and this need only be followed to its origin to expose the neck of the typical vertebral-PICA aneurysm. It is important to remove clot from the proximal and distal vertebral artery, working across the neck of the aneurysm in order to gain appreciation of the configuration of the vertebral artery and the width of the neck. We have often found it necessary and useful to narrow the neck of this aneurysm with bipolar cautery, and to use aperture clips to enclose and protect the PICA and the twelfth nerve in the aperture to gain control of this aneurysm. It should be stressed again that dissection and exposure of aneurysms of the vertebral artery necessitate working between the filaments of the lower cranial nerves. This must be done gently and carefully to prevent their injury and the concomitant, disabling postoperative complications (Fig. 172-12).[9]

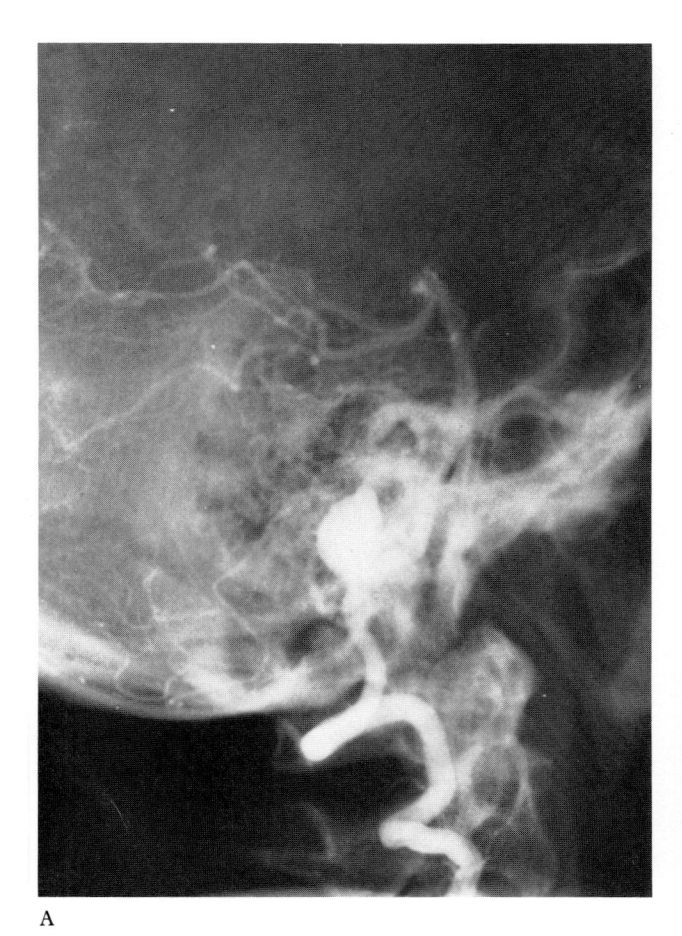

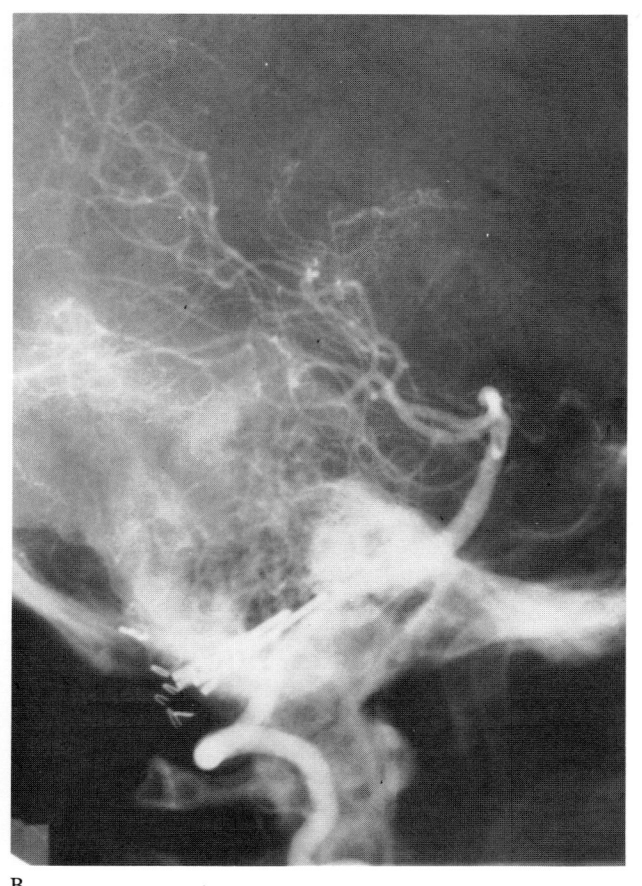

Figure 172-12 *A.* Lateral vertebral angiogram showing a partially thrombosed giant vertebral-PICA aneurysm. *B.* This aneurysm was secured with tandem clips, maintaining the patency of the vertebral artery and the PICA.

Transoral-Transclival Approaches to Basilar Trunk and Vertebrobasilar Aneurysms

These approaches are mentioned only to be condemned. Many years ago we attempted to expose aneurysms of the basilar trunk through the mouth and after removal of the clivus. This approach has many disadvantages. The exposure is always very confining. It almost always places the fundus of the aneurysm between the operator and the parent and branch vessels. Perhaps most importantly, there is real difficulty in obtaining a watertight closure, and the risk of CSF leakage and postoperative meningitis is very high. With refinements of the subtemporal and suboccipital approaches, we have not found it necessary to even consider the transoral-transclival exposure.

Results and Conclusions

A summary of our results over 25 years is given in Tables 172-1 to 172-3. These figures represent an experience that spans our original and, by comparison to today, crude efforts of direct attack on the aneurysms arising from the vertebrobasilar system. Until 1975, the operating microscope was not used routinely; microsurgical techniques were in their infancy, and clip technology was primitive. Moreover, neuroanesthesia and radiology have improved remarkably in the past decade. Nevertheless, our series is cumulative and historical, and the trials, tribulations, pitfalls, and complications of our original experience cannot be disregarded. They are, therefore, necessarily recorded in this summary.

In Table 172-1, small (up to 1.5 cm in diameter) and large (up to 2.5 cm in diameter) aneurysms are grouped and the results of surgical therapy indicated by the site of origin of the aneurysm. It is evident that the majority of the unsatisfactory results have occurred with aneurysms of the terminal basilar artery—a cogent reminder of the vital importance to normal brain function of the P1 perforating vessels. In these average-sized aneurysms in patients of all grades, we have experienced a surgical mortality of 4.6 percent; in the past 5 years and in more than 200 cases, the mortality has been less than 2 percent, with a corresponding decline in morbidity.

Table 172-2 summarizes our results with giant aneurysms (greater than 2.5 cm in diameter) arising from the various sites of the vertebrobasilar vessels. These lesions, because of their size, intraluminal thrombosis, sclerosis and calcification of the wall, incorporation of branch vessels, compression of the brain stem, and the confined space of the region, are clearly more hazardous. In patients harboring these large sacs, we have encountered a 12 percent mortality and 23 percent morbidity, although two out of three poor results were present before surgery and were unaffected by the surgical effort.

Our total experience, until August 1983, for all sizes of aneurysms and in all grades of patients is summarized in Table 172-3. Excellent or good results have been achieved in 82 percent of patients.

At the present time, if a surgical team has complete familiarity with the anatomy, technical experience, and excellence in neuroanesthesia, and pays particular attention to the many small details that encompass aneurysm surgery, it will find that most aneurysms of the vertebrobasilar system are amenable to surgical treatment.

TABLE 172-1 Vertebrobasilar Aneurysms (Small and Large): Results by Site, All Grades

Site*	Number	Excellent	Good	Poor	Dead
Basilar bifurcation	450	312	66	52	20
Basilar–SCA junction	134	107	15	9	3
Basilar–AICA junction	45	31	5	6	3
Vertebrobasilar junction	42	34	4	2	2
Vertebral	128	111	8	2	7
Posterior cerebral	31	22	4	1	4
Totals	830	617	102	72	39
		87%		13%	

*AICA, anterior inferior cerebellar artery; SCA, superior cerebellar artery.

TABLE 172-2 Giant Vertebrobasilar Aneurysms: Results by Site, All Grades

Site	Number	Excellent	Good	Poor	Dead
Basilar bifurcation	90	30	21	27	12
Basilar–SCA junction	36	12	8	10	6
Basilar trunk	31	17	3	6	5
Vertebrobasilar junction	22	11	4	5	2
Vertebral	13	9	3		1
Posterior cerebral					
P1	18	12	2	3	1
P2	15	10	4	1	
Totals	225	101	45	52	27
		65%		23%	12%

TABLE 172-3 Vertebrobasilar Aneurysms (All Sizes, All Grades): Summary of Results

Size	Number	Excellent	Good	Poor	Dead
Small	654	510	72	43	29
Large	176	107	30	29	10
Giant (>2.5 cm)	225	101	45	52	27
Totals	1055	718	147	124	66
		82%		18%	

References

1. Dandy WE: *Intracranial Arterial Aneurysms*. Ithaca, Comstock, 1944.
2. Drake CG: Bleeding aneurysms of the basilar artery: Direct surgical management in four cases. J Neurosurg 18:230–238, 1961.
3. Drake CG: Surgical treatment of ruptured aneurysms of the basilar artery: Experience with 14 cases. J Neurosurg 23:457–473, 1965.
4. Drake CG: Further experience with surgical treatment of aneurysms of the basilar artery. J Neurosurg 29:372–392, 1968.
5. Falconer MA: Surgical treatment of spontaneous intracranial hemorrhage. Br Med J 5074:790–792, 1958.
6. Jamieson KG: Aneurysms of the vertebrobasilar system: Surgical intervention in 19 cases. J Neurosurg 21:781–797, 1964.
7. Logue V: Posterior fossa aneurysms. Clin Neurosurg 11:183–207, 1964.
8. Peerless SJ: Pre- and postoperative management of cerebral aneurysms. Clin Neurosurg 26:209–231, 1979.
9. Peerless SJ, Drake CG: Surgical techniques of posterior cerebral aneurysms, in Schmidek HH, Sweet WH (eds): *Operative Neurosurgical Techniques*. New York, Grune & Stratton, 1982, pp 909–931.
10. Poppen JL: Vascular surgery of the posterior fossa. Clin Neurosurg 6:198–250, 1959.
11. Schwartz HG: Arterial aneurysm of the posterior fossa. J Neurosurg 5:312–316, 1948.
12. Sugita K, Kobayashi S, Shintani A, Mutsuga N: Microneurosurgery for aneurysms of the basilar artery. J Neurosurg 51:615–620, 1979.
13. Tönnis W: Zur behandlung intrakraniellar Aneurysmen. Arch Klin Chir 189:474–479, 1937.
14. Yasargil MG, Antic J, Laciga R, Jain KK, Hodosh RM, Smith RD: Microsurgical pterional approach to aneurysms of the basilar bifurcation. Surg Neurol 6:83–91, 1976.

173

Surgery for Unruptured Intracranial Aneurysms

Duke Samson

Over the past 15 years the importance of surgical treatment of ruptured intracranial aneurysms has become well established in the neurosurgical and neurological literature. The development of modern neuroanesthetic techniques coupled with the use of microscopic visualization and its attendant microsurgical techniques have sharply dropped the mortality and morbidity figures of patients undergoing such treatment well below the levels that can be expected with conservative nonsurgical management of such lesions. In the light of such advances, attention has turned to consideration of surgical therapy for patients harboring incidental or multiple aneurysms that at the time of discovery are unruptured. In large measure because of the paucity of firm data describing the natural history of such lesions, clinicians have varied widely in their enthusiasm for surgical attack on unruptured intracranial aneurysms, especially when such therapy would require a separate operative procedure and when the lesions in question are small in size or located in what are traditionally thought to be relatively inaccessible anatomical sites. In the absence of a randomized prospective study, a definitive resolution of this controversy will not be reached to the satisfaction of all involved; however, a brief review of the pertinent aspects of this issue may serve to provide sufficient information on which to base a rational if not completely scientific approach to this relatively common neurosurgical quandary.

Natural History of Unruptured Aneurysms

Several studies, beginning with the Cooperative Study of intracranial aneurysms and subarachnoid hemorrhage, have attempted to address the important issue of the natural history of the unruptured intracranial aneurysm.[2,5–7,9,23,24] Clinically, the patient population evaluated in these studies falls rather clearly into two separate catagories:

1. Patients with symptomatic unruptured lesions
2. Patients with asymptomatic unruptured lesions

A review of all available data from the Cooperative Study through the present date shows conclusively that the bulk of patients presenting with symptomatic but unruptured aneurysms have routinely undergone surgical procedures, which leaves only a small percentage of patients for evaluation of the natural history of this specific subgroup. In the Cooperative Study follow-up, 28 percent of such patients subsequently died of subarachnoid hemorrhage and an additional 16 percent were functionally disabled by other effects of their intracranial aneurysm.[9] Somewhat surprisingly, no surviving patient was thought to have had a nonfatal subarachnoid hemorrhage from a symptomatic but previously unruptured intracranial aneurysm. In a recent publication 36 percent of patients harboring symptomatic but unruptured aneurysms subsequently suffered subarachnoid hemorrhages, which were fatal to seven of eight.[23] Realizing that both of these small groups of patients represent only a small minority of patients coming to clinical attention with unruptured symptomatic lesions (the bulk having been selected out for a surgical procedure), no statistically valid conclusions about this population can be drawn. It is of interest, however, that of those patients not selected for surgery, over a third suffered a fatal subarachnoid hemorrhage or were disabled by the effects of their intact aneurysm.[9,23]

A larger amount of material is available regarding the natural history of the unruptured asymptomatic intracranial aneurysm, much of which is drawn from the follow-up of subarachnoid hemorrhage patients with multiple aneurysms in whom only the ruptured lesion has been treated.[5,6,11,23] Heiskanen, in evaluating a group of 61 patients with subarachnoid hemorrhage and at least 2 patients with intracranial aneurysms in which only the ruptured aneurysm had been clipped, found in a long-term follow-up period a risk of rehemorrhage of some 21 percent, with a mortality of 12 percent over a period of more than 10 years.[5,6] In a review of the available literature on the subject, Jane and his colleagues speculated that the natural history of an unruptured asymptomatic aneurysm is similar to the natural history of a "healed" ruptured aneurysm, that is, a hemorrhage rate of some 3 to 4 percent per year,[7,24] figures not significantly different from those of Heiskanen or from the previously published statistical study of Bailey and Loeser.[1] Dell, in a second statistical study, has projected a life-time 16 percent risk of subarachnoid hemorrhage for a 20-year-old patient harboring an unruptured aneurysm.[2] All of these studies, then, suggest a relatively low yearly incidence of hemorrhage in the range of 2 to 4 percent for incidental aneurysms, with a cumulative risk that obviously is of considerable significance, especially in younger patients.

Closely tied to the considerations of aneurysmal symptomatology is the parameter of aneurysm size. All available studies beginning with the initial Cooperative Study report have indicated that aneurysms below 5 mm in radiographic diameter are unlikely to be associated either with subarachnoid hemorrhage or with other symptomatology, whereas those 7 mm to 1 cm in diameter are most commonly associated with subarachnoid bleeding and with the production of other symptoms such as cranial nerve palsy, visual loss, and lateralized neurological deficit.[8,9,10,14,23] Moreover, recent studies have demonstrated that large aneurysms greater than 2.5 cm in size are not only frequently associated with significant neurological deficit but also, contrary to previous belief, with frequent and often fatal subarachnoid hemorrhage.[18,20] Therefore by symptomatological and radiographic criteria, unruptured aneurysms greater than 7 mm in radiographic diameter would appear to be those most commonly associated with subsequent subarachnoid hemorrhage or progressive neurological deficit and therefore those most worthy of consideration for prophylactic surgical treatment.

Results of Surgical Therapy

As mentioned previously, the marked improvement in surgical management of ruptured intracranial lesions has rekindled interest in the surgical treatment of unruptured aneurysms in both the symptomatic and asymptomatic categories. As surgical mortality figures from ruptured intracranial lesions approach 5 percent in most aneurysm centers,[3,17,19,21,22] it would not be unreasonable to assume that corresponding figures for unruptured lesions, be they symptomatic or asymptomatic, should be significantly lower than 5 percent. Indeed, small series published throughout the 1970s and early 1980s have suggested this to be the case, with several centers reporting no mortality and very low neurological morbidity in series of 40 to 100 patients undergoing separate surgical procedures solely for obliteration of unruptured intracranial arterial aneurysms.[4,12,13,15,16] Most recently, a retrospective cooperative study of intracranial aneurysm surgery for unruptured lesions was conducted at 12 separate medical centers reporting a total of 107 patients undergoing surgery for this problem.[25] In this series there was no operative mortality and an operative morbidity of less than 7 percent, which suggests that surgical risk in such cases, when handled by experienced aneurysm surgeons, has been brought to an almost irreducible minimum level. My review of publications dealing specifically with unruptured aneurysms to date shows that mortality and morbidity figures are in the range of 1.5 and 7.5 percent, respectively.[12,13,15,16]

Significant Modifiers Affecting the Risk of Surgical Treatment

As every neurosurgeon who deals with ruptured intracranial aneurysms realizes, translation of theoretical concepts to practical technical accomplishments is often studded with problems specific to the individual case under consideration. These particular concerns deal with the peculiarities of the aneurysm itself, the patient's specific condition, and, of not the least importance, the surgeon's own experience and technical competence.

Unruptured aneurysms tend to be located with disproportionate frequency on the internal carotid artery and its proximal branches, the ophthalmic and posterior communicating arteries. Certainly these locations are ones frequently visited by the neurosurgeon in pursuit not only of aneurysms but also of other abnormalities in the parasellar area and therefore represent a familiar anatomical background, which should certainly maximize the opportunity for an optimum surgical result. Such has indeed been the case in the small published series devoted to the surgery of intracranial aneurysms, in which lesions of the internal carotid are associated with the most favorable surgical results.[4,12,13,15,16,25] Less common aneurysm sites such as the anterior communicating artery and the middle cerebral bifurcation are not surprisingly somewhat less favorable terrain, and in dealing with aneurysms of the posterior circulation, technical requirements of the surgical procedure are such that a further increase in the possibilities of intraoperative and postsurgical complications must be expected.

Similarly, aneurysms below 10 mm in size are those most amenable to complete surgical exposure and uncomplicated clip obliteration; as the aneurysm increases in size, in anatomical complexity, and in distortion of surrounding normal anatomy, a concomitant increase in the incidence of operative complications must be expected, especially when dealing with giant aneurysms greater than 2.5 cm in diameter. For adequate obliteration, these latter lesions not infrequently must be opened and evacuated of clot and atheroma to prepare a satisfactory neck for clipping, with the attendant possibilities of embolization or ischemia secondary to temporary occlusion. Furthermore, often a giant aneurysm, because of branch vessels tightly applied to its fundus, requires tedious and extensive microdissection for adequate visualization and subsequent occlusion of its broad, rigid neck. Understandably, the risks of adequate surgical treatment of such lesions must be reasonably estimated as considerably higher than those associated with smaller aneurysms.

Of equal importance in a clinical context is the condition of the patient harboring the unruptured intracranial aneurysm. In this light, serious consideration must be given to the patient's overall clinical status and life expectancy. In general, patients in poor clinical condition from a ruptured intracranial aneurysm should not undergo elective surgery for obliteration of any unruptured intracranial aneurysm until their clinical condition is such as to minimize the risk of a second intracranial procedure. Additionally, patients with other life-threatening disease processes, especially those involving the cardiovascular system, deserve special consideration prior to the recommendation of an elective procedure for the prophylactic elimination of an unruptured asymptomatic lesion, although symptomatic lesions should in general be approached in a more aggressive fashion. Although some studies suggest that symptomatic unruptured lesions most commonly tend to rupture within the initial 6 months of the onset of their symptomatology[23] (and therefore the patient's age at discovery of the lesion is relatively unimportant), other series of asymptomatic unruptured lesions demonstrate that frequently subarachnoid hemorrhage from such lesions may occur 10 or more years following the initial discovery of the aneurysm.[5,6] These reports may encourage recommendations for early surgery in the young healthy patient with a symptomatic lesion as opposed to the older more precarious survivor of a recent subarachnoid hemorrhage who harbors additional unruptured aneurysms.

Finally, as is true of every neurosurgical procedure, the surgeon must modify the results reported in the literature by an accurate evaluation of his own surgical ability. Incidental aneurysms are perhaps not best operated on by incidental aneurysm surgeons. If a frank self-appraisal of the surgeon's own clinical experience and technical expertise does not support prospective operative morbidity and mortality rates in the range of 5 and 1 percent, respectively, the elective obliteration of such lesions in this surgeon's hands may not carry a sufficiently significant improvement over their natural history to warrant their surgical treatment.

References

1. Bailey WL, Loeser JD: Intracranial aneurysms. JAMA 216:1993–1996, 1971.
2. Dell S: Asymptomatic cerebral aneurysm: Assessment of its risk of rupture. Neurosurgery 10:162–166, 1982.
3. Drake CG: Management of cerebral aneurysm. Stroke 12:273–283, 1981.
4. Drake CG, Girvin JP: The surgical treatment of subarachnoid hemorrhage with multiple aneurysms, in Morley TP (ed): *Current Controversies in Neurosurgery*. Philadelphia, Saunders, 1976, pp 274–278.
5. Heiskanen O: Risk of bleeding from unruptured aneurysms in cases with multiple intracranial aneurysms. J Neurosurg 55:524–526, 1981.
6. Heiskanen O, Marttila I: Risk of rupture of a second aneurysm in patients with multiple aneurysms. J Neurosurg 32:295–299, 1970.
7. Jane JA, Winn RH, Richardson AE: The natural history of intracranial aneurysms: Rebleeding rates during the acute and long term period and implication for surgical management. Clin Neurosurg 24:176–184, 1977.
8. Kassel NF, Torner JC: Size of intracranial aneurysms. Neurosurgery 9:466, 1981. (Abstr.)
9. Locksley HB: Natural history of subarachnoid hemorrhage, intracranial aneurysms and arteriovenous malformations: Based on 6,368 cases in the cooperative study, in Sahs AL, Perret GE, Locksley HB, Nishioka H (eds): *Intracranial Aneurysms and Subarachnoid Hemorrhage: A Cooperative Study*. Philadelphia, Lippincott, 1969, pp 37–108.
10. McCormick WF, Acosta-Rua GJ: The size of saccular aneurysms: An autopsy study. J Neurosurg 33:422–430, 1970.
11. McKissock W, Richardson A, Walsh L: Multiple intracranial aneurysms. Lancet 1:623–626, 1964.
12. Mount LA, Brisman R: Multiple intracranial aneurysms (letter). N Engl J Med 281:1307, 1969.
13. Moyes PD: Surgical treatment of multiple aneurysms and of incidentally discovered unruptured aneurysms. J Neurosurg 35:291–295, 1971.
14. Ojemann RG: Management of the unruptured intracranial aneurysm (letter). N Engl J Med 304:725–726, 1981.
15. Salazar JL: Surgical treatment of asymptomatic and incidental intracranial aneurysms. J Neurosurg 53:20–21, 1980.
16. Samson DS, Hodosh RM, Clark WK: Surgical management of unruptured asymptomatic aneurysms. J Neurosurg 46:731–734, 1977.
17. Samson DS, Hodosh RM, Reid WR, Beyer CW, Clark WK: Risk of intracranial aneurysm surgery in the good grade patient: Early versus late operation. Neurosurgery 5:422–426, 1979.
18. Sonntag VKH, Yuan RH, Stein BM: Giant intracranial aneurysms: A review of 13 cases. Surg Neurol 8:81–84, 1977.
19. Sundt TM Jr, Kobayashi S, Fode NC, Whisnant JP: Results and complications of surgical management of 809 intracranial aneurysms in 722 cases: Related and unrelated to grade of patient, type of aneurysm, and timing of surgery. J Neurosurg 56:753–765, 1982.
20. Sundt TM Jr, Piepgras DG: Surgical approach to giant intracranial aneurysms: Operative experience with 80 cases. J Neurosurg 51:731–742, 1979.
21. Sundt TM Jr, Whisnant JP: Subarachnoid hemorrhage from intracranial aneurysms: Surgical management and natural history of disease. N Engl J Med 299:116–122, 1978.
22. Suzuki J, Onuma T, Yoshimoto T: Results of early operations on cerebral aneurysms. Surg Neurol 11:407–412, 1979.
23. Wiebers DO, Whisnant JP, O'Fallon WM: The natural history of unruptured intracranial aneurysms. N Engl J Med 304:696–698, 1981.
24. Winn HR, Richardson AE, Jane JA: The long-term prognosis in untreated cerebral aneurysms: I. The incidence of late hemorrhage in cerebral aneurysm: A 10-year evaluation of 364 patients. Ann Neurol 1:358–370, 1977.
25. Wirth FP, Laws ER Jr, Piepgras D, Scott RM: Surgical treatment of incidental intracranial aneurysms. Neurosurgery 12:507–511, 1983.

174

Inflammatory Intracranial Aneurysms

John G. Frazee

Inflammatory intracranial aneurysms are divided into two forms: bacterial, which have traditionally been called mycotic aneurysms, and fungal, or true mycotic aneurysms. These lesions are uncommon but life-threatening and are often unsuspected until they produce a devastating hemorrhage. Historically, these lesions were fatal whether treated medically or surgically. However, as knowledge has increased we have developed a better understanding of which patients are at risk to develop an aneurysm, of the period for which they are at risk, and of guidelines for treatment. In this chapter I will review the available information about both forms of aneurysm and will outline the current controversies associated with treatment.

Historical Perspective

It appears that Church in 1869 first traced a causal relationship between the formation of an intracranial aneurysm and vegetative endocarditis.[4] Osler first used the term *mycotic* in his "Gulstonian Lectures on Malignant Endocarditis," given in 1885.[15] However, this term was used to refer to any process of infection and did not distinguish between bacterial and fungal infections.

Eppinger was the first to call the aneurysms associated with endocarditis *mycotic embolic*.[6] It has been only recently, most notably with Bohmfalk et al.[3] that the term *bacterial aneurysm* has been defined and substituted for mycotic aneurysm.

In 1923 Stengel and Wolferth reviewed 34 reported cases of bacterial aneurysm.[17] This was followed in 1954 by a report of 16 more by Shnider and Cotsonas.[16] The results were poor, with only 4 survivors from a group of 50 patients. In the most recent comprehensive review, Bohmfalk et al. found 85 reported cases from 1954 to 1978, with 4 of these cases being their own. The largest single hospital experience was reported by Frazee et al. in 1980,[7] bringing the total documented experience since 1954 to 95. The data for this review have been drawn from this group of 95 cases.

Bacterial Aneurysms

Patient Population

The patients reported to have bacterial aneurysms ranged in age from 7 months to 78 years. The age distribution was uniform below the sixth decade and the average age of the patients was 30 years.

When careful histories are obtained from those patients presenting with bacterial aneurysm, a majority of the patients are found to have either congenital heart disease or some other predisposing condition that might lead to bacterial endocarditis, including recent dental work, bronchitis, carious teeth, prolonged labor, and urological surgery.

Incidence

Bacterial intracranial aneurysms are thought to constitute between 6.2 and 29 percent of all intracranial aneurysms.[3] Those patients with bacterial endocarditis appear to have a risk of 4 to 15 percent of forming an intracranial aneurysm.[3] However, these figures are likely to be an underestimate of the true incidence, as some aneurysms are asymptomatic and some patients present with multiple aneurysms.

Bacteriological Studies

All the patients reported were confirmed to have bacterial aneurysms either by the association of an intracranial aneurysm with positive blood cultures and other evidence of bacterial endocarditis or by pathological study of autopsy or surgical specimens. Positive blood cultures were not substantiated in all reports, but of the 54 that were, 36 grew a *Streptococcus* species and 13 grew a *Staphylococcus* species. The remaining patients demonstrated a variety of unusual organisms, including *Neisseria*, *Enterococcus*, and *Pseudomonas*. Other, extra-arterial infections responsible for bacterial aneurysms included meningitis (six patients) and cavernous sinus thrombophlebitis (six patients).

Pathogenesis

In 1968, Nakata et al. published experimental results showing that after the introduction of bacteria into a dog aorta that had been isolated by temporary clamps above the renal arteries and at the aortic bifurcation, vascular wall destruction began in the vasa vasorum.[14] They concluded that stasis and sepsis in the vasa vasorum was a necessary initiating event for the formation of a bacterial aneurysm.

Molinari et al. pointed out that although the original site of infection might be the vasa vasorum, these are rarely present in cerebral arteries, particularly in distal branches where bacterial aneurysms are most likely to form.[11,12] Using experimental dog models with bacterial emboli introduced into the cerebral circulation, they were able to conclude that aneurysms consistently appeared at the site of the infected embolus and that the early changes in the vessel walls appeared in the adventitial layer and involved the media. Their proposal was that in the absence of the vasa vasorum, bacteria could escape through the occluded origins of thin-walled penetrating vessels to the Virchow-Robin spaces and then to the adventitia of a parent vessel. They explained that the aneurysmal enlargement was produced either by pulsation against the necrotic wall of the occluded vessel or by the same pulsation against the weakened wall of the recanalized vessel. This latter process might explain the late appearance of an aneurysm during antibiotic treatment for bacterial endocarditis.

Molinari et al. stressed the short time (1 to 3 days) between the lodging of an infected embolus in the cerebral vessel and an aneurysm formation in animals not treated with antibiotics or infected with virulent organisms. However, they also noted that if dogs were partially treated with an appropriate antibiotic, aneurysm rupture no longer regularly occurred in the 1- to 3-day period, but aneurysms were present when the dogs were killed 7 or 8 days after embolization. These results would suggest that an aneurysm may develop in patients with bacterial endocarditis in as short a period as 1 week even if the patient is treated with appropriate antibiotics.

Clinical Presentation

The neurological symptoms and signs of patients who develop bacterial intracranial aneurysms are variable but are often secondary to either septic embolization, meningitis, or subarachnoid hemorrhage. The first two produce symptoms and signs before aneurysm formation and are infectious processes that may go on to aneurysm formation as noted by Molinari et al.[11,12] The third is a direct result of aneurysm rupture and is frequently associated with disastrous results.

Most authors have expressed concern that there are no early warning signs to herald the aneurysm formation and that it is only subarachnoid hemorrhage which leads to the diagnosis. Thus, unless all patients with bacterial endocarditis undergo cerebral angiography, it is reasoned that the mortality rate cannot be reduced. Our experience suggests that most patients do present with symptoms or signs that herald the formation of a bacterial aneurysm.[7]

It has been reported that 28 to 39 percent of patients with bacterial endocarditis have some form of neurological involvement.[9] As this still constitutes a large population, it is important to select from this group of patients with neurological symptoms or signs those patients who are most likely to be at risk for aneurysm formation. In our review of 13 patients from one institution, each of the cases was noted to be accompanied by premonitory symptoms or signs suggestive of intracranial disease. In six patients who survived, these events initiated angiography. One other patient who survived had early warning symptoms and signs but angiography was not done until she suddenly became hemiplegic. The six patients who died as a direct result of intracranial hemorrhage also had warning symptoms and signs. In two patients the symptoms occurred only a few hours before catastrophic events, and it is doubtful whether early diagnostic procedures would have changed their clinical course. However, the remaining four patients had symptoms and signs days before the catastrophic event, which if correctly interpreted would have led to early angiography and definitive treatment. These results suggest that patients who develop a sudden and severe headache, focal neurological deficits, or seizures should be selected for further study, including angiography. Comparing this set of symptoms and signs with those that have been reported for the population of patients with bacterial endocarditis as a whole, we could expect that 25 to 33 percent of patients with any of these three symptoms and signs would have an angiographically demonstrable intracranial bacterial aneurysm.

Serial Angiography

Several points should be noted from a review of the literature: (1) rupture of a bacterial intracranial aneurysm may occur at any time during a 6-week course of antibiotic therapy; (2) a new aneurysm may appear in subsequent angiograms even though previous angiograms have been negative; (3) new aneurysms may appear after excision of a solitary aneurysm.

These facts emphasize the need for serial angiography throughout treatment for bacterial endocarditis. The experimental literature indicates that aneurysms may be present 7 days after a septic embolus to the brain in subjects treated with antibiotics and as early as 3 days following septic embolization in subjects not treated. The experience of our review suggests that there is a delay (averaging 10 days) from the onset of warning symptoms or signs to a catastrophic hemorrhage or to an angiographic demonstration of a cerebral aneurysm. If we assume that the early symptoms or signs are related to the lodging of the embolus in the cerebral vascular tree, then the time to formation of an aneurysm is similar to that noted in the experimental literature. Therefore, three-vessel cerebral angiography at the onset of symptoms or signs is appropriate, and it seems appropriate to repeat angiography every 7 to 10 days during a 6-week period of antibiotic therapy, even after surgical excision of one aneurysm, if aneurysms are to be detected before rupture. Some authors have suggested that this may be too aggressive an approach, citing reports that aneurysms disappear in some instances or decrease in others on follow-up angiography.[2] In fact, of the 30 patients reported to have undergone more than one angiogram, the aneurysm resolved completely in 13 patients and decreased in size in another 5 (Table 174-1). However, 10 patients showed an enlargement of the original aneurysm or the appearance of a new aneurysm. These aneurysms, therefore, appear to be unpredictable in their course and the use of serial angiography is justified in part by the high mortality rate for rupture of a bacterial aneurysm.

TABLE 174-1 Results of Serial Angiography (30 Patients)

Aneurysm resolution	13
Decreased size of aneurysm	5
Aneurysm enlargement	6
New aneurysm	4
Aneurysm excised	2

TABLE 174-2 Documented Aneurysm Location (63 Patients)

Site	% of Total
Proximal artery	
Intracavernous segment, internal carotid artery	11
Intradural segment, internal carotid artery	21
Distal artery	
Anterior cerebral artery	16
Middle cerebral artery	43
Posterior cerebral artery	9

It is important to point out that a bacterial aneurysm is more likely to be located on the distal arterial tree, with most of these occurring in the distribution of the middle cerebral artery (Table 174-2). Those patients who demonstrate a proximal aneurysm may have developed that aneurysm from cavernous thrombophlebitis, in which case the aneurysm has an intracavernous location, or from infection of a previously present proximal berry aneurysm. It is also noteworthy that multiple aneurysms are not uncommon, having been reported in 17 patients (18 percent).

So far, computed tomography has not been helpful in establishing the diagnosis of bacterial aneurysm other than to show intracranial or intracerebral hemorrhage. The more recent development of digital venous angiography may prove to be a less invasive but adequate means for demonstrating bacterial aneurysms and may in the future be an alternative to the use of serial arterial angiography.

Treatment—Surgical or Nonsurgical

The crux of the controversy surrounding the treatment of patients with bacterial intracranial aneurysms has been whether the risk of surgery is prohibitively high, particularly in light of the fact that many patients have aneurysms that either fail to rupture, become smaller, or disappear. In a review of 45 patients with intracranial bacterial aneurysms, Bingham emphasized that 11 of 21 patients followed with serial angiography had complete resolution of their aneurysms and an additional 6 patients of this group had a decrease in aneurysm size.[2] This led him to suggest serial angiography for all patients with a documented aneurysm. He recommended an operation only if the aneurysm enlarged or did not change in size after 6 weeks of antibiotic therapy. He reported that 3 of 20 patients who received only antibiotic therapy died, and 6 of 25 patients who received combined antibiotic and surgical treatment died. However, he noted that the higher mortality rate associated with operation was not a true reflection of surgical mortality, for these patients were frequently moribund at the time of operation.

Bohmfalk et al. reviewed 85 patients, 45 of whom were included in the Bingham series.[3] They noted that an aneurysm resolved completely in 11 of 25 patients treated with antibiotics alone and followed with serial angiography. This group of patients, as with Bingham's series, was a selected population and excluded the majority of patients (60 of 85, 20 of 45, respectively) who were not followed by serial angiography. Therefore, it is important to emphasize that although intracranial bacterial aneurysms do resolve or decrease in size in some patients, the mortality with antibiotic therapy alone is still high. Bohmfalk and colleagues reported that 20 of 38 patients (53 percent) in this group died. This should be compared with surgical results. Combining the results of 78 patients with known outcome, we find that 34 patients underwent surgical therapy. Of these 16 were electively operated upon, with one death, not directly attributed to the surgery, and 13 underwent emergency surgery with 8 deaths, all of which were secondary to the moribund state of the patient. This gives an overall surgical mortality of 26.5 percent. These data suggest that therapy for patients with bacterial intracranial aneurysms should consist of excision of the aneurysm as well as antibiotic treatment whenever possible.

Proximal and Multiple Aneurysms

The most recent comprehensive review has suggested that nonsurgical treatment for proximal and multiple aneurysms is the best approach, unless there is evidence of aneurysm enlargement.[3] A review of the outcome of 13 patients with proximal aneurysms, excluding those in the cavernous sinus, shows one surgical death in 3 patients and six deaths among 9 patients treated with antibiotics alone (Table 174-3). These groups are too small to allow us to draw conclusions as to the risks of therapy, but the trend seen in those patients treated with antibiotics alone suggests a high mortality for this therapy. It would again lead us toward the conclusion that the best alternative may be surgical intervention accompanied by antibiotic therapy.

The concern for cerebral infarction as a complication of excision of a proximal bacterial aneurysm is reasonable, but there are other approaches that should be examined before relying on nonsurgical therapy alone. These would include clipping of the aneurysm with a superficial temporal to middle cerebral artery bypass or trapping of the aneurysm with or without a bypass. Finally, there is the possibility of wrapping the aneurysm with muscle or muslin, but this would certainly be less than optimal therapy. The use of methyl methacrylate to coat bacterial aneurysms probably would lead to more serious trouble as this would constitute a foreign body in the face of an ongoing infection.

Patients have presented with multiple aneurysms in 17 instances (Table 174-3), 6 of which were treated surgically and 11 nonsurgically. No patient died. It is unclear why

TABLE 174-3 Treatment and Mortality for Proximal and Multiple Bacterial Aneurysms

Treatment	Total Cases	Died
Proximal aneurysms*		
Surgical	3	1
Nonsurgical	9	6
Multiple aneurysms		
Surgical	6	0
Nonsurgical	11	0†

*Treatment and outcome are unknown for one patient.
†Results of treatment for two patients are unknown.

there is no mortality in the nonsurgically treated group. However, with the generally high mortality for the nonsurgical group, these patients should be considered surgical candidates. If multiple aneurysms are unilateral, they should be excised at one operation whenever possible. If they are bilateral, the largest aneurysm or the one presumed to have bled should be excised first. An appropriate recovery period should be allowed and angiography repeated to ensure that the aneurysm is still present before further surgery is planned.

Summary

In view of the serious consequences of a ruptured bacterial aneurysm, the high morbidity and mortality with nonsurgical therapy, the low elective surgical mortality rate, and the rapid appearance of new aneurysms in some patients, aggressive management is indicated for those patients with bacterial endocarditis who develop sudden severe headache, focal neurological symptoms or signs, or seizures. Such patients should undergo cerebral angiography or digital venous angiography every 7 to 14 days. If an aneurysm is identified, it should be excised whenever possible. Finally, patients with proximal or multiple aneurysms should be considered for operation, but their therapy should be more individualized.

Fungal Aneurysms

The first case of fungal aneurysm was reported in 1968[10] and since that time only five such cases have been reported.[1,5,8,13,18] The rarity of this disease is obvious, but the widespread use of cortical steroids and immunosuppressive drugs would suggest that fungal infections, including those of cerebral arteries, will be increasing in number.

In each instance of fungal infection reported to date, the patient died from a severe, sudden, subarachnoid hemorrhage and in each case an autopsy report was available. The age of the patients varied significantly from as young as 11 to as old as 75. The group is too small to draw any conclusions about sex distribution. A primary illness that might have contributed to the formation of a cerebral aneurysm was present in at least four of the five cases. The site of the problem is much different from that of bacterial aneurysms in that it seems to involve the proximal major vessels such as the internal carotid artery or the basilar artery.

In every case except one the infecting organism was *Aspergillus*, the remaining case being due to *Penicillium*. The source of infection was by both direct extension and hematogenous spread. The autopsies demonstrated a marked inflammatory disease of the cerebral vessels with invasion of the vascular wall by the fungus either from the intimal side or from the adventitial side. The vessels showed infiltration by branching hyphae, with severe loss of the normal vascular layers.

Unlike the patients with bacterial aneurysms, these patients appear to lack significant warning symptoms or signs that would suggest intracranial disease. The disease appears to progress rapidly and is quite lethal. To date there is no report of surgical intervention for this problem, yet it would seem that the approach recommended for proximal bacterial aneurysms might be appropriate in this situation if the diagnosis could be made early. In general, however, the outlook is even dimmer for fungal aneurysms of intracranial vessels than for aneurysms of bacterial origin.

References

1. Ahuja GK, Jain N, Vijayaraghavan M, Roy S: Cerebral mycotic aneurysm of fungal origin: Case report. J Neurosurg 49:107–110, 1978.
2. Bingham WF: Treatment of mycotic intracranial aneurysms. J Neurosurg 46:428–437, 1977.
3. Bohmfalk GL, Story JL, Wissenger JP, Brown WE Jr: Bacterial intracranial aneurysms. J Neurosurg 48:369–382, 1978.
4. Church WS: Aneurysm of the right cerebral artery in a boy of thirteen. Trans Pathol Soc Lond 20:109–110, 1869.
5. Davidson P, Robertson DM: A true mycotic (*Aspergillus*) aneurysm leading to fatal subarachnoid hemorrhage in a patient with hereditary hemorrhagic telangiectasia: Case report. J Neurosurg 35:71–76, 1971.
6. Eppinger H: Pathogenesis (Histogenesis und Aetiologie) der Aneurysmen einschliesslich des Aneurysma equi verminosum. Arch Klin Chir 35:1–553, 1887.
7. Frazee JG, Cahan LD, Winter J: Bacterial intracranial aneurysms. J Neurosurg 53:633–641, 1980.
8. Horten BC, Abbott GF, Porro RS: Fungal aneurysms of intracranial vessels. Arch Neurol 33:577–579, 1976.
9. Jones RH Jr, Siekert RG, Geraci JE: Neurologic manifestations of bacterial endocarditis. Ann Intern Med 71:21–28, 1969.
10. Mahaley MS Jr, Spock A: An unusual case of intracranial aneurysm, in Smith JL (ed): *Neuro-ophthalmology*, vol 4. St Louis, CV Mosby, 1968, pp 158–166.
11. Molinari GF: Septic cerebral embolism. Stroke 3:117–122, 1972.
12. Molinari GF, Smith L, Goldstein MN, Satran R: Pathogenesis of cerebral mycotic aneurysms. Neurology 23:325–332, 1972.
13. Morriss FH Jr, Spock A: Intracranial aneurysms secondary to mycotic orbital and sinus infection: Report of a case implicating *Penicillium* as an opportunistic fungus. Am J Dis Child 119:357–362, 1970.
14. Nakata Y, Shionoya S, Kamiya K: Pathogenesis of mycotic aneurysm. Angiology 19:593–601, 1968.
15. Osler W: Gulstonian lectures on malignant endocarditis. Lancet 1:415–418, 459–464, 505–508, 1885.
16. Shnider BI, Cotsonas NJ Jr.: Embolic mycotic aneurysms, complication of bacterial endocarditis. Am J Med 16:246–255, 1954.
17. Stengel A, Wolferth CC: Mycotic (bacterial) aneurysms of intravascular origin. Arch Intern Med 31:527–554, 1923.
18. Visudhiphan P, Bunyaratavej S, Khantanaphar S: Cerebral aspergillosis: Report of three cases. J Neurosurg 38:472–476, 1973.

175

Aneurysm Treatments Other than Clipping

John F. Alksne

Although microsurgical clipping is clearly the treatment of choice for most intracranial aneurysms, other options do exist that the neurosurgeon can consider for special situations. Dott identified these possibilities during his pioneering work on aneurysms in the 1930s and 1940s: namely, suture ligation of the neck, proximal arterial occlusion, wrapping the aneurysm, and filling the aneurysm with a foreign material[5] (Figs. 175-1 and 175-2). A variety of attempts have been made to perfect these methods and there are certain situations in which they offer an advantage either to the patient in terms of outcome or to the surgeon in terms of ease of application. These will be discussed separately.

Suture Ligation of the Neck

Suture ligation of the neck of an aneurysm is actually very similar to clipping from the standpoint of exposure and dissection required. As better and more versatile aneurysm clips have been developed, the use of ligation has decreased because the clip can perform the same function with less manipulation. Nevertheless, situations can arise in which neck ligation is more applicable than clipping. For example, aneurysms of the posterior inferior cerebellar artery that are entangled with the lower cranial nerves may be difficult to clip but easy to ligate. For these situations a curved ligature carrier that can aid in passing the ligature behind the aneurysm is essential. I prefer to use 4-0 silk because it will tie easily and hold the knot without slipping.

It is recommended that the aneurysm be opened after ligation to ensure that the neck is completely occluded. If any bleeding should ensue, it is frequently possible to reinforce the ligature with a clip once the aneurysm has been collapsed.

Proximal Arterial Ligation

In 1956 Logue reported his series of 37 anterior communicating artery aneurysms treated by ligation of one anterior cerebral artery.[9] In his cases he made no attempt to dissect the aneurysm or identify its neck. Likewise, he made no attempt to isolate the arteries distal to the aneurysm for trapping. The rationale for this approach was that it is possible to expose and ligate the anterior cerebral artery with minimal brain retraction or manipulation and with reduced operative morbidity and mortality. Logue believed that by occluding the dominant feeding artery to the aneurysm as determined by preoperative angiography the risk of second rupture would be greatly reduced but that no brain ischemia would occur because of the available collateral. He emphasized that this treatment should only be considered when cross flow through the anterior communicating artery had been demonstrated on preoperative angiograms. He recommended that the occlusion be performed close to the origin of the anterior cerebral artery in order to avoid injury to the perforators. Unfortunately, there is no published long-term follow-up of Logue's patients. However, a subsequent report on a small series by Cook et al. indicates a low incidence of rebleeding (1 of 25 patients) after anterior cerebral ligation.[3]

With the advent of microsurgery and improved methods of reducing brain bulk during retraction, most neurosurgeons do not utilize this technique, although Scott indicates that the procedure was utilized up to 1973[12] and there are still situations in which the dissection of anterior communicating aneurysms is difficult and this method may be useful.

A daring parallel concept for the treatment of vertebrobasilar aneurysms was reported by Drake in 1975.[6] He performed proximal vertebral artery occlusion or basilar artery occlusion in his patients in an attempt to induce thrombosis in otherwise inoperable lesions. He obtained satisfactory results in the majority of the vertebral artery cases in spite of one operative mortality and one fatal rerupture but a generally unsatisfactory outcome in the patients with basilar artery ligation. The long-term usefulness of this method remains to be proved.

Wrapping the Aneurysm

Since Dott's first report of wrapping an intracranial aneurysm with muscle, neurosurgeons have used a wide variety of encasing materials. Selverstone and Ronis introduced the concept of plastic coating in 1958 with the introduction of vinyl copolymers.[13] His technique requires a dry field and the application of the material as a spray to a completely dissected aneurysm. Mount and Antunes[10] modified this technique by first wrapping the aneurysm with muslin as suggested by Gillingham[8] and then reinforcing with polymer. They found that muslin plus plastic was definitely superior to muscle, which degenerated, allowing delayed rupture.

Yashon et al. considered the use of a cyanoacrylate adhe-

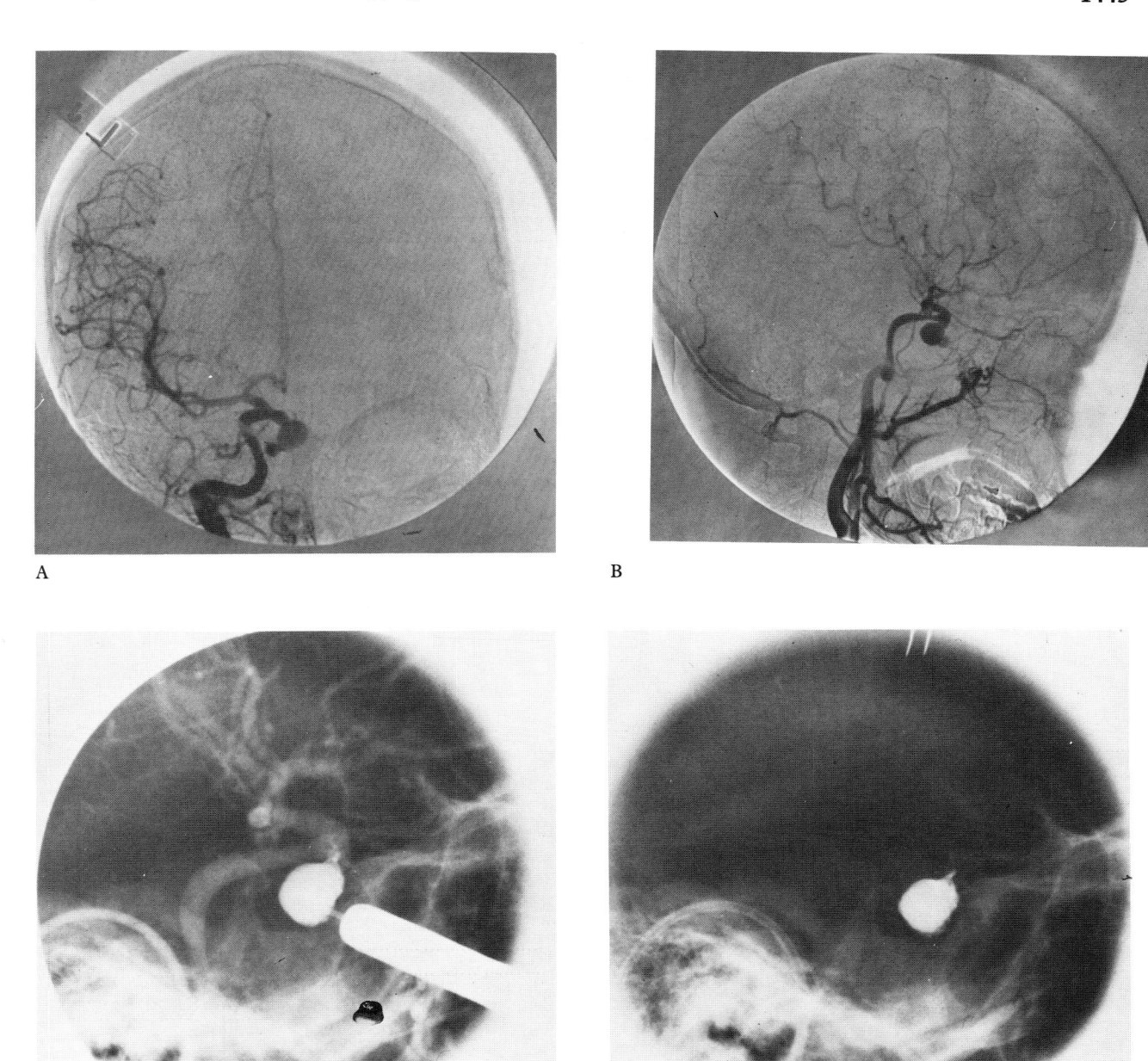

Figure 175-1 Roentgenograms of a 13-year-old girl who presented to the emergency room with massive epistaxis requiring transfusions. *A.* An anteroposterior angiogram shows an aneurysm arising from the internal carotid artery and projecting into the region of the sella turcica. *B.* The lateral angiogram shows the internal carotid aneurysm in the sella with a daughter aneurysm projecting into the region of the sphenoid sinus. *C.* A photograph of the fluoroscopic angiogram made in the operating room shows the magnetic probe, which has been placed stereotactically into the sphenoid sinus adjacent to the internal carotid aneurysm. A short needle projects from the end of the magnetic probe and enters the aneurysm, which has been filled with a radiopaque iron-acrylic mixture. The angiographic contrast medium demonstrates the patency of the carotid artery and its branches. *D.* A lateral x-ray film of the skull shows persistence of the iron-acrylic mixture in the aneurysm. The patient has had no further symptoms from the aneurysm and has returned to normal activities with no neurological deficit.

A

B

C

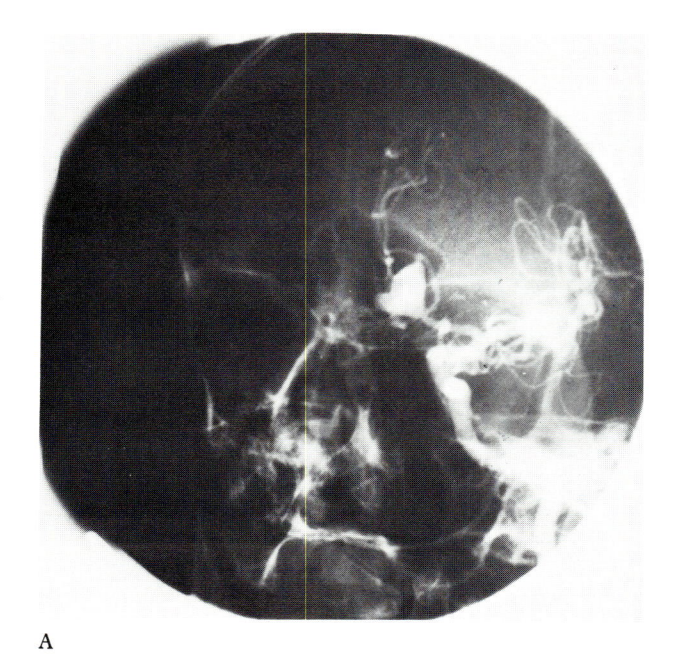

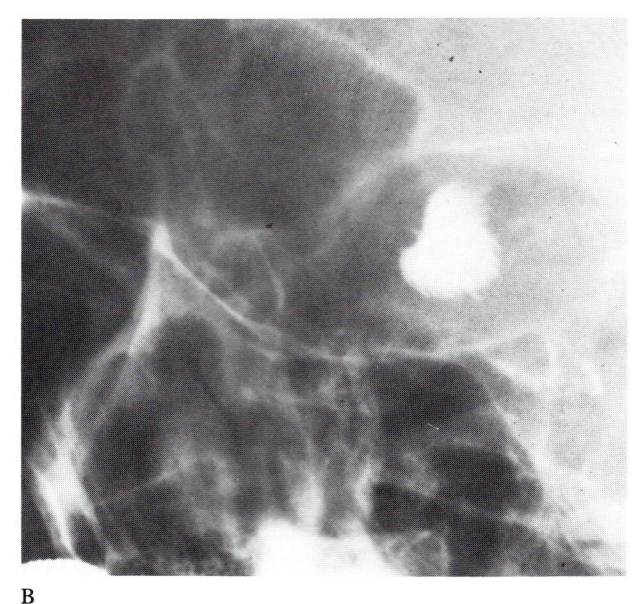

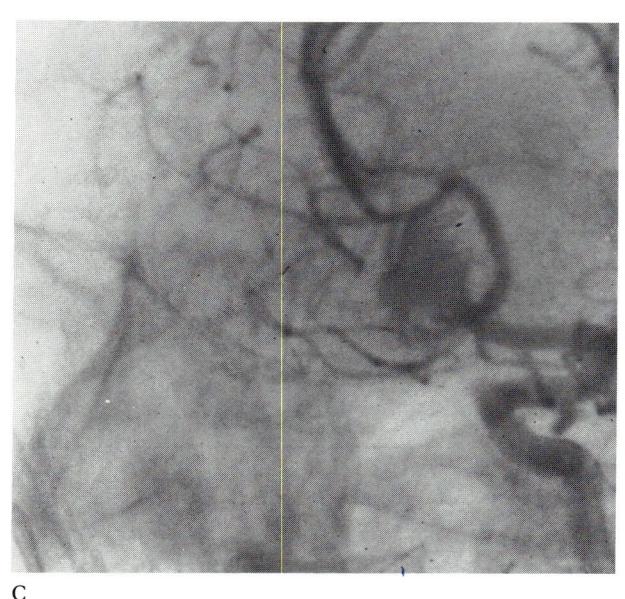

Figure 175-2 Roentgenograms of a 50-year-old man who had a subarachnoid hemorrhage while convalescing from a major myocardial infarction. His cardiac surgeon would not proceed with bypass grafting until his aneurysm was repaired. His neurosurgeon was hesitant to perform a craniotomy because of his compromised cardiac status. Therefore, he was referred for stereotactic thrombosis. *A*. The preoperative angiogram shows a large anterior communicating artery aneurysm. *B*. A postoperative skull film shows the iron-acrylic mixture within the aneurysm; note the radiating pattern of the iron, which follows the magnetic lines of force. *C*. A follow-up subtraction angiogram shows obliteration of the aneurysm with patency of the anterior cerebral artery. The patient subsequently underwent coronary artery grafting and is doing well with no neurological deficit.

sive superior because this material can be applied to a moist field.[16] In addition, they recommended the use of oxidized regenerated cellulose (Surgicel, Johnson & Johnson Products Inc., New Brunswick, N.J.) as a reinforcing matrix. This is my preference because of the ease of application and the availability of materials. However, reports have appeared recently that point out the irritating effects of cyanoacrylate adhesives on neural and vascular tissues.[2] Therefore, it appears preferable to limit the adhesive to contact with the aneurysm fundus where an inflammatory thickening is actually desired. The neighboring blood vessels should be protected from the adhesive by moist Gelfoam (absorbable gelatin sponge, The Upjohn Company, Kalamazoo, Mich.).

Wrapping of an aneurysm is indicated whenever the application of a clip or ligature would compromise essential blood vessels. It is preferable to dissect out the entire aneurysm so that all aspects of the fundus can be exposed because the most common cause of failure after wrapping is hemorrhage from a point of the aneurysm that was not adequately reinforced.

Filling the Aneurysm

The concept of injecting materials into intracranial aneurysms was a natural outgrowth of Dott's original idea of opening an aneurysm and packing it with muscle. The objective of all subsequent efforts has been to obliterate the interior of the aneurysm and thereby render it incapable of further enlargement or bleeding.

Gallagher was the first to report injection through the wall of an aneurysm.[7] He developed an air gun to inject "hog hair" through the intact aneurysmal dome and induce internal thrombosis. All Gallagher's procedures were performed after operative exposure of the aneurysm. There have been no recent reports utilizing this method so one can presume it has been abandoned.

Mullan was the first to develop stereotactic aneurysm thrombosis.[11] He inserted fine wires into the aneurysmal fundus utilizing x-ray control and induced thrombosis by passage of an electric current. This technique was effective for small aneurysms but required multiple electrode insertions for larger lesions. Unfortunately, the induced thrombosis was frequently not permanent.

Alksne and Smith followed Mullan's lead but injected a liquid iron suspension into the aneurysm, which was held in place by a magnet until it solidified.[1,15] Initially the iron particles were suspended in an albumin solution, but subsequently they have been mixed with polymerizing methyl methacrylate to minimize embolization and ensure rapid solidification. Although the stereotactic methods have given encouraging results, they have not gained wide acceptance, probably because of concurrent marked improvements in microsurgical clipping and because of the highly technical nature of the procedures, requiring extensive instrumentation. Nevertheless, the stereotactic methods may be beneficial for some patients who have aneurysms that are not readily treated by conventional means, such as those within the sella (Fig. 175-1), or for those patients who are considered at high risk for open craniotomy (Fig. 175-2).

The idea of treating an aneurysm without craniotomy by approaching the lesion through the arterial system is an intriguing potential refinement of the filling concept. Serbinenko first reported the occlusion of an intracranial aneurysm using a transvascular detachable balloon.[14] Subsequently, Debrun et al. reported a small series of such cases in conjunction with a larger series of carotid-cavernous fistulas.[4] The technical problems of keeping the balloon within the aneurysm and the fear of rupturing the aneurysm by overinflation of the balloon have essentially forced the abandonment of this technique except in very special circumstances. This does not mean that future improvements may not be made that would make the transvascular approach to aneurysms feasible.

References

1. Alksne JF, Smith RW: Stereotaxic occlusion of 22 consecutive anterior communicating artery aneurysms. J Neurosurg 52:790–793, 1980.
2. Chou SN: Use of cyanoacrylates (letter). J Neurosurg 46:266, 1977.
3. Cook AW, Dooley DM, Browder EJ: Anterior communicating aneurysms: Treatment by ligation of an anterior cerebral artery. J Neurosurg 23:371–374, 1965.
4. Debrun G, Lacour P, Caron JP, Hurth M, Comoy J, Keravel Y: Detachable balloon and calibrated-leak balloon techniques in the treatment of cerebral vascular lesions. J Neurosurg 49:635–649, 1978.
5. Dott NM: Intracranial aneurysmal formations. Clin Neurosurg 16:1–16, 1969.
6. Drake CG: Ligation of the vertebral (unilateral or bilateral) or basilar artery in the treatment of large intracranial aneurysms. J Neurosurg 43:255–274, 1975.
7. Gallagher JP: Pilojection for intracranial aneurysms. J Neurosurg 21:129–134, 1964.
8. Gillingham FJ: The management of ruptured intracranial aneurysm. Hunterian lecture. Ann R Coll Surg Engl 23:89–117, 1958.
9. Logue V: Surgery in spontaneous subarachnoid haemorrhage. Br Med J 1:473–479, 1956.
10. Mount LA, Antunes JL: Results of treatment of intracranial aneurysms by wrapping and coating. J Neurosurg 42:189–193, 1975.
11. Mullan S, Raimondi AJ, Dobben G, Vailati G, Hekmatpanah J: Electrically induced thrombosis in intracranial aneurysms. J Neurosurg 22:539–547, 1965.
12. Scott M: Ligation of an anterior cerebral artery for aneurysms of the anterior communicating artery complex. J Neurosurg 38:481–487, 1973.
13. Selverstone B, Ronis N: Coating and reinforcement of intracranial aneurysms with synthetic resins. Bull Tufts N Engl Med Center 4:8–12, 1958.
14. Serbinenko FA: Balloon catheterization and occlusion of major cerebral vessels. J Neurosurg 41:125–145, 1974.
15. Smith RW, Alksne JF: Stereotaxic thrombosis of inaccessible intracranial aneurysms. J Neurosurg 47:833–839, 1977.
16. Yashon D, White RJ, Arias BA, Hegarty WE: Cyanoacrylate encasement of intracranial aneurysms. J Neurosurg 34:709–713, 1971.

SECTION C

Vascular Malformations and Fistulas

176

Intracranial Arteriovenous Malformations

H. D. Garretson

Historical Review

Intracranial arteriovenous malformations were studied and classified as early as the mid-1800s (Luschka, 1854; Virchow, 1863), with the first surgical exposure of an arteriovenous malformation by Giordano occurring about three decades later in 1890.[43,52,72] Fedor Krause attempted to surgically eliminate an arteriovenous malformation by ligating its feeding arteries in 1908,[34] but Olivecrona appears to have been the first to actually completely excise a cerebral arteriovenous malformation (AVM) in 1932 and later a cerebellar AVM in 1938.[17] Except at a few major centers, however, an aggressive surgical approach to the larger examples of these lesions has awaited the major technological advances of neurological surgery, neuroradiology, and neuroanesthesia during the past two decades.

Embryologic Basis of Arteriovenous Malformations

Arteriovenous malformations of the brain are congenital lesions most likely developing during the late somite stages of the fourth week of embryonic life and almost certainly no later than the eighth week. The primary pathological lesion consists of one or more persisting direct connections between the arterial inflow and venous outflow without an intervening capillary bed.

Early in the third week of embryonic life, cells (angioblasts) begin to differentiate from the mesoderm, forming small, syncytial islands.[54,64] These small clumps of syncytial cells develop tiny sprouts that extend to interconnect the cell groups, forming a syncytial plexus. Intercellular clefts appear within the syncytial masses.[49] These clefts fuse to form the primitive vascular lumen. The syncytial cells enveloping these clefts become the endothelium of the new vessels. Proliferative growth of this endothelium links the vascular lumina into a continuous irregular endothelial vascular meshwork over the surface of the developing brain. Further extension of this primitive network, present over the developing telencephalon of human embryos at 4 weeks of age, occurs through endothelial sprouting. Sabin has described a fascinating alternative process for the development of the primitive vascular plexus.[54] She observed the appearance of intracellular vacuoles which coalesced to form the future vascular lumen, with the liquid of the vacuole becoming the primitive plasma. According to this schema, the first primitive vascular lumen is embryologically an intracellular structure, with the syncytial cells containing these interconnected vacuoles forming the primitive vascular endothelium.

The primordial vascular plexus first differentiates into afferent, efferent, and capillary components over the more rostral portion of the embryonic brain. The more superficial portion of the plexus forms larger vascular channels, eventually evolving into the arteries and veins, with the deeper portion resolving into the capillary component more closely attached to the brain surface. Beginning circulation to the brain appears around the end of the fourth week of embryonic life. Arteriovenous malformations arise from persistent direct connections between the future arterial and venous sides of the primitive vascular plexus, with failure to develop an interposed capillary network.

During the sixth and seventh weeks the third pair of aortic arches, together with the dorsal aorta, transform into the primitive internal carotid arteries, with the first and second arches undergoing early involution. The vertebral arteries arise from a longitudinal linkage of the dorsal rami of the intersegmental arteries of the neck during the fourth week. All the original proximal intersegmental artery stalks except the most caudal one atrophy, resulting in a longitudinal vessel taking origin along with the subclavian from the sixth cervical intersegmental artery. The vertebral artery establishes communication with the internal carotids through the basilar artery, which arises independently through the consolidation of two longitudinal vascular channels beneath the brain. This linkage is established by the sixth week of fetal life. Between the sixth and eighth week of fetal life, a compartmentalized brain, dural, and extracranial circulation has been established.[64] By the eighth week of fetal life the major venous sinus pattern of the adult has begun to emerge.

Pathological Classification of Arteriovenous Malformations

The development of cerebral angiography catalyzed interest in and the study of intracranial vascular anomalies, providing the first major new insights into the pathophysiology of these lesions. The first major classification of intracranial vascular malformations, used extensively in the older European literature, consisted of four overall categories: (1) angioma cavernosum, (2) angioma racemosum, (3) angioreticuloma, and (4) angioglioma.[5,18] Angioma racemosum included the subheadings of (a) telangiectasis, (b) Sturge-Weber syndrome, (c) angioma racemosum arteriale, (d) angioma racemosum venosum, and (e) arteriovenous aneurysm. The term "arteriovenous aneurysm" corresponds to our current designation "arteriovenous malformation."

McCormick in 1966 proposed a more clinically oriented categorization into five pathological types: (1) telangiectasia, (2) varix, (3) cavernous angioma, (4) arteriovenous malformation, and (5) venous angioma.[45] Telangiectasias are capillary angiomas, usually small and solitary and most frequently occurring in the pons and the roof of the fourth ventricle. They are only occasionally associated with hemorrhage. A varix is usually quite small and is occasionally invisible grossly, consisting of one or more dilated veins not associated with an arteriovenous shunt. These small lesions, found in either the parenchyma or the leptomeninges, may be associated with hemorrhage, occasionally massive. Cavernous angiomas are dilated sinusoidal vascular anomalies varying in size or diameter from 1 mm up to many centimeters and are occasionally associated with hemorrhage as well as seizures. They occur most often in the cerebrum but may occur in any part of the central nervous system. Brain parenchyma is absent between the sinusoidal vascular spaces. Calcium deposition and hyalinization of the vessel walls are common. Spontaneous thrombosis of either part or all of the lesions may occur. The blood in a cavernous angioma is not arterialized. The term *venous angioma* defines a malformation consisting entirely of veins not associated with an arteriovenous shunt, though otherwise closely resembling an arteriovenous malformation in gross appearance. They occur somewhat more commonly in the spinal cord than in the brain.

The term *arteriovenous malformation*, the primary topic of this section, refers to a congenital maldevelopment of blood vessels, with preservation of one or more primitive direct communications between otherwise normal arterial and venous channels. The malformations are found throughout the central nervous system, occurring most commonly in the cerebral hemispheres, with from 70 to 93 percent found in the supratentorial structures in various reported series.[8,47,51,52] Arteriovenous malformations of the cerebral hemispheres most frequently involve the distribution of the middle cerebral arterial tree, followed in declining frequency by those of the anterior and then the posterior cerebral arteries. Hemispheral arteriovenous malformations can be further subclassified into those involving either one or a combination of the epicerebral, the transcerebral and the subependymal circulations.

The epicerebral circulation consists of short perforating branches arising from the small pial arteries on the cortical surface and penetrating the cortex more or less at right angles to the brain surface (Fig. 176-1).[57] They form a distinct palisade of parallel short arteries of varying length, supplying the superficial, middle, and deep layers of the cortex. These slender cortical arteries show a grapnel-like pattern of branching, spreading outward and back upward toward the cortical surface as they terminate in a capillary bed. The longer transcerebral arteries, averaging 2 to 3 cm in length, traverse the cortex to feed an elongated capillary mesh or plexus paralleling the transcerebral arteries in the white matter. The transcerebral arteries terminate in the periventricular plexus.

Paralleling the arterial pattern, the venous drainage of the epicerebral circulation courses back outward to the veins on the pial surface.[58] The venous drainage of the transcerebral arterial circulation is predominantly inward toward the subependymal venous plexus of the lateral ventricles, though anastomotic connections with and associated flow to the epicerebral veins are also present.

Malformations involving only the transcerebral arteries are not visible on the cortical surface, although it is common to see arterialized venous channels on the pial surface of the cortex as a result of the anastomotic connections between the transcerebral and epicerebral venous drainages.

Pathology

The gross appearance of an arteriovenous malformation is that of a tangled mass of dilated tortuous vessels (Fig. 176-2). Small areas of hemosiderin staining and thickened, milky appearing pia-arachnoid are common in the immediate vicinity of the lesion in older patients. If the transcerebral circulation is involved in the malformation, the lesion presents a characteristic wedge-shaped appearance with the apex of the wedge at the ependymal surface of the lateral ventricle and the base of the wedge parallel to the overlying cerebral convexity (Figs. 176-3 and 176-4). There is a rare but surgically very favorable group of arteriovenous malformations limited entirely to the pial surface of the brainstem.[12]

Arteries emptying into the malformation become passively enlarged with time secondary to the high flow volume resulting from the abnormally low peripheral resistance of the A-V shunt.[11,20,21,23] The venous system draining the shunt similarly undergoes progressive enlargement with increasing tortuosity as a result of the high flow volume and sustained increased venous pressure produced by the arteriovenous shunt. Atrophic changes of the cortex and subcortical white matter in the immediate vicinity of the malformation are also common findings in the older patient. Secondary changes with time have been found in the arterial

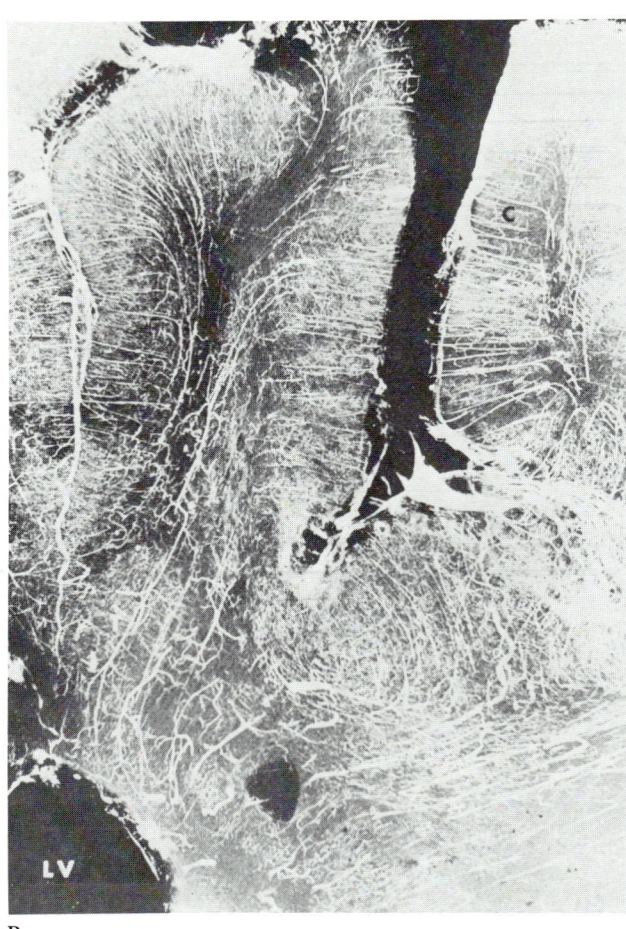

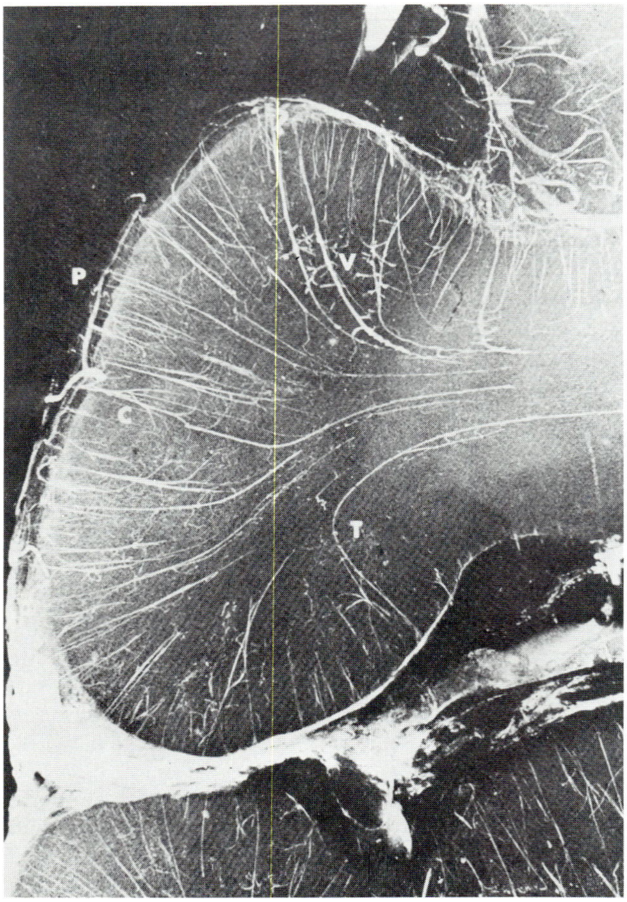

Figure 176-1 *A.* Postmortem radiography of an intra-arterial micropaque barium injection (human cortex, ×11) showing short perforating epicerebral arteries (c) with "grapnel-like" endings, and sweeping curves of the transcerebral arteries (T). Several veins (V) are also filled. P, pial artery. *B.* Convergence of transcerebral arteries (T) on the periventricular vascular plexus (coronal section, ×5). LV, lateral ventricle. (From Saunders et al.[57])

walls of the feeding arteries in the immediate vicinity of the malformation, with collagenous replacement of the normal smooth muscle component of the media.[21] Saccular aneurysms are an associated finding in between 10 and 15 percent of patients with arteriovenous malformations.[29,33,48] Between 60 and 95 percent of these aneurysms occur on arteries hemodynamically related to the arteriovenous malformation.

The external carotid artery may make a significant flow contribution to a cerebral arteriovenous malformation and occasionally may be the sole source of arterial inflow to the lesion.[9,14,53]

Incidence; Age and Sex Distribution

The cooperative study on intracranial aneurysms and arteriovenous malformations suggested that the frequency of intracranial arteriovenous malformations is about one-seventh that of saccular aneurysms.[51] This would indicate that about 0.14 percent of the U.S. population, or approximately 280,000 individuals, harbor one of these lesions in a given year. The majority of lesions become symptomatic by the age of 40 and in most large series show no predilection for either sex. Although occasional reports of familial incidence are found in the literature, the larger series show no familial or genetic predisposition.[1,47,51]

Clinical Features

In adult life the first symptom of an arteriovenous malformation is usually either a hemorrhage or a seizure. These two types of presentation occur with about equal frequency. The average age of onset for epilepsy as the initial symptom is about age 25, with age 30 the corresponding figure for hemorrhage.[17,61] Patients with large arteriovenous malformations are over twice as likely to have seizures in contrast

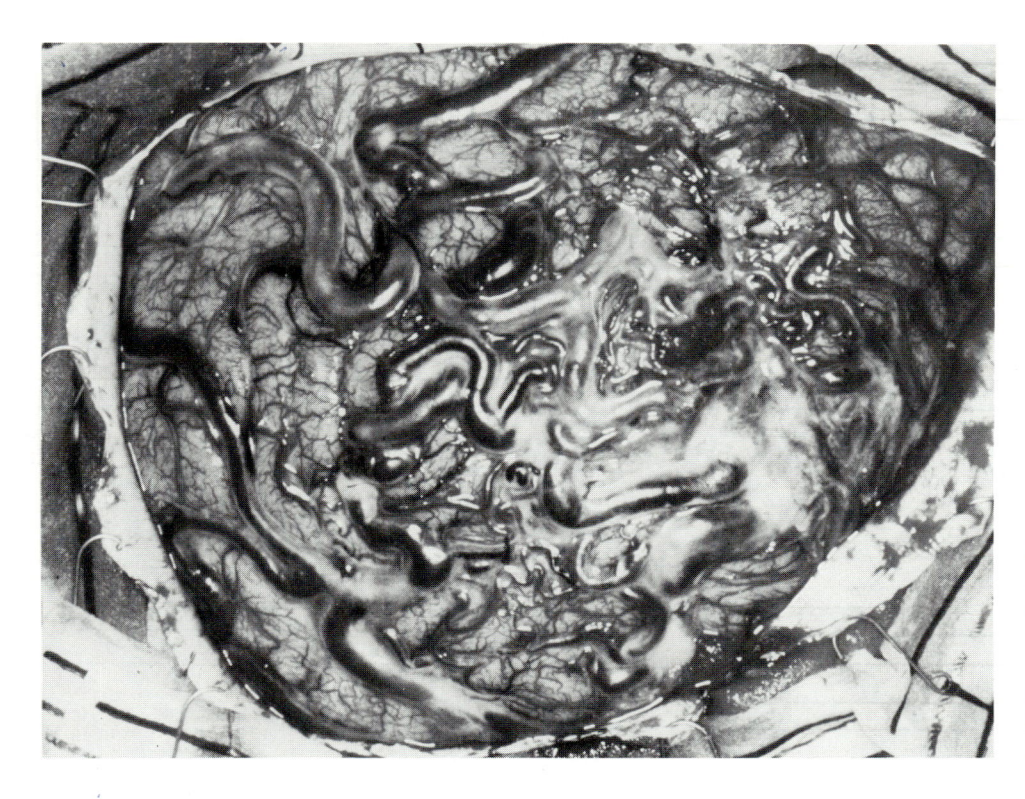

Figure 176-2 A parietal AVM involving both the epicerebral and transcerebral circulations with thickened pia-arachnoid and interstitial scarring from small, old focal hemorrhages.

to hemorrhage as their initial symptom, whereas the reverse is found for small lesions.[73]

The reported incidence of headache from an arteriovenous malformation as an early symptom before the onset of either seizures or a hemorrhage ranges from 5 to 35 percent.[52,65,67] A pseudotumor syndrome secondary to elevated venous sinus pressure from large arteriovenous shunts, particularly if the shunts are near the torcular and transverse sinus, and hydrocephalus as a sequela to previously undiagnosed small subarachnoid hemorrhages are less common as a presenting feature.[70,74] Arteriovenous malformations may occasionally mimic a demyelinating disease or brain tumor, particularly when located in the brain stem or deep basal ganglia.[7] Intellectual deterioration tends to occur with large AVMs in the older age groups. This deterioration appears to be at least partially related to a cerebral steal phenomenon.[16,75]

In children, hemorrhage is seven times more likely than a seizure to be the initial presenting event.[28] An additional common presentation of an arteriovenous malformation in the neonatal period is high-output left ventricular cardiac failure. Detailed hemodynamic studies have shown that right heart failure may evolve as an additional complicating factor secondary to right side overload from the left to right shunt.[37]

The clinical course of an arteriovenous malformation, apart from hemorrhage, is usually one of slowly progressing symptomatology referable to the site of the lesion. The mortality rate from hemorrhage in the cooperative study of 453 patients was 10 percent from the initial bleeding episode, 13 percent from a second, and 20 percent from a third.[51] The risk of recurrent hemorrhage after an initial bleeding episode is between 3.5 and 4.0 percent per year.[13,51,65] The risk of hemorrhage in a patient presenting with cerebral seizures but with no known previous hemorrhage has been variously reported as between 1 and 2.3 percent per year.[17,51] Forster et al. found, in a 15-year average follow-up of 35 patients presenting with epilepsy alone, a 17 percent mortality and 20 percent severe disability secondary to hemorrhage.[17] They further noted that if the patient had had one hemorrhage, there was a 25 percent risk of rebleeding over the next 4 years. If there had been two previous hemorrhages, the risk for further rebleeding was 25 percent within the year following the most recent hemorrhage. A review of 137 patients treated conservatively with a follow-up period ranging from a minimum of 10 years to a maximum of 25 years found only 20 percent of the 137 alive and well at the end of the study. Thirty-seven patients either had died or were severely incapacitated by the arteriovenous malformation.[68]

Vascular malformations presenting during pregnancy pose a special problem. They are more likely to rehemorrhage than those in the nonpregnant patient, with the frequency of rebleeding approaching that of saccular aneurysms.[69] The posthemorrhage mortality and morbidity figures, however, remain significantly lower than those for saccular aneurysms and comparable with those for the nonpregnant individual. Surprisingly, the timing of rebleeding does not appear to peak or parallel the cardiovascular changes in pregnancy. The peak incidence of hemorrhage from AVMs occurs between the fifteenth and twentieth week of pregnancy as compared with the peak incidence of aneurysm rebleeding between the thirteenth and fourteenth week of gestation. Only 2 of 77 AVM hemorrhages during pregnancy in this series occurred during labor. Elective cesarian section at 38 weeks gestation was felt to carry the smallest combined risk to mother and child.

1452   Vascular Diseases of the Nervous System

ning of therapy and assessment of risks to the patient. Computed tomographic (CT) scanning with current fourth-generation scanners is rapidly becoming a common screening technique for the diagnosis of vascular malformations (Fig. 176-6). Angiographically occult AVMs have been found on CT scans. Intracerebral hemorrhage enhancing on CT scan, even when arteriography fails to demonstrate a vascular anomaly, should raise the suspicion of the presence of a small AVM.[6,38] CT scanning does not presently reveal the anatomical detail necessary for surgical planning and does not reliably disclose the presence of associated vascular anomalies such as saccular aneurysms.

In a group of 43 patients with AVMs studied with unenhanced, enhanced, and 1-h postcontrast scans, the precontrast scan was abnormal in 81 percent of patients.[30] Two patients showed a venous angioma on the immediate postcontrast scan, which was not apparent on either the precontrast or the 1-h delayed scan. The 1-h delayed scan revealed one angiographically occult, thrombosed AVM not seen on the precontrast or immediate postcontrast scan. The 1-h delayed scan also showed additional pathological changes in areas adjacent to the lesions shown on the precontrast and immediate postcontrast scans. Delayed high-contrast CT scanning was judged to show no advantage as the routine screening procedure and, if done as a sole procedure, might miss at least some venous angiomas.

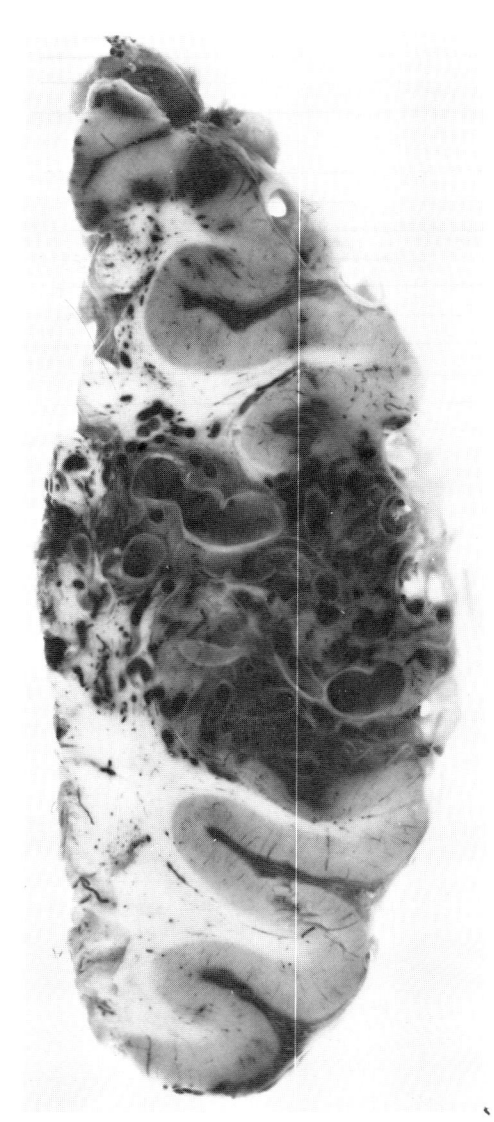

Figure 176-3 Pathological specimen of a well-defined right frontal arteriovenous malformation showing that it tapers as it extends into the white matter toward the lateral ventricle. (From Burger PC, Vogel FS: *Surgical Pathology of the Nervous System and Its Coverings*, 2d ed. New York, Wiley, 1982, p. 415.)

wedge shaped.

Occasional spontaneous disappearance of intracranial arteriovenous malformations has been reported, but this remains a very rare occurrence.[36,56]

Radiology

Cerebral angiography continues to be the definitive study for the assessment of intracranial vascular malformations (Fig. 176-5). Careful bilateral carotid as well as vertebral angiography often demonstrates unexpected crossover or collateral filling of AVMs and is essential for adequate plan-

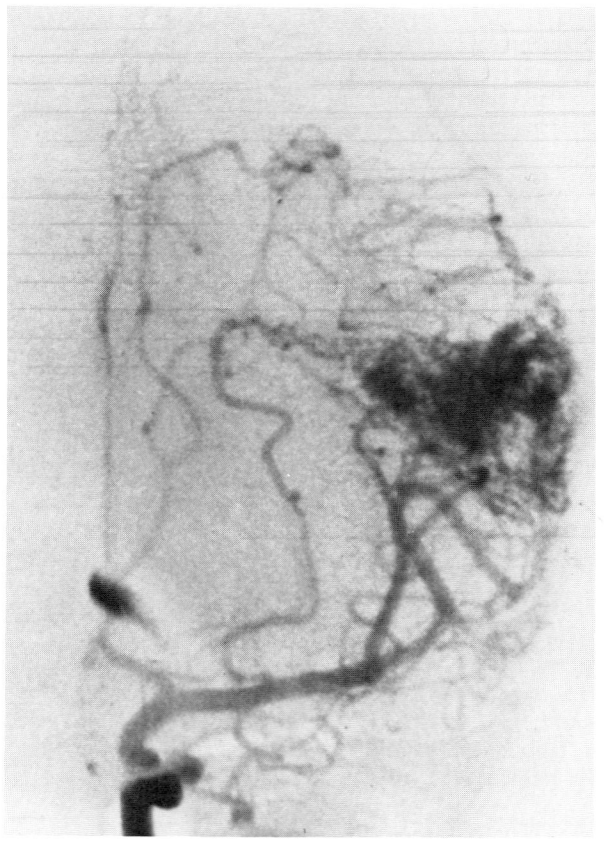

Figure 176-4 Early angiographic phase of a left central prerolandic AVM with a characteristic wedge appearance, involving both the epicerebral and transcerebral circulations.

Intracranial Arteriovenous Malformations

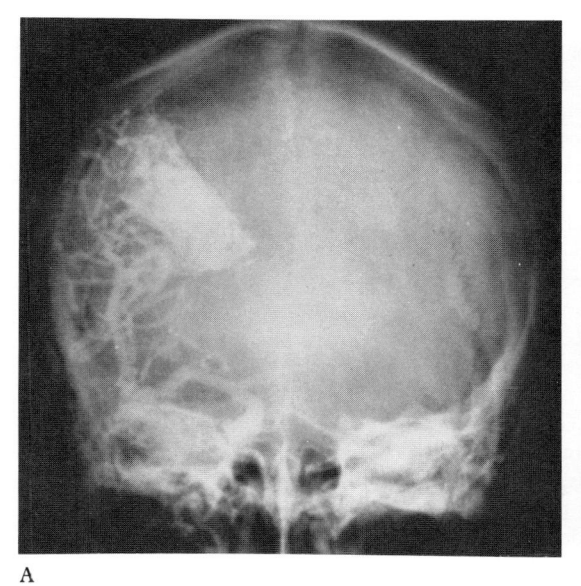

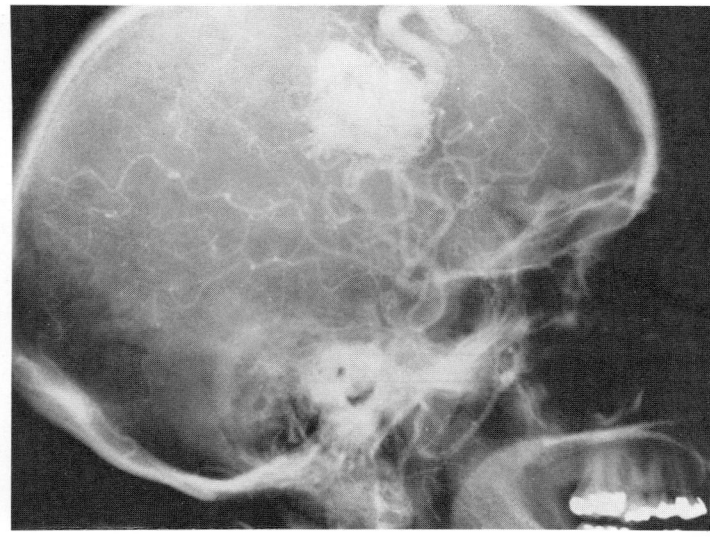

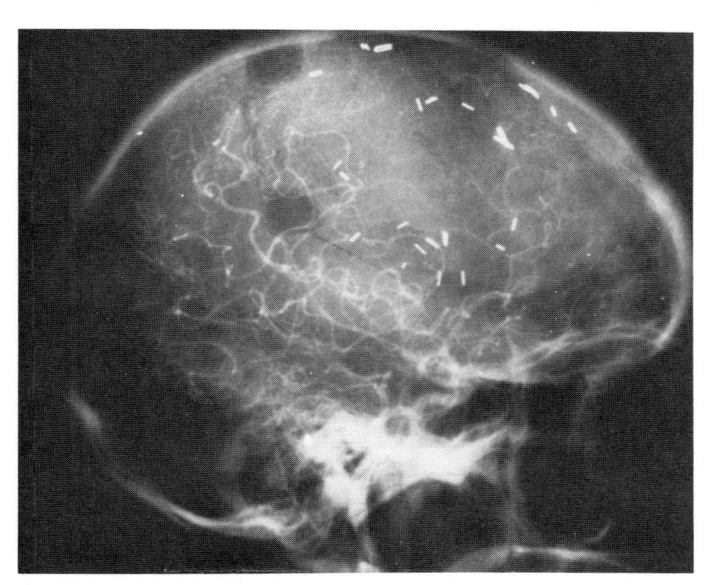

Figure 176-5 Anteroposterior (*A*) and lateral (*B*) views of a right carotid angiogram showing the early filling phase of a right posterior frontal AVM. *C.* A postoperative carotid angiogram to document surgical removal in this neurologically intact patient.

Indications for Operation

The role of surgery in the clinical management of a given patient is based on a composite of the probable natural history of the patient's future clinical course, the risk of surgical management with particular reference to the patient's required occupational or daily activities, and finally, the patient's age. Patients in the older age group with seizures but who are otherwise neurologically intact and without a previous history of hemorrhage have comparatively a smaller cumulative risk of major morbidity and mortality with continued conservative management. An important factor in long-term planning for the younger patient is the problem that seizure foci secondary to AVMs tend to become progressively more resistant to medical management with the passage of time. Although most current surgical series show some reduction in seizure tendency after malformation excision, extirpation of the malformation more importantly may block the further development of medically intractable seizure activity. In the younger patient, as is discussed in more detail below, the risk of mortality or major morbidity with surgery using current techniques is competitive with the 10-year prognosis for lesions that have not bled, and is better than the 5-year prognosis for malformations with a previous history of at least one hemorrhage. Malformations in areas of eloquent function are being found increasingly amenable to a surgical approach, with mortality or major morbidity risks of 10 percent or less.[23,24] Deep lesions involving the internal capsule, thalamus, midbrain, and lower brain stem are still usually found to be inoperable in terms of acceptable risks to neurological function.

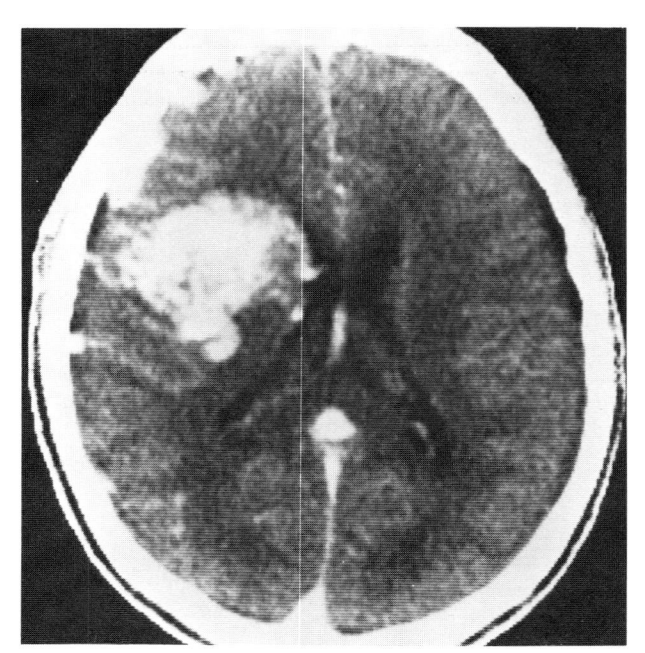

Figure 176-6 An enhanced CT scan showing cortical arterial inflow toward, and engorged cortical and deep venous drainage from, a right frontal AVM.

Assessment of Operability

Key factors in determining operability of a vascular malformation are the location of the lesion, the number and size of feeding arteries to the shunt, and the age of the patient. The size of vessels to the lesion is more important than the number, although a large number of small feeding arteries can make the surgical procedure more tedious. However, if the vessels are not only numerous but large, the hydraulic shock produced by the sudden conversion of a low-resistance high-flow system to a high-resistance low-flow status, with the associated abrupt rise in intraluminal pressure of the already passively dilated proximal arteries, results in major vasocongestion around the margins of the excision.[20,21,50,60] The more proximal arteriolar branches to the normal cortex arising from a parent artery emptying into an A-V fistula have been functioning at a lower-than-normal perfusion pressure since birth or early life. The abrupt obliteration of the low-pressure sump effect of the A-V fistula results in the sudden appearance of an abnormally high pressure head in the parent artery which is delivered to its side branches to the normal cortex. Breakthrough bleeding and massive cerebral swelling around the margins of the excision may occur in association with this phenomenon. Structural changes in the feeding arteries proximal to the AVMs in older patients have been reported, which may interfere with the ability of the proximal artery to return to normal caliber.[21] This decrease in arterial lumen size contributes to the return of peripheral resistance in the proximal vascular tree back toward normal and lowers the intraluminal pressure head at the level of the cerebral cortex. Patients past the fourth decade of life may experience a significantly more stormy course because of these structural vascular changes. Accordingly, if an AVM is to be excised, it is better to excise it at as young an age as is possible.[21,23]

Assessment of operability has been attempted through anatomical grading of AVMs. Luessenhop and Gennarelli proposed a numerical grading of 1 through 4, dependent on the number of feeding arteries of sufficient anatomical size and consistent presence to have acquired generally accepted nomenclature.[40] They have indicated that malformations receiving arterial inflow from four such named vessels are generally inoperable. There appear to be, however, in some series a significant number of exceptions to this rule.

Malformation grading for hemispheral lesions has been suggested.[22] The grading incorporates a letter designation indicating involvement of the epicerebral, transcerebral, or choroidal/subependymal circulations, followed by an Arabic number indicating the number of proximal major (circle of Willis) arterial trunks contributing flow to the malformation, with a final Roman numeral modifier indicating the decade of life of the patient (Table 176-1).[22] The anterior and posterior choroidal arteries are considered as individually counted major vessels, and the ganglionic branches of the middle cerebral are collectively counted as an additional "one." This appears to provide a useful picture or "feel" for individual lesions. Additionally, a surgical index can be derived by assigning a cumulative numerical value to these factors. With this schema, by assigning a value of 1 to 3 for the epicerebral, transcerebral, and choroidal circulation designations, a graded surgical index of increasing difficulty is produced, with a value of between 10 and 12 approaching the upper limits of reasonably safe surgical resectability. For example, a malformation involving both the epicerebral and the transcerebral circulations with flow derived from both proximal anterior cerebral arteries and the ipsilateral middle cerebral artery in a 48-year-old patient would be cataloged as AB:3:IV (10). The inclusion of patient age in the surgical equation for resectability is important for reasons discussed above in this section.

Role of Embolization

Embolization of larger AVMs has become an important therapeutic adjunct to their surgical management.[3,4,10,27,39,41,46,55] The large majority of these lesions to

TABLE 176-1 AVM Classification for Hemispheral Lesions

Arterial Circulation Involved	Specific Major Arterial Feeders Counted	Patient's Age (Decade)
A. Epicerebral	Anterior cerebral	
	Middle cerebral	
	Posterior cerebral	
B. Transcerebral	Anterior choroidal	I–X
	Posterior choroidal	
C. Choroidal	Ganglionic middle cerebral	
	Any additional arterial supply > 2 mm diameter	

date cannot be totally occluded by embolization techniques. Embolization does, however, permit a staged preoperative reduction in size of the arteriovenous shunt, producing significant circulatory readjustment and reducing the degree of hydraulic shock resulting from the final occlusion of the fistula at the time of surgical resection of the lesion. Embolization when practical has largely replaced staged surgical occlusion of the feeding arteries to achieve this effect.[20,60]

Embolic agents are classified as either absorbable or nonabsorbable and as either solid or fluid. Solid embolic agents are injected into the internal carotid or vertebral artery feeding the malformation, relying on the high-volume axial flow characteristics of the circulation to the AVM to carry the solid particles into its nidus. This technique is not satisfactory if the pellets have to leave the parent artery at a sharp angle to enter a branching vessel, such as would be required for a pellet entering the anterior cerebral artery from the internal carotid.

Barium-impregnated silicone spheres in graded sizes from 0.5 up to 3.0 mm in diameter are the most common nonabsorbable, solid embolic agent and are currently the most satisfactory agent for producing graded preoperative reduction in flow through cerebral arteriovenous malformations. Care must be taken to stop the embolization before the flow rate has been so reduced that it is no longer effective in ensuring against passage of pellets into other arterial branches not associated with the malformation. When necessary, pellet embolization can be carried out at several different sessions, staged 3 to 4 weeks apart. Surgery may be safely planned for at an interval of between 3 to 6 weeks after the most recent embolization. Recanalization or establishment of new collateral flow during this time interval has not been seen.[21,23] Gelfoam, cut into 1 × 2 mm strips, impregnated with tantalum powder and soaked in angiographic contrast material has been the most common absorbable solid embolic agent. Although this material is relatively easy to handle, it has been more unpredictable in producing occlusion on the arterial side of the shunt and has no major advantages over the silicone spheres.

Fluid embolic agents employed to date have been nonabsorbable and of either the bucrylate or silicone types. Isobutyl-2-cyanoacrylate (ICBA) is a prototypic material of the bucrylate group. It is a rapidly polymerizing, low-viscosity tissue adhesive which is made radiopaque by the addition of tantalum powder. ICBA polymerizes rapidly on contact with ionic solutions such as blood or normal saline, while a 5% glucose solution will block polymerization. Considerable skill and experience are required in the use of this material. The speed of polymerization and rate of injection must be finely calculated to ensure that polymerization occurs on the arterial side of the malformation. Distal migration of this fluid into the major sinuses has occurred.[13] If the arterial inflow is not arrested by polymerization on the arterial side of the shunt, sudden swelling and rupture of the malformation with major hemorrhage may occur. Bucrylate produces a foreign body giant cell reaction with chronic inflammatory changes not only in the vessel wall but also to a lesser degree in the adjacent brain parenchyma.[71] The long-term effects of this material are not as yet fully known. Occasional malformations have been completely occluded with bucrylate, although the success rate for total occlusion has not been high.

There are several additional technical problems in using this material for attempting occlusion of malformations in areas of eloquent function. Arterial branches to normally functioning eloquent cortex often depart from the parent artery distal to the first arterial branches going to the malformation. Total occlusion of the malformation would, of necessity, require sacrificing these normal branches, with potentially serious neurological sequelae. Additionally, the hardened, noncompressible prongs of bucrylate within an incompletely occluded malformation may significantly increase the difficulty of subsequent safe separation and surgical removal of the malformation from areas of critical function.

Silicone fluid mixtures have occasionally been used instead of bucrylate.[4] The mixture consists of a silastic elastomer containing a filler necessary for vulcanization, and a medical-grade silicone fluid that acts as the diluent to the more viscous Silastic elastomer. These two silicones are mixed to the desired viscosity and tantalum powder added to permit radiographic visualization. A catalyst to produce vulcanization is required. The Silastic is injected just before vulcanization occurs. It has no adhesive properties, so that a complete filling or cast of the vascular lumen is required.

After embolization with attendant reduction in the sump effect of the AVM, occasional patients have been noted to show some improvement in intellectual performance, suggesting the correction of some degree of symptomatic cerebral steal.[75] Wolpert et al. found, however, that embolization had no long-term effect on the progression of neurological symptoms or signs and no effect on seizure frequency.[75] Incomplete occlusion of the malformation by embolization has not reduced or modified the natural history of the lesion with respect to hemorrhage.[42]

Serbinenko in 1974 reported the use of detachable flow-directed balloons on the tips of catheters threaded into the proximal vessels to the malformation.[59] This technique has been a key factor in permitting selective catheterization of these vessels for bucrylate injection but has not been a satisfactory therapeutic occlusive maneuver in and of itself.[66]

Operative Management

Preoperatively, the patient is placed on anticonvulsants to minimize the risk of seizures during the early postoperative period of cerebral vasocongestion and cerebral swelling, even if the patient has no previous history of cerebral seizures. Serum anticonvulsant levels are checked immediately before surgery to ensure that adequate anticonvulsant levels are present. Dexamethasone is started 36 to 48 h preoperatively to help stabilize capillary membrane permeability during the early postoperative interval of hydraulic shock and local tissue reaction to surgical manipulation.

If the malformation lies in or immediately adjacent to the expected location of the motor cortex or major speech centers, the surgical procedure may be carried out under local anesthesia with cortical mapping to ensure accurate localization of the areas of eloquent function and to permit the testing of these functions serially throughout the removal of the malformation.[24,26] In this latter situation, temporary clips are placed on the arterial feeders immediately proximal to the malformation, followed by function testing. The temporary clips are then replaced with permanent ones if no functional impairment has ensued.

Surgical resection should always be carried out under magnification with appropriate microsurgical instrumentation. The dissection plane follows along the immediate margin of the malformation in the thin, gliotic nonfunctional zone between the malformation and the adjacent cortex and white matter. Particular care must be taken in occluding the small, thin-walled endothelial tubules composing the transcerebral venous drainage. These vessels are extremely fragile and, if torn, back-bleed profusely due to the increased venous pressure in the subependymal venous plexus from the A-V shunt. It is essential to avoid pursuing these vessels if unacceptable neurological deficit is to be avoided. Temporary placement of small fluffy cotton pledgets, accompanied by having patience and by moving on to another area of the removal, will normally secure hemostasis of these individual venous bleeding points. Careful positioning of the head so that the major intracranial venous drainage is above heart level is a major factor in reducing venous congestion and attendant blood loss.

Selective identification and occlusion of the arterial inflow to the lesion with protection of the venous drainage as long as possible is important, although Malis advocates using one of the draining veins as a "handle" and a guide to resection when several major draining veins are present. Major reduction in venous outflow before interruption of the arterial inflow must be avoided if malformation rupture with massive bleeding is to be avoided. High-contrast visual dye can be injected intra-arterially to aid in the identification of the feeding arteries to the malformation if the vascular tangle of the malformation makes selective identification of the arterial inflow otherwise difficult.[25] Significant fragility of the lesion persists down to the very end of the resection, making it essential that neither fatigue nor impatience results in a rush or hurry to complete the final stages of the removal.

A grid technique of localization of cortical function for a malformation lying in or adjacent to the central areas has been proposed by Kunc.[35] This technique presupposes a consistent pattern of cortical function with reference to standard anatomical landmarks. Experience with cortical mapping unfortunately has revealed significant deviation in location from the more common patterns of cortical function around the margins of arteriovenous malformations, especially with respect to speech localization. Modern techniques of anesthesiology have made a major contribution to increasing the safety of the surgical approach to, and manipulation of, these lesions. Moderate hypotension during critical periods of surgical resection is well tolerated, even under local anesthesia, and does not interfere with patient alertness and function testing.[26] The general anesthesia technique of jet ventilation can also essentially eliminate brain movement secondary to respiration.[19]

Preliminary experience with surgical lasers used on intracranial vascular lesions is beginning to appear in the literature.[15] At present, the lasers seem to have limited application to the surgery of AVMs. This is particularly true with the CO$_2$ laser, which has relatively poor vessel coagulation ability because of its extremely shallow depth of penetration. The CO$_2$ laser tends to punch holes in the walls of larger vessels. The neodymium:YAG laser is more efficient in achieving hemostasis due to its greater depth of penetration. This laser may, when federally approved for neurosurgical use, provide a useful surgical adjunct for the resection of some AVMs.

Gentle handling of the arteries proximal to the lesions is essential, particularly in the posterior fossa where proximal propagation of clot from the point of arterial occlusion can result in a disastrous outcome for an otherwise technically satisfactory surgical excision. After completion of the resection, the patient's blood pressure should be brought to normal levels and the operative field observed carefully to ensure that hemostasis is complete. Feeding arteries of 1 mm or larger must be securely clipped, if delayed postoperative hemorrhage is to be consistently avoided. Bipolar coagulation alone for these larger vessels is not adequate.

Postoperatively, the patient is nursed with the head of the bed elevated 30 to 40 degrees to maintain optimal venous outflow. It is helpful to maintain the systolic blood pressure between 90 to 110 torr, using a trimethaphan camsylate drip, to minimize the effects of hydraulic shock and attendant hyperperfusion around the margins of the resection during the first 24 h postoperatively. Crystalloids are restricted in order to produce a mild dehydration, with the goal of a serum osmolarity between 295 and 305. Blood volume is maintained with colloid administration. Dexamethasone is continued postoperatively for 8 to 10 days and is then rapidly tapered. Postoperative angiography is essential to confirm that complete removal of the malformation has been achieved (Fig. 176-5C).

Bragg Peak Proton Beam Therapy

Proton beam therapy using the Bragg peak phenomenon has been utilized by Kjellberg et al. for the treatment of inoperable vascular malformations.[32] The optimum lesions for this technique appear to be those deeply situated lesions, preferably some distance removed from the major cortical areas of motor and speech function, with multiple small feeding arteries. Conventional high-energy radiation therapy has not been found to be of significant help in the management of large cortical AVMs, although elimination of smaller, deeply placed lesions has been reported.[31] All forms of radiation therapy appear to require from 7 to 22 months for the disappearance of susceptible malformations.[32,63]

Results

The type of patient screening before surgical referral as well as the aggressiveness of the consulting neurological and neurosurgical units are obvious factors in reported results. In larger series in which over 60 percent of all patients referred underwent surgical extirpation of the lesions, a mortality rate ranging from 7 to 14 percent is found.[2,12,23,44,62] The increasingly widespread use of the surgical microscope and the staged preoperative embolization of the lesions are major factors in the improving mortality and morbidity statistics. Surgical mortality rates now appear to compare favorably with the long-term mortality rates of these lesions managed conservatively in the younger patient. More information with respect to the quality of postoperative survival, as compared to the quality of life with conservative management, is needed. In the few instances where this information is beginning to appear, preliminary indications are that the long-term quality of life is more favorable when surgical extirpation of the lesion has been carried out.

References

1. Aberfeld DC, Rao KR: Familial arteriovenous malformation of the brain. Neurology (NY) 31:184–186, 1981.
2. Albert P: Personal experience in the treatment of 178 cases of arteriovenous malformations of the brain. Acta Neurochir (Wien) 61:207–226, 1982.
3. Berenstein A: Technique of catheterization and embolization of the lenticulostriate arteries. J Neurosurg 54:783–789, 1981.
4. Berenstein A, Kricheff II: Neuroradiologic interventional procedures. Semin Roentgenol 16:79–94, 1981.
5. Bergstrand H, Olivecrona H, Tönnis W: *Gefässmissbildungen und Gefässgeschwülste des Gehirns*. Leipzig, Georg Thieme Verlag, 1936, p 181.
6. Bitoh S, Hasegawa H, Fujiwara M, Sakurai M: Angiographically occult vascular malformations causing intracranial hemorrhage. Surg Neurol 17:35–42, 1982.
7. Britt RH, Connor WS, Enzmann DR: Occult arteriovenous malformation of the brainstem simulating multiple sclerosis. Neurology (NY) 31:901–904, 1981.
8. Chou SN, Erickson DL, Ortiz-Suarez HJ: Surgical treatment of vascular lesions in the brain stem. J Neurosurg 42:23–31, 1975.
9. Dahl RE, Kline DG: Intraparenchymal arteriovenous malformations with predominant external carotid artery contribution. J Neurosurg 41:681–687, 1974.
10. Debrun G, Vinuela F, Fox A, Drake CG: Embolization of cerebral arteriovenous malformations with bucrylate: Experience in 46 cases. J Neurosurg 56:615–627, 1982.
11. Delitala A, Delfini R, Vagnozzi R, Esposito S: Increase in size of cerebral angiomas: Case report. J Neurosurg 57:556–558, 1982.
12. Drake CG: Surgical removal of arteriovenous malformations from the brain stem and cerebellopontine angle. J Neurosurg 43:661–670, 1975.
13. Drake CG: Cerebral arteriovenous malformations: Considerations for and experience with surgical treatment in 166 cases. Clin Neurosurg 26:145–208, 1979.
14. Faria MA Jr: External carotid component of AVMs. [Letter] J Neurosurg 56:740, 1982.
15. Fasano VA: The treatment of vascular malformation of the brain with laser source. Lasers Surg Med 1:347–356, 1981.
16. Feindel W: The influence of cerebral steal: Demonstration of fluorescein angiography and focal cerebral blood flow measurement—pathophysiological aspects, in Pia HW, Gleave JRW, Grote E, Zierski J (eds): *Cerebral Angiomas: Advances in Diagnosis and Therapy*. Berlin, Springer-Verlag, 1975, pp 87–100.
17. Forster DMC, Steiner L, Håkanson S: Arteriovenous malformations of the brain. A long-term clinical study. J Neurosurg 37:562–570, 1972.
18. French LA, Chou SN: Conventional methods of treating intracranial arteriovenous malformations. Prog Neurol Surg 3:274–318, 1969.
19. Frost EAM: Anaesthetic management of cerebrovascular disease. Br J Anaesth 53:745–756, 1981.
20. Garretson HD: Surgical techniques in intracranial vascular malformation surgery. Presented at the Annual Meeting of the Society of University Neurosurgeons, Rochester, MN, May 1975.
21. Garretson HD: Postoperative pressure and flow changes in the feeding arteries of cerebral arteriovenous malformations. Neurosurgery 4:544–545, 1979.
22. Garretson HD: Arteriovenous malformations: Thoughts on classification. Presented at the Annual Meeting of the Society of University Neurosurgeons, Gainesville, FL, May 17, 1980.
23. Garretson HD: Arteriovenous malformations, in Rosenberg RN, Grossman RG, Schochet S, Heinz ER, Willis WE (eds): *The Clinical Neurosciences*. New York, Churchill Livingstone, 1983, pp II:1089–II:1099.
24. Garretson HD, Geevarghese, G: Arteriovenous malformations of the dominant hemisphere. Presented at the Annual Meeting of the American Association of Neurological Surgeons, Miami, FL, April 6–10, 1975.
25. Garretson H, Perot P, Yamamoto YL, Feindel W: Intracarotid Coomassie blue dye as an aid in the surgery of intracranial vascular lesions. J Neurosurg 26:577–583, 1967.
26. Geevarghese KP, Garretson HD: "Alert" anesthesia for craniotomy. Int Anesthesiol Clin 15(3):231–251, 1977.
27. George ED, Pevsner PH: Combined neurosurgical-neuroradiological therapy for cerebral arteriovenous malformation—The Walter Reed protocol, in Smith RR, Haerer AF, Russell WF (eds): *Vascular Malformations and Fistulas of the Brain*. New York, Raven Press, 1982, pp 169–191.
28. Gerosa MA, Cappellotto P, Licata C, Iraci G, Pardatscher K, Fiore DL: Cerebral arteriovenous malformations in children (56 cases). Childs Brain 8:356–371, 1981.
29. Hayashi S, Arimoto T, Itakura T, Fujii T, Nishiguchi T, Komai N: The association of intracranial aneurysms and arteriovenous malformation of the brain: Case report. J Neurosurg 55:971–975, 1981.
30. Hayman LA, Fox AJ, Evans RA: Effectiveness of contrast regimens in CT detection of vascular malformations of the brain. AJNR 2:421–425, 1981.
31. Johnson, RT: Radiotherapy of cerebral angiomas: With a note on some problems in diagnosis, in Pia HW, Gleave JRW, Grote E, Zierski J (eds): *Cerebral Angiomas: Advances in Diagnosis and Therapy*. Berlin, Springer-Verlag, 1975, pp 256–267.
32. Kjellberg RN, Hanamura T, Davis KR, Lyons SL, Adams RD: Bragg-peak proton-beam therapy for arteriovenous malformations of the brain. N Engl J Med 309:269–274, 1983.
33. Koulouris S, Rizzoli HV: Coexisting intracranial aneurysm and arteriovenous malformation: Case report. Neurosurgery 8:219–222, 1981.
34. Krause F: Krankenvorstellung aus der Hirnchirurgie. Zentralbl Chir 35(35):61–67, 1908.
35. Kunc Z: Surgery of arteriovenous malformations in the speech and motor-sensory regions. J Neurosurg 40:293–303, 1974.
36. Kuwahara S, Shima T, Ishikawa S, Uozumi T, Miyazaki M: A clinical study of intracranial AVMs with reference to their enlargement and regression—a follow-up study with angiography and CT scan. Neurol Med Chir (Tokyo) 19:149–161, 1979.
37. Lakier JB, Milner S, Cohen M, Levin SE: Intracranial arteriovenous fistulas in infancy—haemodynamic considerations: A review of 3 cases. S Afr Med J 61:242–245, 1982.
38. Leblanc R, Ethier R: The computerized tomographic appearance of angiographically occult arteriovenous malformations of the brain. Can J Neurol Sci 8:7–13, 1981.
39. Luessenhop AJ: Artificial embolization for cerebral arteriovenous malformations. Prog Neurol Surg 3:320–362, 1969.
40. Luessenhop AJ, Gennarelli TA: Anatomical grading of supra-

41. Luessenhop AJ, Mujica PH: Embolization of segments of the circle of Willis and adjacent branches for management of certain inoperable cerebral arteriovenous malformations. J Neurosurg 54:573–582, 1981.
42. Luessenhop AJ, Presper JH: Surgical embolization of cerebral arteriovenous malformations through internal carotid and vertebral arteries. Long-term results. J Neurosurg 42:443–451, 1975.
43. Luschka H: Cavernöse Blutgeschwulst des Gehirns. Virchows Arch 6:458–470, 1854.
44. Martin NA, Wilson CB: Medial occipital arteriovenous malformations: Surgical treatment. J Neurosurg 56:798–802, 1982.
45. McCormick WF: The pathology of vascular ("arteriovenous") malformations. J Neurosurg 24:807–816, 1966.
46. Merland JJ, Riche MC, Chiras J, Bories J: Therapeutic angiography in neuroradiology: Classical data, recent advances and perspectives. Neuroradiology 21:111–121, 1981.
47. Michelson WJ: Natural history and pathophysiology of arteriovenous malformations. Clin Neurosurg 26:307–313, 1979.
48. Miyasaka K, Wolpert SM, Prager RJ: The association of cerebral aneurysms, infundibula, and intracranial arteriovenous malformations. Stroke 13:196–203, 1982.
49. Moore KL: *The Developing Human: Clinically Oriented Embryology*, 3 ed. Philadelphia, Saunders, 1982.
50. Nornes H, Grip A: Hemodynamic aspects of cerebral arteriovenous malformations. J Neurosurg 53:456–464, 1980.
51. Perret G, Nishioka H: Arteriovenous malformations. An analysis of 545 cases of cranio-cerebral arteriovenous malformations and fistulae reported to the cooperative study. J Neurosurg 25:467–490, 1966.
52. Pool JL, Potts DG: *Aneurysms and Arteriovenous Anomalies of the Brain: Diagnosis and Treatment*. New York, Harper & Row, 1965, pp 326–373.
53. Russell EJ, Berenstein A: Meningeal collateralization to normal cerebral vessels associated with intracerebral arteriovenous malformations: functional angiographic considerations. Radiology 139:617–622, 1981.
54. Sabin FR: Preliminary note on the differentiation of angioblasts and the method by which they produce blood-vessels, blood-plasma and red blood-cells as seen in the living chick. Anat Rec 13:199–204, 1917.
55. Samson D, Ditmore QM, Beyer CW Jr: Intravascular use of isobutyl 2-cyanoacrylate: Part I: Treatment of intracranial arteriovenous malformations. Neurosurgery 8:43–51, 1981.
56. Sartor K: Spontaneous closure of cerebral arteriovenous malformation demonstrated by angiography and computed tomography. Neuroradiology 15:95–98, 1978.
57. Saunders RL, Feindel WH, Carvalho VR: X-ray microscopy of the blood vessels of the human brain. Med Bio Illus 15:108–122, 1965.
58. Saunders RL, Feindel WH, Carvalho VR: X-ray microscopy of the blood vessels of the human brain, Part II. Med Biol Illus 15:234–246, 1965.
59. Serbinenko FA: Balloon catheterization and occlusion of major cerebral vessels. J Neurosurg 41:125–145, 1974.
60. Spetzler RF, Wilson CB, Weinstein P, Mehdorn M, Townsend J, Telles D: Normal perfusion pressure breakthrough theory. Clin Neurosurg 25:651–672, 1978.
61. Stein BM, Wolpert SM: Arteriovenous malformations of the brain. I: Current concepts and treatment. Arch Neurol 37:1–5, 1980.
62. Stein BM, Wolpert SM: Arteriovenous malformations of the brain. II: Current concepts and treatment. Arch Neurol 37:69–75, 1980.
63. Steiner, L: Radiosurgery for arteriovenous malformations. Presented at the Meeting of the Italian Neurosurgical Society, Rome, April 1978.
64. Streeter GL: The developmental alterations in the vascular system of the brain. Contrib Embryol 8:5–38, 1918.
65. Svien HJ, McRae JA: Arteriovenous anomalies of the brain: Fate of patients not having definitive surgery. J Neurosurg 23:23–28, 1965.
66. Taki W, Handa H, Yonekawa Y, Yamagata S, Miyake H, Matsuda I, Handa J, Iwata H, Suzuki M, Ikada Y: Detachable balloon catheter systems for embolization of cerebrovascular lesions. Neurol Med Chir (Tokyo) 21:709–719, 1981.
67. Troost BT, Newton TH: Occipital lobe arteriovenous malformations: Clinical and radiologic features in 26 cases with comments on differentiation from migraine. Arch Ophthalmol 93:250–256, 1975.
68. Troupp H, Marttila I, Halonen V: Arteriovenous malformations of the brain: Prognosis without operation. Acta Neurochir (Wien) 22:125–128, 1970.
69. Tuttelman RM, Gleicher N: Central nervous system hemorrhage complicating pregnancy. Obstet Gynecol 58:651–656, 1981.
70. Vassilouthis J: Cerebral arteriovenous malformation with intracranial hypertension. Surg Neurol 11:402–404, 1980.
71. Vinters HV, Debrun G, Kaufmann JCE, Drake CG: Pathology of arteriovenous malformations embolized with isobutyl-2-cyanoacrylate (bucrylate): Report of two cases. J Neurosurg 55:819–825, 1981.
72. Virchow R: *Die Krankhaften Geschwülste*. Berlin, A. Hirschwald, 3:345–463, 1863–1867.
73. Waltimo O: The relationship of size, density and localization of intracranial arteriovenous malformations to the type of initial symptom. J Neurol Sci 19:13–19, 1973.
74. Weisberg L, Pierce JF, Jabbari B: Intracranial hypertension resulting from a cerebrovascular malformation. South Med J 70:624–626, 1977.
75. Wolpert SM, Barnett FJ, Prager RJ: Benefits of embolization without surgery for cerebral arteriovenous malformations. AJR 138:99–102, 1982.

177
Vein of Galen Aneurysms
A. Loren Amacher

Aneurysms of the vein of Galen are rare. It is impossible to deduce their true incidence, but less than 200 cases have been reported in the world literature. Nevertheless, these lesions have important, frequently dramatic, clinical consequences. They tend to present in stereotyped patterns depending upon the age of the patient. Most often the victim is very young, a neonate or young infant, and the clinical features are those of actual or potential hemodynamic decompensation usually coupled with hydrocephalus. Some authors have used terms such as "spectacular" or "intimidating" to describe their radiological and hemodynamic characteristics. Certainly, the surgeon who undertakes the obliteration of such a lesion must approach the experience with some trepidation.

The 1964 review of these aneurysms by Gold et al. contains the historical perspective.[4] They credit Jaeger, Forbes, and Dandy with the first description of a vein of Galen aneurysm in 1937.

The vein of Galen was investigated by Bedford in 1934, and he showed that sudden occlusion of the structure would not induce hydrocephalus, although the relationship of such an occlusion to raised intracranial pressure remained moot.[2,3]

Anatomy and Embryology

The vein of Galen lies in the sagittal plane just within and then behind the transverse cerebral fissure. It is formed by the confluence of the internal cerebral veins and the basal veins of Rosenthal, a few millimeters above the pineal gland. After a short, upward traverse of 10 to 20 mm, it penetrates the junction of the falx and the tentorium, uniting with the inferior sagittal sinus to form the straight sinus. In its course it sweeps around the posterior inferior aspect of the splenium of the corpus callosum. Usually, venous drainage from the medial deep nuclei and the medial occipital and temporal lobes and the superior cerebellar surface occurs through the galenic system.

According to Padget, the differentiation of the primitive vascular plexuses of the brain into arterial and venous channels occurs between the 20- and 40-mm stages of embryonic development.[10] The primitive arteries and veins of the neural tube arise from separate capillary plexuses. The arteries lie superficial to the veins, and they frequently cross at right angles. Until the 40-mm stage, both types of vessels are simple endothelial channels, and the potential for fistula formation is very real.

The galenic system is thought to originate from veins of choroidal origin, a development of primitive vessels draining the medial telencephalon, the diencephalon, and the metencephalon. Since the size and number of perpendicular crossings of primitive arteries and veins are greatest near the relatively massive embryonic choroid plexuses, it is perhaps not surprising that the niduses of most angiomas are deeply situated.

It is likely that the fistulas that give rise to a vein of Galen aneurysm occur between vessels of choroidal origin. These include branches of the posterior, middle, and anterior cerebral and superior cerebellar arteries.[10] A very high flow arteriovenous shunt develops, and the vein of Galen responds by arterialization of its wall. Unfettered by dural walls, the vein dilates enormously, much more so than the relatively restricted straight sinus. The wall of the vein of Galen aneurysm becomes thick and tough in response to increased flow, pressure, and turbulent flow. Cerebral arterial aneurysms grow thin apically in response to the same factors. Perhaps that explains why vein of Galen aneurysms rupture so seldom.

Classification

There are two types of vein of Galen aneurysm. The distinction is important because therapy is different for each type.

1. **Primary** The arteries noted previously feed directly into the sac of the aneurysm. The arterial feeders are usually huge, and through them the majority of the blood carried by the main-stem vessel may be diverted to the fistula. In cases symptomatic at birth there may be a myriad of small vessel feeders anteroinferiorly as well.[9] Occlusion of all arterial input to the fistula will obliterate the shunt and allow for collapse of the aneurysm. Excision of the sac is unnecessary.

2. **Secondary** The dilated galenic system serves as the venous outflow for an adjacent (very occasionally remote) angioma. Usually the angioma is situated in the medial posterior hemispheres, the superior cerebellum, the brain stem, or the deep ganglionic structures. Often, the inferior sagittal and straight sinuses are greatly dilated as well. With these lesions, the principles of angioma excision apply. The angioma must be obliterated; occlusion of the venous outflow from the lesion leaving the arterial component intact will lead to disaster.[13]

Figures 177-1, 177-2, and 177-3 show the angiographic and computed tomographic (CT) characteristics of primary and secondary vein of Galen aneurysms. This chapter is concerned only with primary aneurysms.

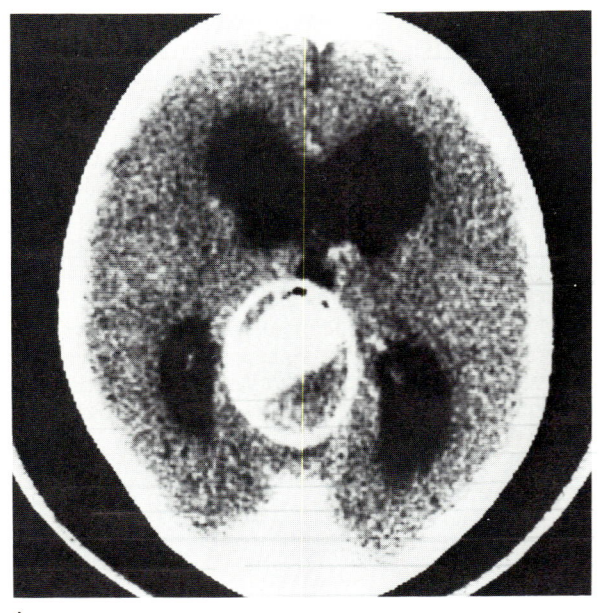

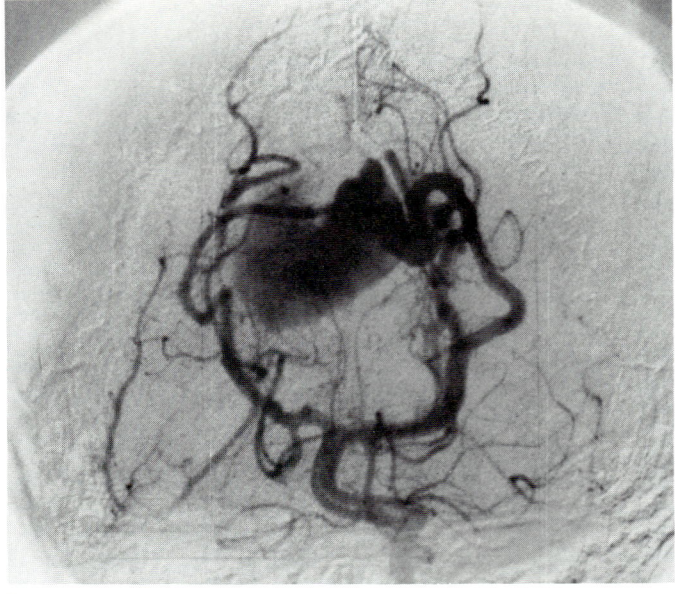

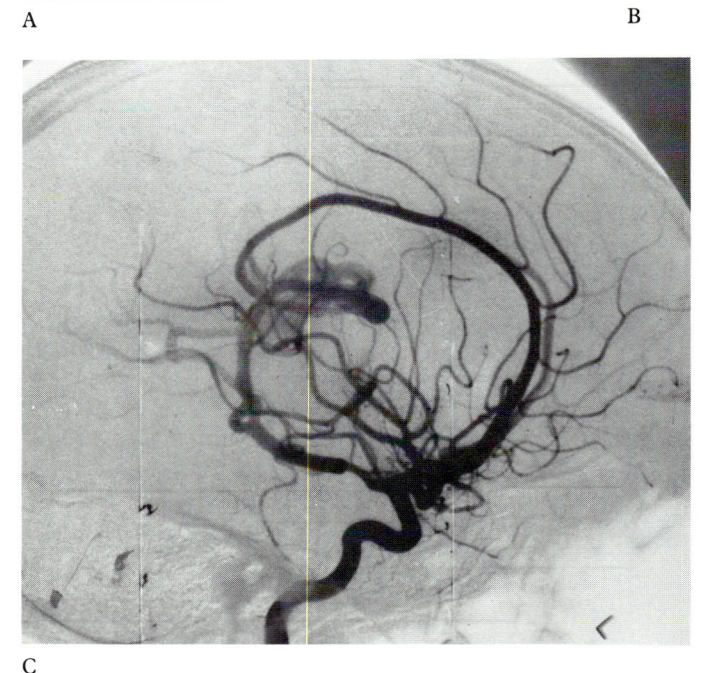

Figure 177-1 A partially thrombosed primary vein of Galen aneurysm. *A.* CT appearance. *B.* Towne's projection from an angiogram of the same aneurysm. Note the very large left posterior cerebral artery with three fistulous connections to the vein of Galen. The right posterior cerebral artery also feeds directly into the vein. *C.* A lateral view from a carotid angiogram showing the sites of fistulous connection.

Clinical and Diagnostic Features

The clinical syndromes associated with primary vein of Galen aneurysms fall neatly into four groupings (Table 177-1) corresponding to the age of the patient at presentation.[1]

Neonatal Group

Almost universally, these children present at or shortly after birth with overwhelming high output, preload heart failure. As much as 80 to 90 percent of the infant's cardiac output may pass through the galenic fistula. Emergency investigation of such a child will show high jugular venous oxygen tension, and an angiogram will reveal the aneurysm. Most commonly there are numerous small feeders into the anterior and inferior aspects of the sac.[5] There is usually a loud cranial bruit of virtually constant intensity. CT scanning with a late-generation machine, with or without contrast, is diagnostic. Recently, positive identification of a vein of Galen fistula by ultrasound and pulsed Doppler echoes has been reported.[11] Continuous (rather than pulsatile) internal jugular blood flow is noted, along with an echo-free shadow in the region of the vein of Galen wherein the flow characteristics are similar to those of the internal jugular vein.

Operative attacks upon these aneurysms in the face of intractable heart failure have been of no avail. The children die postoperatively of heart failure in spite of rigorous cardiac care, even including drastic reduction of circulating

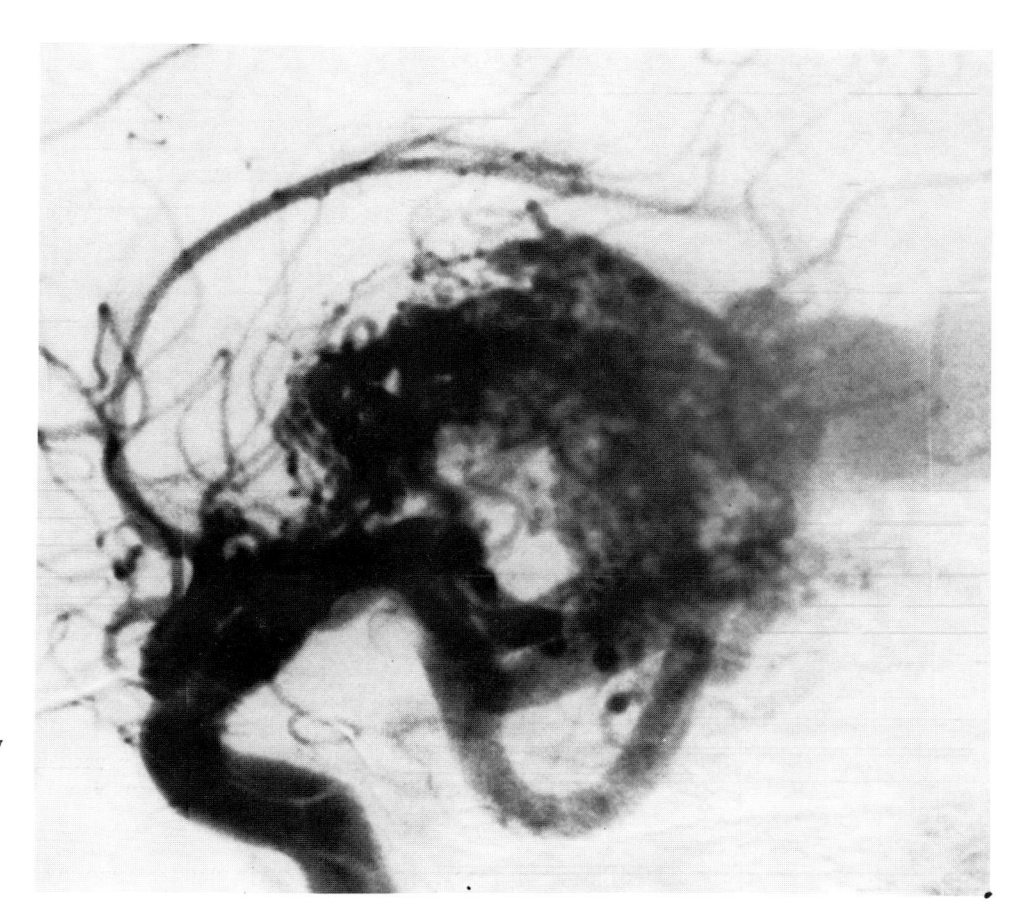

Figure 177-2 Lateral view from a carotid angiogram, showing a secondary vein of Galen aneurysm, draining a bilateral thalamic angioma.

blood volume. Occlusion of the cervical carotid arteries has not helped. Myocardial infarction occurs commonly, due to the low cardiac perfusion, aggravated by any intraoperative hypotension.[5]

Norman and Becker described the postmortem condition of the brain in seven neonates with this lesion.[8] Severe brain damage was seen in all, whether or not an operative procedure had been attempted. Neuropathological findings in-

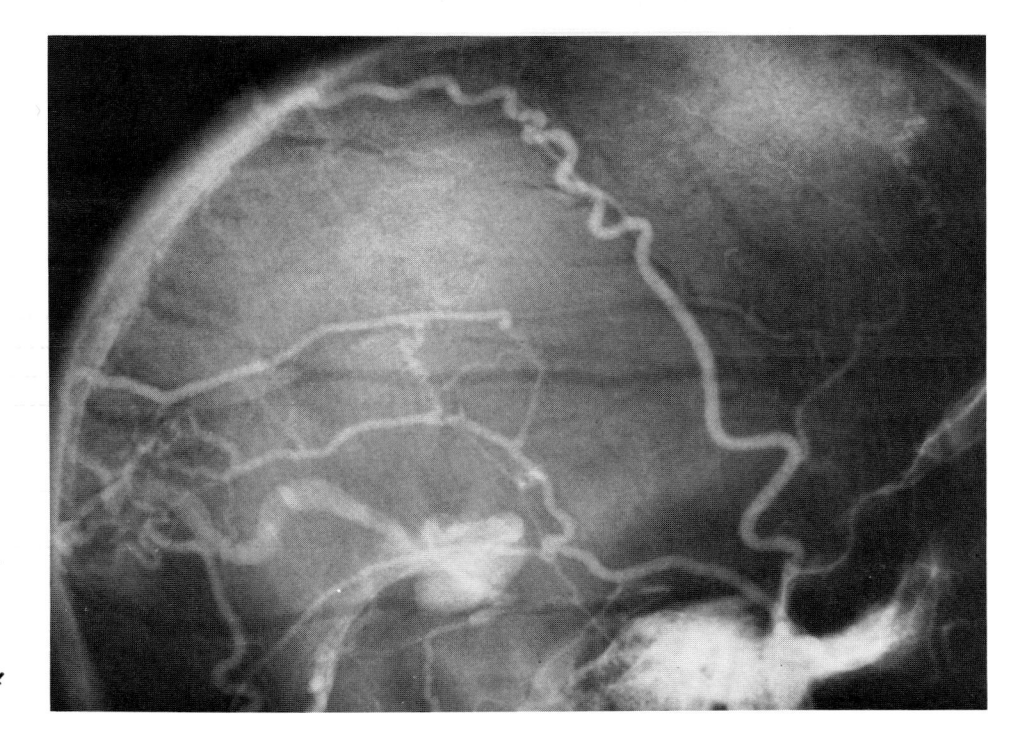

Figure 177-3 Lateral view from an external carotid angiogram, showing a secondary vein of Galen aneurysm draining a tentorial angioma.

TABLE 177-1 Clinical Groupings, Vein of Galen Aneurysms

Group	Presentation	Prognosis
Neonatal	Extreme high-output cardiac failure, usually lethal	Operation very dangerous; usually die of intractable heart failure
Infantile	Borderline cardiac status; early mild heart failure that recovers; hydrocephalus	Need preoperative cardiac assessment; often need CSF shunt
Childhood	Hydrocephalus; may have cardiomegaly; occasional SAH*; occasional pineal mass, ring calcification	Depends upon degree of hydrocephalus
Mature	Headache; pineal mass, ring calcification; SAH*; hydrocephalus	Good

*Subarachnoid hemorrhage.

cluded periventricular leukomalacia, deep parenchymal hemorrhages, numerous very small feeders to the sac, cortical gliosis and subcortical cavitation, and cortical infarction and calcification. They proposed as mechanisms of cerebral damage, arterial steal, ischemia secondary to heart failure, hemorrhagic infarction, compression atrophy, and operative trauma. They concluded that operative correction of the fistula in the neonate was futile, an opinion supported by the case reported by Sivakoff and Nouri; the neonate survived operation for 10 months in a vegetative state and at autopsy showed neuropathological findings comparable with those mentioned above.[11]

Infantile Group

Two patterns are seen in this clinical grouping.

1. The child may have had mild cardiac decompensation neonatally, the condition settling down spontaneously or with treatment; later (1 to 12 months, usually) the patient is found to have craniomegaly because of hydrocephalus. Usually there is a loud bruit over the entire head, but heard best posterolaterally. A CT scan will be diagnostic.
2. The patient has craniomegaly, the cause of the hydrocephalus is discovered by CT scanning, and the chest film frequently shows cardiomegaly. There is no history of cardiac decompensation.

Very occasionally the sac is discovered as a pineal area ring calcification on a plain x-ray film of the skull. The aneurysm may not fill at angiography because of complete thrombosis[6] (unusual in a young child), or it may show the angiographic "target" sign if the periphery of the sac is thrombosed.[12] In this situation, the calcified rim of the aneurysm is separated from the contrast "bull's-eye" by clot—hence the target appearance. Usually the entire sac fills with contrast, often demonstrating the entering jets of contrast and the turbulent currents within.

The ventriculomegaly is usually pronounced, involving the lateral and third ventricles. The implications of this fact are discussed under "Treatment."

Childhood Group

Most cases discovered past the age of 2 years have come to light during the investigation of craniomegaly. Some have presented with subarachnoid hemorrhage. There may be mild cardiomegaly as well. Cranial bruits are usually associated. It must be pointed out that flow bruits are commonly heard with auscultation of the skull or ocular globes of a normal infant or child. These physiological bruits are clearly identifiable as flow phenomena by their maximum systolic intensity over the eyes and temples, and their tendency to go away with minimal pressure over the cervical carotid arteries. In the child, the bruit associated with a vein of Galen aneurysm may be no more intense than a physiological bruit, but it is heard best at the parietal apex or near the midline posteriorly. In the neonate and infant, the bruit usually is much louder, tends to run into diastole, or may be virtually continuous.

Mature Group

In later childhood, adolescence, or young adulthood, the aneurysms present in a variety of ways: subarachnoid hemorrhage, a pineal area mass, headache usually associated with raised intracranial pressure, rim calcification near the pineal region, syncopal attacks resembling those encountered occasionally with colloid cysts of the third ventricle, and hydrocephalus. CT scanning and angiography are diagnostic.

Treatment

The surgeon who takes on the obliteration of a vein of Galen aneurysm must do so with full awareness of the hazards involved. In general, the younger the child, the more risky the procedure. The problems to be considered and anticipated are cardiac hemodynamics, hydrocephalus, operative blood loss, and aftercare.

Cardiac Hemodynamics

Even if no history of early cardiac decompensation is forthcoming, it is wise to have the infant or child assessed by a cardiologist. Of great importance is an accurate calculation of blood volume preoperatively. Infants with a large fistula into the vein of Galen may have a greatly expanded blood volume in response to a very high cardiac output. Sudden occlusion of the fistula, with the accompanying significant increase in peripheral vascular resistance, may precipitate intraoperative and disastrous heart failure. The sudden increase in peripheral vascular resistance produces an afterload for which the myocardium cannot compensate. This, combined with the preload factor of a pathologically large blood volume, induces severe cardiac failure, and immediate reduction of blood volume may not correct the problem even with inotropic stimulation of the myocardium. Precise and intensive cardiac monitoring is essential,[7] intraoperatively and postoperatively. Swan-Ganz catheterization preoperatively is advisable when there is concern that central pressures may rise significantly during surgery.

Management of Hydrocephalus

The aneurysm sac produces hydrocephalus by compression of the midbrain and occlusion of the aqueduct. It is reasonable to hope that release of the compression force produced by the tense, distended aneurysm may allow reopening of the aqueduct, thereby curing the hydrocephalus. Several reported cases support this possibility, but in a significant number of patients subsequent shunting will be necessary.

Although drainage of large ventricles at the time of craniotomy does facilitate a deep midline exposure, the collapse of a thin cerebral mantle is almost certain to lead to subdural fluid accumulation in the early postoperative period. For this reason, precraniotomy shunting of grossly distended ventricles is advisable. One should not wait until the ventricles have returned to normal, however, before getting on with the attack on the aneurysm. To do so simply makes the exposure of the sac more difficult than it need be.

Operative Blood Loss

Except in the young infant, this item should not be a problem. These children have an expanded blood volume to begin with, and some volume reduction may be beneficial for a heart on the verge of preload failure. The aneurysm sac is tough and resilient; it will not burst unless roughly handled. Intentional hypotension to a mean of 40 to 50 torr during dissection of the sac helps reduce sac tension and increases the surgeon's sense of security. But where myocardial ischemia is a risk, hypotension must be eschewed.

Aftercare

The need for careful cardiac monitoring has been stated. Seizures may occur, particularly if the cerebral mantle has sustained injury because it has sagged away from the skull. Persistent subdural effusions may require drainage, and unresolving hydrocephalus must be dealt with.

Surgical Technique

The consensus is that a posterior interhemispheral exposure of the aneurysm is best. The occipital approach along the falx is usually unencumbered, especially if the ventricles are drained of some volume. Magnified vision is essential. Transcallosal approaches are recommended for anteriorly placed fistulas (Figure 177-1C).

The head should be positioned to facilitate exposure and provide a comfortable posture for the surgeon. In infants, the supine position with the head turned 45 degrees to either side is usually satisfactory. In older patients, the park-bench position has advantages, particularly for microscope placement. The semisitting position with the head flexed forward has the advantage of presenting the anatomy in a familiar manner, but may allow collapse of the cerebral hemisphere if the ventricles are large. It is essential to use an exposure that is familiar to the surgeon, lest the three-dimensional anatomy of the region become confused. The subtentorial approach is disadvantageous because the major feeders into the sac will be unnecessarily remote from the point of first contact with the aneurysm.

Usual measures relating to pressure points and prevention of excessive hypothermia are taken. The bone flap should be generous, right to the midline, and placed over the posterior parietal and anterior occipital lobes. Retraction of the occipital pole usually is not necessary.

With the operating microscope and self-retaining retractors, exposure down the falx is gentle and easy. Seldom is there extensive scarring in the vicinity of the sac, though arachnoid bands are encountered. These should be coagulated and divided; it is unlikely that they will contain feeder vessels of small caliber, except in neonates or very young infants.

Figure 177-4 shows the typical appearance of a sac and an entering artery. The feeders should be divided between clips

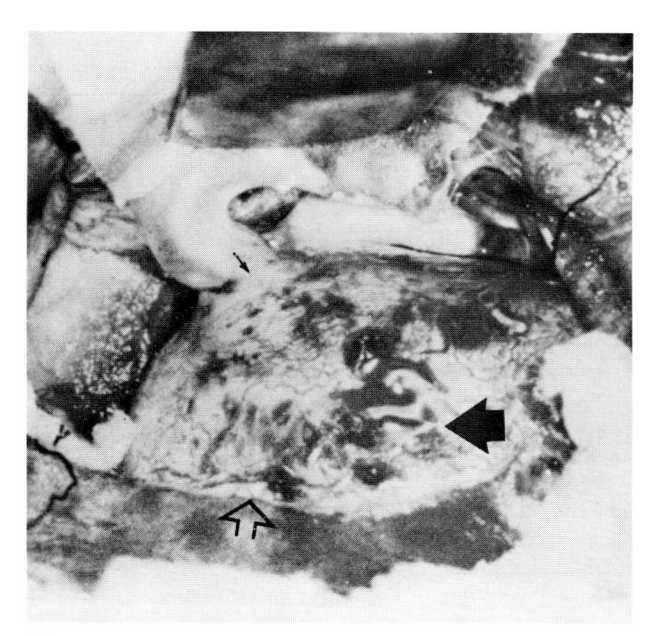

Figure 177-4 Operative photograph of a vein of Galen aneurysm. The small arrow indicates the site of an arterial fistula. The large dark arrow is on the aneurysm. The open arrow indicates the edge of the falx. The occipital lobe is behind the retractor at the top. (From Amacher and Shillito.[1])

far enough from the sac to allow the stumps to serve as handles for rotating the lesion. The arteries should be doubly secured proximally. By gently rolling the sac upward, feeders inferiorly are brought into view. This process is repeated until all the communications on one side have been divided.

Depending upon the size of the sac, the opposite side feeders may be brought into view by rotation of the aneurysm, or by cutting a superiorly based flap in the falx[14] to help in the visualization of those arteries. This latter maneuver is necessary only with a very large sac.

During this process, the anesthesiologist must maintain a strict vigil concerning the cardiac status, especially in young infants. Signs of incipient heart failure must be dealt with immediately and vigorously, including pharmacologic cardiac support, reduction of peripheral vascular resistance, and withdrawal of blood. In some situations it may be safest to desist from further fistula reduction and to plan to return in a few days when cardiac hemodynamics have stabilized. A two-stage procedure is preferable to a dead child. Or the next visible feeder may be occluded by a temporary clip; if cardiac stability persists, it may be divided.[7]

Upon completion of fistula closure, the sac will be soft, largely collapsed, and darker in color. Now a needle may be introduced to collapse the sac further and to determine oxygen tension of the blood in the sac. If all feeders have been divided, there is no need to excise the aneurysm. However, if the sac wall is rigid with calcification or if the lesion is largely or totally thrombosed, partial or total excision for reduction of mass effect is reasonable. There is no excuse for damaging the walls of the posterior hypothalamus and thalamus while attempting a total removal of one of these aneurysms.

If very large ventricles have been drained, they should be re-expanded with core temperature physiological solution before the bone flap is secured. Even so, subdural effusions are likely to occur.

Postoperative angiography is necessary to confirm total closure of the fistula. Very small residual feeders may be watched for a time, as they are likely to disappear.[1]

In small children, the cardiac vigil must be maintained well into the recovery period. Of premier importance is the control of fluid and blood volumes. The surgeon must realize that these patients are at great risk intraoperatively and postoperatively. Better to leave the fistula alone than to approach it with a cavalier attitude.

Embolization Techniques

The remarkable success of the interventional radiologists in reaching and occluding certain deep-seated intracranial vascular lesions has prompted some attacks upon both primary and secondary vein of Galen fistulas. However, no successful obliterations have been reported to this point. Nevertheless, the principles of surgical treatment apply. All arterial feeders must be occluded except, perhaps, very small ones. Angiomatous lesions feeding the vein of Galen must be the target in the secondary fistulas.

The very high flow in the large arterial feeder may sweep away spherules and fast-setting polymers, even using the newest calibrated-leak catheters. Of major concern in such situations is the risk of occluding the outlet of the aneurysm before the feeders are closed. Such an event would be catastrophic for the patient.

The long and tortuous path to the fistula may preclude the use of detachable balloons. In spite of present difficulties, these techniques are evolving. Combined closure of feeders by interventional radiology and surgery may become the preferred approach for many of these lesions in the future.

Prognosis

Previous reviews of the literature have presented a rather somber picture regarding survival and quality of life following surgical treatment of these lesions, particularly in the young.[1,4-6,12,13] Surgical mortality has been 33 percent or higher in the infant and childhood groups,[14] and not a single useful survival has been reported in the neonatal group. Although the majority of cases reviewed were done before the advent of microsurgical techniques and critical care units, Yasargil still experienced a one-third surgical mortality using the operating microscope.[14] In most cases, postoperative deaths have been from cardiac causes, while the poor results have occurred because of residual brain damage from hydrocephalus, vascular steal, or both.

Nevertheless, there is reason for optimism. Several patients, children included, have survived with normal function and intellect. In the most recent report from Toronto, five of eight surgically treated infants are normal.[5] The points of emphasis mentioned throughout this chapter must be observed if good outcomes are to be obtained.

1. For primary vein of Galen aneurysms, the fistula must be obliterated. The sac need not be excised unless a mass effect is to be reduced. Damage to the posterior hypothalamus and thalamus is inexcusable.
2. For secondary dilatations of the galenic system, occurring as venous outflow from an adjacent angioma, the angioma must be the target of the surgeon. The expanded galenic veins will collapse once the primary lesion is removed.
3. Strict attention to cardiac status and hemodynamics is critical during and following surgery. Intractable heart failure is the most sinister threat facing the child.
4. Proper control of hydrocephalus is necessary to optimize the patient's future.

References

1. Amacher AL, Shillito J Jr: The syndromes and surgical treatment of aneurysms of the great vein of Galen. J Neurosurg 39:89–98, 1973.
2. Bedford THB: The great vein of Galen and the syndrome of increased intracranial pressure. Brain 57:1–24, 1934.
3. Bedford THB: The venous system of the velum interpositum of the rhesus monkey and the effect of experimental occlusion of the great vein of Galen. Brain 57:255–265, 1934.
4. Gold AP, Ransohoff J, Carter S: Vein of Galen malformation. Acta Neurol Scand [Suppl] 11:5–31, 1964.

5. Hoffman HJ, Chuang S, Hendrick EB, Humphreys, RP: Aneurysms of the vein of Galen. J Neurosurg 57:316–322, 1982.
6. Lazar ML: Vein of Galen aneurysm: Successful excision of a completely thrombosed aneurysm in an infant. Surg Neurol 2:22–24, 1974.
7. Long DM, Seljeskog EL, Chou SN, French LA: Giant arteriovenous malformations of infancy and childhood. J Neurosurg 40:304–312, 1974.
8. Norman MG, Becker LE: Cerebral damage in neonates resulting from arteriovenous malformation of the vien of Galen. J Neurol Neurosurg Psychiatry 37:252–258, 1974.
9. O'Brien MS, Schecter MM: Arteriovenous malformations involving the Galenic system. AJR 110:50–55, 1970.
10. Padget DH: The cranial venous system in man in reference to development, adult configuration, and relation to the arteries. Am J Anat 98:307–355, 1956.
11. Sivakoff M, Nouri S: Diagnosis of vein of Galen arteriovenous malformation by two-dimensional ultrasound and pulsed Doppler method. Pediatrics 69:84–86, 1982.
12. Smith DR, Donat JF: Giant arteriovenous malformation of the vein of Galen: Total surgical removal. Neurosurgery 8:378–381, 1981.
13. Ventureyra ECG, Ivan LP, Nabavi N: Deep seated giant arteriovenous malformations in infancy. Surg Neurol 10:365–370, 1978.
14. Yasargil MG, Antic J, Laciga R, Jain KK, Boone SC: Arteriovenous malformations of vein of Galen: Microsurgical treatment. Surg Neurol 6:195–200, 1976.

178

Other Cranial Intradural Angiomas

Setti S. Rengachary
Uma P. Kalyan-Raman

Vascular malformations of the nervous system can be divided into four major clinicopathological categories (Fig. 178-1).

1. An *arteriovenous malformation* (AVM, racemose angioma, arteriovenous fistula, cirsoid aneurysm) consists of large feeding arteries, markedly dilated draining veins, and a vascular nidus consisting of tortuous dilated vessels, but no capillary bed. Arterial blood directly shunts into the venous system, resulting in poor tissue perfusion and tissue ischemia.
2. A *cavernous hemangioma* (cavernoma) consists of a honeycomb of vascular spaces containing blood in very sluggish circulation. The blood is essentially stagnant and remains sequestrated in these vascular spaces. As a consequence, sedimentation, thrombosis, calcification, and ossification occur. The feeding artery and the draining vein are quite small and are not usually demonstrable on radiological studies. There is no brain tissue within the malformation.
3. *Capillary telangiectasia* represents a collection of abnormally dilated, varicose capillaries with intervening brain parenchyma.
4. A *venous angioma* is a vascular malformation without an apparent arterial component. It consists of a myriad of small tapering veins arranged in a radial fashion in the deep white matter. These veins drain into a central vein, which in turn empties into a prominent cortical vein or dural sinus. Only the latter three entities are discussed in this chapter.

Cavernous Hemangiomas

Pathological Features

Cavernous hemangiomas may occur virtually anywhere in the central nervous system or peripheral nerves, although the cerebral hemisphere is the most common site (Table 178-1). In some instances they may be multiple,[31] and on occasion they may be associated with similar lesions elsewhere in the body.[36] Familial occurrence is rare.[2,5]

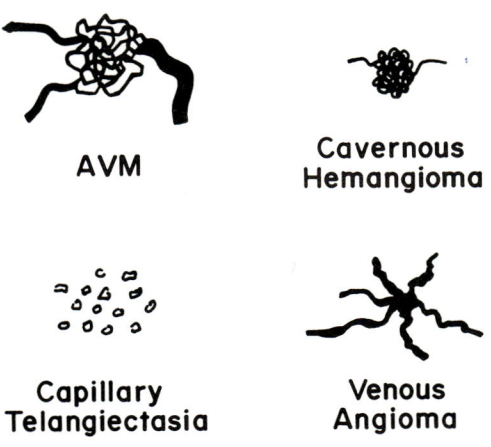

Figure 178-1 Types of vascular malformations that occur in the nervous system. AVM, arteriovenous malformation.

TABLE 178-1 Distribution of Solitary Cavernous Hemangiomas in and around the Nervous System

Cerebral hemispheres: cortical and subcortical areas of the frontal, parietal, occipital, and temporal lobes[33]
Basal ganglia
Diencephalic region[19]
Optic nerve and chiasm[16]
Ventricular system: lateral, third, fourth ventricles; aqueduct of Sylvius; choroid plexus[24]
Pineal region[10]
Pituitary fossa[28]
Middle cranial fossa: extradural;[20] extradural with contiguous extension into the face[22]
Orbit: retro-ocular;[13] retinal[11]
Brain stem
Cerebellum; cerebellum with contiguous extension into the suboccipital region[7]
Cranial nerves (III)[37]
Spinal cord
Spinal root
Spinal epidural space[27]
Vertebral body
Dura mater[18]
Calvarium[38]
Scalp[8]
Peripheral nerve[35]

The size of a cavernous hemangioma is variable, ranging from that of a pinhead to a mass several centimeters across. The majority of lesions when clinically recognized are 1.5 to 3 cm in diameter. The lesion is very well circumscribed, although it lacks a definite capsule (Fig. 178-2). The surface is finely nodular, the nodules representing the external surfaces of the cavernous vessels (Fig. 178-3). The consistency may be soft, firm, or rocky hard depending upon whether the cavernous spaces contain blood, thrombus, organized or hyalinized tissue, calcium deposits, or bone (Fig. 178-4).

The surrounding neural tissue may undergo gliosis and may be stained yellow. The yellow staining is often attributed to "repeated small hemorrhages," but lack of apoplectic events in the clinical history makes this conjecture extremely unlikely. Slow lysis of red cells consequent to their sequestration in the cavernous spaces allows red cell pigments to diffuse out of the lesion into the adjacent tissue. This pigment seems to induce gliosis and may account for the formation of a seizure focus. Experimental studies suggest that chemical compounds containing iron are potent agents in inducing a seizure focus.[4,30] Thus the pathogenesis of seizures in the arteriovenous malformations and cavernous hemangiomas seem to be based on differing mechanisms: in the former it is probably due to ischemia of the neurons as a result of hyperdynamic circulation, low perfusion pressure, and shunting; in the latter it is probably secondary to chemical irritation of the neurons by the iron-containing blood pigments.

Histological sections show a honeycomb of vascular spaces of varying size *without intervening neural tissue except at its very margins*. This is a defining characteristic that distinguishes it from the telangiectasia and the venous angioma (Fig. 178-4). The vascular spaces are lined by a single layer of endothelial cells, supported by collagenous walls. Smooth muscle and elastic tissue are entirely lacking. Thrombosis, organization, hyalinization, calcification, or ossification in the vascular spaces are frequently seen; typical needle-shaped cholesterol crystals may be found in the thrombosed spaces. In the adjacent brain, there may be hemosiderin deposition and gliosis.[17]

Clinical Features

Cavernous hemangiomas may remain clinically silent, being diagnosed incidentally on a computed tomogram (Fig. 178-5) or during a routine autopsy examination of the brain (Fig. 178-2). Headaches, if present, may be vague and poorly defined. "Chronic tension headache" or "migraine variant" are often the admitting diagnoses. Even if a cavernous angioma is found in such instances, a causal relationship may not always be established, since the headaches may remain unaltered even after complete removal of the angioma. A seizure is a frequent presenting symptom. The nature of the seizure

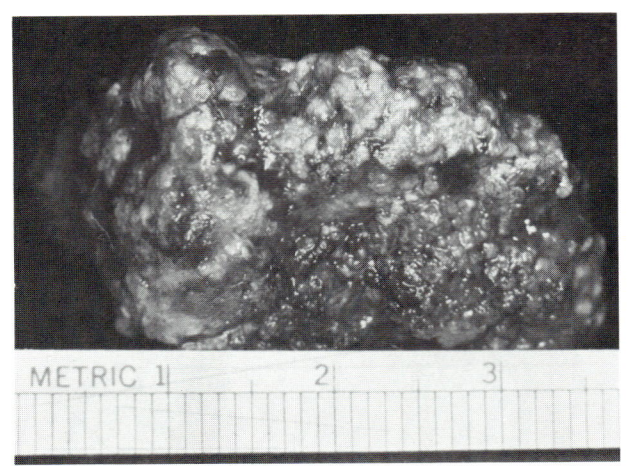

Figure 178-3 The gross appearance of a surgically excised cavernous hemangioma. The surface is finely nodular.

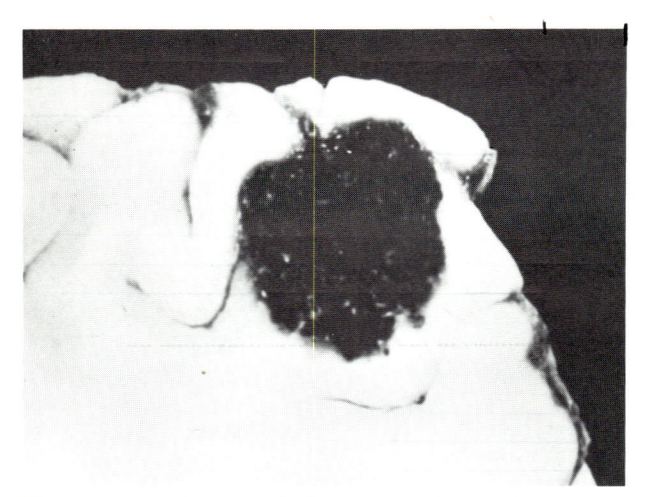

Figure 178-2 A subcortical cavernous hemangioma noted incidentally at autopsy. The lesion is very well circumscribed. (Courtesy of John J. Kepes, M.D.)

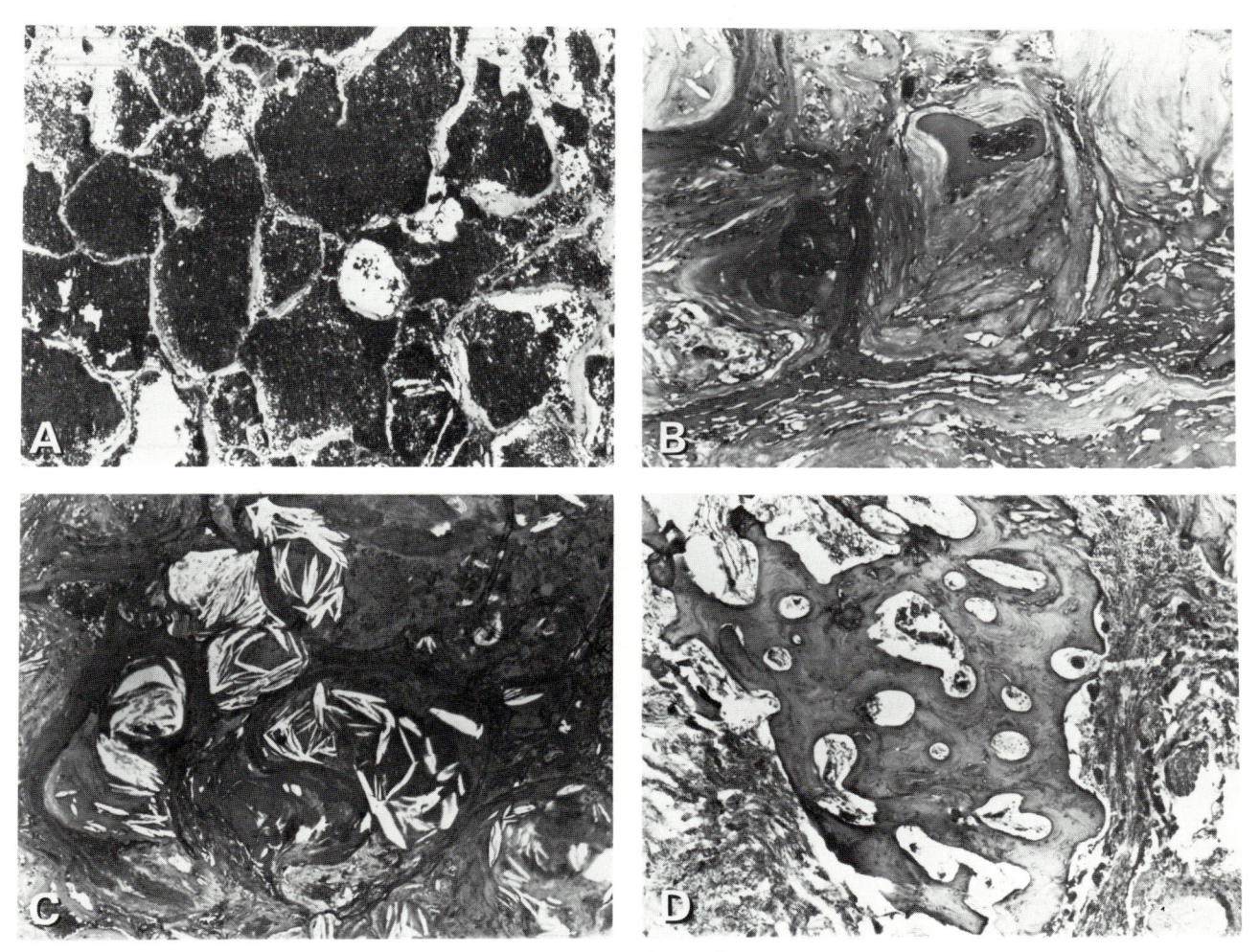

Figure 178-4 Histological appearances of a cavernous hemangioma: *A.* An area showing a honeycomb of vascular spaces without intervening neural tissue. The vascular spaces are lined by a single layer of endothelial cells supported by collagenous walls. *B.* An area showing organization and hyalinization within the vascular spaces. *C.* Typical needle-shaped cholesterol crystals within the thrombosed part of the angioma. *D.* An area of bony metaplasia. (Courtesy of Itaru Watanabe, M.D.)

varies with the location of the angioma.[33] Thus, cavernous hemangiomas around the rolandic fissure induce focal motor-sensory seizures,[25] those located in the temporal lobe (especially in its medial aspect) produce partial complex seizures,[23] and those in the frontal lobe cause generalized seizures. Subarachnoid or intraparenchymal hemorrhage is very uncommon. Increased intracranial pressure from mass effect is likewise exceptional. Certain specific focal symptoms depend upon the anatomical location of the angioma.

Middle cranial fossa cavernous hemangiomas tend to attain a large size before they are clinically manifest. They are usually located extradurally, the dura itself forming a pseudocapsule of the mass.[20] Thought to arise from the cavernous sinus, they surround the structures within it, namely cranial nerves III, IV, V_1, V_2 and VI, and the internal carotid artery. They may involve the bone of the floor of the middle fossa and be contiguous with an angioma of the infratemporal fossa and face.[22] Extension anteriorly into the orbit through the superior orbital fissure (Fig. 178-6) or medially into the sella turcica may also occur.[12] The clinical presentation varies with the extent of the lesion. Headache is common because of the mass effect, distortion of the brain, stretching of the dura, and erosion of the bone. Ocular findings are most common. They may consist of proptosis from retro-orbital extension of the angioma, visual impairment and optic atrophy from direct involvement of the optic nerve, hemianopic field cuts from involvement of the optic chiasm or tract, anisocoria and diplopia due to oculomotor paresis, and papilledema due to increased intracranial pressure. Numbness in the face reflects trigeminal impairment. Encroachment into the sella may lead to panhypopituitarism. The lesion is more frequently seen in women than in men, with a sex ratio of 10:1. The symptoms may precipitate or worsen during pregnancy, presumably as a result of vascular congestion and an increase in the size of the mass. Curiously, most cases of cavernous hemangioma in this location have been reported from Japan.

Cavernous hemangioma in the *pineal region* produces a

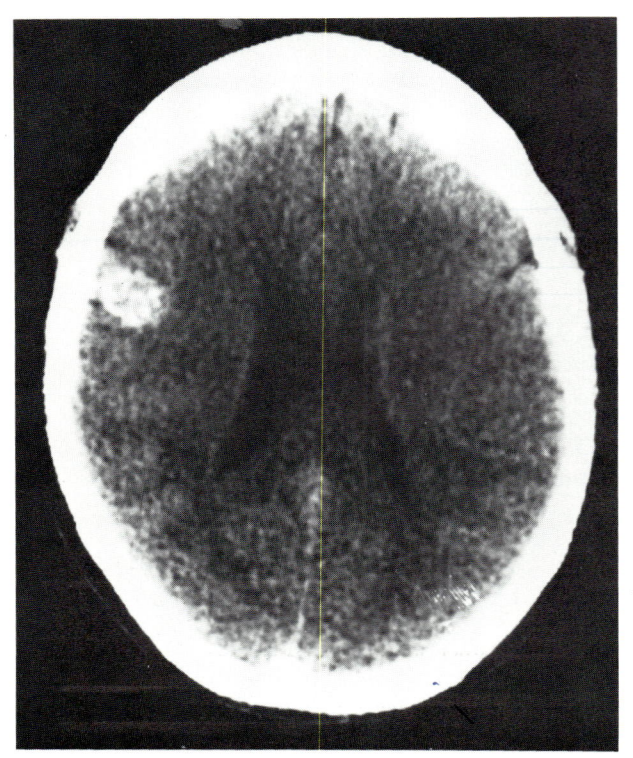

Figure 178-5 The typical appearance of a cavernous hemangioma on a computed tomogram. The lesion is seen as a dense collection of rounded granular densities. There is no edema around the lesion, and there is no mass effect.

typical syndrome characteristic of a mass in this location, consisting of impairment of upgaze and convergence, sluggishly reactive and/or unequal pupils, obstructive hydrocephalus, and papilledema.[10] A distinction from other pineal masses may not be possible even after a complete radiological workup. The occurrence of such benign and curable lesions in this location strengthens the argument for a tissue diagnosis before shunting and radiation therapy are instituted.

A *diencephalic angioma*[19] may delay the onset of puberty, retard growth, and induce obesity, loss of libido, visual field cuts, and memory impairment. Radiological abnormalities may mimic those of a hypothalamic glioma or craniopharyngioma. A single instance of a large cavernous hemangioma of *the pituitary fossa* which was found incidentally at autopsy has been reported.[28]

Cavernous hemangioma occurring exclusively in the cranial or spinal *dura mater* remains clinically silent, as one would expect, and may be discovered incidentally at autopsy.[18] An *intraventricular cavernous hemangioma* may be responsible for intraventricular hemorrhage or cause obstructive hydrocephalus if it is strategically situated at the foramen of Monro or in the aqueductal region.[24]

Cavernous hemangioma rarely occurs in the *retina*,[11] but when it does, it provides the most direct opportunity to study its morphology and hemodynamics through funduscopic visualization. It appears as a mass, resembling a cluster of grapes, lying on the inner retinal surface and protruding into the vitreous. It consists of dilated, rounded, thin-walled saccular blood vessels containing dark-red venous blood. Sluggish circulation through the lesion is evidenced by layering of clear plasma over sedimented erythrocytes in many of the saccules. There is usually no evidence of hemorrhage or exudation. The retinal arteries and veins in the vicinity of the malformation appear to be of normal caliber. Fluorescein angiography demonstrates a significant delay in the perfusion of dye through the lesion. Extravascular leakage of the dye does not occur around the lesion. In some individuals with retinal cavernous hemangioma, there may be similar lesions in the brain (which may or may not be symptomatic) and the skin and there may be a strong family history. In this regard, this oculoneurocutaneous triad resembles other well-known neurocutaneous syndromes (phakomatoses).

A cavernous hemangioma occurring within the *optic nerve, chiasm, or tract* may induce varying degrees of impairment of acuity and visual fields depending upon its exact location and extent.[16] Cavernous hemangioma is the most common benign *retro-orbital* tumor that occurs between the ages of 30 and 49 years. Painless, nonpulsatile proptosis without a bruit is the most common finding.[13] Arising from the muscle cone directly behind the globe, it produces axial proptosis in most instances; if an eccentric position is noted, it is likely to be downward. Indentation of the posterior globe results in (1) hyperopia, which may be partially or totally correctable; and (2) the formation of retinal striae (choroidal folds). Direct compression of the optic nerve or its blood supply results in a field cut of varying types depending upon the location of the mass. A mild disc edema is common.

Giant hemangiomas of the *scalp*[8] present in the newborn as a soft compressible mass with prominent distended veins coursing over it. If the lesion is massive enough, it may result in cephalopelvic disproportion and dystocia.

Calvarial hemangiomas[38] most commonly occur in the parietal or frontal region and occur in females three times as frequently as in males. A long-standing painless bony swelling is the presenting symptom. On palpation, scalp tissues move freely over the hard mass. Roentgenograms of the skull show a well-circumscribed lucent area in the vault of the skull with a honeycomb-like trabeculated appearance. The margins of the lesion do not usually show sclerosis, a point of distinction from intradiploic epidermoids. The outer table is expanded, with the inner table maintaining its normal contour. On tangential views, radial spicules of bone produce a "sun ray" appearance. There is no reactive hyperostosis, in contradistinction to that produced by a meningioma. Angiography reveals delayed circulation through the lesion, with venous puddling. Histological sections show blood-filled cavernous spaces separated by spicules of normal bone.

In cavernous hemangiomas involving *peripheral nerves*,[35] a rounded mass along the course of the nerve may be palpable. Application of pressure on this mass may induce tingling and paresthesias along the sensory distribution of the nerve. A sensory-motor deficit that corresponds to the distribution of the nerve may be detectable. The hemangioma may be entirely intrinsic to the nerve, or it may be a part of more diffuse hemangioma of the soft tissues. When entirely intrinsic, the hemangioma simply splays the nerve fascicles such that total removal by microdissection is possible without having to sacrifice the fascicles.

A hemorrhagic diathesis may be encountered in patients with cavernous hemangiomas. It primarily occurs in infants and young children with a massive angioma involving many tissue planes or large viscera; thus, it is not ordinarily encountered with relatively small hemangiomas that occur in the brain parenchyma. An extensive hemangioma involving the middle cranial fossa, cranial base, and face, however, may lead to such a bleeding diathesis. The disorder may be manifested spontaneously or become evident after an operative procedure. Abnormal bleeding may be based on two pathological mechanisms: (1) a consumption coagulopathy due to extensive spontaneous thrombosis within the malformation, the consumption of platelets, fibrinogen, and other clotting factors, and a generalized bleeding tendency (Kasabach-Merritt syndrome),[34] and (2) a chronic bleeding disorder due to a qualitative platelet defect, the "storage pool disease" of platelets. This syndrome is characterized by minor bleeding episodes, a prolonged bleeding time, the absence of a secondary aggregation in response to adenosine diphosphate (ADP) or epinephrine, and a decreased aggregation response to collagen. The platelets in this clinical setting have a reduction in the level of ADP and a comparatively smaller drop in the level of adenosine triphosphate (ATP), resulting in an ATP/ADP ratio that is significantly higher than in normal platelets. There is a specific depletion of the storage pool of adenine nucleotides from the dense granules of platelets while the metabolically active adenine nucleotides remain unaffected.[14]

Radiological Evaluation

Skull roentgenograms may show an area of faint granular calcification, but generally these are not helpful. Computed tomography is more sensitive than plain roentgenograms in demonstrating calcification.[29] Radionuclide brain scans may show an increased uptake in about three-fourths of the cases but seldom provide specific diagnostic information. Factors determining whether a scan is positive are the size of the lesion and its depth from the cortical surface.

As a general rule, angiography is completely normal even with the use of magnification and subtraction techniques. In contrast to the angiography of arteriovenous malformations, there is usually no evidence of large arterial feeders, an anomalous cluster of blood vessels, or early draining veins. An avascular area in the capillary phase may be discernible. A faint capillary blush or punctate venous puddling may be seen in rare instances. A mass effect is ordinarily absent. Hypervascularity and a mass effect (suggesting the diagnosis of glioblastoma) are demonstrated only in exceptional cases.[26]

Computed tomography is the most sensitive and the most definitive diagnostic test for intracranial cavernous hemangiomas. This is reflected in the increasing reports of this lesion in the recent literature. Routine use of this diagnostic modality has allowed the recognition of symptomatic as well as incidental lesions.

A typical lesion is seen as a well-demarcated hyperdense area consisting of a collection of rounded granular densities (Fig. 178-5). The attenuation values of the lesion approximate those of calcified tissue or blood. Contrast enhancement, although definitely present in the majority of cases, is minimal and is not easily discernible for two reasons: first, cavernous hemangiomas contain stagnant, sequestered blood, virtually excluded from the dynamic parenchymal circulation; second, the inherently high density of the lesion from the presence of blood and calcium obscures the identification of contrast enhancement, unless the actual attenuation values before and after contrast injection are compared. In a minority of cases a mixed hyperdense-hypodense pattern may be observed. The hypodense areas in such instances probably represent caverns containing old lysed blood, hyalinized areas, or cholesterol crystals (Fig. 178-4). Perilesional edema and mass effect from the lesion are conspicuous by their absence. In exceptional cases a poorly defined zone of low density may surround the lesion, representing an area of gliosis or edema.

Cavernous angiomas may be difficult to differentiate from low-grade astrocytomas. The following features are helpful in their differentiation, although no one feature is absolute for either lesion. Astrocytomas, even the slow-growing ones, tend to have a shorter clinical history than cavernous angiomas that are congenital hamartomas. The calcification in astrocytomas may be in the form of granular, nodular, or linear deposits, generally in the center of the tumor. There is a larger area of peripheral soft tissue compared with the central calcified area. Cavernous hemangiomas tend to be uniformly calcified up to the periphery of the lesion. Astrocytomas show peritumoral edema, produce a mass effect, and increase appreciably in size on serial computed tomograms done over a period of time, whereas cavernous angiomas generally do not show edema or mass effect and remain static in size.

Thrombosed arteriovenous malformations may be indistinguishable from cavernous hemangiomas on computed tomograms although their histological features are quite different. A large calcified cavernous hemangioma in the middle cranial fossa may closely simulate a sphenoid ridge meningioma (Fig. 178-6).

Management

There are several indications for surgical excision of an intracranial cavernous hemangioma. The foremost is the need to establish the tissue diagnosis. Although the diagnosis may be suspected from comprehensive radiological studies, it may be impossible to differentiate this lesion from a calcified astrocytoma or oligodendroglioma. Middle cranial fossa hemangiomas cannot be differentiated from sphenoid wing meningiomas. Long-standing seizures are a justifiable indication for removal, although occasional seizures may persist after surgical therapy. In an asymptomatic patient, one may remove a cortical or subcortical lesion with the hopes of preventing the formation of a seizure focus, although such reasoning may be challenged on the grounds that the probability of such a patient developing a seizure focus remains unknown at the time; even if it is known, to justify an operation it should be higher than the probability of a seizure

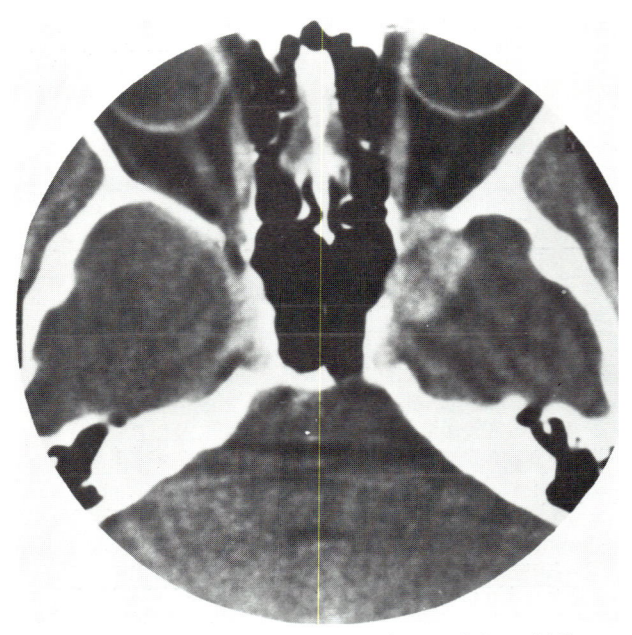

Figure 178-6 A cavernous hemangioma of the middle cranial fossa arising in the region of the cavernous sinus, simulating a meningioma. The lesion extends through the widened superior orbital fissure into the orbit. (Courtesy of David G. Harper, M.D.)

from a surgical scar. The fact that these lesions may be removed with surprising ease with minimal bleeding and minimal tissue dissection should be taken into account in the decision-making process. The risk of spontaneous hemorrhage from the lesion is a valid indication, although this risk is quite small. The location of the lesion in a strategic area such as the pineal region, the diencephalon, or the cavernous sinus region, or the presence of a significant neurological deficit, may mandate its operative removal.

In the planning for the operative removal of a cavernous hemangioma, it is helpful to precisely localize and mark the lesion site on the skin surface, utilizing computed tomography. This is especially important for a subcortical lesion because the cortical surface may appear quite normal at operation, without gyral widening or increased vascularity. Unnecessary subcortical exploration may thus be avoided. The most helpful clue to the presence of the cavernous angioma is the invariable yellow staining of the cortical or subcortical area around the lesion. The lesion itself is usually calcified, hard, and nodular, but almost always the nidus of the lesion is surrounded by a soft, gelatinous, deeply yellow stained zone of gliotic tissue. The lesion literally appears to float within this soft reactive tissue (Fig. 178-7). Dissection around the lesion through this adventitious tissue is surprisingly easy, with minimal or no bleeding. Even deep lesions that appear to be in the basal ganglia may be removed with relative ease. Wherever possible, the reactive hemosiderin stained tissue around the malformation should be removed along with the angiomatous nidus to minimize the incidence of postoperative seizures.

For lesions located in the pineal region, diencephalic area, or the foramen of Monro region, appropriate operative exposures that are discussed elsewhere in the text should be used. Lesions in the middle cranial fossa pose certain unique problems. The lesions in this location are unusually vascular, being fed by meningeal branches of the external and internal carotid arteries. Attempted resection is usually associated with profuse blood loss. Intimate association of the lesion with the cranial nerves passing through the cavernous sinus, the internal carotid artery, and the optic nerve render these structures vulnerable to damage during surgical resection. Diffuse intravascular coagulopathy is a potential risk after the removal of such a large middle fossa angioma.

The prognosis is very good for patients with a cortical or subcortical cavernous hemangioma. The operative mortality and morbidity risks are slightly higher for lesions in the pineal or foramen of Monro region. Middle cranial fossa cavernous angiomas carry the worst prognosis.

Capillary Telangiectasias

Capillary telangiectasias are malformations composed of pathologically dilated capillaries. Most of these malformations are clinically silent, are not detectable on radiological studies, and are found incidentally at autopsy. They occur most commonly in the pons, near the midline. Other common locations are the cerebral cortex and the paraventricular white matter. On occasion they may be multiple[3] or may occur in association with other vascular malformations such as cavernous hemangiomas; indeed, in some instances transitional forms between telangiectasias and cavernous hemangiomas may occur. In exceptional cases telangiectasias may calcify and may be diagnosed as hemangioma calcificans[32] in the plain roentgenograms. In an unusual case, the medulla oblongata was extensively involved with this malformation, which resembled a sieve. The patient, who died of lymphosarcoma, had had a progressive unexplained neurological deficit for several years prior to death.[9] Massive hemorrhage

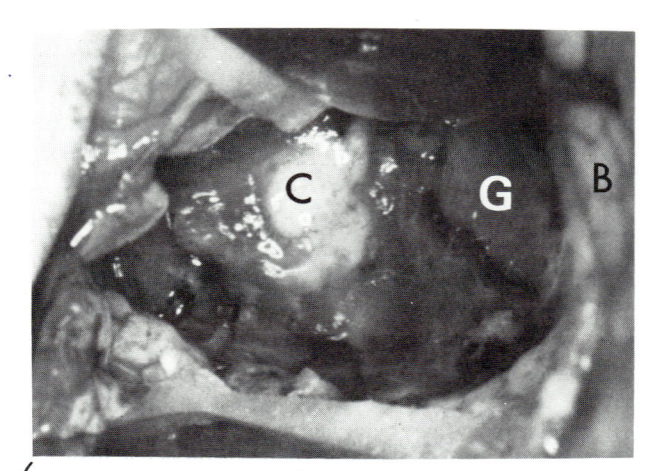

Figure 178-7 The typical appearance of a cavernous hemangioma exposed surgically: C, densely calcified cavernous hemangioma; G, a gelatinous gliotic area, stained deeply yellow, surrounding the malformation; B, the cortical brain surface.

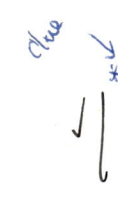

Other Cranial Intradural Angiomas

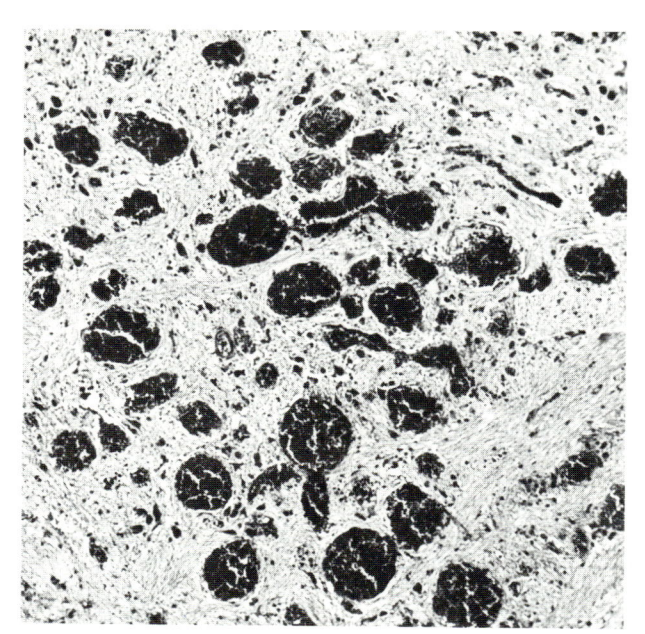

Figure 178-8 Capillary telangiectasia. The lesion consists of pathologically dilated capillaries with intervening brain parenchyma.

→ areas of 'petechial' hemorrhage.

from capillary telangiectasia into the brain parenchyma has been reported; the source of bleeding in such instances may be missed unless biopsy of the wall of the hematoma is undertaken.

On gross inspection, the malformation appears as poorly defined punctate pink foci resembling an area of petechial hemorrhage. No dilated arteries or veins are seen leading to or from the malformation. Microscopically, the lesion consists of a group of variably dilated and varicose capillaries. In contrast to cavernous hemangiomas, there is intervening brain parenchyma (Fig. 178-8). This parenchyma generally appears normal, without evidence of gliosis, necrosis, and recent or remote hemorrhage.

Venous Angiomas

A venous angioma may be defined as a vascular malformation without an obvious arterial component.[21] Generally it is clinically silent, often diagnosed only incidentally on a contrast-enhanced computed tomogram or cerebral angiogram. Subarachnoid hemorrhage or a seizure disorder may occur but is exceptional. Most venous angiomas are located in the frontal or parietal lobe in the supratentorial space, or deep in the cerebellar white matter in the vicinity of the vein of Galen.

The appearance of a venous angioma on a cerebral angiogram has been described as a 'caput medusae,' a hydra, spokes of a wheel, a spider, an umbrella, or a sunburst. The lesion consists of a myriad of small tapering veins arranged in a radial fashion in the deep white matter. These veins converge into a relatively large and centrally located draining vein, which in turn may empty into a larger cortical vein or a dural sinus (Fig. 178-9). Or the large collecting vein may drain into a subependymal vein in the wall of the lateral ventricle. Opacification of this anomalous venous network generally occurs in the venous phase of the arteriogram; the arterial and capillary phases are usually normal even with magnification and subtraction techniques. Early filling of the venous angioma in the arterial or capillary phase occurs infrequently. The large transcerebral draining vein remains opacified through the late venous phase. The circulation time is within the normal range. No evidence of a mass effect is apparent unless the malformation has bled into the cerebral parenchyma.

A contrast-enhanced computed tomogram recapitulates the appearance seen on an angiogram.[15] The large draining vein is seen as a serpentine density, while the nidus of the malformation resembles the spokes of a wheel. A venous angioma may be visualized as a focal area of increased uptake in the venous phase of a dynamic radionuclide brain scan.

On histological examination, the vessels composing a venous angioma contain smooth muscle and elastic tissue,

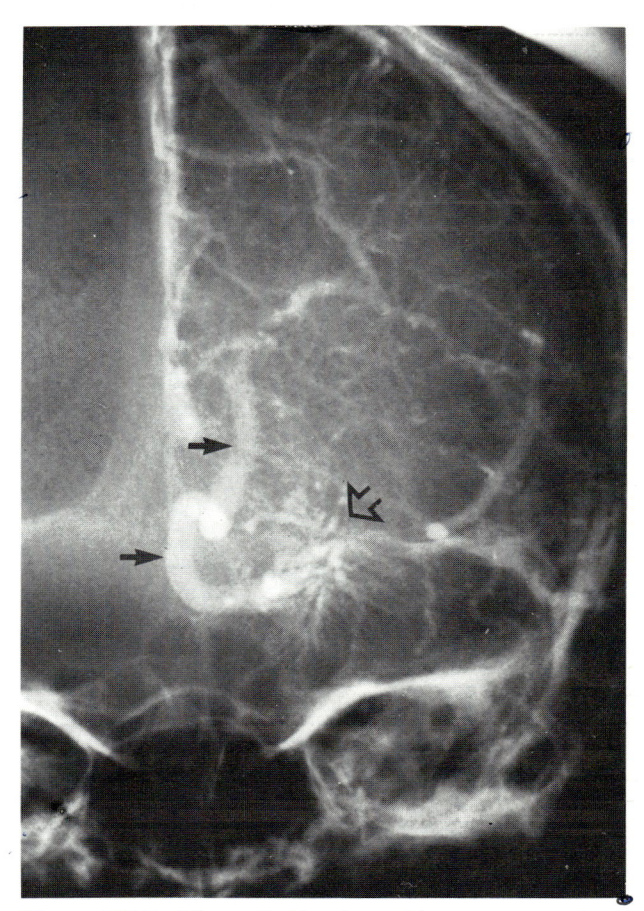

Figure 178-9 The typical angiographic appearance of a venous angioma. The angioma consists of a myriad of small tapering veins arranged in a radial fashion in the deep white matter (*open arrow*). A prominent large cortical vein drains the malformation (*solid arrows*). (Courtesy of K. Arjunan, M.D.)

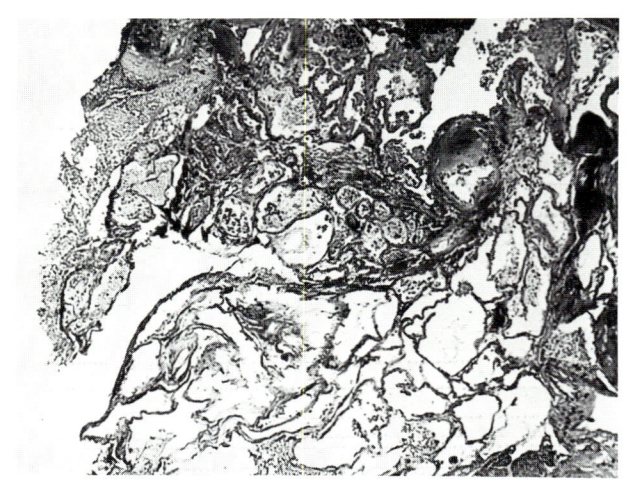

Figure 178-10 The histological appearance of a third ventricular venous angioma.

but to a much lesser extent than in arterial walls. Hyalinization and thickening of the vessel walls are common (Fig. 178-10). As with arteriovenous malformations and telangiectasias, but unlike cavernous hemangiomas, neural parenchyma is found between the vascular elements of this malformation.

Since most venous angiomas are clinically silent and the risk of subarachnoid hemorrhage is quite small, a conservative approach is mandated if such a lesion is found incidentally on a cerebral angiogram. Their deep location and the necessity to remove large segments of normal brain parenchyma along with the malformation further dictate a conservative approach unless bleeding is documented from the malformation or an intractable seizure disorder is causally related to it. Berenstein and Choi have recently reported direct percutaneous puncture of these lesions under fluoroscopic control and the in situ embolization with 95% ethanol; they reported significant improvement in all patients so treated.[1]

Cryptic Vascular Malformations

The cryptic vascular malformations are a heterogeneous group of small angiomatous malformations (telangiectasia, venous angioma, cavernous hemangioma, arteriovenous malformation) that, although angiographically occult, is detected by computed tomography or at autopsy.[6] The failure of opacification during arteriography may be explained by small size or lack of arterial feeders, or by thrombosis within the malformation. A cryptic vascular malformation may induce seizures, mimic neoplastic lesions in computed tomograms, or produce spontaneous intracerebral hemorrhage. The following features characterize intraparenchymal hemorrhage from a cryptic vascular malformation: (1) occurrence in a relatively young individual; (2) absence of known predisposing factors such as hypertension, trauma, blood dyscrasia, etc.; (3) apoplectic onset with headaches; (4) delayed onset of loss of consciousness except with a hemorrhage occurring within the brain stem; (5) location of the bleeding usually in the periventricular white matter, ventricle, or the brain stem; and (6) absence of a demonstrable aneurysm, arteriovenous malformation, or other vascular lesion in the angiogram.

References

1. Berenstein A, Choi IS: Treatment of venous angiomas by direct alcohol injection. AJNR 4:1144, 1983 (abstr).
2. Bicknell JM, Carlow TJ, Kornfeld M, Stovring J, Turner P: Familial cavernous angiomas. Arch Neurol 35:746–749, 1978.
3. Burke EC, Winkelman RK, Strickland MK: Disseminated hemangiomatosis. Am J Dis Child 108:418–424, 1964.
4. Chusid JG, Kopeloff LM: Epileptogenic effects of pure metals implanted in motor cortex of monkeys. J Appl Physiol 17:697–700, 1962.
5. Clark JV: Familial occurrence of cavernous angiomata of the brain. J Neurol Neurosurg Psychiatry 33:871–876, 1970.
6. Cohen HCM, Tucker WS, Humphreys RP, Perrin RJ: Angiographically cryptic histologically verified cerebrovascular malformations. Neurosurgery 10:704–714, 1982.
7. Dandy WE: Venous abnormalities and angiomas of the brain. Arch Surg 17:715–793, 1928.
8. De Klerk DJJ, Northover RC: Giant haemangiomas of the scalp. S Afr Med J 55:59–62, 1979.
9. Farrell DF, Forno LS: Symptomatic capillary telangiectasis of the brainstem without hemorrhage: Report of an unusual case. Neurology 20:341–346, 1970.
10. Fukui M, Matsuoka S, Hasuo K, Numaguchi Y, Kitamura K: Cavernous hemangioma in the pineal region. Surg Neurol 20:209–215, 1983.
11. Gass JDM: Cavernous hemangioma of the retina. Am J Ophthalmol 71:799–814, 1971.
12. Harper DG, Buck DR, Early CB: Visual loss from cavernous hemangiomas of the middle cranial fossa. Arch Neurol 39:252–254, 1982.
13. Harris GJ, Jakobiec FA: Cavernous hemangioma of the orbit. J Neurosurg 51:219–228, 1979.
14. Khurana MS, Lian ECY, Harkness DR: "Storage pool disease" of platelets. JAMA 244:169–171, 1980.
15. Lotz PR, Quisling RG: CT of venous angiomas of the brain. AJNR 4:1124–1126, 1983.
16. Manz HJ, Klein LH, Fermaglich J, Kattah J, Luessenhop AJ: Cavernous hemangioma of optic chiasm, optic nerves and right optic tract. Virchows Arch [Pathol Anat] 383:225–231, 1979.
17. McCormick WF: The pathology of vascular ("arteriovenous") malformations. J Neurosurg 24:807–816, 1966.
18. McCormick WF, Boulter TR: Vascular malformations ("angiomas") of the dura mater. J Neurosurg 25:309–311, 1966.
19. Mizutani T, Goldberg HI, Kerson LA, Murtagh F: Cavernous hemangioma in the diencephalon. Arch Neurol 38:379–382, 1981.
20. Namba S: Extracerebral cavernous hemangioma of the middle cranial fossa. Surg Neurol 19:379–388, 1983.
21. Numaguchi Y, Kitamura K, Fukui M, Ikeda J, Hasuo K, Kishikawa T, Okudera T, Uemura K, Matsura K: Intracranial venous angiomas. Surg Neurol 18:193–202, 1982.
22. Pásztor E, Szabó G, Slowik F, Zoltán J: Case report: Cavernous hemangioma of the base of the skull. J Neurosurg 21:582–585, 1964.
23. Penfield W, Ward A: Calcifying epileptogenic lesions. Arch Neurol Psychiatry 60:20–36, 1948.

24. Pozzati E, Gaist G, Poppi M, Morrone B, Padovani R: Microsurgical removal of paraventricular cavernous angiomas. J Neurosurg 55:308–311, 1981.
25. Pozzati E, Padovani R, Morrone B, Finizio F, Gaist G: Cerebral cavernous angiomas in children. J Neurosurg 53:826–832, 1980.
26. Rao VRK, Pillai SM, Shenoy KT, Radhakrishnan VV, Mathews G: Hypervascular cavernous angioma at angiography. Neuroradiology 18:211–214, 1979.
27. Richardson RR, Cerullo LJ: Spinal epidural cavernous hemangioma. Surg Neurol 12:266–268, 1979.
28. Sansone ME, Liwnicz BH, Mandybur TI: Giant pituitary cavernous hemangioma. J Neurosurg 53:124–126, 1980.
29. Savoiardo M, Strada L, Passerini A: Intracranial cavernous hemangiomas: Neuroradiologic review of 36 operated cases. AJNR 4:945–950, 1983.
30. Sypert GW, Willmore LJ: A new model of post-traumatic epilepsy: Iron cations. Presented at the 28th Annual Meeting of the Congress of Neurological Surgeons, Washington, D.C., September 28, 1978.
31. Tindall RSA, Kirkpatrick JB, Sklar F: Multiple small cavernous angiomas of the brain with increased intracranial pressure. Ann Neurol 4:376–378, 1978.
32. Vaquero J, Manrique M, Oya S, Cabezudo JM, Bravo G: Calcified telangiectatic hamartomas of the brain. Surg Neurol 13:453–457, 1980.
33. Voigt K, Yasargil MG: Cerebral cavernous haemangiomas or cavernomas. Neurochirurgia (Stuttg) 19:59–68, 1976.
34. Wacksman SJ, Flessa HC, Glueck HI, Will JJ: Coagulation defects and giant cavernous hemangioma. Am J Dis Child 111:71–74, 1966.
35. Wood MB: Case report: Intraneural hemangioma: Report of a case. Plast Reconstr Surg 65:74–76, 1980.
36. Wood MW, White RJ, Kernohan JW: Cavernous hemangiomatosis involving the brain, spinal cord, heart, skin and kidney. Staff Mtgs Mayo Clin 32:249–254, 1957.
37. Wright GP: Discussion: The pathology of spontaneous intracranial hemorrhage. Proc R Soc Med 47:689–693, 1954.
38. Wyke BD: Primary hemangioma of the skull: A rare cranial tumor. AJR 61:302–316, 1949.

179
Dural Arteriovenous Malformations
Alfred J. Luessenhop

The first description of an arteriovenous malformation (AVM) confined to the dura was probably that of Sachs in 1931. This was followed by additional descriptions by Tönnis in 1936 and Röttgen in 1937. Another case, clearly post-traumatic and demonstrated by angiography, was described by Fincher in 1951, and in the same year Verbiest first described a dural malformation involving the posterior fossa.[25]

Subsequently, with the further development of cerebral angiography, many more cases were reported with detailed descriptions of the pathological anatomy and physiology, and at present, close to 200 cases are recorded in the literature. Today the dural AVMs are regarded as relatively rare. Their incidence may be approximated by the frequency with which they appear relative to AVMs involving primarily the brain. In reported series, this has ranged from 10 to 15 percent. The estimated number of patients with cerebral AVMs in the United States is approximately 280,000.[16] Hence, the number of cases with AVMs confined to the dura may range from 28,000 to 42,000 in the United States. However, if these lesions are acquired and spontaneous resolution is common, as most evidence now suggests,[3,11] their prevalence must be considerably less.

Most of the earlier reported cases were managed by ligation of the external carotid artery or appropriate branches. Success varied, particularly when the predominant symptom was an annoying bruit. An intravascular approach, using flow-directed emboli, was introduced by Luessenhop in 1960,[17] and, subsequently, this was modified to a selective catheter technique by Djindjian.[6] More recently, the need for extensive isolation of the involved dural sinuses has become evident, and surgical techniques for the isolation or sacrifice of the major sinuses, as described by Hugosson and Bergstrom in 1974,[12] are frequently employed.

Embryology, Pathology, and Pathogenesis

Embryologically, the circulations of the brain and its coverings, including the dura, skull, and scalp, are united. Hence, it can be anticipated that arteriovenous communications developing in one of these layers may have vascular participation from any or all of the adjacent layers. Also residual vascular communications may enlarge in fistulas acquired later. Angiographically, at least 20 percent of AVMs residing solely within the cerebral hemispheres continue to have some dural arterial participation. Also, isolated examples of direct shunts between cerebral arteries and adjacent dural sinuses, as well as cerebral lesions supplied solely by dural arteries, have been described. Finally, extensive lesions involving the scalp, skull, dura, and brain are known. However, most commonly the AVMs are restricted to the brain or one of the covering layers, and hence, they can be categorized according to this primary anatomical site. Those with significant vascular participation from adjacent layers may be considered variants.

Consideration of the pathology and probable pathogenesis of the dural AVMs requires exact knowledge of the normal vasculature of the dura and its sinuses. The normal arterial supply of the intracranial dura is shown in Fig. 179-1. In the anterior fossa, dural branches from the anterior and posterior ethmoidal arteries arise from the ophthalmic artery. For the middle fossa, the middle meningeal and the accessory meningeal arteries are the main source of supply. The middle meningeal divides into an anterior and a posterior division, and these pass to the region of the sagittal sinus and anastomose with meningeal arteries from the opposite side over the sinus. (The main source of supply for the tentorium and dura of the posterior fossa are branches of the meningohypophyseal trunk arising from the internal carotid artery, dural branches from the posterior auricular artery, anterior and posterior dural branches from the ascending pharyngeal artery, and two dural branches from each of the vertebral arteries as they pierce the dura.) Finally, the occipital arteries have dural branches passing through the occipital bone and supplying generous portions of the dura of the posterior fossa. Potential anastomoses with the muscular branches of the vertebral arteries and ascending cervical arteries exist and become prominent in extensive dural fistulas. Along the margins of the venous sinuses, there are multiple arteriovenous communications which normally are too small for angiographic detection.

The dural AVMs may be classified according to the major venous sinus involved. These are the sphenoparietal sinus along the lesser wing of the sphenoid bone,[2] the cavernous sinus,[21] the superior and inferior petrosal sinuses, the straight sinus, the inferior occipital sinus,[5,10,13,22] the transverse sinus with its continuation into the sigmoid sinus,[14,22,23] and the anterior sagittal sinus.[4,7,26] The posterior portion of the sagittal sinus is less frequently involved, and in general, involvement of the sagittal sinus is mostly restricted to lesions which are clearly traumatic in etiology and associated with fractures in the lateral walls of the calvarium.

Angiographically, the lesions appear as multiple, direct shunts between the enlarged dural arteries and their collat-

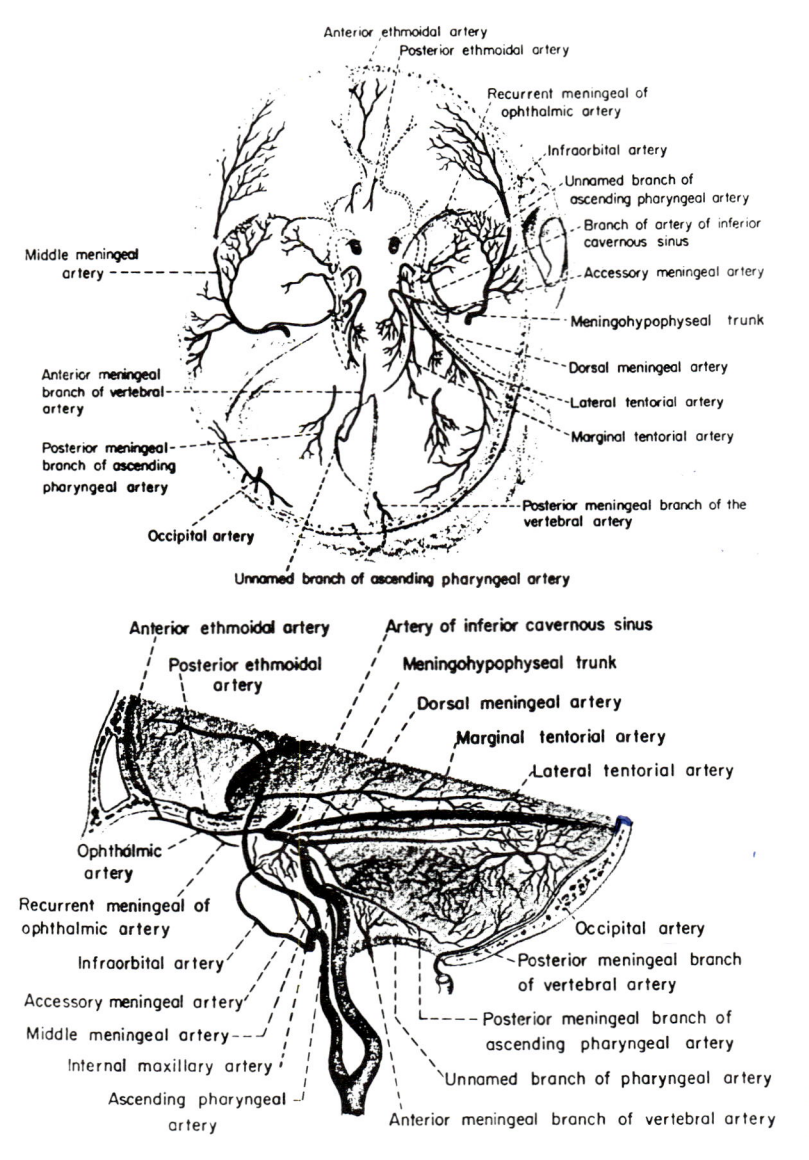

Figure 179-1 Arterial supply to the dura of the cranial base. (From Houser et al.[10])

erals passing directly to the walls of the involved sinuses (Figs. 179-2 and 179-3).[1,5,10] This is in contrast to the cerebral AVMs in which the sites of direct shuntings are less obvious angiographically and the bulk of the lesion is a closely packed network of pathological vascular channels referred to as a nidus. Occasionally, there is enlargement of the involved sinus or aneurysmal enlargement of an immediately adjacent pial vein. Retrograde flow is frequently seen in the sinuses and veins when the fistulas are extensive. This correlates with associated increased intracranial pressure which is probably secondary to an elevated pressure transmitted to all the draining sinuses.[13,20,21] When the venous drainage includes the deep venous system with enlargement of the great vein of Galen, obstructive hydrocephalus may ensue.

Microscopic examination of sections at the fistulous sites reveals a network of dysplastic tortuous vascular channels attached to or incorporated into the dura. There are no specific microscopic features favoring either a congenital or acquired etiology.[3,11]

Many of the dural fistulas are clearly traumatic in origin, because they become symptomatic after a significant head injury or are immediately adjacent to a fracture. Further, a preponderance of evidence suggests that the majority, if not all, of the remaining lesions are acquired.[1,3,11] Evidence for this stems from the following: (1) Initial clinical presentation is mostly during mid-life, and presentation during early childhood or infancy is rare. (2) There is a high incidence of spontaneous resolution, particularly for the lesions involving the cavernous sinus.[18] (3) Angiographically, there is a frequent association with abnormalities of the involved sinus. These may be either complete thrombotic occlusion or irregularities in the sinus walls consistent with an organizing or recanalizing thrombotic process.[3,8,11] (4) Fistulas have been demonstrated in patients in whom some years before angiography demonstrated a normal dural vasculature.[3]

On the basis of the above, the proposed mechanism is that an inflammatory or thrombotic process within a major sinus leads to partial or total occlusion and subsequent opening of the pre-existing, minute arteriovenous fistulas in the sinus walls. Following recanalization of the sinus, the fistulas persist. Spontaneous resolution, which is far more common than in cerebral AVMs, may result from renewed thrombosis of the sinus or reclosure of the fistulas.[3,11] This mechanism may be extended to include those few cases noted in infancy or childhood by assuming that there is damage to the sinuses, particularly the transverse and sigmoid sinuses, during parturition. However, there are rare cases with extensive dural involvement and hyperostosis of the skull for whom a congenital etiology still seems likely.

Clinical Features

Because of wide variability with respect to the degree of arterial shunting and the sinuses primarily involved, symptomatic presentation also varies widely.[1,21–23] However, a common feature is spontaneous bleeding, which may be subarachnoid, subdural, or, in rare instances, intracerebral. Headache and a subjective bruit are also common irrespective of the anatomical location. In approximately two-thirds of the reported cases, the transverse and sigmoid sinuses are principally involved. Most of the remaining one-third involve the cavernous sinus and adjacent sinuses of the middle fossa. Primary involvement of the sagittal sinus of the anterior fossa or the posterior portions of this sinus is rare.[4,7,26]

For the fistulas involving the cavernous sinus, the patients are predominantly women over the age of 40. The presenting symptom is usually head pain localized to the orbit or to the frontal or temporal regions. The most common findings are dilated conjunctival veins and mild proptosis with an associated sixth nerve palsy. Marked proptosis with chemosis is seen only occasionally. A bruit may not be present subjectively or objectively, and as a rule, ocular pulsations are absent in contrast to those encountered with internal carotid-cavernous fistulas.

For fistulas involving the petrosal or sphenoparietal sinus, the usual initial complaint is an annoying bruit, and on examination this may be the only finding. Most of these cases are related to preceding head trauma.[2,5]

For the dural fistulas involving the transverse and sigmoid sinus, the presenting symptom may be a bruit and an occipital headache. Occasionally there is an associated increase in intracranial pressure with papilledema and visual failure.[15] A bruit can be detected over the mastoid region on the involved side in nearly all cases.[1,5,10,13,14,22]

For the rare fistulas involving the superior sagittal sinus wholly or partly, bruit is generally not a symptom, and the patient may remain asymptomatic unless subarachnoid hemorrhage ensues.

Radiological Features

Nearly all the extensive fistulas will show some changes in plain skull films. These changes include prominent vascular markings of the meningeal vessels and an enlarged foramen

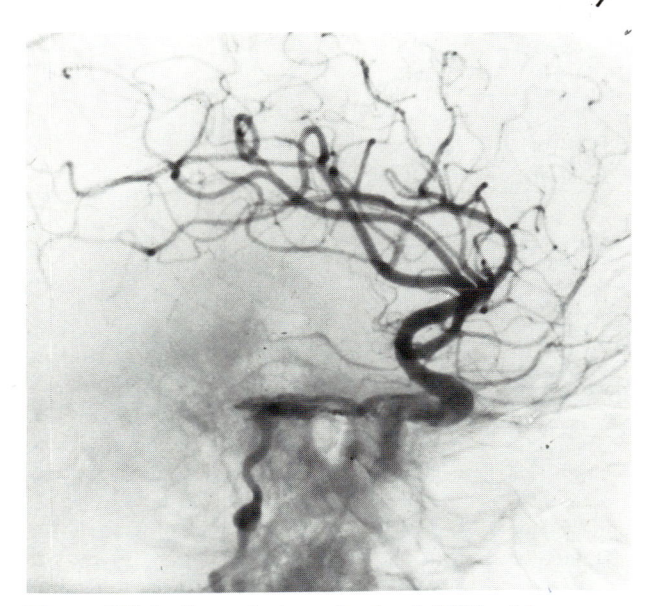

Figure 179-2 Lateral view of a dural AVM with branches of the meningohypophyseal trunk draining into the inferior petrosal sinus.

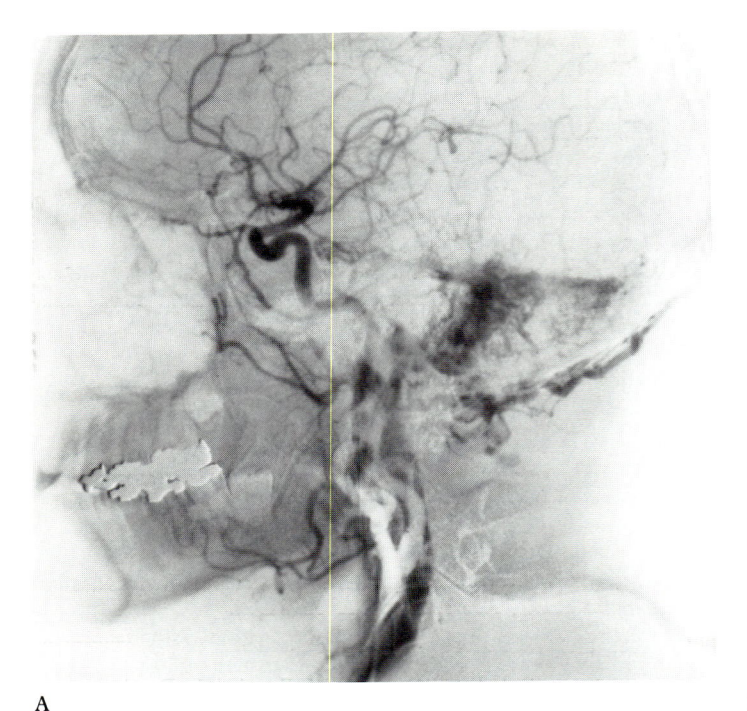

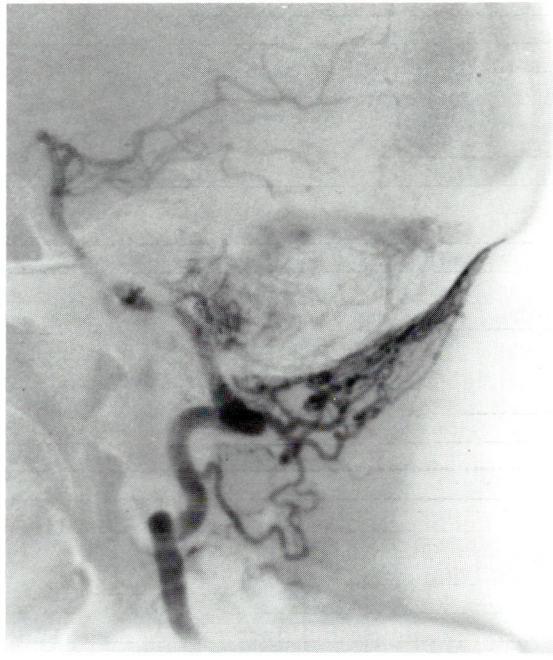

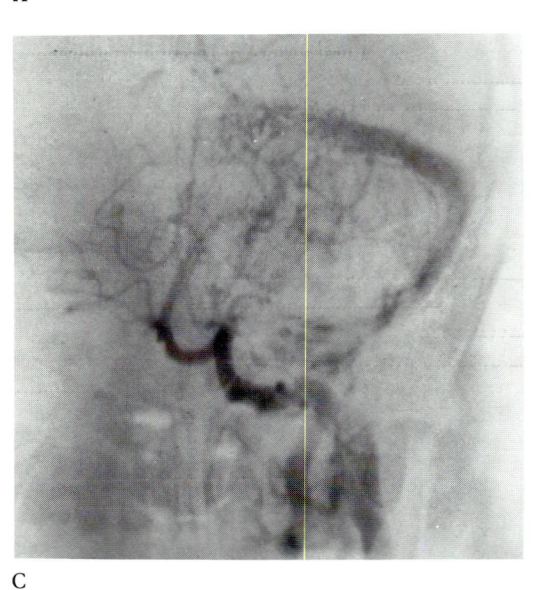

Figure 179-3 A dural AVM of the transverse sinus. *A.* A lateral view from a carotid angiogram shows arterial participation from the meningohypophyseal trunk and the middle meningeal and occipital arteries. *B.* A lateral view from a vertebral angiogram shows the participation of dural branches of the vertebral artery and muscular branches anastomosing with the occipital artery. *C.* An anteroposterior view from the vertebral angiogram.

spinosum when the middle meningeal artery is principally involved. In very extensive lesions, there may be hyperostosis of portions of the calvarium under which most of the fistulas reside. However, definitive diagnosis requires angiography. Selective bilateral external carotid angiography and vertebral angiography with subtraction technique are essential for most cases. In addition to defining the extent and degree of arterial shunting to the involved sinus, irregularities within the sinus wall, occlusion of the sinus, and retrograde flow to pial veins can be demonstrated.

Natural History

Most of the dural AVMs become symptomatic in patients over the age of 40, and the patients are predominantly females, particularly in cases where lesions involve the cavernous sinus. Many cases follow significant head injury, becoming symptomatic weeks to months thereafter, and others may follow a variety of systemic illnesses that might be associated with venous thrombosis.[3] Overall, there is an insufficient number of cases followed for a long period of time to formulate a natural history useful for accurately guiding treatment. But, in general, the larger lesions tend to persist and frequently lead to increased intracranial pressure or obstructive hydrocephalus, which, in turn, may progress to blindness and multiple associated neurological abnormalities. For the smaller lesions, spontaneous resolution occurs not infrequently, particularly for the cavernous sinus group.

All lesions are capable of spontaneous bleeding, but the yearly rate for this, once diagnosis is established, is not known.

Treatment

Considering the variability of the dural arteriovenous fistulas with respect to size, extent, and sinuses involved, it is obvious that one surgical technique may be entirely effective in some cases but totally ineffective in others. Because the natural history is not perfectly known, extensive high-risk surgery may not be rational for certain lesions where the symptomatology is relatively minor. Simple ligation of the external carotid artery or one or two of the branches implicated may suffice if the only clinical problem is an annoying bruit. An intravascular approach with particle embolization, or infusion with polymerizing plastics, may be effective in other cases, depending upon the anatomy. The intravascular approach has generally been effective for the acquired lesions involving the cavernous sinuses,[9,19,20,24] but for the extensive lesions, particularly those involving the transverse and sigmoid sinuses, the intravascular approach generally falls short. Surgical isolation of the entire length of these sinuses, including removal of most of the mastoid, may be necessary.[11,12]

There are very extensive lesions which even this radical surgery has failed to cure. These include the extensive fistulas of the posterior sagittal, transverse, and sigmoid sinuses with participation of the upper cervical arteries, including muscular branches from the vertebral arteries and ascending cervical arteries. At present, it seems most logical to proceed in those cases in which surgery becomes mandatory with the simplest, low-risk procedure first, advancing to more radical procedures as the clinical situation requires.

References

1. Aminoff MJ: Vascular anomalies in the intracranial dura mater. Brain 96:601–612, 1973.
2. Bitoh S, Arita N, Fujiwara M, Ozaki K, Nakao Y: Dural arteriovenous malformation near the left sphenoparietal sinus. Surg Neurol 13:345–349, 1980.
3. Chaudhary MY, Sachdev VP, Cho SH, Weitzner I Jr, Puljic S, Huang YP: Dural arteriovenous malformation of the major venous sinuses: An acquired lesion. AJNR 3:13–19, 1982.
4. Dardenne GY: Dural arteriovenous anomaly fed by ethmoidal arteries. Surg Neurol 10:384–388, 1978.
5. Debrun G, Chartres A: Infra and supratentorial arteriovenous malformations: A general review. About two cases of spontaneous supratentorial arteriovenous malformation of the dura. Neuroradiology 3:184–192, 1972.
6. Djindjian R, Cophignon J, Théron J, Merland JJ, Houdart R: Embolization by superselective arteriography from the femoral route in neuroradiology: Review of 60 cases. I. Technique, indications, complications. Neuroradiology 6:20–26, 1973.
7. Handa J, Shimizu Y: Dural arteriovenous anomaly supplied by falcine artery. Neuroradiology 6:212–214, 1973.
8. Handa J, Yoneda S, Handa H: Venous sinus occlusion with a dural arteriovenous malformation of the posterior fossa. Surg Neurol 4:433–437, 1975.
9. Hardy RW Jr, Costin JA, Weinstein M, Berlin AJ Jr, Gutman FA: External carotid cavernous fistula treated by transfemoral embolization. Surg Neurol 9:255–256, 1978.
10. Houser OW, Baker HL Jr, Rhoton AL Jr, Okazaki H: Intracranial dural arteriovenous malformations. Radiology 105:55–64, 1972.
11. Houser OW, Campbell JK, Campbell RJ, Sundt TM Jr: Arteriovenous malformation affecting the transverse dural sinus—an acquired lesion. Mayo Clin Proc 54:651–661, 1979.
12. Hugosson R, Bergstrom K: Surgical treatment of dural arteriovenous malformation in the region of the sigmoid sinus. J Neurol Neurosurg Psychiatry 37:97–101, 1974.
13. Kosnik EJ, Hunt WE, Miller CA: Dural arteriovenous malformations. J Neurosurg 40:322–329, 1974.
14. Kuhner A, Krastel A, Stoll W: Arteriovenous malformations of the transverse dural sinus. J Neurosurg 45:12–19, 1976.
15. Lamas E, Lobato RD, Esparza J, Escudero L: Dural posterior fossa AVM producing raised sagittal sinus pressure: Case report. J Neurosurg 46:804–810, 1977.
16. Luessenhop AJ: The natural history of cerebral arteriovenous malformations, in Wilson CB, Stein B (eds): *Cerebral Arteriovenous Malformations*. In press.
17. Luessenhop AJ, Kachmann R Jr, Shevlin W, Ferrero AA: Clinical evaluation of artificial embolization in the management of large cerebral arteriovenous malformations. J Neurosurg 23:400–417, 1965.
18. Magidson MA, Weinberg PE: Spontaneous closure of a dural arteriovenous malformation. Surg Neurol 6:107–110, 1976.
19. Mahaley MS Jr, Boone SC: External carotid-cavernous fistula treated by arterial embolization: Case report. J Neurosurg 40:110–114, 1974.
20. Manaka S, Izawa M, Nawata H: Dural arteriovenous malformation treated by artificial embolization with liquid silicone. Surg Neurol 7:63–65, 1977.
21. Newton TH, Hoyt WF: Dural arteriovenous shunts in the region of the cavernous sinus. Neuroradiology 1:71–81, 1970.
22. Newton TH, Weidner W, Greitz T: Dural arteriovenous malformation in the posterior fossa. Radiology 90:27–35, 1968.
23. Obrador S, Soto M, Silvela J: Clinical syndromes of arteriovenous malformations of the transverse-sigmoid sinus. J Neurol Neurosurg Psychiatry 38:436–451, 1975.
24. Suzuki J, Komatsu S: New embolization method using estrogen for dural arteriovenous malformation and meningioma. Surg Neurol 16:438–442, 1981.
25. Verbiest MH: L'anévrisme artérioveineux intradural. Rev Neurol (Paris) 85:189–199, 1951.
26. Waga S, Fujimoto K, Morikawa A, Morooka Y, Okada M: Dural arteriovenous malformation in the anterior fossa. Surg Neurol 8:356–358, 1977.

180

Surgical Anatomy of the Cavernous Sinus

Dwight Parkinson

The cavernous sinus was so named by Winslow because he thought it resembled in structure the corpus cavernosum of the penis.[12] He should have known better because the two structures serve no similar purpose, and nature does nothing in vain. Nevertheless, the name has persisted.

I have been unable to find any reference to the embryology of this area. For instance, we do not know whether the gasserian ganglion starts as a separate structure with its own dural and arachnoid development as do other ganglia, and in turn, grows forward and backward to its ultimate connections. We do not know whether the dura of the middle fossa divides to form the medial and lateral walls of this space or whether the medial wall forms as a separate structure.

Grossly and microscopically, the walls fuse inferiorly and superiorly. Unlike the walls of the other intracranial sinuses, the two walls of the so-called cavernous sinus are nowhere near of equal thickness, the lateral wall being several times thicker than the medial, which is in many areas closer to the arachnoid in structure. In the adult male, this entire space measures 2½ cm in length by 2 cm in maximal height. The width is determined largely by the diameter of the internal carotid (Fig. 180-1).

Arteries

The curvature of the carotid siphon varies tremendously. The carotid is fixed at its point of entry into this space known as the cavernous sinus, and it is fixed at its point of exit; between, it hangs relatively freely.

The first and most consistently present artery to leave the carotid within this space is the meningohypophyseal, which leaves from the midline of the carotid just at or just proximal to the apogee of the first forward curve.[3] It trifurcates immediately into divisions of nearly equal caliber which run for 2 or 3 mm adherent to the surface of the carotid, often giving the appearance of three separate vessels arising at some distance from each other (Fig. 180-2). If the specimen is fixed before dissection, this impression is enhanced.

The three divisions are (1) the tentorial artery, (2) the dorsal meningeal artery, and (3) the inferior hypophyseal artery. The tentorial artery leaves the meningohypophyseal trunk in a posterolateral direction, giving off minute branches to supply the third and fourth nerves before entering the tentorium between the two dural leaves just beneath the entrance of the fourth nerve.[1]

The dorsal meningeal artery leaves the meningohypophyseal trunk in a posteroinferior-medial direction, going back and around the dorsum and anastomosing directly with its fellow from the opposite side as well as supplying numerous smaller indirect anastomoses up and down the dorsum and the clivus, eventually anastomosing with meningeal branches of the cervical arteries and the vertebrobasilar meningeal vessels.

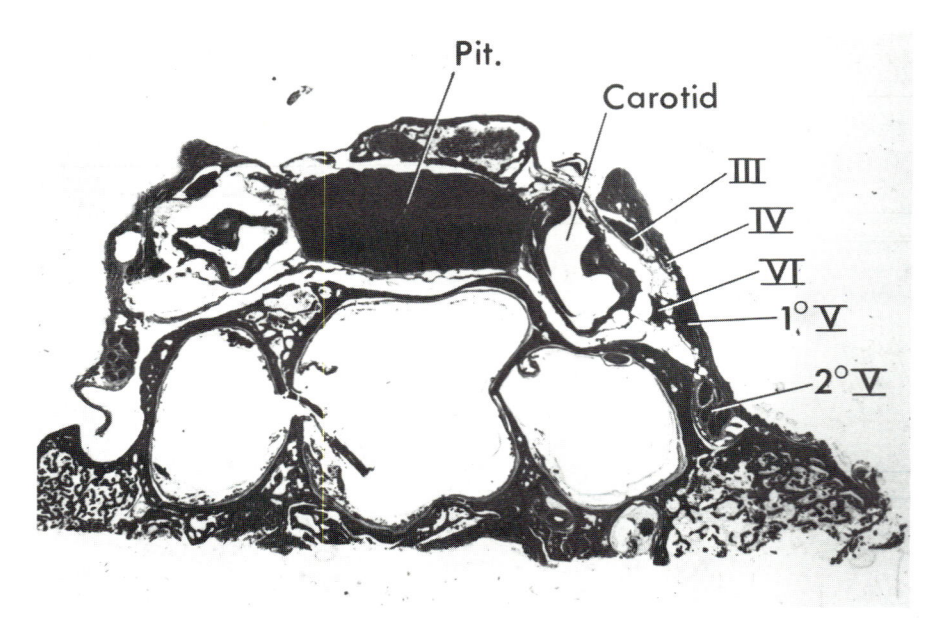

Figure 180-1 Coronal cross section at the center of the pituitary (Pit.). The two carotid arteries show atheromatous plaques in their upper and lateral aspects. The third division of V has already departed through the foramen ovale posterior to the plane of this section. Between VI and the wall of the carotid artery can be seen three venous channels in cross section, and another in longitudinal section beneath them and above the bone. On the left, just lateral to 1°V is a large venous channel in the lateral dural wall. On both sides, adipose tissue is visible just below and medial to III and IV. The space between IV, VI, and 1°V is a part of the triangular space, and widens posteriorly. (Modified from Parkinson and West.[9])

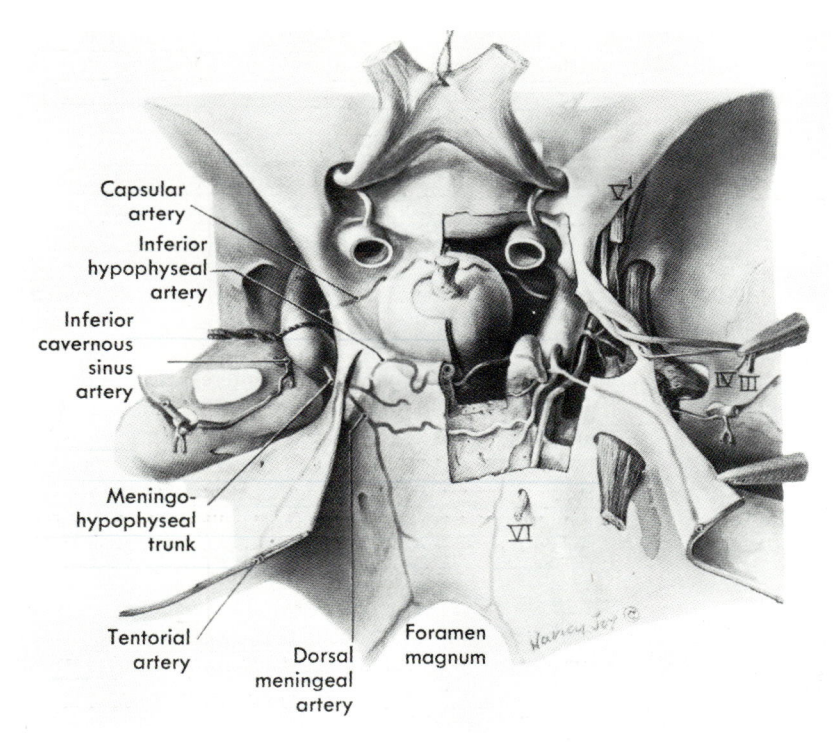

Surgical Anatomy of the Cavernous Sinus

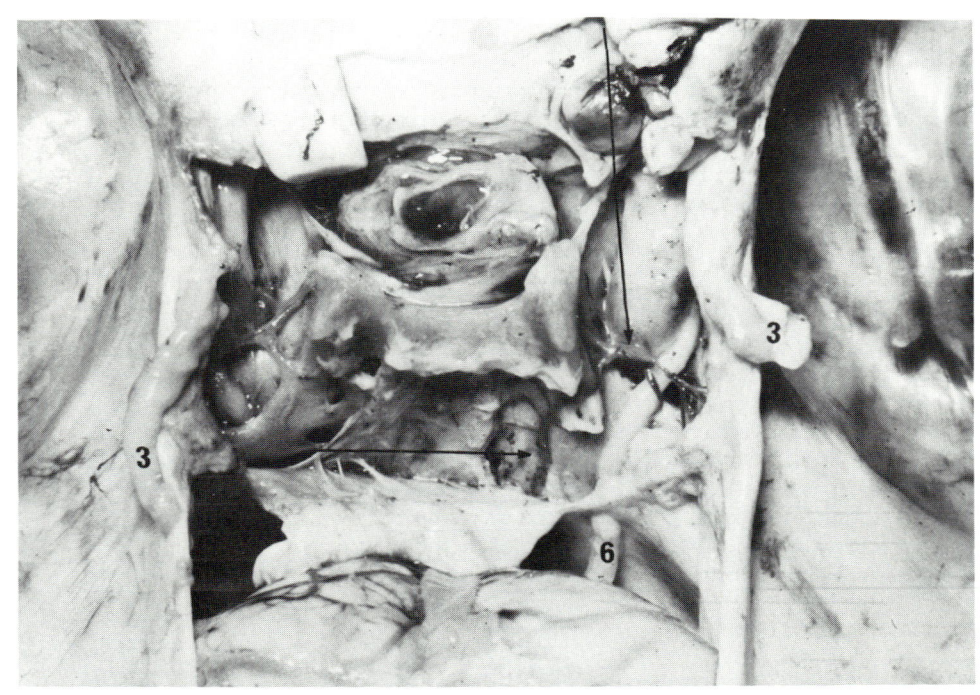

Figure 180-2 *A.* A drawing from multiple cadaver dissections, showing the relationships between the arteries, cranial nerves, and dural coverings in the lateral sellar space (cavernous sinus). *B.* A cadaver dissection in similar perspective. The third cranial nerves (3) are hanging out laterally over the free margin of the tentorium. The sixth cranial nerve (6) is visible coming from the brain stem on the right, up through Dorello's canal, then turning around the carotid artery beneath the branches of the meningohypophyseal trunk, which is indicated by the descending thin vertical arrow. The right tentorial artery leaves from this point and goes to the right across the sixth nerve, sending a small branch down to the sixth nerve, but then branches again just before entering the tentorium. The left meningohypophyseal trunk is less completely exposed, but the inferior hypophyseal artery and dorsal meningeal arteries are visible in their proximal portions. The right dorsal meningeal artery (*horizontal arrow*) is visible throughout a considerable length descending along the clivus, which has been exposed by cutting the dura and reflecting it backward and downward. (From Parkinson.[3])

The third division is the inferior hypophyseal artery, which goes medially and slightly anteriorly from the meningohypophyseal trunk. It divides as it approaches the posterior floor of the sella, supplying the posterior hypophysis and the dura around the posterior clinoid. It anastomoses directly with its fellow from the opposite side (Fig. 180-2). The entire meningohypophyseal complex is above the sixth nerve. In the few instances where we have had an opportunity to view a persistent trigeminal artery, it has been below the sixth nerve.[7]

The second artery, slightly less constant, departs about ½ cm further along from the inferior lateral aspect of the carotid artery. It runs down over the sixth nerve beneath the gasserian ganglion which it supplies along with the structures of the inferior cavernous sinus and its coverings. This is the artery of the inferior cavernous sinus, and it anastomoses directly with branches of the meningeal vessels coming through the foramen spinosum.[3]

McConnell's capsular artery is the least common of the carotid branches and departs 2 or 3 mm further along from the inferior medial aspect and runs directly across the floor of the sella and anastomoses with its opposite number. The paucity of branches and the short length and comparatively large caliber would indicate that its function is more anastomotic than nutrient when present. When not present, its distribution to a greater or lesser extent will be taken over by branches from the meningohypophyseal artery, usually the inferior hypophyseal division, as is also the distribution of the artery of the inferior cavernous sinus when absent.

Veins

Our surgical experience and angiographic interpretation originally led us to suspect that the cavernous sinus is not a trabeculated venous space with an artery running through it, but instead, a plexus of veins.[4,5] Hamby[2] suggested that this is probably a plexus of veins; and Taptas,[11] in an article on the dural covering, made this isolated statement many years ago although the article had no supporting documentation. Solassol et al. found the venous structure in this region to be a plexus in embryos.[10] Our injection preparations formed from below (i.e., via the jugular vein) have consistently shown a plexus of veins in the parasellar region.[5,8] These veins differ significantly from the classic concept of a trabeculated sinus in that the carotid artery is incompletely surrounded.

The cavernous sinuses differ from the other intracranial sinuses in at least three respects. First, the pattern is of different configuration from specimen to specimen, and even from side to side in the same specimen. Second, the channels are multiple. Third, there is no distinct lateral border that one can indicate as the edge of a sinus as in all the other cerebral sinuses (e.g., note the superior sphenoidal sinus in Fig. 180-3A). Recently, we have been injecting this space in a retrograde fashion through the orbital vein, and so far, our findings are similar, i.e., multiple venous channels incompletely surrounding the carotid artery, varying in pattern from patient to patient and from side to side, and extending without any distinct lateral border out into a continuity with the veins of the middle fossa (Fig. 180-3).

Nerves

The third and fourth cranial nerves enter the roof of this space and carry with them an arachnoid sleeve (Figs. 180-1 and 180-2). They remain in the same relative position to each other throughout their course on the way to the superior orbital fissure, with a much thinner layer of dura medially and inferiorly. The sixth nerve enters low down through Dorello's canal and courses upward and laterally around the carotid. Aside from the sympathetics, it is the only cranial nerve which is truly within this space. The fifth nerve enters from the posterior fossa through a large opening which resembles a pocket that might be formed by invaginating a three-fingered hand through the dura and the arachnoid. The invaginated portion is known as Meckel's cave, and it contains the gasserian ganglion and the first portions of the three divisions of the fifth cranial nerve. The dura is exceedingly thin between the fifth nerve and this space (Fig. 180-1). The relationship of the gasserian ganglion and its three branches to the arachnoid and dura differs from the relationship of the third and fourth nerves entering the same coverings only in the size of the sleeve or compartment. The third and fourth nerves coming in from above and the sixth nerve and first division of the fifth coming from below, all converging at the superior orbital fissure, outline a triangular space[3] with its base posteriorly and its apex anteriorly (Figs. 180-1, 180-2, and 180-4).

In addition to the cranial nerves, the sympathetic nerves enter this space. Usually, one to three nerves from the superior sympathetic ganglion pass up parallel but not adherent to the internal carotid artery through the base of the skull to the parasellar region. En route, and within the parasellar region, they undergo minimal branching and rejoining, forming a very modest plexus. At frequent intervals, they send fibers to the wall of the carotid artery, but there is nothing to indicate in the gross that any structures are supplied by sympathetic nerves coming from the wall of the carotid. The largest residual of the ascending sympathetic nerves or nerve joins the sixth nerve, runs with it for several millimeters, and then departs and joins the first division of the fifth, just before its departure through the superior orbital fissure[6] (Fig. 180-4).

Connective Tissue

In a coronal cross-section through the middle of the pituitary, the cavernous sinus is roughly triangular (Fig. 180-1 and 180-2). Superiorly, the medial wall is formed by the lateral aspect of the pituitary and its coverings. Inferiorly, the medial wall is formed by the roof of the sphenoid sinus. The superior wall of this space is a very thin layer of dura extending from the upper layer of the pituitary laterally to the thickened forward extension of the tentorial margin. Laterally, the wall of this space is formed by the dura extending up from the floor of the middle fossa (Fig. 180-1). Anteriorly, this space twists 45 degrees and tapers to a narrow horizontal triangle constituting the superior orbital fissure and becomes progressively tightly packed with nerves, fat, and the superior orbital vein. Posteriorly, it tapers to a twisting, curving slit formed by the lateral and medial surfaces curving to join and become the superior and inferior surfaces of the tentorium. The posterior and inferior wall is formed (or reinforced) by the dura sweeping off the dorsum and the clivus to turn up and under, thus becoming the inferior surface of the tentorium. The dura is much thicker superiorly and laterally as a prolongation from the tentor-

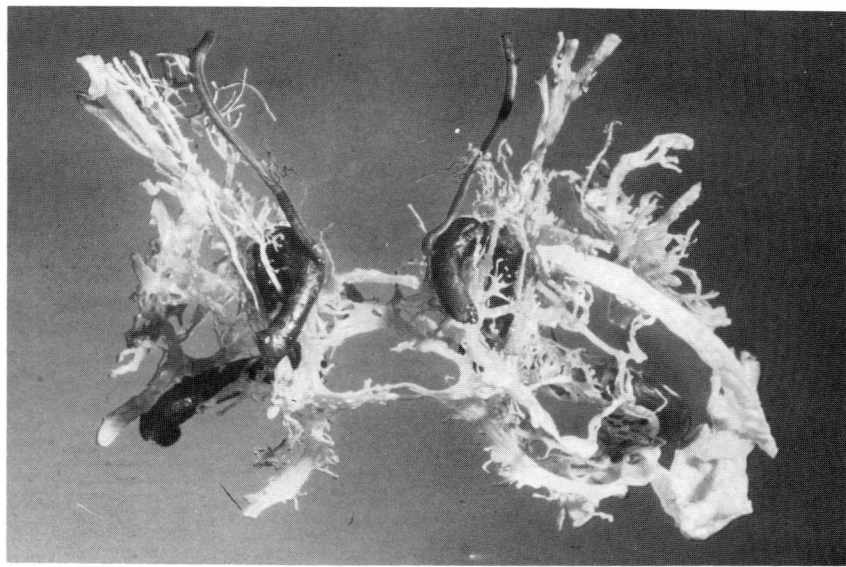

Surgical Anatomy of the Cavernous Sinus

Figure 180-3 *A.* A corrosion specimen with the carotid siphon (*dark*) and the venous channels (*light*) on each side. The two ophthalmic arteries are visible running upward and forward. Lateral to each are the superior orbital veins and branches. Running down and to the right is a clearly demarcated superior sphenoidal sinus. Note the smooth, distinct lateral borders over a considerable length, and the complete absence of any such in the parasellar region. The pituitary fossa is outlined with connecting venous channels. The venous channels around the carotid artery in the lateral sellar region are in no way different from the venous channels along the floor of the middle fossa or out into the orbit. They do not completely surround the carotid nor do they form a "discrete single sinus" or even a trabeculated sinus. They are multiple venous channels forming a plexus. *B.* The same specimen viewed from the right. Note the plexus of veins incompletely surrounding the carotid artery in the region of the carotid canal. Next, note that the carotid artery in the parasellar region is incompletely surrounded by venous channels, and in particular, note that no one of these channels could justifiably be called a sinus as distinct from any other venous channels in the region. This photograph should be compared with photographs in our other publications of the venous anatomy which emphasizes the fact that no two specimens show any similarity in venous pattern in the parasellar region (nor any evidence of a lateral margin that could be indicated as the edge of a "sinus"). Thus, this region is inconsistent in its venous pattern as compared to the other cerebral sinuses, has no distinct lateral margin, and is not a single channel. (From Parkinson and West.[9])

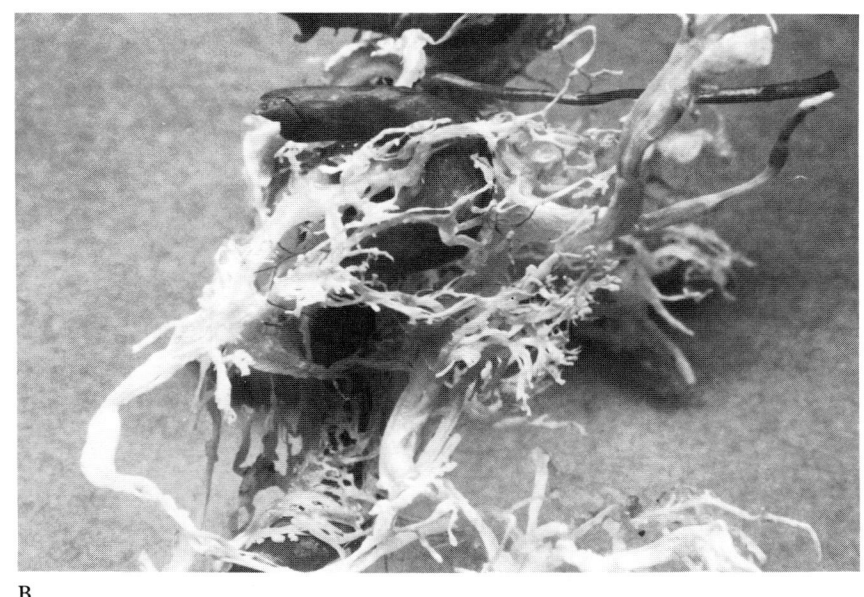

ium to both the anterior and posterior clinoids (Figs. 180-1 and 180-2). There is a small, canoe-shaped groove between these two extensions. The third and fourth nerves enter in this groove carrying a sheath of arachnoid (Figs. 180-1 and 180-2).

Thus, in addition to the carotid artery and the sixth nerve which lie relatively free in this space, there are numerous small branches of the sympathetic nerves as well as the branches of the carotid artery and their subsequent subdivisions, plus exceedingly thin-walled venous channels. As the lateral wall of this parasellar space is pulled outward, all these structures stretch, and in the case of the venous walls, may fenestrate. Aside from these structures, we have found nothing that would resemble the alleged trabeculae. The fat, which is constantly present within this space, is not always grossly evident (Fig. 180-1).

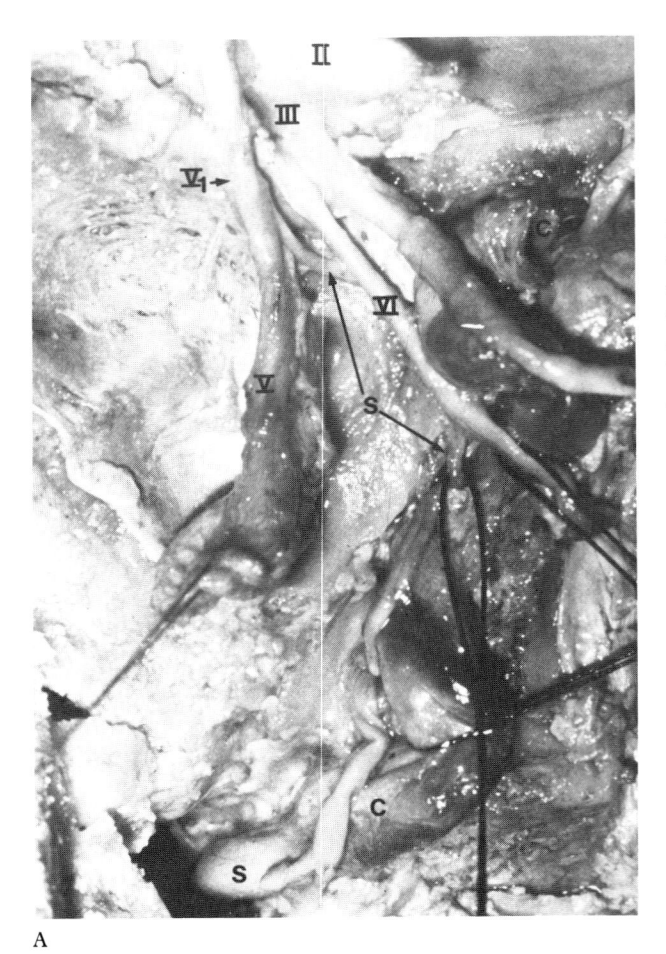

Figure 180-4 *A.* An extensive dissection of the left parasellar space: (II) cut end of the left optic nerve above the clinoid, which has been removed; (III) third cranial nerve converging with the sixth cranial nerve (VI) and the first division of the fifth (V$_1$), at the superior orbital fissure. The gasserian ganglion (V) has been turned down and out and held with a suture. The carotid artery (C) has a suture drawing it to the right just as it comes through the carotid foramen, and its cut end is visible just above the third cranial nerve, where it comes up beneath the clinoid, which has been largely removed in this specimen. The letter s designates the superior sympathetic ganglion at the bottom drawn up through the carotid foramen. From this ganglion one can trace the sympathetic nerve up to the arrows at the right and left of the uppermost letter s. These arrows point to the sympathetic nerve joining the sixth and then leaving it to join the first division of the fifth. Just beneath this left arrow tip is the second division of the fifth nerve going through the foramen rotundum. *B.* A diagram of the structures shown in *A.* (From Parkinson et al.[6]) *C.* A diagram of the sympathetic connection from the superior ganglion to the sixth nerve (VI) and then from VI to the first division of the fifth (V). The triangular space is also outlined by VI, the first division of V below, and the third (III) and fourth (IV) nerves indicated as dotted lines above. (From Parkinson and West.[9])

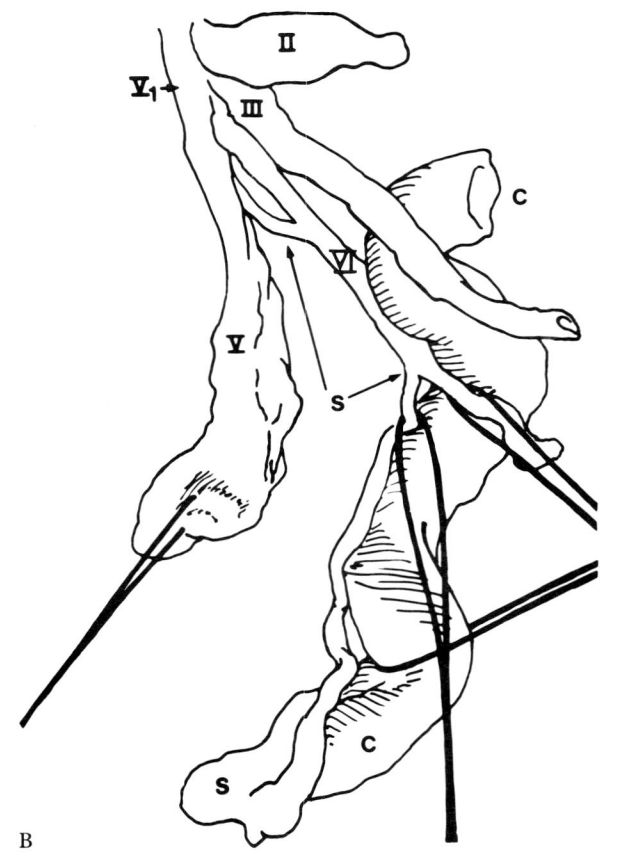

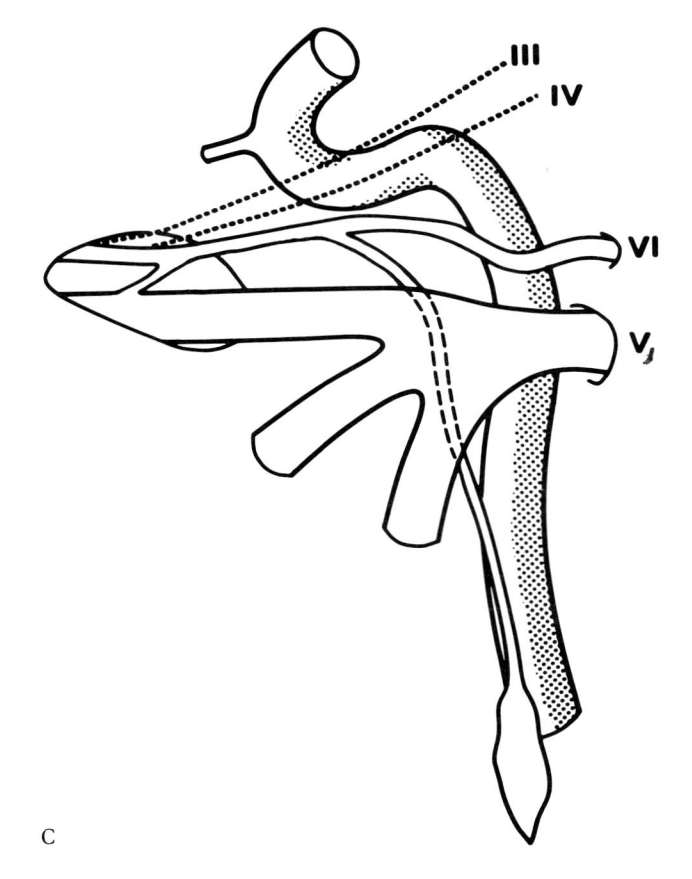

References

1. Bernasconi V, Cassinari V: Caratteristiche angiografiche dei meningiomi del tintorio. Radiol Med (Torino) 43:1015–1026, 1957.
2. Hamby WB: *Carotid-Cavernous Fistula*. Springfield, Ill. Charles C Thomas, 1966.
3. Parkinson D: Collateral circulation of cavernous carotid artery: Anatomy. Can J Surg 7:251–268, 1964.
4. Parkinson D: A surgical approach to the cavernous portion of the carotid artery: Anatomical studies and case report. J Neurosurg 23:474–483, 1965.
5. Parkinson D: Transcavernous repair of carotid cavernous fistula. J Neurosurg 26:420–424, 1967.
6. Parkinson D, Johnston J, Chaudhuri A: Sympathetic connections to the fifth and sixth cranial nerves. Anat Rec 191:221–226, 1978.
7. Parkinson D, Shields CB: Persistent trigeminal artery: Its relationship to the normal branches of the cavernous carotid. J Neurosurg 40:244–248, 1974.
8. Parkinson D, Shields CB, Hunt B: Venous anatomy in the parasellar region. Presented at a poster session, American Association of Anatomists, Vancouver, British Columbia, April 1–6, 1978.
9. Parkinson D, West M: Lesions of the cavernous plexus region, in Youmans JR (ed): *Neurological Surgery*, 2d ed. Philadelphia, Saunders, 1982, pp 3004–3023.
10. Solassol A, Zidane C, Slimane-Taleb S: Les veines du sinus caverneux du foetus human de quatre mois. CR Assoc Anat 149:1009–1015, 1970.
11. Taptas JN: Etiologie et pathogenie des exophtalmies d'origine vasculaire, dites exophtalmies pulsatiles. Arch Opht (Paris) 10:22–50, 1950.
12. Winslow JB: *Exposition Anatomique de la Structure du Corps Humain*. London, Prevost, 1732, vol 2, p 31.

181
Carotid-Cavernous Fistulas and Intracavernous Aneurysms

Sean Mullan

Carotid-Cavernous Fistulas

Historical Review

Pulsating exophthalmos due to an arteriovenous fistula has been a recognized surgical problem since Traver's diagnosis and treatment by common carotid artery ligation in 1809.[5] Nélaton by 1856 recognized clearly that the problem lay in the cavernous sinus rather than in the orbit.[5] In the subsequent 100 years a multitude of case reports appeared indicating that common carotid ligature, which frequently failed, carried a significant morbidity, and that internal carotid closure, though it had a higher success rate, had an even more serious morbidity problem. In addition, proximal ligation by either method, though usually yielding an initial improvement or cessation of symptoms, was not infrequently followed by a later recrudesence. By 1932, Gardner added the intracranial carotid ligature, thereby apparently isolating the fistula.[5] In 1942, Adson added ligation of the ophthalmic artery in an attempt to secure an even better isolation.[5] In 1965, Parkinson clearly described the carotid branches in the cavernous sinus that contributed to or were responsible for the re-establishment of the fistulous flow (together with a branch in the petrous region) when all else had been ligated.[13]

As early as 1931 it was recognized that arterial ligation had significant limitations which demanded a better solution. In that year Brooks reported on opening the internal carotid artery and floating a long thin strip of muscle into the fistulous sinus.[3] The problem with this technique was the difficulty in choosing the exact size of embolus which was small enough to pass into the cavernous sinus but large enough not to float on through, into one of the many venous exits from the sinus, leaving the body of the sinus and the remaining exits unobstructed. There was also the risk, in low-flow fistulas, that the embolus would be carried into the cerebral vessels. Ipsilateral internal carotid ligature after the embolus was floated was added to the procedures, and these methods and their variations continued intermittently until the 1960s.

A preliminary intracranial carotid clip was introduced to prevent intracranial embolization but did not always hold.[12] Arutiunov et al. used a restraining thread attached to the embolus, anchoring its proximal end in the neck, and they closed the artery.[1] Black et al. did the same but left the artery open and demonstrated that it remained angiographically patent 6 months later.[2] Others used a variety of embolic material other than muscle, including absorbable gelatin sponge, polyurethane sponge, methyl methacrylate, and plastic-covered steel balls, with reports of isolated success.[2]

Hamby's book in 1966[5] and Morley's in 1976[8] contain the essence of the arterial ligation experience. The common carotid procedure cured one of Hamby's six patients. The remaining five had a total of sixteen procedures before two further obliterations occurred. None of Morley's three fistulas was sealed initially, but two closed later. All three suffered serious subsequent visual loss.

Two of Hamby's twelve patients were cured by internal carotid ligature. In subsequent operations upon the others, there was one death. Of Morley's seven patients, three fistulas were immediately sealed, but two patients became blind and one became hemiparetic. Two fistulas closed later, but both patients lost vision and one became hemiparetic.

Trapping the internal carotid intracranially and extracranially sealed the fistula in 17 of Hamby's 18 cases. In seven of Morley's eight patients in this category the fistula was sealed, but all patients had visual loss. One had a transient hemiparesis. The eighth died.

One of Hamby's muscle embolization patients was initially asymptomatic but later developed recurrence. Three patients had initial intracranial surgical occlusion of the carotid and ophthalmic arteries, followed by embolization and then by triple occlusion of the internal, external, and common carotid arteries in the neck. Among Morley's seven patients, four fistulas were sealed, but one patient lost vision. Two of the remaining three developed visual loss, and one of these had a hemiparesis.

Morley then went on to treat eight more patients by total intracranial and extracranial arterial ligation plus stuffing of the intracavernous carotid artery with macerated muscle introduced through an intradural arteriotomy proximal to the intradural clip. There were no hemispheric or ophthalmic complications or deaths. Hamby's own results were much better than those he quoted from the antecedent literature and those subsequently reported by Stern et al. in 1967, who recognized that an excellent success rate of closure was then being achieved but that the morbidity and mortality of that achievement left much to be desired.[16]

The problems were that a common carotid ligation was largely ineffectual because of the wide collateral, and an internal carotid ligation stressed both the hemisphere and the retina in that the fistula stole directly from their remaining arterial sources. A simple trapping procedure placed the retina in exceptional hazard because the fistula stole from the ophthalmic artery. A trapping procedure that also included the ophthalmic artery, left intact, as did all the other procedures, the intracavernous carotid branches. These could, in time, form a rich anastomosis with the dural arteries bilaterally and restore the volume of the leak. In addition, a rete mirabile could easily develop around the internal carotid artery in the neck distal to its occlusion.

Hamby clearly recognized that thrombosis of the cavernous sinus was essential for cure. Parkinson, in 1965, reported his detailed study of the intracavernous anatomy and designed a direct approach to the intracavernous carotid in order to obliterate the exact site of the fistula.[13] This was through a horizontal incision in the posterior cavernous sinus between the third and fourth nerves above and the sixth below. The problem is that the operation demanded cardiac arrest, a procedure in which, up to the present, there remains an unavoidable mortality factor. The author, working on thrombogenic techniques since 1960, sealed fistulas by deliberate thrombosis of the cavernous sinus while sparing the carotid artery, and in 1979 reported upon 33 cases without mortality and virtually without morbidity.[9,10]

Prolo and Hanbery in 1971 initiated an entirely new approach by sealing the actual lumen of the fistula from within the artery using an inflated balloon catheter inserted from the neck.[14] This, in one simple procedure, solved the technical problem of fistula closure without incurring a fistulous drain upon the hemisphere or upon the retina. In most patients the fistula has induced a compensatory delivery of extra blood to the ipsilateral hemisphere and retina, and these patients tolerate immediate and permanent carotid closure much better than do normal patients without a fistula. There is not yet enough collected experience on this method, but the author is not aware of any reported mortality. However, the possibility of a very low morbidity factor in terms of hemiplegia remains. In addition, the loss of a single carotid artery is undesirable at any age, because in later years a progressive atherosclerosis may demand all the collateral that is possible. The theoretical problem of balloon closure while sparing the carotid was solved by Serbinenko in 1974[15] and by Debrun somewhat later by the development of the detachable balloon which, if successfully placed, will enter the fistula and seal it, leaving the carotid intact. Success in this placement depends upon the size of the fistulous opening, and can be either high or low according to selection.[4]

The existence of dural arteriovenous shunts supplied primarily by dural arteries which drain into the cavernous sinus rather than by the internal carotid artery itself has been clearly recognized since the communication by Hayes in 1963.[6] These fistulas have lent themselves to treatment by selective embolization of the external carotid artery. The existence of dural fistulas supplied by both external and internal carotid contributions has not had such wide recognition. These require obliteration of the cavernous sinus.

Pathological Types

There are basically two types of fistulas, traumatic and spontaneous. The traumatic fistula can arise from direct puncture by a penetrating foreign object, but it has even been known to follow an unusually vigorous attempt to clear out a carotid thrombus using a balloon catheter. Usually, closed head injuries which produce fistulas are quite severe. They occur in high-speed automobile accidents or in an extensive fall, but a small group results from direct crushing of the skull, as occurs when a jacked-up automobile falls off its support. Arterial branch avulsion would seem inadequate to explain the large opening that frequently permits entrance of a balloon catheter. It is uncommon to see a penetrating spicule of bone in the x-ray films. The relatively large size of these fistulas would correlate with the previous existence of an unruptured aneurysm, but there is nothing that could further confirm such an idea. The exact mechanism of traumatic fistulas is usually unclear. Classically they are supplied exclusively by the internal carotid artery, but some (particularly the crush group) may be liberally supplied by both the external and internal carotid arteries.

Hamby believed that the spontaneous fistulas are mostly the result of ruptured intracavernous aneurysms. We have several very clearly documented cases, including one patient whose aneurysm was known to exist before rupture. Obrador et al. have shown an aneurysm to be present at autopsy although it was not visualized in the clinical angiograms.[12] Thus, the failure to demonstrate aneurysms in the majority of spontaneous fistulas does not negate the traditional idea that they are due to ruptured aneurysms (except in those instances where a demonstrable dural AVM exists). Hamby considered pregnancy as a precipitating factor but found that only 2 of 27 women had a relationship to pregnancy. One developed a fistula 2 weeks before and the other 4 days after delivery. Dandy, quoting Sadler, reported a relationship in 17 of 41 cases, and Walker gave a 25 to 30 percent figure.[5] We have not observed any.

The other large, or possibly larger, group of spontaneous fistulas is that of the pericavernous dural arteriovenous malformations. These fistulas are not widespread malformations such as are seen in the cerebral substance but rather appear as multiple arterial channels feeding into a single site of leak such as is sometimes seen at other dural sites following a known penetrating injury. Most are supplied exclusively by the external carotid branches (unilaterally or bilaterally), but there is a well-defined smaller group which is, in fact, supplied by both the external and internal carotid branches. Dural AVMs occur predominantly in older females. Whether the AVMs develop primarily at that age or whether they are an exacerbation of an asymptomatic condition which has been present for many previous years is not known.

Most series record a preponderance of young males in the traumatic group and of older women in the spontaneous variety. Of Hamby's 42 patients, 15 were male, and 27 were female. In his group, 19 of the fistulas were spontaneous, and 23 were traumatic. In our series of 50, 27 were females, and 23 were males. In our group, 28 of the fistulas were due to trauma, 10 were due to dural arteriovenous malformations, 4 were due to definite aneurysms, 7 were due to suspected aneurysms, and 1 was associated with fibromuscular dysplasia. Of the 10 patients with dural AVMs, 9 were female.

Once a leak of any type develops, its progress depends upon the site, the size of the leak, the specific venous arrangement of that individual sinus, and the blood pressure. Since virtually all cavernous sinuses communicate freely with the opposite side, through anterior and posterior channels in the pituitary fossa and through the basilar plexus behind the posterior clinoid, most large fistulas will eventually show bilateral signs, although as a rule, the ipsilateral side predominates. Rarely, and we have one example, the fistula is so situated that it jets across to the opposite side and the signs are more prominent contralaterally. If there is no good posterior exit from the sinus, then the ocular signs will be prominent from even a small fistula; and if there is hypertension, they may be prominent from even a very small fistula. However, if the exit drainage is predominantly posterior, then orbital signs may be minimal even with a relatively large leak. If there is no anterior drainage, and we have one example, there are no signs referable to the orbit. In these cases of absent or defective anterior drainage, the signs will be those of cavernous nerve pressure, more commonly the sixth, but including total ophthalmoplegia.

The presenting symptom may be a subjective bruit, but more commonly in the spontaneous variety it is an appearance of reddening, or chemosis, or protrusion of the eye. When severe, the eye is immobilized by venous distension and edema, and it may not be possible to know how much of this is due to this orbital distension and how much to nerve paralysis. Further progress is very variable. It may take days, weeks, or months to become significant or to endanger eyesight, but it should be noted that in the acute traumatic case, sight may irreversibly disappear within a few days. We have not seen it disappear within hours but could contemplate such a possibility. The acute mechanism is a low retinal arterial pressure plus a high venous pressure which causes retinal ischemia. In the very chronic variety sight is not endangered by retinal ischemia but by the slow onset of a cataract or glaucoma. We have not observed a post-traumatic fistula to disappear spontaneously. The milder dural arteriovenous malformation group has a reputation for spontaneous disappearance. We have seen this happen twice. We have also observed two patients with relatively mild fistulas suddenly develop very severe exacerbation while awaiting resolution.

As a rule, carotid-cavernous fistulas do not cause hemiplegia or endanger life. It is probable that in a few, with acute head injury, the condition exacerbates the existing cerebral damage, leading to death in the acute stage. In those who present later with hemiplegia or intellectual defect since the time of the accident, the degree to which the fistula contributed to the hemispheric impairment is unknown. Devastating nose bleeds are rare but can occur acutely or in the chronic stage.

Late subarachnoid hemorrhage is also a rather rare complication in the more chronic variety. We have encountered two, one of which proved fatal. This experience, together with the severe exacerbation in two patients in whom no treatment was advised and with the well-known risks of cataract and glaucoma, has led us to have less faith in watchful waiting than we initially possessed.

Surgical Anatomy of the Cavernous Sinus

Although anatomical studies of the normal cavernous sinus clearly show multiple venous channels with multiple intervening septa, it would appear that in the chronic cavernous fistula these septa disappear. Probably the single most direct channel of exit enlarges and obliterates the others by compression. We have repeatedly inserted 80 or more feet of thrombogenic wire into a single site from which the coil filled the entire radiologically visible cavity rather than remaining confined to a single compartment. In the acute traumatic fistula in which the volume of leak may be high but in which the cavernous sinus may not yet be greatly distended, it would appear that multiple channels persist, making packing somewhat more difficult. In all cases there is a functional barrier created by the carotid artery itself, dividing the sinus into an anteroinferior lateral segment and a posterosuperior more medial segment. The communication between these two is mostly medial to the artery, but it may be lateral or both. Figures 181-1 and 181-2, derived largely from McGrath's study,[7] outline some of the essential central

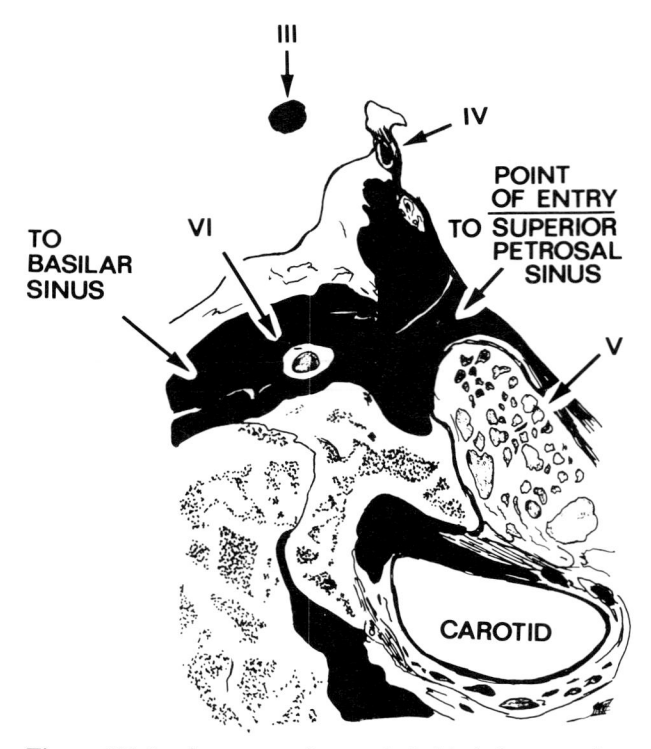

Figure 181-1 A cross section made behind the posterior clinoid at the point of entry of the superior petrosal sinus into the cavernous sinus shows the carotid as it is about to begin its first ascending limb as well as nerve VI, which will immediately swing laterally behind the ascending carotid. Nerve IV is protected by dura, and III has not yet entered the dura.

relationships that must be understood in surgical packing of the fistula. In the distended fistulous sinus the relative relationships are somewhat disturbed by this distension, the third and fourth nerves being more dorsally displaced and the ophthalmic and maxillary nerves being thinned out, separated, and laterally displaced. The convenient surgical routes of access for packing are the anteroinferior lateral corner at the point of entry of the ophthalmic vein and the posterosuperior region at the point of entry of the superior petrosal sinus. If there is not a tortuous carotid loop at the junction of its horizontal and anterior ascending limbs, then the space between the ophthalmic and maxillary divisions of the fifth nerve consists of a distended venous channel without arterial or neural content. The carotid artery is high and medial. The maxillary nerve is inferior, and the sixth lies under cover of the ophthalmic division, being separate from the venous channel by a very thin barrier (Fig. 181-3A).

Posterosuperiorly (Fig. 181-4) the third nerve has not yet entered the dura at the point of surgical access, which is behind the posterior clinoid at the point of entry of the superior petrosal sinus into the cavernous sinus. This is essentially the most posterior extent of Parkinson's triangle.[13] The fourth nerve lies very close to the line of the free margin of the tentorium and can be avoided by keeping lateral to that line. At this point it is still within the dura and is well protected. The nerve at risk is the sixth, which at this point is passing forward and laterally around the posterior margin of the carotid artery, separated from a venous channel by a very thin barrier. If thrombogenic material is directed downward and laterally, it could easily injure this nerve. A direct medial packing would get into the basilar sinus but would not block the fistula. If the direction is forward and slightly medial the packing will enter the sinus medial to the ascending limb of the carotid, but at the same time at a level high enough to avoid the sixth nerve.

Radiological Considerations

For all patients complete selective, subtracted, bilateral, internal and external carotid and vertebral angiography is essential (transfemoral). A lateral tube which automatically takes stereoscopic views is desirable.

Preoperative

The primary objective in examination of the internal carotid fistula is to find the exact site of the leak. This is best accomplished in the lateral view using subtraction technique. The critical factor is the frequency of exposure. The conventional machine with 3 frames per second is too slow. Six frames per second are much more likely to reveal the very early appearance of the contrast medium within the sinus, but probably much of this problem will be solved by digital angiography (using arterial injection) which will give 30 or more frames per second. There are, in addition, sup-

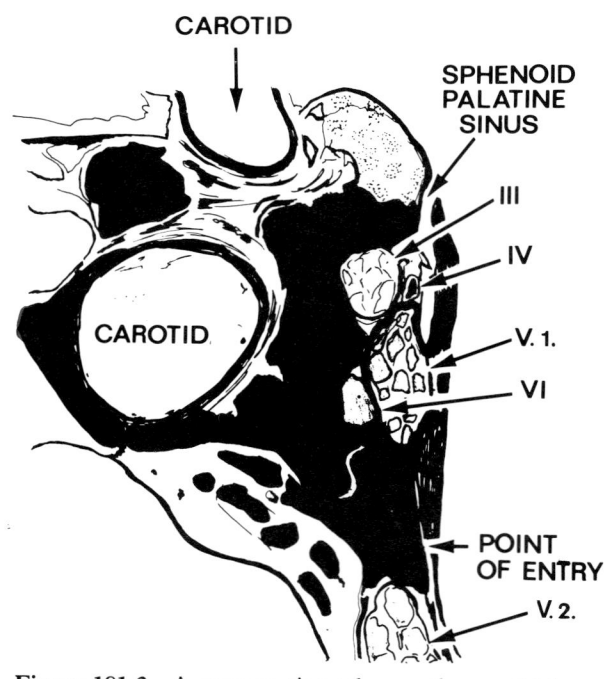

Figure 181-2 A cross section taken as the carotid has entered its second ascending limb at the level of the anterior clinoid. Nerves III and IV remain relatively protected, but VI is swinging medially under the limited protection of the first division of V.

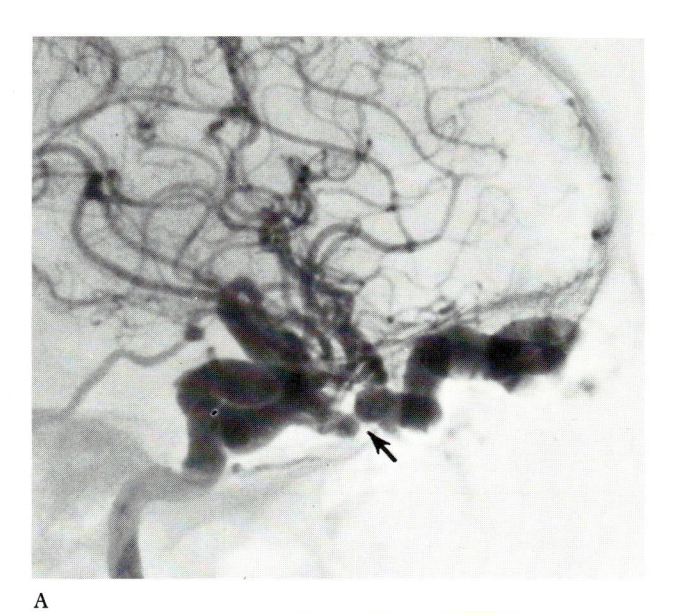

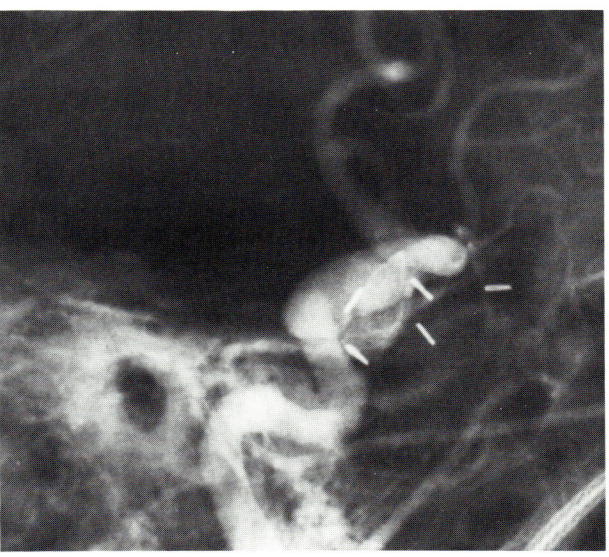

Figure 181-3 Lateral views of a carotid angiogram. *A.* The arrow indicates the constriction between the ophthalmic vein and the cavernous sinus which is the site of entry. This fistula drains entirely anteriorly. *B.* The fistula was entered at the most anterior clip. Initial packing did not eliminate the entire fistula. The residual was thrombosed by wire inserted at a point equidistant from the four adjoining markers. The choice of wire was a matter of convenience. Further packing with conventional material would also have been effective.

plementary methods of slowing the flow into the fistula to accomplish this same end. Manual ipsilateral compression of the carotid artery during a vertebral, or an opposite carotid, injection will give a relatively slower retrograde filling of the carotid, up to its point of leak into the sinus. (Fig. 181-5). A double lumen ipsilateral balloon catheter in the internal carotid will block the artery by means of the balloon and permit slow injection of contrast through the distal port, again showing the exact point at which the fistula opens into the sinus. The stereoscopic pictures are especially useful when looking at those fistulas with deep medial extension into the sphenoid and ethmoid sinuses. The anteroposterior projection is less useful than the lateral but may also be of value for these deep medial extensions. Since obliteration of the carotid artery is avoided, specific cross-flow studies to determine collateral blood supply are not required.

For dural AVM fistulas the prime goal is to identify all the feeding vessels and trace them through into the final venous phase. Here, especially in patients with bilateral signs, the anteroposterior views and the lateral stereo views are both most important. A right lateral arteriogram might show a blush apparently in the right cavernous sinus area, but the stereoscopic views could show that it was in the left sinus, and the anteroposterior views could trace the right arterial pathways across the midline to the left sinus. Still later, stereoscopic views could show the right cavernous sinus filling, and the late anteroposterior films would demonstrate that this was effected by the intercavernous venous plexus. Such an angiographic study would direct therapy to the site of leak which was in the left sinus.

Intraoperative Radiography

Single roentgenograms in the arterial phase are required, and serial exposures offer no advantage. A ceiling-mounted x-ray unit with the patients's head placed laterally is suitable. It is important in outlining the carotid artery in relation to its dural markers that the position of the tube does not

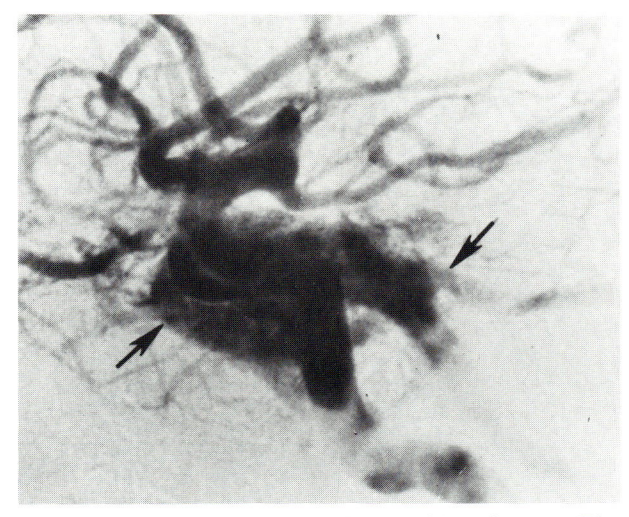

Figure 181-4 A lateral view of a carotid angiogram. The arrows indicate points of entry posterosuperiorly and anteroinferiorly. This fistula drains mainly posteriorly, and the posterosuperior chamber is packed first. The ophthalmic veins are only slightly enlarged.

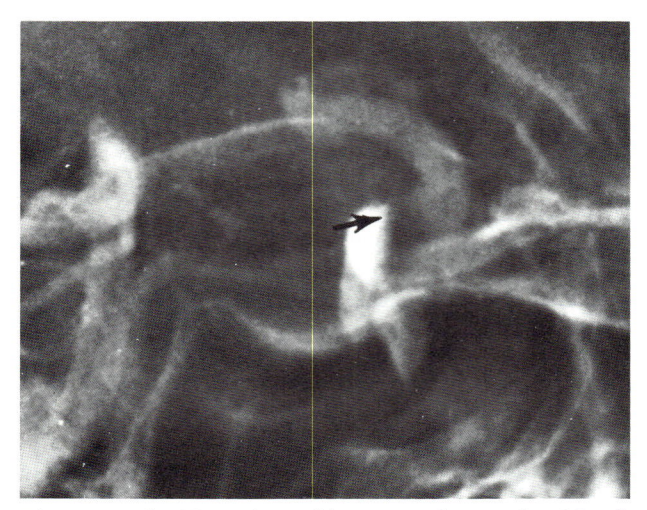

Figure 181-5 Manual carotid compression on the side of the fistula during vertebral injection discloses the site of the fistula (*arrow*).

change during the course of the thrombosis, or this will alter the marker-carotid relationship. A portable radiography unit is adequate, but the possibility of movement and therefore of error must be guarded against.

Surgical Therapy

Since a carotid-cavernous fistula only rarely poses a threat to life or to hemispheric function, its treatment should not deliberately include a surgical manipulation which involves either. For this reason all forms of trapping, with or without concomitant embolization, and direct obliteration under cardiac arrest, though effective, are outmoded. This leaves some form of balloon occlusion or direct venous occlusion, for those fed by the internal carotid, and selective embolization of external carotid feeding vessels, for those fed exclusively by the external circulation, as the currently available methods of choice. The exact decision depends upon the type of the fistula and upon the resources and experience available to the surgeon.

Acute traumatic fistulas, usually in the young and especially in males, have, as a rule, a high fistulous volume. Frequently the entire carotid flow is captured by the fistula, and none enters the brain. The opening is large enough to accept a detachable balloon catheter which flows into it easily. This is the method of choice. A problem arises if the balloon will not enter the fistula but remains in the carotid. If detached at the site of leak, it will cure the fistula at the expense of sacrificing the artery. The exact incidence of complications of leaving such a balloon in situ is not known. Spread of a thrombus distal to the balloon and deflation of the balloon followed by its distal migration are possible hazards but have not been reported. Mere occlusion of a fistulous carotid, while leaving the fistula open, results, according to Hamby, in a death rate which is 50 percent (or less than) that of occlusion of a nonfistulous carotid (as for aneurysm). This is due to the previous establishment of a circulatory compensation mechanism under the stress induced by the fistulous leak. With the fistula sealed by the balloon the ischemic complication rate should be even lower. However, as long as any mortality or morbidity exists, the surgeon must look at alternatives. If he cannot seal the fistula without arterial occlusion, and if he has the skills and resources to carry out a direct venous occlusion, then he should weigh the hazards of both methods and elect that which carries the lower risk. The sinus occlusion procedure, which almost invariably spares the carotid, is theoretically superior in its preservation of all vessels into the atherosclerotic years.

Fistulas which are exclusively filled by external carotid arteries, either unilateral or bilateral, may be occluded by transfemoral selective external carotid branch embolization. If the operator does not feel confident of doing this without incurring some risk of reflux embolization of the internal carotid artery, then the procedure may be carried out by direct puncture of the exposed external carotid after its temporary operative occlusion. The use of liquid embolization rather than solid embolization material must still be regarded as under clinical trial and is therefore reserved for those centers staffed by those with special interest and skills.

Direct venous occlusion of the carotid sinus is the treatment of choice for

1. Small-volume fistulas (which will not accept a balloon) supplied by the internal carotid artery.
2. All fistulas in patients in whom occlusion of a carotid artery might pose any ischemic hazard, e.g., patients with advanced age, known atheroma on the opposite side, history of ischemic episodes, or very poor response to the Matas transcutaneous carotid compression test. (It should be recognized that a patient who fails this test while the fistula remains open may not suffer any problem when the fistula is closed at the same time the carotid is occluded.)
3. Patients with combined internal and external carotid filling. The flow could be diminished by external embolization, but since occlusion of the sinus will take care of both types of feeder, embolization is in most instances redundant.
4. Late recurrent fistulas following previous carotid ligation and trapping methods.
5. At least one side of true bilateral independent fistulas in order to run no risk of blocking both carotid arteries.

Technique of Direct Venous Thrombosis

The essentials are good anatomical detail and a relaxed brain. Preoperative angiography reveals the site of leak exactly and directs the thrombogenic endeavor toward that point. If the fistulous connection is clearly into the anterior inferior sac, then that compartment will be thrombosed first. This can be done in most instances by an extradural approach in which the ophthalmic vein is opened as it enters the dura from the inferior orbital fissure. The major advantage of entering the sinus from the extradural site is that this approach precludes any possibility of damage to the artery.[10]

When the fistula is in the posterior superior compartment, it is entered by an intradural approach which demands an exact radiographic knowledge of the position of the carotid relative to the cavernous dura before packing commences. When the fistula causes both compartments to fill simultaneously, or if the minor compartment persists after obliteration of the major compartment, then both must be packed. It is best to prepare for both approaches in all instances (Fig. 181-4).

Good brain relaxation is accomplished by placing the patient in the lateral position with the head slightly down to facilitate gravity retraction of the temporal lobe, by placing an indwelling lumbar catheter for drainage of CSF (except in the elderly) and by using 500 ml of 20% mannitol.

Anteroinferior Compartment

A good arterial line is established in the superficial temporal artery by means of a cut-down catheter which enters the artery in a retrograde manner as far as possible. If very well anchored, a 1-cm penetration may be adequate. Papaverine relaxation will facilitate catheterization. The superior thyroid and occipital arteries are possible alternatives, and it is probably better to use one of them than to allow a transfemorally introduced catheter to lie in the carotid for several hours. Next, through a relatively small temporal flap, with bone removed very far anteriorly, the dura is mobilized from the anterior wall and from the medial wall of the middle fossa until the foramen rotundum is reached. This lies on the medial wall of the middle fossa rather than on the floor, unlike the foramen ovale. The inferior and superior orbital fissures lie medial and superior to it. The very thin bone between these, which constitutes both the medial wall of the middle fossa and the lateral wall of the apex of the orbit, is drilled out (Fig. 181-6). Bone bleeding is controlled by bone wax. The periorbita comes immediately into view, and the superior ophthalmic vein is seen beneath it in the larger and more chronic fistula, as it moves downward and laterally. It joins the smaller inferior orbital vein while still in the orbit, and the combined vein, following the direction of the inferior vein, then enters the cavernous sinus through a relatively narrow neck by way of the inferior orbital fissure. This neck remains narrow despite massive bulging of both vein and sinus. The inferior orbital fissure contains no nerves (Figs. 181-3A and 181-7A).

Thrombogenic material is prepared. This consists of many thin triangular wedges of dry Gelfoam (absorbable gelatin sponge, The Upjohn Co., Kalamazoo, Mich.) about 15 to 20 mm long and 5 to 8 mm wide at the base. About half of these wedges are coated with a few light strands of fluffy cotton to give the Gelfoam strength, and a surface to grip, when wet. Otherwise it may become soggy and get blown out by the intracavernous pressure. In addition, short strips of oxidized cellulose are added. These three materials, Gelfoam, Gelfoam with cotton backing, and oxidized cellulose, provide different consistencies and are used at different stages.

A small incision about 3 mm wide is made at the site of venous entry, and packing is begun with Gelfoam. When some pressure is needed to push the packing material further along, then the other firmer materials come into use. If the opening in the vein is not wide enough, the packing may be introduced erroneously into an extravenous space and never come into contact with the fistulous opening. It may also come into contact with the sixth nerve. If the direction is not accurate, packing may be mistakenly directed into the orbit. The site of entry is occluded between insertions by a wide-bore sucker covered by a small pad of wet fluffy cotton. This restricts egress and sucks up that blood which escapes.[10]

If the ophthalmic vein is not visible beneath the periorbita, it can usually be located by aspiration using a 28-gauge needle. If that fails, then a decision is made to enter into the subdural space, retract the brain, visualize the anterolateral wall of the cavernous sinus, and make an opening in it far anteriorly immediately above the maxillary nerve exit. Be-

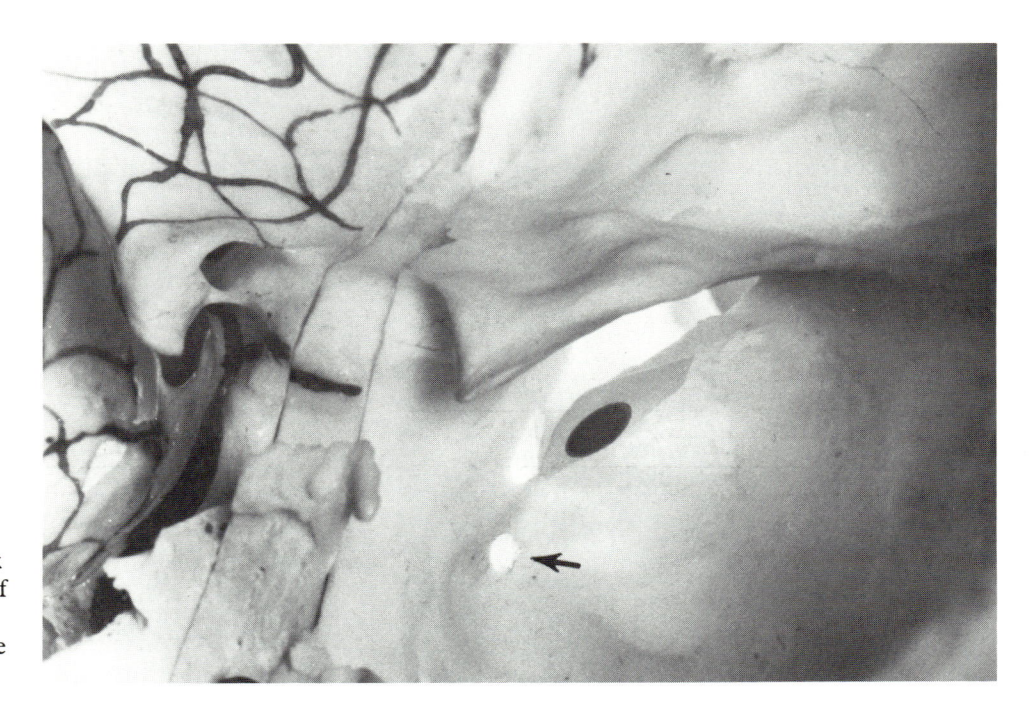

Figure 181-6 Oblique view of the right middle fossa of the skull. The arrow indicates the foramen rotundum. The black dot marks the thin shelf of bone that should be removed in order to find the ophthalmic vein.

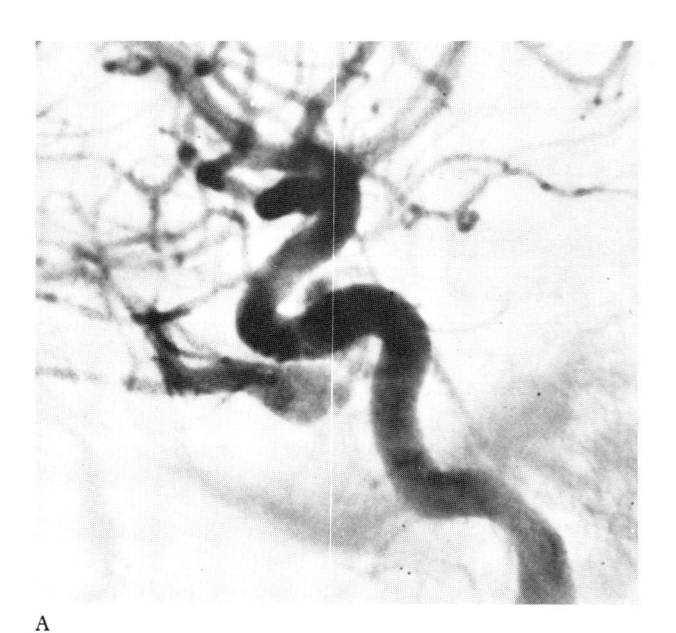

Figure 181-7 Left carotid angiograms. *A.* A lateral view, showing internal carotid filling of an anterior fistula. Note the large superior ophthalmic and small inferior ophthalmic veins, which join in the orbit to enter the cavernous sinus through the inferior orbital fissure. *B.* A lateral view, showing filling of the fistula by the external carotid artery. *C.* An anteroposterior view of the external carotid injection, showing secondary filling of the right cavernous sinus. *D.* A small pack, inserted at the point shown by the clip, sealed the fistula.

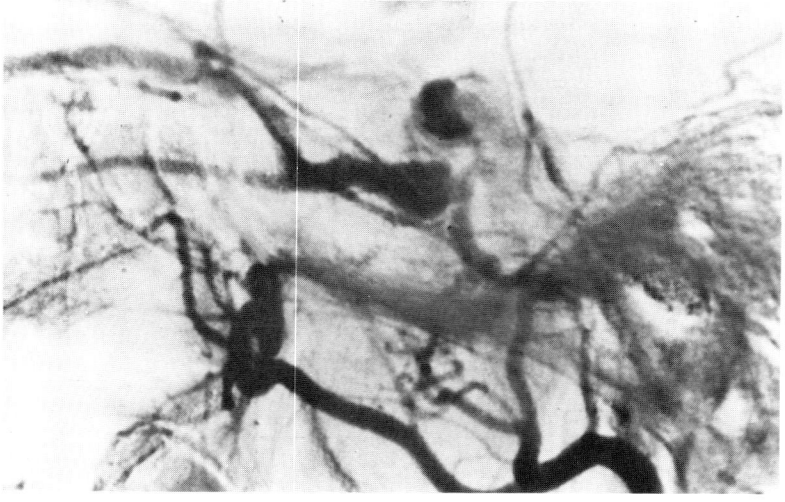

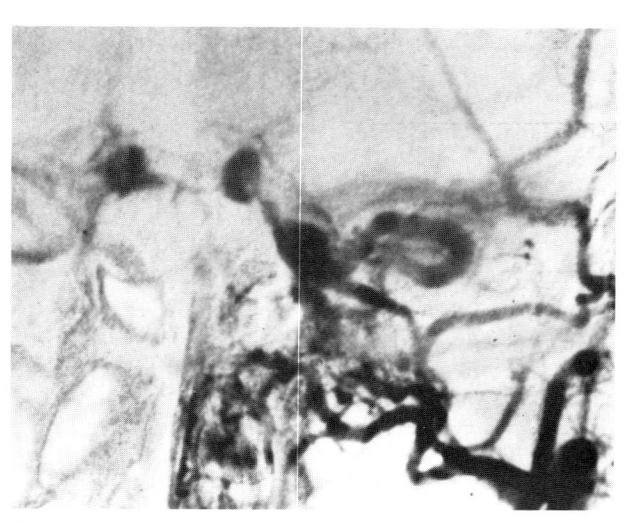

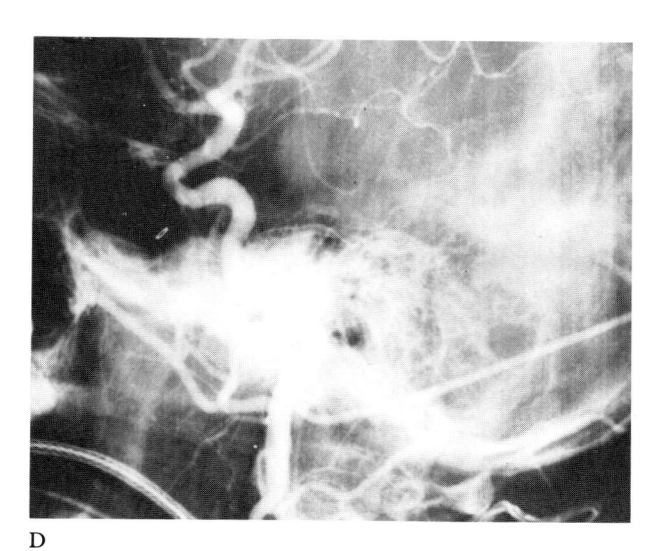

fore carrying out this last step, several small metal clips are sewn onto the cavernous dura to mark the presumed course of the carotid. Arteriography is then performed through the retrograde temporal catheter (8 to 10 ml of contrast medium), and the defined relationship of the artery (from which one may also deduce the presumed course of the sixth nerve) to the dural markers is examined. The incision, about 3 mm long and parallel to the maxillary fibers, is then made at an anteroinferior point which will be free from both artery and nerve.

Packing continues slowly, using the firmer cotton-covered Gelfoam and oxidized cellulose to push the semisolid Gelfoam further back toward the fistula, the tips of the introducing forceps rarely penetrating more than a few millimeters into the sinus. The degree of pressure used is an arbitrary one, and is one which the operator believes the sixth nerve will tolerate, if in contact. When bleeding ceases, some of the more recently introduced packing may be removed in an effort to reduce any possibility of nerve pressure as a clot forms and swells within the tight confines of the sinus. Serial angiogram films may be needed during the packing process to determine closure of fistula and absence of compression against the carotid. If, subsequent to obliteration of the anterior inferior compartment, there is persistent filling of the posterior superior compartment, then one proceeds to deal with it (Figs. 181-2, 181-3, and 181-7).

Posterosuperior Compartment

With the relaxed brain gently retracted, the third and fourth nerve points of entry are located, and their course along the free margin of the tentorium is outlined. The superior petrosal sinus may be visible or may be located by needling at the junction of the petrous bone with the tentorium. Usually one must carry the incision forward into the cavernous sinus because the superior petrosal is generally too small to carry a large volume of packing. Therefore dural markers, angiography, and definition of the arterial course are necessary before the incision is made. Here the sixth nerve as it winds laterally around the first ascending limb of the carotid is at risk. Packing is therefore directed anteriorly, medial to the artery and rather high toward the roof. Initially both the third and fourth nerves are encased in the roof and are not likely to be injured. It is only when they come lateral to the carotid that they clearly emerge from the wall and are unsupported and vulnerable. The site of entry is, in fact, the most posterior limit of Parkinson's triangle. Packing and serial angiography proceed until the fistula is entirely obliterated (Figs. 181-1 and 181-4).

The experienced surgeon may use stereotactic copper needles or thrombogenic wire to simplify the technique of thrombogenesis, but except in some unusual cases with far medial extension into the ethmoid and sphenoid sinuses, thrombogenic wire is not necessary. Electric current is not used and is neither necessary nor desirable. It will hasten thrombogenesis but might cause arterial spasm and possibly some nerve damage (Fig. 181-3B).[10,11]

Occlusion by a transcutaneous transjugular venous balloon catheter was effective in sealing a fistula in one of five attempts. Our two attempts to catheterize the sinus percutaneously through the ophthalmic vein were unsuccessful. Further efforts by these currently available transvenous techniques are probably not justified, unless the inferior petrosal sinus looks unusually favorable.

Technical Problems

If one seals the venous exits from the sinus, but fails to place thrombogenic material in apposition to the site of leak, then one merely converts a fistula into an aneurysm—which may, in fact, make some symptoms such as cavernous nerve palsy temporarily worse. The problem is dealt with by adding more thrombogenic material. An initial subtotal closure occurred in five instances and may be related to a more persistent septate division than is the rule. It is more likely to be encountered in the recent high-volume post-traumatic cases than in the more chronic variety. Temporary sixth nerve palsy occurred in two patients. Carotid spasm occurred in two but was asymptomatic.[10]

Problems in Judgment

An initial experience with 30 patients had led us to believe that surgical treatment was not a matter of urgency, but the last 20 have outlined some of the problems of delay. There have been four patients in whom a delay was serious. An alcoholic patient with multiple injuries from a road accident was blind in the right eye, comatose for 3 weeks, and had a fistula on the left. While an improvement in the state of infected gluteal wounds was awaited, she suddenly lost sight in the left eye, which did not return following successful fistula closure. A schizophrenic youth shot himself in the left ear, developing a CSF fistula and a carotid-cavernous fistula. The CSF fistula was not immediately repaired, and he died of meningitis before the carotid fistula could be dealt with. An elderly lady developed a small post-traumatic fistula which her physician elected not to treat. A few months later she had a massive subarachnoid hemorrhage. Closure of the fistula 3 weeks later while she was still in coma did not improve her, and she eventually died. A fourth patient, a disturbed youth who was the victim of an attempted homicide, did not wish to tolerate a balloon placement under local anesthesia. The initial venous thrombosis attempt did not completely close the fistula, but he would not consent to further surgery until after the eye went blind.

Bilateral Fistulas

Most severe fistulas, if permitted to develop long enough, will drain copiously into the opposite cavernous sinus and give bilateral symptoms. They are, however, truly unilateral. A few patients with traumatic fistulas (3 of 50 in our series) have had independent bilateral fistulas. In such cases, each side is treated separately and sequentially.

Extensive dural AVMs often have bilateral symptoms because of cavernous drainage to the opposite side. A few may even have bilateral feeding vessels, but the leak is usually on one side only and all arterial channels are directed to that side. Drainage may then affect both eyes. Unilateral cavernous thrombosis relieves the bilateral symptoms. We have seen two patients with independent bilateral dural AVMs which drained separately into each cavernous sinus. One was treated bilaterally, and one was treated unilaterally, the opposite side being asymptomatic.

Results

In all instances except when blindness was already present, vision has been restored. Proptosis and bruit have always been relieved. Cranial nerve palsies have resolved usually within a few months, but one patient with a third nerve palsy took 9 months. There were no operative infections and no late symptoms or signs that could be definitely attributed to the procedure. One child had a postoperative seizure 6 months later, but whether this was related to her trauma or to her operation is uncertain. No patient developed hemispheric damage. One patient died of meningitis before fistula occlusion. One died of antecedent subarachnoid hemorrhage and coma despite occlusion. Two died subsequently of unrelated causes.

Intracavernous Aneurysms

Symptoms and Natural History

Intracavernous aneurysms present with retro-orbital pain or with diplopia, as a result of third, fourth, or sixth nerve palsy. Being protected by the dura, they very rarely burst intracranially; I have only encountered one proven case and one suspected case. They may burst into the cavernous sinus, but this too is infrequent. Most commonly they simply enlarge, resulting in a complete ophthalmoplegia. Classically the third nerve palsy does not give a dilated pupil because the sympathetic fibers, which dilate the pupil, are also paralyzed. Pain and progression of symptoms tend to be episodic, lasting days, weeks, or even months, indicating episodes of distension rather than a uniformly steady expansion. Progression can be entirely painless although this is uncommon. The condition, especially in older women, may be bilateral.

Treatment

Treatment of the unilateral case traditionally consists of internal carotid ligation. This can be done perfectly safely in a graduated manner under anticoagulation in those patients who have an adequate collateral. Adequacy is initially determined by the patient's ability to tolerate ipsilateral manual carotid compression. Patients with a totally defective collateral will experience ischemic symptoms in about 9 or 10 s. If the patient can tolerate 30 s without symptoms, then he can probably tolerate graduated internal carotid artery occlusion. An adequate filling of the ipsilateral anterior and middle cerebral arteries should then be demonstrated angiographically via the opposite carotid or by the vertebral while the ipsilateral carotid is compressed. Lastly, in those centers where xenon washout blood flow determinations are available, defective flow on either side will warn against internal carotid occlusion.

Technique of Occlusion

Through a high oblique cervical incision at least one finger breadth below the angle of the jaw (to spare seventh nerve fibers), under local or general anesthesia, the internal carotid artery is exposed and a Selverstone clamp is applied. The clamp is left in the fully open position. Three days later when heparinization will not cause any possibility of hematoma in the recent wound, the patient is fully heparinized. The clamp is fully closed. If symptoms do not develop, a xenon blood flow measurement is done (if available). If the flow remains within normal limits, the clamp should be set one-half turn short of full occlusion. The next day it is set at one-quarter turn short, and on the third day it is fully closed. These 2 days allow the distal internal carotid to decrease in diameter in proportion to flow. When heparinization is then discontinued, clotting occurs in a constricted vessel. This prevents embolization which (rather than ischemia) is the main problem with internal carotid ligation. If clotting occurred in a full-caliber internal carotid, then when it constricted over the next day or 2, it would squeeze out its contents as an embolus (Fig. 181-8).

If the xenon-determined cerebral blood flow was decreased out of the normal range (for that particular blood flow apparatus), then occlusion would be more gradual and would be based upon daily flow determinations. If flow determinations are not available, ophthalmoplethysmography may give a useful indication. In general, without the reassurance of an adequate flow it is best to slow complete occlusion by an extra 2 days. If symptoms develop at the initial trial closure, it might not be possible to effect a closure,

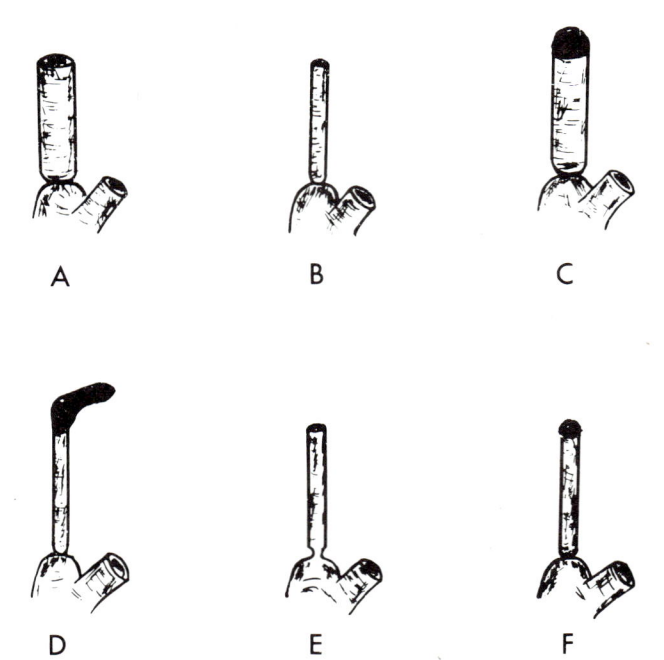

Figure 181-8 Diagrams of vascular shrinkage. *A*. An occluded vessel shrinks to the diameter shown in *B*. If it contains a clot (*C*), it will extrude the clot when it constricts (*D*). If it is permitted to constrict before clotting (*E*), there is no extruded clot in the final stage (*F*).

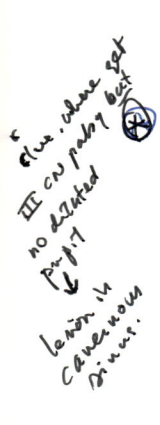

Carotid-Cavernous Fistulas and Intracavernous Aneurysms   1493

although a very graduated program of 1 to 2 weeks could be successful.

In all instances when occlusion is complete, heparinization is continued for 2 further days. If symptoms develop during the graduated occlusion or within these 2 days, the clamp is opened fully. It may then be slowly closed again when all symptoms have disappeared. We have only had to do this once after occlusion had been completed. The transient symptoms disappeared.

We have followed patients angiographically during graduated occlusion without heparinization. The aneurysm will clot off completely in the half-turn open position within a few days, but the clot will slowly disappear (by lysis rather than by embolization) if the clamp is opened (Fig. 181-9). It is quite clear that once occlusion is complete and heparinization is stopped, the aneurysm will thrombose in like manner.

If the patient could not tolerate internal carotid occlusion, common carotid occlusion could be considered. It will certainly lower pressure within the aneurysm for months or years, but it will not thrombose it.

For those patients who do not tolerate initial carotid occlusion and for those with contralateral atherosclerotic disease, a preliminary extracranial-intracranial bypass procedure should be done. The clamp is placed at the same time and is closed to the half-turn mark (if tolerated) as soon as the patient awakens in order to encourage patency within the anastomosis. Full closure is best guided by blood flow measurements and may take several days. Heparinization is not used because of the recent craniotomy. In one of our patients full closure took 2 weeks despite an apparently satisfactory bypass. When bilateral aneurysms are present, one might treat the side with presenting symptoms if the symptoms, especially pain, are serious enough. This may be done with or without a bypass, depending upon the collateral. The remaining side is untreated.

Not infrequently in older patients it is possible to accept unilateral or even bilateral ophthalmoplegia rather than accept any risk of hemiplegia or of death. I have followed one such patient for 20 years. She keeps her upper lid raised on one side by a "crutch" attached to her glasses and lives a satisfactory life.

Alternative Methods

The goal of obliterating these aneurysms while preserving carotid blood flow remains desirable. Three methods have received some attention. They are (1) transcarotid placement of a detachable balloon, (2) transdural placement of a detachable balloon, and (3) transdural placement of needle or wire thrombogenic material. A problem with detachable balloons is that in the distended state they continue to exert pressure upon the cavernous nerves and thereby may not relieve symptoms. A transcarotid balloon is difficult to place, and a misplaced one would simply obstruct the carotid. Not enough transdural balloons have been placed, nor followed long enough to evaluate the method adequately.[11] Transdural wire or needle thrombosis is effective for the smaller aneurysms (Fig. 181-10). The very large aneurysms have too large a neck (Fig.181-9B), and this would permit the thrombus to spread into the carotid lumen.[10] It might be speculated at this time that a greater familiarity with the surgical anatomy of the cavernous sinus and an ability to control its venous channels may permit the surgeon to enter the sinus (without cardiac arrest) and surgically clip some of the small aneurysms before they reach the giant size which makes them so difficult to treat.

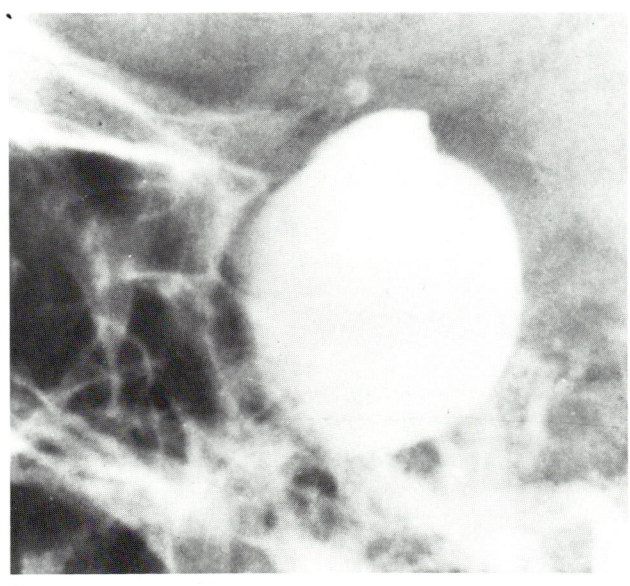

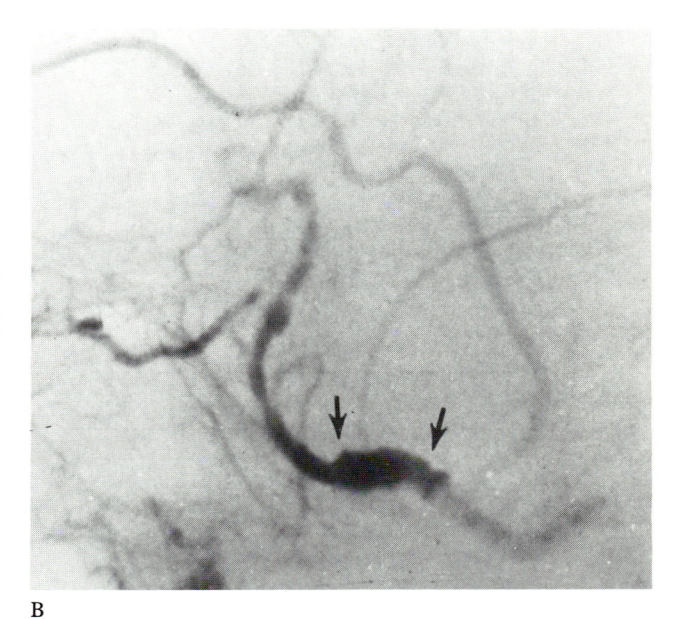

Figure 181-9 Giant cavernous aneurysm. *A.* Those with a pointing irregularity may be more liable to intradural hemorrhage. *B.* The subtotal clamp has caused thrombosis of the aneurysm. Note the very wide neck indicated by the arrows.

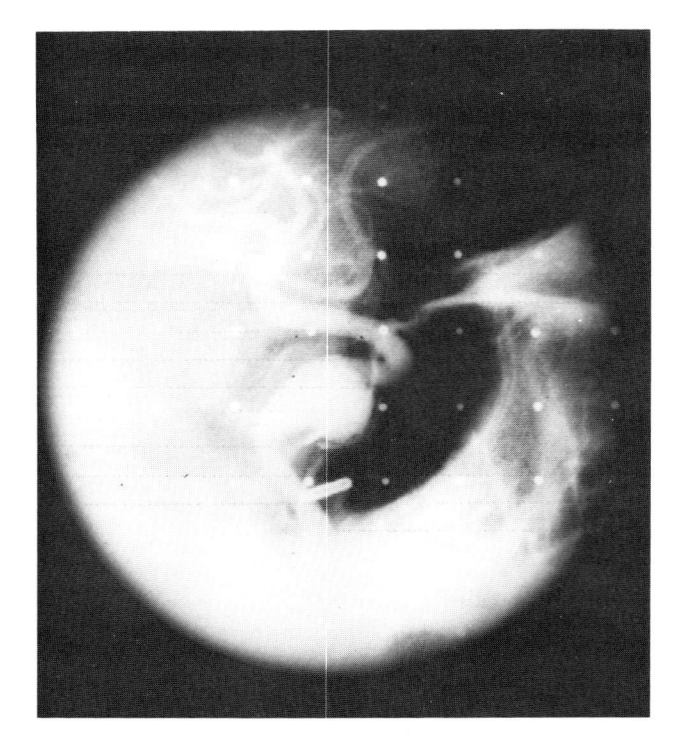

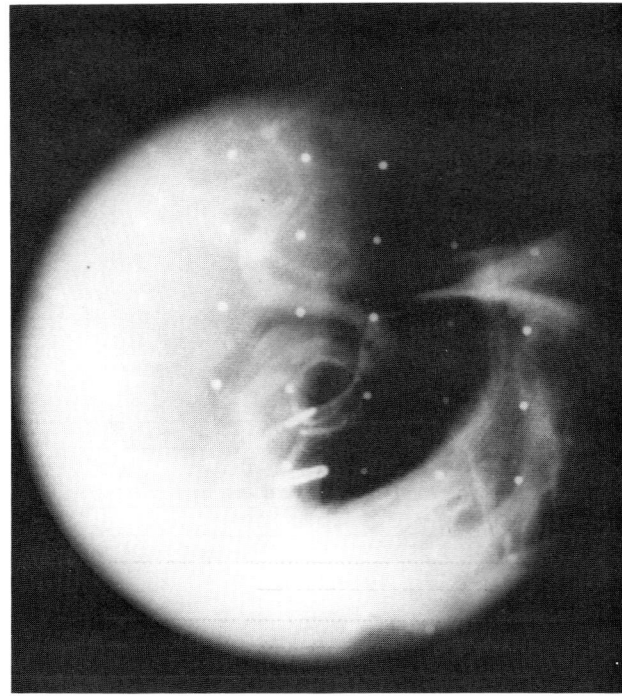

Figure 181-10 Intraoperative angiogram of a small cavernous aneurysm with overlying dural markers. *A.* Before treatment. *B.* The aneurysm has been occluded by phosphor bronze wire inserted at the anterior end of the superior clip.

References

1. Arutiunov AI, Serbinenko FA, Shlykov AA: Surgical treatment of carotid-cavernous fistulas. Prog Brain Res 30:441–444, 1969.
2. Black P, Uematsu S, Perovic M, Walker AE: Carotid-cavernous fistula: A controlled embolus technique for occlusion of fistula with preservation of carotid blood flow: Technical note. J Neurosurg 38:113–118, 1973.
3. Brooks B: Discussion of paper by Noland L, Taylor AS. Trans South Surg Assoc 43:176–177, 1931.
4. Debrun G, Lacour P, Vinuela F, Fox A, Drake CG, Caron JP: Treatment of 54 traumatic carotid-cavernous fistulas. J Neurosurg 55:678–692, 1981.
5. Hamby WB: *Carotid-Cavernous Fistula.* Springfield, Ill, Charles C Thomas, 1966.
6. Hayes GJ: External carotid-cavernous sinus fistulas. J Neurosurg 20:692–700, 1963.
7. McGrath P: The cavernous sinus: An anatomical survey. Aust NZ J Surg 47:601–613, 1977.
8. Morley TP: Appraisal of various forms of management in 41 cases of carotid-cavernous fistula, in Morley TP (ed): *Current Controversies in Neurosurgery.* Philadelphia, Saunders, 1976, pp 223–236.
9. Mullan S: Experiences with surgical thrombosis of intracranial berry aneurysms and carotid cavernous fistulas. J Neurosurg 41:657–670, 1974.
10. Mullan S: Treatment of carotid-cavernous fistulas by cavernous sinus occlusion. J Neurosurg 50:131–144, 1979.
11. Mullan S, Duda EE, Patronas NJ: Some examples of balloon technology in neurosurgery. J Neurosurg 52:321–329, 1980.
12. Obrador S, Gomez-Bueno J, Silvela J: Spontaneous carotid-cavernous fistula produced by ruptured aneurysm of the meningohypophyseal branch of the internal carotid artery: Case report. J Neurosurg 40:539–543, 1974.
13. Parkinson D: A surgical approach to the cavernous portion of the carotid artery: Anatomical studies and case report. J Neurosurg 23:474–483, 1965.
14. Prolo DJ, Hanbery JW: Intraluminal occlusion of a carotid-cavernous sinus fistula with a balloon catheter: Technical note. J Neurosurg 35:237–242, 1971.
15. Serbinenko FA: Balloon catheterization and occlusion of major cerebral vessels. J Neurosurg 41:125–145, 1974.
16. Stern WE, Brown WJ, Alksne JF: The surgical challenge of carotid-cavernous fistula: The critical role of intracranial circulatory dynamics. J Neurosurg 27:298–308, 1967.

182
Spinal Arteriovenous Malformations

Ayub Khan Ommaya

Although arteriovenous malformations (AVMs) of the spinal cord are hamartomatous in nature, we do not usually include such lesions as cavernous angioma and telangiectasis among the AVMs. In the following account of these lesions I will refer only to abnormal connections between arteries and veins, without intervening capillaries, located in the spinal cord and its leptomeninges. In this sense, other than the anatomical constraints of spinal cord structure, spinal AVM is comparable to cerebral AVM with only a few differences.

Advances in the surgical treatment of neural disorders are usually preceded or associated with improvements in diagnostic techniques that lead to greater understanding of such diseases. The contributions of Egas Moniz (carotid angiography), Walter Dandy (pneumoencephalography), and G.N. Hounsfield (computed tomography) created a virtual revolution in the diagnostic basis of modern neurosurgery. Application of such advances in diagnostic technique, as a general rule, have always been much slower for diseases of the spinal cord as compared with those of the brain. Vascular diseases of the spinal cord are no exception. Thus, it was not until 1969 that the first English language monograph on the subject, *Selective Arteriography of the Spinal Cord*, was published; this described our earliest experiences with arteriovenous malformation of the spinal cord.[5] The work of R. Djindjian in France had begun somewhat earlier, and although these pioneering efforts on the vascular radiology of the spinal cord began in the early 1960s, it was not until the 1970s that the diagnostic and therapeutic aspects of the vascular diseases of the spinal cord (especially AVMs) became well understood.

These developments are well summarized in a number of publications, the most notable being the excellent monographs of R. Djindjian et al.[4] and Aminoff,[1] and the text edited by Pia and Djindjian.[14] This chapter cannot provide the type of detail available in these texts, and therefore I will confine my effort to a summary of my experience in the diagnosis and surgical treatment of 104 cases of such lesions culled from over 200 cases of nontraumatic myelopathy directly referred as suspected arteriovenous malformations of the spinal cord and studied between 1961 and 1980 at the Clinical Center of the National Institutes of Health and between 1980 and 1983 at the George Washington University Medical Center. All of the 104 cases in this series were studied with selective spinal angiography. Table 182-1 lists the discharge diagnosis of 201 cases of nontraumatic myelopathy, of which 104 were proved to have an AVM.

Terminology and Classification

Arteriovenous malformations or angiomas of the spinal cord are congenital abnormal clusters of blood vessels formed as a developmental anomaly of the spinal circulation. Turnbull has described four stages in the development of the spinal vascular system, and it is at the end of the second or "initial" stage (third to sixth weeks) that maldevelopment leads to persistence of thin-walled tortuous vessels with poorly developed media and elastica, primitive capillary and precapillary channels, and abnormal arteriovenous shunts typically seen in an AVM.[16] These lesions were first described in reports by Hebold in 1885 and by Gaupp in 1887, who picturesquely called them "hemorrhoids of the pia mater" and recognized them as a source for subarachnoid hemorrhage.[8,9]

AVMs are usually classified according to their regional localization by selective spinal angiography into three groups: cervical, thoracic, and thoracolumbosacral. Based on an angiographically analyzed series of 150 cases, Michael Djindjian has given overall regional percentages of 14 percent for cervical (C1-T1), 22 percent for thoracic (T2-6), and 64 percent for the largest group of thoracolumbosacral AVMs (T7 to cauda equina).[3] These figures are in rough agreement with our own series of 104 cases in which we have also observed an equivalent contribution of blood supply to the AVM from posterior arteries in 48 percent and from both anterior and posterior vessels in 52 percent. Our data also confirm the observation that more rostral AVMs have more anterior blood supply while the caudally placed AVMs have more posteriorly derived vascular inputs. M. Djindjian's observations in association with his father (R. Djindjian) at the Lariboisiere Hospital in Paris with Rey and Houdart on the classification of intramedullary AVMs form an important contribution with great surgical significance, and the reader is referred to this work for further details.[3,4,13]

TABLE 182-1 Discharge Diagnosis in 201 Patients Referred with Myelopathy Due to Suspected AVM (1965 to 1981)

Spinal arteriovenous malformation	104
Nontraumatic myelopathy of unknown origin	34
Intradural spinal tumor	24
Astrocytoma	12
Ependymoma	4
Hemangioblastoma	4
Neurofibroma	4
Cervical or lumbar spondylosis or disc herniation	20
Syringomyelia	12
Motor neuron disease	2
Multiple sclerosis	2
Chronic arachnoiditis	2
Cholesteatoma of posterior fossa	1

Our first radiological classification of AVMs recognized three basic types: the single, coiled, unbranched type I lesion, commonly seen in adults; the less common plexus or "glomus" type II lesion; and the variable, rapid-flow, type III lesion with multiple feeding arteries often seen in younger patients and hence termed the *juvenile* type.[5] From the surgeon's point of view, a division of all spinal cord AVMs into low-flow and high-flow lesions is a simple rubric to separate the surgically easy, mainly extramedullary low-flow cases from the surgically difficult and often intramedullary, high-flow lesions. High-flow AVMs are completely visualized by selective angiography in less than 5 s, whereas low-flow AVMs require much longer times for contrast clearance. Table 182-2 is a summary of the main features of our current classification.

Incidence

In neurosurgical series, the incidence of spinal AVM ranges from a low of 3.3 percent in the preangiography era to a figure of 40 percent of all CNS vascular malformations after the introduction of selective angiography.[13] These figures certainly show that spinal AVMs are not rare lesions, but in view of the absence of adequate epidemiologic data and the relative paucity of cases in published series, the true incidence is not known. However, it is reasonable to expect that at least 10 percent of vascular space–occupying lesions of the spinal cord will be AVMs.[11]

In our series, males were preponderant (79 percent), whereas incidence for age was approximately equal from the second to the sixth decade. The incidence of high-flow AVMs in adults was approximately one-fourth that of the low-flow AVMs, which clearly are much more commonly seen in individuals over 18 years of age.

Pathogenesis of AVM Effects on the Spinal Cord

In an earlier publication we discussed the pathogenesis of AVM symptoms and signs, and we questioned the significance of the factors of mechanical compression by the venous bulk of the lesion and vascular diversion ("steal").[10] These and other more significant factors such as decreased arteriovenous (AV) pressure gradient, bleeding, and progressive thrombosis are further discussed in the contributions of M. and R. Djindjian,[3,4] Pia and Djindjian,[14] and Aminoff.[1] The consensus would point to a variable contribution of five factors causing spinal cord ischemia: increased venous pressure, mechanical pressure by bulky arterialized veins, subarachnoid hemorrhage, and thrombotic phenomena. It is our current view that steal is the least likely to be effective in causing cord ischemia but that it may also play some role. The variable contribution of these factors may explain the often unpredictable response to embolization of feeders, which cures the steal without relieving the compression, as well as the genesis of so-called Foix-Alajouanine disease as a thrombotic end stage in the life of an untreated AVM, as first suggested by Pia and Djindjian.[14] The etiology of thrombosis in an AVM is unknown, but that it occurs is unequivocally certain. The role of increased extramedullary venous pressure has been hypothesized by

TABLE 182-2 Spinal Angiomas or Arteriovenous Malformations (AVMs) of the Spinal Cord

Low-Flow AVM	High-Flow AVM
Synonyms	
Type I AVM*	Type II (glomus)*
Single coiled vessel	Type III (juvenile)*
Angioma racemosum venosum (Wyburn-Mason)	Angioma racemosum arteriovenosum (Wyburn-Mason)
Angioma racemosum (Krayenbühl et al.)	Arteriovenous malformation with multiple feeders
Long dorsal malformation (Malis)	
Location of Nidus	
Extradural and/or dural	Extradural and/or dural
Subdural and subarachnoid	Subdural and extramedullary
Combined types	Combined types
Usual Level of AVM†	
Thoracic-lumbar-sacral	Cervical-thoracic-lumbar

*Ommaya et al. Note: Type II (glomus) AVM occurs most often in the cervical cord or at the cervicomedullary junction.
†Levels are indicated in sequence of most to least common site.

Aminoff et al.[2] These authors postulate a sequence of high venous back pressure causing a reduced intramedullary AV pressure gradient, which in turn causes reduced blood flow leading to spinal cord ischemia either directly or indirectly via intravascular thrombosis. Although a number of authors dismiss the role of mechanical compression, extensive experience by numerous authorities confirms our own findings of bulky AVMs acting as space-occupying lesions; furthermore, in the book by Pia and Djindjian pathological evidence is clearly reviewed to show both cord and root compression.[13]

Clinical Diagnosis

The most striking clinical fact about the AVM of the spinal cord is the protean nature of its natural history, making early diagnosis (within 6 months of the first symptom) very difficult. Thus in 60 percent of our 104 cases, 2 years or more had elapsed. Increasing awareness of AVM as a cause of progressive nontraumatic myelopathy has, however, improved early recognition in the past 10 years of our more than 20-years experience with these lesions. Thus, among the first 45 of the 104 patients referred to us, only 17 were recognized as AVM cases within 1 year of symptom onset, and 19 were not properly diagnosed until 3 to 15 years after the original symptoms appeared. Within the past 10 years, however, 47 patients were diagnosed within 2 years of onset. Difficulty of early diagnosis is often related to the insidious character of the onset of the initial symptoms and signs.

The most common deficits to appear first are either motor or sensory or both (80 percent), with pain as a frequent component in nearly half the cases. Disturbances of sphincteric and sexual functions as initial signs were less common (9 percent). The acute onset of any or all of these symptoms and signs, usually due to subarachnoid hemorrhage, occurred in only 11 percent of our cases. The clinical course is almost invariably progressive, but in 32 percent of our cases the progression displayed a fluctuating intensity, a characteristic feature described by many authors and the possible causes of which are well detailed in the monograph by Aminoff.[1]

It is obvious from the above that there is no unique constellation of symptoms and signs that is pathognomonic of spinal cord AVM. In our series, the shortest history was one of sudden severe back pain and paraplegia, with the final diagnosis established in less than 1 week. The longest delay between symptom onset and diagnosis was 16 years in a patient misdiagnosed as having motor neuron disease. The differential diagnosis includes all the disease categories listed in Table 182-1, with multiple sclerosis and motor neuron disease being the commonest mistakes.

We have previously drawn attention to the value of cutaneous angiomatous lesions in suspecting and localizing spinal cord AVMs (in 19 percent of cases), particularly when a Valsalva maneuver causes enhancement of the color intensity of such skin lesions.[7] This maneuver can also exacerbate other symptoms and signs of the AVM. Trauma, pregnancy, increase of body temperature, overeating, postural changes, and muscular effort are additional factors that may precipitate or aggravate AVM symptoms.[1] One of our patients, a successful fund-raiser for a well-known university, presented with three episodes of postprandial transient paraplegia that spontaneously reversed 4 to 6 h after the meal. Only two patients in our series had audible bruits over the AVM; both had extensive dural, extradural, and extraspinal components.

Radiological Diagnosis

Since the early work reported in 1969 and 1970 from Paris and Bethesda, the numerous contributions on this subject have elaborated in considerable detail on the techniques and efficiency of selective spinal angiography, and the reader is referred for such details to these sources.[1,4,5,13] Although angiography is essential for the precise understanding of the surgical anatomy and subsequent surgical therapy planning as well as postoperative evaluation, it should be remembered that myelography remains the major screening method for AVM. Plain x-ray films were only occasionally useful in our series (6 percent positive versus 94 percent negative findings). The finding of bony erosions in vertebral elements and interpedicular space widening in patients with motor or sensory deficits in the lower extremities is certainly a useful diagnostic clue. Myelography, on the other hand, was positive in 97 percent of our cases and diagnostic for AVM in 86 percent, showing the characteristic serpiginous filling deficits. The necessity for *complete* myelographic examination of the cord, including its dorsal aspect, has been repeatedly emphasized, not only for exact diagnosis but also to provide the necessary localization of the AVM that precedes angiographic delineation of its vascular details. It should be obvious that without myelographic guidance, spinal angiography of *all* the cord blood supply would be required—a most tedious task fraught with risk. Moreover, in our series we have not had a single case in which an entirely normal myelogram was found in an AVM case, and a negative myelogram (of a *total* nature) is conclusive in ruling out AVM. It is, therefore, recommended that selective spinal angiography not be done in patients with a suspected AVM whose myelograms show no abnormality whatsoever. On the other hand, cases with abnormal myelograms *not* clearly diagnostic of AVM but with *clinical* evidence of a progressive clinical course (e.g., a case with "localized arachnoiditis") should be examined angiographically. The relative contributions of the three major modes of radiological investigation of AVM are shown in Table 182-3.

Interpretation of spinal angiograms, as of myelograms, must be based on a clear understanding of normal intraspinal structure. Selective angiography was successful in demonstrating the lesion in 98 percent of our cases. Failure to show by angiogram an AVM that has been suspected both clinically and myelographically suggests a bad prognosis. Results of surgical removal of such "nonfilling" AVMs in our series were not attended by any significant benefit to the patient. Spinal angiography is a time-consuming procedure, and a careful examination of the blood supply and vascular anatomy of a large AVM may require two or even three angiographic sessions. It is our practice to protect the patient during such investigations with dexamethasone.

Surgical Treatment and Results

In the course of two decades of neurosurgical experience the author has tested and used all the various modes of surgical therapy for AVM. These include arterial ligation for certain low-flow lesions,[12] microsurgical total excision for both low-flow and certain high-flow lesions,[11] and embolization in collaboration with Doppman[6] and Davis, both as a preoperative maneuver and as a sole or supplementary mode of therapy. As discussed below, each of these methods alone or in combination has to be mastered by the neurosurgeon who wishes to provide optimal management to all patients with spinal cord AVM.

The evolution of microsurgical technique in neurosurgery led by the pioneering efforts of Donaghy and Yasargil has resulted in a consensus that the nidus or true shunt zone of the spinal cord AVM should be resected in toto whenever possible. Pia, in a comprehensive survey of the operative treatment of AVM of the spinal cord, including his own extensive experience, has emphasized that the operative technique for resection is not new and was first carried out in 1927 by Berthes based on the first myelographic demonstration of an AVM, with significant clinical improvement after surgery.[13] In our own series, dorsally placed low-flow lesions with a primarily posterior blood supply as well as glomus-type high-flow lesions in the cervical and cervicomedullary zones were amenable to total resection even where significant intramedullary extensions were present. Anteri-

TABLE 182-3 Radiological Diagnosis

	Positive, %	Negative, %
Plain spine films*	6	94
Myelography†	97	3
Arteriography‡	98	2

*Widening of interpedicular space and bone erosions.
†Six did not show typical serpiginous defects. Four had complete blocks. Two of the negative myelograms suggested arachnoiditis only, with subsequent positive angiography.
‡Six studies were incomplete.

orly located or "global" lesions (invariably of the high-flow type) were not usually amenable to total resection, and partial resections and arterial ligation with and without embolization were the alternative procedures undertaken. Intramedullary lesions of the nonglomus or juvenile type with a major supply from the anterior spinal artery are usually not totally resectable, but partial resections are often quite useful in causing neurological improvement in patients with a short history.

The results of treatment in the author's personal series of 104 cases are summarized in Table 182-4. The patients have been divided into three groups according to the type of therapy used as the primary method of management. The results shown were based on clinical evaluation at a minimum of 1 year after the primary procedure. The category of result titled "unchanged" means that the previously progressive myelopathy was arrested but not reversed. This effect on the myelopathy was clear-cut in group I patients but often was temporary in group II and group III patients followed up over 3 to 4 years. Delayed resumption of progressive myelopathy was especially noted in patients over the age of 60 in whom all results were qualitatively less satisfactory.

Our best results were obtained in low-flow lesions situated over the dorsum of the spinal cord where total resection and intradural or dural-extradural interruption of the nidus produced almost equally good results. In high-flow lesions, total resection achieved within the first year of lesion presentation (by history) also produced good results, especially in the cervical cord, provided that myelopathy was noted to be minimal and was present for less than 6 months. Our worst results occurred in patients in whom angiography (often repeated) failed to reveal the myelographically diagnosed AVM, in patients with progressive myelopathy of more than 12 months duration, and in patients with high-flow lesions in whom total resection of the nidus was not achieved. The critical role of symptom duration on the result of treatment was clearly shown in our 64 group I patients, among whom 50 who recovered almost completely were all operated upon within the first year after the onset of symptoms.[13]

The course of recovery after surgical treatment was often quite variable, as illustrated by the following five case histories.

Case no. 68 in our series underwent a total excision of a low-flow intradural dorsally placed AVM fed by the iliolumbar arteries bilaterally. Only slight improvement was noted 1 year postoperatively, but this continued so that after 5 years the patient was completely normal and has remained thus during the subsequent 5 years.

Case no. 80 (age 55) also had a low-flow thoracic AVM completely resected, with immediate worsening of his neurological deficits postoperatively. However, after 3 years he had improved significantly, and 6 years postoperatively he showed marked restoration of neurological function. This type of delayed improvement after an initial worsening was never seen in patients who underwent intradural arterial ligation with or without subtotal AVM resection.

Case no. 72 (age 44) underwent "arterial" ligation of all angiographically demonstrated feeders of a low-flow thoracolumbar AVM. The immediate postoperative improvement was steadily maintained, and when last seen 4 years after surgery, he was working full time. The return of neurological deficits then led to discovery of a missed dural component, resection of which returned full recovery to the patient.

Case no. 76 (age 64), on the other hand, also had a low-flow thoracolumbar AVM and received similar surgical treatment, but in spite of significant improvement maintained beyond the first year, he showed progressive deterioration starting at 3 years and ending in complete paraplegia 11 years postoperatively. Repeat myelography and angiography showed no recurrence of the AVM. Significant cord shrinkage and arachnoiditis suggested a Foix-Alajouanine syndrome secondary to delayed thrombotic and ischemic changes in an intermedullary component of the AVM.

Case no. 92 (age 32) had a prodromal history of "migraine" with vivid fortification spectra culminating in the sudden onset of quadriplegia. A high-flow cervicomedullary junction AVM with significant intramedullary and extramedullary components was resected under hypothermia and total circulatory arrest of 45-min duration. The patient made an excellent recovery, which persisted for over 3 years. Return of lateralized spastic hemiparesis and arm-shoulder pain led to the discovery of dural components missed at the first angiographic study, and surgical removal of this dural nidus led to the return to full activity of the patient.

Microsurgical Technique for Total Excision

In spite of the best radiographic data, it is important to note that true operability of a difficult spinal cord AVM can be determined only when the lesion is inspected at operation. It is crucial, therefore, that the exposure should be carried out with meticulous attention to hemostasis. It is the practice of the author to use an air-powered rongeur for completion of the bone work, exposing the dura as widely as possible without removal of the facet joints. It is not necessary to expose more of the dura than is necessary, i.e., precisely the area over the main mass of the AVM or the so-called nidus of the lesion. It is true that in certain cases the draining veins are so inextricably entwined that a large exposure is necessary, but careful review of the angiograms will usually result in a smaller field of exposure. At this stage, the microscope is introduced and the dura is carefully examined, particularly in the lateral recesses and along the roots to exclude dural components of the AVM. A dural opening in the midline is

TABLE 182-4 Results of Therapy

Types of Therapy	Total Number of Patients	Improved	Unchanged	Worse
Microneurosurgical total resection	64	50	12	2
Arterial ligation ± partial resection	28	16	8	4
Embolization	12	2	9	1
Totals	104	68 (65.4%)	29 (27.9%)	7 (6.7%)

then performed; the arachnoid is preserved and the escape of CSF is prevented at this stage.[13]

After the dura is tacked up to the muscles with retaining sutures, the arachnoid is opened in the midline and in turn is tacked up to the dural edges using small metal clips. In the "easy" case, a dorsally placed lesion lies primarily in the subarachnoid space, and sharp dissection is used to cut arachnoidal bands holding the lesion to the cord. Arterial feeders are sought (the surgeon is guided by the angiographic data) and divided between clips with bipolar coagulation of the cut ends. Arterial feeders can usually be identified as they enter the dural sheath in the lateral gutter. The cut end of the artery attached to the AVM is then used as a "handle" to aid in the further subarachnoidal dissection and removal of the AVM mass in toto. It should be emphasized that what is resected in toto is only the nidus and it is not necessary to remove the often voluminous draining veins. This is especially true of the so-called dural AVM, the nidus of which may be quite small and simple coagulation or interruption of the transdural shunt may be quite successful.[15] If the lesion has subpial and intramedullary extensions, these can be pursued using a combination of bipolar coagulation to shrink bulging vascular components and both sharp and blunt dissection with microprobes and dissectors. Intramedullary AVMs fed mainly from the anterior spinal artery or by anteriorly placed vessels such as the vertebral artery branches to the anterior spinal artery, as seen in one of our cases, will have to be approached via a careful median myelotomy and extraction from within the cord, with careful attention to preservation of the anterior spinal artery as described by Yasargil et al.[18] Although this is often possible in the cervical region, where high-flow lesions tend to be more compact and of the glomus type, more caudally placed thoracolumbar lesions may be only subtotally resectable because of extensive and diffuse anterior intramedullary portions.

Our increasing experience with these lesions over the past decade and a half has not eased the difficulties one faces with these highly variable lesions. Resection of a dorsally placed low-flow extramedullary lesion, whether dural or subdural, and with exact correspondence of angiographic and surgical anatomy, is usually quite easy. The high-flow AVM with major intramedullary and anteriorly placed components and dense cicatricial attachments to normal structures remains a major challenge to the neurosurgeon, and although increasing experience frequently converts the "impossible" to the merely "difficult" case, the hazards to the patient are correspondingly much greater. Our only mortality in this series occurred in such a case (no. 82 in our series), in which after a subtotal resection of a very large and diffuse lesion under total circulatory arrest and 30 min of hypothermia, death occurred due to cardiac tamponade by a hemopericardium. A similar procedure with a much more compact AVM at the cervicomedullary junction (case 92, above), causing quadriplegia and respiratory failure, was, however, successfully treated under deep hypothermia (16°C) and total circulatory arrest for 45 min.

We believe that embolization is an effective preoperative technique to facilitate surgical resection of difficult lesions. It probably works by converting high-flow to low-flow lesions. It may be the only recourse in patients with previous incomplete surgery with severe arachnoiditis that makes further surgery hazardous. In a few low-flow cases with a few or even solitary feeders, embolization may well succeed in effectively occluding and preventing revascularization of the lesion, and in experienced hands may be considered as part of the angiographic session. Recent advances in catheter and embolic material technology may well expand the contribution of embolization to the improved management of such lesions. In particular, the use of controlled intraoperative obliteration of flow in complicated high-flow lesions with quick-setting polymers may be a useful addition to our armamentarium.

References

1. Aminoff MJ: *Spinal Angiomas* (with contributions by V Logue and BE Kendall). Oxford, Blackwell Scientific Publications, 1976.
2. Aminoff MJ, Barnard RO, Logue V: The pathophysiology of spinal vascular malformation. J Neurol Sci 23:255–263, 1974.
3. Djindjian M: Le Traitement Chirurgical des Angiomes Intra-Medullaires. Thesis, U Paris, 1976.
4. Djindjian R, Hurth M, Houdart R: *L'angiographie de la Moelle Epiniere* (English text by L Kricheff). Baltimore, University Park Press, 1970.
5. Doppman JL, DiChiro G, Ommaya AK: *Selective Arteriography of the Spinal Cord*. St Louis, Warren H Green Inc, 1969.
6. Doppman JL, DiChiro G, Ommaya AK: Percutaneous embolization of spinal cord arteriovenous malformations. J Neurosurg 34:48–55, 1971.
7. Doppman JL, Wirth FP Jr, DiChiro G, Ommaya AK: Value of cutaneous angiomas in the arteriographic localization of spinal cord arteriovenous malformations. N Engl J Med 281:1440–1444, 1969.
8. Gaupp J: Casuistische Beiträge zur pathologischen Anatomie des Rückenmarks und seiner Häute. Beitr Pathol Anat 2:510–524, 1887.
9. Hebold O: Aneurysmen der kliensten Rückenmarkgefässe. Arch Psychiatr Nervenkr 16:813–823, 1885.
10. Kaufman HH, Ommaya AK, DiChiro G, Doppman JL: Compression vs. "steal": The pathogenesis of symptoms in arteriovenous malformations of the spinal cord. Arch Neurol 23:173–178, 1970.
11. Ommaya AK: Arteriovenous malformations of the spinal cord, in Youmans JR (ed): *Neurological Surgery*, 1st ed. Philadelphia, Saunders, 1973, pp 852–862.
12. Ommaya AK, DiChiro G, Doppman J: Ligation of arterial supply in the treatment of spinal cord arteriovenous malformations. J Neurosurg 30:679–692, 1969.
13. Ommaya AK: Surgery for arteriovenous malformations of the spinal cord, in Ransohoff J (ed): *Modern Technics in Surgery*. Neurosurgery Installment VI. New York, Futura, 1984.
14. Pia HW, Djindjian R (eds): *Spinal Angiomas: Advances in Diagnosis and Therapy*. New York, Springer-Verlag, 1978.
15. Symon L, Kuyama H, Kendall B: Dural arteriovenous malformations of the spine: Clinical features and surgical results in 55 cases. J Neurosurg 60:238–247, 1984.
16. Turnbull IM: Blood supply of the spinal cord, in Vinken PJ, Bruyn GW (eds): *Handbook of Clinical Neurology*, vol 12. Amsterdam, North Holland, 1972, pp 478–491.
17. Wirth FP Jr, Post KD, DiChiro G, Doppman JL, Ommaya AK: Foix-Alajouanine disease: Spontaneous thrombosis of a spinal cord arteriovenous malformation. Neurology 20:1114–1118, 1970.
18. Yasargil MG, DeLong WB, Guarnaschelli JJ: Complete microsurgical excision of cervical extramedullary and intramedullary malformations. Surg Neurol 4:211–224, 1975.

183

Spontaneous Intraspinal Hemorrhage

Hugh S. Wisoff

Spontaneous intraspinal hemorrhage is an uncommon event, most frequently heralded by the apoplectic onset of back pain. Hematoma formation in the epidural, subdural, and subarachnoid spaces causes compression of the underlying neural elements. Spontaneous hemorrhage and hematoma formation also occur within the parenchyma of the cord unassociated with trauma, vascular lesions, or tumors. Bleeding in the three extramedullary compartments may be caused by lumbar puncture and epidural anesthesia.

Spinal Epidural Hemorrhage

Spontaneous hemorrhage in the spinal epidural space has been reported in approximately 100 patients. This entity was first described by Blauby in 1808 according to Mayer.[14] Scholarly reviews of the subject were published in 1972 by Jellinger[13] and in 1976 by Bruyn and Bosma.[6] The true incidence is unknown: undoubtedly many cases are not reported. Bleeding without hematoma formation and compression of neural structures is not generally reported. In 1963, Gold reported five cases from our institution seen during a 2-year period.[9] We have not encountered more than one case every 5 or more years since his report.

Trauma as the cause of spinal epidural hematoma is likewise exceedingly unusual. Approximately 100 additional patients have been reported in whom a spinal epidural hematoma was associated with vertebral fracture, significant injury without fracture (including birth injury), lumbar puncture (usually associated with a coagulopathy secondary to a blood dyscrasia, anticoagulants, alcoholism and liver disease, etc.), and spinal epidural anesthesia. Other rare causes include vascular anomalies of the epidural space and hemangioma of the vertebra.

The term *spontaneous* in the context of this chapter includes those cases in which the onset is associated with activities of daily living: lifting, pulling, coughing, straining at stool or during micturition, dressing, shaving, turning over in bed, and trivial trauma. Arteriosclerosis and hypertension are reported frequently, particularly in the aged. Coagulopathy secondary to primary hematologic disorders is frequent; 25–30 percent of cases are associated with anticoagulants.[28] It has also been associated with pregnancy.[26]

Spontaneous spinal epidural hematoma is twice as common in males of all ages than in females. It is reported from early childhood to the eighth decade of life and is most frequent in the middle and older age groups. The lesion may occur at any spinal level. It is usually localized to two or three segments, although it may extend over eight to ten or more segments. In childhood, it is more common in the cervical and upper thoracic regions.

The hematomas are virtually always restricted to the posterior aspect of the epidural space, may be thicker on one side, and may extend into the lateral gutters. An anteriorly located hematoma was reported by Phillips et al. in a 21-year-old man, extending from T2 to T6.[18] Jackson's oft-quoted case report, frequently referred to as the first description of this entity, also described an anteriorly located hematoma: "The whole cervical portion of the spine, but particularly anteriorly and to the left side, was imbedded in an oblong clot of dark venous blood outside the membranes."[12]

The spinal epidural space is truly an intradural space between two leaves of the spinal dura mater. The cranial dura mater splits into two laminae at the foramen magnum: the internal lamina forms the dural sac; the external lamina lines the inner wall of the bony spinal canal. The external lamina is clearly defined in infants but rarely distinguishable in adults. The space external to the internal lamina of the spinal dura mater (between the two laminae) is the epidural space by traditional usage. The anterior portion of the dural tube is closely approximated to the bony canal and is fixed to the posterior longitudinal ligament by connective tissue strands. The posterior spinal epidural space is filled with fatty tissue which extends laterally to surround the nerve roots. The posterior epidural space is thinnest in the thoracic region; it may be as wide as 14 mm in the lumbosacral area and 3 to 6 mm in the cervical region. Small arteries and a complex venous network traverse the epidural fat. Large-caliber longitudinal veins run in the anterolateral epidural space, anastomose from side to side through an anterior and posterior transverse network, and contribute to the internal vertebral plexus which anastomoses in turn with the external vertebral plexus. The epidural venous plexus anastomoses via the segmental veins with the inferior vena cava and azygos and hemiazygos veins.

The internal lamina of the spinal dura mater is supplied by two types of arterial networks originating from lateral spinal arteries: a longitudinal-oriented network on the posterior surface which is more prominent in the cervical and lumbar regions and small vascular clusters in the thoracic region.

The consensus of most authors is that spinal epidural hemorrhage is venous in origin. The lack of valves is a unique feature of the epidural venous plexus. This permits reversal of flow in the system and allows sudden increases in pressure during activities of normal daily living. This mechanism has been promulgated to explain spontaneous hemorrhage. Such an explanation is not satisfactory: one would expect this disorder to be much more common. Spontaneous rupture of a cryptic vascular malformation in the epidural fat or on the external surface of the dural tube seems more likely. Failure to identify the lesion is probably related to its destruction during the hemorrhage.

Premonitory symptoms are not associated with spontaneous epidural hemorrhage except in those cases with an identifiable local lesion such as a hemangioma of a vertebra, a vascular anomaly, or a vertebral or epidural neoplasm. The initial back pain is localized at the level of the lesion, and radicular pain may occur simultaneously with the episode of bleeding or develop minutes to hours later. Signs of neural compression appear rapidly in most cases. Chronic symptoms are most frequently associated with lesions involving the cauda equina.[3] Lack of pain is rare; pain was absent in Jackson's autopsy-proven case report of a 14-year-old girl.[12] In a few cases there has been temporary remission of symptoms attributed to improvement between repeated episodes of small hemorrhages. On rare occasions, up to 2 weeks have elapsed between the onset of bleeding and the signs of myelopathy.

The differential diagnosis of spontaneous epidural hemorrhage includes all those disorders causing acute back pain with spinal cord and root dysfunction. Spinal epidural abscess most closely approaches bleeding in its onset and fulminant signs, but it is usually associated with symptoms of sepsis. Herniation of a thoracic intervertebral disc is uncommonly associated with the acute onset of paraplegia. Chronic epidural hematoma in the lumbar region mimics the symptoms of intervertebral disc herniation. Epidural and vertebral tumors most commonly have preceding back pain, though an apoplectic onset of pain and paraplegia is encountered with vertebral collapse and angulation. Dissecting aneurysm of the aorta, with rupture into the spinal canal, is associated with prominent cardiovascular signs. Spinal subdural hematoma is identical in onset and clinical symptomatology.

The cerebrospinal fluid (CSF) is usually clear and acellular; the protein content is generally increased. Bloody CSF is associated with coagulopathies and bleeding into more than the epidural space; it may result from myelomalacia of the cord and portends a poor prognosis.

The evaluation and treatment of patients with the acute onset of back pain and progressive neural dysfunction must proceed on an emergent basis. Recovery from spinal epidural hematoma is independent of age. Useful motor recovery occurs in less than 50 percent of patients if paralysis persists longer than 36 h.[15]

Plain x-ray films are usually normal. Myelography is the diagnostic study of choice. Both lumbar and lateral C1-2 puncture may be necessary. The use of water-soluble metrizamide usually allows the study to be performed without turning the patient. The myelographic picture is most commonly that of a complete extradural-type block, infrequently an incomplete block, and rarely an elongated defect with an irregular indented appearance. Anterior or posterior compression of the contrast column on frontal projections may suggest an intramedullary tumor; the lateral projection shows the true nature of the extramedullary process, shows its anterior or posterior location within the spinal canal, and helps with proper surgical planning.

High-resolution computed tomographic (CT) scanning has demonstrated reported cases of spinal epidural hematoma. Nuclear magnetic resonance (NMR) scanning, with even greater definition of intraspinal structures than that produced by CT scanning, holds forth additional promise as a diagnostic aid. The NMR T_1 and T_2 values of blood may result in a specific diagnosis. Logistical considerations generally militate against spinal angiography unless a vascular anomaly is a serious consideration.

Treatment consists of prompt evacuation of the clot and decompression of the dural tube, usually by laminectomy. A rare anteriorly situated thoracic hematoma was localized by myelography and CT scanning by Phillips et al. and treated successfully through a costotransversectomy.[18] There have been isolated cases of recovery without operation, after diagnosis by myelography, that have been associated with anticoagulants and hemophilia. It has been theorized that cure might follow seepage of blood through the lumbar puncture needle tract. Percutaneous aspiration of a hematoma has been suggested but never reported.

Spinal Subdural Hemorrhage

Spontaneous spinal subdural hemorrhage is distinctly less common than bleeding in the spinal epidural space. Sixteen cases of spontaneous spinal subdural hematoma have been reported since Schiller et al. described a 16-month-old boy with hemophilia whose lesion was verified at laminectomy in 1948.[23] One other case report was associated with hemophilia, eight with anticoagulants,[21] and six without any known coexisting disorder. All other reported cases have been associated with trauma, including lumbar puncture in patients with hematologic disorders or receiving anticoagulants.[7]

Russell and Benoit reviewed the subject of spinal subdural hematoma in 1983.[21a] They stated that historical precedence should be given to Potts in 1910[19a] and Harris in 1911[10a] rather than Schiller et al.[23] for the first description of the entity. Potts' patient recovered after laminectomy and excision of a posteriorly situated thoracic subdural "cyst." The description of the lesion is compatible with a chronic subdural hematoma. It is unclear to me whether the chronic lumbar hematoma in Harris' operated case was subdural or subarachnoid in location.

The spinal subdural space, in contradistinction to the cranial subdural space, does not normally contain bridging veins. Only extremely small veins are found on the surface of the spinal dura. It has been assumed that spontaneous bleeding in the subdural space originates from a radicular vessel. It has been postulated that a sudden rise in intravascular (venous) pressure might cause rupture of a vessel crossing the subdural space. Weinstein suggested: "... The occasionally observed bridging vessel from the pia of the spinal cord or the arachnoid of the caudal nerve roots to the dura is the responsible vascular channel."[25]

Spontaneous spinal subdural hematoma is most commonly located in the lower thoracic or thoracolumbar region; only one case was reported in the cervical canal.[20] Clinical presentation is either acute, indistinguishable from that of an epidural hematoma, or chronic, taking weeks to months for the development of paraplegia.[5] The acute presentation is usually associated with pain in a radicular distribution in addition to back pain. The CSF is usually clear and acellular; the protein content is generally increased. Bloody CSF is suggestive of primary subarachnoid hemorrhage and secondary rupture of the arachnoid. Spontaneous hemorrhage into both the subarachnoid and subdural spaces has been associated with anticoagulants and hemophilia. Lumbar puncture is frequently "dry" because of collapse of the subarachnoid space secondary to the frequent low thoracic or thoracolumbar location of the clot. Cisternal or lateral C1-2 puncture may be necessary for diagnostic myelography.

The myelographic appearance of subdural hematoma may not be distinguishable from that of an epidural hematoma. The myelogram usually demonstrates a complete block, which is suggestive of an intradural extramedullary tumor, and less often of a filling defect or displacement of the contrast medium to one side. Zilkha and Nicoletti, in their discussion of a post-traumatic lumbar subdural hematoma, stated: "In rare cases of subdural lesions in which the contrast column is displaced to the opposite side, the ipsilateral axillary pouches of the nerve roots may remain in the normal position. In these instances the diagnosis of subdural lesion may be made."[27]

A chronic spinal subdural hematoma develops membranes identical in appearance to those encountered in the cranial cavity.[5,10] A remittent clinical course reminiscent of cranial subdural hematoma was reported in one patient who presented 18 days after the onset of symptoms.[1]

Treatment is by laminectomy and drainage of the hematoma. A clearly identifiable anatomical abnormality to account for the subdural hemorrhage has not been described in any of the "spontaneous" cases. Excellent postoperative recovery was reported in four patients (two associated with anticoagulants and two "spontaneous"), minimal to partial recovery was reported in five patients (including Schiller's case), two patients on anticoagulants had the diagnosis made at autopsy, and five patients died postoperatively (including the one with a cervical lesion) or remained paraplegic.

Spinal Subarachnoid Hemorrhage

Spontaneous spinal subarachnoid hemorrhage constitutes less than 1 percent of all cases of subarachnoid hemorrhage. The clinical manifestations were first described by Michon in 1928: "*Le coup de poignard rachidien*" (stab in the spine).[16] A clearly defined anatomical abnormality is usually demonstrable when bleeding is associated with an arteriovenous malformation, aneurysm[24] (including mycotic aneurysm), coarctation of the aorta with dilatation of collateral intraspinal vessels,[2] and neoplasms (e.g., ependymoma, glioblastoma multiforme, hemangioblastoma, meningioma, neurofibroma, schwannoma, endometriosis, meningeal sarcoma, and meningeal carcinomatosis). However, trauma, including lumbar puncture, particularly in patients receiving anticoagulants or with disorders of the coagulation mechanism, accounts for the bulk of cases with primary spinal subarachnoid hemorrhage and subarachnoid hematoma formation, the latter causing compression of the intraspinal neural elements.

Rare causes of spontaneous spinal subarachnoid hemorrhage include systemic lupus erythematosis, the Sjögren syndrome, periarteritis nodosa, and generalized toxi-infective diseases (e.g., typhoid fever); hemophilia and anticoagulant usage are somewhat more common.[11] No identifiable lesion or coagulopathy was determined in two cases reported by Plotkin et al., both of whom were treated by laminectomy for evacuation of subarachnoid hematomas.[19]

The onset of symptoms is apoplectic (*le coup de poignard rachidien*) with back pain referred to the site of bleeding. If the hemorrhage originates in the cervical region, the symptoms may mimic bleeding originating in the intracranial cavity because of the rapid spread of blood into the cranial subarachnoid space. (Failure to identify a cranial source of subarachnoid hemorrhage should alert the clinician to the possibility of a spinal origin of the bleeding.) Pain extends up and down the back with the spread of blood in the subarachnoid space, associated with signs of meningeal irritation. Pain and paresthesias in the lower limbs develop rapidly if the original site of the bleeding is in the low thoracic or thoracolumbar region. Bleeding into the parenchyma of the cord produces signs of an acute myelopathy.

The clinical differentiation of spinal subarachnoid hemorrhage from other apoplectic events involving the intraspinal contents is difficult. The development of a spinal subarachnoid hematoma, sufficient in size to cause medullary compression, is rare because dilution of the blood by CSF and defibrination by the normal pulsations of the fluid presumably prevent thrombus formation. When bleeding is massive and rapid or normal dilution is mechanically impeded, by tumor or arachnoidal adhesions, a frank hematoma may form more readily. Back pain followed by rapidly progressing paraparesis, a sensory level, meningismus, and a "dry" lumbar puncture characterize the clinical picture of a subarachnoid hematoma.

Myelography via the lumbar route is frequently impossible because of failure to obtain CSF. Introduction of the contrast medium via a cisternal or C1-2 puncture is necessary under such circumstances. A small subarachnoid clot may appear as a nonspecific intradural extramedullary lesion. With increasing size, the clot envelops and displaces the cord with apparent widening of the cord shadow. The myelographic picture may mimic an intramedullary tumor. Capping of the contrast column on frontal and lateral views is the key radiographic feature that points to the extramedullary location of the clot. An intramedullary tumor with exophytic extension or hemorrhage may produce similar findings. Differentiation of a subarachnoid hematoma from a subdural or epidural hematoma is possible because the latter produces extra-arachnoidal myelographic defects. The epidural hematoma tends to displace the axillary pouches, whereas the subdural hematoma may not.[8]

If the etiology of the subarachnoid hematoma is not found at laminectomy, myelography should be repeated postoperatively and spinal angiography performed if an arteriovenous malformation or aneurysm is a significant consideration. The urgent nature of the clinical problem when associated with hematoma formation and compression myelopathy does not usually permit spinal angiography as an emergent preoperative undertaking.

Aneurysms of the spinal cord are rare, and are most commonly associated with arteriovenous malformations. Rupture invariably produces signs of myelopathy. Aneurysms in the high cervical region have been demonstrated during vertebral angiography. Vincent reported successful clipping of an aneurysm, which had bled, arising from the anterior spinal artery at the C1-2 level.[24] Five additional cases were found in a review of the literature: two aneurysms of the anterior spinal artery (T6 and T8, unruptured), one from a C4 radicular artery (unruptured), and ruptured aneurysms of a posterior spinal artery at C1-2 and artery of Adamkiewicz at T6.[24]

Treatment is directed toward decompression of the spinal cord via laminectomy and evacuation of the hematoma. Plotkin et al. reported full recovery following laminectomy in a 48-year-old man for evacuation of a thoracic hematoma, but an 81-year-old man remained totally paraplegic after evacuation of a thoracolumar hematoma.[19] Treatment of an underlying hematologic disorder or coagulopathy is indicated in those patients with bleeding without hematoma formation.

Spinal Intramedullary Hemorrhage

Spontaneous spinal intramedullary hemorrhage (hematomyelia) is very rare, after excluding obvious causes such as an arteriovenous malformation, an aneurysm, a neoplasm, and an injury. The few reported cases, after exclusion of the above, have been associated with anticoagulants, hemophilia, and syringomyelia.

Brandt reported a 65-year-old woman who developed paraparesis 2 days after the development of interscapular pain, progressing to a complete T4 sensory-motor paraplegia over the ensuing 3 days. The myelogram showed a complete block at T2. (The reproduced myelographic pictures suggested an intramedullary tumor to me.) The cerebrospinal fluid was clear and colorless. The preoperative diagnosis was epidural hematoma. A coagulated intramedullary hematoma was removed via laminectomy and myelotomy. No vascular anomaly was identified intraoperatively. Postoperative angiography was not performed. The patient made no neurological recovery.[4]

Schenk reported the case of a 21-year-old man with known hemophilia whose low cervical intramedullary hemorrhage was operated on, and at autopsy there were signs that the bleeding had taken place into a pre-existing syringomyelic cavity. Schenk reported that Tellegen in 1850 gave the first clinical description of spontaneous hematomyelia.[22]

Gowers' syringal hemorrhage was first described by him, and anecdotal reports followed. Perot et al. reported a 39-year-old man who developed a cervical hematomyelia, perhaps related to injury, and whose symptoms and myelogram 6 years earlier were compatible with syringomyelia. The patient improved after myelotomy and evacuation of the intramedullary clot.[17]

Hemorrhage into a pre-existing syringomyelic cavity is possibly related to abnormal vascular channels in its walls. The finding of such abnormal vessels in autopsy studies led to the suggestion that syringomyelia is related to an intramedullary arteriovenous malformation.

References

1. Anagnostopoulos DI, Gortvai P: Spontaneous spinal subdural haematoma. Br Med J 1:30, 1972.
2. Banna MM, Rose PG, Pearce GW: Coarctation of the aorta as a cause of spinal subarachnoid hemorrhage: Case report. J Neurosurg 39:761–763, 1973.
3. Boyd HR, Pear BL: Chronic spontaneous spinal epidural hematoma: Report of two cases. J Neurosurg 36:239–242, 1972.
4. Brandt M: Spontaneous intramedullary haematoma as a complication of anticoagulant therapy. Acta Neurochir (Wien) 52:73–77, 1980.
5. Brandt RA: Chronic spinal subdural haematoma. Surg Neurol 13:121–123, 1980.
6. Bruyn GW, Bosma NJ: Spinal extradural haematoma, in Vinken PJ, Bruyn GW (eds): *Handbook of Clinical Neurology*, vol 26, *Injuries of the Spine & Spinal Cord*. Amsterdam, North-Holland, 1976, pp 1–30.
7. Edelson RN: Spinal subdural hematoma, in Vinken PJ, Bruyn GW (eds): *Handbook of Clinical Neurology*, vol 26, *Injuries of the Spine & Spinal Cord*. Amsterdam, North-Holland, 1976, pp 31–38.
8. Frager D, Zimmerman RD, Wisoff HS, Leeds NE: Spinal subarachnoid hematoma. AJNR 3:77–79, 1982.
9. Gold ME: Spontaneous spinal epidural hematoma. Radiology 80:823–828, 1963.
10. Guthikonda M, Schmidek HH, Wallman LJ, Snyder TM: Spinal subdural hematoma: Case report and review of the literature. Neurosurgery 5:614–616, 1979.
10a. Harris W: Two cases of spontaneous haematorrhachis, or intrameningeal spinal haemorrhage—one cured by laminectomy. Proc R Soc Med 5:115–122, 1911.
11. Henson RA, Croft PB: Spontaneous spinal subarachnoid haemorrhage. Q J Med 25:53–66, 1956.
12. Jackson R: Case of spinal apoplexy. Lancet 2:5–6, 1869.
13. Jellinger K: Traumatic vascular disease of the spinal cord, in Vinken PJ, Bruyn GW (eds): *Handbook of Clinical Neurology*, vol 12, *Vascular Diseases of the Nervous System, Part II*. Amsterdam, North-Holland, 1972, pp 556–630.
14. Mayer JA: Extradural spinal hemorrhage. Can Med Assoc J 89:1034–1037, 1963.
15. McQuarrie IG: Recovery from paraplegia caused by spontaneous spinal epidural hematoma. Neurology (NY) 28:224–228, 1978.
16. Michon P: Le coup de poignard rachidien. Symptome initial de certaines hémorragies sous-arachnoidiennes. Essai sur les hémorragies méningées spinales. Presse Med 36:964–966, 1928.
17. Perot P, Feindel W, Lloyd-Smith D: Hematomyelia as a complication of syringomyelia: Gowers' syringal hemorrhage: Case report. J Neurosurg 25:447–451, 1966.
18. Phillips TW, Kling TF Jr, McGillicuddy JE: Spontaneous ventral spinal epidural hematoma with anterior cord syndrome: Report of a case. Neurosurgery 9:440–443, 1981.
19. Plotkin R, Ronthal M, Froman C: Spontaneous spinal subarachnoid hemorrhage. Report of 3 cases. J Neurosurg 25:443–446, 1966.
19a. Potts CS: Intradural cyst of the spinal meninges removed by operation. Recovery of the patient. Remarks on the location of

the spinal centers for testicular sensibility. J Nerv Ment Dis 37:621–625, 1910.
20. Reynolds AF Jr, Turner PT: Spinal subdural hematoma. Rocky Mt Med J 75:199–200, 1978.
21. Russell N, Maroun FB, Jacob JC: Spinal subdural hematoma in association with anticoagulant therapy. Can J Neurol Sci 8:87–89, 1981.
21a. Russell NA, Benoit BG: Spinal subdural hematoma: A review. Surg Neurol 20:133–137, 1983.
22. Schenk VWD: Haemorrhages in spinal cord with syringomyelia in a patient with haemophilia. Acta Neuropathol (Berlin) 2:306–308, 1963.
23. Schiller F, Neligan G, Budtz-Olsen O: Surgery in haemophilia: A case of spinal subdural haematoma producing paraplegia. Lancet 2:842–845, 1948.
24. Vincent FM: Anterior spinal artery aneurysm presenting as a subarachnoid hemorrhage. Stroke 12:230–232, 1981.
25. Weinstein PR: Comments. Neurosurgery 5:616, 1979.
26. Yonekawa Y, Mehdorn HM, Nishikawa M: Spontaneous spinal epidural hematoma during pregnancy. Surg Neurol 3:327–328, 1975.
27. Zilkha A, Nicoletti JM: Acute spinal subdural hematoma: Case report. J Neurosurg 41:627–630, 1974.
28. Zuccarello M, Scanarini M, D'Avella D, Andrioli GC, Gerosa M: Spontaneous spinal extradural hematoma during anticoagulant therapy. Surg Neurol 14:411–413, 1980.

SECTION D

Hypertension

184

Neurogenic Hypertension

Jack M. Fein

Arterial hypertension is one of the most pervasive health problems in society. It affects over 23 million people in the United States and is responsible for pathological changes in virtually every organ system. Despite its importance, a specific cause for arterial hypertension is found in less than 10 percent of cases.[9] After thorough evaluation of patients for occult lesions which might produce elevation of blood pressure, essential hypertension i.e., hypertension in which the cause remains elusive constitutes the bulk of cases. Since Cushing's earliest observations, the role of the central nervous system in the regulation of systemic blood pressure has been recognized. Significant insights into central neurogenic mechanisms have now accumulated from a variety of physiological, pharmacological, and anatomical studies. Such studies and more recent clinical observations suggest that in addition to a role in the normal regulation of blood pressure, abnormalities of the central nervous system may also play a role in the etiology of essential hypertension. Of particular interest in this regard are observations which indicate that neurogenic hypertension may be induced by arterial compression of the left lateral medullary region. Microvascular decompression procedures in this region have restored normal blood levels in a number of patients with presumed neurogenic hypertension.

Physiology and Pathophysiology

A large body of evidence supports the role of the nervous system in modulating blood pressure levels to meet environmental stresses. Physical and psychosocial stresses as well as operant conditioning are effective means of elevating blood pressure.[1] Electrical stimulation of the cortex, bilateral lesions of the anterior hypothalamus, and bilateral lesions of the nucleus tractus solitarius (NTS) elicit hypertension which is species-dependent. Lesions of the anterior third ventricle region attenuate most types of experimentally induced hypertension. The area around the NTS in the medulla is of particular interest. Baroreceptor information from the carotid sinus and aortic bodies, carried through the ninth and tenth cranial nerves, is distributed here, through synapses in the paramedian and lateral reticular formations and in the parahypoglossal area of the medulla. The caudal part of the NTS and its enlarged midline cell mass, the pars commissuralis, probably form the primary medullary center for the baroreceptor reflex. The efferent component of this reflex arc is carried in vagal parasympathetics, which originate in the dorsal motor nucleus of the vagus nerve and have a negative inotropic and chronotropic effect on the heart. The baroreceptor reflex, therefore inhibits sympathetic outflow. When the inhibitory system is "deafferented," peripheral vascular resistance increases and systemic hypertension results.[2] Further details of these brain stem systems are described in several excellent reviews.[3,11]

Generalized intracranial hypertension may lead to the Cushing response, which is mediated by pressure and stretch-sensitive neurons located between the obex and the facial colliculus in the floor of the fourth ventricle. More specific lesions of the posterior fossa capable of involving these medullary centers are known to produce systemic arterial hypertension. Tumors of the fourth ventricle and cerebellum,[4] syringomyelia involving the NTS, and bulbar poliomyelitis[9] have all been associated with labile hypertension. In more recent reports, neurovascular compression of the lateral medulla has been associated with hypertension,[7,8] leading to anatomical studies of this relationship.

Neurovascular Anatomy

Postmortem studies were carried out to clarify the relation of the posterior inferior cerebellar artery (PICA) and vertebral artery to the ninth and tenth nerve root entry-exit zones in 31 patients.[5] In 28 cases the left vertebral artery was larger than the right vertebral artery; in 3 cases they were of equal size. The left PICA was larger than the right PICA in 27 cases, equal to it in 3 cases, and smaller in 1 case. The first segment of PICA normally forms a loop with its convexity

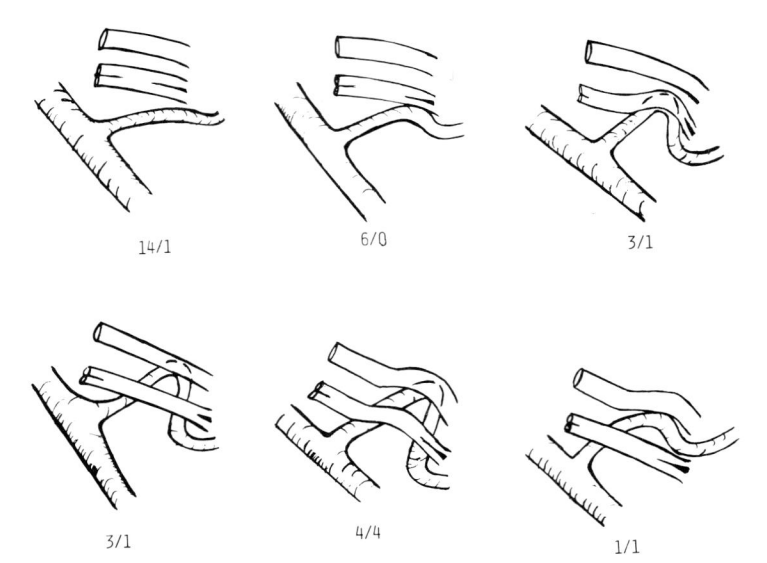

Figure 184-1 Relation of the left vertebral artery and PICA origin to the left ninth and tenth cranial nerve roots as seen on a left lateral view of the brain stem. The number of cases in which there is no contact (*left*), simple contact (*center*), or compression (*right*) is indicated in the numerator, and the number of patients with antemortem hypertension is given in the denominator. (From Fein.[6])

inferiorly placed and traverses the lateral surface of the brain stem just inferior to the tenth nerve. Figure 184-1 shows the relation of the left posterior inferior cerebellar artery to the left ninth and tenth nerve root entry-exit zones in the 31 brains examined. There was compression of the tenth nerve in three cases, compression of both the ninth and tenth nerves in four cases, and compression of the ninth nerve in one case. On the right side, the vertebral artery and the PICA were less prominent, and only three significant variations were seen (Fig. 184-2). The right PICA passed freely from the vertebral artery to the lateral surface of the brain stem without coming into contact with the ninth or tenth nerves in 27 cases, while in 4 cases there was contact but no compression of the nerves.

Eight of the 31 patients were hypertensive. The pertinent clinical information and pathoanatomical correlations are given in Table 184-1. Neurovascular compression of the left ninth nerve root entry-exit zone was found in 16 percent of autopsies. Patient 1 had systolic hypertension but no neurovascular contact or compression. There was simple contact with the ninth and tenth nerve roots in Patient 3; there was tenth nerve root compression in Patient 2. In the other five patients, compression of the ninth nerve was seen. In four patients this was associated with tenth nerve root compression as well. Neurovascular contact or compression in the hypertensive patients was restricted to the left side.

Watt and McKillop described four variations in the relation of the PICA to the lower cranial nerve roots.[12] Most commonly the PICA passed under the tenth nerve, but two of the variations they described produced compression of the ninth nerve root. Watt and McKillop's photographs and drawings do not permit any inference of a specific relation between the arterial loops and the root entry zones.

Surgical Observations

Observations in nine hypertensive patients, eight of whom underwent posterior fossa surgery, are of interest. In this series of patients with vertebrobasilar aneurysm or occlusive disease, compression of the lateral medulla by either the aneurysm or an ectatic arterial loop was found. Reversal of long-standing hypertension was temporally related to the relief of neurovascular cross compression of the root entry-exit zone of the left vagus and/or glossopharyngeal nerves.

Table 184-2 lists the clinical features and diagnostic studies in the nine patients with neurovascular hypertension.

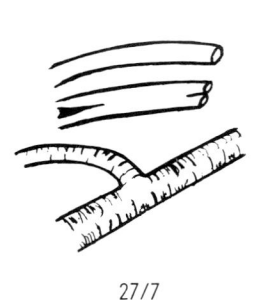

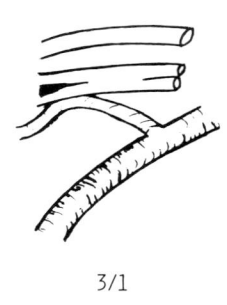

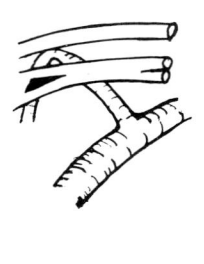

Figure 184-2 Relation of the right vertebral artery and PICA origin to the right ninth and tenth cranial nerve roots as seen on a right lateral view of the brain stem. The number of cases in which there is no contact (*left*), simple contact (*center*), or compression (*right*) is indicated in the numerator, and the number of patients with antemortem hypertension is given in the denominator. (From Fein.[6])

Neurogenic Hypertension

TABLE 184-1 Postmortem Analysis of Neurovascular Compression in Eight Patients with Antemortem Hypertension

Patient No.	Sex	Age	NVC	BP Range, mmHg	Clinical History	Rx
1	F	71	No	160/65–180/80	? Essential hypertension	Methyldopa
2	M	60	X$^+$	160/80–190/90	TIA, MI	Methyldopa
3	F	68	IX & X	140/80–160/90	Hepatic failure	?
4	M	72	IX & X$^+$	160/90–180/100	Gastrectomy	?
5	F	73	IX & X$^+$	170/90–120/110	MI	?
6	M	64	IX & X$^+$	190/110–230/210	Stroke	Methyldopa, reserpine
7	M	69	IX & X$^+$	140/80–180/100	MI	Methyldopa
8	M	61	IX$^+$	150/90–170/100	MI	Methyldopa

NVC, neurovascular compression; BP, blood pressure; TIA, transient ischemic attack; MI, myocardial infarction.

Seven of the nine patients were males. Their age range was 35 to 72 years, and the average age was 51.3 years. Hypertension had been present 1 week to 4 years prior to admission. In all patients, neurological symptoms referable to the posterior fossa led to angiographic study. In six patients, occlusive cerebrovascular lesions in the vertebral circulation led to posterior fossa craniectomy for occipital artery–PICA bypass. In three patients an aneurysm of the vertebral artery or vertebrobasilar junction was seen on angiography. Surgical exploration revealed an ectatic arterial loop invaginating the region of the ninth and tenth nerve entry-exit zones in the patients with cerebrovascular disease. In two patients (Patients 4 and 5) an aneurysm indenting a wide area of the left lateral medulla was found. In one patient (Patient 6) a large aneurysm of the vertebrobasilar junction compressing the left lateral medulla was found at autopsy.

The clinical course and operative findings of Patients 4 and 9 are instructive.

Patient 4

Hypertension began in a 57-year-old woman in February 1968 (Fig. 184-3) and was never adequately treated. In August 1969 she had an acute subarachnoid hemorrhage. Admission examination disclosed a left peripheral facial palsy and a decreased gag reflex bilaterally. Angiography (Fig. 184-4) disclosed a large aneurysm of the left vertebral artery proximal to the origin of the left PICA.

Surgical exploration disclosed a larger aneurysmal mass indenting the left lateral medulla between the hypoglossal nerve and the midpontine region. The neck was identified at its origin from the vertebral artery and was ligated with a size 0 silk suture. The aneurysmal mass was subtotally resected, allowing some residual fibrous adhesions to remain on the brain stem. The patient's hypertension resolved immedi-

TABLE 184-2 Clinical Features of Nine Patients with Neurovascular Hypertension

Patient No.	Age	Sex	BP Range (mmHg) Preoperatively	Drug Treatment	Neurological Symptoms	Angiogram
1	42	M	170/90 to 200/100	Methyldopa 500 mg PO qid		Stenosis of intradural portion of left vertebral artery
2	35	M	210/130	Methyldopa 500 mg PO qid	Ataxia, dysmetria	Stenosis of left intradural vertebral artery
3	48	M	160/100	Methyldopa	Gait ataxia, nystagmus, dysmetria	Left vertebral origin stenosis, right vertebral occlusion at C1
4	57	F	190/125		SAH, left seventh nerve palsy, ↓ gag reflex	Left vertebral–PICA aneurysm
5	49	M	210/120	Chlorthalidone	SAH, lethargic, left seventh nerve palsy, ↓ gag, right hemiparesis	Fusiform left vertebral aneurysm
6	72	M	220/110	Infusion of sodium nitroprusside	Progressive lower cranial nerve palsy	Large vertebrobasilar aneurysm
7	53	F	250/120	Chlorthalidone	TIA posterior fossa	Left vertebral stenosis and ectasia
8	49	M	190/100		TIA posterior fossa	Left PICA occlusion
9	57	M	210/120	Methyldopa	TIA anterior and posterior circulation	Left internal carotid and left vertebral occlusion

BP, blood pressure; PICA, posterior inferior cerebellar artery; SAH, subarachnoid hemorrhage; TIA, transient ischemic attack.

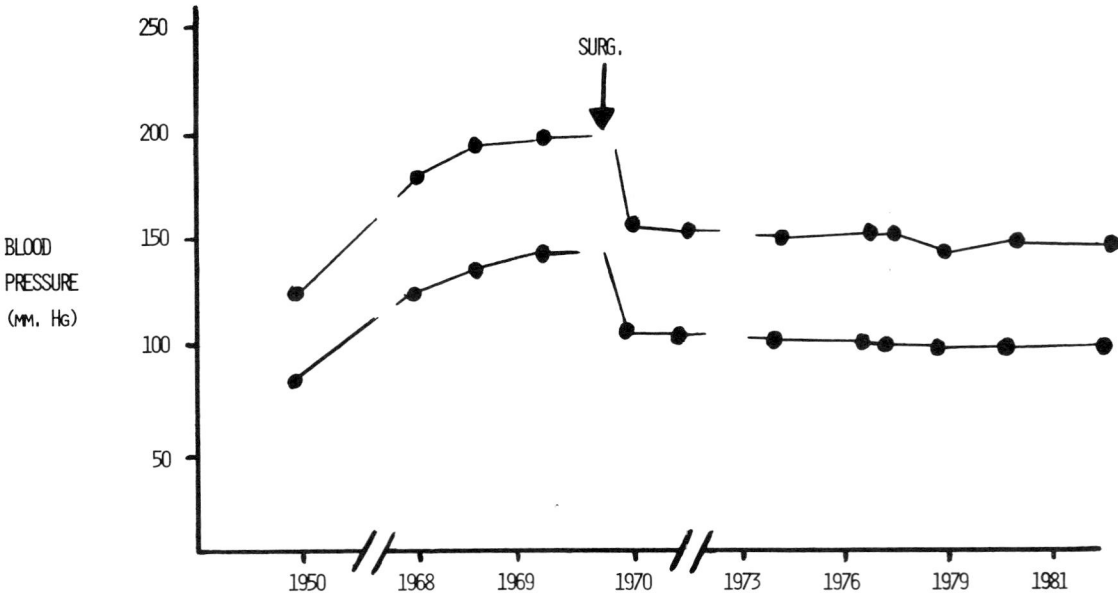

Figure 184-3 Case 4. Blood pressure record of a 57-year-old woman known to have normal blood pressure in 1950. In 1968 her blood pressure was 160/110 mmHg. One year later subarachnoid hemorrhage secondary to a large left PICA aneurysm occured. (From Fein.[6])

ately, and she has remained normotensive for the past 11 years.

Patient 9

Precordial pain began in this 57-year-old male in June 1971, at which time a subendocardial infarction was diagnosed. His blood pressure was 180/106, and he was placed on a regimen of propranolol, methyldopa, and diet. His compliance with this regimen was poor, and his blood pressure ranged between 180/95 and 230/115 over the next 4 years; at the end of that time he developed transient weakness and dysphasia. He refused angiography and was started on aspirin gr. X, PO, bid. In August 1980 he had an episode of severe stance and gait ataxia, which resolved spontaneously. In December 1980 he had another episode of ataxia, which again resolved with no residua. Workup at that time included a CT scan interpreted as normal. Angiography (Fig. 184-5) disclosed a high-grade stenosis of the left vertebral artery near the origin of the PICA. Posterior fossa craniectomy was carried out on January 22, 1981. Preoperatively his resting blood pressure ranged between 180/95 and 220/120.

At operation an ectatic loop of the left PICA was seen invaginating the left lateral medulla and the axillae of the ninth and tenth nerves (Fig. 184-6). This was mobilized from under the nerves and was used as a recipient artery in an occipital artery–PICA anastomosis. His blood pressure immediately after the operation was 170/96 and within 3 days had fallen to 140–150/90. It has remained below 150/92 with no medication over a 2-year follow-up period.

The intraoperative and postoperative course of the nine patients is reviewed in Table 184-3.

The experience of Jannetta and Gendell with a group of hypertensive patients who underwent posterior fossa surgery for other problems is also of interest.[8] Pulsatile compression of the left lateral medulla was seen in 51 of 53 hypertensive patients operated upon on the left side. This compression was not seen in 50 normotensive patients oper-

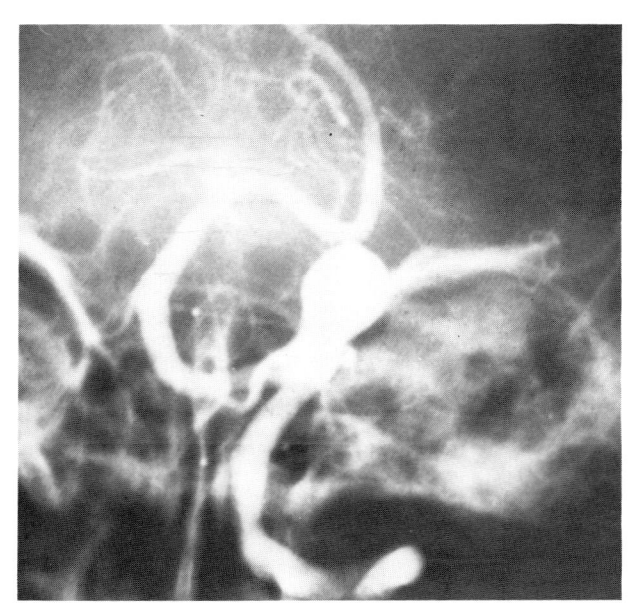

Figure 184-4 Cerebral angiogram (Case 4), anteroposterior view, showing a large aneurysm at the left PICA origin. (From Fein.[6])

Neurogenic Hypertension

TABLE 184-3 Intraoperative and Postoperative Course in Nine Patients with Neurovascular Hypertension

Patient No.	Surgical Findings	Procedure	Postoperative Course
1	Vermian branch of left PICA ectatic, impinging on left tenth nerve root entry zone	Ectatic portion mobilized from nerve root axilla; occipital-PICA anastomosis	Normotensive, off medicine 5 years
2	Vermian branch of PICA in left tenth nerve root entry zone	Loop mobilized; occipital-PICA anastomosis	Normotensive 9 years
3	Left PICA ectatic, elevating ninth and tenth nerve roots at entry zone; compression of left lateral medulla	Occipital-PICA anastomosis	Normotensive 12 years
4	Aneurysm indenting left lateral medulla	Aneurysm neck ligated	Normotensive 14 years
5	Vertebral artery fusiform aneurysm compressing left lateral medulla	Aneurysm mobilized from brain stem, coated and wrapped	Normotensive 7 years
6	Considered inoperable		Progressive hypertension and brain stem failure
7	Ectatic loop PICA in ninth and tenth nerve root entry zones	Loop mobilized; occipital-PICA anastomosis	Normotensive 4 years
8	PICA branch enlarged in ninth nerve root entry zone	Loop mobilized; occipital-PICA anastomosis	Normotensive 5 years
9	Thrombotic loop	Loop mobilized; occipital-PICA anastomosis	Normotensive 2 years

ated upon on the left side and 25 normotensive and 7 hypertensive patients operated upon on the right side. Vascular decompression of the left ventrolateral medulla was attempted in 42 of the 53 patients. Relief of the hypertension resulted in 32 patients and improvement in 4 patients.

Hypertension may be induced by a variety of functional disorders, as well as by specific organic lesions of the nervous system. There is suggestive evidence that arterial pulsatile lesions which involve the left lateral medullary region may be among those organic causes. Surgical

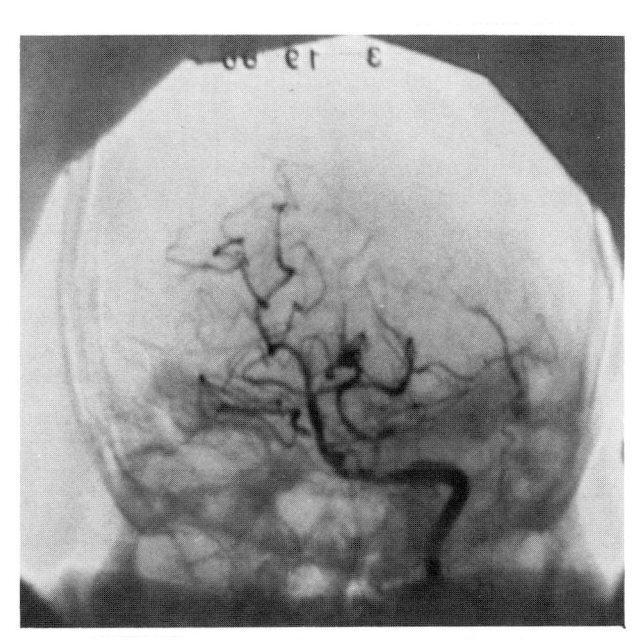

Figure 184-5 Vertebral angiogram (Case 9) demonstrates a high grade stenosis of the left vertebral artery. The PICA branches are thin and ectatic.

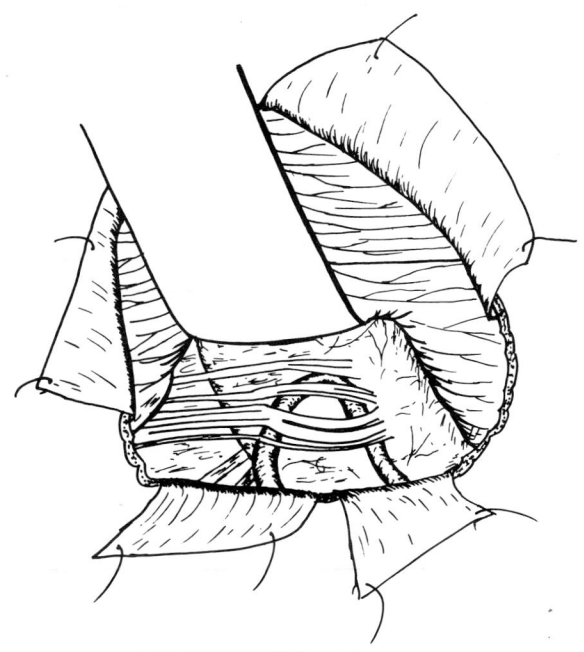

Figure 184-6 Intraoperative sketch of a posterior fossa craniectomy for occipital artery–PICA bypass. A large ectatic loop of the left PICA had insinuated itself into the axillae of the rootlets of the ninth and tenth nerves. Pulsations were directed against the nerve root entry zones of these nerves.

decompression of this region by mobilizing the arterial lesions away from the brain stem effectively reduces the hypertension. At the present time the significance of such lesions in hypertensive patients is unclear. Angiotomographic diagnosis of these lesions has been unsatisfactory, and observations are therefore limited to patients who underwent posterior fossa procedures for other reasons. Further observations along these lines are necessary in order to understand the significance of neurovascular compression as a cause of systemic hypertension.

References

1. Baumann H, Martin G, Urmantscheeva TG, Degen G, Wolter F, Chasabova WA, Gurk C, Hinays I, Läuter J: Neurophysiologische Mechanismen der arteriellen Hypertonie unter chronisch-experimentellem Emotionalstress. Acta Biol Med Ger 35:889–913, 1976.
2. Dejong W, Palkovits M: Hypertension after localized transection of brainstem fibres. Life Sci 18:61–64, 1976.
3. Dickinson CJ: *Neurogenic Hypertension.* Oxford, Blackwell, 1965.
4. Evans CH, Westfall V, Atuk NO: Astrocytoma mimicking the features of pheochromocytoma. N Engl J Med 286:1397–1399, 1972.
5. Fein JM: Microvascular anatomy of the glossopharyngeal and vagus nerves. Presented at the Annual Meeting of the Congress of Neurological Surgeons, Houston, Texas, October 1980.
6. Fein JM: Hypertension and the central nervous system. Clin Neurosurg 29:666–721, 1982.
7. Fein JM, Frishman W: Neurogenic hypertension related to vascular compression of the lateral medulla. Neurosurgery 6:615–622, 1980.
8. Jannetta PJ, Gendell HM: Clinical observations on etiology of essential hypertension. Surg Forum 30:431–432, 1979.
9. Julius S: Classification of hypertension, in Genest J, Koiw E, Kuchel O (eds): *Hypertension: Physiopathology and Treatment.* New York, McGraw-Hill, 1977, pp 9–12.
10. McDowell FH, Plum F: Arterial hypertension associated with acute anterior poliomyelitis. N Engl J Med 245:241–245, 1951.
11. Miura M, Reis DJ: The role of the solitary and paramedian nuclei in mediating cardiovascular reflex responses from carotid baro- and chemoreceptors. J Physiol (Lond) 223:525–548, 1972.
12. Watt JC, McKillop AN: Relation of arteries to roots of nerves in posterior cranial fossa in man. Arch Surg 30:336–345, 1935.

185

Spontaneous Intracerebral Hemorrhage

Thomas B. Ducker

One of the most devastating forms of cerebrovascular disease is spontaneous intracerebral hemorrhage (bleeding into the parenchyma of the brain without coincident trauma). Despite a wealth of literature spanning well over 100 years of vigorous research into the etiology and treatment of this type of stroke, its mortality remains over 50 percent and more than three-fourths of the survivors are left with moderate to severe disabilities.

Neurosurgeons have led the struggle to find a satisfactory means of alleviating the morbidity attending this form of stroke since Harvey Cushing's pioneering efforts around the turn of the century. Charles Bagley published a paper in 1932 in which he divided intracranial hemorrhage into subarachnoid and intracerebral.[1] Intracerebral bleeding was divided into deep and superficial. It was Bagley's belief that only superficial hemispheric hematomas "may be helped surgically."[1] In 1933, Penfield reported two cases of spontaneous intracerebral hematoma operated on successfully.[11] By the end of World War II, a variety of reports had appeared on the subject of the surgical management of intracerebral hemorrhage.

Cushing and Bagley depended on clinical history, neurological examination, and lumbar puncture for the diagnosis and localization of the intracerebral hematoma. Penfield suggested the use of transcerebral ventriculography. By the mid-1950s cerebral angiography became the diagnostic method of choice, thereby offering a considerable advance in accuracy.

Numerous uncontrolled and retrospective studies have been reported in the literature over the last 25 years, each vigorously advocating one or another type of treatment. However, despite all these efforts, McKissock et al. stated after reporting a randomized prospective clinical study on conservative versus surgical therapy, "We have clearly made no contribution to the treatment of primary intracerebral hemorrhage by surgery,"[9] and the controversy still rages over the best treatment for this devastating form of stroke. Further study on treatment modalities is warranted at this time. An interesting treatment modality was presented as late as 1981 by Zhong-Xiu: "Traumatic and non-traumatic hematomas were treated with traditional Chinese herbs. All of the cases obtained a good result. Symptoms and signs improve in about three days. . . . They returned to their work about one to two months after treatment."[16]

Epidemiology

According to the National Survey on Stroke, spontaneous intracerebral hemorrhage accounts for 6.3 to 12 percent of all new strokes occurring in the United States each year.[15] Of all intracerebral hemorrhages, 67.9 percent are fatal. The average annual incidence for intracerebral hemorrhage in the United States is 9 per 100,000 population. Seventy to ninety percent of all cases are hypertensive. Two-thirds of cases occur between the ages of 45 and 75, and almost one-half between 55 and 75. Men have a 5 to 20 percent higher incidence than do women. There is a higher incidence in blacks than among whites, perhaps corresponding to a higher incidence of hypertension in that subset of the population.[15]

Pathology and Etiology

Epidemiologically, 70 to 90 percent of spontaneous intracerebral hematomas are associated with hypertension. In most autopsy series, the figure is 50 to 60 percent, while in most clinical series, the figure is about 40 percent. Although McCormick and Rosenfield found hypertension alone as the contributing etiology in only one-fourth of their 144 autopsy cases, there is little doubt that hypertension is the most frequently associated disease in those cases of spontaneous intracerebral hematoma in which there is no other apparent etiology.

The pathogenesis of hypertensive intracerebral hemorrhage has long been disputed. Cruveilhier and Virchow had divided intracerebral hemorrhage into two types in the first half of the nineteenth century. One type included blood clots surrounded by damaged brain, and the other, softened, necrotic brain into which hemorrhage had occurred. In 1814, Rouchoux postulated that the softening (i.e., infarction) was the primary event, and that pericapillary bleeding then led to the hematoma in most cases. In 1918, Rosenblath proposed that a noxious stimulus elaborated by the kidney might lead to angionecrosis, infarction, and secondary hemorrhage. Westphal and Bar proposed the theory of angiospasm. Schwartz believed that vessel wall damage sustained in a hypertensive crisis might lead to capillary leakage with a hematoma resulting from the confluence of these diapedetic hemorrhages, a theory supported by Mertlu. A laboratory model of intracerebral hematoma induced in monkeys given cerebral vasodilators during the vasoproliferative phase 5 days after cerebral infarction following middle cerebral artery occlusion was provided by Laurent et al. in 1976.

In 1868, Charcot and Bouchard published a famous paper on "miliary aneurysms" discovered in the walls of intracerebral hematomas shortly after death in 84 cases.[3] The significance of these microaneurysms was questioned for almost a century when in 1967 Cole and Yates studied the brains of 200 subjects, 100 hypertensives and 100 normotensives.[4] These researchers found aneurysms measuring 0.05 to 2.0 mm in 46 percent of the hypertensives and only 7 percent of the normotensives. Among hypertensives with intracerebral hemorrhages, 86 percent had microaneurysms. The locations of the microaneurysms corresponded closely to the relative sites of origin of the hematoma. The microaneurysms were found in the hemispheres, mainly in the basal ganglia but also in the white matter; a few were also found in the pons and cerebellum.[4]

As early as 1941, Anders and Eicke found that hyalinosis (deposition of hyalin material into the media of small cerebral arteries with secondary constriction of the lumen and destruction of the wall) correlated closely with intracerebral hemorrhage. Many authors have subsequently redocumented the findings of "hypertensive fibrinoid angiopathy," "angionecrosis," "arteriosclerosis," or "hyaline necrosis" among patients with hypertensive intracerebral hematoma. That hypertension can induce such changes in small vessels was proved in the Goldblatt model by Murhead et al. and in hypertensive rats by Ooneda et al.

Zülch has found hyaline arteriosclerosis in association with virtually all hypertensive intracerebral hemorrhages. In the majority of cases, small aneurysms of a variety of types are also present. Zülch postulates that hyaline degeneration of the vessel wall coupled with increased proximal pressure secondary to distal stenosis or occlusion, as well as the measurable high pressure normally present in the proximal lenticulostriate system, may lead to rupture of the arterioles at their points of greatest weakness, with or without definite microaneurysms. This most usually occurs at the bifurcation points near the "knee" of the lenticulostriates. This culmination of pathogenetic theories is the most widely accepted today.

Common Anatomical Sites

The location of an intracerebral hemorrhage may suggest the most likely etiology of the bleeding. Hypertensive intracerebral hemorrhage occurs most frequently in the basal ganglia, especially the putamen, the internal capsule, or the external capsule. Lobar hemorrhages are more likely associated with tumors, arteriovenous malformations, or coagulopathies, but not predictably. Of those hemorrhages in which hypertension is the only apparent associated illness, 80 percent occur above the tentorium and 20 percent below. Jellinger has averaged 11 separate series of hypertensive intracerebral hematomas and found that 64 percent occur in the basal ganglia, 13 percent in the hemispheric white matter, 10 to 12 percent in the pons and midbrain, 12 percent in the cerebellum, and 11 percent in the thalamus.[12]

Among ganglionic hematomas, the majority do occur in the distribution of the lateral lenticulostriate branch of the middle cerebral artery (Charcot's *artere de l'hémorrhagie cérébrale*), although a significant proportion occur more medially. It has long been known that the blood in an intracerebral hemorrhage frequently dissects along planes and often displaces rather than destroys the surrounding brain. Ganglionic hemorrhage frequently extends in an anterior posterior plane, whereas thalamic hemorrhage frequently extends laterally. The incidence of intraventricular hemorrhage in some series is as high as 60 percent overall.

Brain stem hemorrhages usually originate at the junction

of the tegmentum and basis pontis at the border zone between the areas of distribution of the ventral perforating and dorsal lateral arteries. Cerebellar hemorrhages usually originate near the dentate nuclei.

Clinical Presentations

According to the 1981 National Survey of Stroke, 72 percent of all intraparenchymal hemorrhages present with coma and over 8 percent with stupor. Among noncomatose patients, Walker relates that 60 percent are hemiplegic, 43 percent have "speech difficulties," 13 percent have pupillary abnormalities, and 16 percent have seizures. Two-thirds of patients with intraparenchymal hemorrhages are disoriented, almost one-third are vertiginous, and one-fourth have "abnormal sensations." In the Harvard Stroke Registry, 60 percent of hematoma patients had a headache before, during, or after the onset of their neurological deficit, but only 33 percent with the onset; 51 percent had vomited.[15]

Ganglionic (especially putaminal) hematomas tend to produce symptom complexes which vary according to the specific location of the mass. Hier et al. noted that small putaminal hematomas often produce only moderate hemimotor or hemisensory defects, whereas moderate-sized hemorrhages may produce the classic syndrome of flaccid hemiplegia, hemisensory defect, lateral gaze preference, homonymous hemianopsia, and aphasia. Massive hemorrhages produce coma, bilateral extensor plantar responses, fixed dilated pupils, absent eye movements, papilledema, and rapid demise.[12]

When compared with putaminal hemorrhages, thalamic hemorrhages may present similarly, but the hemisensory deficit may be more severe, a small hematoma may be associated with a more profound disturbance of consciousness, and extraocular movement disorders may be more complex. Paralysis of upward gaze and skew deviation may be commonly seen in thalamic hemorrhage.

Lobar intracerebral hematoma is differentiated from deeper hemorrhage by a much lower incidence of coma and a much higher incidence of seizures and headache. Ropper and Davis described four discrete clinical syndromes according to the lobar location of the clot. Dense hemiparesis and gaze preference rarely occur in lobar hemorrhage.

Large pontine hemorrhages present with coma, but smaller hemorrhages, now commonly seen with CT scanning, are less devastating. Virtually all patients with brain stem hemorrhage suffer extraocular movement defects, especially paralysis of ipsilateral conjugate gaze or ocular bobbing, usually demonstrated by abnormal oculocephalic or oculovestibular testing. The pupils are usually small but are reactive to bright light. A variety of cranial nerve palsies, as well as variable degrees of extensor posturing, are often present.

In cerebellar hemorrhage, consciousness is not usually lost with the onset of symptoms, although coma may ensue within 48 h. The most common mode of presentation is severe headache (especially suboccipital); vomiting occurs in 75 to 100 percent of cases. Over one-half of the patients will complain of dizziness (not necessarily true vertigo) and the inability to stand or walk. Unlike pontine hemorrhage, there is a notable absence of hemiplegia or hemisensory defect. Before the onset of stupor or coma, the majority of the patients will manifest prominent cerebellar signs with both truncal and/or ipsilateral appendicular ataxia and hypotonia. At least half will display horizontal gaze palsy on the ipsilateral side, occasionally with contralateral deviation. The pupils are either normal or small and reactive. Horizontal nystagmus ipsilaterally is frequently noted, and as the level of consciousness sinks, a peripheral facial palsy and depressed corneal reflex frequently ensue ipsilaterally. There is a notable absence of vertical gaze abnormalities until late in the course. McKissock et al. have suggested that the triad of constricted and reactive pupils, periodic respirations, and gaze palsy are useful in diagnosing cerebellar hemorrhage.[9]

CT Appearance

There can be little doubt that the computed tomographic scanner has revolutionized diagnosis in intracranial hemorrhage. With the presently available machinery, clots of 1 cm or less can routinely be visualized in their exact anatomical location viewed in multiple two-dimensional planes. The hematoma appears as a high-density lesion (70 to 80 HU) in the acute phase and initially has no surrounding low-density area or contrast enhancement unless there is an associated vascular anomaly.

Ventricular extension or primary ventricular hemorrhage presents with variable attenuation values dependent on the ratio of blood to CSF. Laun et al. have found that blood must account for at least 15 percent of the ventricular volume in order to be visualized by CT. A small amount of blood localized to one small ventricular compartment may be easily visualized, whereas the same blood volume spread diffusely throughout the ventricular system may not.

Regardless of etiology, intracerebral hematomas undergo progressive pathological alterations with time. These changes, which are well established pathologically, produce corresponding changes in CT images. Dolinskas et al. found that "the density of intracerebral hematomas decreases an average of 0.7 EMI units per day" and that "the dense portion of the hematoma decreases in size by an average of 0.65 mm per day."[6] However, it should be remembered that the decrease in mass effect was delayed beyond the decrease in the size of the hematoma in all cases in which mass effect was present.

Kendall and Radue reported that a low-density ring appears around every intracerebral hematoma within 6 h. This ring increases in width over the next 24 to 48 h and likely represents surrounding brain damaged by the precontracted hemorrhage. Laster et al. described six stages in the resolution of an intracerebral hematoma as defined by CT criteria. Stage I lasts 1 to 10 days, during which the hematoma is of high density, well marginated, surrounded by a thin peripheral lucency, and not enhanced with contrast. In stage II, from 3 to 20 days, the hematoma shows decreasing density, less distinct margins, a wide surrounding lucency with the beginning of the "ring sign," and contrast enhancement of the inner part of this lucent zone. During this stage, the enhancement may be attenuated by the administration of steroids. In stage III, from 18 to 64 days, the hematoma is isodense, but still has an enhanceable ring sensitive to steroid administration. At 35 to 70 days, stage IV, the hematoma is lucent with a steroid-modifiable enhancing ring. Stage V occurs between 42 and 84 days, and at this point, the contrast-enhanced ring can no longer be modified by steroids. Finally, in stage VI, enhancement no longer occurs, steroids produce no change, and only a lucent cavity remains at 82 to 240 days. It has been proposed that the steroid-modifiable enhancement occurs as a result of the breakdown of the blood-brain barrier, whereas the nonmodifiable enhancement marks "luxury perfusion" associated with the development of vascular granulation tissue. Intraventricular blood clears considerably faster than intraparenchymal blood and is rarely present after 14 to 21 days.

The most underutilized capability offered by computed tomography in the management of an intracerebral hematoma is the ability to assay quantitatively the planimetric dimensions of the mass. As early as 1975, Steiner and others in Stockholm devised a method for accurately estimating the volume of an intracerebral clot with the use of a complex equation.[14] More recently, software programs for estimating the volume of a hematoma have become more widely available, and in the future, specific volume criteria may become important in therapeutic decision making.

Although it is likely that the hematoma volume producing dire neurological consequences will vary depending on location, rate of formation, mechanism of formation, and other factors, it is nonetheless likely that quantitative volumetric analysis offers a significant step forward in the management of this condition. At the 1982 International Intracranial Pressure Conference in Japan, Tazawa et al. presented their findings relating the size of the hematoma to intracranial pressure changes in patients with hypertensive intracerebral hemorrhage. Their results indicate that the critical level of maximum diameter of a hematoma associated with increasing intracranial pressure is approximately 4 cm.

Cerebral Angiography

As little as 5 years ago, new papers on the angiographic diagnosis and classification of primary intracerebral hematoma were still appearing. At present, however, the role of angiography lies in the establishment of the etiology of an intracerebral hematoma rather than in revealing its existence or location within the brain. Although the CT scan can often predict the etiology of an intracerebral hematoma, it will often fail to demonstrate a significant percentage of small aneurysms, angiomata, and occasional tumors.

Complete cerebral angiography on every patient who has intracerebral hematoma would undoubtedly improve our premortem diagnostic accuracy, and yet even this aggressive measure leaves significant room for error. Many authors have commented on the fallibility of angiography. Cerebral angiography tailored to each patient individually is indicated in every case in which an invasive surgical procedure is contemplated. Preoperative knowledge of the cause of the hemorrhage may drastically alter the planned surgical or medical approach to a given patient. Conversely, in those patients in whom surgery is deemed inadvisable, invasive diagnostic studies are rarely indicated. The risks of angiography are well established, especially in elderly and hypertensive individuals. The most beneficial timing of angiography has not been established. One's position on this question must be directly tied to his or her position on the timing of surgery, a question still debated vigorously. Postoperative angiography seems indicated only when there is doubt about the success of the operation in the extirpation of the lesion or when the results of such a study would influence the future therapeutic regimen.

Surgical Therapy

Historically, the surgical literature has been predominantly concerned with hemispheric intracerebral hemorrhage.[8] In 1965, Cuatico et al. reported a surgical series of 102 cases, re-emphasizing the importance of the level of consciousness on surgical outcome.[5] They suggested that surgery was the treatment "par excellence" for what they termed "medullary" hematomas which are equivalent to lobar intracerebral hematomas. Conversely, in ganglionic intracerebral hematoma, they found surgery beneficial only in rare cases without significant depression of the sensorium and with only "partial" or "borderline" destruction of the nuclear structures. They also found better results with normotensives than with hypertensives and with cases whose progression was subacute rather than acute and devastating. Surgical mortality has been reportedly higher among comatose patients (54 to 77 percent).[5]

In their review more than 10 years ago, Ransohoff et al. suggested that all patients who (1) require artificial means to support blood pressure or respiration, (2) have focal neurological deficits associated with "rapid progressive deterioration of consciousness," (3) need to be stabilized on medical regimens, or (4) have medical contraindications to surgery should be excluded from surgical consideration.[13] Restating that position "in a more positive fashion," only those patients "who survive the initial ictus without an early massive neurologic deficit" and who subsequently deteriorate or fail to improve were treated surgically.[13] Pasztor et al. restated the risks concurrent with age in hypertensives over 50.[12]

Despite the bias against operation in ganglionic/thalamic hematoma, a high percentage of intracerebral hematomas are hypertensive in etiology and a high percentage of hypertensive intracerebral hematomas are ganglionic/thalamic in location. The Japanese have faced this issue most squarely. Kanaya et al., through a retrospective study, found that among patients who were "alert," "confused," or "somnolent," the results of treatment were good and differed little regardless of treatment modality. For patients who were "stuporous" or "semicomatose without signs of herniation," surgical results were significantly better than medical. They also reported that the majority of the surgical survivors were left independent in activities of daily living, whereas the medical survivors were left "totally disabled" in 11 of 18 cases.[12]

Brain stem hemorrhages have been divided into three

categories based on CT appearance. Group A have hematomas entirely within the pons and less than 1 cm in diameter. Group B have hematomas entirely within the pons but more than 1 cm in diameter, and Group C have hematomas which extend beyond the borders of the pons and are associated with ventricular hemorrhage and hydrocephalus. Sano and Ochiai concluded from their experience in comparing surgical treatment with medical treatment of these groups of patients that there are no indications for direct surgical attack on hypertensive pontine hematoma, but that brain stem hematomas in nonhypertensives under 40 should be evacuated in an effort to extirpate the suspected cryptic angioma to prevent rebleeding. In all cases, associated hydrocephalus should be treated with ventricular drainage.[12]

Concerning cerebellar hematomas, several authors agree that operative treatment should be accomplished in the acute phase, within 24 h, to obtain a good result. It seems that surgery is indicated in the majority of cases of cerebellar hematoma diagnosed very early.

Sano and Yoshida evaluated a series of 39 cases of cerebellar hematoma, 30 associated with hypertension and 9 with cryptic angiomas. The mean age of the hypertensive group was 64 years. Among the hypertensives, 27 percent were fully conscious, 33 percent were drowsy, 20 percent were stuporous, and 2 percent were comatose. Eighteen of the thirty patients were operated on, with one-half of the operations done within 48 h of onset. The overall operative mortality was 39 percent and correlated well with the preoperative level of consciousness. Of the eleven survivors, seven were left well or with minimal disabilities and four were left moderately or severely disabled. The quality of survival was also directly correlated with the preoperative level of consciousness. Among patients with hypertensive hemorrhages treated conservatively, one comatose patient died, three of five stuporous or drowsy patients survived with varying amounts of disability, and six awake patients recovered completely. Several authors have emphasized that patients undergoing successful evacuation of cerebellar hematomas are frequently left with little neurological deficit.

The major contribution by the Japanese to the study of surgery for intracerebral hematomas concerns the appropriate time for surgery. In 1932, Bagley suggested 2 weeks after the onset as the proper time.[1] Penfield suggested that the earlier the operation, the smaller the residual disability might be.[11] In the 1940s, French surgeons operated during the first week. In the controlled trial published by McKissock et al. in 1961, they concluded that early surgery offered no statistical benefit over conservative treatment.[9]

Mitsuno et al. have taken the stand that "24 to 48 hours after onset is the ideal time" to operate on the hypertensive intracerebral hematoma.[12] Over the years that followed, several authors reported conflicting statistics on the timing, suggesting times from 24 h to 10 days as being optimal.

Following these conflicting opinions, Kaneko et al. in 1977 reported 38 consecutive cases of laterally situated hypertensive intracerebral hematomas operated upon within 7 h of the ictus.[7] At the time of surgery, 35 of the 38 were stuporous or comatose. Of these 38, 12 showed virtually complete recovery, 12 were left independent with mild disability, 10 needed partial care at home, 1 was bedridden, and 3 died. The authors postulated that these excellent results were related to the removal of the hematoma before edema could form and a secondary cerebral insult could transpire. In 1981, this same group reported similar findings on 100 cases operated upon within 7 h. Both Suzuki and Kaneko have accumulated several hundred cases now and think that immediate operative removal in properly selected patients definitely improves the outcome and lessens morbidity and mortality—a view now widely held in Asia.[12]

The results of intracranial pressure monitoring in the management of intracerebral hematoma, as reported by Papo et al., tend to support early operation, for it is only in this group that intracranial pressure was more than transiently improved by surgery.[10] Despite this, Pia has written in 1980 that "operating on hypertensive hematomas during the first day has no effect and has been completely abandoned in Europe."[12]

The criteria used at our university for surgical treatment utilize both the position and the size of the hematoma (Figs. 185-1 and 185-2).[2] If the hematoma is lobar, the treatment can be surgical removal; if the hemorrhage is ganglionic, operation can be carefully done through the sylvian fissure; and if the hemorrhage is deep thalamic or has ventricular extension, rarely is an operation performed. Size criteria used are based on the amount of intracranial space occupied by the hematoma: i.e., if this is 0 to 4 percent of the supratentorial space, surgery is rarely indicated; if 4 to 8 percent of the space is occupied by hematoma and there is associated clinical instability or deterioration, the patient is a candidate for surgery; if the value is 8 to 12 percent, the patient is a definite operative candidate; and if it is more than 12 percent, he will most likely die and surgery may not be of benefit. The strongest indication to operate is a patient with an altered level of consciousness and a deteriorating neurological status despite maximum medical therapy.

By utilizing both the anatomical site and the size of the hematoma, guidelines to therapy are possible. Supratentorially, a fairly large (10 percent) lobar hematoma should be removed immediately in most cases. Conversely, a small (4 percent) thalamic hemorrhage is rarely considered for a major operation; the patient may be monitored and treated with an intraventricular catheter. Large cerebellar hematomas usually need immediate removal. Conversely, small pontine hemorrhages require no operative intervention. If we operate, we favor the immediate (Japanese) approach.

Prognosis

Despite major advances in the diagnosis of intracerebral hematoma consequent to the advent of computed tomography, major improvements in surgical techniques consequent to the advent of the operating microscope, and major advances in medical therapeutics, the morbidity and mortality of spontaneous intracerebral hematoma remain unacceptably high. With the possible exception of lobar hemorrhage secondary to a vascular anomaly, the mortality rate is about 50 percent and the combined morbidity mortality rate is 70 to 80 percent.

The mortality increases with the size of the hematoma and with ventricular rupture. The level of consciousness on

Spontaneous Intracerebral Hemorrhage

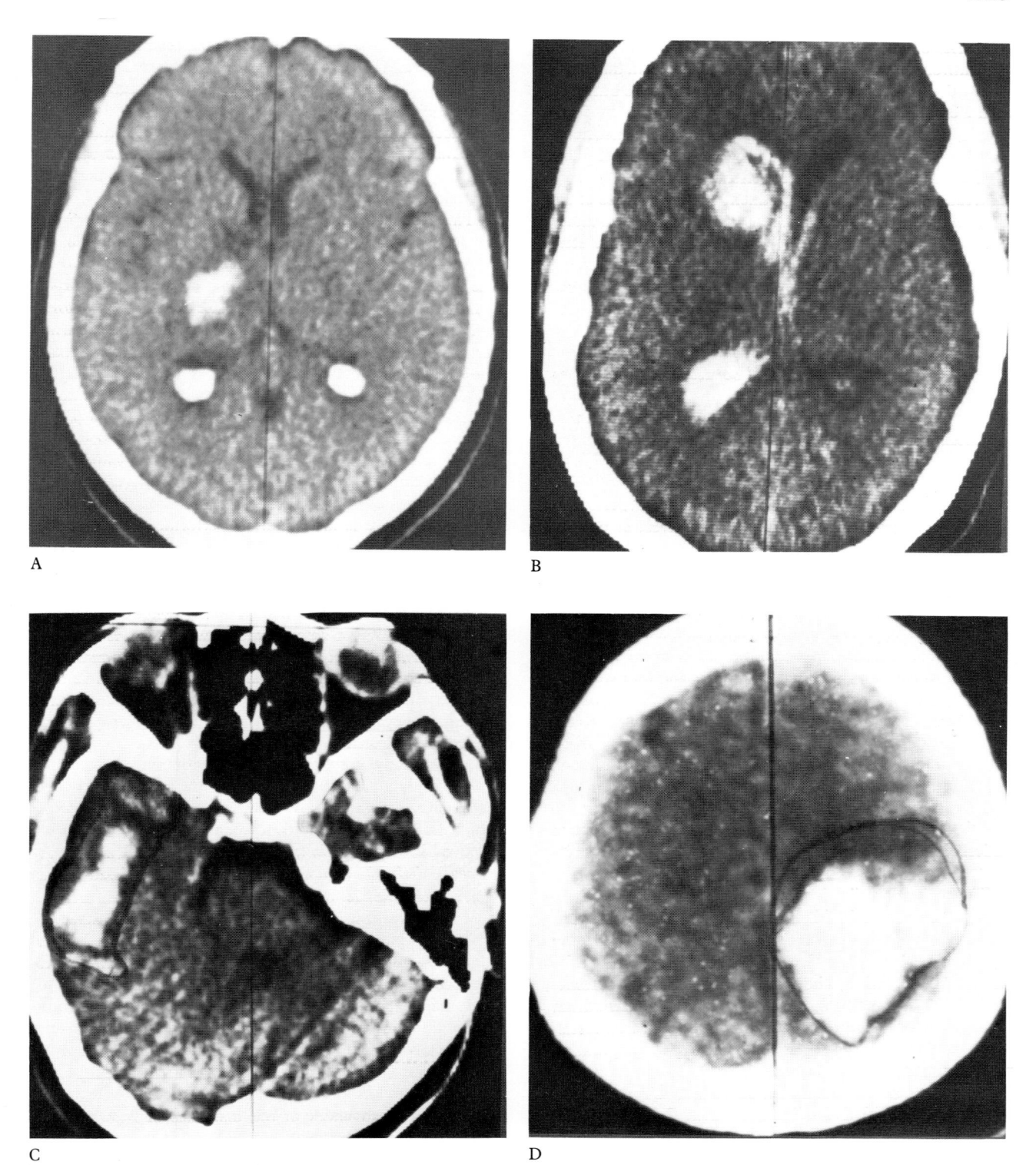

Figure 185-1 The CT scans of four patients who did not require an urgent operation show the types of hemorrhage that can be managed medically. *A.* A small thalamic and internal capsular hypertensive hemorrhage which would not require operative removal. *B.* A small- to medium-size caudate nuclear hypertensive hemorrhage with ventricular spill which can usually be handled without operative care. *C.* A temporal lobe hemorrhage which is small and not associated with a significant shift or brain stem compression (but which may be associated with a middle cerebral artery aneurysm). *D.* A moderate parietal lobe hypertensive hemorrhage which can be removed if the patient is unstable or deteriorates.

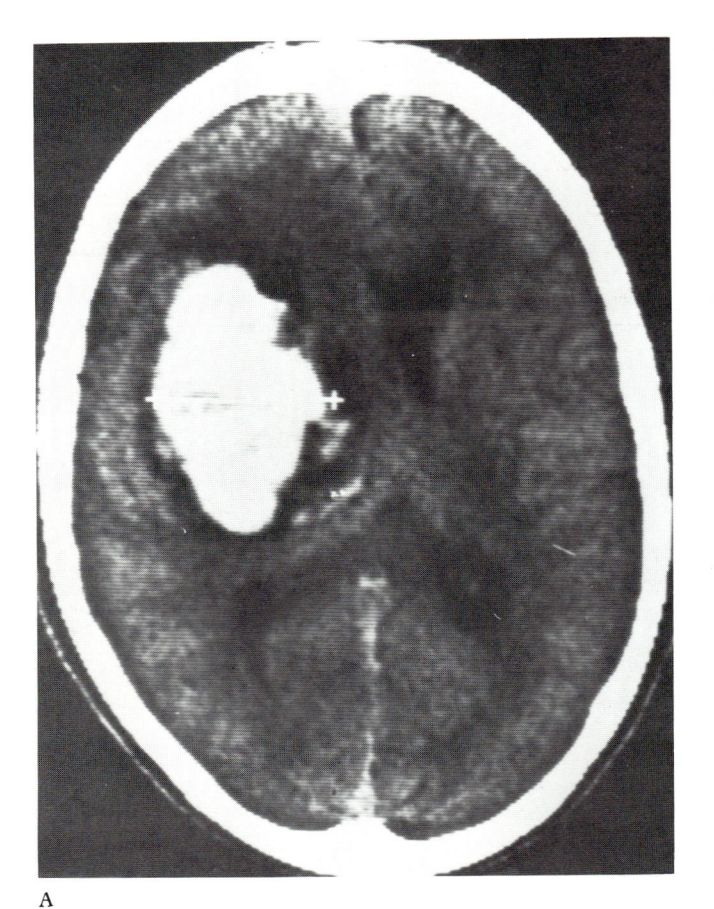

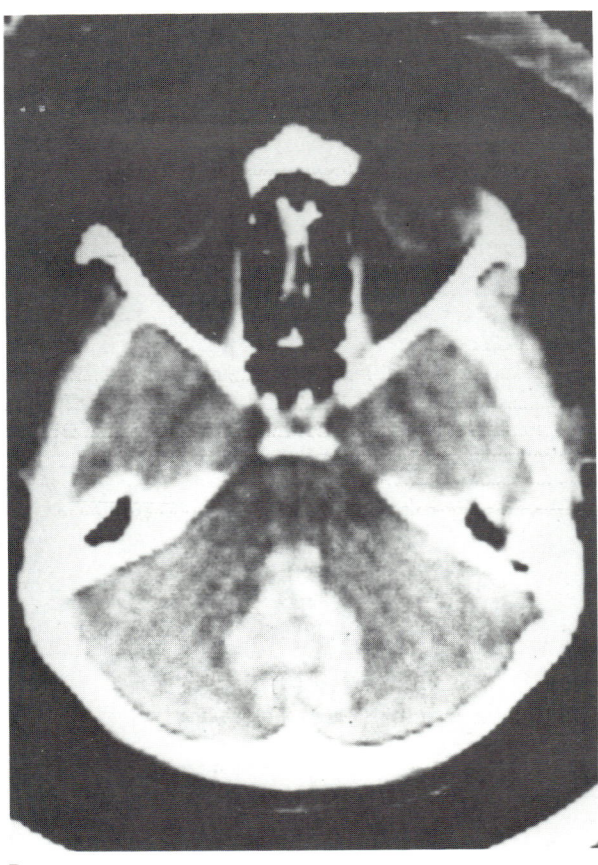

Figure 185-2 The CT scans of two patients who required urgent (emergency) operative care. *A.* A large hypertensive hemorrhage which is in the lentiform nuclear area lateral to the internal capsule in a patient with neurological deterioration who was treated immediately with a trans-sylvian approach with removal of the hematoma and coagulation of the bleeding lenticulostriate vessel. *B.* A large hypertensive midline cerebellar hemorrhage which obstructs the fourth ventricle and which was readily removed surgically.

admission and the location of the mass are far more important than is the etiology per se. Acute inpatient mortality is generally between 40 and 50 percent for the hypertensive intracerebral hemorrhage. It appears that increasing age, thalamic involvement, and delayed definitive care raise the mortality rate.

Few long-term studies have been done on survivors of hypertensive intracerebral hemorrhage. McKissock et al. reported a 6-month follow-up in which 2 percent of the survivors were able to return to work and 16 percent continued to be partially disabled.[9] In a recent study by Douglas and Haerer, a 2½-year follow-up was done. In their series, 57 percent of the patients died either in the hospital or during the follow-up period. Of the remaining 43 percent, approximately 39 percent were ambulatory at follow-up. Their data also revealed that unlike patients with aneurysms, hypertensives rarely, if ever, experience rebleeding. In their study, the worst prognosis was in the 30- to 40-year-old age range; these patients were almost all severely hypertensive black males.

Conclusion

The major controversy concerning the hypertensive intracerebral hemorrhage remains the best means of therapeutic management. Well-controlled, randomized (by therapeutic modality) studies need to be carried out to ascertain the best treatment for these patients. Medical regimens including steroids, ICP monitoring, osmotic agents, control of hypertension, and antifibrinolytics need to be examined carefully for benefit. The timing and indications for surgery also need careful study so that precise guidelines can be developed. Reduction in the morbidity and mortality from this devastating form of stroke is the goal of the treatment, and only through adequate research can this goal be obtained.

Humiliated by our lack of precise scientific data, we must nevertheless practice the art of medicine. Aggressive operative care applied appropriately can undoubtedly help certain individual patients. We have presented our current guidelines which we think give our patients the best possible care.

References

1. Bagley C Jr: Spontaneous cerebral hemorrhage: Discussion of four types, with surgical consideration. Arch Neurol Psychiatry 27:1133–1174, 1932.
2. Cahill DW, Ducker TB: Spontaneous intracerebral hemorrhage. Clin Neurosurg 29:722–779, 1982.
3. Charcot JM, Bouchard C: Nouvelles recherches sur la pathogénie de l'hémorrhagie cérébrale. Arch Physiol (Paris) 1:110–127, 643–665, 725–734, 1868.
4. Cole FM, Yates PO: Pseudo-aneurysms in relationship to massive cerebral hemorrhage. J Neurol Neurosurg Psychiatry 30:61–66, 1967.
5. Cuatico W, Adib S, Caston P: Spontaneous intracerebral hematomas: A surgical appraisal. J Neurosurg 22:569–575, 1965.
6. Dolinskas CA, Bilaniuk LT, Zimmerman RA, Kuhl DE, Alavi A: Computed tomography of intracerebral hematomas. AJR 129:681–688, 689–692, 1977.
7. Kaneko M, Koba T, Yokayama T: Early surgical treatment for hypertensive intracerebral hemorrhage. J Neurosurg 46:579–583, 1977.
8. Luessenhop AJ, Shevlin WA, Ferrero AA, McCullough DC, Barone BM: Surgical management of primary intracerebral hemorrhage. J Neurosurg 27:419–427, 1967.
9. McKissock W, Richardson A, Taylor J: Primary intracerebral haemorrhage: A controlled trial of surgical and conservative treatment in 180 unselected cases. Lancet 2:221–226, 1961.
10. Papo I, Janny P, Caruselli G, Colnet G, Luongo A: Intracranial pressure time course in primary intracerebral hemorrhage. Neurosurgery 4:504–511, 1979.
11. Penfield W: The operative treatment of spontaneous intracerebral haemorrhage. Can Med Assoc J 28:369–372, 1933.
12. Pia HW, Langmaid C, Zierski J (eds.): *Spontaneous Intracerebral Hematomas: Advances in Diagnosis and Therapy*. Berlin, Springer-Verlag, 1980.
13. Ransohoff J, Derby B, Kricheff I: Spontaneous intracerebral hemorrhage. Clin Neurosurg 18:247–266, 1971.
14. Steiner L, Bergvall U, Zwetnow N: Quantitative estimation of intracerebral and intraventricular hematoma by computed tomography. Acta Radiol [Suppl] (Stockh) 346:143–154, 1975.
15. Weinfeld, FD (ed): *The National Survey of Stroke*. Stroke 12, Suppl 1, 1981, pp 1–91.
16. Zhong-Xiu C: Treatment of intracranial hematoma with traditional Chinese herbs (short communication). Neurochirurgia [Suppl] 24:93, 1981.

SECTION E

Coagulopathies and Vasculopathies

186

Coagulopathies Causing Intracranial Hemorrhage

Justin W. Renaudin
Ralph P. George

Etiology

Hemostasis involves three basic elements: vessel wall, platelets, and coagulation factors. In this discussion, a coagulopathy will be defined as a disorder of blood coagulation involving plasma coagulation factors or platelets. The discussion will focus chiefly on the more common coagulopathies that result in intracranial hemorrhage (ICH). Rare disorders of coagulation which include inhibitors of coagulation factors or qualitative platelet abnormalities that do not result in ICH as frequently will be covered only briefly. Vasculopathy is the subject of another chapter.

The process of blood coagulation is complicated, and even after many decades of study, remains incompletely understood. It has been described in detail in an earlier chapter. Briefly, a vessel is injured, and a reaction of platelets with the injured endothelial and subendothelial tissues results. The formation of plasma (intrinsic) thromboplastic activity follows. Prothrombin is converted to thrombin in the presence of thromboplastin and calcium. Finally, fibrinogen is converted to fibrin in the presence of thrombin.

Anticoagulation Therapy

The most commonly used anticoagulants are warfarin and heparin. Warfarin retards the synthesis of vitamin K dependent factors (factors II, VII, IX, and X). The effects of warfarin are not immediate, and the prothrombin time will lengthen to a therapeutic level over a couple of days. The maintenance dose is titrated against the desired prothrombin times, usually 1½ to 2 times the control. Warfarin is taken orally and is used on a long-term, outpatient basis. Among the many drugs which enhance the effect of warfarin are alcohol, aspirin, and cimetidine.

Heparin is administered either intravenously or subcutaneously. It is used on a short-term, inpatient basis and can usually be neutralized promptly with protamine sulfate. It acts as an anticoagulant at several points along the coagulation sequence. There is individual variation in response with most of the anticoagulants, and one needs to monitor treatment carefully. Patients receiving heparin are followed with activated partial thromboplastin time (APTT) determinations. The effect of heparin is short-lived, a matter of 4 to 8 h, whereas it customarily requires 3 to 5 days before the effect of warfarin is eliminated.

Pharmacologic anticoagulants have prevented many deaths from thrombosis and embolism. Conversely, they have resulted in some very serious complications. ICH is far more common in patients treated with warfarin than with heparin.[5]

Blood Dyscrasias

Thrombocytopenia is a common hematologic abnormality. A reduction in the number of circulating platelets may be due either to decreased production of platelets by the bone marrow or increased destruction or trapping of platelets. Most of the platelets are released by megakaryocytes in the bone marrow. The platelet life-span as estimated by isotope labeling is about 9 days. A large array of drugs, various chemical and physical agents, and several diseases may cause a reduction in the number of platelets. Generally, so long as the platelet count exceeds 60,000 per cubic millimeter, no untoward hematologic complications will ensue. Once the platelet count falls below 20,000 per cubic millimeter, the patient is distinctly at risk for hemorrhage.

Qualitative platelet disorders may be inherited or acquired. Von Willebrand's disease is an inherited hemostatic defect due to the lack of von Willebrand's factor (vWF) necessary for proper platelet function.[3] Aspirin will inhibit platelet aggregation to a significant degree and is such a commonly used drug, it deserves mention. The inhibitory effect of aspirin lasts for the life-span of the platelet. Von Willebrand's disease and its variants, as well as aspirin, will prolong bleeding times, but I have no personal experience with these conditions causing ICH.

Hemophilia is an inherited hemorrhagic disease due to a deficiency of a clotting factor. In the cases of hemophilia, 85 percent are factor VIII deficient (hemophilia A). Factor IX deficiency accounts for about 14 percent (hemophilia B). The "hemostatic" level is about 30 percent, and abnormal bleeding usually ceases if the factor level is 30 percent or greater.

The liver is the main site of synthesis of the large majority of plasma coagulation factors. Therefore, a coagulopathy may be present in various types of severe liver disease; the alcoholic with severe liver disease may be further burdened with thrombocytopenia and is particularly at risk for intracranial bleeding.

In leukemia, ICH accounts for about one-half of the serious bleeding episodes. ICH is more likely to develop in leukemic patients with very high leukocyte counts, and more so in granulocytic than lymphocytic leukemia. Leukostasis in the small cerebral vessels and disruption of the vessel wall is a serious risk in patients with white blood counts greater than 100,000 per cubic millimeter. Thrombocytopenia, from mild to severe, has been observed in 90 percent of the leukemic patients with ICH. Other coagulation abnormalities may be observed in patients with leukemia.

Clinical Presentation

As a general rule, hereditary coagulation factor deficiencies—hemophilia A and B—are more apt to present at a younger age and exclusively in males. A history of episodes of hemarthrosis is common.

Thrombocytopenic patients frequently manifest petechial hemorrhages. With the exception of acute idiopathic thrombocytopenia purpura, which is more common in children, thrombocytopenia is usually observed in the adult population.

In some instances of ICH associated with a coagulopathy, the hemorrhage is caused by trauma that may not necessarily be severe, or even noticed. The history may provide useful clues that a coagulopathy exists. The neurological symptoms and signs of ICH are similar in patients whether or not they have a coagulopathy. This merits emphasis, since patients suspected of ICH will have CT scans performed, and if indicated, an operative procedure may follow promptly. A screening survey for the patient with a possible coagulopathy and unable to give a history would include a complete blood count with a quantitative platelet count, prothrombin time, APTT, and bleeding time. Failure to recognize a coagulopathy before operation might lead to difficult, if not uncontrollable, bleeding during the operative procedure.

A review of the literature of published figures indicates that subdural hematoma is far more common than intracerebral hematoma in patients receiving anticoagulants. This has been the observation of Iizuka[2] and Silverstein[4] in large reviews. The most frequent presenting symptom is headache, and this must be regarded seriously in any patient on anticoagulants. The presence of arterial hypertension, poorly controlled anticoagulation, and repeated episodes of trauma are important aspects of the history.

The incidence of ICH in patients with thrombocytopenia is between 1 and 4 percent. Bleeding may be intracerebral, subdural, or subarachnoid in location. Intracerebral bleeding is the most common.

Central nervous system bleeding is the leading cause of death among hemophiliacs. In an 11-year study from 1965 to 1976, there were 65 patients with ICH in a population of 2500 hemophiliacs.[1] Among this population, 2100 were factor VIII deficient and 400 were factor IX deficient. The most common presenting symptom was headache or vomiting. Of the 65 patients, the mix of sites for ICH was fairly evenly divided among the subdural, subarachnoid, and intracerebral spaces. Of these patients, two-thirds were under 18 years of age; of this group, one-half of the patients were under 3. A symptom-free interval of greater than 24 h with a mean of 4 ± 2.2 days was noted in one-half of their patients with central nervous system trauma. This is frequently seen in patients with subdural hematoma, hemophiliac or not, but this longer latency period observed in some instances of intracerebral bleeding underlines the incidence of indolent bleeding in the hemophiliac population. Recurrent CNS bleeding will occur in 26 percent. The vast majority of patients with ICH had factor levels less than 2 percent.

In patients with severe liver disease, the alcoholic represents the high-risk portion of this population. The coagulation abnormalities and thrombocytopenia are contributing factors to the known increased incidence of ICH in the alcoholic.

ICH in the leukemic patient is most commonly intracerebral; the subarachnoid space is the next most common, and the subdural space is the least common. Of the patients with intracerebral bleeding, almost half will demonstrate multiple sites (Fig. 186-1).

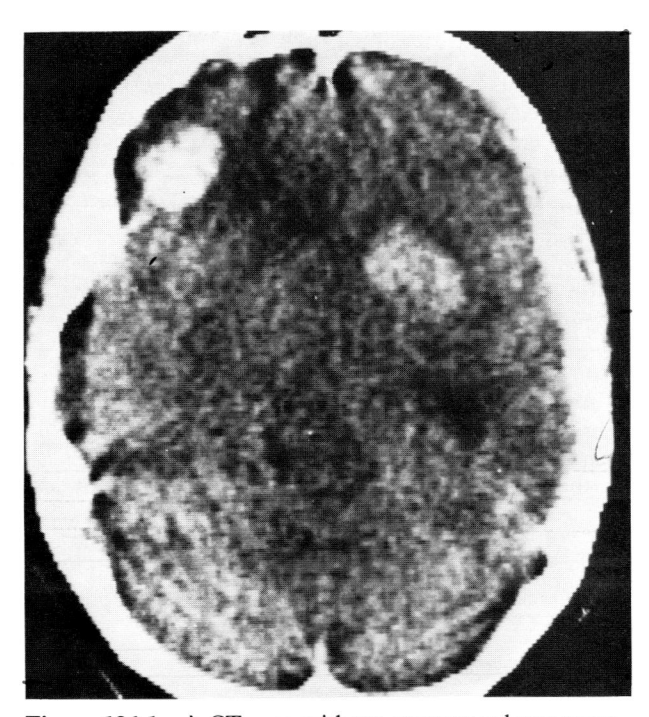

Figure 186-1 A CT scan without contrast enhancement, showing multiple hemorrhages in a patient with acute granulocytic leukemia. There were two more hematomas in other CT sections. The white blood cell count was 326,000 per cubic millimeter, and the platelet count was 29,000 per cubic millimeter.

Hematologic Therapy

Some of these disorders are complex, and a close liaison with an expert in hematology is mandatory.

In patients receiving warfarin, the anticoagulant is stopped immediately, and vitamin K_1 is administered. If necessary, fresh frozen plasma may be given.

Thrombocytopenic patients may be treated with random donor platelet units, and one unit of platelets should theoretically increase the platelet count of a 70-kg man approximately 10,000 per cubic millimeter. In practice this is rarely obtained. Patients in whom the thrombocytopenia is due to immunologic disturbances may benefit from corticosteroids. Some of these patients are candidates for splenectomy, and surgical consultation will be in order.

Factor VIII and factor IX assays are available in most large hospital laboratories and are essential to the diagnosis and regulation of treatment in the hemophiliac. In classic hemophilia, the factor VIII level should be raised to 100 percent for operations and maintained at least at 30 to 50 percent for 2 weeks after the ICH and operation. For factor VIII deficiency, lyophilized concentrates or cryoprecipitates are available. The concentrates have a greater level of factor VIII per unit of volume and are used more frequently in the critical situation.

Treatment of factor IX deficiency involves the same principles as the treatment of factor VIII deficiency. Konyne [factor IX complex (human), Cutter Laboratories, Berkeley, Calif.] is prepared commercially from plasma pools of large numbers of donors. In addition to the high concentration of factor IX, the concentrate contains factors II, VII, and X.

Hematologic treatment of coagulation factor abnormalities in severe liver disease may be very frustrating. Vitamin K_1 should be administered, and fresh frozen plasma or Konyne may be transfused. There are risks involved with either. Coexisting thrombocytopenia is treated with platelet transfusion.

Thrombocytopenia in leukemic patients is managed with platelet transfusions.

Surgical Therapy

In treating patients with operable intracranial lesions, the neurosurgeon should establish a close working relationship with the hematologist. If the patient's condition will tolerate the procedure, and no contraindication exists, any (except trivial) subdural or epidural hematoma should be evacuated. The timing of the operative procedure requires collaboration with the clinical laboratories and the blood bank. The clinical laboratories must ensure that clotting factors and platelet counts have reached at least acceptable levels. The blood bank must be prepared to meet estimated surgical requirements of whole blood, packed red blood cells, coagulation factors, and platelets.

The site, size, side, and shift measurements will influence the management of an intracerebral hematoma. Serial clinical examinations and CT scans are beneficial, and if an operation is indicated, coordination with the hematologist, clinical laboratories, and blood bank is paramount.

Silverstein has recommended that anticonvulsants be administered to hemophiliacs with ICH, whether they are operated upon or not.[4] Without anticonvulsants, the incidence of seizures in hemophiliacs with ICH is slightly over 50 percent. The margin of safety in these patients is low, and prophylactic anticonvulsant treatment is recommended. Hemophiliacs must be maintained for 2 weeks after operation with factor VIII or factor IX concentrates so that the levels are maintained at 30 percent or higher.

Results

Many factors will influence the results. Among these are the severity of the underlying disease and the location of the intracranial hemorrhage. The intracranial hemorrhage associated with anticoagulant therapy has been found to be more frequently subdural than intracerebral, and the results have been favorable in about two-thirds of these patients.

The mortality from ICH in the hemophiliac population is 34 percent.[1] Among the patients reported by Eyster et al., of the group that died, one-fourth had inhibitors to the deficient factor. Of the hemophiliacs who survived, half showed motor impairment, mental retardation, or seizure disorders. The other half demonstrated no neurological deficit.[1]

The results of treatment are poor in patients with chronic severe liver disease or leukemia.

References

1. Eyster ME, Gill FM, Blatt PM, Hilgartner MW, Ballard JO, Kinney TR, and the Hemophilia Study Group: Central nervous system bleeding in hemophiliacs. Blood 51:1179–1188, 1978.
2. Iizuka J: Intracranial and intraspinal hematomas associated with anticoagulant therapy. Neurochiurgia (Stuttg) 15:15–25, 1972.
3. Miale JB: *Laboratory Medicine, Hematology*, 6th ed. St Louis, Mosby, 1982.
4. Silverstein A: Neurological complications in patients with hemorrhagic diathesis, in Vinken PJ, Bruyn GW (eds): *Handbook of Clinical Neurology*, vol 38. Amsterdam, North-Holland, 1979, pp 53–91.
5. Snyder M, Renaudin J: Intracranial hemorrhage associated with anticoagulation therapy. Surg Neurol 7:31–34, 1977.

187
Vasculopathies
Setti S. Rengachary

A host of heterogeneous pathological processes affects blood vessels. Attempts at classification of various vascular disorders are hampered by poor understanding of the etiology and pathogenesis of many of them.[5] Current knowledge leads to the classification proposed in Table 187-1. Imperfect as the table may be, it provides an overview of the spectrum of vascular disorders. The emphasis in this chapter is on those miscellaneous vascular disorders which are not discussed elsewhere in the text and which are of some relevance to the nervous system.

Temporal Arteritis

Temporal arteritis is a vasculopathy of unknown etiology affecting the elderly, past the age of 50.[7] It involves mainly the branches of the external carotid artery. When diagnosed early, the disease may be treated effectively with steroids, and blindness, a dreaded complication of the disease, may be averted.

Numerous synonyms have been used to describe this syndrome, but none is satisfactory. Thus the terms "temporal arteritis" and "cranial arteritis" are topographically too restrictive, because in some individuals larger extracranial vessels such as branches of the aorta may be affected. "Giant cell arteritis" may be a misleading term, since giant cells are not always found, nor is their presence necessary to establish the histological diagnosis if other criteria are met; even if found, they are not exclusive to this disease. Similar criticisms may be leveled against such terms as "arteritis of the aged," "granulomatous arteritis," and "polymyalgia arteritica."

Certain notable paintings from around the fifteenth century depicting individuals with very prominent temporal arteries and other external features suggestive of temporal arteritis have not escaped the attention of present-day rheumatologists.[3] Notable among them are Jan Van Eyck's *The Virgin with the Canon* (1436) and Pieri di Cosimo's *Portrait of Francesco Gamberti* (1505) (Fig. 187-1).

Hutchinson was the first to describe this disease in 1890. His patient was an octogenarian who presented with inflamed, tender temporal arteries. Hutchinson believed that the disease was caused by a tight-fitting hat. Horton et al. reported seven cases in 1932. They emphasized the importance of headache and jaw claudication in this syndrome and presented the histological findings for the first time. Numerous additional reports have appeared since then, especially from North America and Europe, emphasizing other facets of the disease such as the occurrence of blindness, the association with polymyalgia rheumatica, and the involvement of larger systemic arteries.

TABLE 187-1 A Classification of Vasculopathies

I. Degenerative arteriopathies:
  A. Atherosclerosis
  B. Monckeberg's medial calcific sclerosis
  C. Arteriolosclerosis
    1. Proliferative
    2. Hyaline
II. Systemic necrotizing vasculitides:
  A. Classic polyarteritis nodosa
  B. Allergic granulomatous angiitis (Churg-Strauss)
  C. Granulomatous angiitis of the nervous system
  D. "Overlap syndrome" (features of polyarteritis nodosa and of allergic granulomatosis)
III. Hypersensitivity vasculitides:
  A. Drug-related vasculitides
  B. Henoch-Schönlein purpura
  C. Serum sickness and serum sickness-like reactions
  D. Vasculitis associated with malignancy (especially lymphoid neoplasms)
IV. Wegener's granulomatosis
V. Giant cell arteritides:
  A. Temporal arteritis
  B. Takayasu's arteritis
VI. Neoplastic angioendotheliomatosis
VII. Specific disorders associated with vasculitis:
  A. Arteritis associated with lupus erythematous
  B. Arteritis associated with rheumatoid arthritis
  C. Arteritis associated with acute rheumatic fever
  D. Arteritis associated with scleroderma
  E. Arteritis associated with sarcoidosis
VIII. Miscellaneous:
  A. Amyloid angiopathy
  B. Thromboangiitis obliterans
  C. Vasculopathy induced by x-irradiation
  D. Neoplastic encirclement or invasion of vessels
  E. Moya moya disease
IX. Infectious arteritides:
  A. Bacterial
  B. Tuberculous
  C. Syphilitic (meningovascular and gummatous)
  D. Yeast, fungal, parasitic, viral, and rickettsial
    1. Actinomycosis
    2. Aspergillosis
    3. North American blastomycosis
    4. Candidiasis
    5. Cladosporiosis
    6. Coccidioidomycosis
    7. Cryptococcosis
    8. Histoplasmosis
    9. Nocardiosis
    10. Mucormycosis
    11. Cysticercosis
    12. Viral
    13. Rickettsial

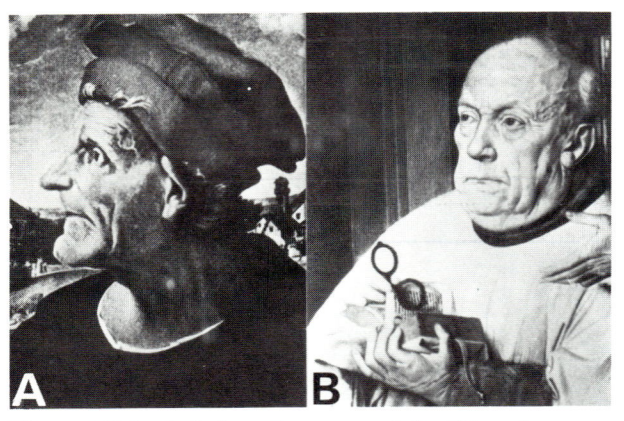

Figure 187-1 Paintings from around the fifteenth century depicting individuals with the appearance suggestive of temporal arteritis. *A. Portrait of Francesco Gamberti* by Pieri di Cosimo, 1505 (Rijkmuseum, Amsterdam). *B.* Canon Vander Paele in Jan Van Eyck's *The Virgin with the Canon*, 1436. (Groeningemuseum, Bruges, Belgium.)

Temporal arteritis appears to be more prevalent in northern climates and in persons of Scandinavian descent; it is quite uncommon in Orientals, Blacks, and American Indians. An incidence of 2.4 per 100,000 per year for the general population and 17.4 per 100,000 per year for those over the age of 50 and a prevalence rate of 133 per 100,000 in the later age group have been recorded in Olmstead County, Minnesota. Of the affected individuals, 65 percent are women. The highest incidence occurs in individuals over 70 years of age. There have been sporadic reports of familial aggregation of the disease, suggesting a genetic influence; yet no HLA type consistently identifies the disease.

Clinical Features

The onset may be abrupt, but quite frequently vague constitutional symptoms such as fatigue, malaise, weight loss, or low-grade fever have been present for weeks to months before a definitive diagnosis is made. "Occult malignancy," "fever of unknown origin," or "depression" is often the admitting diagnosis. Severe boring headaches localized to the temporal regions are seen as an initial symptom in 90 percent of the affected individuals. Variations in the nature and location of the headache are sufficiently common to warrant a high index of suspicion of temporal arteritis in any elderly individual with the onset of a new headache. Scalp pain may be present, especially around the superficial temporal or occipital artery, which may worsen with combing the hair, wearing a hat, or laying the head on a pillow. The superficial temporal artery may be swollen, nodular, tender, and pulseless. Jaw claudication after chewing is thought to be pathognomonic of the disease. It results from involvement of the facial artery; less commonly, claudication in the tongue ("tongue angina"), pharyngeal muscles, calf, or arm may occur. Rarely, gangrene of the scalp, tongue, or an extremity may set in due to vascular occlusion.

Visual symptoms are present in 25 to 50 percent of affected individuals, but permanent visual loss has been recorded in only 5 to 10 percent of patients. Patients generally have systemic symptoms for several weeks or months before visual symptoms set in. Although abrupt blindness frequently occurs, a history of amaurosis fugax, scintillating scotomata, or transient diplopia often precedes the onset of blindness. Visual loss is a reflection of ischemia of the retina or optic nerve secondary to involvement of the ophthalmic, posterior ciliary, or less commonly the central retinal artery. Rarely, cortical blindness may occur from infarction of the calcarine cortex. Funduscopic examination will show evidence of ischemic optic neuropathy with a swollen pale disc, small hemorrhages, and a few retinal cotton-wool patches. These features coupled with pallor of the opposite disc constitute the "pseudo Foster-Kennedy syndrome." In cases of central retinal artery occlusion, the retinal vessels appear obliterated, the disc is swollen, and the macula appears cherry red. In retrobulbar ischemic neuropathy, the fundus may appear normal.

Involvement of the contralateral eye can occur within a few days or weeks. Blindness, once it occurs, usually is irreversible; thus the primary goal in management is the prevention of blindness with prompt treatment with corticosteroids once the diagnosis is suspected or established. Extraocular muscle palsy or ptosis may occur due to involvement of the vasa nervorum of the cranial nerves supplying these muscles.

A forme fruste variant is "occult" temporal arteritis. The patient presents with the sudden onset of blindness without any other associated symptoms although a temporal artery biopsy is positive for arteritis.

The aorta or its major branches may be involved with giant cell arteritis. Involvement of the subclavian, axillary, and brachial arteries may produce claudication in the arm, bruits over the major arterial trunks, and decreased pulses. The common or internal carotid artery may be tender, swollen, and cordlike. Aortic dissection or rupture has been reported. Although the renal arteries may be involved, the renal parenchyma is rarely affected, thus differentiating this from polyarteritis nodosa. Occasional instances of myocardial infarction from coronary arteritis have been reported.

Polymyalgia Rheumatica

This symptom complex[2] occurs in about half of the patients with temporal arteritis; it may begin before the symptoms related to arteritis develop, or occur concurrently with them or develop after they appear. Polymyalgia rheumatica consists of arthralgias and myalgias in the neck, shoulder, and hip girdle associated with an elevated sedimentation rate. The symptoms are maximal on arising in the morning. The muscles are not tender to palpation. Muscle enzymes and electrical and histological studies of the muscles are normal. Inflammatory synovitis of the affected joints, which perhaps explains the clinical symptomatology, may be demonstrated with radionuclide scanning and with histological examination. In about a third of the patients with polymyalgia rheumatica, temporal artery biopsy will show evidence of arteritis in the absence of specific clinical symptoms related to the arteries.

Vasculopathies

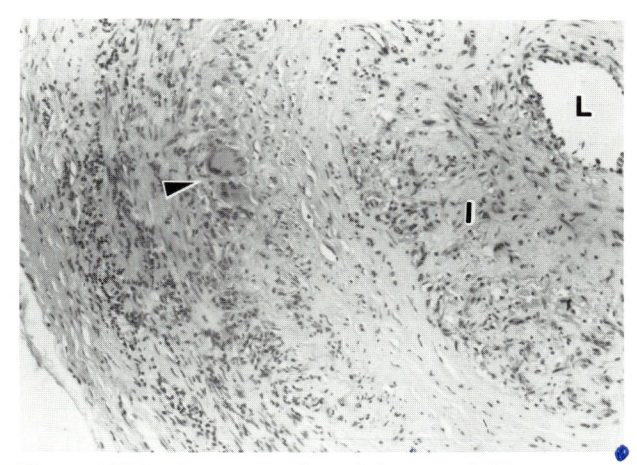

Figure 187-2 A cross section of the superficial temporal artery showing features characteristic of temporal arteritis: narrowing of the lumen (L), fibrous thickening of the intima (I), giant cells (*arrowhead*) at the usual site of the internal elastic lamina, and diffuse mononuclear infiltration of the media and adventitia. (Courtesy of Venkata R. Challa, M.D.)

Pathology

Any one or a combination of the following features may be found (Fig. 187-2): (1) disruption of the internal elastic membrane; (2) the presence of Langhans giant cells in the region of the internal elastic membrane; (3) an inflammatory infiltrate consisting of lymphocytes, eosinophils, plasma cells, and, less frequently, neutrophils through all layers of the vessel wall; and (4) intimal proliferation and thrombosis. The giant cells are not always present; their presence is unrelated to prognosis.

Some have hypothesized that the damage to the elastin in the arterial wall is the primary inciting factor and that the mononuclear inflammatory response along the disrupted internal elastic membrane represents an autoimmune reaction to elastin. Involvement primarily of extracranial branches of the carotid artery, which are rich in elastin, lends some support to this hypothesis.

Laboratory Data

The erythrocyte sedimentation rate (Westergren) is consistently elevated (usually greater than 50 mm/h), although occasional cases of biopsy-proven temporal arteritis with a normal sedimentation rate have been reported. Mild normochromic or hypochromic anemia with hemoglobin values in the range of 9 to 12 g/dl is common. The leukocyte count is usually normal, but mild elevation may occur. Serum protein electrophoresis reveals an increase in α-2 globulin and fibrinogen. Hepatocellular dysfunction may be reflected in an increase in serum glutamic oxaloacetic transaminase and alkaline phosphatase levels. A liver biopsy may show granulomatous hepatitis.

Diagnosis

Selective arteriography of the superficial temporal artery has been recommended in the past: (1) to diagnose the disease solely on the basis of angiographic abnormalities or (2) to identify pathological segments of the affected artery to aid in the selection of a biopsy site since in about 30 percent of patients "skip lesions" occur. Practical experience with arteriography, however, has been disappointing. No pattern of angiographic abnormality typical for giant cell arteritis has been found. The findings consist of nonspecific segmental narrowing of the vessel, a finding representative far more often of atherosclerosis than giant cell arteritis in a geriatric population. Temporal arteriography is not a substitute for temporal artery biopsy.

Temporal artery biopsy is the most crucial and most specific diagnostic study. At least 3 to 5 cm of the artery should be removed to make sure that representative pathological segments are included in the specimen. Before biopsy of the artery is undertaken, careful attention must be paid to the clinical data to make certain that the patient is not dependent upon the superficial temporal artery as a major collateral channel in perfusing the brain due to occlusion of the internal carotid artery in the neck, or that the patient may not require this artery for bypass grafting for the same reason.

Treatment

Corticosteroid therapy should be instituted as soon as the diagnosis is suspected or established. If the clinical history and findings are suggestive of temporal arteritis, blood is drawn for a sedimentation rate and electrophoresis, the patient is started on 45 to 60 mg of prednisone daily in divided doses, and temporal artery biopsy is scheduled for the next elective day. One should not postpone the therapy with steroids until arterial biopsy is completed, because a few days of steroid therapy does not materially alter the histological appearances of the lesion. Symptoms dramatically respond, and the sedimentation rate drops rapidly with prednisone. The effective starting dose should be continued until the clinical symptoms and laboratory data have normalized. This generally takes 3 weeks to a month. Thereafter, the prednisone dosage is tapered gradually to a maintenance level of 15 to 25 mg daily. Therapy should be monitored with clinical evaluations and sedimentation rate determinations. Occasional exacerbations may require a temporary increase in the dose of the steroid. Therapy may have to be continued for 6 months to 2 years. Alternate-day steroid therapy has been shown to be not as effective as daily therapy. Once visual loss sets in, it is not generally reversed by steroid therapy. In patients with polymyalgia rheumatica without vascular signs or symptoms, treatment with nonsteroidal anti-inflammatory drugs may be adequate. Long-term steroid therapy may be associated with certain well-known complications, for example, osteoporosis and compression fracture of a vertebra, the development of cushingoid features, gastrointestinal bleeding, aseptic necrosis of the femoral head, steroid myopathy, and an increased requirement for insulin in diabetics, to cite a few.

Although the symptoms of this disease are effectively controlled with steroid therapy, the length of survival remains unaffected with therapy.

Takayasu's Arteritis

Takayasu's arteritis (synonyms: pulseless disease, aortic arch arteritis, obliterative brachiocephalic arteritis, reversed coarctation syndrome), a rarer form of giant cell arteritis, is named after a Japanese ophthalmologist who described the ocular manifestation of the disease. There are many similarities and differences between temporal arteritis and Takayasu's arteritis (Table 187-2).

Takayasu's disease has a strong predilection for young women (10 to 45 years), with a female to male ratio of 7:1. Although reported from throughout the world, most cases have been from Japan. The etiology of the disease is unknown, but the demonstration of high titers of antiaorta antibodies in a significant number of proven cases suggest an autoimmune process directed against the aorta and its major branches. Typically the arch of the aorta and its major branches, the brachiocephalic, common carotid, and subclavian arteries, are afflicted. In a third of the patients, there may be evidence of involvement of the descending thoracic and abdominal aorta and their branches.

The histology of the affected vessel is one of granulomatous panarteritis. In the early stages, granulomatous inflammation with infiltration of lymphocytes, plasma cells, reticular cells, and multinucleate giant cells occurs at the junction of the media and adventitia. The inflammation then spreads through the thickness of the vessel wall. Lymphocytic infiltration and endothelial proliferation occur around the vasa vasorum. The elastic fibers and the smooth muscles in the media undergo necrosis and are replaced by collagen fibers. In the end stages, fibrosis of the media and adventitia and thickening of the intima lead to severe stenosis of the affected vessel. Thrombotic occlusion of the lumen occurs terminally. Ectatic dilatation and aneurysm formation from weakening of the vessel wall from scarring occur infrequently.

Early prodromal symptoms include asthenia, lassitude, weight loss, vague musculoskeletal pain, arthralgias, pain over the involved arteries, and low-grade fever. As the stenosis of the arteries occurs, symptoms and signs of ischemia

TABLE 187-2 Comparison of Two of the Giant Cell Arteritides

	Temporal Arteritis	**Takayasu's Arteritis**
Epidemiology	Disease of the elderly (50–90 years); slightly higher preponderance in women; more prevalent in northern climates, especially in persons of Scandinavian descent; quite uncommon in Orientals, blacks, and American Indians.	Disease of young women and children (10–45 years); male to female ratio is 1:7; although reported from all over the world, most cases are from Japan.
Arteries involved	Typically involves branches of the external carotid artery; involvement of the ophthalmic, posterior ciliary, or central retinal artery leads to blindness; the aorta or its branches may sometimes be involved.	Typically involves the arch of the aorta and its major branches; less commonly the abdominal aorta and its branches may be involved.
Pathology	Granulomatous panarteritis; disruption of the internal elastic membrane is an early feature; inflammatory infiltrate consists of lymphocytes, eosinophils, plasma cells, Langhans-type giant cells, and less frequently neutrophils through all layers of the vessel wall.	Histological changes are virtually similar to those of temporal arteritis except for the following subtle differences: infiltration by giant cells is less common in Takayasu's arteritis; in general, temporal arteritis begins in the media, whereas Takayasu's arteritis begins at the junction of the media and adventitia.
Etiology	Thought to be an autoimmune process directed against the elastic lamina of the arteries.	An autoimmune process directed against the aorta and its major branches; high titers of antiaorta antibodies support this hypothesis.
Clinical manifestations	Prodrome consisting of malaise, fatigue, loss of appetite, and anemia, followed by headaches. Half of the patients have manifestations of polymyalgia rheumatica. Blindness is a dreaded complication.	Prodromal symptoms are present but may not be striking. Symptoms and signs related to decreased blood flow to the head and upper extremities: vertigo, syncope, convulsions, dementia, trophic changes in the skin and mucous membranes of the head, impaired or absent pulses in the upper extremities, bruit in the neck.
Laboratory data	Elevated sedimentation rate; mild anemia; increase in α-2 globulin and fibrinogen. Evidence of hepatocellular dysfunction. Temporal artery biopsy may show pathognomonic changes.	Elevated sedimentation rate; aortography may show stenosis or occlusion of the aortic arch or its major branches; results of arterial biopsy are pathognomonic.
Treatment	Dramatic response to steroid therapy. The disease is self-limited.	Moderate response to steroid therapy; the disease is usually relentlessly progressive; surgical excision of a stenotic segment and grafting may be necessary.

Vasculopathies

of the head and upper extremities set in. These include dizziness, syncope, visual impairment, convulsions, dementia, and claudication in the upper limbs. All symptoms seem to worsen with activity. The upper limbs may feel cool and be pulseless. Bruits may be heard over the root of the neck. Trophic changes consisting of atrophic skin over the face and scalp, alopecia, loss of teeth, and ulcerations of the lips and the tip of the nose may occur in the late stages. The patient may assume a stooped, head-low position in an attempt to improve the blood supply to the head. Hypertension that occurs in about half of the patients may be from narrowing of the thoracic or abdominal aorta, rigidity of the aortic wall, or renal artery involvement. To detect the hypertension, the blood pressure has to be recorded from the legs.

The erythrocyte sedimentation rate is elevated, a normochromic, normocytic anemia may be found, and α-2 globulin, fibrinogen, and γ-globulin values may be elevated. Aortography may show segmental stenosis or occlusion. Biopsy of the affected vessel confirms the diagnosis.

Steroids are helpful in suppressing the early systemic symptoms and reducing the inflammation of the affected arteries. The response to steroids, however, is not as striking as in temporal arteritis.

After collagenization occurs, surgical measures to resect or bypass a stenotic segment should be resorted to. The disease is relentlessly progressive. Death usually occurs from congestive heart failure or a cerebrovascular accident. The roles of anticoagulants, vasodilators, and cytotoxic drugs in this disease remain to be elucidated.

Primary Cerebral Amyloid (Congophilic) Angiopathy

Primary cerebral amyloid angiopathy, as the name implies, is a clinicopathological entity characterized by deposition of amyloid substance in the walls of cerebral and leptomeningeal vessels.[10] It is thought to be a variant of Alzheimer's disease. The following distinguishing characteristics justify its separation into a distinct nosological entity: (1) Patients with amyloid angiopathy may not present with dementia; (2) senile plaques may not be found with amyloid angiopathy; and (3) most patients with Alzheimer's disease do not have vascular deposition of amyloid.

Amyloid was originally thought to be a starchlike substance because of its characteristic reaction with iodine, but recent chemical analysis indicates that it is a protein. The nature of the protein varies in different disorders where amyloid deposition occurs, thus accounting for different types of amyloid. The amyloid protein that is deposited in the central nervous system is believed to be the light chain component of γ-globulin. In central nervous system amyloidosis, the viscera are spared; the reverse occurs in systemic amyloidosis with a few exceptions.

The cardinal clinical manifestation of amyloid angiopathy is dementia, although as stated earlier, a subset of patients may exhibit an exception to this rule. The clinical and radiological features may on occasion simulate the low-pressure hydrocephalus syndrome, but cerebrospinal fluid shunting fails to reverse the symptoms. Operative procedures on the brain in patients with cerebral amyloid angiopathy carry a higher than usual risk of postoperative hemorrhagic complications. This is attributed to the inability of amyloid-laden vessels to contract normally. Another complication of neurosurgical interest is the occurrence of spontaneous intracerebral hematomas. The occurrence of nontraumatic intracerebral hemorrhage in a normotensive elderly dement should arouse a suspicion of cerebral amyloid angiopathy. The extent of bleeding varies from small petechiae to massive intracerebral hematomas (Fig. 187-3). These hemorrhages are usually multiple in both time and location. In contrast to the hypertensive hemorrhages which occur predominantly in the basal ganglia, pons, or cerebellum, hematomas from amyloid angiopathy tend to be near the cortical surface in the parietal or occipital area. It is estimated that amyloid angiopathy accounts for 2 percent of all spontaneous intracerebral hematomas in adults. Weakening of the vessel wall due to the deposition of amyloid is thought to precipitate rupture of cortical vessels; occurrence of fibrinoid necrosis and microaneurysms in hypertensive individuals further potentiates the problem.

Cases of amyloid angiopathy reported from the United States are of the sporadic form. A familial form has been described from Japan and Europe. A notable example was reported by Gudmundsson et al. from Reykjavik, now designated as the "icelandic form" of amyloid angiopathy. In their study, a survey of a family tree consisting of 117 individuals through four generations showed that 22 suffered from cerebral hemorrhage. In contrast to the sporadic form, the patients were young at the time of their death, were not demented, and lacked senile plaques. In a recent report of 23 well-documented cases of amyloid angiopathy from the Mayo Clinic, Okazaki et al. emphasized the frequency of multiple ischemic cerebral lesions in their patients. The clinical picture was one of transient ischemic attacks, single or multiple strokes, or dementia. Dementia in amyloid angiopathy is thought to be due to the presence of senile plaques. Numerical correlations have been made between the senile plaques and dementia.

There are no specific diagnostic tests, other than brain biopsy, to establish the diagnosis of cerebral amyloidosis.

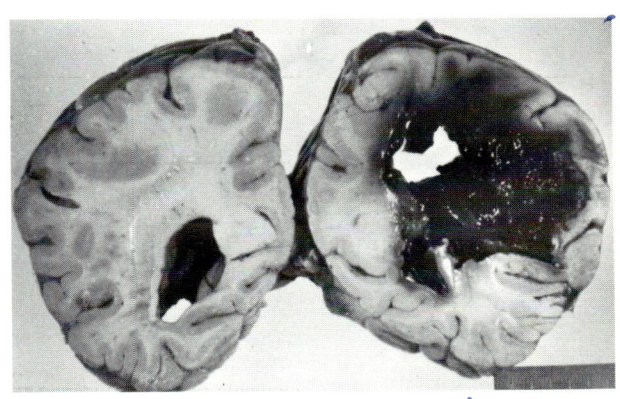

Figure 187-3 An intracerebral hematoma with rupture into the ventricular system in a patient with amyloid angiopathy.

The histological diagnosis of amyloid angiopathy is made from certain specific tinctorial properties. With the hematoxylin and eosin stain, uniformly pink staining hyaline amyloid material may be seen in the vessel wall. The outline of the vessel may be fuzzy and indistinct due to the spread of the amyloid infiltrate into the adjacent neuropil. Sections stained with crystal violet will show evidence of metachromasia. With the Congo red stain, a deep purplish red staining of the vessel may be noted; when the same section is viewed under polarized light, a greenish yellow birefringence will be apparent (Fig. 187-4). With electron microscopy, characteristic filamentous amyloid fibrils measuring 90 to 95 mm in diameter may be noted in the vessel wall and the adjacent perivascular extracellular space (Fig. 187-5).

Vasculopathy Associated with Drug Abuse

Numerous intracranial complications are known to occur among drug abusers. These are attributable to "behavioral toxicity," pharmacologic toxicity, or infectious complications. Behavioral toxicity refers to the irrational acts committed by the drug abuser under the influence of the drugs which may lead to physical injury to himself such as a high-speed automobile accident, drowning, or a fall from a height. Infectious complications resulting from the injection of drugs under unsterile conditions may lead to bacterial endocarditis, septic emboli, infectious intracranial vasculitis, aneurysms, subarachnoid hemorrhage, and brain abscess.

A noninfectious necrotizing vasculopathy with histological features similar to polyarteritis nodosa involving multiple organ systems including the brain has been reported among drug abusers. Since most abusers use multiple drugs, it is hard to incriminate a single agent in the induction of vasculopathy, but amphetamine or metamphetamine seems to be the most likely causal agent.[6,12] The clinical picture may be one of acute intracerebral hemorrhage or ischemic cerebrovascular stroke. A computed tomogram may confirm the

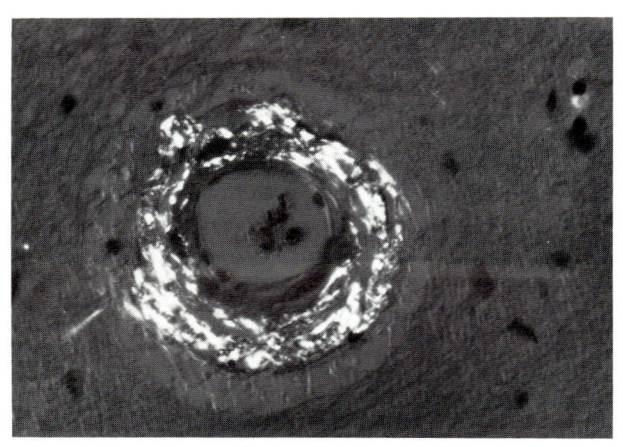

Figure 187-4 An amyloid-laden blood vessel in a section stained with Congo red and viewed with polarized light to show the birefringence of the amyloid.

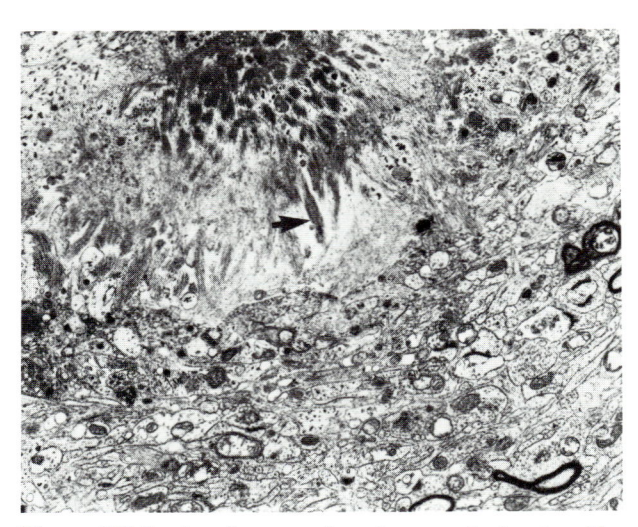

Figure 187-5 An electron microphotograph showing filamentous amyloid fibrils in the perivascular extracellular space (*arrow*).

presence of a hematoma in the brain parenchyma or ventricular system, and a cerebral arteriogram may show beading from segmental luminal irregularities, indistinctness of vessel outlines, microaneurysm formation, or arterial spasm or thrombosis. Histological examination of the involved arteries may show fibrinoid necrosis with cellular infiltration.

Drug-induced vasculopathy responds to steroid therapy with reversal of the abnormal features seen on arteriography. An intracerebral hematoma may need to be removed surgically.

Transverse myelopathy may occur with narcotic abuse (morphine or heroin). The extent of abuse may range from a single exposure to many years of addiction. Symptoms referable to the spinal cord generally appear on resumption of narcotic use following a period of enforced abstinence in a prison or hospital. This sequence of antigenic sensitization and challenge suggests a hypersensitivity reaction to the narcotic or adulterant. In a typical sequence, an addict goes to sleep or becomes comatose after self-administration of the drug. It is thought that during this interval he may become severely hypotensive from the effect of the drug, although this is not well documented. He awakens to find that he is unable to move his legs or void. Neurological examination indicates a transverse myelopathy involving the midthoracic cord with flaccid weakness of muscles, an atonic bladder, and absent muscle stretch reflexes. Over a period of days to weeks the weakness may improve, or it may remain unchanged, progressing to spastic paraplegia. The cerebrospinal fluid may show mild pleocytosis and an increase in protein content. Myelogram may either be normal or show widening of the spinal cord. In the instances where the latter is mistaken for a tumor, biopsy has yielded only necrotic tissue. In autopsy specimens, necrosis is frequently restricted to the gray matter, although segmental infarction in the distribution of a spinal artery may occur. On rare occasions vasculitis involving the small arteries and arterioles with fibrinoid necrosis and proliferating thickening of the vessel wall may be present. Doubly refractile foreign particles seen in histological sections may represent adulterants present in black market drugs. Involvement of the midthoracic segment of the spinal cord is attributed to marginal blood supply in this "watershed" region which presumably is reduced to ischemic levels with severe hypotension after intravenous opiate administration. Associated vasculopathy may further compound the ischemia.

Neoplastic Angioendotheliomatosis

Neoplastic angioendotheliomatosis is a rare and unique form of vascular malignancy, probably of endothelial origin, which affects smaller arteries, arterioles, capillaries, and veins of virtually every organ system in the body.[1,11] Malignant transformation and intraluminal proliferation of vascular endothelial cells result in packing of vascular lumina with neoplastic cells, with resultant impediment to blood flow, and tissue ischemia (Fig. 187-6). The malignant cells remain confined to the lumina; extravascular invasion or distant metastasis is unusual. The disease is relentlessly progressive and is invariably fatal. The longest known survival after the onset of symptoms is 32 months.

Since the original description of the Viennese authors Pfleger and Tappiner in 1959, who documented the cutaneous manifestations of the disease, numerous case reports have appeared in the literature to allow this disease to be recognized as a distinct clinicopathological entity. Strouth and his associates were the first to emphasize the nervous system manifestations of the disease. Although vascular involvement is generalized, with virtually no tissue being spared, the clinical manifestations broadly fall under two equally frequent classes representing primarily cutaneous central nervous system involvement. Adrenal gland involvement in a few cases has resulted in an addisonian syndrome.

Although most patients have been in their fifth through eighth decades at the time of the onset of symptoms, no age group is exempt; the sexes are affected about equally. The most frequent and dominant symptom of central nervous system involvement is confusion and rapidly progressing dementia. Although certain specific intellectual faculties appear to be involved in the initial phases, relentless progression of the multi-infarct syndrome leads to global dementia. Lethargy and stupor may set in in the later stages, ultimately culminating in coma. Superimposed on this background of intellectual impairment are numerous focal neurological symptoms and signs such as transient ischemic attacks with brief episodes of paralysis, numbness, or blindness. A strokelike syndrome with the sudden onset of hemiparesis may occur. Dysphasia and abulia have been reported. Seizures are not uncommon. Infarction of the spinal cord may result in the sudden onset of a flaccid paraplegia. Thus, the rapid clinical progression of an array of generalized or multifocal neurological symptoms and signs with negative laboratory data and virtually nondiagnostic radiological tests frustrates the clinician, who feels helpless until a tissue diagnosis is established by brain biopsy. Indeed in many instances, an antemortem diagnosis had not been made.

The cerebrospinal fluid protein level is frequently elevated, but the cytology has been consistently negative. If the computed tomograms show any abnormality at all, it consists of low-density areas in the brain parenchyma consistent with infarction, in rare instances the infarction may be massive or hemorrhagic and may produce a mass effect. The cerebral arteriograms do not show any changes; in an isolated instance a picture of arteritis has been seen.

The leptomeningeal vessels are most frequently affected. The vessels are filled with hyperchromatic tumor cells with a high nuclear to cytoplasmic ratio. The nuclei are large and vesicular with prominent nucleoli. Unlike angiosarcoma, there is no tendency to the formation of solid tumor and no vascularization of the tumor tissue, and metastasis is very rare. In some vessels, the tumor cells merely fill the lumen which is lined by the non-neoplastic endothelial lining of the blood vessel wall. Fibrin deposition occurs between tumor cells. An inflammatory reaction consisting of plasma cells and lymphocytes occurs around the adventitia of the vessels. Transmural invasion of neoplastic cells is of rare occurrence. Thrombosis of vessels may occur. Areas of infarct around the blood vessels denote irreversible tissue ischemia, which is the basis of the clinical symptomatology.

The immunoperoxidase technique has failed to demonstrate factor VIII related antigen (an endothelial cell marker) on the neoplastic cells. This is thought to be due to dedifferentiation during the process of malignant transformation. However, an ultrastructural marker for endothelial cells, the Weibel-Palade body, has been frequently observed in the neoplastic cells. Histocytochemical studies have shown that the neoplastic cells have lost their oxidative enzymatic activity compared with that of their normal counterparts. An attractive hypothesis regarding the pathogenesis of this entity is that it results from the inappropriate secretion of a substance resembling the tumor angiogenesis factor.

The prognosis is dismal. Frequently the definitive diagnosis is made late in the clinical course of the disease, if at all. Steroids have offered transient symptomatic relief in some instances, and combination chemotherapy on rare occasions has induced a remission, but survival is generally measured in months.

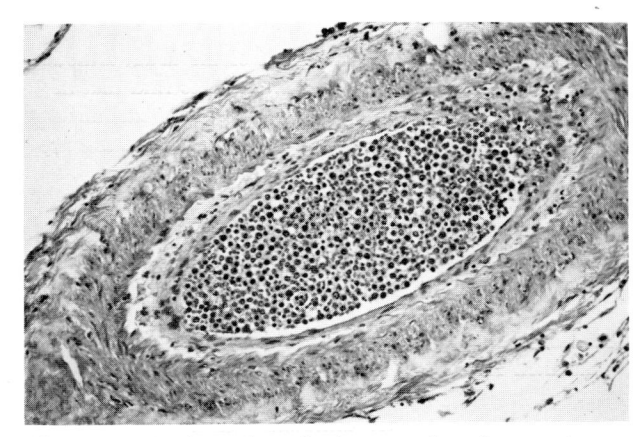

Figure 187-6 A section of a leptomeningeal artery in a patient with proven angioendotheliomatosis. The vessel is occluded by malignant cells. The endothelial cells appear normal, indicating secondary accumulation of tumor cells at this site. (Courtesy of Bernd W. Scheithauer, M.D.)

Granulomatous Angiitis

Granulomatous angiitis in an uncommon noninfectious necrotizing vasculopathy of unknown etiology affecting predominantly or exclusively the central nervous system.[4,8] Extracerebral vessels are rarely affected. Although frequently fatal and not diagnosed until after death, there are recent reports of cases, diagnosed on the basis of surgical biopsy, that have been successfully treated.

The disease presents as a diffuse or multifocal encephalopathy or transverse myelopathy. It generally affects middle-aged or elderly adults, with no predilection for sex or race. The onset is characterized by confusion, loss of memory, disorientation, and intellectual impairment. Progressive impairment of consciousness occurs as the disease progresses. Focal cerebral manifestations and seizures may be present during the course of the disease. About 15 percent of the reported cases have been associated with lymphomas (usually of the Hodgkin's type) and *Herpes zoster* infection (usually in the trigeminal distribution), suggesting a causal relationship to these entities. Indeed patients with granulomatous angiitis harboring lymphomas improve from their vasculopathy if the lymphoma is brought to remission with no specific therapy directed toward the angiopathy. In patients with *Herpes zoster* ophthalmicus, the virus is thought to spread along the first division of the trigeminal nerve to the internal carotid siphon and its proximal branches, inducing focal granulomatous angiitis. Contralateral hemiplegia may result. Spread through the subarachnoid space is thought to result in diffuse angiitis.[9] A causal relationship to the zoster virus is suspected but not proved.

Small arteries, arterioles, and venules less than 200 μm in diameter are generally affected. Leptomeningeal vessels are especially involved. Histological changes include fibrinoid necrosis of the vessel wall, and a variable inflammatory infiltration consisting of polymorphonuclear leukocytes, lymphocytes, epithelioid-appearing histiocytes, and multinucleated foreign body or Langhans-type giant cells. The segmental vasculitis may be associated with parenchymal ischemic or hemorrhagic infarcts.

Computed tomographic scans show multiple areas of poorly defined nonenhancing low-density lesions. Cerebral arteriograms shows signs of vasculitis which are nonspecific.

References

1. Beal MF, Fisher CM: Neoplastic angioendotheliosis. J Neurol Sci 53:359–375, 1982.
2. Chuang TY, Hunder GG, Ilstrup DM, Kurland LT: Polymyalgia rheumatica: A 10 year epidemiologic and clinical study. Ann Intern Med 97:672–680, 1982.
3. Dequeker JV: Polymyalgia rheumatica with temporal arteritis, as painted by Jan Van Eyck in 1436. Can Med Assoc J 124:1597–1598, 1981.
4. Faer MJ, Mead JH, Lynch RD: Cerebral granulomatous angiitis: Case report and literature review. AJR 129:463–467, 1977.
5. Fauci AS, Haynes BF, Katz P: The spectrum of vasculitis: Clinical, pathologic, immunologic, and therapeutic considerations. Ann Intern Med 89 (Part 1):660–676, 1978.
6. Harrington H, Heller HA, Dawson D, Caplan L, Rumbaugh C: Intracerebral hemorrhage and oral amphetamine. Arch Neurol 40:503–507, 1983.
7. Huston KA, Hunder GG: Giant cell (cranial) arteritis: A clinical review. Am Heart J 100:99–107, 1980.
8. Kolodny EH, Rebeiz JJ, Caviness VS Jr, Richardson EP Jr: Granulomatous angiitis of the central nervous system. Arch Neurol 19:510–524, 1968.
9. MacKenzie RA, Forbes GS, Karnes WE: Angiographic findings in herpes zoster arteritis. Ann Neurol 10:458–464, 1981.
10. Rengachary SS, Racela LS, Watanabe I, Abdou N: Neurosurgical and immunological implications of primary cerebral amyloid (congophilic) angiopathy. Neurosurgery 7:1–9, 1980.
11. Wick MR, Scheithauer BW, Okazaki H, Thomas JE: Cerebral angioendotheliomatosis. Arch Pathol Lab Med 106:342–346, 1982.
12. Yu YJ, Cooper DR, Wellenstein DE, Block B: Cerebral angiitis and intracerebral hemorrhage associated with methamphetamine abuse. J Neurosurg 58:109–111, 1983.

Part VIII

Trauma

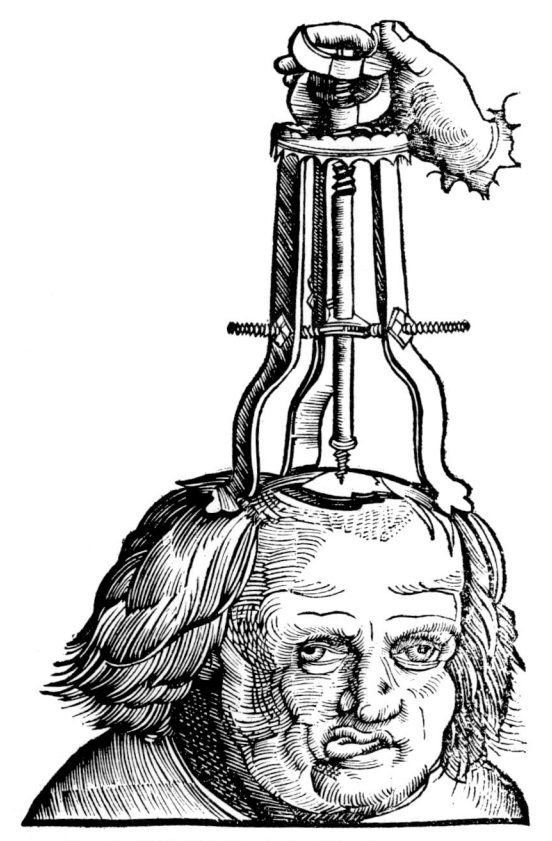

von Gersdorff H. *Feldtbuch der Wundartzney*. Strassbourg, J Schott, 1517. An illustration showing the method of elevating depressed skull fractures. Right third and twelfth nerve palsies and left facial weakness are present.

SECTION A
Cranial Trauma

188
Biomechanics of Head Injury

Thomas A. Gennarelli
Lawrence E. Thibault

How mechanical energy injures the head has been of interest to physicians for centuries. Gradually a picture has emerged that now permits a comprehensive understanding of the causes of many types of head injury. In this chapter we will review the state-of-the-art knowledge of the mechanical events that result in the numerous varieties of head injury that we encounter clinically.

To understand how an individual mechanical input to the head results in a particular type of head injury, one must consider multiple factors. First, the nature, the severity, and the site and direction of mechanical input to the head are important. The manner in which the head responds to that input will determine what structures are injured and to what extent they are injured. Finally, the total injury produced by mechanical trauma depends not only on the primary mechanical damage but also on the complex interaction of pathophysiological events that follow. This chapter will concern only the primary mechanical events.

In general terms, primary head injuries include three distinct varieties, each having a unique set of mechanical etiology (Table 188-1). *Skull fracture* can occur with or without damage to the brain, but is itself usually not an important cause of neurological disability. Injuries to the vascular or neural elements of the brain and its coverings cause neurological dysfunction and can be readily divided into two categories, each of which has, for the most part, different mechanistic causes. *Focal injuries* result from localized damage and account for approximately 50 percent of all hospital admissions for head injury.[1,3a] The cortical contusions, subdural hematomas, epidural hematomas, and intracerebral hematomas that constitute focal injuries are responsible for two-thirds of head injury associated deaths.[4] *Diffuse brain injuries* are associated with widespread brain damage. This damage may be principally functional, as in the case of concussive injuries, or may be structural, as seen in prolonged traumatic coma unassociated with mass lesions, a condition recently termed *diffuse axonal injury*.[2,3a,6] Diffuse brain injuries account for approximately 40 percent of hospitalized head-injured patients and for one-third of the deaths, and are the most serious cause of persisting neurological disability in survivors.

Mechanisms of Injury

The types of mechanical loading of the head are numerous and complex.[9] Input can be either slow (static loading) or, as more commonly occurs, rapid (dynamic loading). Static loading implies that the injury forces are applied gradually, usually over 200 ms or longer. This is comparable to a slow squeezing effect, and if sufficient force is applied, serious multiple skull fractures result. After the skull has absorbed as much energy as it can withstand, it begins to crush, the brain itself becomes compressed and distorted, and serious or fatal brain injury occurs. Static loading is so uncommon that it will not be discussed in further detail.

The most frequent type of mechanical input is dynamic input. Here the injury forces act in less than 200 ms, and in most cases in less than 50 ms. As will be seen later, the duration of the input is a critical factor in determining which type of head injury occurs. Dynamic loading can be of two types, impulsive loading and impact loading. *Impulsive loading* occurs when the head is set into motion (or when the moving head is stopped) without the head being struck. These conditions occur not infrequently, as when a child is shaken by the shoulders or when a blow occurs to the body in such a manner that the head moves violently (blows to the

TABLE 188-1 The Primary Head Injuries

Skull Fractures	Focal Injuries	Diffuse Injuries
Linear	Contusions	Concussion
Depressed	Coup	Mild
Basilar	Contrecoup	Classical
	Intermediate	Diffuse axonal injury
	Hematomas	Mild
	Extradural	Moderate
	Subdural	Severe
	Intracerebral	

face or impact to the chest or thorax). In these circumstances, there is no impact to the cranium, and the resulting head injuries are caused solely by the inertial forces that result from head acceleration or deceleration.

Impact loading is the more frequent type of dynamic loading and usually causes acceleration of the head (inertial effects), as well as many regionalized effects known as contact phenomena. The inertial effects can be minimal in certain impact conditions if the head is prevented from moving when it is struck. The contact phenomena are a complex group of mechanical events that occur both near and distant from the point of impact. The magnitude and importance of these contact phenomena vary with the size of the impacting device and with the magnitude of force of the impact. Immediately beneath the point of impact there is localized skull deformation, with inbending of the skull surrounded by outbending of the skull peripheral to the impact site. If the degree of local skull deformation is significant, penetration, perforation, or fracture of the skull occurs. Additionally, shock waves that travel at the speed of sound propagate throughout the skull from the point of impact, as well as directly through the brain substance. The shock waves cause local changes in tissue pressure, and if these result in sufficient brain distortion, brain damage results.

The strains induced by the inertial (acceleration-deceleration) or by the contact (skull bending, shock waves) loading are the ultimate and proximate causes of injury. Three types of strain can occur: compression, tension, and shear. The type of injury that results from a particular circumstance is determined by the type and location of the induced strains and by the tissue's ability to withstand those particular strains. Strain is best understood as the amount of deformation that the tissue undergoes as a result of mechanical loading. Tensile strain, for example, is the amount of elongation that occurs when a material is stretched. If a column of rubber 10 cm in length becomes 11 cm long when stretched, it has undergone a 10 percent tensile strain. A glass column under the same load may become only 10.1 cm long, a 1 percent strain. The inherent properties of these two materials are different, not only in how much strain occurs under given loading conditions but also with regard to how much strain is necessary to cause failure (breakage) of the material. Thus the rubber column may tolerate a 20 percent strain before it breaks, while the glass column may break at 0.5 percent strain. In this example the glass rod would have broken, but the rubber column would not have, even though the rubber underwent a greater strain. In addition, biological tissues are viscoelastic; that is, their tolerance to strain changes with the rate at which the mechanical load is applied. Characteristically, biological tissues withstand strain better if they are deformed slowly rather than quickly; that is, they become more brittle and will break at lower strain levels under rapidly applied loads.

The three principal tissues involved in head injury vary considerably in their tolerances to deformation; bone, for example, is considerably stronger than vascular or brain tissue. It therefore requires more force to obtain injurious levels of strain. However, bone shares with vascular and brain tissue the common property of being more able to withstand compressive strains than shear strains, with a tensile strain tolerance somewhere in between. For bone there is proportionately less difference between the three strain tolerances, whereas for brain there is a considerable difference in its ability to withstand compression and shear. Since brain is virtually incompressible and since it has a very low tolerance to tensile and shear strain, the latter two types of strain are the usual causes of brain damage. The same is true for vascular tissue. Whether vascular or brain tissue damage occurs depends on the exact properties of these two tissues. As we will see later, vascular tissue tends to fail under more rapidly applied loading conditions than does brain tissue, and situations exist that, depending on the type of input to the head, can cause relatively pure injury to the vascular elements or to the neural elements within the head.

Mechanistic Causes of Head Injuries

Most head injuries are due to one of two basic mechanisms, contact or acceleration. Contact injuries require that the head strike or be struck, irrespective of whether the blow causes the head to move afterward. Acceleration injuries result from violent head motion, irrespective of whether the head moves because of a direct blow or not (Table 188-2).

Contact Injuries

Contact injuries, in general, are caused by forces that occur during impact. These injuries result solely from contact phenomena and have nothing whatever to do with head motion or head acceleration or deceleration. Since most impacts also set the head into motion, these injuries rarely occur clinically in pure form; more frequently, contact injuries have superimposed acceleration (inertial) injuries. Many times, however, the injuries received by a patient are predominantly contact-related. Contact injuries can therefore be viewed as injuries that would occur if the head were prevented from moving.

Contact forces are twofold in nature: effects that occur locally at or near the impact and effects that occur remote from impact. In both instances, contact injuries cause focal injuries; contact forces do not cause diffuse brain injury (concussion or primary traumatic unconsciousness).

TABLE 188-2 Mechanistic Types of Head Injury

Contact Injuries*	Acceleration Injuries†
Skull deformation injuries	Surface strains
Local:	Subdural hematoma
Skull fracture (linear, depressed)	Contrecoup contusion
Extradural hematoma	Intermediate coup contusion
Coup contusions	Deep strains
Remote:	Concussion syndromes
Vault and basilar fractures	Diffuse axonal injury
Shock wave injuries	
Contrecoup contusion	
Intracerebral hematoma	

*Blow to head necessary; head motion not necessary.
†Direct blow to vault not necessary; head motion necessary.

Local Contact Effects

Injuries due to the local effects of contact forces comprise most linear and depressed skull fractures, epidural hematomas, and coup contusions.

The occurrence of skull fracture depends on the material properties of the skull, the magnitude and the direction of impact, the size of the impact area, and the thickness of the skull in various areas.[8] When an object strikes the head, local skull inbending occurs, and the resulting skull deformation causes a compression strain on the outer table and a tensile strain on the inner table. Since bone is weaker in tension than in compression, sufficient inbending causes a fracture to begin in the inner table. It will then propagate along lines of least resistance from the impact site. The length of the fracture and its direction depend on the thickness of the skull at the impact site. A sufficiently small impactor will focus the impact energy at the impact site and is more prone to cause a depressed fracture or skull perforation, whereas a larger object distributes the impact force over a wider area and is less likely to cause fracture.

The epidural hematoma can be viewed as a complicated variety of skull fracture in which the dural vessels are torn. The mechanical failure of these vessels can occur as a fracture propagates across the vessel, or the vessel may be injured without fracture if there is sufficient skull bending to tear it.

Coup contusions occur beneath the site of impact under certain conditions. Such contusions are due to either direct injury to the brain beneath an area of skull inbending or negative pressures that develop when an area of skull inbending rapidly snaps back into place. The former mechanism causes highly focused compressive strains, whereas the latter subjects the brain surface to very high tensile strains; in either case these strains are sufficient to cause tissue failure of the pial and cortical vessels and of the brain tissue itself. The localized contusion that results is therefore a mixture of vascular and brain disruption. Brain laceration is an extension of the same phenomena, where skull inbending is sufficient to perforate the brain tissue.

Remote Contact Effects

Contact phenomena can cause injury remote from the impact site by two mechanisms: skull distortion and shock waves. Both contribute to vault fractures that occur away from the impact site, to basilar skull fractures, and to contrecoup and the so-called intermediate coup contusions.

Remote vault fracture can occur if the impact occurs over a thick portion of the skull. Local inbending has little effect, but the skull bends out around the impact zone, putting the outer table under tension and the inner table under a compressive strain. If this area of outbending is in a thin area of the skull, a fracture begins in the outer table some distance from the point of impact. The fracture will again propagate along the line of least resistance, usually, but not always, toward the impact site. Often the line of least resistance is not over the vault, and the various characteristic types of basilar skull fracture occur.

Shock waves begin from the point of impact and travel rapidly in all directions from it. Those that spread through the skull contribute to skull distortion and the ensuing basilar and remote vault fractures. Other shock waves spread through the brain in several microseconds and, like waves in water, may reflect from the opposite side of the head and reverberate within the brain. If the shock waves are amplified by this reverberation, the resulting strains may be sufficient to exceed the brain's tolerance. Damage to vascular or brain tissue at sites of strain concentration would result. Although this thesis has been used to explain the genesis of intermediate and contrecoup contusions, the role of shock waves in causing local brain damage has been a matter of debate. It has been argued that because these waves travel exceedingly rapidly through the brain, their effects are so quickly dissipated that they are not an important injury mechanism.

Acceleration (Inertial) Injuries

Inertial loading of the head, whether caused by impact or by impulsive loading, accelerates or decelerates the head. From the mechanical point of view, acceleration and deceleration are the same physical phenomenon and differ only in direction. Thus the effects of accelerating the head in the sagittal plane from posterior to anterior are exactly the same as the effects of decelerating the head from anterior to posterior.

Head acceleration results in compressive, tensile, and shear strains that cause structural damage by one of two mechanisms. First, acceleration damage can be due to differential acceleration of the skull and the brain. This well-known phenomenon occurs because the brain is free to move within the skull and because it lags behind the skull for a brief moment after acceleration begins. The result is that the brain moves relative to the skull and the dura, causing strain on the subdural bridging veins. This is the mechanism that causes most subdural hematomas. Furthermore the movement of the brain away from the skull creates regions of low pressure (tensile strain) which if sufficiently intense cause contrecoup contusions. The second way that acceleration is injurious is that it produces strains within the brain itself. This is the mechanism for diffuse brain injuries (the concussion syndromes and diffuse axonal injury) and the so-called intermediate coup contusions. In diffuse brain injuries that are associated with structural damage, the acceleration loading causes sufficient strains within the brain so that the brain tissue itself is injured; in the case of intermediate coup contusions, the vascular tissue tolerances are exceeded.

The type of acceleration damage that occurs depends on the type of acceleration, the amount of acceleration, the direction of head motion, and the duration of the acceleration load. Three *types of acceleration* can occur: (1) translational acceleration occurs when the brain's center of gravity (roughly the pineal gland) moves in a straight line, (2) rotational acceleration occurs when there is movement about the center of gravity without the center of gravity itself moving, and (3) angular acceleration occurs when components of translational and rotational acceleration are combined. Here there is movement of the center of gravity in an angular manner. Rotational acceleration is a virtual impossibility in clinical situations since it requires that the head must pivot around an axis that goes through the pineal region. This would mean that the whole body swings around the head. However, rotational acceleration may occur, namely with motion in a horizontal plane. Similarly, purely translational acceleration is uncommon, since this type of movement is very unphysiological, except perhaps in the case of acceleration in the superoinferior direction that results from a pure vertex impact. Because of the head-neck anatomy, angular acceleration is the most common type encountered clinically, the center of angulation most often being in the lower cervical spine. The exact location of the center of angulation determines the proportion of translation and rotation that the brain undergoes. As the center of angulation moves higher up the cervical spine, there is a greater rotational component, and when the center of angulation moves lower, there is proportionately more translational acceleration. Knowing the type of acceleration is important since it has been shown that concussive injuries do not occur if the head is not accelerated[3] or if it undergoes a purely translational acceleration,[9] but that concussion readily occurs when the head experiences angular acceleration.[9] Although it does not produce concussion, translational acceleration is injurious and can produce various focal injuries including cortical contusion, intracerebral hematoma, and subdural hematoma. It is not surprising, therefore, that situations exist where substantial brain damage has occurred without loss of consciousness.

However, considering the three types of head acceleration, angular acceleration is not only the most frequent, but the most injurious. Except for skull fracture and epidural hematoma, virtually every known type of head injury can be produced by angular acceleration.[1]

The amount of acceleration damage also depends on the magnitude of the acceleration loading. However, because of the viscoelastic nature of biological tissue, the response of the tissue is determined not only by the acceleration magnitude, but also by the rate at which the acceleration occurs. The acceleration magnitude can be viewed as proportional to the amount of strain delivered to the brain and the acceleration rate to the strain rate. The rate of acceleration varies inversely with the duration for which the acceleration is applied if the acceleration magnitude is constant, and varies directly with the acceleration magnitude if the acceleration duration is constant.

Three zones of interest are encountered as acceleration duration increases at a constant amount of acceleration. First, at very high strain rates (short acceleration durations) the properties of the brain are such that much of the acceleration effects are damped, and as a consequence, the brain actually experiences very little strain. Therefore, extremely high accelerations are required to produce injury. The second zone begins as the acceleration duration is increased slightly. Less damping occurs, and therefore it requires less acceleration to produce injurious strains within the head. However, the strain that occurs under these conditions is confined to the surface, since the acceleration is present for such a short time that the strains cannot penetrate deeply. The types of injury that can be produced in these circumstances are those at the brain surface, notably subdural hematoma. As the duration of acceleration increases further, the third zone begins; less of the inertial effects are damped, and the resulting strains are able to propagate deeper into the brain. This can cause axonal injury and result in prolonged traumatic coma.

Strain rate also increases if, for constant acceleration duration, the acceleration magnitude is increased. In the first zone described above, the strain rate is already so high that increasing it further adds little to the injury pattern. In the second zone, vascular tissues at the brain surface are already jeopardized, and so increasing the strain rate further can exceed the vascular tissue tolerance and cause damage where none existed before or can increase the number of disrupted vessels. In the third zone, where strain rate produces damage to brain tissue but is insufficient to produce vascular damage, increasing the acceleration magnitude can increase the strain rate sufficiently to cause vascular damage.

Therefore, acceleration damage to the brain can be of several types, depending on the amount of acceleration, the duration of acceleration, and the rate at which acceleration is applied to the head. *Structural damage* to superficial vascular tissue, especially to bridging veins and pial vessels, occurs in high strain rate conditions (short acceleration duration), whereas brain tissue, principally axonal, damage occurs in lower strain rate, longer pulse duration circumstances. An intermediate zone exists in which both vascular damage and axonal damage occur. *Functional damage* without gross tissue disruption occurs at lower levels of strain, as is seen in cerebral concussion.

Injuries and Their Mechanisms

This section summarizes the injury mechanisms for each of the several types of clinically important head injuries.

Skull Fracture

Linear Fracture Linear fractures occur solely because of the contact effects due to impact. Acceleration (inertial) effects play no role. A linear fracture is caused by an impacting surface that is of intermediate size; it has to be sufficiently large so that skull penetration does not occur and sufficiently small so that the contact phenomena are not distributed widely over the head. Acceleration injuries may be superimposed, if substantial head motion occurs after impact.

Depressed Fracture Depressed fractures are similar to linear fractures except that the impacting surface is smaller. The contact phenomena are more focused, allowing skull perforation.

Basilar Fracture Basilar fractures are due to the remote effects of skull impact. Stress waves that propagate from the impact point or changes in skull shape due to impact cause them.

Epidural Hematoma

Epidural hematoma, like skull fracture, is not related to head acceleration. Vascular disruption occurs because of contact-related skull fracture or contact-related skull deformation.

Contusions

Coup Contusions Contusion beneath the site of impact is caused by local tissue strains that arise from local skull inbending. In order for such localized effects to occur, the impacting surface must be relatively small and hard. The failure of pial vessels most likely occurs because of high tensile strains that are produced when the focally depressed skull rapidly returns to its normal configuration.

Contrecoup Contusions Superficial focal areas of vascular disruption remote from the site of impact occur principally because of acceleration (inertial) effects. Brain motion toward the impact site causes tensile strains to occur at an area opposite from impact; if the tensile strains that result are larger than the vascular tolerance, contusion results. However, unlike coup contusions, impact is not necessary for contrecoup contusion to occur; the term *coup* is therefore a misnomer, since the critical mechanism is acceleration (or deceleration) and not impact. In situations where the head undergoes impulsive loading, contrecoup lesions occur solely because of the acceleration effects. If impact causes considerable skull distortion (due to stress waves), tensile strains can also occur remote from impact and cause contusional damage, but the predominant mechanism for contrecoup contusions is head acceleration.

The relative proportion of coup versus contrecoup contusions depends on the response of the head to impact, that is, on how much of the impact energy is converted into head motion. A hard, small impact surface (hammer blow) tends to produce focal skull deformation with underlying coup contusion, but since much of the energy is dissipated at the impact site, there is little head acceleration and consequently little or very small contrecoup contusion. On the other hand, a softer, larger impact surface (as seen in falls) results in less focal injury beneath the point of impact; more energy is converted into setting the head into motion. In this case a large contrecoup contusion results, the coup lesion being smaller or not present. It has been stated that coup lesions predominate if the head is accelerated, and contrecoup contusions predominate if the head is decelerated. This may be a useful clinical saw, but it is true only to the extent that *most* clinical situations in which the head is accelerated are injuries from small, hard impactors (assaults), and *most* deceleration injuries occur against broad surfaces (falls) or against softer surfaces (padded auto interiors). Thus most "acceleration" injuries have a greater proportion of contact phenomena and less acceleration than do "deceleration" injuries, where the proportion is usually reversed.

Intermediate Coup Contusions This name has been given to vascular disruptions on brain surfaces that are not adjacent to the skull. Although the mechanism of these lesions has not been extensively studied, it is likely that the lesions are due to strain concentrations that result from impact-generated stress waves. In some instances, however, brain movement due to acceleration effects may cause focal loading against internal bony or dural elements. This may be the mechanism for inferomedial temporal lobe (against the tentorium or petrous ridge) or cingulate (against the falx) intermediate coup contusions.

Intracerebral Hemorrhage/Hematoma

Large traumatic intracerebral hematomas are often associated with extensive cortical contusions; these can be viewed as contusions in which larger, deeper vessels have been disrupted. Smaller hematomas that are not associated with contusion probably occur because of stress wave concentration due to impact or because of acceleration-induced tissue strains (tensile and shear) deep within the brain. Deep, medial, or paracentral small hemorrhagic lesions seen in prolonged coma are undoubtedly due to tissue and vascular tears at areas of strain concentration due to acceleration effects.

Subdural Hematoma

Three varieties of acute subdural hematoma (SDH) are found clinically. The first two can be called complicated SDH—SDH associated with contusion and SDH associated with cortical laceration. These result from contact or acceleration effects that cause the primary lesion. The third type of SDH is most frequent and is due to disruption of surface vessels, usually bridging veins, and results entirely from inertial, and not from contact, forces. Because of the sensitivity of the bridging veins to high strain rate conditions and because of their superficial location, SDH results from head accelerations that produce short-duration, high-strain rate loading.[5] These conditions are best met in falls where the head strikes a broad surface; there is a distributed loading of the head so that little of the energy is dissipated by focal skull injury, and the deceleration causes tensile and shear strains of high strain rate to occur at the brain-skull interface. Not infrequently, subdural hematoma is associated with diffuse axonal injury (DAI; see below) because the mechanism of these two injuries is similar and often the two coexist. This explains those cases where SDH is small but the underlying brain damage is great.

Cerebral Concussion

All gradations of concussion (transient neurological dysfunction due to trauma) are produced entirely by inertial forces. That is, brain motion causes these injuries, not the contact forces associated with impact. Therefore, for concussion to occur as an isolated injury, contact forces must be minimal. Often this is not the case, and the contact forces then may compound the concussion with contact injuries, most commonly skull fracture and contusion.

Diffuse Axonal Injury

Axonal damage appears to be the pathological substrate of prolonged traumatic coma and, like cerebral concussion, is solely due to inertial effects and not to contact phenomena.[6] The amount and location of axonal damage probably determine the severity (duration and depth) of injury and depend on the magnitude, duration, and rate of onset of acceleration. DAI is produced by longer acceleration loading and loading with more gradual onset than loading which produces acute SDH. Thus DAI is most common when the head is impulsively loaded or where impact occurs with relatively soft broad objects, such as occurs in accidents involving motor vehicle occupants. In fact, although both DAI and SDH are acceleration injuries, there is a marked difference in their causes. Almost all cases of DAI, especially its severe form, arise from vehicular injury (impact to padded dashboards, resilient windshields, energy-absorbing steering columns, etc.) where acceleration duration is long. Conversely, most cases of acute SDH occur because of falls or assaults where the impact duration is short and the deceleration abrupt.[3a]

Characteristic patterns of injury have been described and document areas where brain tissue tears or microscopic damage to axons occur.[2,7] The location of the damaged axons in DAI determines the specific neurological sequela of the injury and is very dependent on the direction in which the head moves during injury. Current data suggest that coronal plane head movement is much more injurious than sagittal plane movement.[6]

References

1. Adams JH, Gennarelli TA, Graham DI: Brain damage in nonmissile head injury: Observations in man and subhuman primates, in Smith W, Cavanagh JB (eds): *Recent Advances in Neuropathology*. Edinburgh, Churchill Livingstone, 1982, pp 165–190.
2. Adams JH, Graham DI, Murray LS, Scott G: Diffuse axonal injury due to nonmissile head injury in humans: An analysis of 45 cases. Ann Neurol 12:557–563, 1982.
3. Denny-Brown D, Russell WR: Experimental cerebral concussion. Brain 64:93–164, 1941.
3a. Gennarelli TA: Head injury in man and experimental animals: Clinical aspects. Acta Neurochir (Wien) [Suppl] 32:1–13, 1983.
4. Gennarelli TA, Spielman GM, Langfitt TW, Gildenberg PL, Harrington T, Jane JA, Marshall LF, Miller JD, Pitts LH: Influence of the type of intracranial lesion on outcome from severe head injury. J Neurosurg 56:26–32, 1982.
5. Gennarelli TA, Thibault LE: Biomechanics of acute subdural hematoma. J Trauma 22:680–686, 1982.
6. Gennarelli TA, Thibault LE, Adams JH, Graham DI, Thompson CJ, Marcincin RP: Diffuse axonal injury and traumatic coma in the primate. Ann Neurol 12:564–574, 1982.
7. Grcevic N: Topography and pathogenic mechanisms of lesions in "inner cerebral trauma." Rad Jazu (Med) 402/18: 265–331, 1982.
8. Gurdjian ES, Lang WA, Patrick LM, Thomas LM (eds): *Wayne State University Symposium on Impact Injury and Crash Protection: Impact Injury and Crash Protection*. Springfield, Ill., Charles C Thomas, 1970.
9. Ommaya AK, Gennarelli TA: Cerebral concussion and traumatic unconsciousness: Correlation of experimental and clinical observations on blunt head injuries. Brain 97:633–654, 1974.

189
Pathophysiology of Head Injury

A. John Popp
Robert S. Bourke

Craniocerebral trauma may produce direct impact injury to the brain with parenchymal contusion and laceration or with shearing of myelinated pathways in the white matter of the cerebral hemispheres and brain stem. These primary injurious processes may set in motion a train of secondary alterations in brain metabolism, intracranial hemodynamics, and brain water compartmentation which evolve during the hours following head injury. A satisfactory outcome for the head-injured patient requires recognition and successful treatment of these derangements. In addition, these evolving pathophysiological processes can produce changes in the intracranial pressure-volume relationship with resulting intracranial hypertension and transtentorial and subfalcine brain herniation. Despite the apparent diversity of these derangements in brain physiology, the magnitude of the insult to the brain parenchyma is ultimately dependent on the degree of hypoxic/ischemic injury sustained by the neurons therein.

The skein of problems cited above may be further complicated by the systemic manifestations of head trauma which include abnormalities of water balance and hormonal function that follow hypothalamic or hypophyseal injuries. In this chapter we will present an overview of cerebral and systemic pathophysiological changes following head trauma; the dynamic interaction between altered intracranial hemodynamics, cerebral metabolism, brain oxygen tension, traumatic brain edema, and increased intracranial pressure is emphasized. The other chapters on cerebral edema, increased intracranial pressure, cerebral blood flow, and normal cerebral metabolism serve as useful background for this chapter.

Cerebral Metabolism and Head Injury

The final common pathway of neuronal injury after head trauma is impairment of the delivery of oxygen and cellular metabolic substrates, especially glucose, to cellular sites.

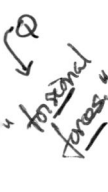

Decreased tensions of tissue O_2 may result from deficient oxygenation of blood by altered pulmonary function, inadequate delivery of oxygen to the brain by altered blood flow, or inadequate oxygen delivery to neurons secondary to focal, scattered increased diffusion path lengths due to brain edema. Cellular hypoxia results when there is a deficient amount of oxygen necessary for maintaining aerobic glycolysis. In this state of deficient O_2 delivery and tissue hypoxia, anaerobic glycolysis predominates; only 2 mol of ATP are formed for 1 mol of glucose consumed. In contrast, when O_2 is not limited, 38 mol of ATP are generated from the consumption of 1 mol of glucose. Thus, tissue oxygen deprivation severely limits the generation of ATP which is necessary for maintenance of brain energy requirements.[12]

An experimentally useful indicator of early cellular hypoxia is the increased amount in the mitochondria of reduced (unoxidized) cytochromes and electron transport coenzymes, especially nicotinamide adenine dinucleotide (NADH). Failure to meet mitochondrial needs for molecular oxygen leads to inadequate transfer of electrons generated by glucose metabolism; energy production fails. Studies in animals have demonstrated an increase in NADH within 5 s of ischemia. When O_2 is not limited, pyruvate produced by glycolysis enters the Krebs cycle for full oxidation and metabolism, but oxygen deprivation shifts pyruvate from the tricarboxylic acid cycle to the generation of lactate with a partial oxidation of the electron transport mechanisms and limited production of high-energy phosphate (pyruvate + NADH + H$^+$ → NAD + H$_2$O + lactate).

Cerebral O_2 and CO_2 Tension

The brain is totally dependent on continued supplies of oxygen and glucose. As an organ the brain represents approximately 2 percent of adult body weight; it receives approximately 20 percent of the cardiac output and utilizes approximately 15 to 20 percent of all oxygen and glucose consumed by the entire body per unit time. Furthermore, approximately 80 percent of glucose and oxygen used by the brain is consumed by the gray matter therein. Contrary to expectation, the average minimal distance between capillaries is greater in the cerebral cortex than in the myocardium and even the gastrocnemius muscle. Oxygen gradients between widely spaced capillaries are, therefore, normally large in the cerebral cortex. Pathological factors which alter oxygen delivery to the arterial end of its capillary will magnify these gradients and diminish the O_2 in cerebral venous blood. For instance, a correlation is to be drawn between brain venous partial pressure (Pv_{O_2}), determined from blood drawn from the sagittal sinus, and the functional neurological state. Thus, under normal circumstances Pv_{O_2} = 34 to 38 torr; when Pv_{O_2} decreases to 17 to 19 torr (critical threshold) following arterial hypoxemia, humans lose consciousness although full restitution of consciousness is expected with the return of Pv_{O_2} to normal values by adequate oxygenation of arterial blood.

A distinction is to be drawn between an alteration in integrated neurological functions (unconsciousness) as occurs dramatically under conditions of moderate and reversible hypoxia (above) and analyses of chemical constituents reflected in a simplified manner by the potential energy charge (representing the high-energy phosphates available for the brain) which may be almost normal despite a profound change in integrated neurological function. The problems in equating particular tissue metabolic parameters with integrated neurological functions are unfortunately manifold and complex. However, one major limitation is the treatment of brain as a uniform tissue rather than an aggregate of many interrelated tissues, each of which has different sensitivities to lack of oxygen and glucose as might occur in brain hypoxia and ischemia. A further reduction of the Pv_{O_2} from the critical threshold (17 to 19 torr) to the lethal threshold (12 torr) may be associated with cellular death and a reduction in the energy charge.

Neurons with an established vulnerability to hypoxic/ischemic insult are localized to the following sites: cerebral cortical pyramidal cells in layers 3, 5, and 6; hippocampal pyramidal cells in areas h$_1$, h$_3$, h$_4$, and h$_5$; cerebellar Purkinje cells, and focal scattered cells in the basal ganglia and thalamus. These are also anatomical sites of hypoxic/ischemic insult to neurons following clinical head injury. It is not clear why a particular cluster of neurons is more susceptible than neighboring cells to a broad insult affecting all. Studies of head injury have shown that acceleration/deceleration head injury yields a shearing injury to some neural structures. Associated are also evolutionary changes providing a hypoxic/ischemic insult in a focal scattered fashion in the brain. Furthermore, regional free radical formation and acidosis may add further to focal membrane insult.

Oxygen (O_2) reaches the neuron by the process of simple diffusion. O_2 tension at the neuronal level is dependent on the partial pressure of O_2 in the capillary, O_2 consumption by the tissue, the diffusion coefficient of O_2, and the diffusion path length.

The classical model of tissue-capillary geometry which would affect cellular O_2 levels is Krogh's cylinder model[11] (Fig. 189-1, top panel). Oxygen tensions at the mid intercapillary distance which is the farthest point from a single nutrient capillary are lowest because of the greater diffusion distance from the capillary source. A number of different pathological conditions occur following head injury which may influence O_2 delivery to neurons within a particular cylinder of CNS parenchyma. For example, if O_2 delivery to the capillary level is abnormal because of pulmonary dysfunction or because of poor perfusion of the cerebral capillary, then the profile of tissue levels which reflect diffusion of O_2 from capillary to neuron will be correspondingly lower. Were the diffusion path length from capillary to neuron lengthened, as occurs in cerebral gray matter edema (Fig. 189-1, bottom panel), then levels of O_2 delivered to neurons at the most distant points of the cylinder might be low enough to produce neuronal death. If O_2 consumption increased as it does with convulsions, particularly in states where O_2 delivery is tenuous, then altered O_2 diffusion might not supply the neuron with adequate levels of O_2 needed for cellular survival. Modest increases in cerebral cortical tissue water content have been shown to alter distances between capillaries[1] (Fig. 189-2).

Carbon dioxide and hydrogen ions have a significant influence on O_2 availability to cerebral cortical tissue.[13] These

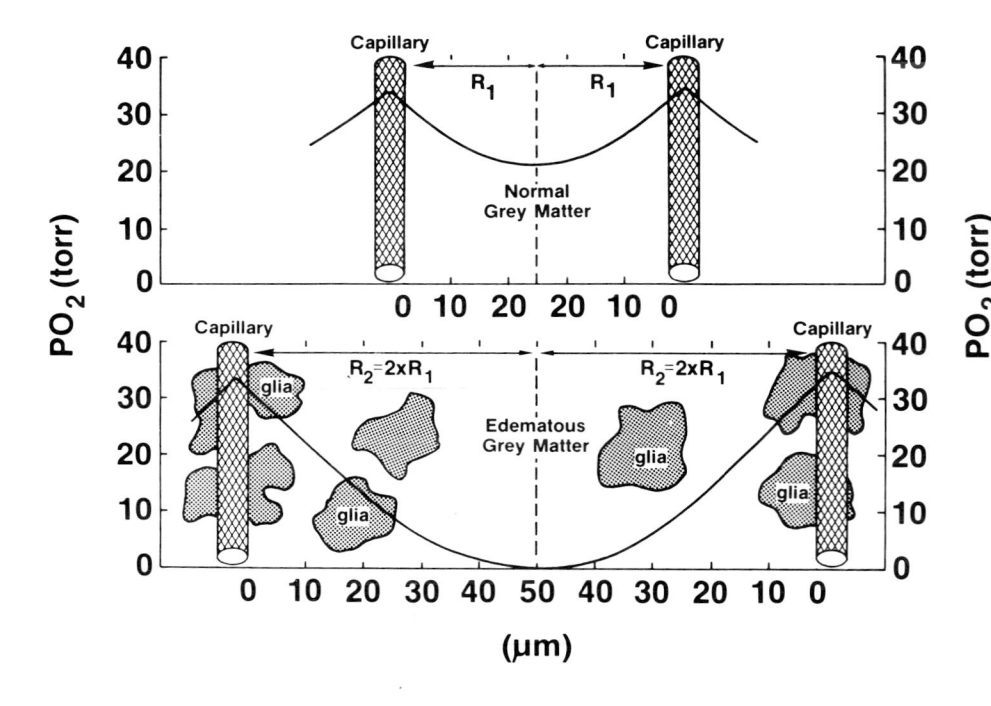

Figure 189-1 Krogh's cylinder[11] represents the idealized relationship of the cerebrocortical vasculature to the cerebral cortex with oxygen gradients in normal (*top panel*) and edematous (*bottom panel*) gray matter at the venous end of the capillary. An increase of the intercapillary distance with an increase in the O_2 diffusion path length produced by gray matter astrocytic swelling is associated with lower levels of tissue O_2 in the mid intercapillary region. Decreased capillary O_2 or poor capillary perfusion would result in a lower capillary baseline O_2 level superimposed on this figure.

influences include the effect of tissue pH on local cerebral blood flow (CBF) and the effect of pH on the affinity of hemoglobin for oxygen. CO_2 and H^+ also have an effect on the glycolytic pathway and might be expected to produce intracellular acidosis. Intracellular pH, however, appears to be well regulated despite increases in tissue CO_2 and H^+.

The mechanism in normal brain for protection against the deleterious effects of hypoxemia is increased CBF induced by increased tissue P_{CO_2} and decreased tissue pH. Increased local blood flow under conditions of hypercarbia and tissue acidosis is altered to a variable extent in injured brain. Despite these changes in local CBF, dissociation of O_2 from hemoglobin (Bohr effect) is facilitated by the acute effect of tissue acidosis.

There is a relative paucity of knowledge of the effect of CO_2 on brain metabolism. However, marked hypocapnia ($Pa_{CO_2} < 20$ torr), as would occur in marked hyperventilation, is associated with decreased CBF, increased tissue lactate levels, and increased lactate-pyruvate and NADH-NAD^+ ratios. These factors have suggested that hypocapnia causes tissue hypoxia. However, this is an area of some dispute since the energy charge potential [E.C. =

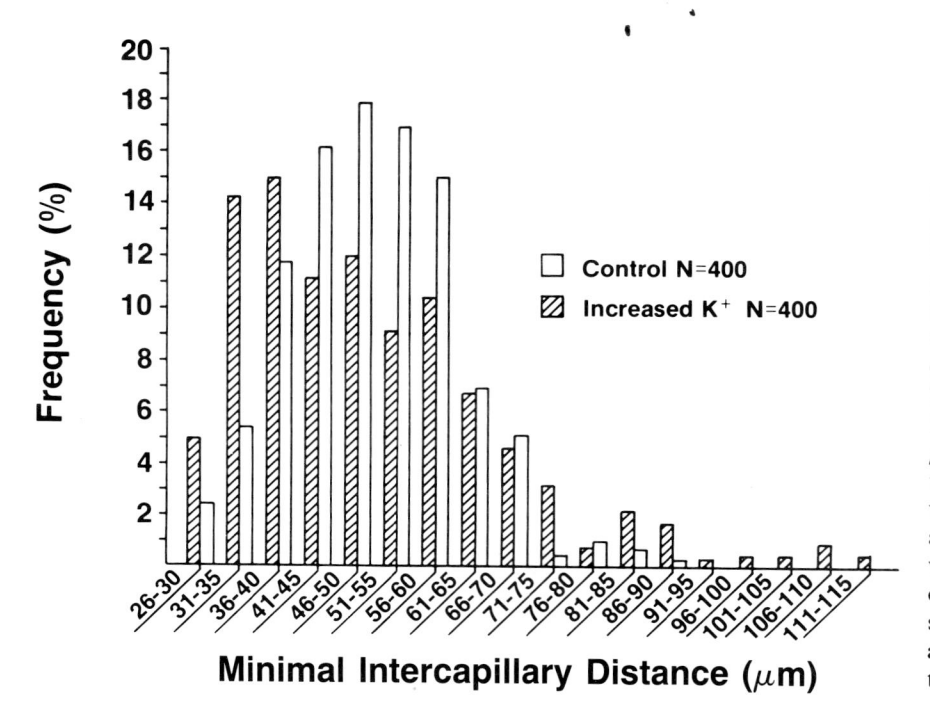

Figure 189-2 A frequency histogram reflecting minimal intercapillary distances (MID) following 14 percent swelling of the cerebral cortex predominately limited to astrocytes therein, by exposure to increased levels of extracellular K^+.[1] The mean MID value for controls is 50 μm with a maximum value of 87 μm; 2.5 percent of values for MID were greater than 70 μm. The mean value for experimental MID was also 50 μm; however, the maximum value was 115 μm, and 10 percent of the values exceeded 70 μm. This supports the concept that modest astroglial swelling substantially alters tissue microgeometry.

(ATP + 0.5 ADP)/(ATP + ADP + AMP)] which reflects energy stores is normal. Furthermore, hypocapnia with alkalosis promotes increased tissue levels of lactate, pyruvate, α-ketoglutarate, and glutamate. These findings suggest a pH effect on a rate-limiting glycolytic step, the phosphofructokinase reaction, rather than a primary effect of limited O_2 availability to tissue sites. Hypocapnia following hyperventilation does diminish CBF and pH-dependent unloading of O_2 from hemoglobin; nevertheless, the degree to which increased tissue levels of lactate following hypocarbia are a reflection of tissue hypoxia must be questioned and requires further investigation. Current evidence suggests that increased tissue lactate levels following shunting of added glucose to anaerobic glycolytic pathways may be a greater insult to brain tissue than that which follows hypocarbia.

Intracranial Hemodynamics Following Head Injury

Cerebral blood flow measurements taken early after human head injury have demonstrated a wide range of values from 20 ml per 100 g brain per min to 65 ml per 100 g brain per min. There appears to be no correlation between early blood flow measurements and clinical outcome. Acutely, head trauma produces impairment of cerebrovascular autoregulation either locally with isolated injury or diffusely with more severe injury and may result in diffuse vasodilatation and an increase in intracranial blood volume, particularly in children. Responsiveness of the cerebral vasculature to varying partial pressures of arterial CO_2 is also initially impaired but not totally lost in areas of dysautoregulation.[9] In this disordered state, the brain vasculature is a mosaic of varying responsiveness to the factors which control CBF: those vessels with normal autoregulatory function maintain normal cerebral blood flow and those vessels with varying degrees of dysautoregulation exhibit patterns of CBF which are dependent on ambient cerebral perfusion pressures.

In the injured brain the effect of intracranial pressure (ICP), cerebral perfusion pressures (CPP), and mean systemic arterial blood pressure (MAP) are critically involved in determining cerebral blood flow (CPP = MAP − ICP). Extreme elevation of intracranial pressure may exceed MAP and prevent nutritive cerebral blood flow. This has been demonstrated angiographically with the absence of blood flow to the intracranial vasculature. In patients with more modest degrees of ICP elevation, changes in CPP in regions of normal autoregulatory function will have little effect on CBF as long as CPP is maintained at 40 to 50 torr or higher. Below this perfusion pressure, CBF decreases, the A-V$_{O_2}$ difference increases, and neuronal injury may occur. In areas of dysautoregulation, decreases in CBF are directly related to decreases in CPP resulting from raised ICP and/or decreased MAP. In severe craniocerebral trauma with elevation of ICP, total vasomotorparalysis of the cerebral vasculature may occur. This is a prognostically ominous finding.

After the acute phase of head injury, patients remaining in coma have a decreased CBF and a reduced cerebral metabolic rate (CMRO$_2$). There appears to be a correlation between low CBF, low CMRO$_2$, and poor outcome in this chronic state.

Traumatic Brain Edema

Brain edema is a frequent concomitant of serious head injury.[2] Cerebral edema is defined as an expansion of the extravascular fluid compartment in the brain. Klatzo divided brain edema into two types: vasogenic and cytotoxic.[5] Vasogenic edema refers to transvascular leakage of solutes and water into the extracellular space, and cytotoxic edema refers to intracellular fluid expansion in response to the cellular toxins or injury.

Vasogenic edema occurs predominantly in the extracellular spaces of the brain, and as implied by the term *vasogenic*, the origin of this swelling is from abnormalities of the injured vasculature. The blood-brain barrier has been localized to the cerebral capillary endothelium. Cerebral capillary interendothelial tight junctions usually restrict net movement of larger molecular weight proteins from the capillary lumen into the extracellular compartment of the central nervous system. Following head injury an alteration in barrier restriction of proteins and other solutes occurs. This may be a mechanical failure of tight junctions or an increase in capillary endothelial pinocytotic activity, either of which may be the source of protein-rich vasogenic edema fluid.

The edema fluid from the damaged blood-brain barrier spreads from the site of focal injury and appears to collect preferentially in the white matter, often at a significant distance from the site of injury. White matter appears to be predominantly involved because of the structural arrangement of parallel laminated fibers and because of the greater size of the extracellular space, which requires less hydraulic pressure to distend this area. Gray matter, on the other hand, is more compact with a smaller extracellular space, and greater force is required for the accumulation of fluid in the extracellular space of the gray matter. Movement of vasogenic edema fluid from the site of injury into white matter is due to tissue hydraulic forces. Edema fluid in white matter moves by bulk flow of solute-rich fluid rather than by simple diffusion of solutes with an osmotic equivalent of water. The degree and speed of the development of vasogenic edema are affected by several factors including the duration of injury to the blood-brain barrier and an increase in the transvascular pressure gradient, as would occur with elevated systemic arterial pressure. Resolution of vasogenic edema appears to occur as a result of fluid resorption into the vascular compartment and by transependymal movement of edema fluid into the ventricular system.

Klatzo's original concept of cytotoxic edema was based on the development of cellular swelling secondary to exposure to toxic substances. In head injury, cytotoxic edema has been taken to indicate intracellular accumulation of fluid resulting *de novo* from injury to the brain. Unlike vasogenic edema which appears to involve the white matter, cytotoxic post-traumatic brain swelling involves principally astrocytes in the gray matter. Since gray matter occupies approximately one-half of the volume of the brain, altered fluid compartmentation of gray matter appears to be of major biological significance. Astroglial cells in gray matter occur at strategic sites in perineuronal and pericapillary loci. Swelling of astrocytes may extend the diffusion path length for oxygen and necessary solutes in transit from cerebral capillaries to neurons (Fig. 189-1). In this circumstance, neurons which have survived the initial traumatic injury and alterations in the intracranial hemodynamics and cerebral metabolism might be irreversibly injured by gray matter edema. Thus, in cytotoxic edema the emphasis is on abnormal fluid compartmentation in astroglial cells in critical locations rather than on the mass effect produced by generalized intracranial hypertension which is usually associated with vasogenic edema. The effects of both major types of edema are additive, and treatment must be directed toward both control of abnormalities of intracranial pressure and treatment of gray matter astroglial edema.

Post-traumatic astroglial swelling appears to be initiated by the hypoxic/ischemic release of intracellular potassium into the extracellular space and potassium-induced secondary release of various neurotransmitters into the extracellular compartment (Fig. 189-3). The result of transmitter-astroglial interaction is net uptake of Cl^- with cation and water by astroglial cells triggered by specific neurotransmitters.[1]

The effects of brain edema may be manifested in different forms after head injury. In a patient with a small cerebral contusion, brain edema may be limited to the perifocal area of injury, or if there is a major vasogenic component, edema may involve the majority of white matter of the hemisphere bearing a focal injury. In the instance of a focal contusion, resultant brain edema superimposes a significantly larger effective mass on the injured brain than the focal brain injury itself. This may produce a worsening in neurological condition, with the development of hemiparesis, speech dysfunction, or convulsions, or the occurrence of a herniation syndrome.

Differential pressures within the brain secondary to the mass effect of edema can produce herniation of brain tissue beneath dural folds that compartmentalize the intracranial cavity. Herniation appears to be an attempt to compensate for the development of significant pressure gradients within a swollen brain limited by a cranial compartment of fixed size. Once brain tissue has herniated, the circulation of the tissue generally is compromised and the degree of swelling due to ischemia increases and perpetuates the ongoing pathological processes. Specific herniations of the cingulate gyrus, the uncus of the parahippocampal gyrus, and tonsilar herniation are well known to the neurological surgeon and constitute a serious problem requiring immediate treatment.

Intracranial Pressure

Intracranial pressure is often elevated after serious head injury.[6-8] A distinction should be drawn between the effects of elevated ICP associated with damaged brain and elevated ICP associated with normal brain. Intracranial hypertension by itself may not be harmful, as exemplified by patients with pseudotumor cerebri who may have ICPs > 40 torr with little clinical neurological dysfunction. However, ICP of the same magnitude with contused brain and altered cerebrovascular autoregulation, incipient hypoxic/ischemic injury, and cerebral edema may result in diminished local cerebral perfusion pressure, a cycle of further vasomotor paralysis, increasing edema, and death.

The intracranial compartment in adults is of fixed volume and normally contains three major incompressible constituents: blood, CSF, and brain parenchyma. Any process which acutely or subacutely alters the dynamic steady-state relationship between these three intracranial constituents by increasing the volume of one of these intracranial constituents will increase intracranial pressure when compensatory mechanisms fail (Fig. 189-4).

Initially after brain injury, increases in ICP are dampened by reduction in volume of intracranial CSF. This occurs by displacement of CSF from the intracranial compartment into the spinal compartment with distension of the spinal dura. Other factors which may be involved in com-

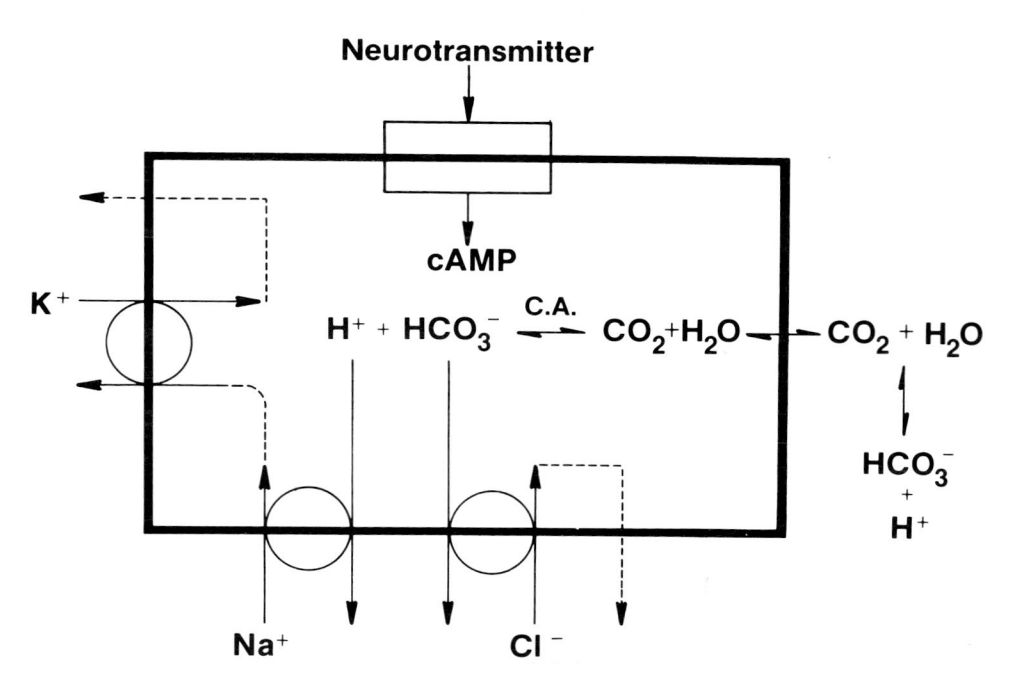

Figure 189-3 Model of astroglial cell showing K^+-dependent release of neurotransmitters which trigger Cl^-/bicarbonate exchange and Na^+/H^+ exchange.[1] Net accumulation of intracellular NaCl accompanied by an osmotic equivalent of water establishes astroglial swelling stimulated by cyclic AMP alteration in a net ion flux initiated by neurotransmitter-astroglial interaction.

Figure 189-4 A depiction of the intracranial pressure/volume relationship,[6-8] showing the changes in intracranial pressure occurring with the addition of volume (intravascular blood, CSF, edematous brain, hematoma) to the intracranial compartment. In segment A, following additions to intracranial volume, compensatory mechanisms, including displacement of CSF to the spinal compartment and collapse of intracranial venous channels, maintain ICP at normal levels. Segment B represents failure of compensatory mechanisms to fully accommodate even small additions of volume to the intracranial compartment. Some reserve remains, however, since further collapse of venous channels may occur, and CSF absorption increases as intracranial pressure increases. Segment C represents the final phase of decompensation with an elevated baseline intracranial pressure. The presence of progressive cerebrovascular vasomotor paralysis in this phase initially produces plateau waves associated with neurological deterioration. Ultimately sustained high elevations of ICP occur which are unresponsive to any treatment modality.

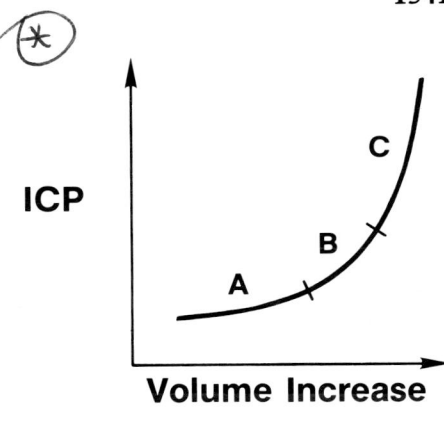

pensation are increased CSF resorption (CSF resorption increases as intracranial pressure increases) and compression of venous channels with a decrease in intracranial venous blood volume. This phase of compensation may be regained or maintained in patients with increasing ICP by withdrawal of CSF if a ventricular catheter is in place. During this phase the intracranial volume-pressure relationship indicates no change in ICP with an increase in the volume added to the intracranial compartment (Fig. 189-4). The elastance of the intracranial compartment (which can be estimated by the change in ICP produced by incremental additions of fluid to the intracranial compartment) is low. Intracranial compliance, the inverse of elastance, is high during the compensatory phase. These two properties are a reflection of the "tightness" of the brain in the intracranial compartment. Therefore, high intracranial compliance indicates that additions to cranial blood volume, CSF, or brain parenchyma may occur without substantial increase in intracranial pressure.

As compensatory mechanisms which dampen initial increases in ICP fail, intracranial compliance decreases and elastance increases. During this phase the baseline ICP may only be slightly increased or normal, but small increases in intracranial volume produced by vasodilatation, CSF obstruction, or increased edema will produce dramatic increases in ICP. This early phase of decompensation can be reversed by various modalities used to treat intracranial hypertension: antiedema agents; elevation of the head of the bed to decrease intracranial venous volume; or hyperventilation to decrease Pa_{CO_2} and produce vasoconstriction in responsive vessels, resulting in decreased intracranial arterial blood volume.

As ICP continues to increase, compliance decreases further, and treatment modalities are less successful in controlling further elevations in ICP. Episodic increases of ICP lasting for fractions of an hour may occur on an already elevated base: these plateau waves are correlated with deterioration of neurological status. The final stage in the decompensation of protective mechanisms occurs when complete vasomotor paralysis of the cerebral vasculature develops. In this phase there is no responsiveness to treatment modalities, and the elevation of ICP is sustained. The development of vasomotor paralysis is ominous.

When a progressive decrease in intracranial compliance occurs, it is necessary to consider that readily correctable secondary processes may magnify diminished compliance initially due to damaged brain. First, rapidly developing, surgically correctable space-occupying lesions are more poorly tolerated than slowly evolving mass lesions which do not exceed the time constants of, or functional capacity of, compensatory mechanisms. Second, obstruction of the CSF pathways may accelerate decompensation either by blocking displacement of CSF into the spinal dural sac or by producing hydrocephalus which adds to mass effect. This, too, is surgically correctable. Lesions obstructing venous outflow or treatment modalities which increase venous pressure such as PEEP (positive end expiratory pressure) may diminish compensatory reserve and result in raised intracranial pressure. Finally, the critical end result of post-traumatic intracranial hypertension is hypoxic/ischemic injury and death of neurons which have survived the initial injury only to fall prey to an insufficient cerebrovascular perfusion pressure. CPP is determined by the mean arterial pressure minus the intracranial venous pressure which closely correlates with the ICP. Patients with ICP elevation and cardiovascular instability are at significantly greater risk than their counterparts with ICP elevation and normal cardiovascular function. Maintenance of a CPP > 40 torr with well-oxygenated blood by maintenance of a satisfactory cardiac output helps to ensure that the patient who is potentially salvageable will not succumb to injury because of regionally insufficient cerebral perfusion. The physician managing a patient with progressive loss of intracranial compliance should repeatedly re-evaluate the causes of reduced compliance, many of which are medically and surgically treatable.

Abnormalities of Systemic Water Balance and Hormonal Function

Lesions in the hypothalamus, pituitary stalk, and pituitary gland have been described at autopsy of patients sustaining fatal head injury.[4] Injuries of the hypothalamus, pituitary stalk, and pituitary gland appear to result from various mechanisms; the hypothalamus and stalk lesions are usually secondary to the shearing stresses of an oscillating brain following impact. Pituitary injury may be secondary to infarction following damage to the hypothalamic-hypophyseal portal (HHP) system. Fractures involving the sella turcica are not necessary concomitants of either clinical or autopsy-proven lesions of the hypothalamic-hypophyseal system.

Abnormalities of water balance, either diabetes insipidus (DI) or the syndrome of inappropriate antidiuretic hormone (SIADH) secretion, are the commonest manifestations of hypothalamic-hypophyseal dysfunction occurring after head injury. DI follows direct injury of the supraoptic-paraventricular hypothalamic nuclei or injury to the pituitary stalk with damage of the axons carrying ADH to the neurohypophysis.

Polyuria is usually the first clue of the presence of DI; other manifestations include polydipsia, low urine specific gravity, and elevated plasma osmolality. Most patients with polyuria after head injury may be assumed to have ADH deficiency if concomitant urine and serum osmolalities are less than 300 mosmol/kg and greater than 300 mosmol/kg, respectively, but further testing may be necessary to confirm the diagnosis. Post-traumatic DI may be permanent, but more frequently only transient polyuria occurs. In awake patients with an intact thirst mechanism, oral intake will often maintain fluid balance. In comatose patients, diagnosis may be difficult before the development of severe dehydration. Early treatment includes fluid replacement and vasopressin; care must be taken to avoid water intoxication when vasopressin begins to inhibit urinary loss of water. Water intoxication can augment pre-existing cerebral edema; systemic volume depletion from DI can be associated with a reduction of MAP and an eventual decrease in CPP. Hence, systemic water balance must be carefully monitored since it may have a major role in determining clinical outcome in patients with a noncompliant brain. Patients with incomplete chronic loss of ADH may be treated with sulfonylureas which potentiate the effect of ADH on the kidney tubules.

Patients with SIADH characteristically present with the following features: low serum sodium level (< 130 meq per liter), low serum osmolality value (< 280 mosmol per liter), a urinary sodium level > 20 meq per liter, and a urinary osmolality level higher than plasma osmolality level. These characteristics help separate SIADH from other causes of hyponatremia after head injury. The effects of profound hyponatremia (< 120 meq per liter) include nausea, vomiting, confusion, seizures, lethargy, and coma. Presumably these effects are produced by water intoxication, with intracellular swelling and raised intracranial pressure. Systemic hypo-osmolality may be magnified by the use of renal and osmotic diuretics and rehydration with saline-poor fluid. Rapid shifts of body Na$^+$ are poorly tolerated. Fluid restriction is the treatment for asymptomatic or mildly symptomatic patients with a serum Na$^+$ value > 125 meq per liter. For symptomatic patients or patients with a serum Na$^+$ value < 125 meq per liter, fluid restriction should be augmented by infusion of 3% or 5% NaCl in calculated amounts (6 ml of 5% hypertonic saline per kilogram of body weight will raise serum Na$^+$ 10 meq per liter). Recently, some patients who fulfill the criteria of SIADH have been found to have a decreased blood volume. This would suggest that in those patients ADH secretion was not "inappropriate" but rather was responding in a normal fashion to hypovolemia.

Symptomatic hormonal dysfunction after head injury is far less common than abnormalities of systemic water balance and usually is not identified until long after the occurrence of the injury. In general, hormonal dysfunction appears to occur after trauma because of interruption of the HHP system producing pituitary ischemia. In some instances, however, intrinsic hypothalamic lesions appear to be causative, presumably due to deficiency of various releasing factors. Deficiencies of nearly all the adenohypophyseal hormones have been reported. DI may be associated with the presence of anterior pituitary dysfunction but may be masked by TSH and ACTH insufficiency. The subsequent use of glucocorticoid therapy in these patients will produce polyuria and polydipsia.

Following injury, corticotropin releasing factor is liberated from the median eminence, causing release of ACTH, which in turn stimulates cortisol secretion from the adrenal gland. Normally, an increased level of serum cortisol would inhibit further production of ACTH by negative feedback, thereby reducing cortisol production. After head injury, however, there is a loss of the normal circadian pattern of ACTH secretion and a loss of responsiveness in the negative feedback mechanism. Dexamethasone suppression tests have demonstrated that the negative feedback loop often remains intact after head injury, but it appears to be set at a higher level, accounting for lack of inhibition of ACTH by higher levels of circulating cortisol.[14] Steroidal-related negative nitrogen balance results.

Systemic Manifestations of Head Injury

Isolated head injury may evoke changes in other organ systems which, if unrecognized and untreated, may lead to further compromise of the patient. Trauma, including head injury, is associated with increased sympathetic activity and increased levels of circulating catecholamines due to adrenal medullary stimulation. The magnitude of this response in isolated head injury is directly related to the severity of the brain injury. It is presumed that increased blood catecholamines are responsible for the hypermetabolic state observed after head injury manifested by hypertension, tachycardia, increased cardiac output, and excessive caloric consumption with the development of a negative nitrogen balance.[3] In addition, a form of pseudodiabetes mellitus may occur, primarily due to the effect of catecholamines on the release of glucose from the liver.

Increased levels of circulating catecholamines may have a deleterious effect on certain target organs, especially the heart and lungs. Myocardial injury in the form of cytolysis and subendocardial hemorrhage occurs after human head injury, and similar abnormalities have been described in the experimental animal following the infusion of norepinephrine. These findings may explain the presence of arrhythmias, EKG changes, and decreased cardiac output observed in some patients after head injury. In the presence of intracranial hypertension these derangements of cardiac function might produce a lower mean systemic arterial pressure and cerebral perfusion pressure and could worsen the severity of the cerebral injury.

Lung dysfunction may also occur as a systemic manifestation of isolated head injury. The ensuing discussion will focus on "neurogenic" pulmonary dysfunction and not on lung dysfunction occurring concomitantly with head injury as a result of aspiration, lung contusion, or hemothorax/pneumothorax.

"Neurogenic" pulmonary dysfunction may occur within minutes after head injury with associated alveolar and tracheobronchial flooding by a blood-tinged protein-rich fluid. This precipitously developing aberration of lung function, termed *neurogenic pulmonary edema*, is uncommon and is generally associated with life-threatening head injuries or other catastrophic intracranial processes. The syndrome is associated with decreased lung compliance, and the chest x-ray film demonstrates diffuse infiltration of the lung parenchyma (white lung). The rapid development of hypoxemia is the most serious manifestation of this disorder. Timely endotracheal intubation and mechanical ventilation delivering an increased fraction of inspired oxygen (Fi_{O_2}) under conditions of positive end expiratory pressure can succeed in preventing a dangerously low Pa_{O_2} which could further impair the delivery of oxygen to an injured brain.

More commonly, pulmonary dysfunction after head injury is delayed in development. It is unknown whether this represents a less serious form of the fulminant variety described above or is an entirely different entity taking from 24 to 48 h to develop.[15] The principal manifestation of the delayed onset type of pulmonary dysfunction is a gas exchange abnormality in the absence of overt pulmonary edema either on chest films or by auscultation. Lung compliance is usually normal, and normal or low extravascular lung water determinations have been documented. Evaluation of ventilation and perfusion compartments of the lung using multiple inert gases of varying solubility has demonstrated areas of the lung with poor perfusion and normal ventilation (increased dead space) and normal perfusion and poor ventilation (increased intrapulmonary shunt).[10] The presence of continued perfusion of areas of the lung with deficient ventilation results in hypoxemia, which is often difficult to correct even using PEEP and an increased Fi_{O_2}. Since the lung compliance is normal, PEEP-related injury to the alveoli (barotrauma) is much more likely to occur in patients with delayed onset pulmonary dysfunction than in patients with fulminant pulmonary edema.

The etiology of pulmonary dysfunction after isolated head injury has been the source of controversy. One theory of origin is based on the postinjury hyperdynamic state: hypertension with increased peripheral vascular resistance produces an increased left ventricular afterload resulting in increased left atrial pressure and pulmonary capillary pressure with resultant lung edema. Animal experiments and studies in humans, however, have shown that pulmonary capillary wedge pressure is not necessarily elevated when post-head-injury pulmonary edema occurs. In humans, this observation does not fully rule out the peripheral hemodynamic theory since significant cardiovascular hemodynamic changes may occur immediately after head trauma, producing ongoing capillary leakage before the start of hemodynamic monitoring.

Another purported etiology for post-head-injury pulmonary dysfunction is the direct effect of circulating catecholamines or sympathetic stimulation on lung microvasculature, resulting in increased vascular permeability. A third general theory concerning the etiology of post-head-injury pulmonary dysfunction advocates injury of the lung vasculature by substances released from platelet and fibrin microaggregates occurring in post-head-injury intravascular coagulation. This cause, if operative, is unlikely to account for the fulminant variety of pulmonary dysfunction since a longer time course would be necessary to produce dysfunction by humoral factors.

A final systemic manifestation of head injury is disseminated intravascular coagulation which occurs as a subclinical or clinically significant coagulopathy in approximately 50 percent of head-injured patients. The brain is rich in tissue thromboplastin which enters the systemic circulation following significant brain injury, activating the extrinsic clotting cascade. The result in extreme cases has been termed a "consumptive" coagulopathy since the clotting factors normally present have been activated and utilized by the presence of brain thromboplastin. Catastrophic hemorrhage may occur in these extreme cases. The diagnosis can be made by the presence of a prolonged clotting time and increased prothrombin time and the presence of fibrin degradation products. Treatment is by transfusion of fresh frozen plasma and other blood products as needed.

References

1. Bourke RS, Kimelberg HK, Nelson LR, Barron KD, Auen EL, Popp AJ, Waldman JB: Biology of glial swelling in experimental brain edema. Adv Neurol 28:99–109, 1980.
2. Cervós-Navarro J, Ferszt R (eds): *Brain Edema: Pathology, Diagnosis, and Therapy*. New York, Raven Press, 1980.
3. Clifton GL, Ziegler MG, Grossman RG: Circulating catecholamines and sympathetic activity after head injury. Neurosurgery 8:10–14, 1981.
4. Crompton MR: Hypothalamic lesions following closed head injury. Brain 94:165–172, 1971.
5. Klatzo I: Neuropathological aspects of brain edema. J Neuropathol Exp Neurol 26:1–14, 1967.
6. Langfitt TW: Increased intracranial pressure. Clin Neurosurg 16:436–471, 1969.
7. Miller JD: Volume and pressure in the craniospinal axis. Clin Neurosurg 22:76–105, 1975.
8. Miller JD, Becker DP, Ward JD, Sullivan HG, Adams WE, Rosner MJ: Significance of intracranial hypertension in severe head injury. J Neurosurg 47:503–516, 1977.
9. Overgaard J, Tweed WA: Cerebral circulation after head injury. Part I: Cerebral blood flow and its regulation after closed head injury with emphasis on clinical correlations. J Neurosurg 41:531–541, 1974.
10. Popp AJ, Shah DM, Berman RA, Paloski WH, Newell JC, Cooper JA, Rahm RL, Gottlieb ME, Bourke RS, Malik AB: Delayed pulmonary dysfunction in head-injured patients. J Neurosurgery 57:784–790, 1982.
11. Purves MJ: *The Physiology of the Cerebral Circulation*. Cambridge, Cambridge University Press, 1972.
12. Siesjö BK: Cell damage in the brain: A speculative synthesis. J Cerebral Blood Flow Metab 1:155–185, 1981.
13. Siesjö BK, Folbergrova J, Messeter K: Acid-base and energy metabolism of the brain in hypercapnia and hypocapnia, in Nahas G, Schaefer KE (eds): *Carbon Dioxide and Metabolic Regulations*. New York, Springer-Verlag, 1974, pp 233–249.
14. Steinbok P, Thompson G: Serum cortisol abnormalities after craniocerebral trauma. Neurosurgery 5:559–565, 1979.
15. Yen JK, Rhodes GR, Bourke RS, Powers SR Jr, Newell JC, Popp AJ: Delayed impairment of arterial blood oxygenation in patients with severe head injury: Preliminary report. Surg Neurol 9:323–327, 1978.

190
Pathology of Closed Head Injury
William F. McCormick

Closed head injury has reached epidemic proportions in Western societies due both to the tremendous carnage engendered by our poorly controlled vehicular traffic and to the rising violence of citizens against each other in times of social unrest. The variety and severity of the types of closed head injury encountered will differ considerably from one study population to the next. Those physicians and paramedical personnel who deal primarily with vehicular-generated CNS trauma will see a spectrum of lesions that will be different from those seen by physicians who usually deal with patients who have sustained accelerative-type head injuries from blows to the head. Furthermore, medical examiners and coroners will see a spectrum of lesions considerably different in both type and severity from those usually encountered by hospital-based physicians. Several types of direct brain stem lesions are rarely seen in hospital populations but are relatively common in a medical examiner's population due to their almost universally rapid lethality. Other types of lesions, such as some of the cranial nerve disorders secondary to closed head trauma, have been little discussed or studied by pathologists. Many are infrequently lethal, and detailed evaluation of these injuries utilizing usual autopsy procedures is difficult.

Two other major changes in our understanding of closed head injury have occurred in recent years: the appreciation that the brain of an infant or young child responds very differently from that of an older child or an adult[8,33,36,40,42,58] and the concept of "diffuse impact injury."[1-5,19,21,40,49,52,53] These two areas of rapidly expanding knowledge will be discussed in some detail in this chapter.

Two difficulties commonly discouraging the study of the pathology of head trauma are the fact that a lethal injury normally will bring the decedent to the attention of the coroner or medical examiner rather than to the hospital-based (academic) pathologist or neuropathologist[1,2,40] and the all too frequent reluctance on the part of hospital pathologists to become involved in cases with a high probability of litigation.

It is critical that as much information as possible be available to the pathologist regarding the probable physical mechanisms responsible for the production of the head wound—whether the head injury resulted from the decedent being in a vehicular crash, or being hit with a hard object (pipe, brick), or being involved in a fall, etc. The often exceedingly complex patterns of vehicular trauma, with their multiple accelerative- and decelerative-type injuries, have been stressed previously. The pattern and extent of soft tissue injuries to the face and head and neck should be known by the pathologist before completing the evaluation of the injuries of the skull and brain and their pattern. The extent, distribution, and type of skull fractures, if present, should be known in detail (not just that a skull fracture was or was not present). The naive belief that the type of head injury can be determined with any degree of precision with the examination of a formalin-fixed brain should be vigorously corrected.

It should be kept in mind that the pathologist, like the clinician, is subjected to a number of constraints when examining a cadaver. These constraints make it difficult at times to carry out as thorough an examination as both the clinician and the pathologist might desire. While this is less often true in cases that involve trauma victims than in cases that involve other types of patients (due to the legal nature of the problem), there are still imperatives not to blatantly disfigure the body or to extensively delay the completion of the autopsy. Perhaps an even more serious problem is the pressure brought by police and attorneys to render a final report in an unrealistically short time. In order to do the most accurate evaluation possible, the autopsy findings must be documented thoroughly with photographs, x-ray films, and diagrams, when applicable.

The pathologist of record should personally carefully examine the soft tissues and bone and the skull as well as the brain. It is highly desirable to remove (or closely supervise the removal of) the brain and spinal cord. The pathologist should see that the dura is stripped from the base of the skull so that careful evaluation of otherwise hidden skull fractures can be made. The paranasal sinuses and the petrous portion of the temporal bones should be opened and examined for bleeding into these structures. It is particularly important that careful examination, with as little manipulation as possible, be made of the cranial-cervical junction and of the upper cervical spine and cord. This is an area that is not well examined in the great majority of autopsies. An attempt should be made to carefully estimate the volume of blood in membrane hematomas (epidural or subdural); all clots should be weighed and the weight recorded. Careful evaluation of midline shifts and hernias should be made in the fresh state, but the fresh brain should not be dissected further. The brain weight should be recorded in the fresh state (without the dura attached to the brain). The weight of the brain changes with fixation, and the amount of change is quite variable and unpredictable in any given case. All handling of fresh material should be done with great care. There are very few lesions that can be seen in the fresh, unfixed brain that are not seen more clearly with better delineation in a properly fixed specimen.

The necessity of utilizing "special stains" in the detailed evaluation of brain trauma cases should be understood by all. These, of necessity, increase the interval between death and the completion of the report, just as they appreciably

Pathology of Closed Head Injury

increase the cost in both time and consumable supplies. An accurate assessment of diffuse impact injury is not possible with only the routine hematoxylin- and eosin-stained sections.

The variety of lesions, both focal and diffuse, that can be found in patients sustaining closed head injury is far greater than was appreciated for many years. Moreover, the correct interpretation of the causative factors and the sequence of events in the pathogenesis of these various lesions is changing. The organization of this chapter will be somewhat different from the classical presentations of the neuropathology of trauma, and an attempt will be made to group the majority of brain lesions into one of three major headings: focal, diffuse, and secondary.

Soft Tissue Injuries of the Head and Neck

Careful evaluation and recording of all soft tissue injuries of the head and neck are important in the evaluation of patients with head trauma. Some of these injuries, such as periorbital ecchymoses and postauricular ecchymoses (Battle's sign), are well-known indicators of orbitofrontal and petrous basilar skull fractures, respectively. Both periorbital ecchymoses and Battle's sign can develop very rapidly, but both, especially the postauricular ecchymoses, may be delayed for several days. All wounds (abrasions, lacerations, and contusions) should be described as to size, freshness, and location, using carefully defined anatomical landmarks. The hair of the head will often largely or partially obscure scalp lesions; the hair should be carefully shaved away from such lesions, allowing their clear delineation. The patterns of soft tissue injuries often suggest the type as well as the location and direction of various forces applied to the head.[18,40]

A significant number of patients who sustained closed head injury will have facial fractures. These are generally neither easily nor well examined at autopsy. Their primary significance, in so far as closed head trauma is concerned, is that they may be associated with severe or fatal hemorrhage, either externally (exsanguination) or internally, drowning the patient. Nasogastric tubes can enter the cranial cavity through such compound facial and basilar skull fractures. Peripheral cranial nerve injuries can result from soft tissue injuries to the head and face. These are usually clinically obvious, and the pathological lesion is that of a traumatic nerve contusion or avulsion. Retinal hemorrhages are often present in cases of closed head injury, particularly in children; retinal hemorrhage may be one of the few physical findings in battered children. Small, apparently innocuous wounds in the soft tissues can represent entrance wounds of penetrating objects. These often have been sutured or taped closed without the realization that a retained foreign body or severe intracranial injury could exist.

While a contusion, laceration, or incision of the soft tissues of the face or head is an indication of trauma to that area and is thus helpful in localizing the impact area, the extent of these lesions is often not a good indication of the seriousness of the intracranial (particularly brain) lesions.

SkullRactures

A skull fracture is a laceration of bony tissue. It indicates significant trauma to the head (skull), but in and of itself it is not lethal. The likelihood of a fracture being produced varies with the site and area of impact, but is largely dependent on the force applied. In my material, slightly over 80 percent of patients with fatal closed head injuries have an associated skull fracture.

A simple working classification of skull fractures is "open," "closed," "linear," or "depressed," followed by qualification as to extent, location, bony fragmentation, and degree of bone fragment displacement. The proximity of a fracture to the underlying envelopes and the brain itself is important to note, as it explains some of the causes of membrane hematomas, fracture contusions, and cranial nerve and vascular lacerations.

1. *Linear* (bursting) fractures are the type most commonly seen in severe head injury and are caused by outbending of the bone at a distance from the impact site as a result of general deformation of the skull (Fig. 190-1). These fractures typically run toward the point of impact but may not reach the impact area. 2. *Depressed* (bending) fractures are due to more localized forces, and may be stellate, comminuted, etc. (Figs. 190-2 and 190-3). 3. *Diastatic* fractures are linear fractures along suture lines resulting in separation of the cranial sutures (Fig. 190-4). Because of the structure of the calvarium with its soft diploe separated by relatively rigid outer and inner tables, depressed (bending) fractures resulting from short-duration forces of limited strength can leave the outer table intact while producing marked fracturing of the inner table.

It is sometimes possible to demonstrate a precise impact point in even an extensive depressed comminuted fracture if the skull is reconstructed. The lines of fracture usually radiate out from the apex of the cone of deformation and may be surrounded by a circular ring or concentric rings (Fig. 190-5). When a fracture is evaluated along with the overlying soft tissue injuries, very accurate localization of impact sites

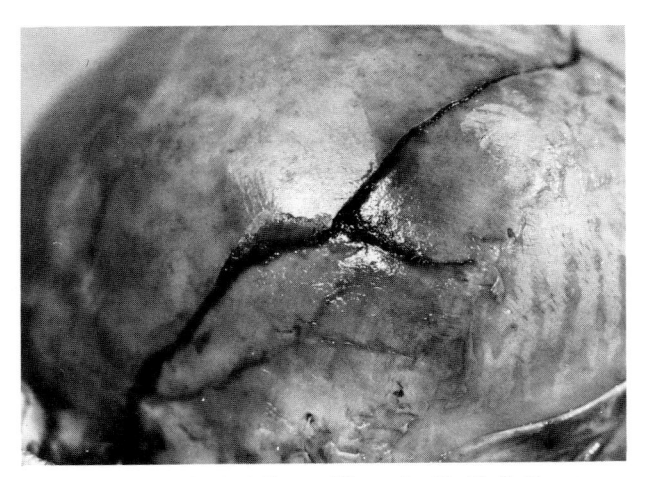

Figure 190-1 Typical linear ("bursting") skull fracture secondary to outbending of the bone at a distance from the impact site.

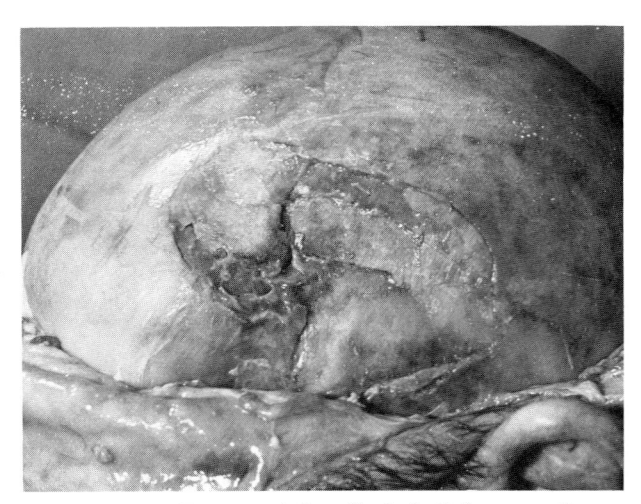

Figure 190-2 Depressed (bending) skull fractures from a localized blow to the side of the head.

can sometimes be determined. However, the general pattern of a skull fracture is not always highly predictive of impact site. Impacts to the chin or occiput, for example, can produce hinge fractures of the base of the skull identical in appearance to those produced by lateral crushing-type injuries (Fig. 190-6).[22] While anatomical features, such as bony buttresses and much thinner "plates," influence fracture patterns, the strength (magnitude) of the forces is paramount. Gurdjian et al. have noted that the same amount of force (energy) can produce different fractures in different people and that once sufficient energy has been absorbed to produce one linear fracture, very little additional energy can produce massive skull destruction (Fig. 190-7).[20] The force needed to produce a fracture varies with the area of skull involved, its thickness, the integrity of the overlying soft tissues, etc., but may be as little as 5 ft · lb.[20] It must be kept in mind that severe and fatal brain injuries can occur in the absence of external evidence of trauma.

Crushing skull injuries often result in direct cranial injuries due to extension of fractures across basilar foramina.

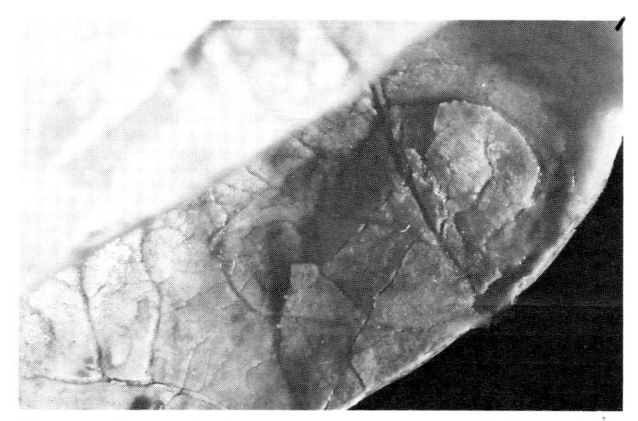

Figure 190-3 The inner surface of the skull from the patient with the depressed skull fracture seen in Fig. 190-2, illustrating the displacement of fragments of the inner table without complete separation.

Russell and Schiller demonstrated experimentally that bilateral crush produces bilateral, or occasionally unrelated, separation of the petrous bone from the greater wing of the sphenoid and from the temporal squama along the petrosquamous fissure.[50] The carotid canal is typically opened. The tegmen tympani is fractured in about half the cases, and the tympanic membranes may be torn. Fractures often extend across the dorsum sellae (Fig. 190-6). A transverse "hinge" fracture running in the direction of compression results. Such crushing injuries are seen in patients whose heads have been overrun by vehicles. While this pattern is typical of lateral compression, impacts to the chin or skull base can result in identical fractures, as seen in Fig. 190-6.[22]

Fractures extending through the cribriform plate into the paranasal sinuses, or through the petrous portion of the temporal bones breaking through the mastoid air cells or eustachian tube, can give rise to cerebrospinal fluid (CSF) leaks. Such CSF leaks are encountered only if the dura is lacerated as well. They are of primary importance as a route of spread of bacteria intracranially.

In the circumstance of a fracture of the calvarium, if during the brief period of time the fractured inner table opens and if the dura and underlying brain are lacerated, leptomeninges and/or brain can become trapped within the fracture line, giving rise to a "growing" fracture. This uncommon event occurs almost exclusively in children; the great majority are less than 3 years of age. These fractures are usually parietal in location and are almost always associated with significant underlying brain damage.[29,38,51]

Depressed skull fractures may lacerate the dura and underlying brain. The resulting problems are essentially those of the direct brain wound; the question of whether all depressed fractures should be elevated is beyond the scope of this chapter.

Brain Injuries

The traumatic lesions within the brain will be discussed under three headings: focal, diffuse, and secondary. Focal lesions are those that manifest themselves structurally in a limited area and are the direct result of trauma to the tissues. Diffuse injuries are those that are manifested over either all or a very large portion of the brain and are the result of very widespread shearing or rotational-type forces. Secondary lesions are those that result as a consequence of dynamic changes within the brain initiated by either focal or diffuse brain injury, usually ischemic in nature. A few patients will have all three types of brain lesions present, many will have two, and a few will have exclusively or overwhelmingly the first or second type.

Focal lesions of the brain include membrane hematomas (epidural and subdural hematomas and subarachnoid hemorrhages), parenchymal contusions and lacerations, intraparenchymal hematomas (including "burst" or "pulped" temporal or frontal lobes), direct cranial nerve lacerations and contusions, direct lacerations and contusions of the brain stem, and direct lacerations of major intracranial vessels (dural sinuses, arteries, veins). Diffuse impact injuries are

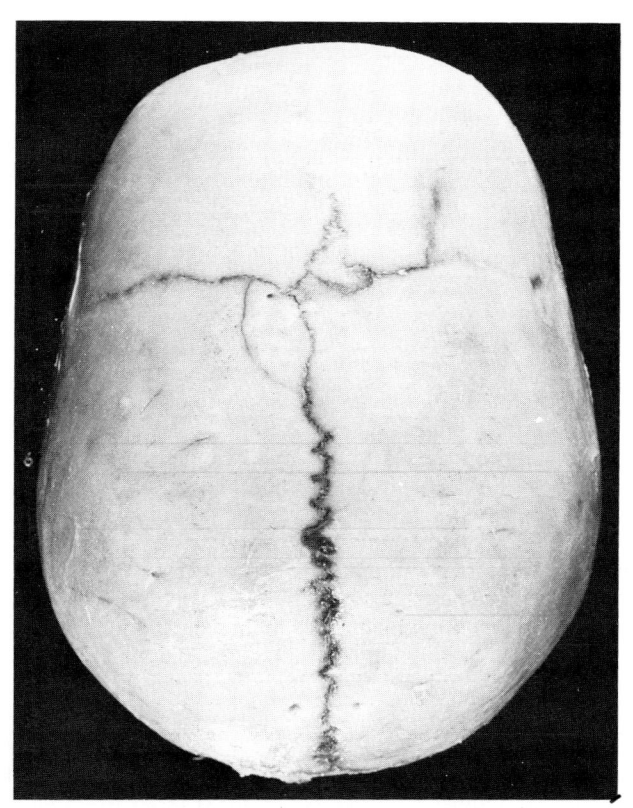

Figure 190-4 Diastatic fracture with extension of a linear fracture into the coronal suture and hemorrhage into the slightly separated suture. Focal diastatic fracturing of a metopic suture is also seen.

those with alterations that are predominantly microscopic but include focal necrosis (hemorrhagic or ischemic) and tears of the corpus callosum and hemorrhagic necrosis of the dorsolateral quadrants of the rostral pons. Associated with those two macroscopic features of diffuse impact injury are reactive axons ("Stritch" lesions) and microglial clusters

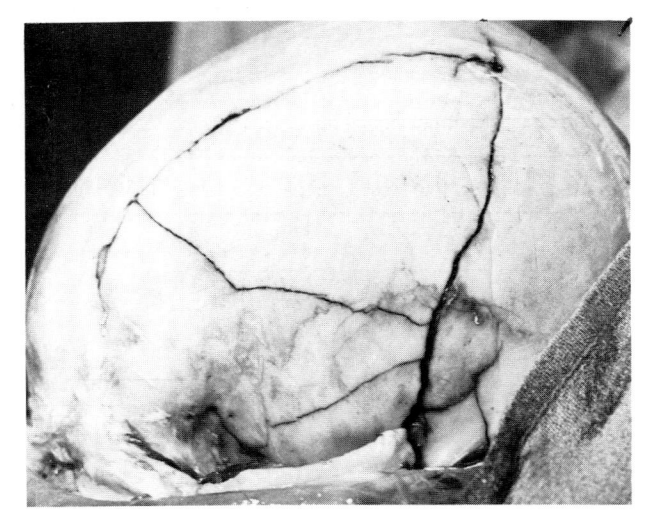

Figure 190-5 Linear ("bursting") fractures with concentric rings encircling the area of impact.

("stars"). The most common secondary lesions resulting from trauma are due to vascular disruptive events secondary to brain hernias and to hypoxic/ischemic complications of closed head injury resulting from severe hypotension with perfusion failure.

Focal Brain Lesions

Intracranial Hemorrhages

Four major categories of traumatic intracranial hemorrhage must be considered. The accumulation of blood between the calvarium and the dura results in epidural (or extradural) hematomas. Bleeding between the dura and the arachnoid gives rise to subdural hematomas, whereas bleeding into the subarachnoid space itself gives rise to the typical subarachnoid hemorrhage. Of these, the subarachnoid hemorrhage is by far the most common in patients who sustain closed head trauma, but is rarely in and of itself lethal, nor is it often as focal as epidural and subdural hemorrhages tend to be. These three types of hemorrhages are considered "membrane" hemorrhages. The fourth type of traumatic intracranial hemorrhage is the intraparenchymal hematoma, including what has been called "burst" or "pulped" lobes.[4]

Epidural (Extradural) Hematomas

These lesions are overwhelmingly most commonly traumatic in origin and represent collections of the blood between the calvarium and the dura, which has been stripped from the overlying bone by both the direct trauma and the hydrostatic force of the blood. Although usually encountered as acute lesions, chronic epidural hemorrhages do occur and are being recognized and described with increasing frequency.[24,25,40] Epidural hematomas are typically located in the temporal or frontal regions associated with an overlying skull fracture. The association of a skull fracture with an epidural hematoma occurs in 75 to 90 percent of patients.[12,18,21,33,40] These hemorrhages most often arise from lacerations of branches of the meningeal arteries by fractured bone edges. The ultimate size of these hematomas is dependent on several variables, including the tightness of adherence of the dura to the inner table of the skull, the depth of the incorporation of the meningeal arteries into the inner table of the skull, and the size of the meningeal artery lacerated. Associated traumatic lesions of the brain, once considered relatively uncommon, are quite frequent in my material,[40] as well as that reported in several other series. These coexisting lesions include subdural hematomas, cortical contusions, and cortical lacerations. The association of traumatic lesions in the brain with epidural hemorrhage has been seen in about one-third of my cases.[40]

The blood within the typical epidural hematoma is clotted, in contrast to the subdural hematoma where the blood often is a mixture of liquid and clotted blood. True encapsulation of epidural hematomas can occur in the more chronic forms, as in chronic subdural hematomas. Larger epidural hematomas, particularly those occurring in the temporal

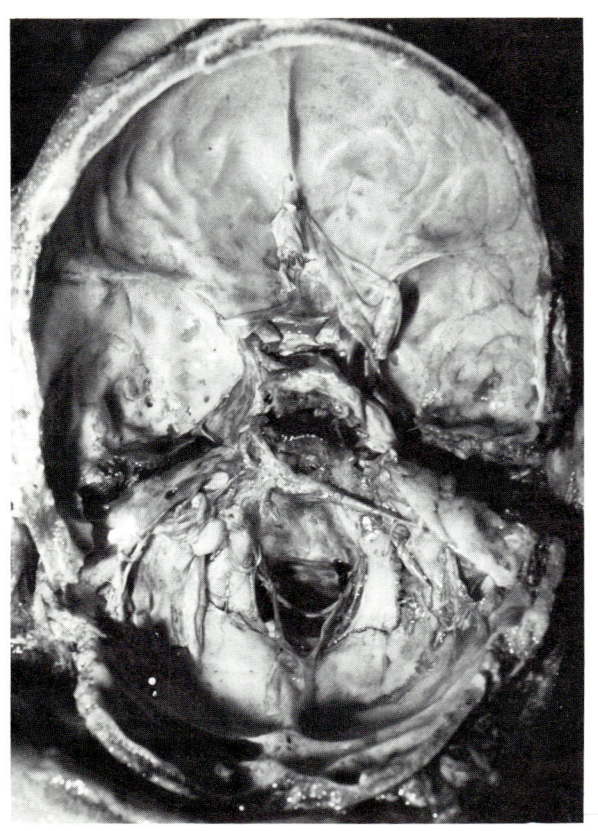

Figure 190-6 Massive "hinge" basilar skull fracture with extension through the sella turcica, complete separation of the petrous bone from the greater wing of the sphenoid, and separation of the temporal squama at the petrosquamous fissure. This pattern of skull fractures can be produced by either lateral crushing injuries or impact to the chin or occiput.

region, tend to be distinctly lens-shaped; those that occur in the posterior fossa tend to be more flattened in configuration. Epidural hematomas due to the laceration of dural sinuses or of the veins of the diploe tend to be relatively thin and much less lens-shaped. Organization of an epidural hematoma occurs if the volume is insufficient to produce brain herniation. Such hematomas may so completely organize as to appear as fibrous plaques along the external surfaces of the dura.[24,27,40]

Subdural Hematomas

Hemorrhage occurring into the dura-arachnoid interface produces subdural hematomas. These are far more common than epidural hemorrhages and are less often clearly the result of head trauma. Moreover, acute subdural hematomas are much more likely to be associated with other, often very significant, focal brain lesions (contusions, lacerations).[1,21,33,40,46,55] This high association with serious brain wounds is at least partially responsible for the frequently quoted mortality rate of as high as 60 to 70 percent in series of patients with acute subdural hematomas.[40]

Subdural hematomas can be subdivided into acute, subacute, and chronic forms, but this division is quite arbitrary and may have little or no special pathological significance.[46] Some authors have used very discrete time intervals for these three types, designating those that produce symptoms within 3 days of the initiating trauma as acute, those whose symptoms begin between 3 days and 3 weeks after trauma as subacute, and those with the onset of symptoms after 3 weeks as chronic.[46] Practically, acute subdural hematomas are so often associated with skull fractures and very significant underlying focal traumatic brain lesions that they should be considered separate from the chronic subdural hematomas, as the chronic varieties are much less commonly associated with clear evidence of significant closed head trauma. (Subdural hematomas may arise from a variety of nontraumatic causes—ruptured saccular aneurysms with lacerations of the arachnoid, blood dyscrasias, etc.[40,47])

One of the problems that pathologists are often asked to address is our estimation of the age of a subdural hematoma. Estimates are based on the degree of lysis of the erythrocytes, the degree of formation and organization of encapsulating neomembranes, and the amount of resolution or extension of the hematoma (Figs. 190-8 and 190-9).[21,40] The use of computed tomography has considerably expanded our knowledge of the evolution of these membrane hematomas. Table 190-1 summarizes the sequence of events in the histological aging of subdural hematomas. It is tempting to be overly precise in the histological aging of subdural hematomas. The timing of events given in this table are as accurate as I can make them, but presuppose adequate material for examination.

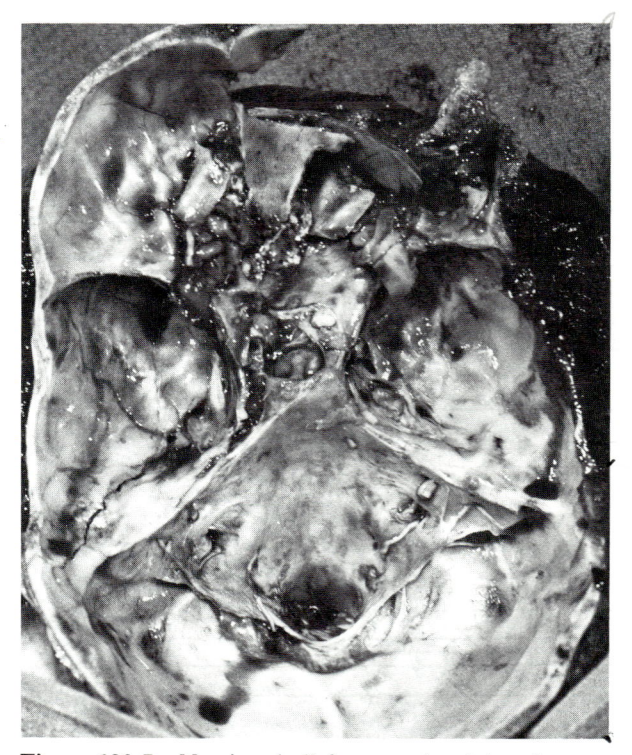

Figure 190-7 Massive skull fractures involving the vertex and base. Once there has been sufficient energy to produce one linear fracture, very little additional force is required to produce such massive bone shattering.

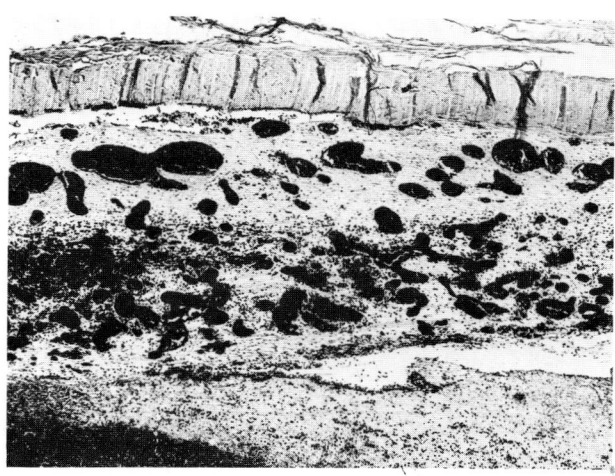

Figure 190-8 Chronic subdural hematoma membranes showing markedly vascular granulation tissue and hemorrhage. At this stage the hematoma membranes are considerably thicker than the overlying dura. This hematoma was 7 weeks old by history. (Trichrome; × 14.)

Subarachnoid Hemorrhage

Bleeding into the subarachnoid space is the most common "lesion" resulting from closed head trauma.[40] It is often trivial, although it may be truly massive. It can be found in the absence of cortical contusions or lacerations, but significant degrees of subarachnoid hemorrhage are almost always associated with cortical contusions. Depending on the size and type of the vessels lacerated (veins, venules, arteries, arterioles), the accumulation of blood within the subarachnoid space may become so extensive as to produce mass lesions. More commonly, subarachnoid hemorrhage may impede the normal circulation of the cerebrospinal fluid, blocking the exit of the CSF from the ventricular system or impeding its absorption by packing the pacchionian granulations over the vertex of the brain (Fig. 190-10). Such a blockage of cerebrospinal fluid passage or absorption can give rise to increased intracranial pressure with resulting brain herniation and secondary brain lesions. This is an example of how focal traumatic brain lesions, often of themselves rather trivial, can result in serious secondary brain lesions.

Contusions and Lacerations

Contusions are bruises of the neural parenchyma and are always traumatic. Most commonly involving the crown of a gyrus (Fig. 190-11), they tend to be wedge-shaped, with the apex extending into the neural parenchyma.[1,2,21,33,35,40] They represent extravasation of erythrocytes about small lacerated vessels within the neural parenchyma (Fig. 190-12). In a simple contusion, the pial-glial membrane is intact. If this membrane is disrupted, a *laceration* is produced. While contusions occur in the absence of lacerations, lacerations are almost always associated with contusions.

Contusions have commonly been classified into one of six types, depending on their spatial relationship to trauma or a specific anatomical structure.[40] These are *coup*, *contrecoup*, *intermediate coup*, *gliding*, *herniation*, and *fracture* contusions. Coup contusions are those that occur beneath the immediate area of impact. Contrecoup contusions are those that are thought to be confined to areas remote from and most often in a straight line with the impact site on the other side of the brain. The distinction between coup and contrecoup contusions appears less sharp now than in the past. The principle reasons for this lack of clear differentiation have been well summarized by Adams et al., who note that frontal and temporal contusions are the predominant ones regardless of the site of head impact.[2]

While the classification of contrecoup contusions still has some utility in a consideration of the distribution of lesions following closed head injury, too great an emphasis on the distribution of contrecoup contusions should not be made. The concept of the intermediate coup contusion has arisen primarily from the publications of Lindenberg and Freytag, who described them as occurring within the neural parenchyma between the impact site and the opposite side of the brain.[33,35,36] These often occur along areas of intermediate tissue density. At least some of those contusions classically called intermediate coup are quite clearly due to secondary vascular phenomena, largely tearing of thalamostriate and of thalamoperforating arteries. I think that true intermediate coup contusions do occur in the sylvian fissure where the temporal and frontal cortices may be forcibly "slapped" against each other during the transmission of the force from one side to the other (Fig. 190-13). Gliding contusions have been described as those that occur at the vertex of the brain and are produced by a rostral to caudal movement of the

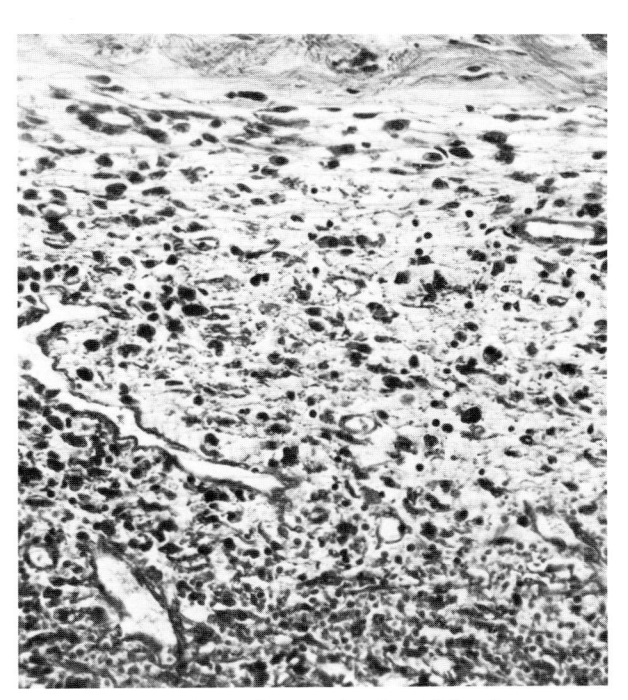

Figure 190-9 Photomicrograph of a subdural membrane showing numerous capillaries, erythrocytes (both intact and lysed), and hemosiderin-laden macrophages entrapped in the vascular granulation tissue. (H&E; × 76.)

TABLE 190-1 Microscopic Features of Subdural Hematomas

Time after Injury	Clot	Dural Side	Arachnoid Side
0–36 h	Erythrocytes intact	Fibrin	Fibrin
36–60 h	Erythrocytes intact	A few fibroblasts at the dural junction	Fibrin
4–5 days	Erythrocytes lysing, with a few pigment-laden macrophages	Fibroblastic layer 2 to 5 cells thick	Fibrin
1–2 weeks	Erythrocytes lysing; angiofibroblastic invasion of clot	Fibroblastic layer 10 to 15 cells thick	May be a single layer of flat, epithelioid-like cells
2–3 weeks	Clot breaks up; vascular sinusoids ("giant capillaries") apparent	Fibroblastic layer now up to one-half the thickness of the dura	Fibroblastic membrane and rare capillaries
3–4 weeks	Vascular sinusoids well developed		
4–6 weeks	Liquefied clot	Fibroblastic membrane equal to the dura in thickness; pigment-laden macrophages	Well-formed membrane; relatively avascular
½–3 months	There is compaction and fibrosis of the membranes of both the dural and the arachnoid sides. There are large capillaries early, and there are often secondary hemorrhages.		
3–12 months	The neomembranes become fused, consist of more mature fibrous tissue, and contain numerous pigment-laden macrophages. Beyond 3 months, it is not possible to give a very accurate approximation of the age of the hematoma.		
Beyond 1 year	The neomembrane forms a distinct, fibrous connective-tissue layer which closely resembles the adjacent dura mater. Occasionally calcification and/or ossification can appear after approximately 3 years.		

brain during decelerative injuries. Unlike the typical contusion, these do not tend to involve the surface of the gyrus as much as the deeper layers of the cortex, with extension into the convolutional white matter (Fig. 190-14).[2,40] The herniation contusion is produced by the sudden forcing of a portion of the brain against a rigid opening, most often the incisura of the tentorium. These contusions are thus seen along the medial portion of the temporal lobes (unci and hippocampi) in the great majority of cases (Fig. 190-15). They occur at the moment of brain impact and are not the type of herniation necrosis that is seen so commonly following relatively long-standing transtentorial herniation. Fracture contusions are coup contusions that lie immediately under the fracture line. The term *fracture contusions* is usually restricted to those contusions immediately under a bursting fracture and does not include the contusions and lacerations that occur under a depressed skull fracture. Typical coup, contrecoup, and gliding contusions have been produced in the experimental monkey model discussed by Adams et al.[8]

Contusions are the classical and primary hallmark of brain trauma. However, they may be totally absent in patients who have sustained severe and even lethal closed head injury.

The characteristic gross appearance of a contusion (of all types except the so-called gliding contusion) is an area of hemorrhage beneath the pia, extending into and usually through the cortex into the convolutional white matter. Contusions tend to be roughly wedge-shaped and are most often located over the crowns of gyri rather than involving the banks or depths of gyri within sulci. When the patient has survived for a significant period of time, there is breakdown of erythrocytes and the directly traumatized neural parenchyma with phagocytosis of the debris. This ultimately results in an area of tissue shrinkage with depression of the area of the old contusion below the adjacent surface (Fig. 190-16). The overlying leptomeninges are often discolored by hemosiderin pigment and may be adherent to the underlying shrunken brain. The ability of the pathologist to accurately guess the age of a contusion is quite limited. Acute inflammation is very transient. Lysis of erythrocytes is evident within 48 to 72 h, and macrophage infiltration increases in amount from 24 h to several weeks. Reactive glio-

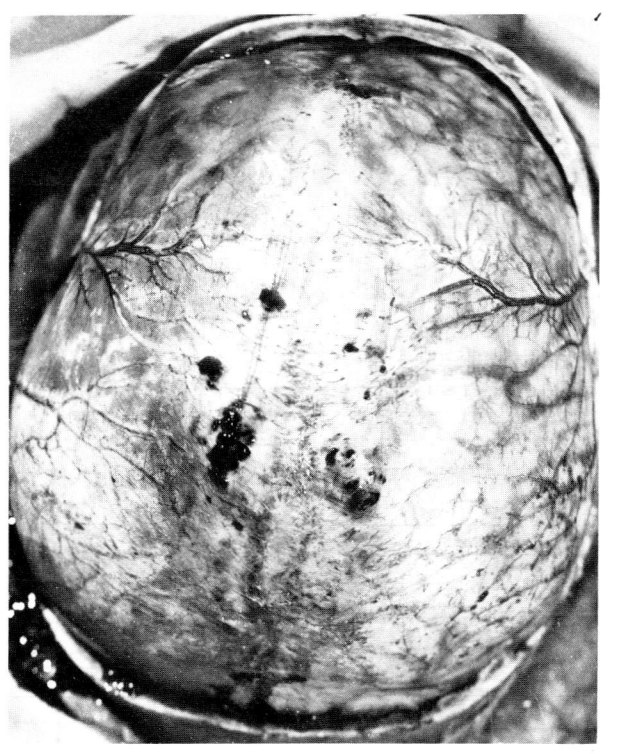

Figure 190-10 The pacchionian (arachnoid) granulations are distended by packed erythrocytes in a patient with a traumatic subarachnoid hemorrhage.

Pathology of Closed Head Injury

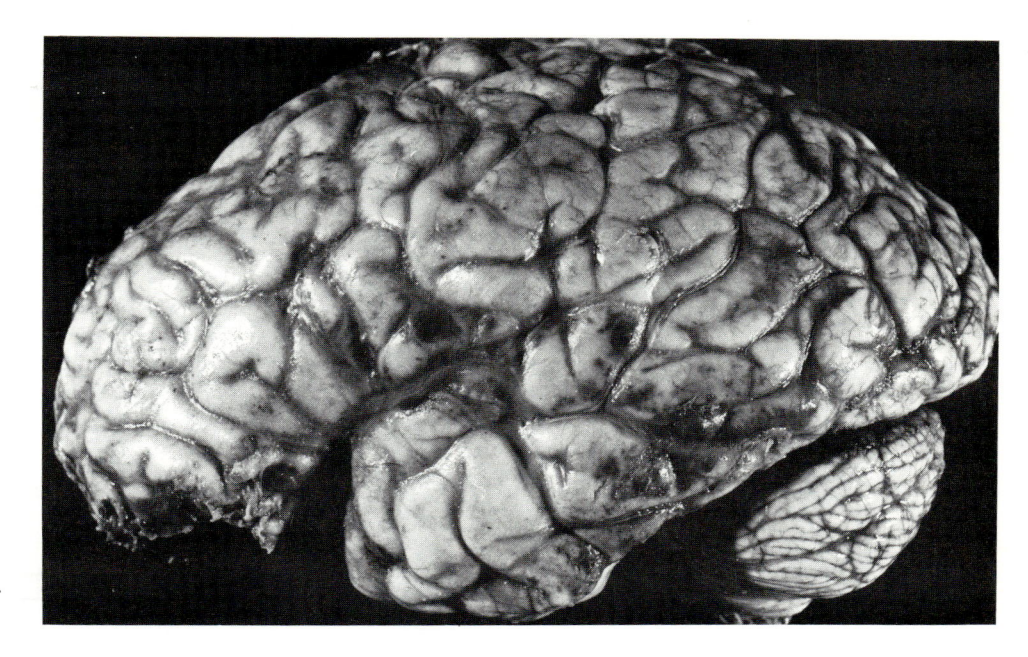

Figure 190-11 Lateral surface of the left cerebral hemisphere, showing numerous fresh cortical contusions involving maximally the crowns of the inferior frontal and temporal gyri.

sis can be seen as early as 48 h about a contusion, and it increases with the passage of time. After several months, it is no longer possible to estimate the age of a contusion. The white matter surrounding a contusion is swollen and microscopically pallid and fenestrated.[40] Reactive axons can be seen within the convolutional white matter surrounding a contusion in a remarkably short time (Fig. 190-17), having been clearly demonstrated in some of our cases within 2 or 3 h of the time of injury.[33,40] Homogenizing necrosis of neurons, manifested by cell shrinkage with hypereosinophilia of the cytoplasm and pyknosis of nuclei, can be seen within 6 h of the injury and becomes truly conspicuous within 18 to 24 h. Capillary endothelial swelling begins early and increases with the passage of time. It is usually quite prominent in contusions of 48 to 72 h or older. It is not uncommon to find small foci of mineral within the neural parenchyma and encrusting neuronal and glial cell bodies and processes in old contusions. This phenomenon is rarely seen in contusions of less than a month's age.[40]

Finally, it is important to understand that patients who die immediately following massive head trauma may have minimal bleeding into the neural parenchyma. Such cases are rarely seen in hospital practices, but are relatively common in medical-legal services that deal with large numbers of massively traumatized vehicular-injured patients.

Brain *lacerations* are physical disruptions of the brain integrity at the macroscopic level. They are often but not invariably associated with obvious contusions and can occur in virtually any part of the brain including the brain stem. (The so-called pontomedullary tear or rent, an example of such a

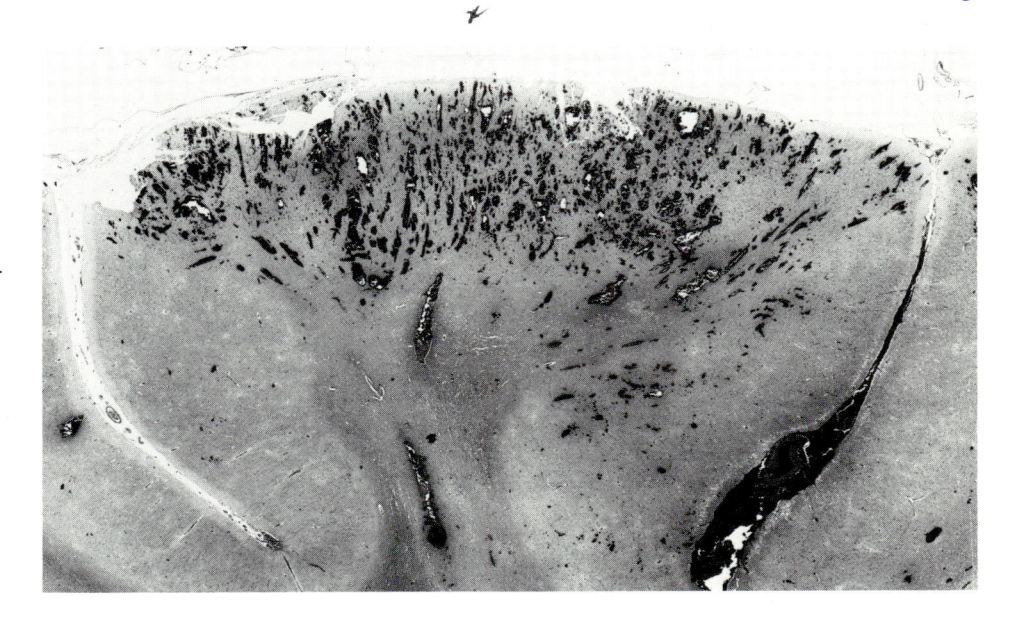

Figure 190-12 Photomacrograph of an acute cortical contusion with minute foci of pial laceration and pallor of staining (early ischemic necrosis) of the adjacent cortex. Note the location of this typical traumatic lesion at the crown of the gyrus and its approximately wedge shape. (H&E; × 6.)

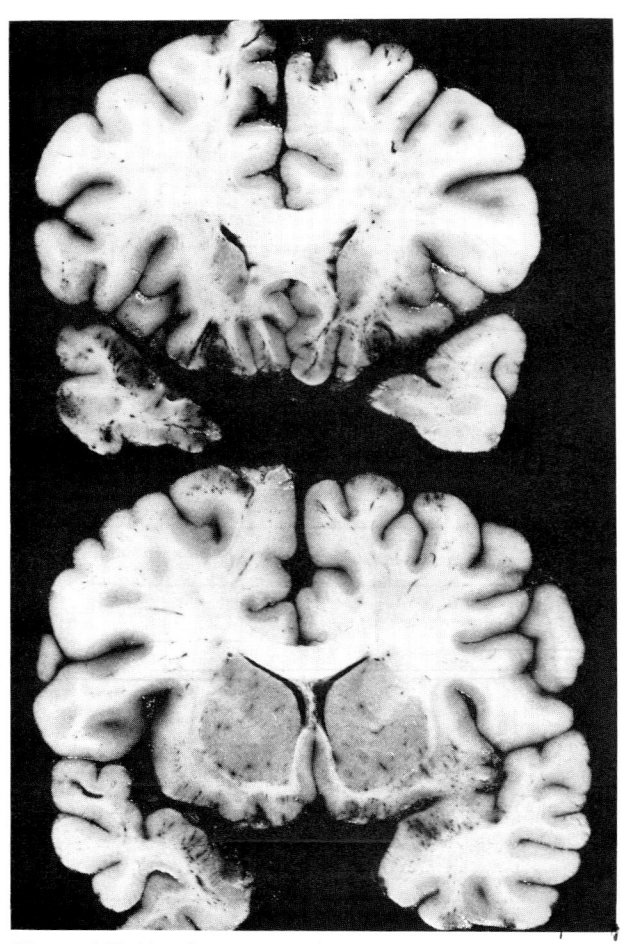

Figure 190-13 Acute contusions in the temporal and frontal gyri in the sylvian fissure. These are sometimes called intermediate coup contusions.

brain laceration, will be discussed under Direct Brain Stem Trauma.)

Intraparenchymal Hemorrhages

Hemorrhages within the parenchyma of the brain forming discrete hematomas, as distinct from contusions with diffusion of blood into the neural parenchyma, occur most commonly in the cerebral hemispheres, with the majority lying in the frontal and temporal lobes (Figs. 190-18 and 190-19). Intraparenchymal brain hemorrhages are often multiple, with patients harboring two or more hematomas of varying size. The overall prevalence of intraparenchymal brain hemorrhages in closed head trauma patients reported in the literature varies from less than ½ percent to approximately 9 percent.[40,48] In the last 110 cases of fatal closed head trauma on my service, 24 have had a massive intraparenchymal hematoma, multiple in 10 and solitary in 14. The high prevalence of massive hematomas (22 percent) in my material reflects its origin from an autopsy series. Clinically derived series of intraparenchymal hemorrhages have, as would be expected, a much lower prevalence rate.

In the great majority of massive traumatic intraparenchymal brain hemorrhages, cortical contusions and lacerations are also present. The great majority of traumatic hemorrhages are "lobar" in distribution and uncommonly ganglionic unless arising in obvious extension from severely contused and lacerated cortex.[21,33,40,48] A significant number of patients with intraparenchymal hematomas will also have membrane hemorrhages, most commonly acute subdural hematomas and subarachnoid hemorrhage. Epidural hemorrhages may be present in these patients, but are relatively uncommon.

Adams et al. have discussed the entity which they call "burst lobes" and have made a distinction between them

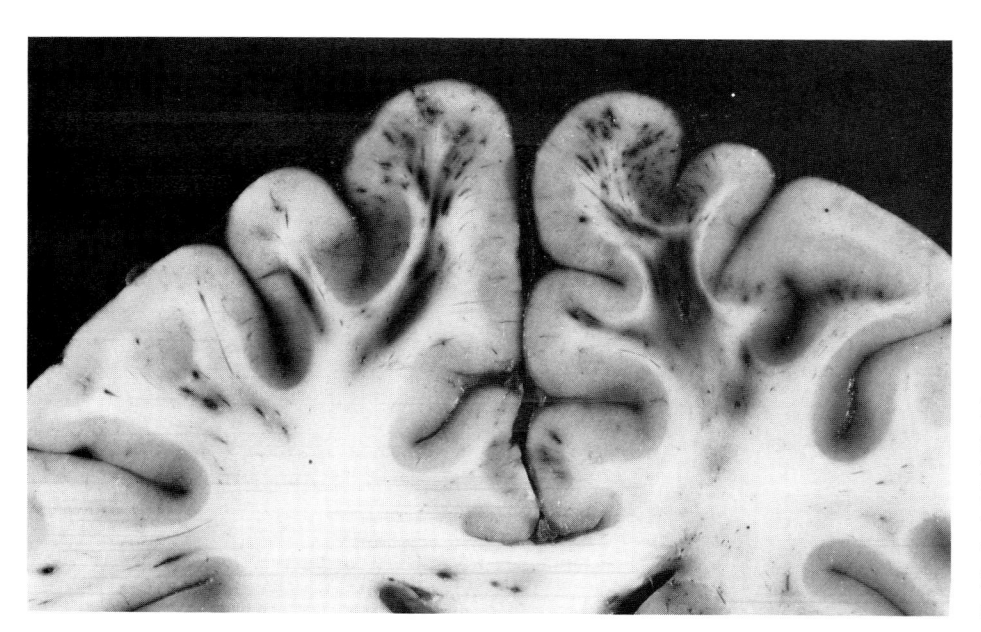

Figure 190-14 A gliding contusion involving the superior frontal convolutions. The hemorrhage has not extended to the pial surface of the cortex and is most prominent in the convolutional white matter.

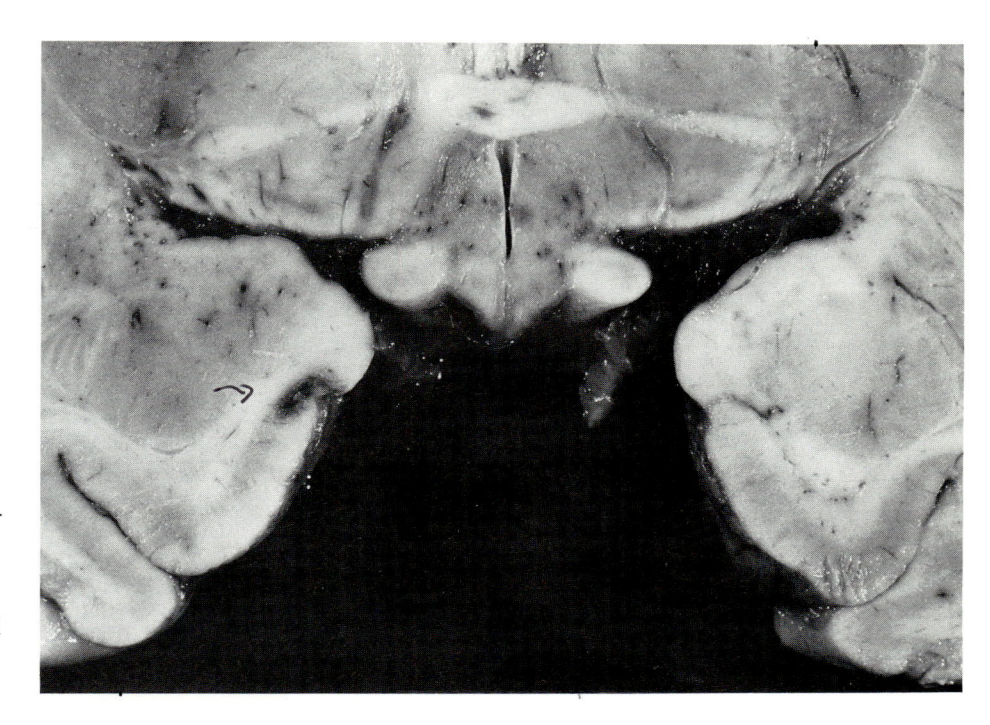

Figure 190-15 Typical herniation hemorrhagic contusion of the left uncus at the point of impaction at the tentorium cerebelli. A much smaller and less hemorrhagic groove is present on the right.

and traumatic intraparenchymal hematomas (Fig. 190-20).[1,4] This distinction is based on whether or not the intraparenchymal hematoma is in direct continuity with overlying lacerated, contused brain, which in turn is in continuity with an acute subdural hematoma. "Burst lobes" should be distinguished, in my opinion, from true hematomas.

The rapidity with which intraparenchymal hematomas accumulate following head trauma has been of considerable interest to a number of investigators. With the advent of computed tomography, it has been possible to observe serially the progress of hematoma development and resolution. It is now clear that many hematomas not present within the first few hours following head trauma will develop subsequently. This observation is also substantiated by the observation that victims dead on the scene or who die within an hour or two will have massive intraparenchymal hematomas far less often than those patients who have survived for a significant period of time.

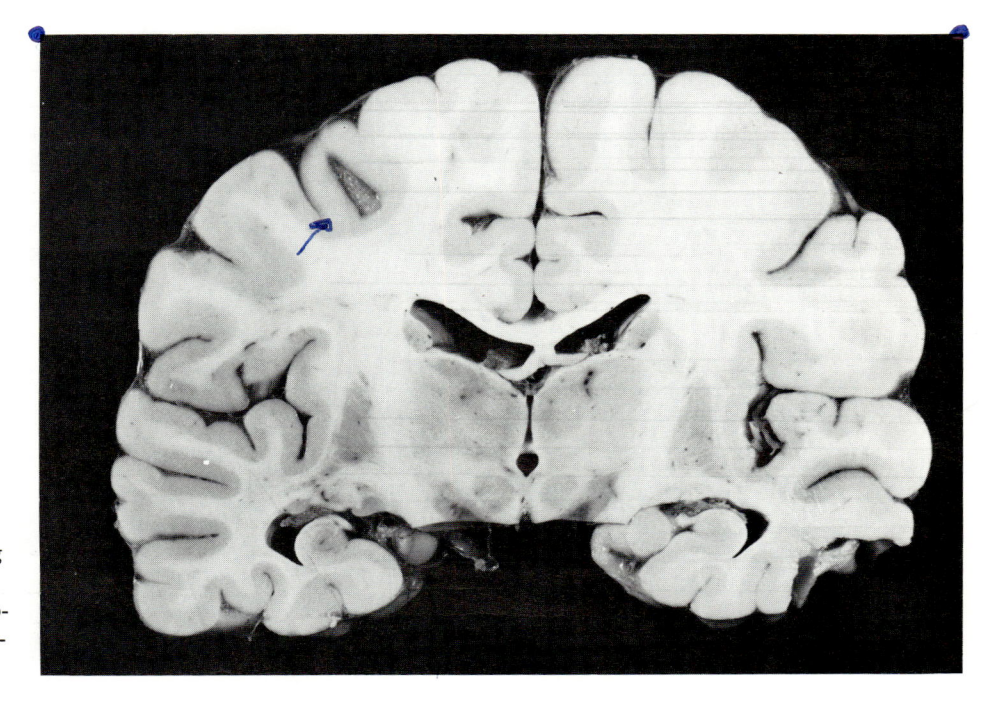

Figure 190-16 Remote contusion in the right middle temporal convolution showing the roughly cone-shaped area of necrosis and tissue loss typical of an old, resorbed contusion.

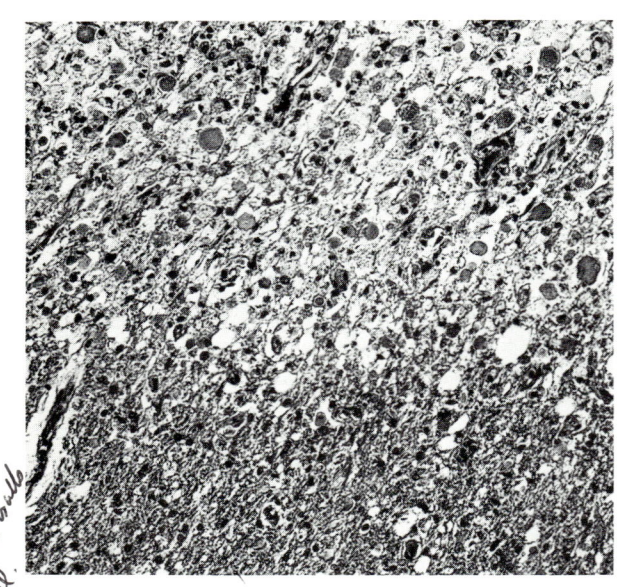

Figure 190-17 Photomicrograph through a small subacute contusion illustrating the numerous reactive axonal balls secondary to axonal transection. This contusion is approximately 120 h old. (Bodian; × 160.)

Delayed post-traumatic hematomas (Bollinger's "Spätapoplexie") have been of interest for a number of years. These hematomas typically become symptomatic a week or more after the traumatic event. Although these hematomas once were considered rare, computed tomography has demonstrated that the delayed development of even massive intraparenchymal hematomas occurs more frequently in trauma patients than had been appreciated.[7,28,32,33,48]

The association of disseminated intravascular coagulation (DIC) with closed head trauma is becoming increasingly evident.[40,41,57] This DIC is apparently triggered by tissue thromboplastins derived from neural parenchymal destruction and is probably responsible for hematoma development from small contusional hemorrhages.

Another type of coagulopathy often encountered in patients with closed head injury is that associated with alcohol intake.[10,17,40] It has been demonstrated that alcohol imbibition has a direct effect on blood clotting,[16] and statistical evidence suggests that it plays a major role in the development of intraparenchymal hematomas in some trauma victims. Of the 24 decedents with massive intraparenchymal hematomas in my material referred to previously, 16 were alcoholics and had alcohol in their blood at the time of hospitalization.

Both intraparenchymal hematomas and typical contusions of the coup-contrecoup type are much less often seen in infancy and early childhood than in adulthood. The most typical alterations found at autopsy in infants dying of closed head injuries are fresh membrane hemorrhages, slitlike intraparenchymal hemorrhages (most frequent in the frontal white matter dissecting along the radiations of the medullary veins),[1,2,21,36,40] and diffuse, often severe brain swelling.[8,33,36,40,42] Less frequently encountered lesions in the brains of such infants are focal areas of decreased density

(ischemia) in arterial border zones, particularly between the distributions of the posterior and middle cerebral arteries; tears of the corpus callosum, usually with minimal associated hemorrhage; and small areas of subependymal hemorrhage with or without intraventricular extension.[40] Acute subdural hematomas are common and should alert the physician to the probability of trauma even in the absence of other external stigmata. They are a common finding in battered children and may be caused by shaking.

The typical slitlike frontal white matter hemorrhagic lesions have been described by Lindenberg and Freytag as "contusional tears."[36] They noted that these tears are largely confined to the white matter with little or no extension into either the overlying cortex or the ventricular system. The amount of blood associated with these small tears is often small, and with the passage of time, only a smooth-walled cleft remains (Fig. 190-21).

In summary, traumatic intracerebral hematomas are relatively common, being reported in 1 to 3 percent of patients in clinical series and up to 25 percent of closed head victim

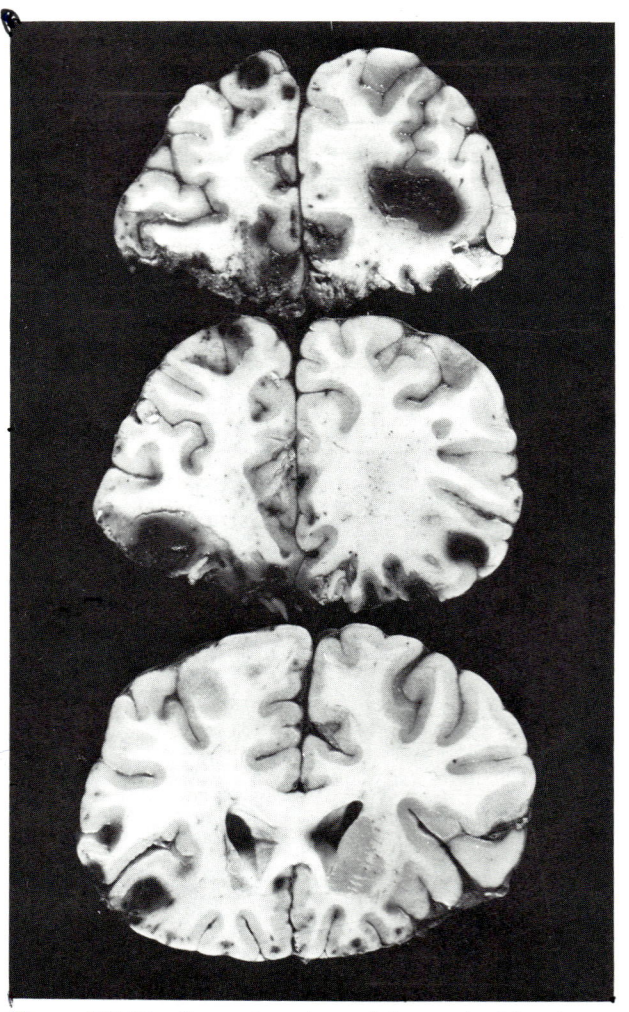

Figure 190-18 Coronal sections of the cerebral hemispheres through the frontal lobes revealing multiple fresh cortical contusions, maximal in the orbital frontal gyri, and a portion of a right frontal hematoma.

Direct Brain Stem Trauma

Contusions and lacerations of the brain stem occur most commonly in association with traumatic lesions elsewhere in the brain (i.e., as a part of more diffuse injury).[1-6,10,21,40,45,49] However, they can occur as essentially solitary lesions as a result of head trauma.[10,21,37,40,45]

One of the primary reasons that the existence of isolated direct brain stem trauma has been questioned is the origin of the cases available for study. Primarily on the basis of the experimental work of Ommaya and Gennarelli, Rosenblum et al.[49] have summarized the reasons for this debate over the existence of primary ("isolated") brain stem lesions in the absence of cerebral hemispheric lesions. Extensive direct brain stem trauma is so typically incompatible with life that victims of such a lesion do not live long enough to be admitted to a hospital and thus are not examined by hospital-based or academic pathologists.[40] It is only when significant material from medical examiners is available for examination

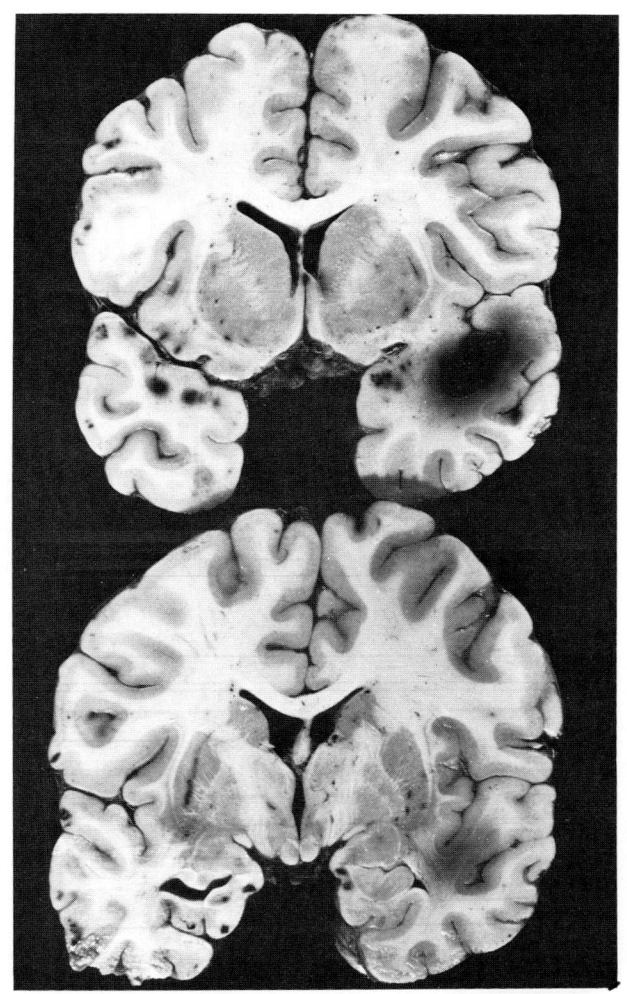

Figure 190-19 Same brain as seen in Fig. 190-17, demonstrating a second independent right temporal hematoma. Small "intermediate coup" contusions are evident in the temporal lobes in the mouth of the sylvian fissure on the right. Herniation contusions are evident in the herniated unci in the bottom section.

deaths in autopsy series. They are often associated with acute subdural hematomas, this association being seen in over 50 percent in some series. They are associated with decelerative-type head injuries in the great majority of cases, are often multiple, and are typically "lobar," with frontal and temporal locations predominating. They are only rarely confined to the basal ganglia/internal capsule areas. Massive traumatic intraparenchymal hematomas are associated with a coexisting skull fracture in 80 to 90 percent of patients. Contusions, either coup or contrecoup, are conspicuous in the brains of the great majority of patients with traumatic hematomas. Their absence, particularly in a patient with a ganglionic hemorrhage, should strongly suggest that the origin of the hematoma is from a cause other than trauma. The gross and microscopic changes seen in traumatic intraparenchymal hematomas seem similar in all respects to hematomas of equal size due to causes other than trauma.

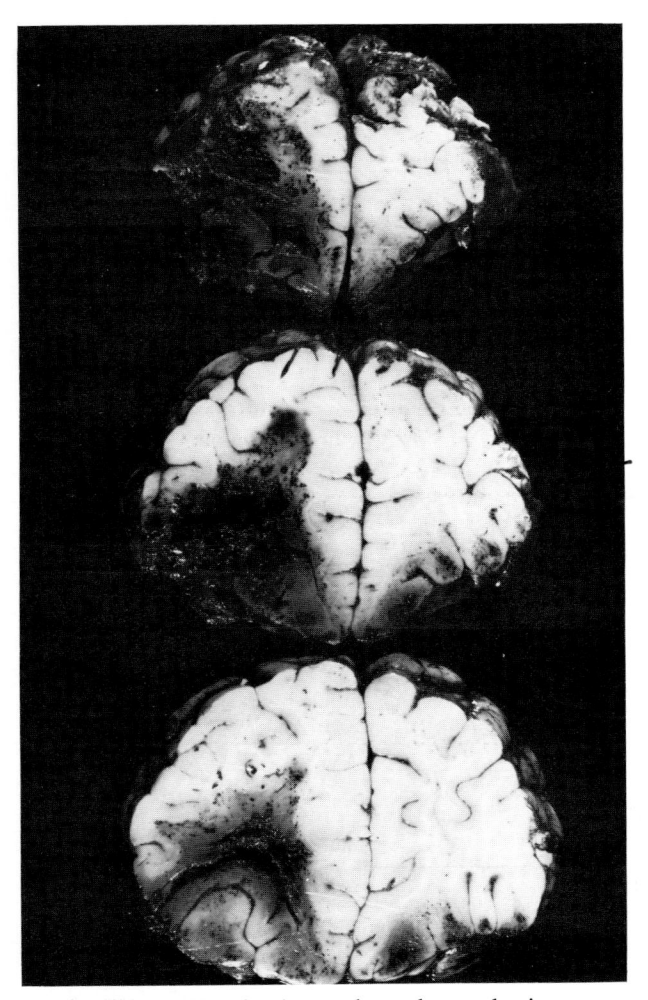

Figure 190-20 Massive hemorrhage, hemorrhagic necrosis, and pulpification of the right frontal lobe (left side of photograph) in a patient with a "pulped" or "burst" frontal lobe. Acute contusions are prominent in the orbital-frontal gyri on the opposite side.

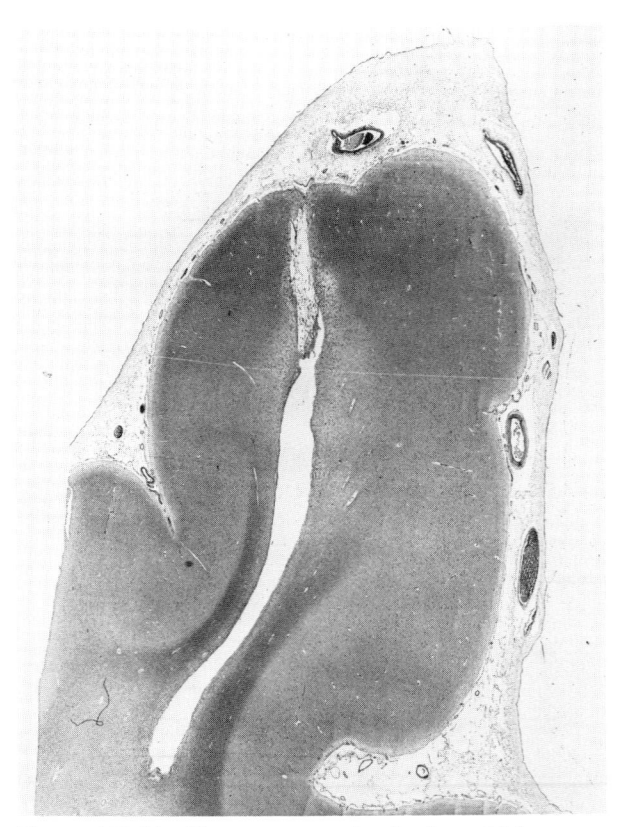

Figure 190-21 Photomacrograph of a frontal lobe revealing an old, slitlike cavity resulting from a closed head injury in an infant who survived for 3 months. A minimal amount of blood remains in this linear cavity. Unlike many of these lesions, this one extended through the cortex. (Trichrome; × 6.)

that many cases of the extensive direct traumatic brain lesions will be found.

While direct isolated brain stem trauma is far more common in forensic pathology cases, a significant number of patients with this type of trauma have survived for sufficient periods of time to reach a hospital. Indeed, Pilz et al. have described a patient who survived for 26 days following head trauma and who was found to have a large pontomedullary rent.[45] This lesion, the pontomedullary tear or rent, is now so well known that most pathologists associated with an active trauma service will have encountered it (Figs. 190-22 and 190-23). Among the larger series of reported cases are those by Lindenberg and Freytag[37] with 21 cases, Britt et al.[6] with 24 cases, Hardman[21] with 12 cases, and my own material with 12 cases.[40] The great majority of these patients, over 95 percent in the series mentioned above, have had a skull or upper spinal fracture. These pontomedullary junction tears are most often due to marked hyperextension of the head on the neck, most often with trauma directed to the brow with the legs and torso bending forward over the temporarily immobile head.[21,37,40,45] It is of great interest to note that Adams and his colleagues have been able to produce pontomedullary rents in monkeys subjected to severe angular acceleration of very short duration.[2]

Another distinct but considerably less commonly observed and described form of direct brain stem trauma is laceration, either focal or massive, at the mesencephalic-pontine junction (Figs. 190-24 and 190-25). In my own material, such separations have been found in 4 patients in the same study population that contains 12 decedents with pontomedullary rents. Britt et al. had 8 patients with such mesencephalic-pontine junction lacerations as compared with their 24 with pontomedullary rents.[6]

A third distinct type of primary traumatic brain stem lesion is the traumatic laceration or even complete separation (transection) of the medulla from the upper cervical spinal cord. Britt et al. reported that 1 of 41 patients with primary brain stem injury demonstrated this type of lesion.[6] I also have had only 1 patient with complete spinal-medullary separation, a young man who sustained trauma to the left side of his neck in a motorcycle accident.[40] This type of lesion is quite common in dead-at-the-scene trauma victims and has been produced in experimental animal models.[56] Indeed, it appears to be one of the more common types of lethal lesions and is due to separation of the atlas from the skull.[56]

Rosenblum and his colleagues have described variable-sized hemorrhagic and nonhemorrhagic necrotic lesions in the mesencephalon in 88 percent of a series of 26 brains from patients dying from head trauma.[49] All patients had survived for "several days or more." These lesions were not considered to be "secondary" to transtentorial herniation and were thought to have occurred at the moment of impact,

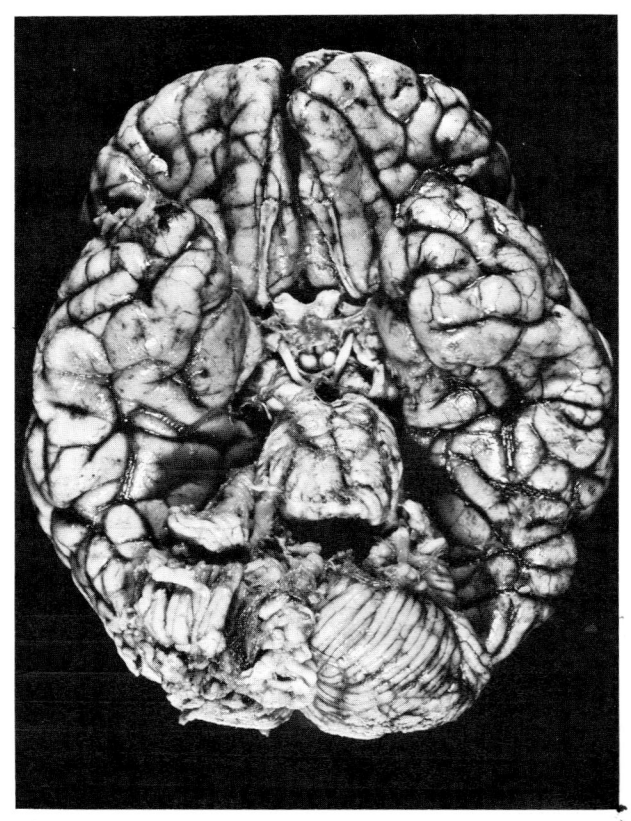

Figure 190-22 Ventral surface of the brain in a patient who sustained a brow impact with hyperextension of the body over the fixed brow. There is deep laceration at the junction of the pons with the rostral medulla.

Pathology of Closed Head Injury

tients with increased intracranial pressure and cerebral contusions. They are not typical secondary brain stem hemorrhages. I do not presently consider these as primary brain stem traumatic lesions but rather a combination of diffuse impact and secondary ischemic injury or, in some patients, a form of secondary vascular lesion (Fig. 190-26). (See below.) Regardless, their documentation by the Rosenblum group is an important contribution to our expanding knowledge of the lesions found in head trauma.

Adams and his colleagues have, in the past, maintained that traumatic brain stem injuries do not occur in the absence of diffuse brain injury. Adams et al. state, "In a personal series of 600 brains from patients dying as a result of head injury, we have never identified a primary traumatic lesion in the brain stem in isolation: when one was present,

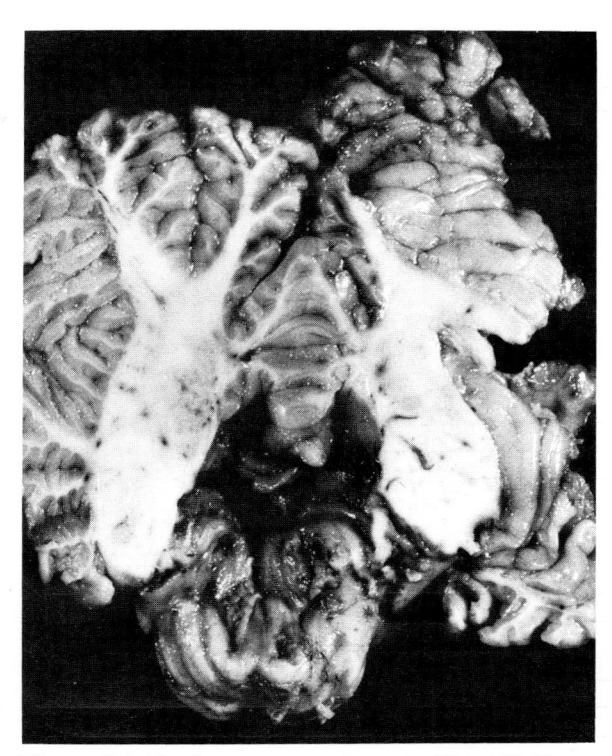

Figure 190-23 Same case as shown in Fig. 190-22. Section of the pons and cerebellum at the level of the pontomedullary separation. A relatively small amount of hemorrhage is typically seen in this area of laceration.

thus being primary lesions. Typically confined to the tegmentum or the lateral or superior margins of the mesencephalon and rostral pons, they show a "spectrum of ages" in agreement with the time lapse between trauma and death rather than all being fresh as in secondary brain stem hemorrhage (Figs. 190-26 and 190-27). They were found in patients without elevated ICP and in patients without gross evidence of brain herniation. These authors summarized their findings and interpretations as follows:.

> We can say that brain stem lesions, particularly of the midbrain, are extremely common in fatal closed head injury, that they are readily found at autopsy, that they can be detected with MEPs during life, and that their presence or absence provides a prognostic indicator at least as accurate [as] or better than other clinical findings. We agree that midbrain lesions rarely occur in "isolation" (that is, in the absence of hemispheric lesions). The almost universal occurrence of hemispheric damage when brain stem damage is present is consonant with the concept of a centripetal spread of forces in closed head injury with resultant "primary" midbrain damage. However, the primary midbrain lesions are common rather than rare, and this fact should not be obscured by the argument concerning the presence or absence of "isolated" brain stem lesions.[49]

I have also found such minute lesions in a number of my 110 cases, but with less frequency and more typically in pa-

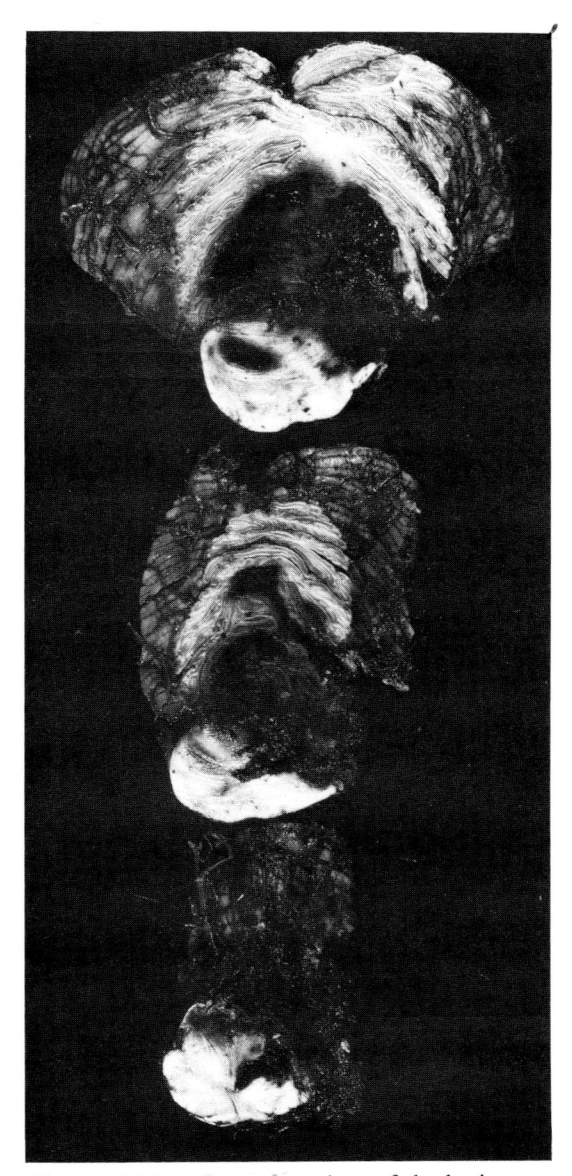

Figure 190-24 Coronal sections of the brain stem and cerebellum through the mesencephalon (*bottom section*) and rostral pons (*middle and upper sections*) showing extensive laceration and hemorrhage in and about the rostral brain stem.

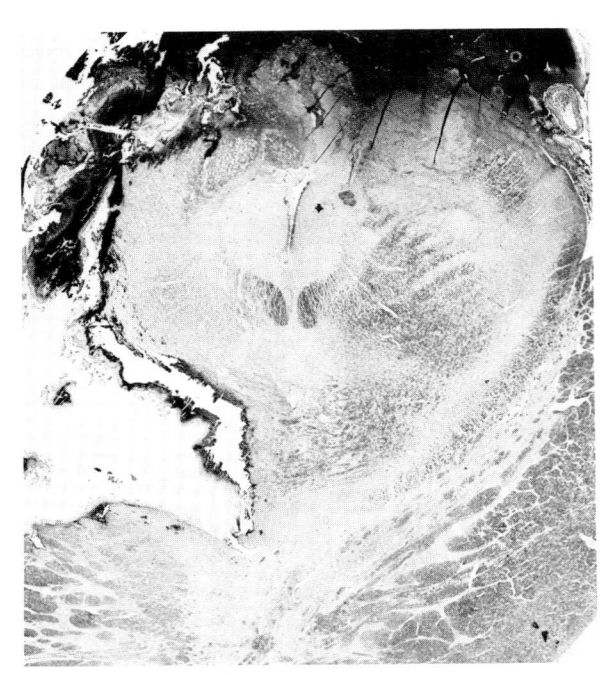

Figure 190-25 Photomacrograph of a typical mesencephalic and rostral pontine laceration in a patient with mesencephalic-pontine separation. This patient lived approximately 1½ h following the injury with ventilatory and circulatory assistance. (Trichrome; × 7.)

there was always evidence of DAI (diffuse axonal injury)."[2] Interestingly, in the same paper they record one patient with a pontomedullary separation (among "several hundred" fatal head injuries) and state, "There is little doubt that these lesions occurred at the time of injury, and it would appear that this is one—and possibly the only—type of primary damage to the brain stem that may occur in isolation." As now amply documented, this statement is not correct. Table 190-2 summarizes the types of brain stem trauma.

Direct Cranial Nerve Injuries

Contusions, laceration, and/or avulsions of cranial nerves can occur either as isolated lesions or, more commonly, as part of more severe and diffuse brain damage. We have en-

TABLE 190-2 Traumatic Brain Stem Lesions

I. Primary brain stem injury
   A. Direct focal injury
      1. Fracture lacerations and contusions
      2. Pontomedullary separations
      3. Medullocervical separations
      4. Mesencephalic-pontine separations
   B. Diffuse impact injury (Strich lesions), including gross hemorrhagic necrosis of the dorsolateral pons.
II. Secondary brain stem injury due to herniations (including rare lateral medullary infarcts due to entrapment of the posterior inferior cerebellar artery)

countered patients with nerve avulsions involving one or more of almost all the cranial nerves.[40] Undoubtedly the most common traumatic cranial nerve lesion is contusion, sometimes to the point of destruction, of the olfactory bulbs and tracts occurring in patients with orbital frontal damage, often associated with orbital plate fractures. Optic nerve and chiasm lacerations have been reported in patients both with and without basilar skull fractures, usually following severe frontal head trauma. Traumatic lesions of the optic chiasm are often associated with hypothalamic injury.

Heinze has described laceration and partial avulsion of the third cranial nerves.[23] I have seen the same type of injury in one patient with mesencephalic-pontine laceration. Far more commonly encountered in trauma victims is hemorrhage and necrosis of the third nerves secondary to transtentorial herniation.

Lacerations and avulsions of the fourth, fifth, sixth, seventh, and eighth cranial nerves have been described (Figs. 190-28 to 190-30).[23,40,50,54] With all these injuries, basilar skull fractures are the rule. The separation of the occipito-sphenoid synchondrosis has been observed to result in direct abducens nerve injury.[54] Petrous fractures, especially those that run perpendicular to the long axis of the petrous portion of the temporal bone (transverse fractures), are quite apt to involve portions of the seventh and eighth cranial nerves. Such fractures are most often secondary to frontal or occipital impacts and are considerably less common (on the order of one-fifth as frequent) than the longitudinal petrous fractures resulting from lateral head impacts.

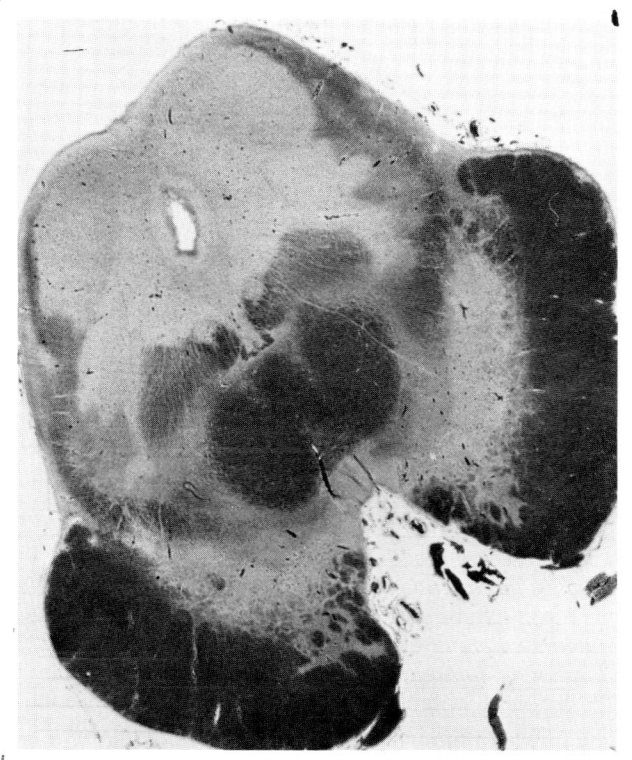

Figure 190-26 Photomacrograph of the mesencephalon of a patient with an extensive acute infarct in the tectum and periaqueductal gray matter. The patient survived 8 h. (Luxol fast blue—PASH; × 3.)

Pathology of Closed Head Injury

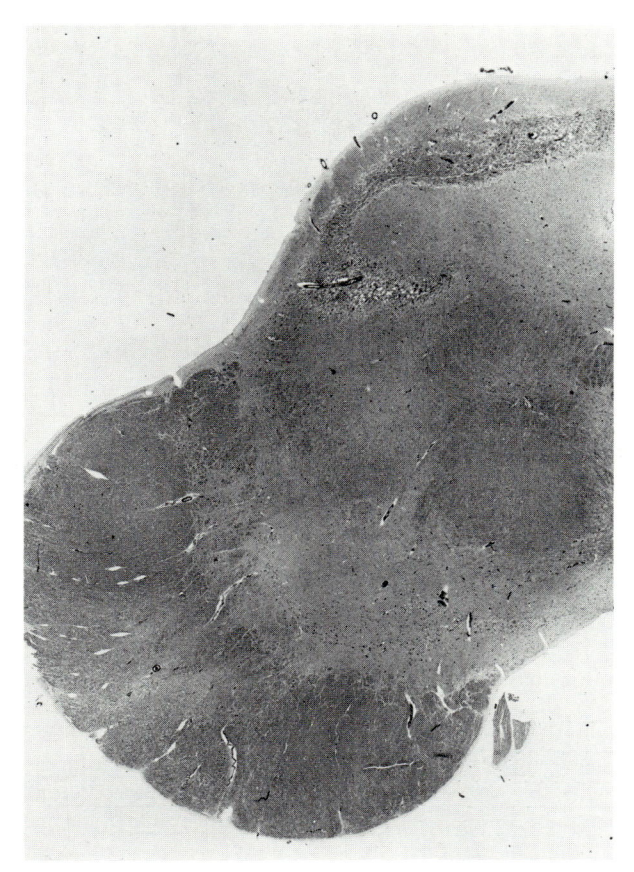

Figure 190-27 Mesencephalic tectal necrosis with features of both diffuse impact and secondary vascular injury. There were typical diffuse impact injuries in the pons and corpus callosum. (Luxol fast blue—PASH; × 7.)

Traumatic cranial nerve injuries are undoubtedly more common than the literature would suggest. Very few pathologists make examinations detailed enough to reveal them.

Direct Arterial Trauma

Another form of focal direct traumatic intracranial lesion is one in which vessels, arteries, veins, and dural sinuses are lacerated, avulsed, or thrombosed. Traumatic carotid-cavernous fistulas have been described extensively during the past 150 years and have been estimated to occur in as many as 1 to 2 percent of patients sustaining severe head injuries.[40] Typically associated with a basilar skull fracture that traverses the cavernous sinus, they are most often the result of a frontotemporal impact, with the fracture extending through the sphenoid bone.

Traumatic aneurysms of the intracranial arteries are also well known, although distinctly uncommon.[26,40,43,44] These have been divided into both "true" and "false." "True" traumatic aneurysms occur when the artery wall is lacerated but not completely penetrated. "False" aneurysms result when there has been mural rupture and organization of the surrounding hematoma, with the interior of the hematoma communicating with the penetrated artery. The false types are the more common. Traumatic aneurysms were described as occurring in five anatomical locations by Jackson et al.: scalp, adjacent cranial vault, arteries traversing the cranium, intracranial arteries, and meningeal arteries.[26] Only the latter two will be of concern in this presentation. The majority of traumatic aneurysms have been found to occur on superficial branches of the middle cerebral arteries, followed in frequency by the peripheral branches of the anterior cerebral arteries. Traumatic aneurysms have been found on

Figure 190-28 Complete avulsion of the third cranial nerve with a hematoma in the parenchyma along the nerve root. Note the wedge-shaped area of acute infarction in the left dorsolateral quadrant of the mesencephalon and focal hemorrhages into the dorsal aspect of the left cerebral peduncle, together with myelin pallor in much of the left peduncle. The patient survived 2 days.

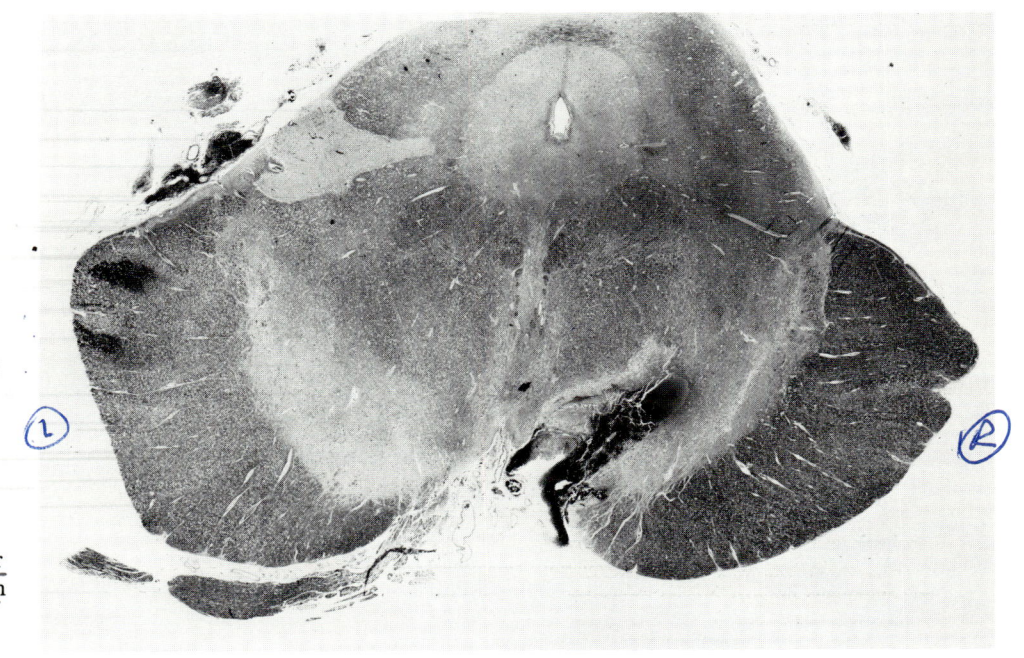

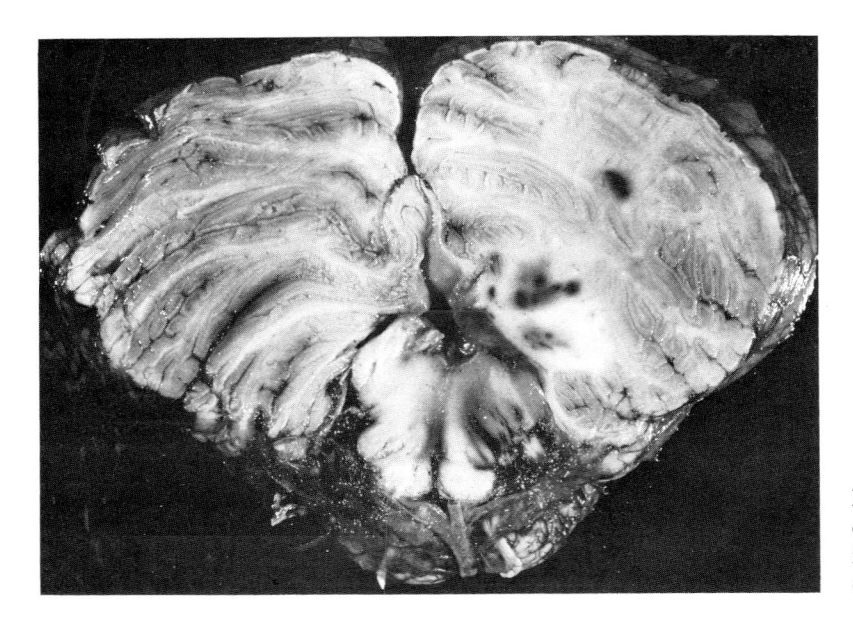

Figure 190-29 Section of the medulla and cerebellum showing hemorrhages extending into the medulla at the point of avulsion of cranial nerve roots.

other arteries, including the anterior choroidal, posterior cerebral, vertebral, superior cerebellar, and posterior inferior cerebellar. When traumatic aneurysms occur in their usual location on a peripheral branch of either the middle or anterior cerebral artery in an area of known trauma, they are not too likely to be confused with the far more common nontraumatic saccular ("medial defect," "congenital") aneurysm. Difficulty in differentiation can occur when a major artery at the base of the brain contains the aneurysm in a patient with severe head trauma. At times, resolution of the etiology of the aneurysm is possible only with detailed microscopic examination and a critical review of all clinical and anatomical evidence. Those features that have been found to be most useful in differentiating traumatic from nontraumatic saccular aneurysms are (1) the location of the aneurysm at a peripheral branch of an intracranial artery and usually not at a bifurcation point, (2) the absence of a demonstrable neck to the aneurysm, (3) an irregular contour of the aneurysm sac, and (4) a delay in angiographic filling and emptying of the aneurysm sac.[43] Many arteries (perhaps the great majority) with a traumatic aneurysm will have multiple discrete injuries to the artery wall adjacent to but separate from the tear that produced the aneurysm.[44] Finally, it should be noted that because of the relative frequency with which both saccular aneurysms and trauma occur in our population, patients with both nontraumatic saccular aneu-

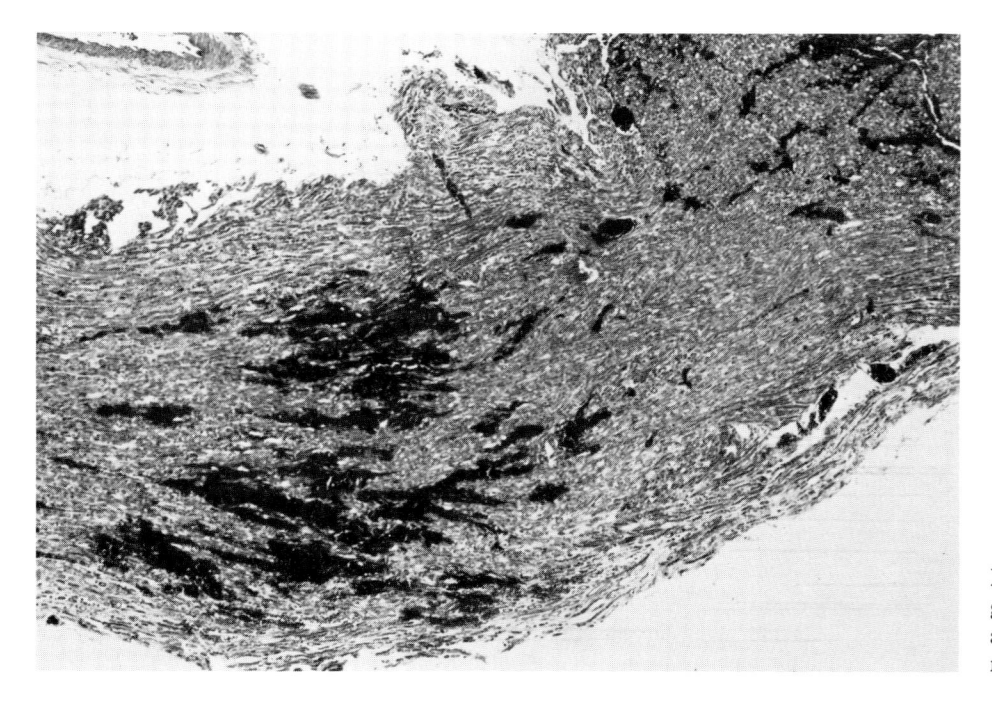

Figure 190-30 Photomicrograph of hemorrhage into an acutely traumatized cranial nerve root. (Trichrome; × 60.)

rysms and significant closed head trauma will be seen. While this problem has been recently addressed in several publications[39] and will not be discussed extensively in this chapter, it has been found that it is unlikely that closed head trauma will cause rupture of a pre-existing saccular aneurysm.

Thrombosis of major intracranial and extracranial cervical vessels secondary to trauma is well known. The initiating trauma may be quite trivial. The event leading to the production of the occluding thrombus is thought to be an intimal tear resulting from stretching of the vessel over a bony prominence. The most common sites of thrombotic occlusion in the internal carotid artery are a few centimeters above the carotid bifurcation and in the carotid canal at the base of the skull. Traumatic rupture of the vertebral artery with high lateral neck injuries is being reported with increasing frequency. Traumatic thrombosis of the vertebral arteries also occurs, most commonly at the C5-6 interspace, at the atlantoaxial joint, or at the atlanto-occipital joint. A rare form of intracranial artery occlusion secondary to head trauma is entrapment of the basilar artery in a transclival fracture, the basilar artery becoming displaced into the fracture at the moment of the impact. When the fracture line closes, the artery becomes entrapped and occluded within it. Traumatic thrombosis of the dural sinuses occurs less commonly than thrombosis of either the carotid or the vertebral artery in the neck.

Direct laceration of cerebral arteries and veins occurs commonly in many forms of closed head injury. Lacerations of smaller branches or tributaries are almost invariably seen in patients with acute subdural hematomas with their associated cortical lacerations and contusions and are obviously the origin of the subdural and subarachnoid hemorrhages seen in these patients.

Pituitary and Hypothalamic Lesions

Traumatic lesions of the pituitary and hypothalamus are common consequences of closed head injury. Clinically, syndromes of diabetes insipidus or hypopituitarism, ranging from severe panhypopituitarism to selective deficiency of a single pituitary hormone, may be observed. Over two-thirds of patients dying with closed head injury will be found to have structural abnormalities in the hypothalamus and pituitary if these areas are carefully examined.[40] In the combined studies of Daniel and Treip,[15] Ceballos,[9] Kornblum and Fisher,[31] and McCormick,[40] involving a total of 434 trauma victims, pituitary lesions were found, consisting most often of hemorrhages into the posterior lobe (Fig. 190-31) or infarction in the anterior lobe (Fig. 190-32), with a smaller number of cases of anterior lobe hemorrhage or stalk hemorrhages and lacerations. Posterior lobe hemorrhage was recorded in 160 cases (37 percent) and anterior lobe infarction in 74 (17 percent). In the last 110 cases of closed head injury on my service, a pituitary lesion of some type (severe capsular hemorrhage, hemorrhage within the stalk, posterior lobe hemorrhage, or anterior lobe infarction) has been found in 94, or 85 percent.

Lesions of the hypothalamus are also common, having been found in slightly over 42 percent of 106 patients with closed head injury studied by Crompton.[13,14] In the group of 106 patients, the pituitary was examined in only 53, of whom 14 (28 percent) had lesions. In the last 110 cases of mine, 22 had grossly evident lesions within the hypothalamus (Fig. 190-33), but an additional 6 patients had microscopic damage consisting of severe neuronal ischemia, focal minute perivascular hemorrhages, and tissue rarefaction (Fig. 190-34). Adams et al. state:

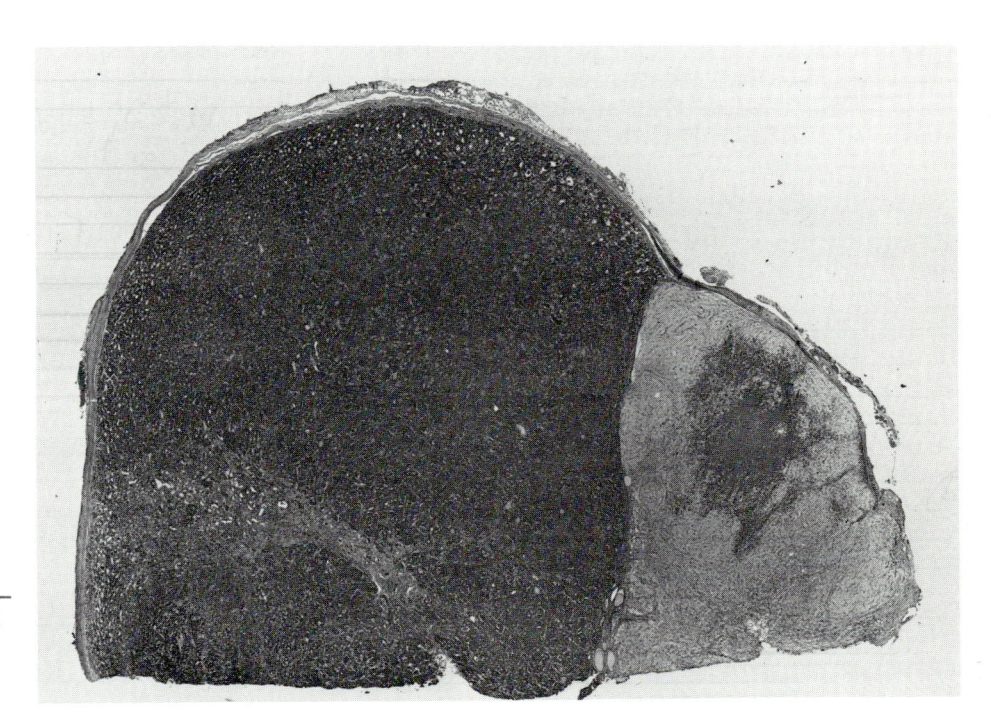

Figure 190-31 The pituitary gland with an acute focal posterior lobe hemorrhage in a case of acute closed head trauma. (H&E; × 10.)

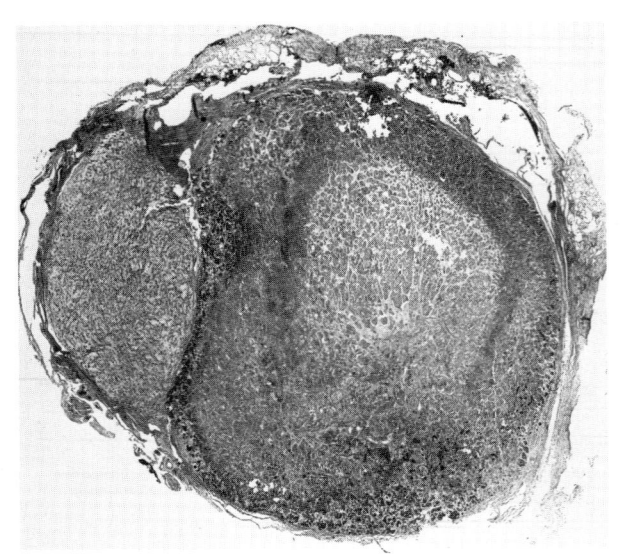

Figure 190-32 Extensive acute infarction of the anterior pituitary in a patient who died of acute head trauma. (Trichrome; × 9.)

There is no doubt that the pituitary stalk can occasionally be torn at the time of head injury, this invariably leading to massive infarction of the anterior lobe of the pituitary gland, but our own study suggests that most of the damage sustained by the hypothalamus and the pituitary stalk is secondary to raised intracranial pressure, a shift and distortion of the brain. We examined the pituitary glands routinely and have found infarcts of varying size in the anterior lobe in about 40 percent of fatal head injuries.[2]

Their contention that the pituitary and hypothalamic lesions are most often secondary to elevated intracranial pressure rather than to the direct consequence of trauma is difficult to refute in many cases; clearly some are. We have seen some patients who had no significant increase in intracranial pressure and who at the time of autopsy manifested little or no evidence of secondary ischemic brain lesions but who had

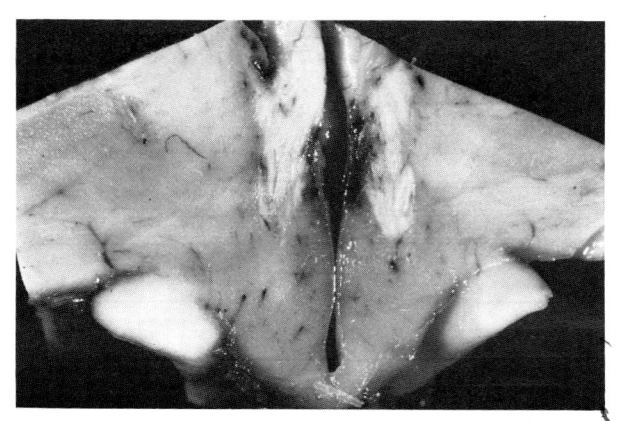

Figure 190-33 Cross section of the brain at the level of the optic tracts, mammillothalamic tracts, and hypothalamus revealing hemorrhagic necrosis of the anterior hypothalamus.

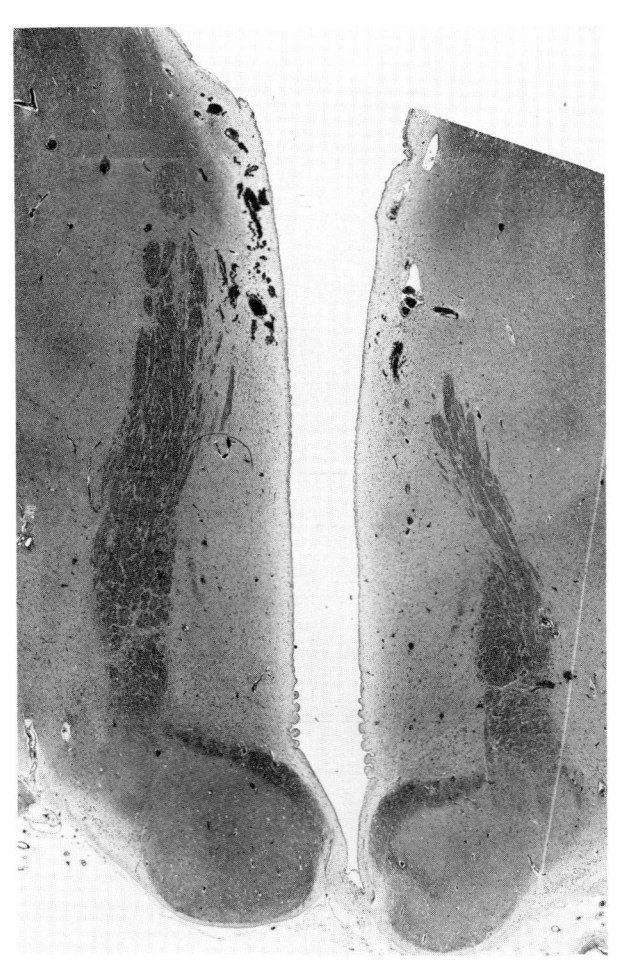

Figure 190-34 Section of the hypothalamus at the level of the mamillary bodies in a patient who died of closed head trauma. Note the small fresh petechial hemorrhages present in the subependymal region. Gross damage to the hypothalamus was not noted in this patient. (H&E; × 6.)

had some pituitary hemorrhages and necrosis. It is my impression that direct damage to this system is more common than Adams et al. would suggest, but I concur with their belief that a significant number (if not the majority) are totally or partially secondary to increased intracranial pressure and secondary ischemic events. Thus, hypothalamic and pituitary lesions are very common in patients with severe closed head injury but rarely, if ever, occur in isolation; they are part of a spectrum of multifocal brain damage. Of 106 patients studied by Crompton, skull fractures were present in 82 percent. In the 110 patients in my own current material, skull fractures were present in 86 percent.

Diffuse Impact Injury (Diffuse Axonal Injury)

The area of perhaps the most rapid expansion in both interest and knowledge has to do with widespread damage to the brain secondary to trauma and not presenting as localized

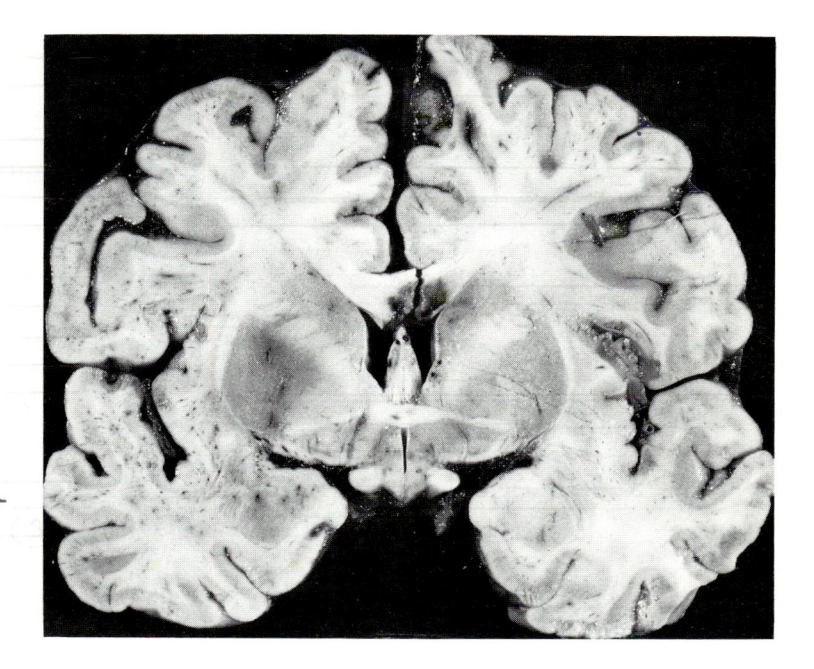

Figure 190-35 Hemorrhagic necrosis in the body of the corpus callosum seen in a section taken at the level of the anterior commissure. There is also conspicuous hemorrhagic necrosis secondary to a herniation contusion in the left uncus. This type of callosal lesion is a typical component of diffuse impact injury but can be found in some patients without other evidence of diffuse impact injury.

injuries or as a consequence of herniation and perfusion failure. This type of injury, referred to by Adams et al.[1,5] as "diffuse axonal injury," was first clearly delineated by Strich.[52,53]

The brains of patients dying with diffuse impact injury (DII) may show minimal gross alterations at the time of their examination. Microscopically, characteristic lesions consisting of reactive axonal swellings secondary to distraction ("shearing") of nerve fibers (Fig. 190-17), scattered microglial clusters ("stars"), and debris-laden macrophages are found. Many brains with DII have hemorrhagic and/or necrotic lesions in the corpus callosum (Figs. 190-35 to 190-38) and in the dorsolateral quadrant of the rostral pons (Figs. 190-39 to 190-41).

Adams et al. compared many of the major findings in 45 patients with diffuse impact injury with those from 132 patients with other types of head injury.[2] They found that rotational accelerations were more constantly a factor in the production of DII than of focal brain lesions. None of their patients with diffuse impact injury had a lucid interval,

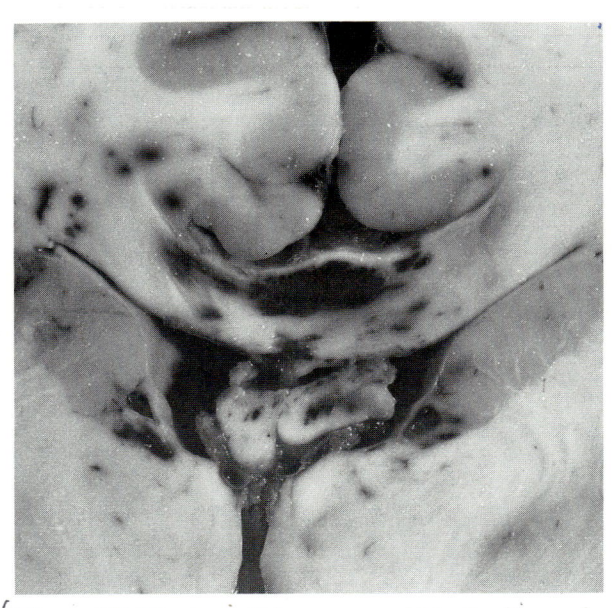

Figure 190-36 A small hematoma within the fibers of the body of the corpus callosum in a patient without other stigmata of diffuse impact injury. This patient sustained a fall with impaction at the vertex of the head.

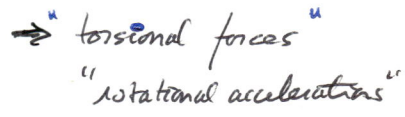

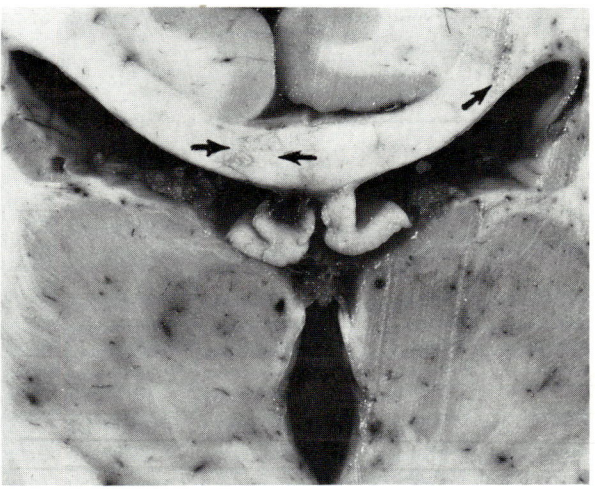

Figure 190-37 Area of ischemic (anemic) necrosis to the left of the midline in the body of the corpus callosum and along the right border (*arrows*). This patient died approximately 72 h after sustaining a closed head injury.

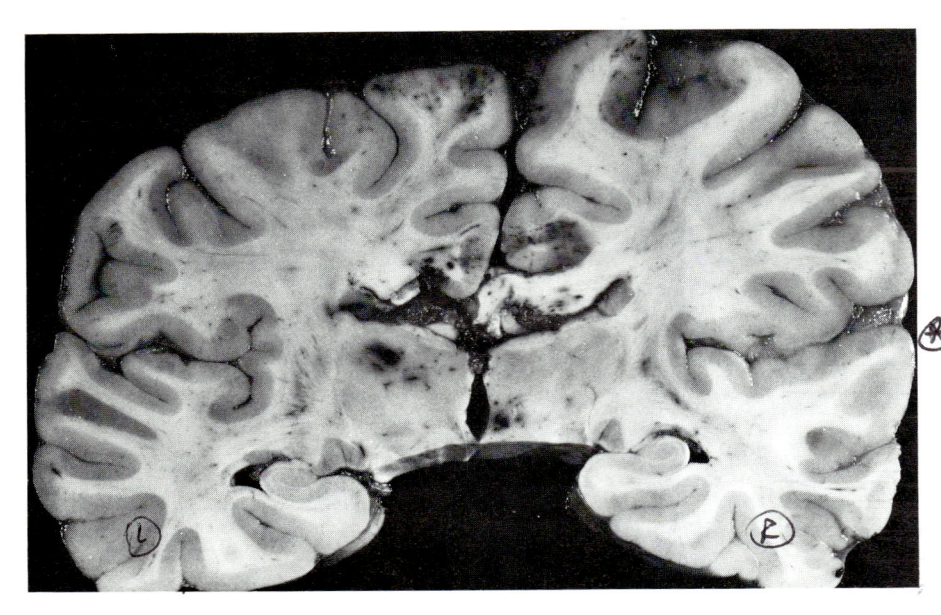

Figure 190-38 Hemorrhage and necrosis with transection of the body of the corpus callosum. There are associated hemorrhagic lesions in the cingulate and superior frontal gyri and small hemorrhages in the left thalamus and right hypothalamus. The impact was to the frontal vertex.

whereas nearly half of their patients with focal brain lesions did. Fractures of the skull were considerably less often encountered in the DII patients than in those with focal injury patterns (29 versus 86 percent). They found no difference in either the amount or prevalence of hypoxic brain damage between the two groups, nor did there appear to be a significant difference in the presence of brain swelling—in spite of the fact that there was elevation of intracranial pressure in 86 percent of the patients with focal brain lesions and only 56 percent of the patients with diffuse impact injury. There was a striking difference in the "mean total contusion index" between DII patients and the focal injury cases, with an index of 8.3 for the diffuse impact injury patients and 17.8 for the trauma patients with other types of head injury.

Of the three "classical" lesions seen in the diffuse impact injury, focal necrosis and/or hemorrhage in the corpus callosum was the first to be clearly delineated, although not then recognized as a part of the pattern now recognized as DII (Figs. 190-35 to 190-38).[1-5,21,30,33,34,40] The 1955 publication of Lindenberg et al. was perhaps the paper most instrumental in introducing the concept of significant callosal lesions in closed head injuries to the American audience.[34] Fifteen percent of the patients reported in that publication were noted to have gross callosal lesions. The prevalence of gross callosal damage in my own closed head trauma material is approximately 30 percent. Microscopic lesions within the corpus callosum are far more common, having been said to occur in 100 percent of the cases examined by Strich.[52]

Originally described as hemorrhage (Fig. 190-36), hemorrhagic necrosis (Figs. 190-35 and 190-38) and anemic necrosis (Fig. 190-37) by Lindenberg et al., these gross callosal lesions range in size from minute and barely visible to those that involve the great majority of the corpus callosum. These callosal lesions are considered to be due to lateral stretching of the corpus callosum due to dorsoventral flattening of the head at the moment of impact. A constant relationship between the presence of gross callosal tears and skull fractures has not been noted. Focal contusion- and laceration-type injuries in adjacent structures (fornix, cingulate gyri, septum pellucidum, caudate nuclei, and dorsal thalamus) are commonly present (Fig. 190-38).

The second classical gross finding in patients with diffuse impact injury is hemorrhagic necrosis in the dorsolateral quadrant of the rostral pons in and adjacent to the brachium conjunctivum (Figs. 190-39 to 190-41). This lesion was once considered to be the result of direct impaction of the pons against the incisura of the tentorium,[27] but it is now vigorously maintained by Adams et al.[1-5] that this is an indirect lesion associated with diffuse impact injury, a conclusion that I now share. These brain stem lesions vary considerably in size and conspicuousness. In patients with a short survival period, the lesions are almost always hemorrhagic, sometimes appearing as discrete hematomas. With the passage of time, the hemorrhagic malacia resorbs, leaving only hemosiderin-stained shrunken malacic areas (Fig. 190-41).

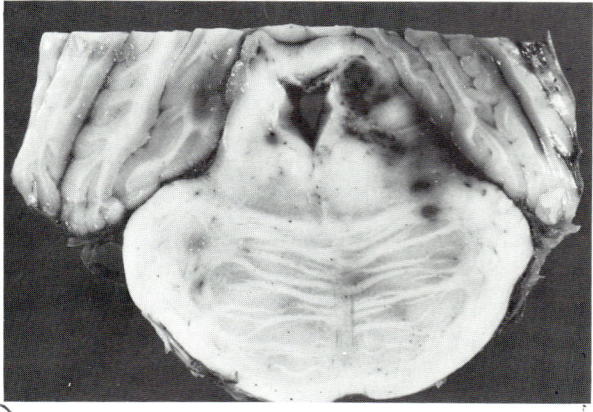

Figure 190-39 Typical gross appearance of the areas of hemorrhage and hemorrhagic necrosis in the dorsolateral aspect of the rostral pons seen in patients with diffuse impact injuries.

Pathology of Closed Head Injury

At the moment of injury, stresses induced by movements of the head are sufficient to injure numerous axons throughout the brain, and it is clear from the experimental studies that contact phenomena are not essential in the pathogenesis of these injuries. Rather the head must undergo appropriate acceleration in particular directions to cause DAI. If the injury is of sufficient magnitude, many axons are physically disrupted, and small vessels—presumably capillaries—may also be torn. Thus, tissue tears appear in the corpus callosum, rostral brain stem and are characterized by the presence of small hemorrhages and axonal retraction balls. Invariably other axons must be injured and appear abnormal, but may not be completely disrupted; this may be represented by tuberosities on axons, where axonal damage is minimal, by the Fink-Heimer technique. Later, microglia migrate into the areas of axonal damage (microglial stars); and still later degeneration of the myelin associated with the destroyed axons leads to the production of lipid stainable by the Sudan dyes and the Marchi technique. Total brain mass is subsequently reduced and an atrophic appearance of the brain ensues.[2]

Secondary Post-Traumatic Brain Lesions

The brains of victims of fatal closed head trauma typically confirm a variety of vascular/ischemic lesions that are secondary to increased intracranial pressure, herniation-

Figure 190-40 Photomacrograph of the rostral pons showing an area of hemorrhage in the dorsolateral quadrant in a patient with diffuse impact injury. (Trichrome; ×8.)

The third lesion characteristic of the triad making up diffuse impact injury is the reactive axonal swelling from tearing of the axon. Reactive axonal "retraction" balls are most easily seen with silver impregnation techniques and increase in prominence with prolonged survival time. Retraction balls can be found within a very short interval following disruption of the axon (Fig. 190-42), having been demonstrated to occur in less than 3 h.[33,40] Degeneration of the corticospinal and corticobulbar tracts may become so advanced that these tracts appear very pallid when stained with Luxol fast blue or silver preparations (Figs. 190-28 and 190-41).

Experimental observations coupled with observations on human material have led Adams and his colleagues to delineate a sequence of events giving rise to diffuse impact injury.

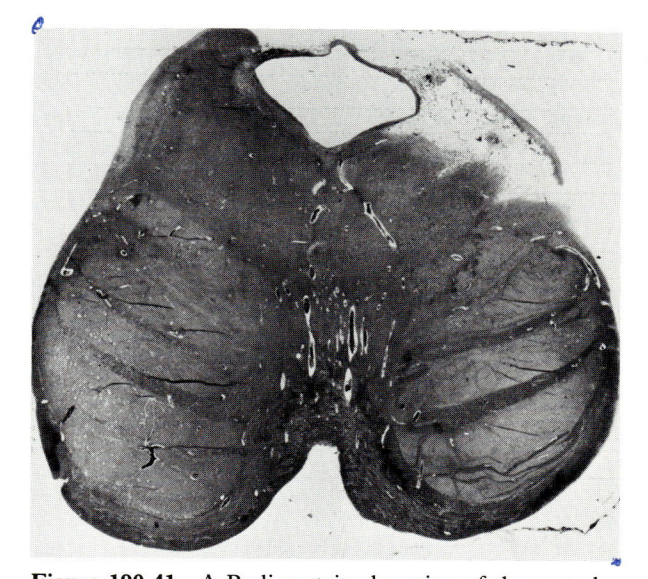

Figure 190-41 A Bodian-stained section of the rostral pons showing a remote cavitary dorsolateral quadrant lesion in a patient with diffuse impact injury and prolonged (120-day) survival. There is marked pallor of staining of the corticospinal and corticobulbar tracts bilaterally. Microscopically, large numbers of reactive axonal swellings were still present in these long tracts. (×5.)

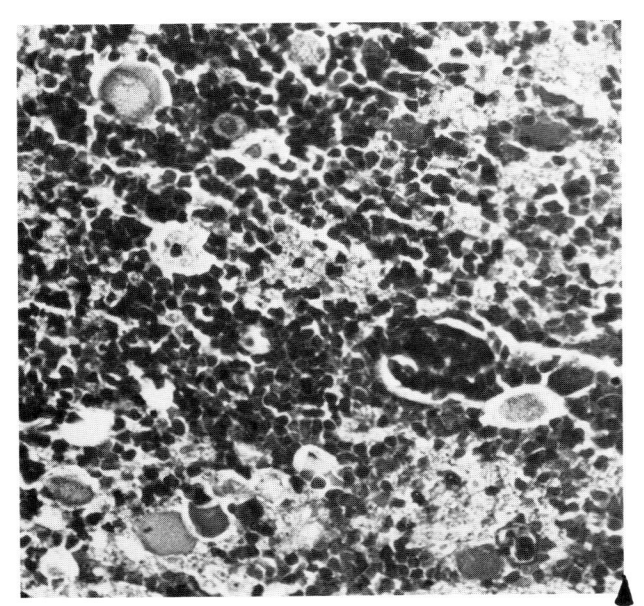

Figure 190-42 Photomicrograph at the base of an acute contusion showing several reactive axonal swellings embedded in fresh hemorrhage. (Trichrome; × 420.)

induced vascular occlusions, or systemic hypotension.[1-5,19,33,40] Morphologically, these alterations differ in no important respect from ischemic/anoxic lesions in nontraumatized brains. They occur in arterial border zones and terminal perfusion beds, in the hippocampi (especially Sommer's sector) (Fig. 190-43), and in the Purkinje layer of the cerebellum. An example is the herniation-induced necrosis in the distribution of the calcarine branch of the posterior cerebral artery (Fig. 190-44). When the cerebral cortex is involved, maximal damage is evident along the banks and in the depth of the sulci rather than over the crown of the gyrus. Areas of brain necrosis may be wedge-shaped, with the base of the wedge at the cortical surface and the apex deep within the parenchyma. Both cortex and convolutional white matter are involved, with some extension into the central white matter in the larger and necrotic lesions. Both grossly and microscopically, these wedge-shaped areas of necrosis resemble typical infarcts.

Adams et al., in examining the brains from a series of patients who had had careful monitoring of their intracranial pressure before death, observed that pressure necrosis in the hippocampal area ("parahippocampal gyri") occurred in the brains of all patients who had an intracranial pressure greater than 40 mmHg and in the majority of the patients in whom the intracranial pressure had been between 20 and 40 mmHg; this change was absent in those patients who had had an intracranial pressure below 20 mmHg.[2] Adams et al. also noted, as have many others, that in the clear majority of patients with increased intracranial pressure there were also hemorrhages and hemorrhagic softenings (secondary or Duret hemorrhages) in the mesencephalon and pons (Fig. 190-45).

Focal ischemic lesions occurring in arterial border zones are commonly encountered in patients who clinically manifested episodes of systemic hypotension and in patients who developed ventilatory compromise secondary to aspiration airway occlusion. Discrete wedge-shaped border zone malacic foci may be unilateral but are more frequently bilateral and occur most commonly between the anterior and middle cerebral artery perfusion beds. Quite similar appearing areas of anoxic tissue necrosis are found at the terminal perfusion beds of the middle cerebral artery in a significant number of patients.

In addition to the very focal anoxic/ischemic lesions, diffuse hypoxic changes ranging from widespread homogenizing necrosis of neurons to widespread pseudolaminar necrosis of the cortex are seen in some patients (Figs. 190-46 and 190-47). In their 1978 study of ischemic brain damage in patients with closed head trauma, Graham et al. found anoxic/hypoxic lesions in 70 of 151 patients.[19] These were described as severe in 29, moderate in 35, and mild in 6 patients. Additionally, 68 of these 151 victims of fatal closed head injury had focal ischemic lesions. Only 13 (8.6 percent) of the patients had neither anoxic nor ischemic brain damage. The location of the hypoxic damage in this series was the hippocampus in 80 percent, basal ganglia in 79 percent, and cerebellum in 44 percent. In a published report of 56 autopsied cases of closed head trauma from my service, it was noted that among the 25 that died in less than 48 h of injury, 17 had diffuse homogenizing necrosis of neurons throughout the brain, 6 had a progressive mass effect, 1 (an infant) had a diffuse massively swollen and congested brain, and 1 had a massive direct pontine laceration secondary to a transclival fracture.[10] In contrast, examination of the brains of 31 patients who survived for greater than 48 h after their injury revealed similar diffuse homogenizing necrosis of neurons in only 6, all of whom were deeply comatose from the time of injury and who undoubtedly would have died in the immediate post-trauma period if not for complete ventilatory support and pressor agents. The remaining 25 patients had only focal lesions, meningitis, severe suppurative bronchopneumonia with sepsis, or massive gastrointestinal bleeding with exsanguination. Among these 25 patients with greater than 48-h survival, 7 died as the result of progressive mass effect and had secondary brain stem hemorrhages from their hernias. All of the patients with diffuse homogenizing

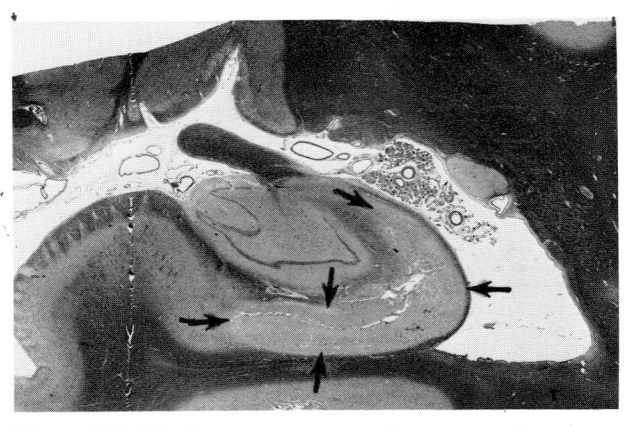

Figure 190-43 Acute sector necrosis as a secondary ischemic/anoxic lesion in a patient with closed head trauma. The swollen, pale necrotic sector is outlined by arrows. (Luxol fast blue—PASH; × 4.)

Pathology of Closed Head Injury

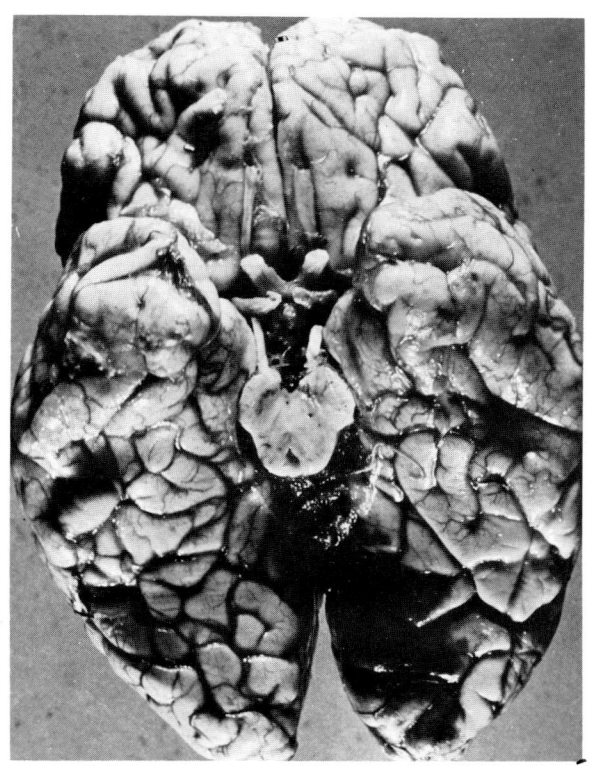

Figure 190-44 Calcarine artery distribution infarction secondary to lateral transtentorial herniation is a common secondary vascular lesion in head trauma patients.

necrosis of neurons had a measured elevation of their intracranial pressure.

The presence of many of the secondary vascular lesions in the brain stem in patients dying of closed head trauma is so well known as to preclude a detailed discussion in this chapter. Most often taking the form of hemorrhage with surrounding hemorrhagic necrosis, these lesions are due to displacement of the brain stem with occluding/shearing effect on the paramedian and short circumflex arteries at the time of transtentorial brain herniation (Fig. 190-45). This is most commonly seen in patients with significant elevations of their intracranial pressure. While the lesions are most commonly overtly hemorrhagic, severe localized pale infarction of the brain stem can occur in patients with transtentorial herniation.

Generally, small ischemic lesions are found in the mesencephalon in many patients with fatal closed head injury. Rosenburg et al. think they occur at the moment of impact.[49] I consider them to be a secondary ischemic event or part of a diffuse impact injury.

Focal discrete infarctions of the brain in specific arterial territories constitute a relatively common and well-known complication of increased intracranial pressure and brain herniations in trauma patients. The best known of these is undoubtedly the hemorrhagic infarction occurring in the distribution of the posterior cerebral artery following lateral transtentorial herniation (Fig. 190-44). Infarcts in the perfusion beds of the anterior choroidal, posterior inferior cerebellar, and posterior choroidal arteries are also encountered. Table 190-3 summarizes the major types of secondary posttraumatic brain damage encountered.

A complication of fatal closed head injury found in many autopsies is fresh subendocardial hemorrhage along the intraventricular septum of the left ventricle (Fig. 190-48).[10,40] These hemorrhages range in extent from a few millimeters to 5 to 6 cm and in thickness from only a few erythrocytes to 3 mm. The hemorrhages are known to be associated with conduction defects in the ECGs of patients when the appropriate studies are carried out during life. Such subendocardial hemorrhages were noted in 16 of the 56 patients dying of closed head injury in a previous report from this laboratory.[10] In the past 110 autopsies on patients dying with closed head injury, the hemorrhages have been observed in 38. The etiology and the pathogenesis of these hemorrhages are not clear. The hemorrhages are not confined to head trauma, being frequently encountered in patients with any mass in the brain (neoplasm, hematoma) with herniation, and in patients with massive subarachnoid hemorrhage from a ruptured saccular aneurysm. It is possible that these hemorrhages are due to subendocardial ischemia secondary to the marked vasoconstrictive effect of norepinephrine which is known to be circulating in greatly increased amounts in patients with closed head trauma.[11]

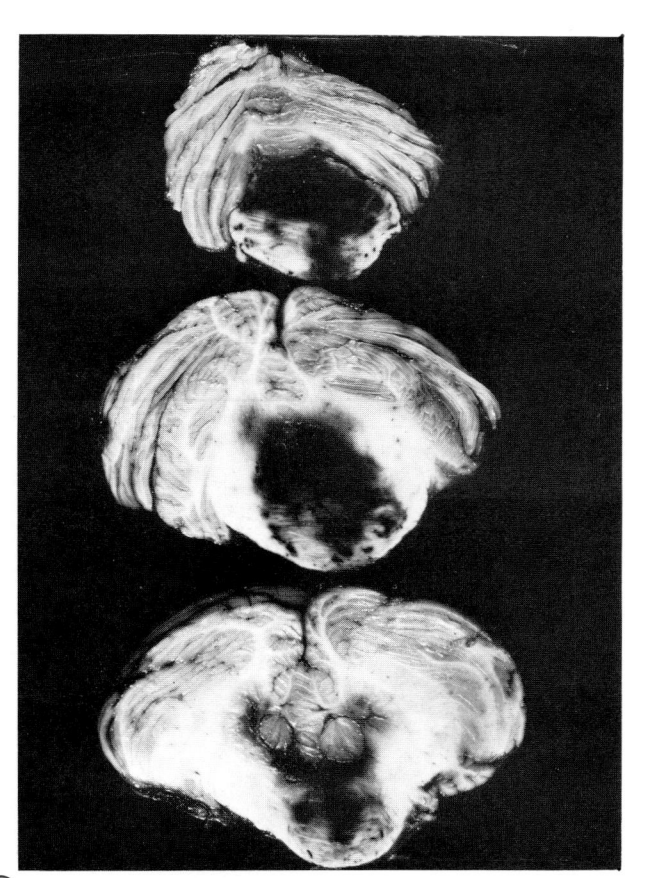

Figure 190-45 Typical extensive secondary (Duret) brain stem hemorrhages associated with transtentorial herniation. These are not direct (primary) brain stem lesions in trauma patients.

TABLE 190-3 Secondary Post-Traumatic Brain Damage

1. *Medial temporal (parahippocampal) necrosis*—caused by vascular compression in the brain as it is displaced against the tentorial edge during transtentorial herniation in a patient with elevated intracranial pressure (ICP)
2. *Focal infarction due to specific artery compression*—caused by transforaminal arterial compressions, the best known and most common being the calcarine infarcts due to posterior cerebral artery compression during lateral transtentorial herniation
3. *Border zone infarcts and focal hypoxic damage*—caused by circulatory failure secondary to systemic hypotension ("pump failure") or direct traumatic arterial thrombosis or laceration
4. *Diffuse ischemic necrosis of neurons* in patients who die rapidly (approximately 48 h) with increased ICP
5. *Secondary brain stem (Duret) hemorrhages*—caused by transtentorial herniation in patients with elevated ICP

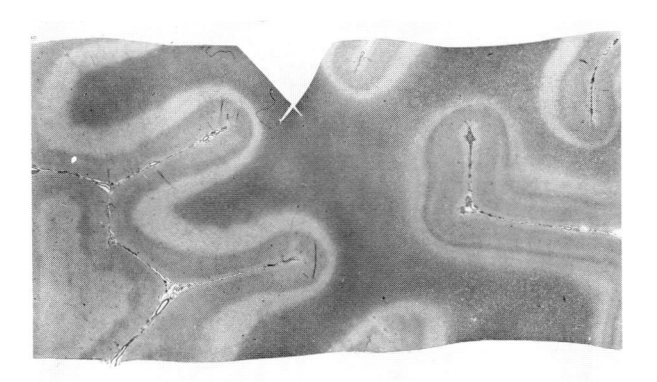

Figure 190-47 Photomacrograph of a cerebral section showing early cortical necrosis and severe convolutional white matter pallor. (Luxol fast blue—PASH; × 3.)

Interpretation of Closed Head Injury: Problems and Pitfalls

A number of major practical problems confront the physician who attempts to interpret traumatic brain lesions. These problems include the attempt to be overly precise in guessing the age of a given lesion; unfounded dogmatism in rendering an opinion without regard to historical data on how the injury occurred; and the attempt to classify every lesion without proper consideration of the clinical features, including intracranial pressure measurements, hypotensive episodes before death, aspiration episodes, etc. It is necessary for the pathologist to be forceful in withstanding exces-

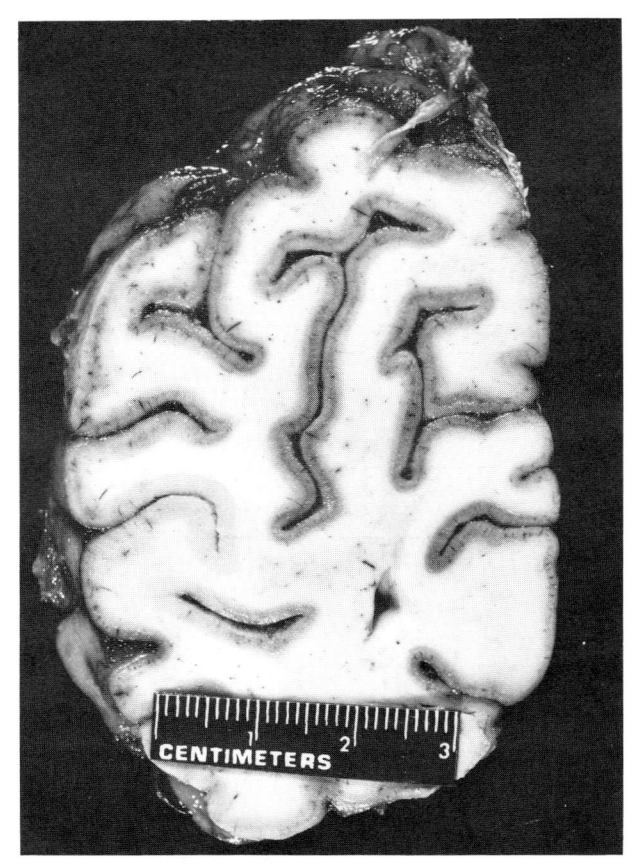

Figure 190-46 Diffuse "anoxic decortication" in a head trauma patient who survived 5 days following an episode of severe circulatory collapse.

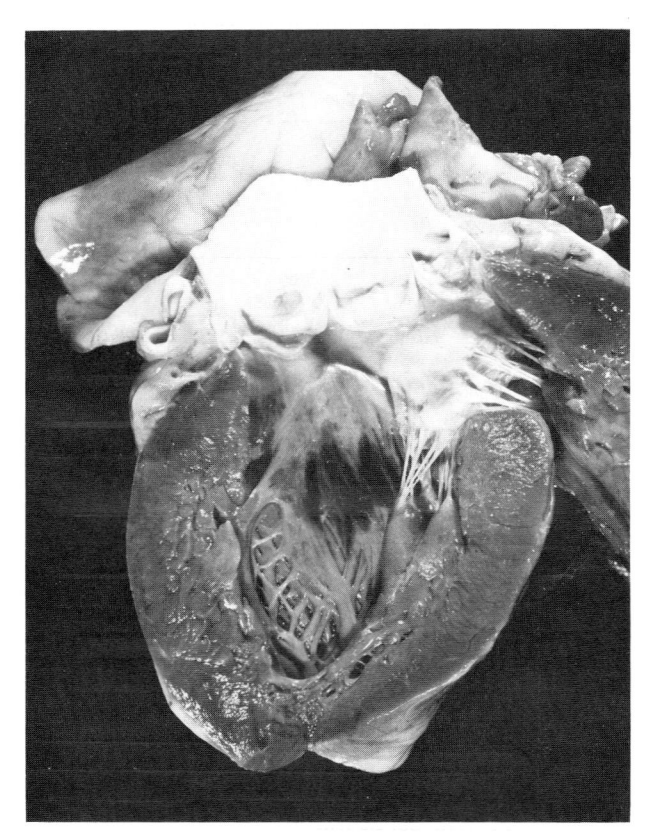

Figure 190-48 Acute subendocardial hemorrhage in the left ventricle of the heart along the interventricular septum. These lesions are found in about two-thirds of patients dying with acute closed head injuries.

sive pressures made to render a detailed opinion before the completion of all studies. It is the unfortunate situation in many forensic services that brains from trauma victims are examined and cut in the fresh state and a final opinion rendered without microscopic (or even detailed gross) examination. This is a major error, and one that has been responsible for retarding the advancement of our knowledge about the pathology and pathophysiology of head trauma. It is also important to remember that different and totally unrelated disorders may be present in the brain of a patient dying with head trauma; trauma in no way precludes the occurrence of natural disease.

References

1. Adams JH: The neuropathology of head injuries, in Vinken PJ, Bruyn GW (eds): *Handbook of Clinical Neurology*, vol 23. Amsterdam, North-Holland, 1975, pp 35–65.
2. Adams JH, Gennarelli TA, Graham DI: Brain damage in nonmissile head injury: Observations in man and subhuman primates, in Smith WT, Cavanagh JB (eds): *Recent Advances in Neuropathology*, no. 2. Edinburgh, Churchill Livingstone, 1982, pp 165–190.
3. Adams JH, Graham DI, Murray LS, Scott G: Diffuse axonal injury due to nonmissile head injury in humans: An analysis of 45 cases. Ann Neurol 12:557–563, 1981.
4. Adams JH, Graham DI, Scott G, Parker LS, Doyle D: Brain damage in fatal non-missile head injury. J Clin Pathol 33:1132–1145, 1980.
5. Adams JH, Mitchell DE, Graham DI, Doyle D: Diffuse brain damage of immediate impact type: Its relationship to "primary brain-stem damage" in head injury. Brain 100:489–502, 1977.
6. Britt RH, Herrick MK, Mason RT, Dorfman LJ: Traumatic lesions of the pontomedullary junction. Neurosurgery 6:623–631, 1980.
7. Brown FD, Mullan S, Duda EE: Delayed traumatic intracerebral hematomas: Report of three cases. J Neurosurg 48:1019–1022, 1978.
8. Bruce DA, Alavi A, Bilaniuk L, Dolinskas C, Obrist W, Uzzell B: Diffuse cerebral swelling following head injuries in children: The syndrome of "malignant brain edema." J Neurosurg 54:170–178, 1981.
9. Ceballos R: Pituitary changes in head trauma (analysis of 102 consecutive cases of head injury). Ala J Med Sci 3:185–198, 1966.
10. Clifton GL, McCormick WF, Grossman RG: Neuropathology of early and late deaths after head injury. Neurosurgery 8:309–314, 1981.
11. Clifton GL, Ziegler MG, Grossman RG: Circulating catecholamines and sympathetic activity after head injury. Neurosurgery 8:10–13, 1981.
12. Cordobés F, Lobato RD, Rivas JJ, Muñoz MJ, Chillón D, Portillo JM, Lamas E: Observations on 82 patients with extradural hematoma: Comparison of results before and after the advent of computerized tomography. J Neurosurg 54:179–186, 1981.
13. Crompton MR: Hypothalamic lesions following closed head injury. Brain 94:165–172, 1971.
14. Crompton MR: Hypothalamic and pituitary lesions, in Vinken PJ, Bruyn GW (eds): *Handbook of Clinical Neurology*, vol 23. Amsterdam, North-Holland, 1975, pp 465–469.
15. Daniel PM, Treip CS: Lesions of the pituitary gland associated with head injuries, in Harris GW, Donovan BT (eds): *The Pituitary Gland*, vol 2. London, Butterworths, 1966, pp 519–534.
16. Eichner ER: The hematologic disorders of alcoholism. Am J Med 54:621–630, 1973.
17. Flamm ES, Demopoulos HB, Seligman ML, Tomasula JJ, Descrescito U, Ransohoff J: Ethanol potentiation of central nervous system trauma. J Neurosurg 46:328–335, 1977.
18. Gordon A, Maloney AFJ: Blunt head injury, in Mason JK (ed): *The Pathology of Violent Injury*. London, Edward Arnold, 1978, pp 197–217.
19. Graham DI, Adams JH, Doyle D: Ischaemic brain damage in fatal non-missile head injuries. J Neurol Sci 39:213–234, 1978.
20. Gurdjian ES, Webster JE, Lissner HR: The mechanism of skull fracture. J Neurosurg 7:106–114, 1950.
21. Hardman JM: The pathology of traumatic brain injuries. Adv Neurol 22:15–50, 1979.
22. Harvey FH, Jones AM: "Typical" basal skull fracture of both petrous bones: An unreliable indicator of head impact site. J Forensic Sci 25:280–286, 1980.
23. Heinze J: Cranial nerve avulsion and other neural injuries in road accidents. Med J Aust 2:1246–1249, 1969.
24. Hirsh LF: Chronic epidural hematomas. Neurosurgery 6:508–512, 1980.
25. Iwakuma T, Brunngraber CV: Chronic extradural hematomas: A study of 21 cases. J Neurosurg 38:488–493, 1973.
26. Jackson FE, Gleave JRW, Janon E: The traumatic cranial and intracranial aneurysms, in Vinken PJ, Bruyn GW (eds): *Handbook of Clinical Neurology*, vol 24. Amsterdam, North-Holland, 1976, pp 381–398.
27. Jellinger K, Seitelberger F: Protracted post-traumatic encephalopathy: Pathology, pathogenesis and clinical implications. J Neurol Sci 10:51–94, 1970.
28. Kaufman HH, Moake JL, Olson JD, Miner ME, duCret RP, Pruessner JL, Gildenberg PL: Delayed and recurrent intracranial hematomas related to disseminated intravascular clotting and fibrinolysis in head injury. Neurosurgery 7:446–449, 1980.
29. Kingsley D, Till K, Hoare R: Growing fractures of the skull. J Neurol Neurosurg Psychiatry 41:312–318, 1978.
30. Komatsu S, Sato T, Kagawa S, Mori T, Namiki T: Traumatic lesions of the corpus callosum. Neurosurgery 5:32–35, 1979.
31. Kornblum RN, Fisher RS: Pituitary lesions in craniocerebral injuries. Arch Pathol Lab Med 88:242–248, 1969.
32. Koulouris S, Rizzoli HV: Delayed traumatic intracerebral hematoma after compound depressed skull fracture: Case report. Neurosurgery 8:223–225, 1981.
33. Lindenberg R: Trauma of meninges and brain, in Minckler J (ed): *Pathology of the Nervous System*, vol 2. New York, McGraw-Hill, 1971, pp 1705–1765.
34. Lindenberg R, Fisher RS, Durlacher SH, Lovitt WV Jr, Freytag E: Lesions of the corpus callosum following blunt mechanical trauma to the head. Am J Pathol 31:297–317, 1955.
35. Lindenberg R, Freytag E: The mechanism of cerebral contusions: A pathologic-anatomic study. Arch Pathol Lab Med 69:440–469, 1960.
36. Lindenberg R, Freytag E: Morphology of brain lesions from blunt trauma in early infancy. Arch Pathol Lab Med 87:298–305, 1969.
37. Lindenberg R, Freytag E: Brainstem lesions characteristic of traumatic hyperextension of the head. Arch Pathol Lab Med 90:509–515, 1970.
38. Lye RH, Occleshaw JV, Dutton J: Growing fracture of the skull and the role of computerized tomography: Case report. J Neurosurg 55:470–472, 1981.
39. McCormick WF: The relationship of closed-head trauma to rupture of saccular intracranial aneurysms. Am J Forensic Med Pathol 1:223–226, 1980.
40. McCormick WF: Trauma, in Schochet SS Jr (ed): *Clinical Neurosciences*, vol 3. New York, Churchill-Livingstone, 1983, pp 241–283.
41. Miner ME, Kaufman HH, Graham SH, Haar FH, Gildenberg PL: Disseminated intravascular coagulation fibrinolytic syn-

drome following head injury in children: Frequency and prognostic implications. J Pediatr 100:687–691, 1982.
42. Ordia IJ, Strand R, Gilles F, Welch K: Computed tomography of contusional clefts in the white matter in infants: Report of two cases. J Neurosurg 54:696–698, 1981.
43. Parkinson D, West M: Traumatic intracranial aneurysms. J Neurosurg 52:11–20, 1980.
44. Paul GA, Shaw CM, Wray LM: True traumatic aneurysm of the vertebral artery: Case report. J Neurosurg 53:101–105, 1980.
45. Pilz P, Strohecker J, Grobovschek M: Survival after traumatic ponto-medullary tear. J Neurol Neurosurg Psychiatry 45:422–427, 1982.
46. Ramamurthi B: Acute subdural haematoma, in Vinken PJ, Bruyn GW (eds): *Handbook of Clinical Neurology*, vol 24. Amsterdam, North-Holland, 1976, pp 275–296.
47. Rengachary SS, Szymanski DC: Sudural hematomas of arterial origin. Neurosurgery 8:166–171, 1981.
48. Rivano C, Borzone M, Carta F, Michelozzi G: Traumatic intracerebral hematomas: 72 cases surgically treated. J Neurosurg Sci 24:77–84, 1980.
49. Rosenblum WI, Greenberg RP, Seelig JM, Becker DP: Midbrain lesions: Frequent and significant prognostic feature in closed head injury. Neurosurgery 9:613–620, 1981.
50. Russell WR, Schiller F: Crushing injury to the skull: Clinical and experimental observations. J Neurol Neurosurg Psychiatry 12:52–60, 1949.
51. Sekhar LN, Scarff TB: Pseudogrowth in skull fractures of childhood. Neurosurgery 6:285–289, 1980.
52. Strich SJ: Diffuse degeneration of the cerebral white matter in severe dementia following head injury. J Neurol Neurosurg Psychiatry 19:163–185, 1956.
53. Strich SJ: Shearing of nerve fibres as a cause of brain damage due to head injury. Lancet 2:443–448, 1961.
54. Summers CG, Wirtschafter JD: Bilateral trigeminal and abducens neuropathies following low-velocity, crushing head injury: Case report. J Neurosurg 50:508–511, 1979.
55. Tandon PN, Prakash B, Banerji AK: Temporal lobe lesions in head injury. Acta Neurochir (Wien) 41:205–221, 1978.
56. Unterharnscheidt F: Neuropathology of rhesus monkeys undergoing $-G_x$ impact acceleration, in Ewing CL, Thomas DJ, Sances A Jr, Larson SJ (eds): *Impact Injury of the Head and Spine*. Springfield, Ill., Charles C Thomas, 1983, pp 94–176.
57. Van der Sande JJ, Emeiss JJ, Lindeman J: Intravascular coagulation: A common phenomenon in minor experimental head injury. J Neurosurg 54:21–25, 1981.
58. Zimmerman RA, Bilaniuk LT, Bruce D, Dolinskas C, Obrist W, Kuhl D: Computed tomography of pediatric head trauma: Acute general cerebral swelling. Radiology 126:403–408, 1978.

191

Neurological Evaluation of a Patient with Head Trauma: Coma Scales

Victoria Neave
Martin H. Weiss

Epidemiology

Interest in the evaluation and treatment of trauma has escalated over the past few decades as the significant morbidity and mortality attendant to trauma have become apparent. Indeed, trauma is now reported to be the leading cause of death in the United States for persons 1 to 44 years of age.[22] In up to 75 percent of trauma-related deaths, head injuries contribute significantly to the demise of the victim.[6] In addition to the significant mortality caused by head injury, devastating physical and functional morbidity is frequently associated with the sequelae of brain injury. No complete national statistics are available for head trauma in the United States, but a prospective study of all admissions and deaths due to head trauma was conducted in San Diego County in 1978.[13] The overall incidence of head injury was found to be 300/100,000, with an overall mortality of 24/100,000; a 7.5 percent case fatality rate was noted. The death rate in males exceeded that in females, and proportionate mortality rates emphasized the striking importance of head injury as a cause of death before age 30. Furthermore, 65 percent of fatalities occurred at the scene of the accident or enroute to a medical facility. Therefore, only one-third of head injuries severe enough to lead to death were evaluated and treated by a physician. It is toward these patients that intensive investigations into improved methods of assessment and therapy are being directed.

Comparison of head injury statistics from the United States with those from other countries is complicated by the different methods and terminologies used in recording trauma information. In Great Britain, however, fatalities secondary to head trauma are specifically identified; an incidence of 200/300,000 with a mortality incidence of 9/100,000 has been reported.[9] The apparent lower case fatality rate is attributed to the assumption that fewer minor head injuries are seen and admitted to the hospital in the United States.

Neurological Assessment

A prompt and systematic evaluation of a head-injured patient is mandatory for appropriate localization of major lesions and for the establishment of therapeutic priorities. The resuscitation of a multiply injured patient is described in another chapter. A detailed neurological examination will frequently establish the principal site of any existing intracranial lesion and indicate the urgency and proper approach to therapy. Obviously, the extent of the neurological evaluation will depend on the type and degree of cerebral injury sustained and the patient's ability to cooperate with the examiner. The examination of the unconscious or poorly cooperative patient is tailored to place more emphasis on objective observations of the responses obtained from known external stimuli. The complete evaluation should include a well-documented assessment of the state of consciousness, motor abilities, pupillary characteristics, eye movements, and vital signs. Despite its limitations, and the development of sophisticated diagnostic tools such as computed tomography and the measurement of evoked potentials, the neurological examination remains the most important factor in the rapid assessment of the extent and severity of cerebral injury and is of vital importance in the subsequent monitoring of improvement or deterioration of the neurological status with the passage of time.

General Examination

The initial assessment of the patient should include notation of any superficial wounds of the scalp or face, asymmetry of orbital or facial structures signifying potential fracture sites, cerebrospinal fluid leakage, and neck or back injuries. Important clues about the underlying site and nature of injury can frequently be elicited. It is well recognized that ecchymosis and swelling over the mastoid process (Battle's sign), hemotympanum, and otorrhea are associated with basilar skull fractures involving the petrous portion of the temporal bone. CSF rhinorrhea, which results from a fistulous communication between the subarachnoid space and the nasal cavity either through the cribriform plate and ethmoid sinuses or through the frontal or sphenoid sinus, is a potential complication of fractures of the floor or ventral surface of the anterior cranial fossa. Periorbital ecchymosis (raccoon eyes) may also be associated with fractures of the anterior cranial vault; direct orbital trauma must be excluded. Examination of the extremities should include an assessment of the degree and symmetry of spontaneous movements. A static position of abduction and external rotation of a lower extremity may reflect paralysis of that limb, and further evidence of paraplegia or hemiplegia should be sought. Hip and femoral neck fractures may result in similar abnormal positioning of the extremity and must be ruled out radiographically.

A myriad of autonomic dysfunctions have been described in the scenario of cerebral injury. The classical Kocher-Cushing reflex of hypertension and bradycardia in response to increased intracranial pressure generally signifies a catastrophic intracranial event and is thought to reflect compression or ischemia of a restricted pressor area lying just ventral to the floor of the fourth ventricle.[19] Vomiting, yawning, and hiccuping may be noted and indicate a relatively intact brain stem.[5]

Normal respiration, which is classically described as arising from within the reticular formation of the lower brain stem and cervicomedullary junction, is in reality a sensorimotor act integrated by neurogenic influences arising from nearly every level of the brain.[1] Several characteristic abnormalities of respiratory pattern have been attributed to specific sites of neural dysfunction, thereby contributing to the evaluation of the level of injury.[4,5,19] Cheyne-Stokes respirations (CSR) have been ascribed to discoordination of the neural structures lying deep in the cerebral hemispheres or diencephalon. The emergence of CSR in patients with suspected supratentorial mass lesions may provide a valuable sign of incipient transtentorial or central herniation.[19] A pure central neurogenic hyperventilation is rare, and such a respiratory pattern requires a search for a metabolic or hypoxic cause, although it has been associated with dysfunction of the rostral brain stem tegmentum. Apneustic and ataxic patterns reflect injury to the respiratory control mechanism located at pontine and dorsomedial medullary levels. In addition to trauma, multiple metabolic and toxic states are also capable of producing or potentiating profound alterations in respiratory patterns. Therefore, when metabolic and traumatic abnormalities occur concomitantly, the accuracy of using breathing patterns as a means of localizing neural dysfunction is in doubt.

State of Consciousness

Consciousness has been defined as the state of total awareness of self, and unconsciousness or coma as the total absence of awareness even with external stimulation.[19] In between consciousness and coma exist a continuum of altered states of consciousness to which a bewildering number of terms have been applied, such as lethargic, clouded, stuporous, and semicomatose. As these terms have different meanings for different examiners, the interpretation of the exact state of consciousness utilizing these labels is exceedingly difficult. Numerous investigators have proposed various definitions and scales for the assessment of mental status, including the Glasgow coma scale which will be discussed in detail later in the chapter.[15,17,19,21,23] All have agreed that the terminology should be specific and that observations should be related to objective responses by the patient to reproducible external stimulation. Despite this basic ideological agreement, the existing methods for assessing mental status still differ widely from institution to institution.

The physiology of altered states of consciousness has been investigated extensively. In 1949, the ascending reticular activating system (ARAS) was first described by Moruzzi and Magoun and identified in their laboratory animals as lying within the center of the brain stem, extending from the midbrain into the hypothalamus and thalamus.[16] Current thinking concurs with their explanation of distinctive arousal effects induced by ARAS stimulation of the cerebral cortex, with alteration of consciousness resulting from depression or injury to the ARAS projections. The midbrain and pontine areas critical to consciousness in humans have been identified as lying in the paramedian tegmental zone ventral to the ventricular system, extending from the lower third of the pons to the posterior hypothalamus.[19] The long axons of the ARAS ascend primarily in the central tegmental tract of the brain stem.[16] The location and extent of interruption of these pathways necessary to produce disruption of cerebral activation and loss of consciousness are not known. Numerous other pathological states aside from direct brain injury may produce or potentiate depressed consciousness; for example, alcoholic or pharmacologic intoxication may exist concomitantly with the head trauma. Therefore, the state of consciousness of a patient taken as an isolated factor is not as useful in determining the anatomical location of injury as some of the other parameters to be discussed. However, when the level of consciousness is integrated with the findings from the rest of the neurological examination, it can provide important substantiation of the degree and level of cortical and upper brain stem function.

If the patient is alert and able to communicate, the mental status examination should be extended to test for higher cognitive functions including memory, concentration, and abstract thinking. Memory loss is a frequent sequela to head trauma and can be divided into retrograde amnesia (memory loss for events occurring before the injury) and antegrade amnesia (signifying loss of memory from the time of injury to the return of conscious remembrance). The latter is also termed post-traumatic amnesia and usually covers a longer time period than retrograde amnesia, which tends to improve with neurological recovery.

Motor Response

As with every aspect of the neurological examination, the assessment of skeletal muscle function will depend to some extent on the patient's ability to cooperate with the examiner. In an awake and responsive patient, muscle tone can be evaluated by testing the passive range of motion of the extremities; muscle strength can be ascertained by voluntary movement against a resistance. The following scale may be used for numerical documentation of strength:

5/5 Normal strength
4/5 Can be overcome with counterresistance
3/5 Antigravity movement only
2/5 Muscles contract, but cannot overcome gravity
1/5 Trace twitch
0/5 No movement

Evaluation of the motor abilities of the uncooperative or unresponsive patient consists primarily of observing the characteristics and strength of the skeletal muscle response to various external stimuli, usually noxious. It is imperative that the nature of the stimulus and the exact motor functions observed be documented to allow for subsequent comparison. Motor reactions to painful stimuli are generally described as localizing, flexor, or extensor.

Abnormal flexor posturing (frequently referred to as decorticate posturing) is characterized by adduction and retraction of the shoulders, flexion at the elbows, and pronation of the forearms.[5] The lower extremities may take a flexor or extensor position. This abnormal posture is classically produced in cats who have undergone cerebral hemispherectomies and is thought to reflect a more rostral and less severe supratentorial injury than does the extensor position.[5,19]

The extensor response (decerebrate posturing) consists of extension of all limbs and opisthotonus. The head is thrown back; the arms are extended at the elbows and are pronated, with palmar flexion of the wrist and fingers; and the legs are rigidly extended, with strong plantar flexion of the feet. Lesions producing extensor rigidity have been produced in animals by transection of the midbrain between the inferior and superior colliculi.[19] In humans, lesions from the pons to the midbrain have been described in association with abnormal extension.[5] Plum and Posner have reported that extension of all extremities correlates best with deeper and more severe but still supratentorial dysfunction, whereas extension of the arms with flexion of the legs reflects pontine injury.[19] While abnormal extensor posturing is generally assumed to occur solely in comatose patients, alert patients with decerebrate rigidity have been described. This emphasizes the different anatomical locations of those neural structures which regulate consciousness and those which subserve motor function.[3]

Diffuse flaccidity without any response to noxious stimuli is commonly associated with severe intoxicant states, such as with alcohol, barbiturate, or narcotic overdose, but has also been described with pontomedullary injury. Traumatic myelopathy with resultant flaccid quadraplegia must also be considered. The other parameters assessed in the neurological examination should provide information for differentiation.

The presence of paralysis of an extremity or extremities should be noted and can be of significant value in localization of the lesion, especially when concomitant cranial nerve abnormalities occur. The most frequently recognized combination is that of a dilated pupil on one side with a contralateral hemiplegia signifying uncal herniation ipsilateral to the paretic oculomotor nerve. In a small percentage of cases the contralateral cerebral peduncle will be injured initially from compression against the contralateral tentorial edge (Kernohan's notch), resulting in hemiplegia ipsilateral to the dilated and nonreactive pupil. In an unconscious patient, a paresis or plegia may be recognized by an asymmetrical motor response to a noxious stimulus. Paralysis following acute cerebral events is usually flaccid, resulting in a difference in muscle tone which can be appreciated by the examiner. Twitching and fasciculations of widespread muscle groups subsequent to cerebral hemorrhage presumably stem from anoxic injury to the descending corticospinal tract or compression of the cerebral peduncle and represent the period of denervation before flaccidity.[5]

Pupils

Because pupillary pathways are relatively resistant to metabolic insults, the presence or absence of the pupillary light reflex is generally held to be the single most important distinguishing feature between structural and metabolic cerebral dysfunction although fixed and dilated pupils have been noted in fulminant hepatic encephalopathy. Pupillary size represents the balance of opposing tonic forces consisting of the pupilloconstrictor parasympathetic and pupillodilator sympathetic influences. Denervation of either system results in the unopposed action of the intact pathway, and characteristic pupillary abnormalities will be apparent and provide site-specific information regarding the injury. A constantly changing dominance of sympathetic or parasympathetic tone influenced by both external and internal stimulation maintains the pupil in the awake person in constant motion through a small range; this phenomenon is known as hippus.

The exact site of origin of the descending pupillodilator fibers in the sympathetic system is not known, but they are believed to reside in the paraventricular and posterolateral nuclei of the hypothalamus because electrical stimulation of these areas produces ipsilateral pupillary dilatation.[7,19] Hypothalamic outflow descends uncrossed through the tegmentum of the midbrain and pons, assumes a lateral position in the medulla, and terminates in the intermediolateral cell column at the C8 to T2 cord levels. Second-order preganglionic fibers exit the cord and pass through the inferior and middle cervical ganglia to synapse in the superior cervical ganglion. Third-order oculosympathetic postsynaptic fibers ascend with the internal carotid artery to enter the skull, while fibers serving facial sweating and piloerection follow the external carotid artery and its various branches. The intracranial sympathetic fibers reach the pupillary dilators and the smooth muscles of the upper and lower eyelids by traversing first the ophthalmic artery and then the nasociliary branch of the trigeminal nerve.

The pupillary light reflex pathway involving the parasympathetic system is functionally described as a three-neuron arc. The afferent limb consists of neuronal transmission from the retinal ganglion cell through the optic nerve, chiasm, and tract, terminating medially in the pretectal nuclear area. The pupillomotor afferents as well as the fibers mediating visual reception from the nasal half of each retina decussate at the chiasm and become incorporated in the contralateral optic tract. Intercalated neurons connect the pretectal region with the paramotor pool in the midbrain (Edinger-Westphal complex) via the posterior commissure. The efferent limb of the arc consists of preganglionic parasympathetic neurons joining the oculomotor nerve where the pupillomotor fibers lie just internal to the epineurium.[7] At the level of the superior orbital fissure the oculomotor nerve divides and the parasympathetic fibers follow the branch to the inferior oblique muscle to synapse in the ciliary ganglion. Postganglionic short ciliary fibers penetrate the globe.

Knowledge of the anatomical and physiological characteristics of these opposing systems allows rapid and precise localization of cerebral lesions utilizing the presence or absence of pupillary irregularities. Changes in pupillary size or reactivity frequently constitute the earliest objective warning of incipient neurological deterioration and should be closely monitored by the physician and nursing personnel caring for the patient.

Bilateral miosis, or "pinpoint" pupils, is classically associated with tegmental pontine lesions, either intrinsic to the pons or from external compression secondary to a cerebellar or extra-axial posterior fossa hemorrhage resulting in a physiological disruption of the descending sympathetic fibers. The pupillary light reflex is generally preserved, although examination with a magnifying glass may be necessary to document a response. Bilaterally small pupils also occur with a variety of metabolic encephalopathies and with opiate ingestion. If any question of the latter is raised, the administration of the opiate antagonist naloxone will reverse any opiate effect on pupillary size. The earliest stages of central "downward" herniation may induce bilateral miosis before progressing to the more frequently seen mydriasis.[19]

Unilateral miosis, produced by ipsilateral disruption of the descending sympathetic outflow from the hypothalamus to the globe, is commonly referred to as Horner's syndrome. The diagnosis is substantiated by the lack of pupillary dilatation in a dark environment and associated ptosis, anhidrosis, and relative enophthalmos. Isolated hypothalamic injuries secondary to head trauma are infrequently seen but characteristically produce an ipsilateral Horner's syndrome with complete anhidrosis involving the entire ipsilateral half of the body. Lateral medullary and cervical spinal cord insults result in anhidrosis of the face, neck, and arm on the ipsilateral side. However, absence of sweating induced by interruption of the third-order postganglionic fibers located in the neck or face is variable and is determined by the extent of concomitant injury to both the pupillomotor fibers located near the internal carotid artery and the sweat fibers coursing with the external carotid artery.

Injury to the midbrain region causing varying degrees of dysfunction of both the descending sympathetic fibers and the parasympathetic outflow originating in the tectal region characteristically produces pupils noted to be "midposition" (4 to 5 mm), irregular, and nonreactive. Not infrequently a degree of anisocoria is present which may reflect incomplete function of one or both pathways.

Unilateral, nonreactive mydriasis in head trauma is one of the most ominous and watched for abnormalities, as it commonly heralds transtentorial herniation secondary to an expanding supratentorial mass lesion. In this circumstance, pupillary dilatation typically precedes complete ipsilateral oculomotor palsy because the superficial location of the pupillomotor fibers running with the oculomotor nerve predisposes them to an earlier susceptibility to pressure effects. With progression of the herniation process, a complete picture of bilateral mydriasis and ophthalmoplegia will evolve. The differentiation of unilateral pupillary dilatation indicative of a shift of intracranial structures versus mydriasis related to local and more peripheral oculomotor nerve injury is important. Oculomotor dysfunction may occur from direct orbital trauma, a fracture through the superior orbital fissure, or a traumatic carotid-cavernous fistula. In these circumstances, the pupillomotor and oculomotor fibers seem to be more equally susceptible to injury, and ocular muscle paresis will almost always accompany the mydriasis.

Close examination of the pupillary responses with the "swinging flashlight" test may elicit an afferent pupillary defect or Marcus-Gunn pupil resulting from deafferentation of the optic nerve. Upon performing the test, a paradoxical dilatation of the affected pupil with retention of the normal consensual response will occur with direct exposure to the light source.

Pupillary irregularities have been described with a number of pharmacologic agents and a complete history of all potential drug ingestions must be obtained before assigning a focal neurological etiology to pupillary abnormalities. Atropine or scopolamine ingestion results in fully dilated and nonreactive pupils. Glutethimide poisoning can mimic the midposition and fixed pupils of midbrain lesions. Extreme miosis suggests the presence of systemic opiates. Barbiturate intoxication, if severe, may abolish the pupillary light reflex altogether.

Eye Movements

Asymmetric dysfunction of eye movements more often accompanies structural than metabolic causes of coma and therefore serves as another parameter useful in the evaluation of neurological function in head injuries. In the cooperative patient the range of voluntary eye movements in all fields of vision may be easily tested by asking the patient to follow slow- and fast-moving objects with his eyes. Different maneuvers are utilized for the unresponsive patient. The oculocephalic or doll's eye test is performed by rotating the head in the horizontal or vertical plane from a resting position of 30 degrees up from the supine. In a normal response the eyes maintain their position in space by moving opposite to the rotation of the head. The doll's eye maneuver should not be performed in the setting of suspected or known instability of the cervical spine. In this case, or when there is doubt in the interpretation of doll's eye testing, caloric testing of the oculovestibular reflexes is in order. Conduction of the temperature gradient between the irrigating fluid and the endolymph produces fluid movement within the semicircular canal and thereby stimulates the vestibular arc of the reflex. The endolymphatic motion normally occurs in 20 to 60 s and lasts up to several minutes. A warm irrigating solution produces a rise in endolymph, stimulating an increase in the tonic vestibular activity and causing conjugate deviation of the eyes away from the ear being irrigated. The opposite reaction is noted using iced saline. These manipulations assess the function of supranuclear, internuclear, and infranuclear structures responsible for normal eye movement.

Supranuclear influences arise primarily in the frontal gaze center for conjugate saccadic eye movements (area 8). A contralateral conjugate gaze deviation is observed with stimulation of this area, whereas the adverse is true with destructive lesions of the prefrontal cortex. Impairment of the ability to smoothly perform slow pursuit or tracking eye movements occurs with injury to the parietal and occipital regions serving this function.[19] Descending corticobulbar fibers traverse the genu of the internal capsule, continue in a caudal and medial fashion until decussating in the lower midbrain and upper pons, and eventually terminate in the parabducens nuclear complex of the pontine paramedian reticular formation which represents the brain stem center for ipsilateral conjugate gaze. A disruptive influence in this region will evoke conjugate deviation of the eyes contralateral to the site of the lesion. Internuclear connections between the nuclei involved in ocular motility, the vestibular complex, and the cerebellum occur via the medial longitudinal fasciculus (MLF) lying ventral to the periaqueductal gray matter. This vital tract provides the basis for the normal oculocephalic and oculovestibular reflexes described above and is responsible for the characteristic picture of internuclear ophthalmoplegia when disturbance of the pathway occurs. Since the doll's eye and oculovestibular reflexes are inherent to the brain stem, any ocular deviation produced by a supratentorial lesion will be overcome by stimulating these reflexes.

Injury involving the nuclei or peripheral projections of the oculomotor, trochlear, or abducens nerves results in characteristic infranuclear palsies. Trochlear dysfunction is difficult to detect and evaluate in the comatose patient. A suspicion of an abducens paresis should arise with unilateral esotropia and decreased lateral excursion of that eye upon oculocephalic testing. Convergence of both eyes in the resting position as might be seen with increased intracranial pressure is indicative of bilateral abducens dysfunction. A unilateral exotropia with diminished medial, superior, or inferior movements associated with a variable degree of mydriasis points to an oculomotor nerve abnormality. Bilateral paralysis of adduction results from interruption of ascending fibers in both medial longitudinal fasciculi.

The central projections controlling vertical gaze have not been well delineated. Upward gaze paresis occurs with compressive or destructive lesions involving the pretectal area of the midbrain, posterior commissure, and dorsal midbrain tegmentum.[19] Extensive lesions in this area have been associated with paralysis of downward gaze as well. Skew deviations in a vertical plane not infrequently reflect lesions involving the brachium pontis or dorsolateral medulla on the side of the inferiorly rotated eye or the MLF on the side of the superiorly rotated globe.[20]

Cranial Nerves

Examination of the pupillary size and reactivity and of extraocular movements yields information about the function of cranial nerves II, III, IV, and VI. Cranial nerve I, the olfactory, is impossible to test in the unconscious patient, and any grimacing observed in reaction to a noxious smell such as ammonia reflects stimulation of the trigeminal nerve. In a cooperative patient, the sense of smell is examined by presenting non-noxious odors to each nostril separately. Unilateral or bilateral anosmia is not an infrequent sequela to fractures of the floor of the anterior fossa or extensive contusions of the frontal lobes, probably secondary to avulsion of the olfactory fibers. Fractures through the cribriform plate may be associated with CSF rhinorrhea.

The presence of an afferent pupillary defect indicating retinal or optic nerve dysfunction has already been mentioned. If possible, a visual examination should include an assessment of the visual acuity of each eye, a careful funduscopic examination, and visual field testing which can be accomplished in an acute setting by the confrontation method utilizing a white pinhead or moving finger. Though it is a crude test, one should be able to appreciate gross visual field abnormalities by confrontation. Traumatic lesions involving solely the optic chiasm are uncommon, but occasionally the pathognomonic bitemporal hemianopsia may be noted. Intra-axial involvement of the temporal lobe may produce a contralateral superior quadrantanopsia or "pie in the sky" defect secondary to disruption of Meyer's loop radiations. Unilateral or bilateral occipital contusions, from either direct occipital trauma or a frontal blow to the head producing a contrecoup injury, result in a contralateral homonymous hemianopsia or cortical blindness, respectively. Funduscopy should include recognition of traumatic lesions of the vitreous and retina as well as the blurred disc margins, erythematous optic disc head, altered cup-to-disc ratio, absence of spontaneous venous pulsations, and retinal flame hemorrhages and exudates indicative of papilledema from increased intracranial pressure. A full-blown picture of retinal vein occlusion may be seen with severe intracranial hypertension.

Trigeminal nerve function is assessed by the degree and symmetry of facial sensation, the presence of corneal reflexes, and the strength of the muscles of mastication. In an unconscious patient, stimulation of the face with a pin may produce grimacing, indicating pain sensation, and allows for the observation of facial muscle tone and symmetry (facial nerve testing). In the presence of a peripheral facial nerve paresis, a blink reflex will be absent in the ipsilateral eye with corneal stimulation. However, the ipsilateral Bell's phenomenon and contralateral blink reflex confirm corneal sensation. Injury to any of the three trigeminal subdivisions may occur with fractures through the base of the skull. Ophthalmic division dysfunction concomitant with a dilated pupil and ophthalmoplegia reflects intracavernous or retroorbital injury.

Facial nerve palsies are either central (supranuclear) or peripheral. The differentiation lies in the evaluation of forehead and eyelid motion. Central paresis produces contralateral flaccidity of the lower half of the face. This is distinct from the ipsilateral paresis of all muscles of facial expression seen with peripheral nerve injury. The latter occurs in the setting of acute head trauma usually in association with basilar skull fractures producing a contusion or transection of the facial nerve in the facial canal. Varying degrees of unilateral or bilateral facial paresis may occur with "brain stem contusions." A central type of paresis or plegia can be produced by lesions anywhere from the cortex to the internal capsule to the corticobulbar fibers in the midbrain.

Oculocephalic and oculovestibular reflexes adequately assess the function of the vestibular portion of the eighth cranial nerve. Formal audiometry may be performed to evaluate the cochlear nerve portion in a cooperative patient. Fractures through the jugular foramen may cause injury to the ninth and tenth nerves, resulting in depression of the gag or cough reflexes. The accessory and hypoglossal nerves are difficult to examine acutely in the unconscious patient, and isolated abnormalities are uncommon. However, examination of the tongue may reveal unilateral or bilateral fasciculations or atrophy resulting from hypoglossal nerve injury.

Grading Scales

The overwhelming need for an accurate, consistent, and reproducible system for the neurological assessment of the head-injured patient has been recognized for years. On an individual basis such a system allows for a precise initial evaluation of the patient's status and lends continuity to subsequent monitoring and recording of the neurological examination. On a broader basis, implementation of a universal scale yields data for comparison of presentation and outcome characteristics of patients within similar categories in an attempt to establish early prognostic features. The benefit of differing modes and timing of therapeutic intervention can be assessed in a prospective fashion in multiple medical centers simultaneously, resulting in further knowledge and improvement of existing approaches to treatment. The need for this is evidenced by the continued high rates of morbidity and mortality seen with severe head trauma despite the sophisticated diagnostic and therapeutic modalities available.

To be effective, such a system would have to meet several requirements. To avoid arbitrary terminology and ambiguous staging methods, it must be based on strictly objective criteria with proven inherent reproducibility. A degree of relative simplicity would ensure more consistent results between different examiners. Assignment of numerical values to the various aspects of the scale greatly facilitates record keeping and statistical analysis. Also, emphasis has been placed on the need to establish the anatomical site and physiological mechanism of dysfunction in a comatose patient. Certain clinical aspects of the neurological examination with recognized pathophysiological correlates may be incorporated into the system to achieve this knowledge.

Plum and Posner have stated that the evaluation of the cause and site of dysfunction should be based on the pattern of change in five physiological functions: state of consciousness, respiratory pattern, pupillary size and reaction, eye movements and ocular reflexes, and motor abilities.[19] Teasdale and Jennett, however, proposed that the degree of coma after severe head injury is the most reliable clinical indicator of the severity of cerebral damage and presented a scale to assess the depth and duration of impaired consciousness and coma.[21] Coma was defined as the inability to obey commands, to speak, or to open the eyes, and these three behavioral aspects were incorporated into the Glasgow coma scale, first introduced in 1974 and then revised by the addition of another motor response level in 1977[10,11] (Table 191-1). The sum of the E + M + V values was termed the responsiveness score, and on a numerical basis, coma was defined as all combinations which summed to 7 or less. A score of 9 or more precluded the diagnosis of coma. Additionally, the authors thought that correlations between the responsiveness score and pupillary reactions, eye movements, and breathing pattern were limited, thus influencing them not to include brain stem reflexes in the coma scale.

It was recognized that while the proposed grading method was functional for the initial assessment and monitoring of the patient, it provided no parameters to describe the clinical outcome in terms of physical and mental neurological residua, which, in the final analysis, represent the most significant aspect of head injury for the patient and his family. Therefore, Jennett and Bond introduced the Glasgow outcome scale in 1975 as a complement to the coma scale and to provide a reference resource for a predictive system[8] (Table 191-2). Detailed descriptions of the clinical characteristics of each level were carefully laid down to avoid inappropriate usage of the terminology.

The clinical and predictive value of the Glasgow coma scale and Glasgow outcome scale was initially assessed by a cooperative effort on the part of the neurosurgical services at

TABLE 191-1 Glasgow Coma Scale Teasdale/Jennet 1974

Eye opening (E)
   4—opens eyes spontaneously
   3—opens eyes to voice
   2—opens eyes to pain
   1—no eye opening
Best motor response (M)
   6—obeys commands
   5—localizes to pain
   4—withdraws to pain
   3—abnormal flexor response
   2—abnormal extensor response
   1—no movement
Best verbal response (V)
   5—appropriate and oriented
   4—confused conversation
   3—inappropriate words
   2—incomprehensible sounds
   1—no sounds

Glasgow, Rotterdam, Southern California, and Groningen universities. Jennett et al. reviewed the relationship between the clinical features of brain dysfunction expressed in terms of the Glasgow coma scale and Glasgow outcome scale for 1000 patients and reported a correlation between the best response during the first several days and neurological function at 6 months.[12] For example, a best Glasgow coma scale score of 3 or 4 was associated with a 97 percent incidence of death or persistent vegetative state (PVS), while a best Glasgow coma scale score of 8 during the same time frame resulted in a 25 percent death/PVS rate and a 61 percent moderate disability/good recovery rate. Numerous other investigators have adopted the use of the Glasgow coma scale and Glasgow outcome scale for assessing and reporting their patients with head trauma. Indeed, Langfitt in a review of head injury data in 1978 re-emphasized the need for ongoing data collection and concluded that the Glasgow coma scale "should be adopted by neurosurgical units throughout the world to evaluate their patients with head injuries."[14]

Despite the coma scale's many advocates, numerous valid criticisms have been levied against it, and various amendments have been proposed. Perhaps the most frequently raised point is the absence of any evaluation of pupillary size and reactivity, eye movements, or other brain stem reflexes in the coma scale. Fisher[5] and Plum and Posner[19] have emphasized that assessment of these parameters yields valuable information regarding the site and cause of the altered neurological status. Other investigators concur with the importance of monitoring more than just the degree of unconsciousness for an accurate evaluation. Even Langfitt stated that the status of brain stem reflexes is "probably the most important set of observations that should be recorded in addition to the coma scale."[14]

TABLE 191-2 Glasgow Outcome Scale

1. Good recovery—resumption of normal lifestyle
2. Moderate disability—disabled but independent
3. Severe disability—conscious but dependent
4. Persistent vegetative state—unresponsive and speechless
5. Death

Other problems arise when the patient is unable to speak because of mechanical impediments such as facial fractures or intubation. Eye opening may be hindered by severe periorbital edema or lacerations. As the Glasgow coma scale is heavily weighted toward speech and eye opening, a patient would be placed in a lower category on the basis of extrinsic limitations, resulting in an artificial skew of the neurological assessment.

Several investigators have proposed modifications to the Glasgow coma scale. Yen has devised the Albany Scale, a quantitative scheme for neurological evaluation with a maximum score of 30 points, including scores for mental status, motor response, and pupillary response.[23] A system based on a 5-point scale of level of consciousness using a punched-card file for direct entry of data into a computer data bank has been proposed by Ommaya and Sadowsky.[17] Probably the most exhaustive neurological watch sheet was described by Bouzarth and Lindermuth and includes a 100-point scoring system encompassing vital signs, level of consciousness, speech, reactivity to various stimuli, pupillary function, and motor abilities.[2] The sheet is kept at the patient's bedside, and continual recording of appropriate information is done by nurse and physician personnel. They have pointed out the efficacy of such a system in closely following the patient's status. However, the assessment of the data obtained in terms of prognostic features and the relationship to neurological outcome have not yet been reported. The major objection to this scheme is the complicated nature of the grading scales involved, but the authors have argued that facility with clinical use of the system is easily acquired and reproducibility among different examiners is good.

Adjunctive Diagnostic Modalities

Although the neurological examination provides the most rapid and clinically relevant assessment of a head-injured patient, several adjunctive diagnostic measures are available and should be utilized to facilitate emergency determination of the precise location and nature of the intracranial lesions.

X-Ray Films of the Skull

X-ray films of the skull are generally obtained to ascertain whether a fracture is present. Linear skull fractures have been associated with a 2- to 400-fold increase in the incidence of intracranial hematomas. However, as numerous reviews in the radiological literature have revealed, the actual yield of abnormalities found on skull films is as low as 2 to 3 percent.[11] Investigators are now attempting to establish a set of high-yield criteria upon which the decision to obtain plain x-ray films of the skull can be based. This might include such features as prolonged loss of consciousness, persistent vomiting, a palpable defect, or evidence of a CSF leak. A standard set of criteria has yet to be adopted. Despite their limitations, skull films can establish the presence of a fracture and determine if a depressed portion is present, demonstrate intracranial air indicating an open fracture with an underlying dural interruption, and reveal the presence of a mass effect by the displacement of a calcified pineal gland.

Sutures and vascular markings as well as artifacts produced by dressings over scalp wounds, air trapped in the wound, or foreign objects external to the cranium may be confused for fracture lines. Clinical correlation and knowledge of the normal skull anatomy will usually clear any confusion. Basilar skull fractures suspected on clinical grounds are frequently not seen on plain x-ray films, and polycycloidal tomography may be necessary to demonstrate the fracture. Tangential views of a suspected depressed fracture will further aid in making this diagnosis definitive.

Computed Tomography

The advent and availability of computed tomography have revolutionized the strategy of investigating suspected intracranial lesions. A CT scan of the head not only will reveal the exact site and nature of the lesion but also affords some insight into the status of the surrounding cerebral tissue, enabling the surgeon to formulate appropriate interventions. A myriad of intracranial abnormalities can be appreciated with CT in the head-injured patient. An in-depth discussion of these abnormalities is beyond the scope of this chapter. However, a few characteristic lesions are seen with some degree of frequency.

An extra-axial collection of high density generally represents an epidural hematoma which is easily identified by its lentiform shape and sharp margins contained within suture lines. Subdural hematomas are the most common extracerebral traumatic lesion and form a cap of blood density over the cortical surface. It is not uncommon to see a mass effect with a midline shift greater than would have been predicted from the size of the subdural collection, reflecting the frequent association of cerebral contusions and swelling with subdural hematomas. Cerebral contusion is a diagnosis frequently made when there is CT evidence of an inhomogeneous area of low and high attenuation values associated with a mass effect. Post-traumatic intracerebral hematomas are generally frontal and temporal, multiple in 20 to 33 percent of cases, and associated with the well-recognized syndrome of delayed hemorrhage in up to 7 to 10 percent of severely injured patients.[18] Curvilinear areas of increased density conforming to the basilar cisterns, convexity sulci, or interhemispheric fissure indicate the presence of blood in the subarachnoid space. CT scans may demonstrate distortion of the ventricular system including slit ventricles secondary to diffuse cerebral swelling, a shift from the normal midline position, or hydrocephalus from outflow obstruction secondary to a lesion in the posterior fossa. The presence of intracranial air or foreign bodies and the extent of bony displacement from a depressed skull fracture may be identified.

Angiography

The use of emergency cerebral angiography for the diagnosis of post-traumatic intracranial abnormalities has essentially been eliminated with the advent of CT scanning. However, if a CT scanner is not available, angiography can be an important diagnostic tool for the investigation of space-occupying lesions which produce a shift of the blood vessels from their normal positions. Characteristic findings seen with a supratentorial mass lesion include a lateral shift of the anterior cerebral and pericallosal arteries and the internal cerebral vein, elevation or depression of the middle cerebral artery, and a shift either of the proximal branches of the intracranial internal carotid artery or of the posterior cerebral artery into the posterior fossa indicating transtentorial or central herniation. The presence of an infratentorial mass may be deduced from displacement of vertebrobasilar vascular structures or the upward sweep of the anterior cerebral and pericallosal vessels with bowing of the striothalamic vein characteristic of hydrocephalus. In the present CT era, perhaps the most important role of angiography lies in the definition of vascular injury, particularly the post-traumatic aneurysm or carotid artery occlusion not visualized on CT. We advocate angiography for the evaluation of all penetrating lesions that traverse the vicinity of major intracranial vessels and also for the assessment of acute unilateral hemispheric dysfunction when the initial CT scan is normal.

Ventriculography

Again, this modality for assessing displacement of the midline ventricular system by a supratentorial mass has yielded to the less invasive and more specific computed tomography. In an emergency situation, however, air or metrizamide introduced into the ventricular system via a ventriculostomy will demonstrate the direction of an intracranial shift and therefore will indicate the side of the significant mass lesion.

References

1. Berger AJ, Mitchell RA, Severinghaus JW: Regulation of respiration. N Engl J Med 297:92–97, 138–143, 194–201, 1977.
2. Bouzarth WF, Lindermuth JR: Head injury watch sheet modified for a digital scale. J Trauma 18:571–579, 1978.
3. Bricolo A, Turazzi S, Alexandre A, Rizzuto N: Decerebrate rigidity in acute head injury. J Neurosurg 47:680–698, 1977.
4. De Jong RN: *The Neurologic Examination*, 4th ed. Hagerstown, Md, Medical Department, Harper & Row, 1979.
5. Fisher CM: The neurological examination of the comatose patient. Acta Neurol Scand [Suppl] 36:1–56, 1969.
6. Gissane W: The nature and causation of road injuries. Lancet 2:695–698, 1963.
7. Glaser JS: *Neuro-ophthalmology*. Hagerstown, Md, Harper & Row, 1978.
8. Jennett B, Bond M: Assessment of outcome after severe brain damage: A practical scale. Lancet 1:480–484, 1975.
9. Jennett B, MacMillan R: Epidemiology of head injury. Br Med J 282:101–104, 1981.
10. Jennett B, Teasdale G: Aspects of coma after severe head injury. Lancet 1:878–881, 1977.
11. Jennett B, Teasdale G: *Management of Head Injuries*. Philadelphia, Davis, 1981, pp 95–151.
12. Jennett B, Teasdale G, Braakman R, Minderhoud J, Heiden J, Kurze T: Prognosis of patients with severe head injury. Neurosurgery 4:283–289, 1979.
13. Klauber MR, Barrett-Connor E, Marshall LF, Bowers SA: The epidemiology of head injury. A prospective study of an entire community—San Diego County, California, 1978. Am J Epidemiol 113:500–509, 1981.

14. Langfitt TW: Measuring the outcome from head injuries. J Neurosurg 48:673–678, 1978.
15. Lindgren SO: *Diagnosis and Classification in Head Injuries.* Edinburgh, Churchill Livingstone, 1971, pp 305–307.
16. Moruzzi G, Magoun HW: Brain stem reticular formation and activation of the EEG. Electroencephalogr Clin Neurophysiol 1:455–473, 1949.
17. Ommaya AK, Sadowsky D: A system of coding medical data for punched-card machine retrieval: Part II. As applied to head injuries. J Trauma 6:605–617, 1966.
18. Peyster RG, Hoover ED: CT in head trauma. J Trauma 22:25–38, 1982.
19. Plum F, Posner JB: *The Diagnosis of Stupor and Coma,* 3d ed. Philadelphia, Davis, 1980.
20. Smith JL, David NJ, Klintworth G: Skew deviation. Neurology 14:96–105, 1964.
21. Teasdale G, Jennett B: Assessment of coma and impaired consciousness: A practical scale. Lancet 2:81–83, 1974.
22. U.S. Department of Health, Education, and Welfare: *Facts of Life and Death.* Publication Number (HRS) 74-1222. Rockville, Md, National Center for Health Statistics, 1974.
23. Yen, JK, Bourke RS, Nelson LR, Popp AJ: Numerical grading of clinical neurological status after serious head injury. J Neurol Neurosurg Psychiatry 41:1125–1130, 1978.

192
Computed Tomography in Head Trauma

Chi-Shing Zee
Hervey D. Segall
Jamshid Ahmadi
Michael L. J. Apuzzo
Steven L. Giannotta

Since its clinical introduction in 1973, computed tomography (CT) scanning has become the primary diagnostic imaging procedure in the evaluation of patients following head trauma. With the advent of CT, the roles of skull roentgenography, cerebral angiography, pneumoencephalography, and radionuclide brain scanning have diminished markedly. The relative advantages of CT over these other imaging modalities (including resolution, safety, and economy of time) have made CT an integral part of the evaluation of a trauma patient. The advantages and the pitfalls of CT scanning in the evaluation of patients with head trauma are summarized in Table 192-1.

Technique

Standard transaxial computed tomography is performed with conventional angulation of slices relative to the orbitomeatal line. Our discussion will relate almost exclusively to the axial plane; coronal and sagittal images could be obtained, but these are rarely used in the evaluation of acute traumatic injuries. Since motion is an important problem to be overcome in scanning patients with head trauma, it is advisable to use the fastest scanning available. Newer scanning instruments can complete a slice within a few seconds. Elimination of motion artifacts by using faster slice times outweighs any slight image degradation that may result. Motion can also be minimized by immobilization of the patient's head by means of tapes secured to the head holder. The use of sponge padding surrounding the head holder is an important adjunct in ensuring patient cooperation during the study. Severely head-injured patients who have a depressed level of consciousness are usually intubated before CT scanning so that total immobilization can be obtained by using muscle relaxants. This technique completely eliminates motion artifacts and also lessens the risk of hypoxia during the study.

A complete examination is critical in the evaluation of head trauma. Contiguous CT slices should be obtained, including all areas from the foramen magnum up to the vertex. This technique will allow for accurate intracranial localization of traumatic lesions or foreign bodies as well as complete delineation of multiple lesions.[7]

Computed tomography may be performed with or without the intravenous administration of a water-soluble contrast material. The decision to use this material is dictated by a number of factors, but most importantly by the clinical setting. The majority of acute traumatic intracranial lesions can be adequately assessed without the use of contrast enhancement. However, in certain circumstances contrast enhancement may be most helpful in the CT workup of head trauma. The indications for the use of contrast will be mentioned in subsequent paragraphs.

Injuries to the Skull

In general, we have found that CT is superior to skull roentgenography in the assessment of many depressed skull fractures.[2] The majority of such fractures are located sufficiently low on the calvarium that axial CT studies can depict their extent and severity. Depth of depression can easily be assessed because axial CT involves imaging tangential to

Computed Tomography in Head Trauma

TABLE 192-1 Computed Tomography in Head Trauma

Advantages	Pitfalls
• A noninvasive and rapid procedure.	• Traumatic intracranial aneurysms are likely to be missed.
• Helps define the nature of an acute mass lesion (hematoma, contusion, edema, etc.).	• Other vascular lesions (such as carotid-cavernous fistula or arteriovenous fistula of the scalp) might be missed if contrast enhancement and proper window settings are not used.
• Provides accurate anatomical localization of blood clots or other space-occupying lesions.	• Unable to show findings related to neck vessel injuries initially.
• Anatomical displacements and hydrocephalus resulting from trauma can be identified.	• Depressed skull fractures may be confused with epidural hematomas if expanded windows are not used. (See Figs. 192-2A and B.)
• Delineates bony fractures as well as changes in the sinuses and soft tissues.	• Depressed skull fractures at the vertex may be missed by axial CT scanning.
• In assessing depressed skull fractures it is better than skull roentgenograms except for vertex fractures.	• A lesion or lesions can be missed unless one has obtained a complete series of slices ranging from the foramen magnum to the vertex.
• Sensitive in detecting smaller amounts of intracranial air compared with skull roentgenograms.	• Motion may degrade the images.
• Much better than skull films in anatomical localization of multiple metallic foreign bodies.	• Artifacts can simulate pathological lesions; they may obscure and prevent the identification of some abnormalities.

most areas where depressed fractures tend to occur. Available skull films frequently do not include a projection tangential to the depressed fracture. A special effort would have to be made in many instances to obtain an adequate tangential view, but this is frequently not done.

However, axial CT does have some limitations in the evaluation of depressed skull fractures. Slices with axial orientation may fail to demonstrate vertex fractures. Fortunately, in these cases the vertex depressed fragment can usually be appreciated on skull roentgenograms. A scout view might also show such a fracture, or one could resort to coronal cuts. Overlying metallic foreign bodies may cast artifacts which impair the evaluation of important features underlying the calvarial depression. Motion artifacts may also be a limitation. In these instances, skull films can also be used in a complementary role.

Fractures of the skull base can be appreciated on CT evaluation. Indirect evidence of trauma to the base of the skull may also be visualized. An air-fluid level may be demonstrated in the sphenoid sinus, indicating the presence of blood or cerebrospinal fluid. If the air-fluid level persists or if there is clinical evidence of a CSF leak, this would favor the air-fluid level being of CSF origin. Although the majority of CSF leaks will resolve spontaneously, occasionally we have found the use of intrathecal metrizamide useful in the evaluation of chronic post-traumatic CSF leaks before their surgical treatment.[7]

A critical adjunct in studying trauma to the skull with CT is the manipulation of window widths. The term *window width* refers to the range of attenuation values between the extremes of the gray scale. Any value above the selected window width appears pictorially in peak white; anything below appears in peak black. Thus, a narrow window width will have a smaller range of numerical absorption values between peak white and peak black, whereas a wide window width will have a larger range of attenuation values.

The window level is the point on the numerical scale of attenuation values representing the center of the range occupied by the window width. Like the window width, the window level may be adjusted by controls on the CT console. Without the use of wide window widths, fractures of the skull may in some instances escape detection (Fig. 192-1). We have also encountered cases in which depressed skull fractures mimicked epidural hematomas on scans displayed at standard window widths. Once the window width was expanded, the depressed fragments were easily depicted (Fig. 192-2). Also, depiction of foreign bodies may be improved by changing window widths and window levels.

CT may be superior not only to plain skull x-ray films but also to complex motion tomography, because it can delineate not only bony fractures but also changes in the sinuses and soft tissues. With expanded window widths, fractures of the lamina papyracea, blowout fractures of the orbit, and fractures of the petrous bone can be clearly demonstrated (Fig. 192-3).

Intracranial Mass Lesions

Before the development of CT, angiography was frequently used to evaluate whether a surgically treatable intracranial mass was present. Although angiography can define the size and approximate location of a mass lesion, it cannot be relied upon to differentiate hematoma from other space-occupying lesions which may or may not require surgical evacuation. The ability of CT to differentiate between various attenuation values aids in defining the nature of most mass lesions. Edema, for example, can be distinguished readily from an acute hematoma. Thus, important management decisions can be made much more readily and with more confidence.

The major advantage of CT scanning is that it enables identification of collections of blood in a manner previously not possible. New and Aronow have shown that whole blood with a hematocrit of 45 percent has an average attenuation value of 28 EMI units (old scale, equivalent to 56 HU), which is greater than that for normal brain tissue.[5] Furthermore, these authors have made the interesting observation that high attenuation values of blood are due largely to the protein fraction of hemoglobin. The iron fraction contributes only about 7 to 8 percent of the attenuation value. Attenuation contributed by calcium in serum or red blood cells

1580   Trauma

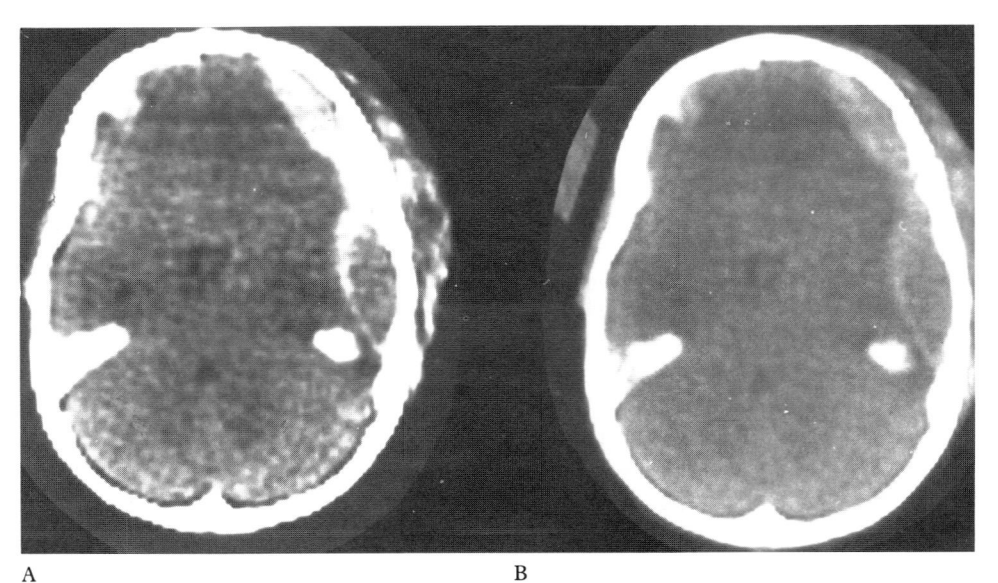

Figure 192-1 Epidural hematomas with an associated linear skull fracture. *A.* Using fairly conventional window width and level settings, two adjacent epidural hematomas are seen. However, a skull fracture cannot be appreciated. *B.* Using a wide window width, a linear fracture involving both the inner and outer tables of the skull is clearly seen. Note also the overlying subgaleal hematoma.

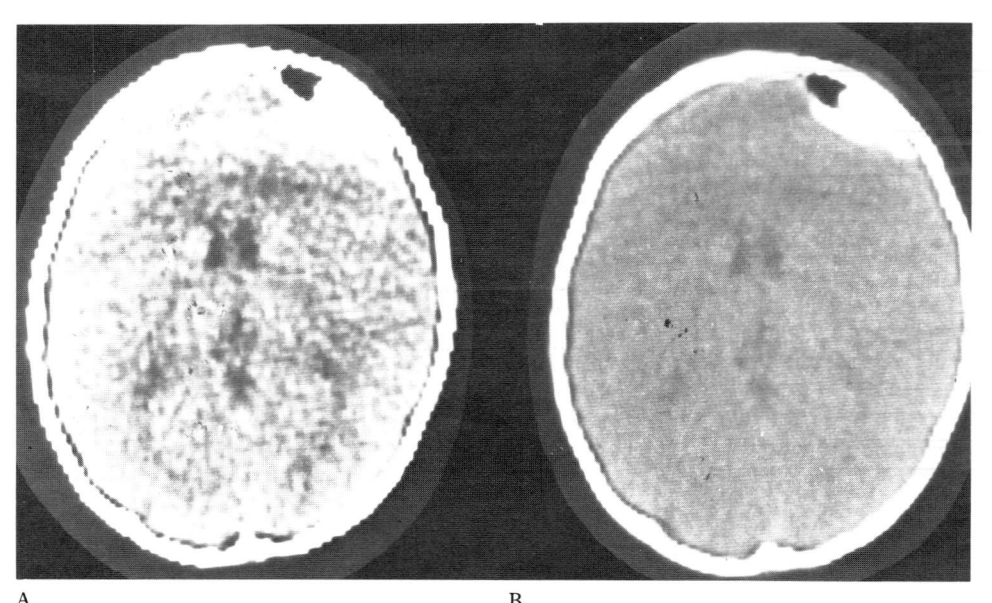

Figure 192-2 Depressed skull fracture mimicking an epidural hematoma. *A.* This scan is depicted utilizing conventional window width and window level settings. It is not possible to tell whether the lentiform high-density lesion in the right frontal region actually represents an epidural hematoma or a depressed skull fracture. The black zone anteriorly represents air (air can enter an epidural blood collection through a scalp laceration or from an air-containing sinus following fracture of the calvarium). *B.* When the same slice is imaged utilizing an expanded window width, it becomes apparent that the abnormal densities seen have much higher values than blood, and are similar to calvarial bone. With the window settings utilized in this example, an epidural hematoma would have appeared in gray tones and not the extreme white density of bone. This image also emphasizes the difference in density of the accompanying low-density area when compared with fluid in the frontal horn. Air has much lower CT values than cerebrospinal fluid and therefore appears much blacker by comparison when images are reprocessed in this manner.

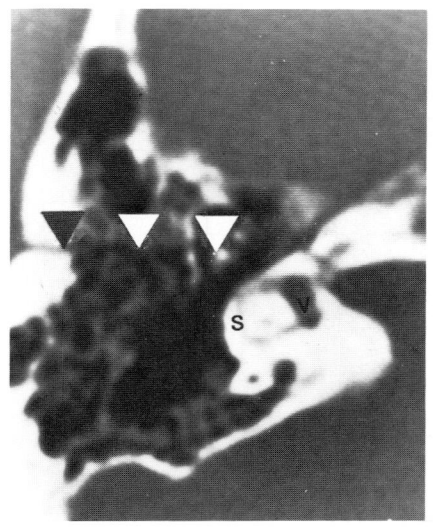

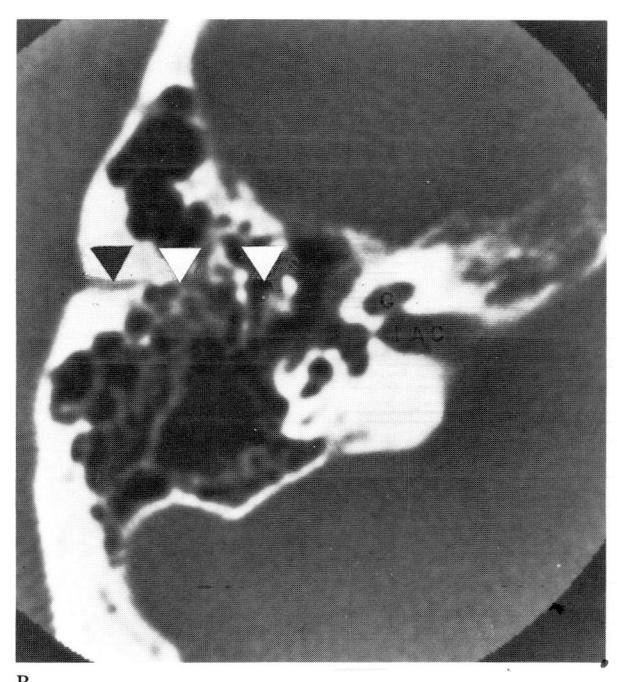

Computed Tomography in Head Trauma

Figure 192-3 Fracture of the petrous portion of the temporal bone shown by CT scanning. *A, B.* Axial high-resolution scans show a longitudinal fracture of the petrous bone, extending into the middle ear cavity (*arrowheads*). The cochlea (C), vestibule (V), lateral semicircular canal (S), and internal auditory canal (IAC) are well seen.

is negligible. In addition, it has been established that there is a linear relationship between hematocrit and radioattenuation.[5]

Accurate anatomical localization of blood clots within the brain is now routine. Extracerebral blood collections can usually be identified as being subarachnoid, subdural, or epidural. Intraventricular blood can be readily appreciated as such (Fig. 192-4). Extra-axial blood collections will be discussed in detail in another chapter.

Acute traumatic hematomas appear within the brain as areas of increased attenuation. These tend to be fluffy, irregular, and poorly marginated compared with "spontaneous" hemorrhages. Frequently, intracranial hematomas in head trauma patients will be multiple and scattered in different areas of the brain. This feature may serve to differentiate traumatic lesions from spontaneous hemorrhages, which are generally solitary.[7]

It has been pointed out that serial scans of patients with intracerebral hematomas frequently show rises in attenuation values of 7 to 14 EMI units in a very short period of time, consistent with clot formation.[5] Thereafter, at a variable rate, there is progressive decrease of attenuation values. The area of increased attenuation within a hematoma usually persists from 1 to 3 weeks. Progressive attenuation of a hematoma occurs first at its periphery and then gradually moves centrally. Eventually, a hematoma may progress through an isodense phase (having the same CT density as adjacent cerebral tissue), ultimately becoming an area of decreased attenuation within the brain. Usually, the density appears less than the normal brain after about 4 weeks.

If intravenous contrast enhancement is utilized, a ring-like area of enhancement surrounding an area of hematoma may be noted from 6 days to 6 weeks after the bleeding has occurred. This disappears approximately 2 to 6 months following the onset of trauma.[11] This ringlike enhancement, a response of the brain to hemorrhage, represents contrast leakage secondary to breakdown of the blood-brain barrier, and should not be confused with neoplasm or abscess (Fig. 192-5).

Usually there is little difficulty in distinguishing a peripherally situated intracerebral hematoma from an extracerebral hematoma. An intracerebral hematoma tends to have its maximum diameter at some distance from the inner table of the skull, whereas an extracerebral hematoma will have its greatest dimension and its edges in close contact with the inner table of the skull.

Contrast infusion can be useful in studying a patient with an isodense subdural hematoma. Enhancement of the underlying cortical vessels can be extremely useful in defining the size of an isodense subdural hematoma. These cortical vessels will appear as a row of punctate dots of enhancement, separated from the inner table of the skull (Fig. 192-6). In other cases of isodense subdural hematoma, a curvilinear continuous line of enhancement may be seen on the inner surface of the isodense collection. This represents enhancement within subdural membranes.[9]

If a CT scan shows no midline shift, no cerebral abnormalities, no evidence of white matter "buckling,"[4] normal size and configuration of the ventricles, and normal-appearing subarachnoid spaces, there is no need to use contrast infusion if the patient's clinical problem is clearly acute head trauma. In evaluating older patients, one may note that the cortical sulci (and, therefore, the adjacent gyri) extend right to the skull's inner table. When this can be observed at multiple levels on CT slices in the head-injured patient, it may be regarded as a sign excluding an isodense subdural hematoma.

Cerebral contusion is a pathological term that implies loss of integrity of cerebral tissue, usually without interruption of the physical continuity of the cerebral cortex or pia. Con-

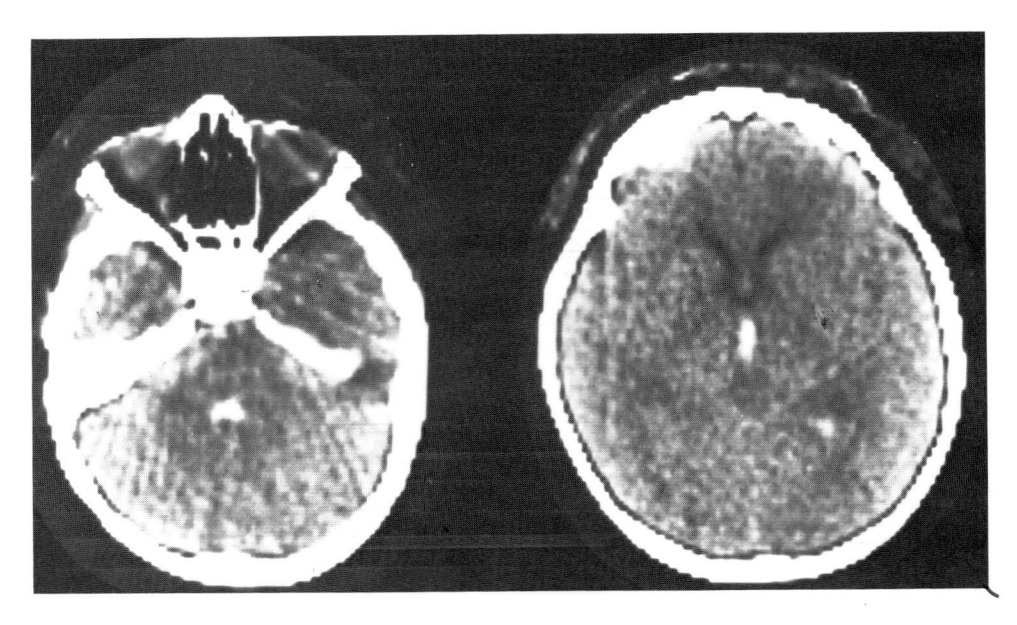

Figure 192-4 Post-traumatic intraventricular hemorrhage. High-density blood is situated within and conforms to the shape of the lateral, third, and fourth ventricles.

tusions are usually found where the dura is not perforated or lacerated. Minor hemorrhages which occur with contusion result from torn or ruptured arterioles, capillaries, or veins. The CT appearance of cerebral contusion may overlap with that of intracerebral hematoma and with cerebral edema, depending on the relative contribution of hemorrhage. Therefore, a contusion may have a combination of high-attenuation areas intermixed with low-attenuation zones, resulting in a "salt and pepper" appearance.[3] As is the case with larger hemorrhages, high-density areas diminish with time. Low-attenuation areas will then remain for a protracted period.

Cerebral contusions are more common in the frontal and temporal regions but can occur anywhere. They may also occur on the side of the brain opposite from the direct blow. This is due to the so-called contrecoup mechanism. Since cerebral contusion involves disruption of vessels, enhancement of the area following contrast infusion might be expected. In fact, some cases of contusion can be isodense on noncontrast scans, and may only be shown as areas of contrast enhancement following the infusion of iodinated material (Fig. 192-7).[9]

Vasogenic cerebral edema occurs when fluid accumulates in the extracellular space. Leakage of edema fluid results from loss of vascular integrity and extravasation of plasma proteins. On CT studies, cerebral edema appears as an area of homogeneously decreased attenuation (15 to 25 HU) which may be accompanied by mass effect. Ventricular compression or obliteration can result. Also, loss of the normal white matter interface may be noted. Cerebral edema is usu-

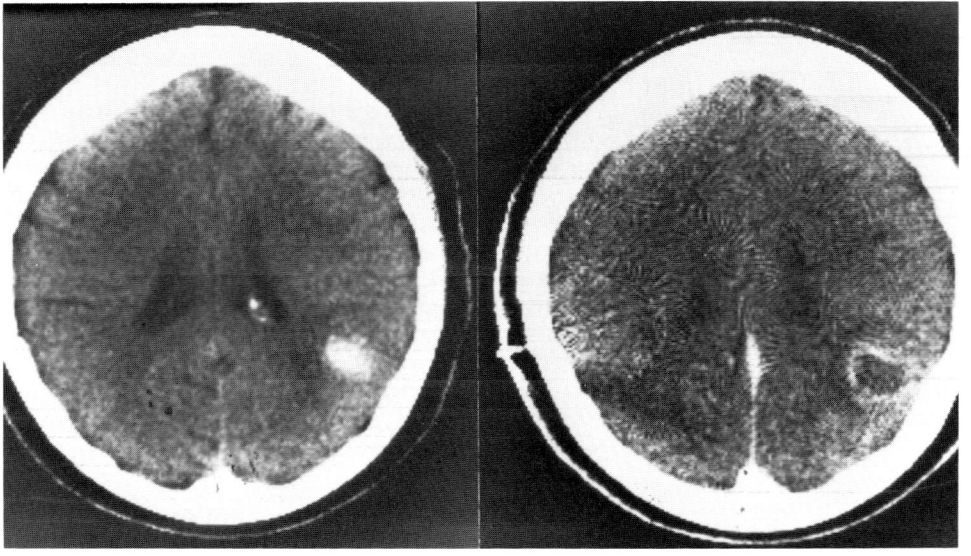

Figure 192-5 Ring enhancement in a resolving intracerebral hematoma. *A.* A post-traumatic intracerebral hematoma is seen in the left parietal region as a high-density area on this CT slice. *B.* A follow-up CT slice (at a very slightly higher level) obtained 2 weeks later shows a ring-like area of enhancement after contrast infusion in the same location as the hematoma (an unenhanced CT scan showed no abnormal densities).

Figure 192-6 An isodense subdural hematoma. *A.* Note the compression of the right lateral ventricle and leftward displacement of the left lateral ventricle. However, the isodense subdural hematoma cannot be seen on this unenhanced slice. (Incidentally noted is ventriculostomy tubing in the body of the right lateral ventricle.) *B.* Following the infusion of contrast material, enhancement of vessels on the cortical surface (*arrows*) and within the sulci can be seen.

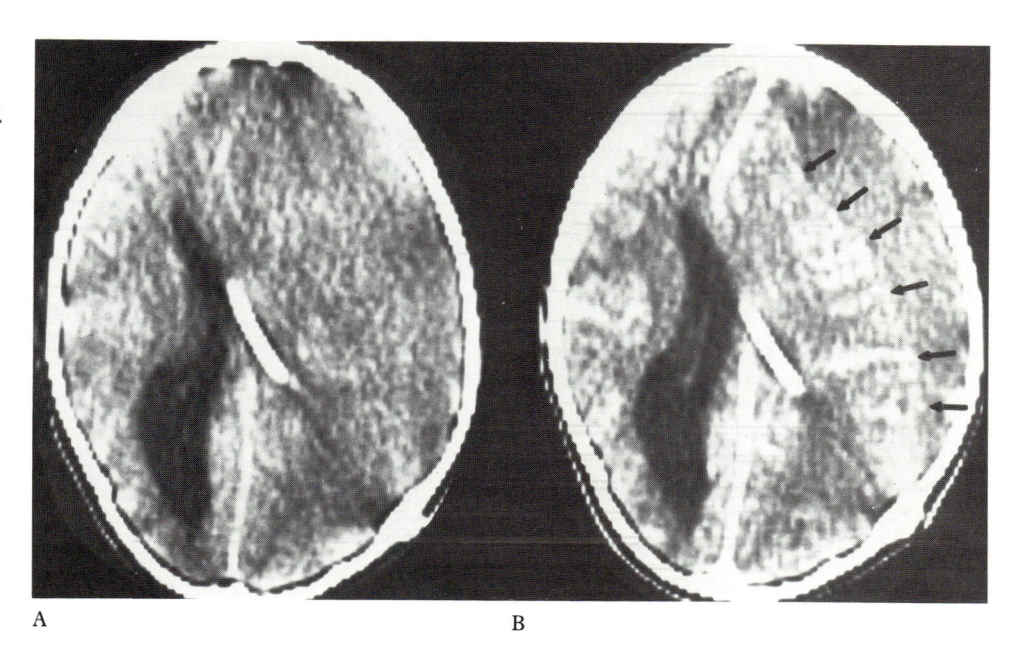

ally most intense at 12 to 24 h following the initial trauma. Edema may be mild and focal or may be multifocal and diffuse. The reader is reminded that low-attenuation areas on CT may also be caused by contusion or by cerebral infarction secondary to a vascular injury suffered during the acute traumatic incident. This topic will be discussed in more detail below.

Acute generalized cerebral swelling manifests itself shortly after trauma.[10] This condition appears primarily in childhood and has certain CT characteristics and pathological features. CT scans show compression or obliteration of the lateral ventricles, the third ventricle, and the perimesencephalic and quadrigeminal cisterns (Fig. 192-8). There is also an increase in the average density of the white matter (of about 3 HU).[10] The slightly increased density seen on CT in this condition appears to be due to hyperemia and correlates with increased regional blood flow as determined by xenon 133 radionuclide measurements. Clinically, almost all patients with acute generalized cerebral swelling are semicomatose or comatose. Many patients will eventually recover with minimal residue. However, intellectual loss, spastic quadriparesis, or death may occur.

Cerebral Herniation

Intracranial shifts of cerebral structures and cerebral herniation may also be identified using CT scanning.[8] The earliest sign of transtentorial herniation is encroachment of the uncus on the lateral aspect of the suprasellar cistern. This is followed then by widening of the ipsilateral crural and ambient cisterns. With more advanced herniation, obliteration of the cisternal spaces at the tentorial level is seen. There may be hydrocephalus of the portions of the ventricular system not directly exposed to mass effect. This is believed to be due to obstruction at the aqueduct or the level of the third ventricle. Thus, dilatation of the temporal horn, atrium, and occipital horn may occur on the side contralateral to the herniation when the alterations are sufficiently severe. Infarction in the posterior cerebral artery distribution can also result from vascular kinking and compression due to tentorial herniation, and may produce CT changes.

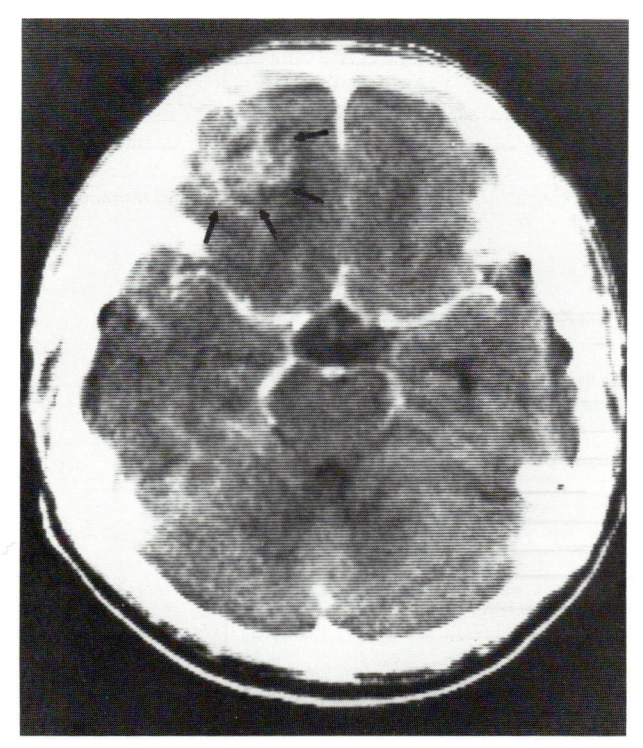

Figure 192-7 An enhancing cerebral contusion. A CT scan following contrast infusion shows a patchy, irregular focus of enhancement within an area of cerebral contusion (*arrows*). An unenhanced CT scan showed no abnormal density.

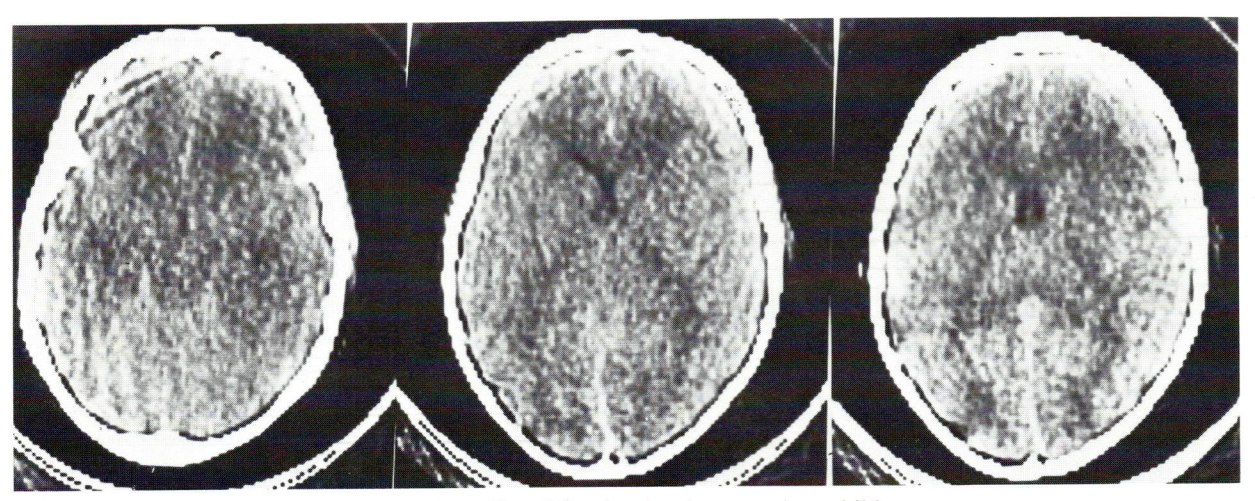

Figure 192-8 Acute generalized cerebral swelling following head trauma in a child. Note the small size of the compressed lateral ventricles and obliteration of the quadrigeminal cistern and the cisterna vena galena magna, due to the bilateral cerebral swelling.

Pneumocephalus

Because of its low attenuation value, air is readily visualized by CT. Pneumocephalus usually results from fractures involving the paranasal sinuses or mastoid air cells, but fractures elsewhere which involve the entire thickness of the cranial vault (scalp, skull, and meninges) may permit air to enter the intracranial space. Air may be seen in the extradural, subdural, or subarachnoid space or within brain parenchyma or the ventricular system (Fig. 192-9). Air is absorbed with time; hence, if pneumocephalus persists, a continuing cerebrospinal fluid leak should be suspected. CT may also dramatically demonstrate small but significant collections of air outside of the intracranial compartment, as well. Figure 192-10 shows an example of orbital emphysema in a patient with a lamina papyracea fracture.

Hydrocephalus

CT can provide a very sensitive index regarding the size of the ventricular system. Following severe head trauma or penetrating injuries, the resulting subarachnoid or intraventricular hemorrhage may, if severe enough, result in a communicating or noncommunicating hydrocephalus. A communicating hydrocephalus which may begin as soon as the first week following the traumatic incident might be revealed by serial CT scanning. Thus, serial CT scanning can give important information regarding the management of hydrocephalus as a sequel of head trauma.

Vascular Lesions

The use of CT in place of cerebral angiography in the neuroradiological evaluation of head trauma clearly has a number of advantages. This practice, however, will result occasionally in the failure to appreciate certain vascular complications of trauma. It is important to be aware that traumatic intracranial aneurysms can be easily missed if CT is the sole study and if angiography is not performed. Before the CT era, during the years 1965 through 1969, nine traumatic cortical aneurysms were diagnosed at our institution.[6] After the advent of CT scanning (during the years 1977 through 1982), only three such aneurysms were found. No other factors have been found to explain these statistics aside from the marked decrease in use of cerebral angiography for head trauma since the emergence of CT.

Rumbaugh et al. reported nine cases of traumatic aneu-

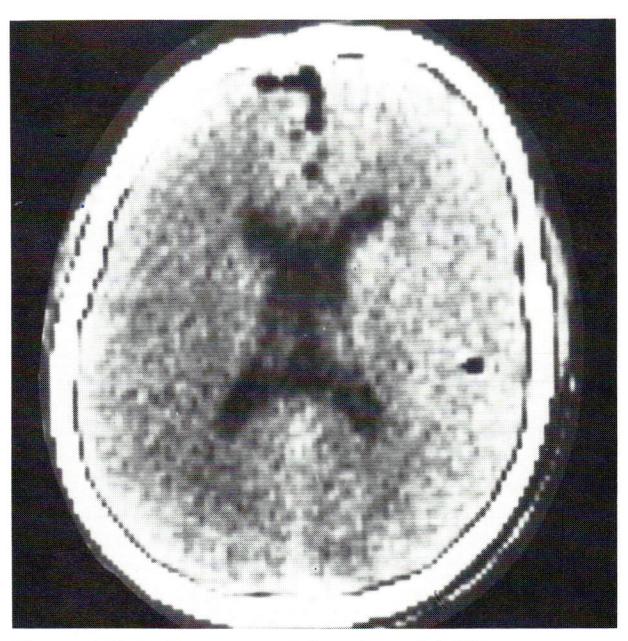

Figure 192-9 Pneumocephalus. An axial CT scan showed air adjacent to the right frontal lobe and extending along the interhemispheric fissure anteriorly. Another small air bubble is seen in the left parietal region.

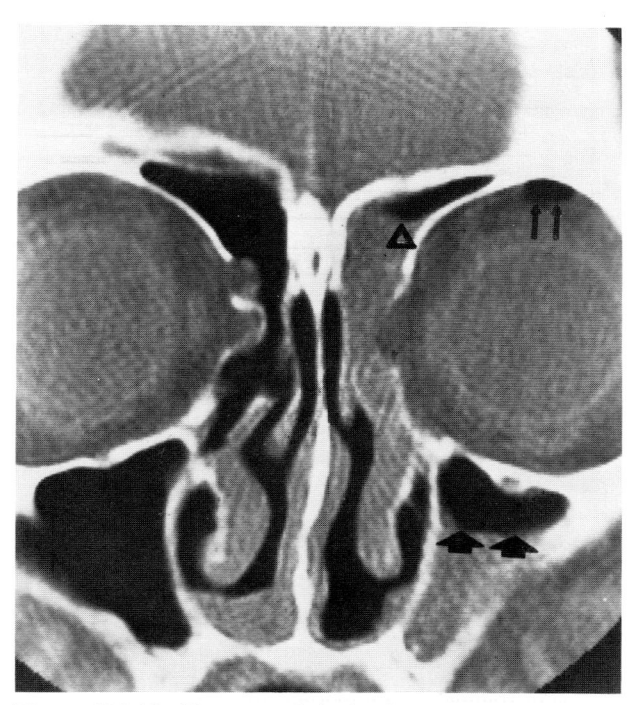

Figure 192-10 Fracture of the lamina papyracea. A coronal CT slice demonstrates an air-fluid level in the left ethmoid sinus (*arrowhead*), orbital emphysema (*small arrows*), and an air-fluid level in the left maxillary sinus (*large arrows*) secondary to a fracture of the lamina papyracea. An air-fluid level is also seen in the inferior nasal cavity below the inferior turbinate and above the hard palate on the right.

rysm, all but one of these cases being associated with a subdural, epidural, or intracerebral hematoma.[6] Four of these cases were associated with skull fracture. The interval between the traumatic episode and the diagnosis of the aneurysm varied between a few hours and 3 weeks.

Figure 192-11A depicts the CT scan of a patient who presented with an area of cerebral contusion following head injury. Two weeks later, a routine follow-up evaluation (Fig. 192-11B) showed a hematoma at the area of the contusion. Because the hemorrhage extended to the surface of the brain, angiography was performed, revealing a cortical aneurysm (Fig. 192-11C). Follow-up CT evaluations are strongly recommended within 3 weeks after injury in patients found to have a skull fracture, intra- or extra-axial hematoma, or contusion. If there is any reason to suspect a traumatic vascular lesion, a cerebral angiogram should be performed. Needless to say, a CT scan should be performed on any patient who deteriorates suddenly after head trauma; however, if that CT scan does not provide diagnostic information, angiography should be considered strongly.

Another vascular complication of head trauma is venous sinus occlusion. While CT scanning may demonstrate dural sinus filling defects, venographic delineation is more sensitive and definitive. Superior sagittal sinus occlusion may present with bilateral hemispheric hemorrhagic infarctions on CT, thus directing one to proceed further with angiography.

Other vascular lesions, such as carotid-cavernous fistula or an arteriovenous fistula of the scalp, might be suspected or even diagnosed with CT if adequate contrast-enhanced studies are obtained and properly scrutinized.[1] Nevertheless, in order to appreciate important anatomical vascular details and to provide information necessary for a surgical approach to treatment, a definitive angiographic study is required.

Some patients may exhibit a profound localized neurological deficit following trauma out of proportion to any abnormalities seen on the initial CT evaluation. These features may also be observed in patients who have sustained a direct or indirect neck injury. In these cases, a high index of suspicion for an underlying vascular injury must be kept in mind, and the clinician must continue to realize the potential pitfalls of CT in evaluating patients with vascular injuries. Blunt trauma to, or sudden distortion of, the neck may cause a thrombus or embolus to form within the internal carotid or vertebral artery which could result in brain infarction. Also, a hematoma in the soft tissues may lead to stenosis or occlusion of the carotid artery by external compression.

Contrast enhancement may add to the information one gets in evaluating vascular lesions associated with head trauma. It is exceedingly important to remember that intracranial hemorrhage may be caused by a primary underlying aneurysm or arteriovenous malformation, or even a neoplasm. Such primary lesions may bleed intracranially, thereby precipitating the event leading to the head injury. Contrast enhancement used judiciously may lead one to suspect an underlying vascular disease as a cause of the traumatic event. Also, a number of other nontraumatic conditions might be revealed by CT. Incidental findings such as venous angiomas have been picked up in otherwise routine evaluation of head trauma patients, again with judicious use of contrast enhancement. Failure to appreciate the possibility of incidental intracranial lesions may have tragic consequences. A case in point relates to a man who had a precontrast and postcontrast CT study following an episode in which there was symptomatology attributed to head trauma. The CT studies were interpreted as normal, and no further studies or neuroradiological examinations were performed, despite the presence of headache and a stiff neck. The patient later died of a ruptured anterior communicating artery aneurysm. A review of the CT studies showed a rounded area of enhancement in the region of the anterior communicating artery. Presumably, had angiography been performed, the correct diagnosis of aneurysm would have been made and the proper treatment would then have been rendered.

The Value of Serial CT Scans

Serial CT scans can be useful in patients with small subdural or epidural hematomas treated conservatively. CT scanning can clearly demonstrate the resolution or enlargement of these lesions.

Occasionally, the occurrence of an intracerebral hematoma may be delayed, appearing days or weeks after the initial traumatic event. Serial CT scans are very useful in detecting delayed intracerebral hemorrhage.

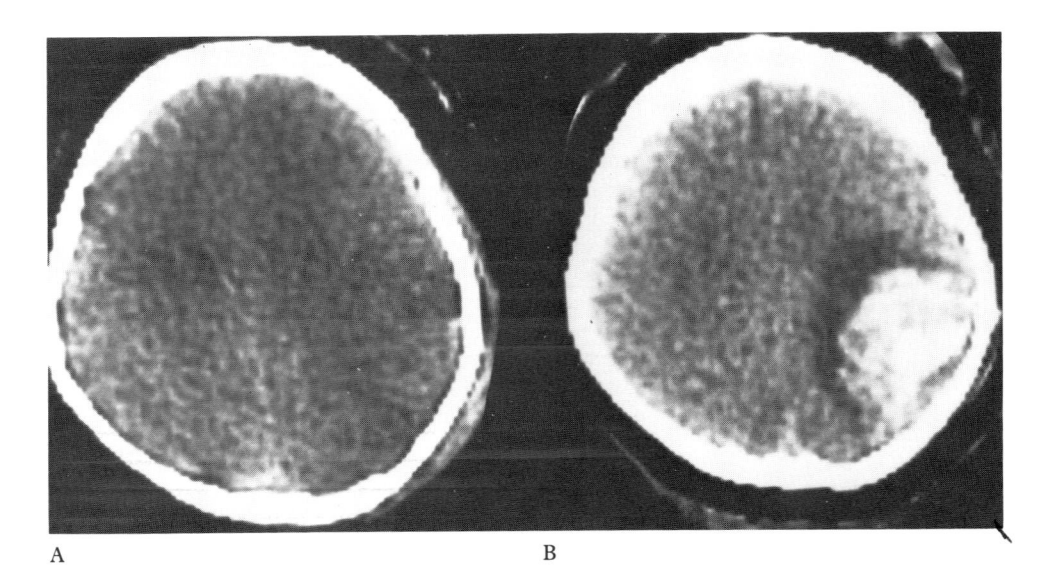

Figure 192-11 Intracerebral hematoma secondary to a traumatic cortical aneurysm. *A.* The initial CT scan following head trauma showed an area of low attenuation in the right parietal region, consistent with cerebral contusion. *B.* A follow-up CT scan 2 weeks later, before discharge, showed an intracerebral hematoma. Note that the hematoma appears to involve the cortical surface, and comes into contact with the calvarium. A low-density area surrounds the higher-density hematoma. *C.* A cerebral angiogram demonstrates a peripheral aneurysm involving a cortical branch of the right middle cerebral artery. This traumatic aneurysm was successfully treated surgically.

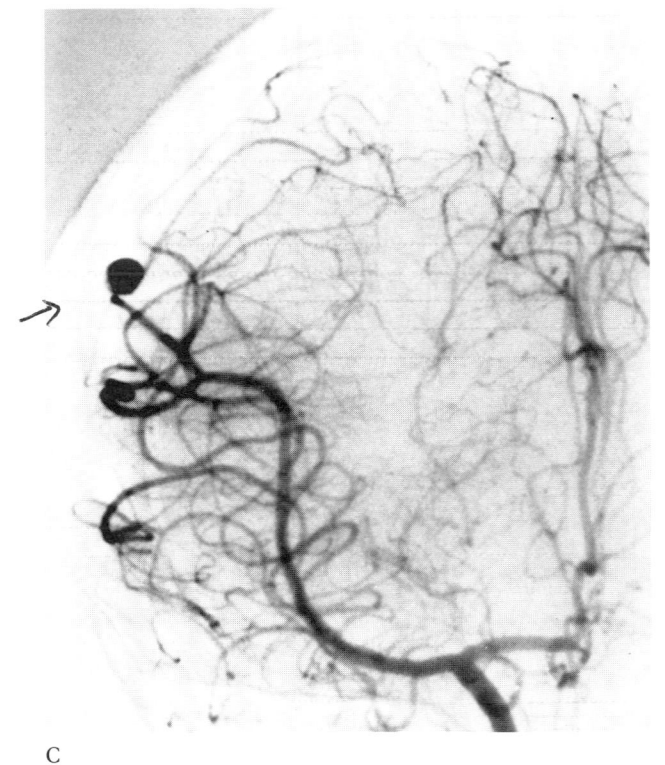

Finally, CT scans are also very helpful in ascertaining whether or not hydrocephalus is developing after head trauma. Other post-traumatic residues involving the brain, such as atrophy, porencephaly, or leptomeningeal cyst formation, can also be detected by late CT scanning.

References

1. Ahmadi J, Teal JS, Segall HD, Zee CS, Han JS, Becker TS: Computed tomography of carotid-cavernous fistula. AJNR 4:131–136, 1983.
2. Cowan BF, Segall HD, Zee CS, Ahmadi J, et al.: Neuroradiological assessment of depressed skull fractures: Axial CT vs skull roentgenography. Presented at the Annual Autumn Meeting of the Western Neuroradiological Society, Coronado, Calif., Oct. 9, 1980.
3. French BN, Dublin AB: The value of computerized tomography (CT) in the management of 1000 consecutive head injuries. Surg Neurol 7:171–183, 1977.
4. George AE, Russell EJ, Kricheff II: White matter buckling: CT sign of extraaxial intracranial mass. AJNR 1:425–430, 1980.
5. New PFJ, Aronow S: Attenuation measurements of whole blood and blood fractions in computed tomography. Radiology 121:635–640, 1976.
6. Rumbaugh CL, Bergeron RT, Talalla A, Kurze T: Traumatic aneurysms of the cortical cerebral arteries. Radiology 96:49–54, 1970.
7. Segall HD, McComb JG, Tsai FY, Miller JH: Neuroradiology in head trauma, in Gwinn JL, Stanley P (eds): *Diagnostic Imaging in Pediatric Trauma.* Berlin, Springer International, 1980, chap 3.

8. Stovring J: Descending tentorial herniation: Findings on computed tomography. Neuroradiology 14:101–105, 1977.
9. Tsai FY, Huprich JE, Gardner FC, Segall HD, Teal JS: Diagnostic and prognostic implications of computed tomography of head trauma. J Comput Assist Tomogr 2:323–331, 1978.
10. Zimmerman RA, Bilaniuk LT, Bruce D, Dolinskas C, Obrist W, Kuhl D: Computed tomography of pediatric head trauma: Acute general cerebral swelling. Radiology 126:403–408, 1978.
11. Zimmerman RD, Leeds NE, Naidich TP: Ring blush associated with intracerebral hematoma. Radiology 122:707–711, 1977.

193

Resuscitation of the Multiply Injured Patient

Paul R. Cooper

The patient with both brain and systemic trauma presents unique challenges and problems; shock, hypoxia, and hypercarbia have adverse effects on survival, and it is now well documented that mortality increases sharply with each additional organ system injured. Only one-fifth of the total number of trauma deaths occur in patients with injuries confined to one body area; in the majority of patients who succumb to the effects of trauma, three or more body areas are involved.[1,7] The superimposition of a brain injury on systemic injury is a particularly lethal combination; brain injury is the cause of death in one-half of multiply injured patients who die.[1] In contrast, cardiac and aortic injuries account for just over 17 percent of deaths and hemorrhage for less than 12 percent.[7]

Overall, about 20 percent of patients with cranial injuries also sustain somatic injuries (Table 193-1). The victims are predominantly males with a median age in the twenties. Motor vehicle accidents or encounters between motor vehicles and pedestrians account for the majority of multiply injured patients and falls for lesser numbers, although the actual frequency of various causes varies according to geography. In urban settings vehicular accidents are less common, and injuries from gunshot wounds, assaults, and falls are more frequently encountered.

Although neurosurgeons do not have the ultimate responsibility for the treatment of patients with systemic injuries, they are closely involved in the initial care of the patient because of the severity of the neurological injury and its bearing on the patient's overall management. This chapter is concerned with the resuscitation of such patients.

Early Management

Ideally upon arrival in the emergency room, a patient will have had an airway established and will be adequately ventilated, with normocarbia and normoxemia. External hemorrhage will have been controlled with direct pressure, and hypotension will have been reversed with a sufficient volume of balanced salt solutions.[9] In practice, however, prearrival care (even when administered at referring hospitals) is less than ideal. Of 100 multiply traumatized patients reported by Hicks et al., 80 percent of the patients with central nervous system injuries did not have a secure airway, 93 percent had an arterial P_{O_2} of less than 65 torr or a P_{CO_2} of greater than 45 torr, and 55 percent had a systolic blood pressure of less than 95 mmHg.[6]

Lindsey[10] has elucidated four principles of emergency management of patients with multiple system trauma: (1) Decisions may have to be made on the basis of limited data and the patient's current status rather than an observed trend. (2) Evaluation is performed simultaneously with treatment and is inseparable from it; the inability to arrive at

TABLE 193-1 Associated Injuries in 209 of 1086 Patients with Cranial Injuries*

Major Associated Injury	Number of Patients
Facial fractures	22
Fracture of extremity	103
Fracture of lower extremity	59
Fracture of upper extremity	39
Fracture of upper and lower extremity	5
Chest injury	29
Pneumothorax	9
Hemothorax	5
Fracture of ribs only	9
Flail chest	5
Intrapulmonary hemorrhage	1
Intra-abdominal injuries	41
Urinary tract injury	5
Multiple visceral injuries	36
Vertebral column injuries	14
Fracture of odontoid process	5
Fracture or dislocation of cervical vertebrae	5
Fracture of thoracic vertebrae	2
Fracture of lumbar and sacral vertebrae	2

*From Clark WK: Trauma to the nervous system, in Shires GT (ed): *Care of the Trauma Patient*, 2d ed. New York, McGraw-Hill, 1979, pp 207–258.

a specific diagnosis must not delay treatment, and a complete examination is an inappropriate way to begin management. (3) The biggest threat to life is dealt with first. (4) In multiple system injuries, the symptoms and signs characteristic of injury to a single system may be obscured. This last point is especially important in managing patients with a depressed level of consciousness from a head injury who have no perception of pain in injured parts of their bodies and who may not develop typical signs of an acute abdomen. Similarly a depressed level of consciousness may be mistakenly attributed to a head injury when depression of central nervous system function results from systemic hypotension and lack of adequate cerebral perfusion.

Upon arrival in the emergency room, those patients who are conscious and breathing adequately need only supplemental oxygen with a mask or nasal catheter. In all others an airway is established using the "simplest and fastest means that will suffice."[10]

Esophageal airways are now frequently inserted at the scene of trauma by paramedical personnel and generally provide for good ventilatory support. They should not be replaced by a more permanent airway until all other aspects of resuscitation are accomplished. Patients will almost invariably vomit after esophageal airway removal, and in order to prevent aspiration, it is essential that an endotracheal airway be inserted and its cuff inflated just before esophageal airway removal.

In patients admitted without an esophageal airway, adequate ventilation can often be established by clearing the mouth and oropharynx of blood, mucus, or false teeth. If the airway is still not satisfactory, an oropharyngeal airway may be sufficient. To insert an oral endotracheal tube, it is often necessary to manipulate the cervical spine. If an unrecognized instability or fracture of the cervical spine is present, intubation may result in spinal cord injury. For this reason oral endotracheal intubation should not be performed until a lateral cervical spine roentgenogram confirms the absence of a subluxation or fracture. If essential, immediate endotracheal intubation may be achieved without manipulating the neck by inserting a nasal endotracheal tube.

In some patients, particularly those with maxillofacial trauma or laryngeal edema, endotracheal intubation may not be possible, and an airway may have to be established by performing a cricothyroidotomy. Incision of the cricothyroid membrane is always preferable to tracheostomy, as the latter is time-consuming, often bloody, and poorly suited to emergency room conditions.

Simultaneous with the establishment of an airway, external bleeding is controlled (generally by direct pressure), and a large intravenous line is inserted. If a superficial vein cannot be found, a subclavian or jugular line should be inserted. Peripheral lines should not be placed in the lower extremities in those patients with bony or soft tissue trauma to the legs lest intravenous fluids extravasate into soft tissue. If it is necessary to do a cutdown, upper extremity veins are preferable, and a sterile small pediatric feeding tube (no. 5 or 8 French) inserted into a peripheral vein will usually be adequate for rapid infusion of intravenous solutions.

If the first intravenous line was not centrally placed, a subclavian puncture is performed, and the intravenous catheter is advanced to lie within the superior vena cava. The central venous pressure is recorded at the midaxillary line in the supine patient and will normally measure from 3 to 8 cmH$_2$O. As long as the central venous pressure is normal or low, a rapid fluid infusion may be continued without fear of overhydration. The central venous pressure is a more important gauge of the adequacy of volume replacement than either the systolic blood pressure or pulse; these latter measurements may be normal in young healthy patients in spite of a large volume loss.

Shock and Volume Replacement

About 13 percent of head-injured patients are reported to present in shock of varying degrees of severity.[25] Survival following hypovolemic shock is related to the duration and severity of the hypotension. Rapid and aggressive treatment of the patient with shock will result in survival of patients who have lost as much as 60 percent of their blood volume.[3] The association of increased intracranial pressure with decreased systemic arterial pressure can result in a narrowing of cerebral perfusion pressure more profound than when either is present alone, and in a corresponding increase in mortality. Indeed the presence of shock in association with severe head injury results in a statistically significant increase in mortality to 83 percent as opposed to 45 percent when head injury is unassociated with shock.[1,3,14,15] Miller et al. studied the relationship of systemic insults (hypotension, anemia, hypercarbia) and outcome in patients who had sustained head injury and found a significant increase in the incidence of unsatisfactory outcome in patients with systemic insults as compared with those without such findings.[13]

Mild shock is defined as that which occurs with blood losses in the range of 10 to 20 percent. Blood pressure may be in the low normal range, and tachycardia may be absent.[9] In patients with a loss of 20 to 40 percent of their circulating blood volume, shock of a moderate degree will exist. By definition, severe shock occurs when greater than 40 percent of the circulating blood volume is lost. In severe shock, compensatory mechanisms consisting of vasoconstriction of the visceral arterial supply are inadequate to provide for adequate cerebral and cardiac blood flow. Failure of central nervous system perfusion will be manifested by a depressed level of consciousness and failure of coronary perfusion (manifested by ischemic changes on the ECG, frank myocardial infarction, or cardiac arrhythmias).

After the insertion of a large-bore intravenous catheter, blood specimens are sent for baseline hematologic studies, electrolyte determinations, typing, and crossmatching. The patient in shock is given a rapid infusion of a balanced salt solution such as Ringer's lactate. The appropriate total volume of infusion and the rate of administration are determined by the patient's initial blood pressure. In patients with mild shock with a blood loss equal to 10 percent of their circulating blood volume, the rapid administration of 2 liters of Ringer's lactate solution will restore the circulating blood volume to normal levels and prevent the depletion of interstitial reserves. In patients with systolic blood pressure of less than 80 mmHg at the time of admission, the volume deficit generally represents 15 to 25 percent of the circulating blood volume, and correspondingly larger amounts of fluid will have to be given.

As the central venous pressure rises to normal levels, the rate of fluid administration may be slowed, and further administration is titrated according to the blood pressure, central venous pressure, and urinary output. Systemic perfusion should be considered adequate when urinary output reaches 50 ml/h or more.

When the initial hemorrhage results in the loss of one-third or more of the circulating blood volume, the red blood cell deficiency will result in inadequate oxygen carrying capacity and necessitate red blood cell replacement in addition to whatever fluids are used for resuscitation.

Although there is general agreement that solutions of balanced crystalloid are appropriate for the replacement of small intravenous volume losses and that red blood cells should be replaced only when the hematocrit descends below 30 percent, there has been considerable controversy over the past 25 years over all other aspects regarding the optimum regimen for replacement of volume lost from hemorrhage. Shires et al. first demonstrated a disproportionate loss of extracellular fluid volume in hemorrhagic shock.[18] He and his co-workers concluded from animal experiments that decreased interstitial fluid volume played an important role in the morbidity and mortality of hemorrhagic shock and that mortality from shock could be improved by restoration of volume with Ringer's lactate alone as opposed to resuscitation with shed blood and Ringer's lactate. Since these studies, however, other investigators have been unable to find a difference in outcome when patients resuscitated with crystalloid are compared with those treated with colloid.[11]

In the head-injured patient with systemic trauma, there is no evidence that either colloid or crystalloid is superior in minimizing traumatic brain edema. Moreover, a critical evaluation of the literature leads one to conclude that even for systemic resuscitation there is little difference between colloid and crystalloid solutions.

Head Injury as a Cause of Shock

Head injury, by itself, does not result in shock except in the most extraordinary circumstances.[8] In children under the age of 2 and, in particular, in infants under 1 year of age who have open sutures, intracranial hemorrhage can lead to a loss of intravascular blood volume large enough to cause shock. A blood loss of a similar magnitude in an adult patient would represent a small percentage of the total circulating blood volume and would not result in shock. In both adults and children, massive blood loss from compound injuries of the dural venous sinuses can result in shock, and these injuries are most commonly seen as a result of gunshot wounds but may also occur with compound skull fractures. Scalp lacerations which transect the superficial temporal or occipital arteries may also result in massive hemorrhage and hypotension. Finally, hypotension may result from injury to medullary cardiovascular centers. This is a preterminal event, and such patients will be apneic and flaccid without brain stem reflexes.

Some Less Common Causes of Shock

Specific injuries and the mechanism by which they result in shock are discussed in the next section. However, there are a number of patients in whom the cause of hypotension is not apparent and in whom shock remains unresponsive (or only transiently responsive) to volume replacement. Continued or hidden blood loss or underestimation of blood loss is the commonest cause for refractory hypotension. Other causes include hypothermia, acid-base imbalance, and hypocalcemia in the patient who has been repetitively transfused. Anesthetic agents or prior therapy with antihypertensive medications may also contribute to hypotension. Of particular interest to neurosurgeons is the contribution of mannitol or other potent diuretics to shock. Ordinarily in the patient with a severe head injury who has not sustained blood loss from a systemic injury, mannitol will have little effect on the systemic blood pressure. However, in the volume-depleted patient who has mobilized maximal amounts of interstitial fluid into the vascular compartment to maintain blood pressure and circulating blood volume, agents such as mannitol or furosemide may cause a rapid and profound hypotension out of proportion to the amount of diuresis they induce. For this reason these agents should be used judiciously in the patient with suspected blood loss and, in particular, in those patients with continuing losses.

Management of Specific Injuries

Management Priorities

In the patient with serious systemic injuries and an altered level of consciousness from a severe head injury, neurosurgeons and general surgeons will sometimes find themselves at cross-purposes regarding management priorities. Patients with a focal neurological deficit or with altered consciousness should have a CT scan before the administration of general anesthesia for the operative management of systemic injuries. In practice, however, this is not always possible. In patients with massive and continuing hemorrhage, even rapid volume replacement with salt solutions or blood may be insufficient to stabilize the systemic blood pressure at satisfactory levels. In such patients, rapid operative control of hemorrhage must take precedence over the definitive neurological diagnosis provided by the CT scan.

The exact point at which diagnostic delay becomes inappropriate and operative intervention mandatory is hard to define and depends upon the exigencies of the specific clinical situation; factors such as the availability of whole blood, the rapidity of CT scanner availability, and the experience of the general surgeon caring for the patient all enter into consideration. As a general rule, when there is serious concern that a surgically treatable head injury is present and the additional delay entailed by a CT scan will result in less than 1 liter additional blood loss in an adult patient, it is probably reasonable to obtain a CT scan.

When a CT evaluation has been deferred and an intracranial mass lesion is suspected, burr holes are placed after systemic hemorrhage and injuries are treated, but before the patient is awakened from general anesthesia. This management strategy will avoid the situation that sometimes occurs after waiting many hours for a patient to awaken from general anesthesia only to realize that an altered level of consciousness is not secondary to anesthesia but to an expanding intracranial mass lesion.

In those patients who have had CT scans showing a mass lesion before the induction of anesthesia, lesions are evacuated as the general surgical procedure is being performed or, if this is not convenient, at the termination of the procedure.

Abdominal Trauma

Blunt Trauma

The evaluation of the patient with blunt trauma to the abdomen poses problems even for one experienced in trauma. In the alert patient, physical examination by itself may be inaccurate in as many as 10 to 20 percent of patients with an acute abdomen. In the obtunded patient diagnosis of injury to intra-abdominal structures is even more difficult, as the examiner is "deprived of the diagnostic information afforded by a careful abdominal examination in a lucid subject."[24] In particular in the patient with spinal cord injury, information provided by physical examination can be totally misleading for the evaluation of abdominal trauma.

For these reasons, diagnostic peritoneal lavage has been advocated for all patients with symptoms or signs of blunt abdominal trauma and in all patients with an altered level of consciousness.[4] Although this policy would seem appropriate for all patients who have sustained a head injury as a result of a vehicular accident, a situation where multiple injuries are frequent, the patient with a head injury sustained by an isolated blow to the cranium or in a minor fall probably does not need lavage.

The value and reliability of peritoneal lavage have been questioned by Meyer and Crass, who note a high incidence of false-positive and indeterminate lavages and advocate that stable patients be followed by serial physical examinations. They believe that lavage is indicated for patients who cannot have serial examinations or those with central nervous system injuries.[12]

The technique of peritoneal lavage has been described in detail.[22] The bladder is first decompressed with a catheter, and an incision is made in the midline down to the peritoneum at a site one-third of the distance between the umbilicus and symphysis pubis. A peritoneal dialysis catheter is advanced through the peritoneum under direct vision. The finding of free blood within the peritoneal cavity is considered an indication for immediate laparotomy. If no blood is found, a liter of Ringer's lactate is introduced through the dialysis catheter into the peritoneum. The lavage fluid is then removed through siphoning. Lavage fluid containing bile, bacteria, greater than 100,000 red blood cells per cubic millimeter, or an elevated amylase level is an indication for laparotomy.

Most recently, abdominal CT scans have been used in the evaluation of patients with equivocal clinical findings, and this modality has been especially useful for the diagnosis of hepatic, splenic, renal, and pancreatic injury.[12]

Penetrating Abdominal Injury

Penetrating abdominal injuries are less commonly seen in association with head injury than are blunt ones. Abdominal stab wounds will penetrate viscera in 30 to 40 percent of cases.[21] The management of abdominal stab wounds is somewhat controversial. In the absence of shock, signs of an acute abdomen, or positive lavage, some authorities advocate 24 h of observation.[23] Others will perform a local exploration of stab wounds and then a laparotomy on all patients who have defects of the anterior abdominal fascia.[12] Eighty to ninety percent of patients will have visceral penetration from gunshot wounds, and laparotomy is mandatory in these patients.

Injury of the Genitourinary Tract; Retroperitoneal Injury

Injury to retroperitoneal structures may result in blood loss which is both massive and obscure and should be considered in all patients who present in shock without apparent cause. If hemorrhage is confined to the retroperitoneal space, abdominal lavage may be negative or equivocal. Signs of trauma to the lower ribs or ecchymosis of the flanks should suggest the possibility of injury to the kidneys or other retroperitoneal structures. Retroperitoneal hemorrhage may be diagnosed by the loss of clarity of the psoas shadows on the anteroposterior abdominal roentgenogram or displacement of the ureters or bladder on the intravenous pyelogram. The abdominal CT scan will provide definitive confirmation of the presence of retroperitoneal hemorrhage, and angiography of specific retroperitoneal structures will define the source of the bleeding.

A urethral injury should be considered if blood is seen at the urethral meatus or if a catheter cannot be passed into the bladder. In such cases a urethrogram should be performed. In the absence of obvious upper or lower urinary tract injury, the presence of microscopic hematuria mandates an intravenous pyelogram, cystogram, and voiding cystourethrogram.[20] Renal arteriography is indicated if there is absence of filling of either kidney on intravenous pyelography.

Musculoskeletal Trauma

Long bone and skeletal fractures are the commonest systemic injuries seen in patients with head trauma.[1,2] Moreover, it is often not recognized that these injuries may result in massive blood loss and shock. The median amount of hemorrhage seen with combined tibial and fibular fractures or open femoral fractures exceeds 2 liters. Closed femoral fractures will commonly result in extravasation of greater than 1 liter of blood into adjacent soft tissues, and pelvic fractures commonly result in an occult blood loss of greater than 2 liters.[3]

Emergency management consists of splinting of apparent fractures followed by roentgenography after the patient's condition is stabilized. Sterile dressings should be applied to compound fractures, and prophylactic antibiotics and tetanus toxoid should be given.

Assessment of peripheral pulses, temperature, and color of the extremities distal to simple or compound fractures is essential. If arterial injury is suspected but the viability of the extremity is not immediately threatened, arteriography is performed. Immediate vascular exploration at the site of a suspected injury is indicated for extremities which are cold, blue, and pulseless.

Thoracic Trauma

One-quarter of trauma deaths occur as a result of thoracic injury. Tachypnea, labored respirations, stridor, cyanosis, and subcutaneous emphysema are the cardinal manifestations.

Pneumothorax

Pneumothorax occurs from entrance of air into the pleural cavity in patients with penetrating chest injuries or from injury to the lung with escape of air into the pleura as will occur with rib fractures which penetrate the pulmonary parenchyma. In patients with a penetrating thoracic injury, the wound is covered with an occlusive airtight dressing to minimize the occurrence of pneumothorax. In patients with suspected pneumothorax (whether the chest is open or closed) who remain in respiratory distress and who have distant breath sounds, a chest tube is inserted into the second intercostal space in the midclavicular line before roentgenograms are obtained. The tip of this tube should be directed superiorly to ensure maximal removal of pleural air.

Tension pneumothorax is a potentially fatal occurrence which results when air escapes from the lung and becomes trapped within the pleural space. As increasing amounts of air accumulate, ventilatory capacity is progressively decreased from pulmonary compression. Tension pneumothorax also leads to compression and shift of mediastinal structures, causing a decrease in venous return and cardiac output which can be rapidly fatal if not treated. The diagnosis of tension pneumothorax should be considered in the patient with an open or closed injury who rapidly develops respiratory insufficiency. Immediate, potentially life-saving treatment consists of aspiration of pleural air with a large-bore needle in the second intercostal space followed by insertion of a thoracotomy tube.

Ventilatory adequacy following chest tube insertion may be assessed by measuring vital capacity. Normal vital capacity should measure between 60 and 80 ml/kg body weight. Mechanical ventilation will usually be necessary when vital capacity falls below 15 ml/kg body weight as a result of pulmonary injury, persistent pleural blood or air, or multiple rib fractures.

Hemothorax

Hemothorax, a collection of blood within the pleural cavity, may result from blunt or penetrating injuries; coexisting pneumothorax may also be present. Hypotension, decreased breath sounds, and dullness to thoracic percussion with signs of respiratory distress should suggest the presence of a hemothorax.

Hemothorax is treated by the insertion of a large-caliber thoracotomy tube into the seventh intercostal space in the midaxillary line. Blood will accumulate posteriorly and inferiorly in the pleural cavity, and the chest tube should be angled in this direction. Removal of blood will result in lung re-expansion; cessation of bleeding will occur in 85 percent of patients after chest tube insertion. Pulmonary bleeding will usually stop without difficulty, as the pulmonary artery pressure is about 15 mmHg. However, bleeding from injuries to the internal mammary, subclavian, or intercostal arteries occurs at systemic arterial pressures and generally will not stop spontaneously. Open thoracotomy is indicated if bleeding exceeds 200 ml/h for 4 h or if total blood loss exceeds 1500 ml.[16] In patients with exceedingly rapid hemorrhage whose hypotension cannot be corrected with infusion of intravenous fluids, emergency room thoracotomy may be necessary.

Cardiac Tamponade

The diagnosis of cardiac tamponade should be considered in the patient who has sustained a penetrating chest wound and who presents with resistant hypotension, a narrow pulse pressure, elevated central venous pressure, and distended neck veins. The heart sounds will be decreased to auscultation, and a pericardial friction rub may be present. Definitive therapy consists of thoracotomy with relief of the tamponade and control of hemorrhage. Emergency treatment of the patient in extremis consists of aspiration of pericardial blood using a no. 18 needle introduced via a subxiphoid approach. Although needle aspiration may be lifesaving, treatment of pericardial tamponade using this modality has a high recurrence rate and high mortality and must be followed by immediate thoracotomy.

Blunt Chest Injury

Blunt chest trauma generally occurs as a result of motor vehicle accidents. Specific injuries include multiple rib fractures with an associated flail chest, traumatic aortic aneurysm, and pulmonary and cardiac contusion. Consequently, the initial evaluation of the patient with blunt chest trauma should include an ECG and a chest film.

A flail chest occurs when two or more contiguous ribs are fractured in at least two places. The fractured segments are effectively detached from the rest of the bony thorax and will move in with inspiration and out with expiration in a paradoxical fashion. This injury interferes with the production of a negative intrathoracic pressure and may result in respiratory insufficiency. Stabilization of the chest wall can sometimes be accomplished if the patient lies on the side of the rib fractures. If respiratory insufficiency persists, endotracheal intubation and positive pressure ventilation are the treatment of choice.

A crushing chest injury with multiple rib or sternal fractures may also produce a traumatic aortic aneurysm. Chest films will show a widened superior mediastinum, left hemothorax, and left to right displacement of the trachea. The definitive diagnosis is made by aortography and will generally show the aneurysm originating just distal to the subclavian artery.

Adult Respiratory Distress Syndrome

Almost one-quarter of patients with severe head injuries have an initial arterial P_{O_2} of less than 60 torr.[19] Most of these patients have hypoxemia secondary to obtundation from their head injury and do not have adult respiratory distress syndrome (ARDS).

In the multiply injured patient, ARDS describes a variety of pulmonary problems which affect patients with serious medical illness or trauma. Dyspnea, tachypnea, or other signs of respiratory insufficiency may appear in the emergency room or in the subsequent hours and days following multiple system trauma. Hypoxemia will be present on ventilation with room air and may persist even when supplemental oxygen or assisted ventilation is provided. The arterial P_{CO_2} will be normal or low. Pulmonary artery pressures measured through a Swan-Ganz catheter will be elevated. The chest film may be normal initially and then show a patchy interstitial edema which may coalesce to give the appearance of a "white lung."

ARDS has a number of causes and may represent a limited response on the part of the lungs to a variety of insults. Among the causes in the multiply injured patient are aspiration of gastric contents, multiple blood transfusions with trapping of platelet aggregates in the lungs, and a reduction of surfactant. The choice of fluids used in resuscitation has been thought to play a role in the production of ARDS, but recent studies show that there is little relationship between the type of fluids used for resuscitation and the frequency of ARDS.[11] In the multiply injured patient who also has increased intracranial pressure, pulmonary edema on a neurogenic basis may be seen in the emergency room. The pathogenesis of this unusual syndrome has not been established with certainty, but it appears that elevation of intracranial pressure causes the pulmonary vascular resistance to be increased; increased lung water content results from passage of fluid across leaking capillaries. Patients will present with massive amounts of frothy sputum, necessitating almost continuous suctioning through an endotracheal tube.

Treatment of the patient with ARDS is designed to keep the arterial oxygen content at 70 torr or greater through the use of supplemented oxygen and mechanical ventilatory support. In overhydrated patients with a pulmonary wedge pressure of greater than 12 torr, the production of a diuresis using furosemide may be an effective treatment. In patients with neurogenic pulmonary edema with an elevated ICP, diuretics and digitalis are ineffective, but the use of mechanical ventilation with a positive end expiratory pressure (PEEP) of 10 cmH$_2$O can result in a rapid relief of symptoms and signs of respiratory distress and improvement of hypoxemia. The use of PEEP in patients with elevated ICP has been a subject of controversy, and there is disagreement over the potential of PEEP to produce or exacerbate elevations of ICP.[5,17] When PEEP is the only means of improving oxygenation in the patient with a brain and systemic injury, the ICP should be monitored, and PEEP should be reduced or discontinued if the ICP rises to dangerous levels.

References

1. Baker CC, Oppenheimer L, Stephens B, Lewis FR, Trunkey DD: Epidemiology of trauma deaths. Am J Surg 140:144–150, 1980.
2. Clark WK: Trauma to the nervous system, in Shires GT (ed): *Care of the Trauma Patient*, 2d ed. New York, McGraw-Hill, 1979, pp 207–258.
3. Clarke R, Fisher MR, Topley E, Davies JWL: Extent and time of blood-loss after civilian injury. Lancet 2:381–386, 1961.
4. Fischer RP, Beverlin BC, Engrav LH, Benjamin CI, Perry JF Jr: Diagnostic peritoneal lavage: Fourteen years and 2,586 patients later. Am J Surg 136:701–704, 1978.
5. Frost EAM: Effects of positive end-expiratory pressure on intracranial pressure and compliance in brain-injured patients. J Neurosurg 47:195–200, 1977.
6. Hicks TC, Danzl DF, Thomas DM, Flint LM: Resuscitation and transfer of trauma patients: A prospective study. Ann Emerg Med 11:296–299, 1982.
7. Hoffman E: Mortality and morbidity following road accidents. Ann R Coll Surg Engl 58:233–240, 1976.
8. Illingworth G, Jennett WB: The shocked head injury. Lancet 2:511–514, 1965.
9. Levison M, Trunkey DD: Initial assessment and resuscitation. Surg Clin North Am 62:9–16, 1982.
10. Lindsey D: Teaching the initial management of major multiple system trauma. J Trauma 20:160–162, 1980.
11. Lowe RJ, Moss GS, Jilek J, Levine HD: Crystalloid versus colloid in the etiology of pulmonary failure after trauma—a randomized trial in man. Crit Care Med 7:107–112, 1979.
12. Meyer AA, Crass RA: Abdominal trauma. Surg Clin North Am 62:105–111, 1982.
13. Miller JD, Sweet RC, Narayan R, Becker DP: Early insults to the injured brain. JAMA 240:439–442, 1978.
14. Newfield P, Pitts L, Kaktis J, Hoff J: The influence of shock on mortality after head trauma. Crit Care Med 8:254, 1980 (abstr.).
15. Olsen WR: Shock and the accident and trauma victim, in Frey CF (ed): *Initial Management of the Trauma Patient*. Philadelphia, Lea & Febiger, 1976, pp 71–93.
16. Oparah SS, Mandal AK: Operative management of penetrating wounds of the chest in civilian practice: Review of indications in 125 consecutive cases. J Thorac Cardiovasc Surg 77:162–168, 1979.
17. Shapiro HM, Marshall LF: Intracranial pressure responses to PEEP in head-injured patients. J Trauma 18:254–256, 1978.
18. Shires T, Coln D, Carrico J, Lightfoot S: Fluid therapy in hemorrhagic shock. Arch Surg 88:688–693, 1964.
19. Sinha RP, Ducker TB, Perot PL Jr: Arterial oxygenation: Findings and its significance in central nervous system trauma patients. JAMA 224:1258–1260, 1973.
20. Thal ER: Initial management of the multiply injured patient, in Cooper PR (ed): *Head Injury*. Baltimore, Williams & Wilkins, 1982, pp 27–41.
21. Thal ER, McClelland RN, Shires GT: Abdominal trauma, in Shires GT (ed): *Care of the Trauma Patient*, 2d ed. New York, McGraw-Hill, 1979, pp 290–348.
22. Thal ER, Shires GT: Peritoneal lavage in blunt abdominal trauma. Am J Surg 125:64–69, 1973.
23. Wilder JR, Kudchadkar A: Stab wounds of the abdomen: Observe or explore? JAMA 243:2503–2505, 1980.
24. Wilson CB, Vidrine A Jr, Rives JD: Unrecognized abdominal trauma in patient with head injuries. Ann Surg 161:608–613, 1965.
25. Youmans JR: Causes of shock with head injury. J Trauma 4:204–209, 1964.

194
Intensive Management of Head Injury

Donald P. Becker
Stephen Gardner

The intensive management of head trauma is directed toward prevention of further damage to an already compromised brain and maintenance of an optimum biological environment to promote cellular recovery in the brain. The unique effects of cerebral injury with the secondary phenomena that result make it crucial that neurosurgeons understand and be able to treat the systemic effects of head injury. The main focus of this chapter is on the early aggressive nonoperative treatment of head injury and its various side effects and complications.

Management of severe brain injury has become increasingly complex, partly as a result of sophisticated electronic and chemical monitoring, improved knowledge about acute severe brain injury, and the general advances in critical care medicine. Patients who expire from head injury commonly suffer from prolonged hypoxia, uncontrolled high levels of intracranial pressure, or untoward systemic events such as cardiopulmonary arrest, hypovolemia, disseminated intravascular coagulopathy, electrolyte imbalance, or renal failure.[3] Appropriate triage of head-injured victims from the scene of an accident to medical center facilities is essential to begin proper aggressive management and to prevent secondary insults. It is now known that the traumatized brain is metabolically deranged and that its cells have increased vulnerability to hypoxic or ischemic insults. Exquisite medical care, providing an environment where partially injured cells receive adequate oxygen and appropriate nutrition, can result in improved patient recovery. This places a great responsibility on the neurosurgeon managing these critically ill patients.

Initial Effects of Head Injury

The initial intracranial and systemic effects of closed head trauma have been carefully evaluated by Ommaya and Gennarelli.[11,25,26] They studied various biological changes seen in graded severity of injury. Alterations of cardiovascular function occur prior to other physiological changes; an initial bradycardia and hypotension are seen, followed by mild elevation of mean arterial pressure. Respiratory irregularity and periods of apnea then can actually precede loss of responsiveness to external stimuli. More severe trauma is necessary to alter consciousness than to change cardiorespiratory patterns, and experimental unconsciousness is related to brain stem trauma with subsequent loss of corneal and pupillary response. Arterial hypertension occurs at the higher injury levels, instead of the hypotension seen at lower levels of trauma.

With increasing levels of injury, loss of consciousness persists longer, and definite focal neurological alterations are seen from involvement of upper brain stem and cortical structures; these are often associated with cortical contusions and ischemic injury of the hippocampus. At the most severe levels of injury, intracranial hematomas, particularly subdural hematomas, occur and result in the worst outcome.

Changes in brain energy metabolism also occur, reflected by CSF acidosis and changes in cerebral blood flow (CBF), as well as the development of cerebral edema and increased intracranial pressure (ICP). Dysfunction of neuroendocrine pathways may occur, and there are major systemic metabolic alterations in response to the physical trauma. Delayed effects of sustained hypoxia, dysregulation of CBF, intracranial hypertension, fat embolism, seizures, and disseminated intravascular coagulation may all occur within the initial 24 h, or may occur later as well.[23]

Initial Management of Acute Closed Head Injury

At the Accident Site and during Transit to the Hospital

Neurosurgeons and all emergency care physicians must realize that comprehensive care of brain-injured patients should begin immediately after trauma and not just on arrival in the emergency room (ER) or intensive care unit (ICU). Systematic, rapid resuscitation must begin at the site of injury and be maintained during each phase of the patient's transport to a definitive neurological care unit. The concern for achieving optimal levels of support for head injuries is well founded as there is a significantly adverse outcome for patients who sustain hypoxia, arterial hypotension, or other systemic compromises that add to the initial morbidity of cranial trauma.[2]

The first echelon of care is to anticipate and prevent further cerebral damage due to pathological systemic physiology, a common occurrence in patients with severe head injury. In such patients, Miller et al. have observed on admission to the ER a 35 percent incidence of hypoxia (Pa_{O_2} of 65 mmHg or less), a 15 percent incidence of arterial hypotension (systolic BP less than 95 mmHg), and a 12 percent incidence of anemia (hematocrit less than 30).[24] As up to 20 percent of trauma victims die as a result of inadequate treatment at the scene or during transport, early recognition of these phenomena and their treatment are crucial to improve outcome.[23] Provision for an optimal internal environment for partially injured neurons will allow improved cellular recovery and patient outcome.[3]

Triage and resuscitation of respiration and blood pressure should proceed simultaneously with the initial diagnostic evaluation. A definitive outline for this has been prepared by the American College of Surgeons [Advanced Trauma Life Support (ATLS)]. Conceptually, using the "ABC" system, where A = airway, B = breathing, and C = circulation, it is aimed at rapidly assessing and initiating those life supports urgently needed, following with more detailed diagnostic examination and adjustment of treatment.

Transport of an unconscious patient should never begin until a patent, functioning airway and adequate ventilation are assured. Transport to a definitive neurological care facility following the resuscitation assessment phase is urgent, but the distance to be traveled is of secondary concern unless shock with uncontrolled hypotension is present and requires stopping at an outlying medical facility to prevent death. Prolonged delays at intermediate hospitals are to be avoided in the face of severe neurological injury that requires immediate and optimal treatment.

It is absolutely necessary that a patent airway be maintained to provide adequate tidal volume, oxygenation and, if necessary, the use of hyperventilation and mild hypocapnia to reduce ICP. Hypoxia and hypercarbia must be avoided as these both lead to increased ICP through vasodilation of the cerebrovascular system. Patients with a Glasgow coma scale (GCS) score of less than 8 (unresponsive to commands and not verbalizing) should receive endotracheal intubation and mechanical ventilatory assistance as soon as possible to achieve proper oxygenation and moderate hypocapnia. Apnea or respiratory arrest followed by irregularity of rate and depth of ventilation is a part of the concussive response, with more severe injuries resulting in prolonged apnea.[26] In some instances, this prolonged apnea may itself be the reason for death at the scene. Apnea of longer than 8 to 10 min in humans treated by intubation and successful respiratory resuscitation can, on occasion, result in a functional recovery.[17]

Care begins with clearing the upper airway of vomitus, blood, or foreign bodies such as false or loose teeth, and using the jawlift or thrust to anatomically align the airway. Immediate oxygenation of inspired air in all patients is necessary since atelectasis, aspiration, or pulmonary contusion may be undetected by the external examination and, despite normal respiratory excursion, can decrease the transfer of oxygen to the blood because of intrapulmonary shunting. Nasal oxygen alone can often raise the Pa_{O_2}, despite a slow voluntary respiratory rate, and it should always be given as a minimum. If a patent airway cannot be obtained with simple oral or nasopharyngeal tubing, the use of an esophageal obturator airway (EOA) or endotracheal tube is indicated. The EOA is inserted into the esophagus, inflated to occlude it, and provides for the use of positive pressure ventilation by ventilator or Ambu bag for lung inflation. Endotracheal intubation requires special skill and, because of frequent misplacement into the esophagus, should be performed only by those qualified to do so. Use of these techniques should be cautiously applied in any unconscious patient or those suspected of cervical spine trauma (injury to or above the clavicles) to preclude potential spinal cord damage.

A surgical alternative to endotracheal intubation is cricothyroidotomy. A linear incision transversely placed across the cricothyroid membrane will allow rapid placement of a small (no. 4 French) tracheostomy tube into the upper airway. It may be used effectively in cases where trauma to the face prevents laryngeal intubation, but should be reserved for patients over 12 years of age and used only by those skilled in the technique.

Most intensive care specialists believe that the best method of mechanical ventilation is volume ventilation under positive pressure. Positive pressure ventilation helps prevent the progressive pulmonary failure often seen in severe injuries and results in early resolution of atelectasis. It also counteracts the potential development of pulmonary edema that can develop as a result of excess catecholamine release that follows on the heels of the brain injury. The early use of intubation and respiratory support also prevents aspiration of gastric contents in a patient who may have a depressed pharyngeal and laryngeal "gag" response, as well as the respiratory insufficiency that can occur in the event of seizure activity or soft tissue swelling of the neck, which could occlude the upper airway. Following intubation, the use of temporary paralysis by administering pancuronium will help in obtaining an artifact-free CT scan and aid in controlling respiration in the combative or restless patient.

Blood pressure can be supported by the placement of multiple (two or more) peripheral intravenous routes and the infusion of balanced crystalloid solution (Ringer's lactate or 5% dextrose and 0.45% saline solution) to achieve a minimum systolic pressure of 100 mmHg. The inflation of a pneumatic antishock garment (PASG), when properly applied, is extremely useful for tamponading intra-abdominal hemorrhage and may also serve as a splint for fractures of the lower extremities or pelvis. In addition to increasing peripheral resistance and "autotransfusing" peripheral blood of the lower extremities centrally to improve circulatory volume and cardiac output, a recent prospective study of 12 patients with severe head injury did not reveal any abnormal increase in ICP with moderate inflation pressures to 45 mmHg in each compartment.[10] These garments have been shown to cause an "autotransfusion" of 200 to 1000 ml of the patient's intravascular volume, and can tamponade hemorrhage at lower extremity, pelvic, or intra-abdominal sites by circumferential pressure. PASG or military antishock trousers (MAST) should not be used in patients with overt cardiac failure or pulmonary edema. Release of PASG should be done only when the blood pressure is stabilized and there exists ample access for fluid support, should it be required.

Maintenance of a "normal" blood pressure is essential to fully evaluate the neurological status. Raising the BP to a normal range may convert "coma" to purposeful responsiveness, totally altering the diagnostic and therapeutic approach. Patients with brain injury almost always have some impairment of cerebral autoregulation. Thus, if the blood pressure falls (even to levels of only 85 or 90 mmHg systolic), CBF may fall pari passu to levels that will not adequately support nerve cell function. Therefore, blood pressure must be maintained above 100 mmHg systolic.

Intensive Management of Head Injury

Prolonged hypotension from brain damage is a preterminal event associated with medullary failure and other signs of brain stem death. The hypotension seen following experimental and human head injury is very transient (less than 3 min) and usually resolves prior to the first clinical evaluation. The most common cause of shock in trauma is the hypovolemia of hemorrhage. Restoring normal volume is crucial to protect the brain and overcome the dysregulation of cerebral blood flow and cerebral vasospasm, which may lead to ischemic infarction of the brain.

Lactic acidosis commonly occurs with hypotension, apnea, and hypercapnia, resulting in a mixed (metabolic and respiratory) systemic acidosis. This can be treated with intravenous (IV) sodium bicarbonate (1 meq per kilogram of body weight, and repeated every 15 min as needed). However, a proper airway with adequate ventilation and blood pressure maintenance will usually quickly correct the acidosis.

Management in the Emergency Room

Following arrival in the ER, the patient should be rapidly assessed using a brief neurological examination while ensuring that airway, ventilation, oxygenation, and BP are stabilized. A lateral x-ray film of the cervical spine should be obtained in all unconscious patients, and those with moderately severe trauma at or above the level of the clavicle. Documentation of the neurological examination provides the baseline for observing change in central nervous system status, and should be continued on a regular and frequent basis.

The immediate evaluation of head injuries requires a systematic approach that defines the problems requiring urgent diagnostic or therapeutic action. Such a system includes neurological evaluation of the level of consciousness as determined by the Glasgow coma scale (eye opening, motor response, and verbal response); pupillary examination for size and reactivity, to assess potential or impending herniation and the status of the upper brain stem; eye movements (either oculocephalic or oculovestibular), to evaluate the midbrain region in the area of the reticular activating system; and motor power using the international five-level scale: normal = 5, moderate weakness = 4, severe weakness (no antigravity function) = 3, trace movement = 2, flaccid = 1. External evaluation of the head may reveal signs of a basal skull fracture such as mastoid ecchymosis (Battle's sign), hemotympanum, periorbital ecchymosis (raccoon eyes), and otorrhea or rhinorrhea.

This examination can be performed in less than 2 min and allows placement of patients into management protocols according to four grades of severity of injury during early resuscitation (Table 194-1). Grade II and grade III patients have had a serious brain injury, reflected by the alteration of consciousness. All grade III patients should have immediate endotracheal intubation and controlled respiration using a slow rate (12 per minute) and adequate tidal volume (15 ml per kilogram of body weight), usually 750 to 1000 ml in adults. This should provide adequate oxygenation and mild hypocapnia. A CT scan to evaluate the possible presence of an intracranial mass lesion is indicated immediately for grade III patients and as soon as possible for grade II patients (the delay should be no longer than 4 h). It should be performed at once in the grade II patient if his or her condition deteriorates to grade III with unresponsiveness to verbal command. The ability to obey commands is a key indicator of the function of the nervous system and a major neurological boundary between moderate and severe intracranial disorders. If CT is unavailable, angiography or air ventriculography should be done to determine the presence of intracranial mass lesions, causing a shift of the midline structures in excess of 5 mm. This is an indication for decompressive craniotomy, as sizable intracranial mass lesions may exist without localizing clinical signs of focal neurological deficit or tentorial herniation, and these patients may suddenly and unexpectedly deteriorate rapidly to an unrecoverable level. Should signs of herniation or mass lesion appear prior to CT scanning, mannitol in a large bolus intravenous dose should be used (1 to 2 g/kg) followed by a single view CT scan at the level of the foramina of Monro across the supratentorial space. If a mass lesion is detected, immediate decompressive craniotomy should be performed without further delay for additional CT scanning. In no case should surgery be delayed beyond 15 min, and an additional bolus dose of mannitol (0.5 to 1.0 g/kg) may be required en route to the operating room (OR).

If transtentorial herniation is not developing, a complete CT scan of the cranial structures should be done, starting at the level of the orbits to allow visualization of possible facial fractures, basal fractures, and pneumocephalus. A noncontrast scan is usually sufficient unless there is a suspicion of a nontraumatic cause of brain damage such as subarachnoid hemorrhage from an aneurysm or arteriovenous malformation, and then a contrast scan is performed.

In all grade II and grade III patients not requiring an immediate craniotomy, the transfer from the CT scanner to the intensive care unit is to be rapid and with close attention to monitoring adequate ventilation and circulatory support.

The measurement of arterial blood gases is useful in adjusting ventilatory therapy to normalize oxygenation and acid-base balance. In acutely head injured patients, the early

TABLE 194-1 Categorization of Patients with Head Injury*

Category	Description
Grade I	Transient loss of consciousness (<5 min); now alert and oriented without neurological deficit; Glasgow coma scale (GCS) rating, 14–15
Grade II	Previous loss of consciousness (>5 min); now impaired consciousness but able to follow at least a simple command; no other neurological deficit; GCS rating, 9–13
Grade III	Previously unresponsive (>5 min); now unable to follow even a single simple command because of disordered level of consciousness; may use words, but inappropriately; pupils may be unequal or nonreactive; motor response varies from localizing pain to posturing or nil; GCS rating, <9
Grade IV	No evidence of brain function (brain death)

*Categories are based on initial evaluation and provide a simple system for triage of patients into a management program appropriate to the degree of their brain injury.

blood pH usually reflects a respiratory alkalosis secondary to hyperventilation, although shock and hypotension or respiratory arrest may cause a metabolic or respiratory acidosis, which, if prolonged, may lead to increased mortality.[5] The studies of McLaurin and King indicated that patients with severe head injuries have a normal or mildly acidotic systemic pH initially, followed by respiratory alkalosis and bicarbonate loss within 24 h.[20] Overall, a primary initial mixed acidosis is replaced by respiratory alkalosis if hypoxia is treated and fluid balance maintained. Despite spontaneous hyperventilation, hypoxia may exist in 30 percent of severely injured patients as a result of ventilation-perfusion inequalities of the lungs resulting from aspiration, atelectasis, pulmonary contusion, or excessive catecholamine sympathetic discharge with vasoconstriction and intrapulmonary shunting.[24] The peripheral vasoconstrictive response may increase peripheral resistance beyond the capacity of left ventricular function, causing left-sided heart failure and subsequent pulmonary edema.[12]

Patients with an undamaged brain may tolerate a Pa_{O_2} level as low as 70 mmHg, but those with cerebral trauma are very sensitive to even moderate hypoxemia (90 mmHg). Gordon and Ponten proposed two reasons for this:

1. Respiratory alkalosis shifts the oxygen-hemoglobin dissociation curve to the left, decreasing effective oxygen transfer to the tissues.
2. Dysregulation of cerebral blood flow and focal vasospasm can create severe relative ischemia and uneven perfusion with the brain.[12]

Both may lead to infarction. Aggressive and timely respiratory support is simple enough therapy to prevent such a severe complication.

Systemic arterial pressure must be measured and recorded at short intervals and kept in a normal range to maintain the cerebral perfusion pressure. MAST trousers, if already applied, may be continued or applied in the OR as indicated. Intravenous fluid infusion continues with balanced crystalloid solution. Hypotonic fluids are to be avoided as they lead to decreased serum osmolality and sodium levels, which can precipitate brain edema. Although extensive edema does not usually occur within the first 24 h, it may be aggravated by the administration of an excess of hypotonic fluid.

A central venous line or pulmonary artery catheter can help determine the intravascular volume status and indicate the adjustments needed to maintain balance and avoidance of fluid overload or dehydration. Hypotension or shock from head injury alone is rare and is usually due to hypovolemia. With the exception of severe hemorrhage from scalp or facial trauma, the source of blood loss will be in the chest, abdomen, extremities, or pelvis.[14] Physical examination and x-ray films of the chest, abdomen, and pelvis may determine the site of hemorrhage, and in all unconscious patients, or those with reduced responsiveness to pain, a diagnostic peritoneal lavage (DPL) should be done. This is a simple technique that has a low incidence of false-positive or false-negative results. Among 225 patients with severe head injuries seen at our institution, Miller et al. found 49 percent with one or more additional systemic injuries, the most common injury being limb fracture (30 percent) or chest trauma (29 percent).[23] Abdominal injuries occurred 17 percent of the time as diagnosed by DPL, and 6 percent of the patients suffered spinal injuries.[22]

Additional studies in the ER include x-ray films of the skull, chest, and all long bones that may be fractured. Arterial blood gases are determined as frequently as the clinical situation dictates, to direct treatment of acid-base imbalance or hypoxia. The central venous line is to be used for evaluation of intravascular fluid volume state. It should not be considered a main infusion site, however, as this is best accomplished through short, large-bore peripheral IV catheters inserted percutaneously or by cutdown. A central venous pressure maintained at 5 to 10 mmH$_2$O is recommended, and patients should not be kept in a hypovolemic dehydrated state.

Venous blood is drawn for laboratory studies, including complete blood count, electrolyte determinations, blood typing and matching, alcohol assay, and coagulation studies. A Foley catheter is placed for urinary bladder drainage, for evaluation of adequate urine flow, and to accommodate increased urinary volume should mannitol be required. Urine is sampled for urinalysis and drug screening. Nasogastric intubation is done to decompress the stomach, prevent aspiration, and detect any gastrointestinal hemorrhage. Based on the hematocrit, CVP, BP, and urinary output, infusion of blood products or crystalloid is used to maintain a systolic arterial blood pressure of at least 100 mmHg.

Management in the Intensive Care Unit

All patients with severe brain trauma, and those postoperative from removal of intracranial hematomas, should be treated in an intensive care unit with a systematic protocol that includes management of respiratory and cardiovascular parameters, intracranial pressure monitoring and control, and cerebral metabolic support.[27]

Hypoxia and hypercapnia must be avoided, and the use of controlled hyperventilation in severe head injury has been shown to produce an improved outcome.[27] The early need for an artificial airway to ensure oxygenation was recognized in 1950 by Echols et al., who recommended tracheostomy.[8] If endotracheal intubation is required beyond 72 h, tracheostomy may be considered, although intubation with a large cuffed tube has been successful for 10 to 12 days without complications.

Controlled ventilation at a slow rate assists in the re-expansion of collapsed alveoli, preventing intrapulmonary shunting due to atelectasis, and allows time for adequate venous return despite positive intrathoracic pressure. The minute volume is adjusted to bring the Pa_{CO_2} level to 25 to 30 mmHg, and the Pa_{O_2} value is maintained above 80 mmHg by adjusting oxygen flow. Medication such as chlorpromazine or morphine may be used to sedate the patient, reduce the effects of noxious stimuli, and "phase" the patient into this respiratory pattern. Pancuronium is a useful neuromuscular blocker, but it should not be used solely to synchronize the patient to the respirator, as it interferes with neurological testing and does not relieve pain from noxious stimuli that may cause an increase in ICP, especially with laryngeal stimulation. Percutaneous catheterization of the radial or dorsalis pedis artery allows for continuous monitoring of BP and easy access for arterial blood gas monitoring. Pulmonary toilet and chest physiotherapy should be used, with bronchoscopy if needed, for removal of mucous plugs. During all pulmonary therapy, careful attention to ICP and systolic arterial pressure is required, as patients with head injury usually have an elevated ICP, and cerebral perfusion pressure may be compromised with increases in ICP, causing further brain damage. Increases in arterial blood pressure may result in ICP increases to dangerous levels in patients who have impairment or loss of autoregulation.

Treatment with controlled hyperventilation is justified for several reasons. It may prevent sudden unexpected hypoxic events and reduce elevated ICP by maintaining a low Pa_{CO_2} with a normal Pa_{O_2}, resulting in a decrease in cerebrovascular volume, while effectively providing adequate oxygen delivery to the brain. When begun early, it tends to deter the development of pulmonary edema and atelectasis by expansion of collapsed alveoli. Additionally, it is effective in relieving the patient of energy-dissipating and exhausting respiratory work during this critical period. The spontaneous, vigorous hyperventilation that is not due to hypoxia may be controlled to the patient's benefit by decreasing muscle fatigue and overwork.

Positive end-expiratory pressure (PEEP) is required for advanced pulmonary insufficiency and pulmonary shunting when the Pa_{O_2} level cannot be brought to normal by increasing inspired oxygen concentration (Fi_{O_2}). Despite the fact that it can decrease cardiac output and increase ICP, PEEP can be used without adverse effect up to a pressure of 10 cmH_2O.[9] Positioning of the patient in a 30 degrees head-upright position is useful if the ICP is above 10 mmHg.

Systemic arterial blood pressure (SAP) should be controlled when hypertensive levels reach over 180 mmHg systolic. Lewelt et al. have shown that abnormalities of cerebral autoregulation correlate with the severity of injury,[18] and Langfitt et al. have demonstrated increased cerebrovascular volume secondary to loss of autoregulation as a prime cause of intracranial hypertension.[16] Furthermore, increases in SAP may contribute to disruption of the blood-brain barrier with extravasation of protein into the extracellular space and the development of cerebral edema.[13] Percutaneous arterial catheterization affords instantaneous monitoring, and control of SAP over 180 mmHg usually can be accomplished with sedatives in small doses. If not, hydralazine or trimethaphan camsylate may be used. Nitroprusside is not recommended when the ICP is elevated because of its cerebral vasodilating effect and potential for causing a further increase in ICP. Swan-Ganz catheterization may be useful in more complicated cases with the potential for pulmonary or cardiac compromise. The information gained will allow for better titration of fluid balance during the acute phase of injury, replacing the CVP line. An adequate hemoglobin (Hb) is necessary for oxygen transport, and patients with hematocrit levels below 30 percent (Hb less than 10 g) should be transfused with blood components as needed. A low hematocrit reduces the oxygen-carrying capacity of the blood, can retard wound healing, and can increase cerebral blood flow, with possible increases in ICP.

Proper fluid balance and maintenance of adequate intravascular volume will help prevent hypotension, intravascular clotting, and electrolyte abnormalities. In multiply traumatized patients, loss of intravascular volume may reduce cerebral perfusion pressure. Davis and Sundt have experimentally demonstrated that with hypovolemic hypotension, it is cardiac output, not SAP, that determines cerebral blood flow.[6] Severe dehydration may predispose to particularly severe electrolyte abnormalities if inappropriate ADH secretion or diabetes insipidus follows head injury, and if sedatives are used in patients with a contracted intravascular volume, sudden episodes of hypotension may occur as a result of their cardiac depressive effects. Cerebral edema should be managed by means other than generalized severe dehydration.

Intravenous fluid infusion should be at the usual maintenance volume. This usually can be started with a 5% dextrose and 0.45% normal saline solution at a rate of 125 ml/h for adults, totaling 3000 ml/day. Central venous pressure is maintained at 6 to 8 cmH_2O, keeping urinary output between 0.5 and 1.0 ml/kg per hour (approximately 30 to 60 ml/h).

Electrolyte imbalance, particularly hyponatremia, is a serious but preventable complication. Abnormalities of serum sodium (below 125 or above 150 meq per liter) and serum osmolarity (less than 260 or above 320 mosmol per liter) should be avoided. Overhydration, per se, will not cause brain edema if the serum sodium value is normal (135 to 145 meq per liter); however, when combined with hyponatremia (less than 130 meq per liter), it can cause edema at brain injury sites. A frequent source of a low serum sodium concentration is SIADH (syndrome of inappropriate antidiuretic hormone), possibly related to hypothalamic trauma. This may occur at any time up to 14 days following injury, and will produce a rapid drop in serum sodium values. Urinary and serum sodium and osmolarity values should be checked to make the diagnosis early (normovolemia with hyponatremia and serum hypo-osmolarity with hyperosmolar urine and increased urine sodium concentration). A low serum sodium value may persist despite sodium loading, and the primary approach to treatment is to eliminate the excess water by fluid restriction. If hyponatremia is severe, serum osmolarity may be raised quickly using 3% NaCl infusion (500 ml over 4 to 5 h) with frequent electrolyte checks. In addition, steroids that increase sodium retention can be given along with furosemide, which will accelerate water excretion. The differentiation of SIADH from the hyponatremia of salt depletion is possible, as none of the signs of hypovolemia (lowered blood pressure, increased BUN) associated with salt depletion exist. A condition frequently confused with SIADH is isotonic fluid loss with hypotonic fluid replacement, during which the preservation of volume takes precedence over tonicity. This is iatrogenic and is preventable by careful monitoring of serum and urine electrolyte levels, nasogastric output, and other fluid intake and output.

Diabetes insipidus is an infrequent but serious result of head injury and may be associated with a poorer prognosis. Treatment requires early diagnosis and administration of vasopressin. It may be difficult to regulate the large volumes of intravenous (IV) fluid required to keep up with urine output. In these patients, vasopressin must be used cautiously as it can cause arterial hypertension with subsequent increases in ICP and excessive fluid retention. A synthetic vasopressive substance, desmopressin (DDAVP), has fewer side effects than vasopressin and may be used as an alternative.[28]

Seizure prophylaxis is a high priority in all moderately or severely head injured patients. Early seizures can be prevented with a 1000-mg loading dose of diphenylhydantoin. This is administered as a 500-mg IV bolus (50 mg/min) along with ECG monitoring, and followed at 6-h intervals with doses of 250 mg IV each × 2. By 24 h, effective plasma levels are usually reached. Maintenance doses of 100 mg IV each 6 to 8 h are continued after loading. In children the loading dose is 10 mg/kg, followed by a maintenance dose of 5 mg/kg. Breakthrough seizures are treated with additional doses of phenytoin if serum levels are determined to be subtherapeutic or with the addition of phenobarbital to the anticonvulsant therapy in doses adequate to achieve therapeutic serum levels (20 to 30 mg/100 ml). Certain individuals appear to hypermetabolize these agents, and interval measurement of serum levels is a method of ensuring adequate prophylaxis. Many neurosurgeons believe that medications should be continued after the acute phase for at least 1 year in the case of severe head injury, and the EEG is useful in determining the need for their extended use.

Pulmonary therapy is aimed at preventing infection and edema while maintaining moderate hypocapnia. Continued or recurrent hypoxia may serve as a warning of an impending acute respiratory distress syndrome and requires prompt preventive measures. In this case, dyspnea, tachypnea, and a decreasing Pa_{O_2} value despite an adequate oxygen supply and assisted ventilation are associated with a normal Pa_{CO_2} value and a chest film showing patchy and fluffy interstitial pulmonary edema that may progress to a total loss of air space. Pulmonary artery catheterization with a Swan-Ganz catheter will reveal a progressively increasing pulmonary vascular pressure despite a relatively normal "wedge" pressure which reflects left atrial function.

The clinical syndrome of acute respiratory distress is probably the result of several factors such as central neurogenic pulmonary edema, shock with aggressive fluid resuscitation, hypoxia, and possibly fat embolism. The IV fluids used in resuscitation have been implicated as a cause; however, there does not appear to be a clear advantage to using colloids over crystalloids.

Treatment of a Pa_{O_2} value less than 70 mmHg should be with an increased Fi_{O_2} and positive pressure volume ventilation with use of PEEP up to 15 cmH$_2$O as long as the ICP will tolerate it. In patients with a pulmonary wedge pressure (PWP) over 15, the use of diuretics and digitalis may be helpful. The differentiation of neurogenic pulmonary edema from ARDS is difficult on clinical grounds, although brain-injured patients with a neurogenic type of pulmonary insufficiency readily respond to therapy.

Fat embolism can be an overlooked cause of ARDS, and although described as occurring in three forms—pure pulmonary, pure cerebral, and systemic with renal and hepatic involvement—it usually is recognized clinically because of its pulmonary effects. The diagnosis can be made on clinical criteria.[15] The syndrome is primarily pulmonary with associated cerebral symptomatology, and the pathological changes include pulmonary edema, hemorrhagic parenchymal necrosis, and fat globules in the alveoli.[7] Petechiae may appear on the chest and in the conjunctivae. Fat embolism is reported to occur in 1 percent of major trauma victims, with the brain being the second most common organ affected.[23]

The most likely causes include fat that is embolized into the venous circulation from traumatized tissue, along with spontaneous lipid droplet formation intravascularly caused by alterations in the blood resulting from the primary traumatic insult. Fat droplets may be formed from existing intravascular free lipids, and this has been shown to occur in nontraumatic conditions.[4]

Regardless of etiology, the pulmonary circulation seems to serve as a filter for circulating fat globules, and this is the primary cause of the pulmonary dysfunction. Early recognition of hypoxia in patients with multiple trauma and long bone fractures allows aggressive early treatment, which may prevent serious complications.

Oxygen therapy with positive pressure, if necessary, combined with adequate intravenous volume replacement, including blood as required, will prevent hypotensive shock and reduce catecholamine release, which contributes to increased lipid metabolism and release. Corticosteroids may reduce the pulmonary effects if given in high doses (at least 16 mg/day of dexamethasone).[1] Therapy designed to improve the microcirculation and reduce plasma lipid levels is controversial. Heparin, intravenous alcohol, and low-molecular-weight dextran have all been used, with mixed and often contradictory results.[15] In general, the best treatment after early recognition appears to be pressurized oxygen therapy to restore alveolar function to normal.

There is evidence that the monitoring of ICP and the management of elevated intracranial pressure in comatose brain-injured patients may significantly improve the outcome of severe head injuries. Intracranial hypertension is a major cause of death in severely head injured patients, and early recognition of an abnormally high intracranial pressure with immediate intervention to return it to normal should be part of any intensive neurological care program. The placement of subarachnoid or intraventricular monitoring devices is discussed in other chapters. Ventricular catheters are preferred by us, subarachnoid bolts being used in patients with very small ventricles, as determined on CT scan, that would be difficult to catheterize.

Generally, ICP values above 20 mmHg in the resting patient are considered abnormally high, and those above 40 mmHg represent very serious and dangerous levels of intracranial hypertension. Controlled ventilation to a hypocapnia level of 25 to 30 mmHg P_{CO_2} is capable of reducing ICP. Additional sedation with morphine sulfate (2 mg/h IV) may be used to reduce agitation and help synchronize respirations with the ventilator. If ICP remains elevated despite normothermia and repositioning of the head at a 20 to 30 degrees head-up posture with avoidance of compression of the jugular venous system, then ventricular drainage is indicated. Ventricular drainage can be set to allow drainage of fluid when ICP elevates above 15 or 20 mmHg. This is done by setting the drainage catheter at 20 to 25 cm above the level of the foramen of Monro. Setting the drainage catheter at this level will prevent ventricular collapse. If this still fails to control ICP, osmotic diuretics (mannitol) in conjunction with loop diuretics (furosemide) may then be employed.

Most prefer to give mannitol as an IV bolus in a dose of 1.0 g/kg of a 20% solution, but some prefer to begin with 0.5 g/kg. Furosemide (0.5 mg/kg IV) may assist the bolus in its effectiveness in lowering ICP. Following the use of diuretics, serum electrolyte and osmolarity values should be checked, as serum values in excess of 320 mosmol per liter preclude further use of osmotic therapy in order to prevent renal damage.

Precipitous increases in ICP unresponsive to therapy should be investigated with a CT scan to detect emergent intracranial hematomas or acute hydrocephalus. If all ventilation, drainage, osmotic, and surgical therapies have been exhausted and ICP remains high, the use of high-dose barbiturate therapy may be indicated in a patient with severe head injury and a GCS score of less than 7 who has no medical contraindication such as liver or renal disease.[19,21] Continuous monitoring of ICP is required to regulate dosage, which can begin with 50 to 100 mg of pentobarbital IV, the EEG being observed continuously. Treatment should continue at least until a burst suppression pattern is obtained on the EEG or the mean arterial blood pressure falls below 80 mmHg. At blood pressures less than this, cerebral perfusion pressure (CPP = MABP − ICP) may be reduced below a level of 40 mmHg, which can cause cerebral ischemia. If the blood pressure tolerates such dosage and burst suppression is obtained, a serum pentobarbital level of 2 to 4 mg/100 ml is maintained using a 1- to 2-mg/kg IV bolus dose each hour. A Swan-Ganz pulmonary artery catheter may be a useful adjunct in determining fluid needs. During active barbiturate therapy, the neurological examination remains less reliable; however, barbiturates in general cause small pupils, and if large, irregular pupils persist, they usually are associated with increased ICP, the development of an intracranial mass lesion with potential herniation, or advanced brain stem dysfunction.

Maintenance of adequate IV fluid balance and oxygenation with a pressure-volume ventilator are critical to prevent the development of pulmonary problems occasionally associated with barbiturate coma. The intermittent use of mannitol may be required in addition to pentobarbital and is permissible provided the serum osmolarity is less than 320 mosmol, and the systolic BP is maintained above 100 mmHg. Treatment is continued for 24 to 48 h after the control of the ICP to less than 20 mmHg, and then the patient is gradually weaned. If the ICP rises again, therapy may be reinstated for an additional 24-h interval prior to weaning. Those patients who cannot tolerate weaning or are unresponsive to barbiturate therapy have a poor prognosis.

Nutritional considerations are important. Feeding via nasogastric tube should not be started before the fourth or fifth day after injury. Total parenteral nutrition (TPN) may be started earlier, and can be quite effective in reducing negative nitrogen balance and generalized inanition. Head-injured patients normally have an elevated metabolic rate, which increases progressively for 1 week to levels as high as 160 to 180 percent of normal. Major trauma and isolated severe head injury usually result in a marked depression of the patient's immune competence. However, properly administered TPN can bring immune responsiveness back toward normal within 2 weeks. There is preliminary evidence that TPN may reduce mortality, and if this proves to be true, it is probably the result of a reduced infection rate. Adults should usually receive between 2200 and 2750 kcal per day. The blood sugar level should not be permitted to rise over 180 to 200 mg/100 ml. Higher levels may contribute to an increased cerebral lactic acidosis, which can further injure the already damaged brain.

Rehabilitation programs should begin during the first week of admission, even while the patient is in intensive care. Nonfractured extremities should be put through a full range of motion repeatedly during each day. Patients who are posturing can have this done during the muscle paralysis and relaxation used for ventilatory control. Many rehabilitation specialists recommend the early institution of controlled visual, auditory, and tactile stimuli, claiming this may hasten and improve recovery. Documentation that this is indeed true remains to be developed, but it certainly cannot be considered detrimental. Careful and gentle, yet direct and honest, family counseling must also begin early in order to prepare the family for an appropriate response to the ordeal ahead.

References

1. Ashbaugh DG, Petty TL: The use of corticosteroids in the treatment of respiratory failure associated with massive fat embolism. Surg Gynecol Obstet 123:493–500, 1966.
2. Becker DP, Miller JD, Ward JD, Greenberg RP, Young HF, Sakalas R: The outcome from severe head injury with early diagnosis and intensive management. J Neurosurg 47:491–502, 1977.
3. Becker DP, Miller JD, Young HF, Selhorst JB, Kishore PRS, Greenberg RP, Rosner MJ, Ward JD: Diagnosis and treatment of head injury in adults, in Youmans JR (ed): *Neurological Surgery*. Philadelphia, Saunders, 1982, pp 1938–2083.
4. Bergentz SE: Studies on the genesis of posttraumatic fat embolism. Acta Chir Scand [Suppl] 282:5–72, 1961.
5. Cook AW, Browder EJ, Lyons HA: Alterations in acid-base equilibrium in craniocerebral trauma: A determinant in survival. J Neurosurg 18:366–370, 1961.
6. Davis DH, Sundt TM Jr: Relationship of cerebral blood flow to cardiac output, mean arterial pressure, blood volume, and alpha and beta blockade in cats. J Neurosurg 52:745–754, 1980.
7. Dines DE, Burgher LW, Okazaki H: The clinical and pathologic correlation of fat embolism syndrome. Mayo Clin Proc 50:407–411, 1975.
8. Echols DH, Llewellyn R, Kirgis HD, Rehfeldt FC, Garcia-Bengochea F: Tracheostomy in the management of severe head injuries. Surgery 28:801–811, 1950.
9. Frost EAM: Effects of positive end-expiratory pressure on intracranial pressure and compliance in brain-injured patients. J Neurosurg 47:195–200, 1977.
10. Gardner SR, Maull KI, Swenson EE, Ward JD: The effects of the pneumatic anti-shock garment on intracranial pressure in man: A prospective study of 12 patients with severe head injury. J Trauma (in press).
11. Gennarelli TA, Segawa H, Wald U, Czernicki Z, Marsh K, Thompson C: Physiological response to angular acceleration of the head, in Grossman RG, Gildenberg PL (eds): *Head Injury: Basic and Clinical Aspects*. New York, Raven Press, 1982, pp 129–140.
12. Gordon E, Ponten U: The non-operative treatment of severe head injuries, in Vinken PJ, Bruyn GW (eds): *Handbook of Clinical Neurology*, vol 24. Amsterdam, North-Holland Publishing Company, 1975, pp 599–626.

13. Häggendal E, Johansson B: On the pathophysiology of the increased cerebrovascular permeability in acute arterial hypertension in cats. Acta Neurol Scand 48:265–270, 1972.
14. Illingworth G, Jennett WB: The shocked head injury. Lancet 2:511–514, 1965.
15. Kramer J, Klawans HL: Fat embolism, in Vinken PJ, Bruyn GW (eds): *Handbook of Clinical Neurology*, vol 24. Amsterdam, North-Holland Publishing Company, 1975, pp 563–574.
16. Langfitt TW, Weinstein JD, Kassell NF: Vascular factors in head injury: Contribution to brain-swelling and intracranial hypertension, in Caveness WF, Walker AE (eds): *Head Injury: Conference Proceedings*. Philadelphia, Lippincott, 1966, pp 172–194.
17. Levine JE, Becker D: Reversal of incipient brain death from head-injury apnea at the scene of accidents. N Engl J Med 301:109, 1979.
18. Lewelt W, Jenkins LW, Miller JD: Autoregulation of cerebral blood flow after experimental fluid percussion injury of the brain. J Neurosurg 53:500–511, 1980.
19. Marshall LF, Smith RW, Shapiro HM: The outcome with aggressive treatment in severe head injuries. Part I: The significance of intracranial pressure monitoring: Part II. Acute and chronic barbiturate administration in the management of head injury. J Neurosurg 50:20–25, 26–30, 1979.
20. McLaurin RL, King LR: Recognition and treatment of metabolic disorders after head injuries. Clin Neurosurg 19:281–300, 1972.
21. Miller JD: Barbiturates and raised intracranial pressure. Ann Neurol 6:189–193, 1979.
22. Miller JD: Physiology of trauma. Clin Neurosurg 29:103–130, 1982.
23. Miller JD, Butterworth JF, Gudeman SK, Faulkner JE, Choi SC, Selhorst JB, Harbison JW, Lutz HA, Young HF, Becker DP: Further experience in the management of severe head injury. J Neurosurg 54:289–299, 1981.
24. Miller JD, Sweet RC, Narayan R, Becker DP: Early insults to the injured brain. JAMA 240:439–442, 1978.
25. Ommaya AK, Gennarelli TA: Cerebral concussion and traumatic unconsciousness: Correlation of experimental and clinical observations on blunt head injuries. Brain 97:633–654, 1974.
26. Ommaya AK, Gennarelli TA: Experimental head injury, in Vinken DJ, Bruyn GW (eds): *Handbook of Clinical Neurology*, vol 23. Amsterdam, North-Holland Publishing Company, 1975, pp 67–90.
27. White RJ: Programmed management of severe head injuries revisited. J Trauma 15:779–784, 1975.
28. Ziai F, Walter R, Rosenthal IM: Treatment of central diabetes insipidus in adults and children with desmopressin: A synthetic analogue of vasopressin. Arch Intern Med 138:1382–1385, 1978.

195

Pediatric Head Injury

Derek A. Bruce
Luis Schut
Leslie N. Sutton

The variations that occur in the mechanical, biochemical, and functional aspects of the brain throughout infancy and childhood are enormous. Thus the spectrum of injuries that can be seen is highly varied, and recovery of function is quite different at each age level. Infants and children are in a position of having to continue their learning and education with a brain that may no longer have the capacity that it was destined to possess, and thus, special problems will be encountered as education and emotional development continue. Those pathological changes and the therapeutic interventions that are specific to the infant and child will be discussed.

Mechanisms of Injury

The incidence of head injury in the pediatric age group is high, and at least 1 out of every 10 children will suffer a significant head injury during the period of childhood. The number of head injuries in the United States appears to be somewhere around 5 million per year. Of these, the majority are minor or scalp lacerations, and less than 10 percent are serious. The type of trauma producing head injury changes from the newborn period to adolescence, ranging from slow constant pressure producing fracture to high-speed motor accidents.

Birth injuries fall into two major categories: injuries produced by the normal forces of labor and delivery and injuries produced by obstetrical instrumentation, usually the inappropriate application of forceps. A prime example of the first type of injury is the Ping-Pong ball fracture, a depressed fracture without swelling or discoloration of the overlying skin. This lesion is produced by steady pressure of the head against the pelvic prominence. Unless small, these lesions usually require elevation. This is done through a small scalp incision near the edge of the fracture. A burr hole is made, and the fracture is elevated by passing a periosteal elevator through the epidural space to beyond the midpoint of the fracture. Other lesions that occur as a result of the normal deformity of the head during delivery are subarachnoid hemorrhage, infratentorial hemorrhage, subdural hemorrhage, and soft-tissue scalp injury (caput succedaneum). These latter injuries usually require no surgical treatment. A patient may present with significant subarachnoid hemorrhage and the onset of hydrocephalus may follow 2 to 3 months later.

Injuries produced by misapplication of forceps show contusion or laceration of the scalp or face; linear or depressed skull fractures can be produced and may be accompanied by dural laceration and epidural, subdural, or intracerebral hemorrhage. Hematomas may occur in the posterior fossa, and the very worst types of injury are associated with basal skull fracture, laceration of the basal sinuses with profuse posterior fossa subarachnoid hemorrhage, and, frequently, hemorrhage from the ear. These injuries are usually rapidly fatal. Stretch injury to the spinal cord at the cervicomedullary junction or stretch injuries of the brachial plexus can also be seen after traumatic delivery.

One major clinical indication of an intracranial mass lesion is the occurrence of seizures in the first 24 h after traumatic delivery. This is an indication for CT scanning. If a depressed fracture is present at the time of delivery, a CT scan should be obtained before surgery to evaluate the underlying parenchymal injury.

In general, no effort should be made to remove contused brain in the neonatal period. The pia-arachnoid is easily stripped from the underlying cortex with the suction tip, and extensive areas of brain ischemia can be produced as a result of surgical intervention. Thus, only frank hematomas should be removed. In general, a conservative, nonoperative approach should be taken to the newborn who shows evidence of having a subdural or parenchymal hemorrhage. The best surgical indication is the progressive deterioration of alertness. Another indication may be seizure activity which is difficult to control and may be helped by evacuation of a surgical mass lesion. Because of the infrequency of these mass lesions and the problems of surgery, anesthesia, and preoperative and postoperative care in this age group, it is suggested that major intracranial surgery in newborns be undertaken in specialized pediatric neurosurgical units. The outlook for babies requiring surgery for intracerebral hematomas in the first few days of life can be very good depending on the location of the hematoma. It has to be realized that hematomas, even in the motor strip, may produce little deficit in the first few months, but the onset of hemiparesis may become noticeable some 6 months later.

After the newborn period, up to 2 years of age, the most frequent cause of head injury, usually minor, is a short fall (e.g., from the bed or changing table). The fall is often onto a carpeted floor. Linear fractures are often seen. These may be extensive and dramatic on plain x-ray films, but are rarely associated with disturbance of consciousness and are usually unassociated with intracranial lesions. Seizures in the first hour following injury are common, and early seizures probably have no prognostic significance. Skull fractures are present in 50 percent of children hospitalized for trauma at our hospital in the first year of life. The early seizures rarely require medication, and the incidence of late seizures in this group of children is well under 1 percent. Most severe head injuries in children under 1 year of age are the result of child abuse.[7] These are usually nonimpact, shaking injuries.[4] They are associated with tearing of the parasagittal bridging veins and acute subarachnoid hemorrhage with blood accumulation in the interhemispheric fissure (Fig. 195-1) and, less frequently, over the hemispheres. The other cause of severe intracranial injury, usually an epidural hematoma, is the occurrence of multiple blows to the head, such as in falls down stairs.

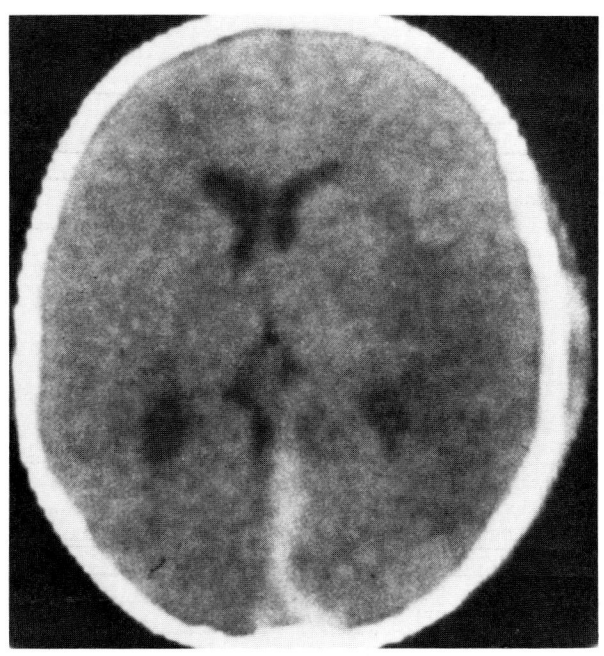

Figure 195-1 A posterior interhemispheric subdural hematoma and decreased density of the right hemisphere secondary to infarction.

The most frequent situation in this age group in which cervicocranial trauma occurs is that in which a child is an unrestrained passenger in an automobile which is involved in an accident. Small children are thrown around in the car and frequently are found apneic under the seats. The cause of death in these children is usually high cervical or cervicomedullary trauma, and not a primary head injury.

After 1 year of age, most minor head injuries are the result of short falls, and most severe head injuries are the result of automobile/pedestrian accidents or falls out of windows (the latter particularly in large urban areas). As the child gets older, major head injuries are more frequently the result of bicycle/automobile accidents. Thus, from infancy to 10 years of age, the major factors producing head trauma are not impact, but acceleration/deceleration forces. Between 10 and 15 years, it is increasingly frequent that the trauma is produced by impact (e.g., falls from bicycles or sports injuries). Unless a mass accumulates, with increased intracranial pressure, and cerebral herniation occurs, the damage done by impact injuries is most frequently local. In contrast, that produced by acceleration/deceleration trauma is almost always diffuse.

Clinical Features

In children and adolescents, a careful history that elucidates the type of injury, height of fall, condition of floor (carpeted or not), initial stage of consciousness (crying or not), occurrence of seizures, and occurrence of apnea must be obtained. A serial history is vital: did the child's general condition improve, stabilize, or worsen; did vomiting ensue; did late seizures occur; etc.? Whenever the history is thought to explain the neurological picture poorly, child abuse must be suspected.

Below the age of 2 years, the Glasgow coma scale (GCS) can be applied only with difficulty. The portion on speech is most easily handled by giving the child a 5, if there is any vocalization at all, and 0 if no crying is obtained. Similarly, eye opening in the severely head-injured child below 18 months of age can occasionally occur in a stereotyped fashion which is not the normal spontaneous eye opening seen in older children, and too much reliance placed on this may lead the examiner to underrate the severity of the child's injury. The motor portion of the examination is applicable after the first few months of life except for the response to command. However, in children, by and large, the GCS gives a good reflection of the initial depth of coma.

In the first few months of life, the neurological examination includes palpation of the fontanels and sutures, examination of the baby for postural changes in tone or clonus, and examination for the presence of primitive reflexes (e.g., the Moro reflex). The presence of spontaneous bicycling movements of the lower extremities is seen in association with major head injuries in this age group and must not be misinterpreted as normal spontaneous motor movements. Vital signs usually reveal a normal blood pressure with tachycardia. Bradycardia is very suggestive of intracranial hypertension in this age group. In the child a necessary part of the examination is visualization of the fundi to seek evidence of retinal hemorrhage as well as papilledema. The presence of retinal hemorrhage, especially in the child under 2 years of age, is extremely suggestive of child abuse. The importance of recognizing this association is that the severity of accumulated injuries may not be appreciated. The child may be thought to be stable, but then a sudden acute deterioration occurs as a result of brain swelling or seizures, producing acute deterioration of the neurological condition, ultimately leading to death. Acute deterioration of consciousness is common in the child after moderate or severe head injury and may be due to seizures or acute brain swelling, or less frequently, to an expanding intracranial clot. Pallor, vomiting, and tachycardia are all extremely common following concussive injury in the child.

Occasionally, hypotension or shock in the small child is due to head injury. This occurs in two situations. The first is in a child under 1 year of age with a large linear skull fracture and an epidural hematoma. The intracranial blood can leak through the fracture, producing an ever-enlarging subgaleal or subperiosteal hemorrhage, which in association with the intracranial blood, may be sufficient to produce anemia and hypotension. The second situation is a head injury occurring in a child with hydrocephalus. In infants and toddlers with functioning shunts, a large amount of intracranial blood may accumulate without much evidence of elevated intracranial pressure (ICP). The ventricular cerebrospinal fluid is displaced down the shunt as the clot accumulates, preventing the usual signs and symptoms of slowly increasing ICP. These children usually present to the emergency room drowsy and irritable with a blood picture suggesting acute blood-loss anemia.

Radiological Evaluation

Skull x-ray films are particularly valuable as a screening procedure in children under 1 year of age with a history of a short fall. Rather dramatic appearing fractures are frequently seen, often crossing suture lines and sinuses. In the absence of evidence on x-ray films of split sutures, and in the presence of a normal neurological examination and soft fontanel, automatic CT scanning is unnecessary. These children rarely develop a delayed chronic subdural or epidural hematoma and rarely have evidence of underlying brain injury. The only late complications are subgaleal hematomas (see elsewhere in this book) and growing skull fractures or leptomeningeal cysts. These latter complications occur only when there is laceration of the dura and contusion of the underlying cerebral cortex.[5] They are uncommon and usually follow an accident in which the level of consciousness was significantly altered. Rather than obtaining routine follow-up x-ray films of the skull, we recommend that these children with extensive linear fractures be re-examined 2 to 3 months after injury. If the area of the fracture site is not enlarged or swollen, then it is unlikely that repeat skull films are necessary. The presence of a persistent fracture line with local swelling suggests a leptomeningeal cyst, and a CT scan is recommended to identify the relationship of the brain to the fracture and the subgaleal swelling. Routine skull films in older children are rarely helpful unless a specific lesion is being sought (e.g., pneumocephalus or a depressed fracture).

Lateral x-ray films of the cervical spine are obtained in all comatose children following head injury, usually before endotracheal intubation. Children most likely to have combined cervicocranial trauma are those who have been unrestrained passengers in an automobile.

The CT scan, as in adults, is the definitive initial study. All unconscious children, all children showing clinical evidence of a deteriorating level of consciousness, and all children with a depressed skull fracture require immediate CT scanning. A persisting or increasing headache over hours or days and persistent vomiting are indications for obtaining a CT scan in a child with minor trauma.

Several CT patterns are unique to the child. The shaken baby typically has a CT scan showing an acute subarachnoid hemorrhage and posterior interhemispheric triangular-shaped subdural hematoma (Fig. 195-1).[9] These hemorrhages are rarely large enough to require surgical evacuation. Areas of low density may be seen on the initial CT scan, and in children, these usually turn out to be major vessel infarctions. Radioisotope perfusion scans usually demonstrate patency of the vessels, suggesting that the infarction was due to distortion and temporary vascular occlusion at the time of injury, transient vascular spasm, or some combination thereof. A herniation syndrome certainly is responsible for infarction in the distribution of the posterior cerebral artery, and it is possible that retroalar herniation of the frontal lobes may result in middle cerebral or anterior cerebral territory infarction.

Diffuse axonal injury is seen on the CT scan in a small percentage of children. This is diagnosed by the finding of small hemorrhages in the head of the caudate nucleus, in the corpus callosum, in the region of the superior cerebellar peduncle, or around the aqueduct. Despite evidence of primary midbrain, periaqueductal hemorrhage, children can make a significantly good recovery (Fig. 195-2). This finding should not be taken as an indication for backing off on therapy. Children with evidence of diffuse axonal injury frequently go on to develop severe brain swelling after 24 h, and ICP monitoring is indicated. Forty to fifty percent of children in coma after head injury will show a primary CT scan pattern within hours of injury which has been described as diffuse cerebral swelling.[2] This pattern has been shown to be associated with an increased cerebral blood flow, and current information suggests that early swelling is associated with vasodilatation and is not due to cerebral edema. Although brain swelling is seen in adults, it is usually unilateral and is frequently underlying an acute subdural hematoma. In children, the swelling is bilateral, rarely associated with any other lesion except primary subarachnoid hemorrhage, and usually unassociated with skull fracture.

Delayed CT scans 7 to 10 days after injury frequently show mild ventricular dilatation and often collections of extracerebral CSF in the frontal areas. These CSF collections do not represent subdural hygromas and do not require surgical drainage.

Management

The initial management of the comatose child is not significantly different from that of the adult.[8] The initial resuscitation fulfills the usual ABC's of management: open and clear the airway, ensure adequate ventilation, and stabilize the circulation. In children it is not necessary to hyperextend the neck to intubate! Gentle pressure on the cricoid cartilage will prevent air from entering the stomach during bagging of the patient before endotracheal intubation and will also prevent regurgitation of stomach contents into the lungs. The timing of the passing of a nasogastric (NG) tube will depend on the level of consciousness of the patient and the type of injury. With severe facial trauma, an NG tube should not be passed until x-ray films of the skull demonstrate that the cranial base is intact. An oral gastric tube may be used in this circumstance, if necessary. In children with a markedly diminished or absent gag response, it is safer to pass the NG tube after an endotracheal tube is in place. In children with a good gag reflex, it is probably safer to pass the NG tube and evacuate the stomach before muscle paralysis and intubation. Intubation of the trachea should be performed (and it would be in the operating room) with hyperventilation using 100% O_2, intravenous injection of thiopental sodium and pancuronium bromide, and then endotracheal intubation. After intubation, moderate hyperventilation to a Pa_{CO_2} level around 25 torr is performed.

Circulatory support with intravenous fluids should never involve the use of 5% glucose in water, and rarely ever one-quarter strength saline, because inappropriate antidiuretic hormone secretion is common in children with severe head trauma. The preferred intravenous solution is 5% dextrose in one-half normal or normal saline, run at one-half to two-thirds the normal maintenance volume. If both shock and

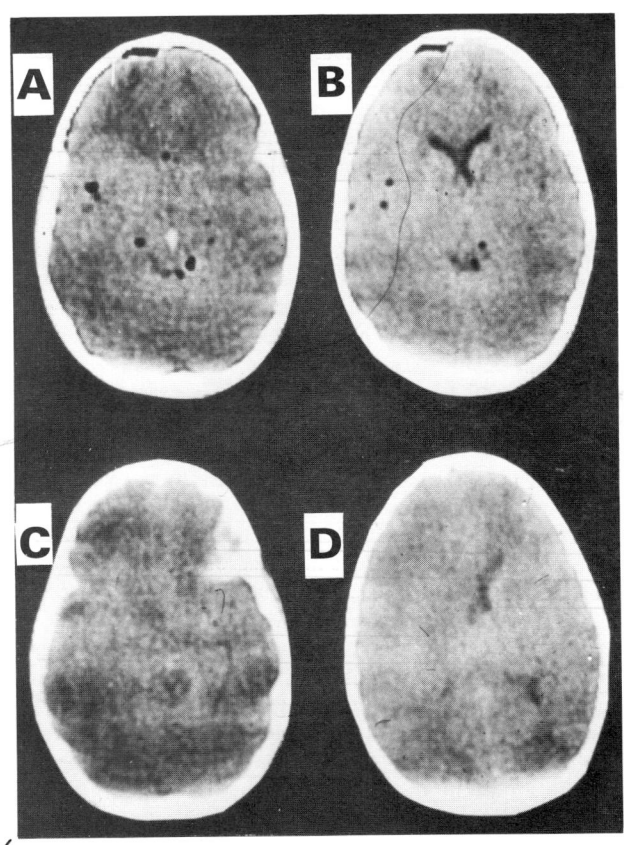

Figure 195-2 CT scans of a 4-year-old child presenting with bilateral fixed and dilated pupils and bilateral decerebrate posturing. *A*, *B*. Scans obtained on the first day show subarachnoid air from a petrous fracture and focal periaqueductal hemorrhage. *C*, *D*. Repeat CT scans at 24 h showing severe brain swelling. This was associated with increased intracranial pressure. This child is now walking independently, but requires special schooling.

coma are present, we suggest the insertion of an ICP monitor during resuscitation, because the large swings in ICP that will occur when large volumes of fluid are infused cannot otherwise be monitored. To establish a good circulation at the expense of an ICP that is equal to blood pressure clearly makes little sense.

In the emergency room, the standard lines for children with a GCS score of 8 or less are a large-bore intravenous line, an arterial line, an endotracheal tube, and (if there is no evidence of perineal trauma) a Foley catheter. In those with a GCS score of 5 or less, an ICP monitor is also inserted. The use of corticosteroids is optional, but if they are used, they should probably be used in megadoses. Mannitol is not used unless the history or the clinical examination suggests an expanding mass lesion (e.g., an epidural hematoma).

The management of epidural hematomas is the same as in adults, except that a craniotomy should always be performed, rather than a craniectomy. Further, the location of the typical epidural hematoma in a child is higher in the parietal region than it is in adults, and the typical low temporal burr hole may miss such a lesion. Acute subdural hematomas usually do not require surgery in childhood. Cerebral contusion, in our opinion, should rarely be operated upon in childhood, and most intracerebral hematomas are small, again not requiring surgical evacuation.

The commonest cause for surgical intervention in the child with a severe head injury is a depressed skull fracture. It has been our practice over the last few years to do a craniotomy, elevate the depressed fracture, and then replace the fracture fragments, wiring them together into the cranium. This has been done even in the face of open compound fractures. It is a valuable way of avoiding the need for a second operation, and with adequate antibiotic coverage, we have not had problems with infection.

In the child less than 1 year old who presents with a bulging fontanel and retinal hemorrhages (i.e., child abuse), the indications for fontanel tap are apnea, decerebrate posturing, or fixed dilated pupils. In these children, rapid intubation and hyperventilation are followed by bilateral fontanel taps with a 20-gauge, short-bevel spinal needle. Often, 10 to 15 ml of bloody CSF, which does not clot, is obtained from either side. This is usually adequate to re-establish ventilation, it frequently brings the pupils down and back to normal responsiveness, and it may improve the decerebrate posturing. CT scanning will then usually show blood in the interhemispheric fissure and brain swelling, but rarely a significant surgical mass lesion. In our experience, it is very rare for these lesions to progress to chronic subdural hematomas, and usually no further subdural taps or surgical intervention is necessary. Children with acute subdural hematomas and subarachnoid hemorrhage frequently develop severe brain swelling, and careful monitoring of ICP is required along with excellent intensive care management to ensure that these children survive with the least possible damage.

The intensive care management of elevated ICP aims at keeping the ICP below 20 torr, or if changes in pupil function are present, at levels below 15 torr.[3] The initial therapy is elevation of the head to 30 degrees with the head kept in the midline, moderate hyperventilation to 25 torr, and muscle paralysis. Muscle paralysis can only be used if the ventilator is equipped with an alarm system. If this is inadequate to control ICP, further therapy will depend upon the findings on the CT scan. In children with diffuse swelling, we prefer to avoid the use of mannitol in the first 24 h if possible. Thus, following hyperventilation to Pa_{CO_2} values as low as 18 to 20 torr, furosemide in doses of 1 mg/kg or ethacrynic acid is given. If this is still inadequate to maintain an ICP below 20 torr, then doses of pentobarbital are used to produce blood levels of 20 to 30 mg per liter. The dose is designed to control the ICP rather than to establish a specific serum level. If despite barbiturate therapy the ICP continues to be a problem, then mannitol is given. In children in whom a midline shift is seen in conjunction with an elevated ICP, mannitol will be used after hyperventilation. If this is ineffective, then once again, barbiturates are used in an effort to lower the ICP (Table 195-1). It is not uncommon in children to see the ICP become elevated again around the third to fifth days. At this time, a repeat CT scan will often show enlargement of the CSF spaces, and now ventricular

TABLE 195-1 Selection of Therapy for Brain Swelling versus Brain Edema

Diffuse Swelling	Brain Edema
Head up	Head up
↓CO_2	Steroids?
Furosemide	Mannitol
Barbiturates	Furosemide
Mannitol	↓CO_2
	Barbiturates

drainage or lumbar punctures may be more than adequate to control the ICP.

Outcome

The mortality rate in children (less than 15 years of age) in coma following head trauma is around 50 percent for those who are flaccid and only 6 to 12 percent for those who are decerebrate. In children with a GCS score above 5, with no evidence of other major trauma or who are not in shock, the mortality should be close to zero. Through the spectrum of severe head injury in childhood (i.e., a GCS score below 8), recovery to independent function should be expected in close to 90 percent of the children.[1,3,6]

References

1. Brink JD, Imbus C, Woo-Sam J: Physical recovery after severe closed head trauma in children and adolescents. J Pediatr 97:721–727, 1980.
2. Bruce DA, Alavi A, Bilaniuk L, Dolinskas C, Obrist W, Uzzell B: Diffuse cerebral swelling following head injuries in children: The syndrome of "malignant brain edema." J Neurosurg 54:170–178, 1981.
3. Bruce DA, Raphaely RC, Goldberg AI, Zimmerman RA, Bilaniuk LT, Schut L, Kuhl DE: Pathophysiology, treatment and outcome following severe head injury in children. Childs Brain 5:174–191, 1979.
4. Caffey J: On the theory and practice of shaking infants: Its potential residual effects of permanent brain damage and mental retardation. Am J Dis Child 124:161–169, 1972.
5. Ito H, Miwa T, Onodra Y: Growing skull fracture of childhood: With reference to the importance of the brain injury and its pathogenetic consideration. Childs Brain 3:116–126, 1977.
6. Mayer T, Walker ML, Shasha I, Matlak M, Johnson DG: Effect of multiple trauma on outcome of pediatric patients with neurologic injuries. Childs Brain 8:189–197, 1981.
7. McClelland CQ, Rekate H, Kaufman B, Persse L: Cerebral injury in child abuse: A changing profile. Childs Brain 7:225–235, 1980.
8. Raphaely RC, Swedlow DB, Downes JJ, Bruce DA: Management of severe pediatric head trauma. Pediatr Clin North Am 27:715–727, 1980.
9. Zimmerman RA, Bilaniuk LT, Bruce D, Schut L, Uzzell B, Goldberg HI: Interhemispheric acute subdural hematoma: A computed tomographic manifestation of child abuse by shaking. Neuroradiology 16:39–40, 1978.

196
Outcome Prediction in Severe Head Injury

Lawrence F. Marshall
Sharon A. Bowers

The prediction of outcome following severe head injury is an area of intense interest. As the salvage rate from severe injuries has improved, it has become increasingly important to try to identify those factors which will predict either a good recovery or an adverse outcome. As resources become more limited, both the scientific and ethical issues regarding prediction will receive even more attention. The two factors which are of greatest significance in determining outcome are the severity of the injury and the age of the patient.

Glasgow Coma Scale

Many methods of neurological assessment are available, but none has been as extensively tested as the Glasgow coma scale (GCS) as a means of rapidly assessing the patient and permitting an early and accurate prediction of outcome.[14] The Glasgow coma scale, which is detailed in a previous chapter, has received widespread acceptance throughout the world. This scale, which assesses eye opening, verbal response, and motor response, is simple and, despite the absence of any specific assessment of brain stem function, yields an early and quite accurate prediction of outcome. The accuracy of the GCS, however, is center-specific, rather than internationally specific. This is probably a reflection of a variety of factors including premorbid condition, the mechanism of injury, and, perhaps, the quality of acute prehospital and hospital care. Nevertheless, patients with GCS scores of 3 through 5 have mortality rates in excess of 60 percent if the score is determined at the time of admission.

As the GCS score rises, there is a precipitous decline in mortality, so that by the time the score is 9 or greater, the mortality rate becomes very low (Fig. 196-1). The exceptions to this are those patients who initially have higher scores and then deteriorate, usually because of a mass lesion. In these patients a high mortality rate is again encountered. In patients with GCS scores greater than 9, death or morbidity usually occurs because of advanced age or complicating conditions.

Abnormalities of Brain Stem Function

The addition of brain stem function tests to the GCS scale adds surprisingly little to initial accurate prediction. This is a reflection of the fact that severe injuries which result in significant primary brain stem injury usually are associated with decerebrate or flexor responses, which by themselves indicate a very poor outcome. In the absence of such abnormal motor movements, however, the assessment of brain stem function becomes much more important in attempting to make an early prediction of outcome.

In patients in whom the initial brain injury is not so severe, but in whom pupillary abnormalities develop because of intracranial hypertension with consequent transtentorial herniation, the prognosis becomes much more grave. The presence of one dilated, unreactive pupil as a result of intracranial hypertension is associated with a mortality of ap-

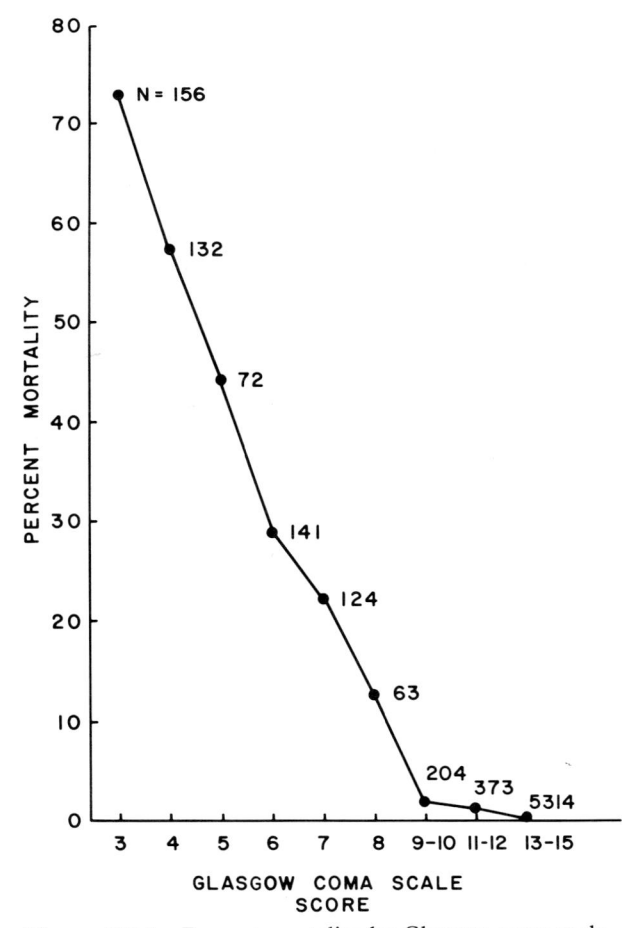

Figure 196-1 Percent mortality by Glasgow coma scale score for hospitalized head-injured patients in San Diego County, 1978–1981.

proximately 50 percent. The presence of bilaterally unreactive pupils is associated with a mortality of greater than 90 percent. The absence of pupillary abnormalities or abnormalities of the oculocephalic responses does not ensure a satisfactory recovery, but the presence of such abnormalities is often ominous.

Effects of Age and Severity of Injury

In patients suffering severe head injury, age and the severity of injury are predominant factors in determining outcome. In younger patients this relationship is extremely strong, as shown in Fig. 196-2. With increasing age, age as an influence begins to predominate, so that by age 45 the curves for age and severity are almost matched for GCS scores of 3 through 7. It is apparent that in patients over the age of 45, the likelihood of significant recovery from an injury in which abnormal motor movements are noted, even for a brief period, is extremely poor.

Abnormalities of the Vital Signs

The predictive power of the Glasgow coma scale is such that the acute influence of shock and hypoxia on neurological function is incorporated into it a priori. The GCS is reduced proportionately by the degree of shock or hypoxia present, and therefore, their presence is reflected in the score. It is important to note, however, that a systolic blood pressure of less than 95 mmHg and a Pa_{O_2} of less than 65 mmHg, when coupled with a GCS score of 7 or less, carry with them an ominous prognosis. If significant intracranial hypertension (intracranial pressure >30 mmHg) is also present, a mortality of almost 100 percent will be observed. Although abnormalities in respiratory function are often seen with severe head injury and complicate its management, their presence is not terribly useful in predicting outcome. Of interest is the observation that bradycardia (defined as a heart rate of 50 or less) at the time of admission is associated with an increased likelihood of death or severe disability of almost four times.

Pathophysiology of the Lesion

The outcome of patients with mass lesions which require operation is generally poorer than that of patients with similar initial neurological function but in whom diffuse injury not requiring surgery is present. This is most likely a product of the deleterious effects of elevated ICP and consequent brain stem distortion. The correlation of outcome with brain shift as seen by computed tomography (CT) scanning supports this hypothesis, as do the numerous clinical reports indicating the poorer outcome of these patients. The observation of Seelig et al. that rapid evacuation of an acute subdural hematoma (i.e., within 4 h) is associated with a remarkably improved outcome in these patients demonstrates that better planning for the care of such patients might materially alter prognosis.[12]

CT Scanning

The influence of CT scanning on neurotraumatology is almost immeasurable. In the area of prediction it has already added considerable power. It is apparent that a shift, while not always correlating with the degree of intracranial hypertension, is an extremely important predictor of outcome. This is particularly true in patients who initially seem to have relatively more moderate injuries.

The preliminary data from the Pilot Phase of the National Traumatic Coma Data Bank showed that a shift was the most important predictor of a poor outcome in patients who talked before their condition deteriorated.[8] It is also apparent from our own experience that shifts of greater than 10 mm are extremely poorly tolerated, and that if such shifts are associated with advanced age, the prognosis is uniformly dismal.

The presence of multiple contusions was initially thought

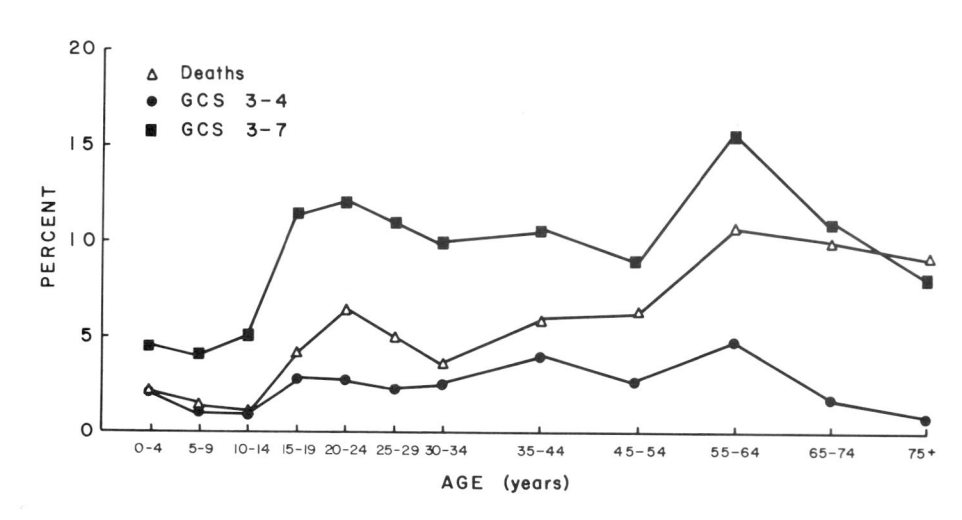

Figure 196-2 The percentages of patients who died, or who had a Glasgow coma scale score of 3 or 4, or of 3, 4, 5, 6, or 7, shown by age (hospitalized head-injured patients in San Diego County, 1978–1981).

to indicate a poor prognosis, but this conclusion is not universally applicable. This is in part a reflection of the difficulty in recording the severity of specific lesions within a particular CT scan, and not necessarily a reflection of the lack of predictive power of scanning per se. Deep contusions, seen as areas of hemorrhage in the deep gray matter, corpus callosum, or internal capsule, are associated with a poor outcome.[2] These contusions appear to represent stigmata of diffuse axonal injury as described by Gennarelli, Adams, and their colleagues.[1,3]

The presence of small ventricles or the absence of ventricles on the initial CT scan (when coupled with ICP measurements) or the absence of the basal cisterns can be used in making predictions, not only of impending difficulty in management of intracranial pressure (ICP), but also prognostically.[13]

The utility of CT scanning in supplementing our clinical assessments to make early and accurate prognoses will be improved as better methods are developed for more specific descriptions of CT abnormalities.

Intracranial Pressure Measurements

ICP monitoring has yielded useful information regarding the pathophysiology of brain injury. It is also apparent that the inability to control ICP will also give very reliable predictive information. In patients in whom the ICP exceeds 30 mmHg at the time of admission, an extremely high death rate can be expected. Furthermore, in patients in whom the ICP exceeds 30 mmHg after the evacuation of hematoma or during the intensive management of diffuse brain injury, the prognosis is markedly worse. Failure to control ICP (i.e., to reduce it to or below 20 to 25 mmHg) has in our experience and the experiences of others been uniformly associated with fatality.[7,9] Whether more specific predictive value for ICP can be found is not yet apparent. What is clear is that the absence of intracranial hypertension, for patients with equally severe injuries, is predictive of a better outcome than that observed in patients who have ICP elevations during their acute course.

Multimodality Evoked Potentials

The use of multimodality evoked responses, including brain stem auditory evoked responses and somatosensory evoked response recordings, has attracted increasing interest as a means of identifying those patients in whom aggressive therapy will be of no avail and also as a means to further delineate the ability of these measurements to aid the clinical examination in predicting outcome. Greenberg and his associates have been at the fore in utilizing these techniques for prediction.[4,5,10,11] They have demonstrated, using a grading system for evoked responses, that significant abnormalities in somatosensory evoked responses are almost always associated with a poor outcome and that approximately 20 percent of patients with head injuries who reach the hospital alive have irreversible brain stem injuries and are likely to die or to do very poorly. By correlating the evoked response data with postmortem examination of both hemispheres and of the brain stem, this group has begun to demonstrate, in a very elegant way, that (1) brain stem injuries are more common as a primary cause of deterioration than was previously thought, (2) deterioration in neurological function from medical complications can be detected by multimodality evoked responses, and (3) a combination of evoked response measurements is more useful than the measurement of one modality alone.

Abnormal brain stem auditory evoked responses are an extremely reliable indicator of a poor outcome, unless brain stem compression is the cause of the abnormality and can be reversed rapidly. However, the presence of intact brain stem auditory evoked responses is a much less useful predictive tool because they tend to be relatively robust, and therefore are unreliable in predicting a good outcome.

In the future, a combination of multimodality evoked responses, with continuous recording of the EEG using computerized techniques, will probably further enhance our predictive abilities. Karnaze et al. have shown that the presence of monotonous, low-amplitude, slow-frequency activity on the somnogram, which is an all-night recording of brain cortical electrical activity, is indicative of an adverse outcome and correlates quite nicely with multimodality evoked response abnormalities.[6]

The Future of Outcome Prediction

As electrophysiological monitoring becomes increasingly more applicable, these techniques, in concert with ICP measurements, CT scanning, and, of course, the clinical examination, will allow for an increasingly improved prediction of the level of outcome. This is very important. As resources become scarce, decisions regarding the length of aggressive support for patients with severe head injuries will need to be determined at the earliest possible time. As the National Traumatic Coma Data Bank begins to develop predictive data from the large number of patients studied, these issues shall be addressed. It is apparent that in patients of advanced age, with GCS scores of 7 or less, the outcome is almost always poor. What is not obvious is what the outcome will be for similar patients who are much younger and in whom the clinical examination clearly is not powerful enough to yield reliable outcome predictions. It is in this group of patients that we must concentrate our efforts in an attempt to identify those factors which will lead us to accurate predictions at the earliest possible time.

An information base which includes the results of the clinical examination, serial electrophysiological assessments, the initial CT scan, and, where indicated, ICP measurements is likely to yield a significant improvement in predictions of outcome for patients in whom the outcome is not obvious from the clinical examination alone. It is important to recognize that prediction requires a very high degree of specificity and sensitivity. It is unsatisfactory to identify all patients who will do poorly but to include in such a group some patients who ultimately will do well. The clinical examination has not been adequate to allow such sensitivity.

Whether the use of the combined techniques described here will achieve the accuracy of prediction required is not yet known. However, such accuracy seems to be an achievable objective.

References

1. Adams JH, Graham DI, Murray LS, Scott G: Diffuse axonal injury due to nonmissile head injury in humans: An analysis of 45 cases. Ann Neurol 12:557–563, 1982.
2. Andrioli GC, Zuccarello M, Trincia G, Pardatscher K, Mingrino S: The significance of cerebral contusions. Presented at the International Conference on Recent Advances in Neurotraumatology, Edinburgh, 1982.
3. Gennarelli TA, Thibault LE, Adams JH, Graham DI, Thompson CJ, Marcincin RP: Diffuse axonal injury and traumatic coma in the primate. Ann Neurol 12:564–574, 1982.
4. Greenberg RP, Becker DP, Miller JD, Mayer DJ: Evaluation of brain function in severe human head trauma with multimodality evoked potentials. Part 2: Localization of brain dysfunction and correlation with posttraumatic neurological conditions. J Neurosurg 47:163–177, 1977.
5. Greenberg RP, Newlon PG, Hyatt MS, Narayan RK, Becker DP: Prognostic implications of early multimodality evoked potentials in severely head-injured patients: A prospective study. J Neurosurg 55:227–236, 1981.
6. Karnaze DS, Marshall LF, McCarthy CS, Klauber MR, Bickford RG: Localizing and prognostic value of auditory evoked responses in coma after closed head injury. Neurology (NY) 32: 299–302, 1982.
7. Marshall LF, Smith RW, Shapiro HM: The outcome with aggressive treatment in severe head injuries, Part II. J Neurosurg 50:26–30, 1979.
8. Marshall LF, Toole BM, Bowers SA: The National Traumatic Coma Data Bank. Part 2: Patients who talk and deteriorate: Implications for treatment. J Neurosurg 59:285–288, 1983.
9. Miller JD, Becker DP, Ward JD, Sullivan HG, Adams WE, Rosner MJ: Significance of intracranial hypertension in severe head injury. J Neurosurg 47: 503–516, 1977.
10. Newlon PG, Greenberg RP, Hyatt MS, Enas GG, Becker DP: The dynamics of neuronal dysfunction and recovery following severe head injury assessed with serial multimodality evoked potentials. J Neurosurg 57:168–177, 1982.
11. Rosenblum WI, Greenberg RP, Seelig JM, Becker DP: Midbrain lesions: Frequent and significant prognostic feature in closed head injury. Neurosurgery 9:613–620, 1981.
12. Seelig JM, Becker DP, Miller JD, Greenberg RP, Ward JD, Choi SC: Traumatic acute subdural hematoma: Major mortality reduction in comatose patients treated within four hours. N Engl J Med 304:1511–1518, 1981.
13. Teasdale E, Teasdale G, Cardoso E, Galbraith S, Graham DI, Adams JIH, Doyle D: CT scan correlations in severe diffuse head injury. Presented at the International Conference on Recent Advances in Neurotraumatology, Edinburgh, 1982.
14. Teasdale G, Jennett B: Assessment of coma and impaired consciousness: A practical scale. Lancet 2:81–84, 1974.

197
Minor Head Injury: Management and Outcome

Rebecca W. Rimel
John A. Jane

Minor head injury can be defined in many ways, ranging from loss of consciousness requiring hospitalization to lacerations of the scalp and face that clearly do not affect the brain. In a study conducted by the National Center for Health Statistics, the total number of injuries to the head occurring in the United States was estimated to be in excess of 8 million per annum.[9] The number of patients who experience loss of consciousness or post-traumatic amnesia (that is, the number of patients at risk for the consequences of minor head injury) may be approximately 1.5 to 2 million per year.

Much energy and many resources have been expended in studying the treatment and eventual outcome of severely head-injured patients. However, the number of surviving patients in this group is quite small when compared with the number of persons sustaining minor head injuries. Data collected on the complete spectrum of head trauma at our institution demonstrate that only a quarter of all injuries fall into the severe group and only one-half of these patients survive their injuries. In contrast, minor head injury, as defined subsequently in this paper, constitutes over 50 percent of all injuries. Many patients after such injuries show a decrease in their ability to perform in everyday life situations. In view of the problems experienced by some patients following what seemed to be an insignificant injury, minor head trauma presents a major health and socioeconomic problem. In light of this, the problem of minor head injury needs to be better defined, the morbidity experienced by these patients quantified, and possible treatment regimens evaluated with the hope of helping patients to better cope with their residual difficulties, and to allow them to resume daily life activities quickly and effectively.

Definition of Minor Head Injury

Changes in the level of consciousness constitute the earliest sign of neurological deterioration following head injury. Unfortunately, meaningful evaluation of this parameter of neurological function has been hampered by the use of unstandardized and purely descriptive terminology. In order to quantitatively designate the severity of head injury and predict outcome, Teasdale and Jennett developed the Glasgow coma scale.[7] Briefly, the Glasgow coma scale (GCS) is a 13-point scale, ranging from 3 through 15, divided into three categories of neurological responsiveness: eye opening, verbal responses, and motor responses. This scale has become a standardized method of grading severity of neurological deficit with reproducibility among observers.[6] A score of 15 is normal.

In 1978 we divided head injury into three categories basic to the Glasgow coma scale. The categories were defined as severe, with a GCS score of 3 to 8 (comatose patients by definition); moderate, with a GCS score of 9 to 12; and minor, with a GCS score of 13 to 15. In a previous report we described the demographics and outcome of patients with minor head injury on the basis of the above GCS criteria.[5] Much of the data reported herein are taken from that report and our ongoing research efforts in this group of patients. Our current data base includes 1800 patients with minor head injury, all of whom have been admitted to our medical center since 1977.

Patients with minor head injuries differ significantly in terms of demographic characteristics from the more severely injured. Patients with minor head injury are slightly younger (mean age, 27), with most being between 11 and 20 years of age. The percentage of males is lower (66 percent) than in the patients with severe injuries. Employment is also correlated with severity in that the patients with minor injuries have a higher job status and lower overall unemployment rate. The group with the highest risk for minor injuries is composed of students. The incidence of previous head injury is 27 percent among the patients with minor injuries compared with 46 percent in the severe group. This poses an interesting question which has been raised by others about the susceptibility of the brain to more severe injuries after multiple insults.

Chronic alcohol abuse and acute intoxication seem to be a somewhat smaller problem in patients with minor injuries but still very prevalent. In our series, 47 percent of the patients with minor injuries were drinking at the time of their injury. The confounding effect of alcohol on the findings of the neurological examination presents a real challenge for the neurosurgeon. However, our preliminary studies indicate that a positive blood alcohol level between 0.01 and 0.20 mg/100 ml only changes the GCS score 1 point. Therefore a positive alcohol level should not be the deciding factor in discharging the patient from the emergency department if the patient has an altered sensorium.

Higher-velocity trauma such as auto accidents and assaults is more prevalent as a cause of severe injuries, whereas falls and sporting accidents account for a larger percentage of the minor injuries. In general, patients sustaining minor injuries are a relatively homogenous group with similar demographic characteristics. Their differences from, and similarities to patients with more severe injuries are not well understood because researchers have focused most of their efforts on understanding severe injury and have elected to subdivide patients into an increasing number of categories. In our preoccupation with subdividing the population, we have overlooked the fact that head injury is a continuum and much can be learned about the epidemiology, treatment, and outcome by looking at the entire spectrum of trauma, much of which has been neglected in the past.

Management of Minor Head Injuries

Most neurosurgeons in the past have thought that recovery from minor head trauma was uneventful. Although there is an admitted incidence of so-called postconcussion syndrome, this is frequently assumed to be of a nonorganic basis. Indeed, there has been a great deal of debate over admission policies for patients with such injuries,[2,3] mainly because of concern over the development of an intracranial hematoma. A review of our own experience has clearly indicated that the problems encountered by these patients are considerable; however, rarely do they require neurosurgical intervention.

Our admission policy for head trauma requires that all patients sustaining trauma that results in loss of consciousness be admitted for observation. At the time of admission, each patient is seen by a member of the neurosurgical staff and given a neurological examination and Glasgow coma scale score. In addition, skull films are obtained. There is a great deal of debate over the value and economic justification of x-ray films of the skull in these patients. In our study, 5 percent of patients with a minor head injury had a skull fracture diagnosed by skull films. Given the difficulty in obtaining an accurate history due to poor patient cooperation or the confounding effects of alcohol ingestion, we think that there is a definite indication for these studies. The potential for the early diagnosis of an epidural hematoma is also possible with the availability of such studies.

Computed tomographic (CT) scans are only obtained in those patients in whom assessment is complicated by a very high blood alcohol level or the use of other drugs, or in patients who deteriorate after admission. The diagnostic benefit of "preventive scanning" cannot be justified in light of the costs.

The issue of admission versus nonadmission of patients with minor head injury has not been resolved. The admission criteria may be based on the individual policy of the neurosurgeon in charge, the emergency department protocol, or the availability of beds. It is mandatory that a minor head injury victim have close supervision for 24 to 48 h following injury. Whether adequate monitoring of the patient's condition can be performed on an outpatient basis may depend on the availability of appropriate personnel such as family or friends, the distance from the hospital, the mechanism of injury, the use of drugs, and a history of previous injuries.

Rigid triage criteria do not exist simply because therapy must be individualized. In addition, the therapeutic and diagnostic resources of different medical communities vary. We have developed the following minor head injury triage classifications; however, they should be viewed only as a flexible guideline[8]:

1. Patients sustaining a scalp injury without symptoms or signs of craniocerebral injury can be safely discharged with appropriate observation instructions. The obvious exceptions include those patients who suffer major blood loss from scalp lacerations and those whose scalp wounds cannot be closed satisfactorily in the emergency department.

2. The debate over admission revolves around the asymptomatic patient whose concussion has resolved by the time of presentation in the emergency department. Such patients are fully ambulatory and conversant, appear to be completely normal according to a neurological exam, and usually complain of little more than a mild headache. Ideally, such patients might be admitted for overnight observation, but alternatively they can be discharged from the emergency department provided they can spend the night near the hospital with a responsible adult who has access to transportation. Both the patient and the adult with whom the patient will be staying should be warned to return to the hospital if increasing headache, vomiting, or obtundation supervenes.

The following patients with minor head injury should always be admitted for observation:

1. Patients with unresolved concussion. Such patients should be admitted for observation until they are fully oriented and can consistently demonstrate normal immediate recall and recent memory. They need not remain in the hospital until the headache resolves provided that the headache is diminishing. Most patients in this category can be discharged within 48 h.

2. Preschool children, even if the results of the neurological examination are normal. Patients in this age group often react atypically to head trauma. Intermittent somnolence, agitation when aroused, and vomiting are seen after both trivial and major injuries. The degree of severity of head injury is usually apparent after a day of observation.

As reflected in the above discussion, it is evident that the issue of admission to the hospital following minor head trauma is of considerable importance. In our current research we are evaluating various treatment alternatives for minor head trauma, one of which is nonhospitalization. By following various cases we can compare hospitalization versus nonhospitalization alternatives as well as community or regional hospitalization versus triage to a major university-based medical center and its possible consequences. In this way, we can address the issue of who should be admitted and the consequences of admission versus nonadmission alternatives on economic and social outcomes.

Outcome Following Minor Head Injury

Patients who sustain minor head injuries are usually discharged from the hospital within 48 h and told to resume normal activity within several days. Until recently the significant morbidity experienced by these patients was unrecognized except for the occasional patient returning for further treatment to the neurosurgeon. The problems experienced by patients with minor head injury are probably not unique to persons sustaining various types of trauma. Often patients are discharged from the hospital after the physical examination shows they have returned to normal, and it is presumed that they return quickly to their previous lifestyle. The patients are unwilling to discuss problems for fear of being accused of malingering. This sequence of events often leads to an accentuation of problems which might have resolved quickly with appropriate counseling.

In our experience with 538 patients with minor head injury, we found that over half were experiencing difficulties with their lives 3 months after injury. The majority of patients had headaches, and more than half of the patients complained of memory deficits. One-third of the patients who were gainfully employed before injury were unemployed 3 months later.[5]

Three reasons for persistent problems after minor injuries bear discussion: (1) residua of organic brain damage produced by the injury; (2) a quest for secondary gain; and (3) psychological reactions to the injury. Most patients in our studies scored lower than their expected norms on standardized neuropsychological testing, with the principal problems being cognitive deficits in the spheres of attention, concentration, memory, and judgment, as described by other authors. This raises the question of the extent to which the intellectual and other impairments demonstrated on the neuropsychological tests in the unemployed patients were due to the consequences of the minor head injury and were responsible, in part at least, for the unemployment of these patients and the extent to which they were a reflection of the large influences that education and motivation seem to have on social functioning.

One of the most important questions still unanswered is the incidence and importance of organic brain damage in patients who are rendered unconscious by a blow to the head. Studies by Jane and Gennarelli et al. have documented organic damage in the monkey following minor head injuries.[1] Two monkeys were injured in the Philadelphia injury apparatus and were both awake 2 min following their injury and appeared normal thereafter. At 7 days, they were perfused. Examination of their brains revealed no abnormality on either gross or cut section, and all stains were perfectly normal. However, when the Fink-Heimer technique for degenerating axons was applied to these brains, striking degeneration was noted in the brain stem reticular formation. These findings support the contention that minor head injury can be associated with organic damage to the nervous system. They also suggest, at least in the acceleration model, that the first injury to occur is in the brain stem rather than in the cortex and that shearing of axons is a major pathological event. A great deal of work remains to be done in this area to further document these findings. With such a model, recovery curves could be developed with respect to organic damage, and the structural effects of multiple injuries could be measured.

A second possible reason for persistent morbidity and failure to return to work is litigation related to the accident itself and compensation for the injuries. In our studies as well as others, evidence does not support the fact that insurance claims or litigation is a significant factor in prolonged morbidity. Nevertheless, the effects of these issues on recovery from minor head injury require further investigation.

The third potential cause for so much disability in these patients and for even greater disability in the unemployed compared with the employed patients is emotional stress caused by persistent symptoms and the psychological response to those symptoms. Patients with minor head injury may sustain organic brain damage that causes problems in attention, concentration, memory, and judgment. For the most part, they recognize these symptoms and are disturbed by them. The disturbance is all the greater because the patient may have been assured at discharge that the injury was inconsequential and that therefore the recovery should be immediate and complete. Neither the patients nor their families understand why they are continuing to have so much difficulty, and the harder the patients try, the more anxious and frustrated they become. In time the patients may become incapacitated by their psychological responses to their injuries even though the organic effects may have largely disappeared.

Conclusions

The relationships between health care practitioners and patients are powerful instruments that can either facilitate or retard patients' social functioning, sense of personal worth or potential, and even motivation or willingness to struggle against demands imposed by illness or injury. Whatever fears or anxieties patients may have during recovery and rehabilitation, how they view themselves in relation to illness or injury, and what confidence they have in their ability to negotiate their social environment may be heavily influenced by the practitioner-patient relationship. Although the treatment of choice is not known for patients with minor head injury, the practitioner must be aware of the sequelae which follow the injury and, where possible, provide the necessary counseling and support. Many have recognized the importance of psychological components in the treatment of these patients and have proposed ways to ameliorate psychological problems, including "active treatment," encouragement, and sympathetic reassurance. It has also been suggested that "better doctoring" throughout the management of patients with minor head injury can prevent considerable morbidity.[2] Although neurosurgeons will continue to be the primary physicians involved in the acute management of head-injured patients, the sequelae experienced by patients after minor head injury might be more efficiently addressed by other physicians, given the large number of patients and the nature of their problems.

Langfitt and Gennarelli discussed the need to "examine the influence of each one of a substantial number of variables on the outcome from head injury before concluding that any one of them is more important than the other."[4] This is true for the complete spectrum of head injury, from the most severe injuries to the minor injuries, the topic of this discussion. A greater understanding of the natural history and evolution of head injury will be gained by evaluating the epidemiology, pathology, and outcome over the entire continuum of injury in clinical and laboratory studies. This, coupled with the large number of patients sustaining minor head injuries and the amount of disability such injuries can cause in the individual patient, makes it imperative that we develop a better understanding of the problem of minor head injury.

References

1. Jane JA, Rimel RW, Pobereskin LH, Tyson GW, Steward O, Gennarelli TA: Outcome and pathology of head injury, in Grossman RG, Gildenberg PL (eds): *Head Injury: Basic and Clinical Aspects* (Seminars in Neurological Surgery Series). New York, Raven Press, 1982, pp 229–237.
2. Jennett B: The problem of mild head injury. Practitioner 221:77–82, 1978.
3. Jennett B, Galbraith SL: Head injury and admission policy. Lancet 1:552, 1979.
4. Langfitt TW, Gennarelli TA: Can the outcome from head injury be improved? J Neurosurg 56:19–25, 1982.
5. Rimel RW, Giordani B, Barth JT, Boll TJ, Jane JA: Disability caused by minor head injury. Neurosurgery 9:221–228, 1981.
6. Rimel RW, Jane JA, Edlich RF: An injury severity scale for comprehensive management of central nervous system trauma. JACEP 8:64–67, 1979.
7. Teasdale G, Jennett B: Assessment of coma and impaired consciousness: A practical scale. Lancet 2:81–84, 1974.
8. Tyson GW, Rimel RW, Winn HR, Butler AB, Jane JA: *Acute Care of the Head and Spinal Cord Injured Patient in the Emergency Department*. Charlottesville, Va, University of Virginia Press, 1978.
9. Wilder CS: *Data from Health Interview Survey*. Rockville, Md, National Center for Health Statistics, Department of Health, Education, and Welfare, 1976.

198

Scalp Injuries

William J. Barwick

The scalp is a specialized structure of skin, muscle, and fascia which is unique. In addition to providing coverage for the cranium, it contains some 100,000 hairs, which in addition to their esthetic value, also provide a form of insulation.

The superficial location of the scalp makes it first in line for injuries to the head by a variety of physical and chemical agents. Injuries to the scalp vary from minor lacerations to total loss, either by scalping or by burning.

The ability to treat severe scalp injuries has been enhanced by recent developments in musculocutaneous flaps and microsurgery. Injuries which would have been fatal 100 years ago can now be handled with relative ease. This chapter will present a general overview of the anatomy of the scalp and the treatment of scalp injuries and defects.

Anatomy

General Considerations

A sound working knowledge of the anatomy of the scalp is necessary to treat scalp injuries effectively. The scalp extends from the supraorbital ridges to the inferior nuchal line. Laterally it extends to the auriculocephalic angle. In most individuals, the scalp is completely covered with hair except for the anterior portion, which is the forehead.

In cross section, the scalp contains five distinct layers (Fig. 198-1). The skin of the scalp is the thickest in the body, making it a good, if infrequently used, donor site for split-thickness skin grafts. Immediately subjacent to this is a layer of dense fibrofatty tissue into which the roots of the hair extend. In the deep portion of this layer are the main blood vessels which supply the scalp. Just beneath this is the galea aponeurotica which forms a continuous layer of tough fascia connecting the anterior, posterior, and lateral parts of the epicranius muscle. The epicranius muscle has two main divisions: the occipitofrontalis and temporoparietalis. Both the occipital and frontal portions of the occipitofrontalis consist of a pair of broad quadrilateral muscles which are continuous with the galea. These muscles act to move the scalp forward and backward. The frontal portion also elevates the eyebrows and wrinkles the skin of the forehead. The epicranius muscle is innervated by branches of the seventh cranial nerve.

The first three layers of the scalp are firmly adherent to one another and may be considered as a single unit. Beneath the galea is a layer of loose areolar tissue. This tissue can be easily separated and is the plane in which scalp flaps are raised and scalp avulsions occur. The final layer is the pericranium, which is firmly adherent to the skull, particularly at the sutures.

Vascular Anatomy

The creation of dependable scalp flaps as well as the repair of avulsion injuries to the scalp requires a thorough knowledge of its blood supply. Blood is supplied to the scalp through terminal branches of the internal and external carotid arteries. Five major arteries enter the scalp on each side, anastomosing freely with each other and with the opposite side (Fig. 198-2). The anterior portion is supplied by the supraorbital and supratrochlear (frontal) arteries, which are branches of the ophthalmic artery. These vessels pass around the supraorbital ridge into the frontalis muscle and supply the skin of the forehead.

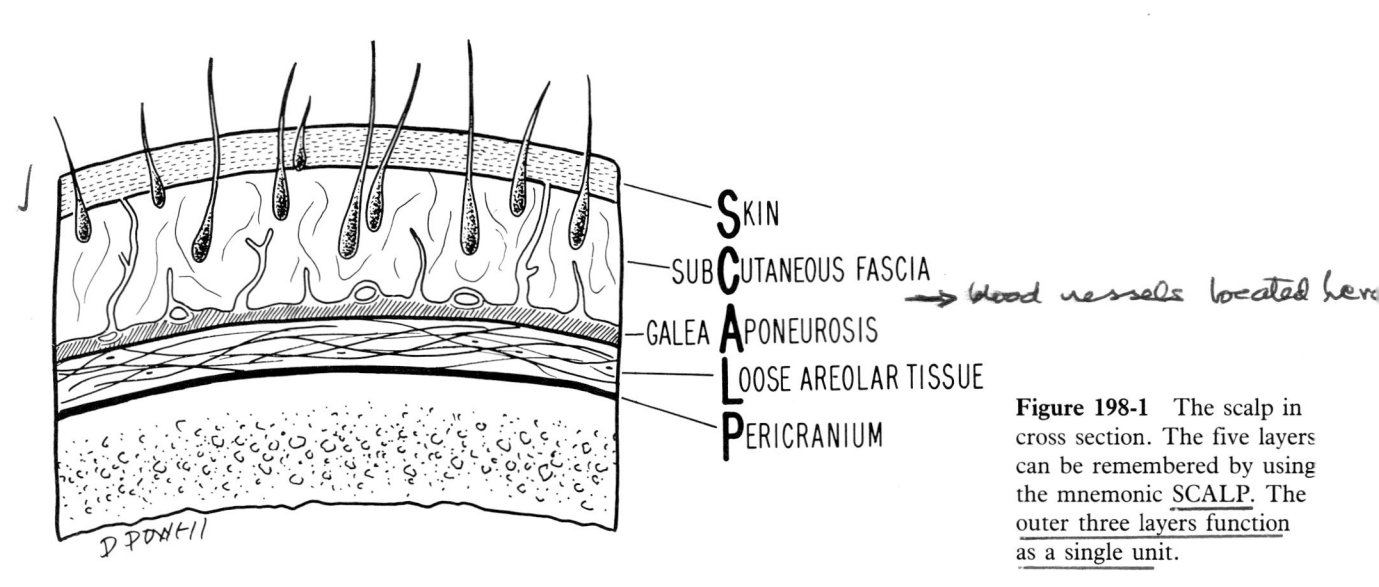

Figure 198-1 The scalp in cross section. The five layers can be remembered by using the mnemonic SCALP. The outer three layers function as a single unit.

Scalp Injuries

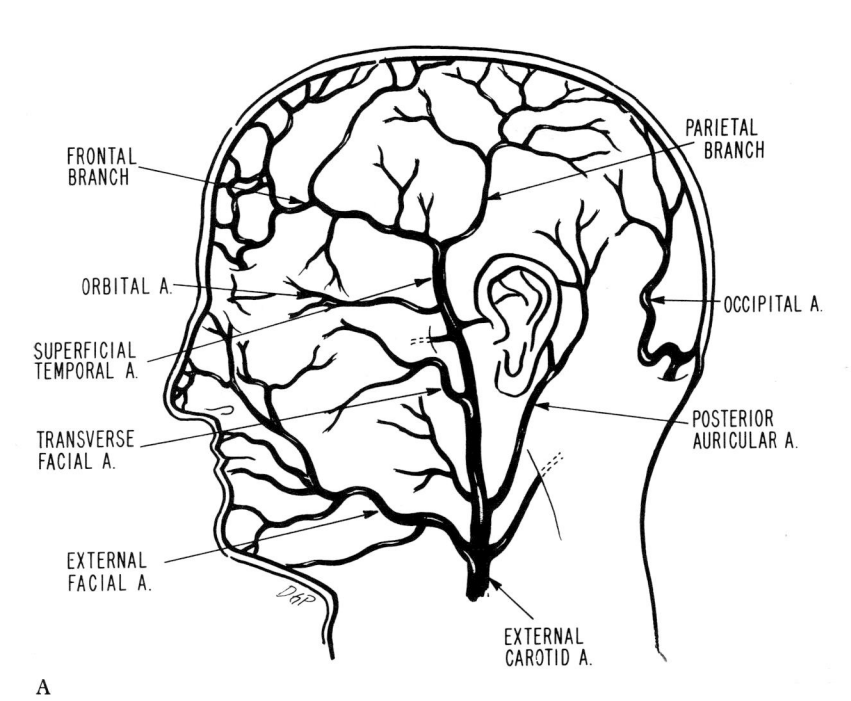

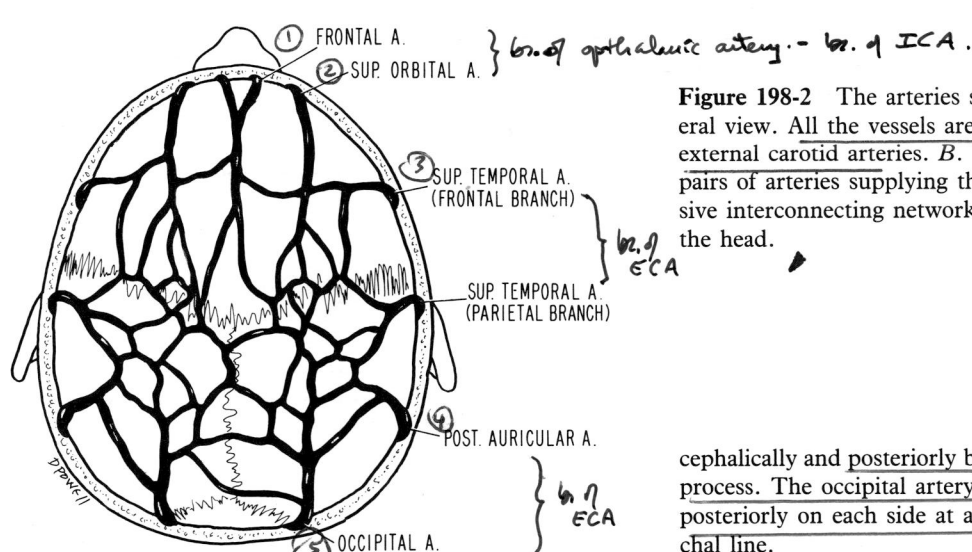

Figure 198-2 The arteries supplying the scalp. *A.* Lateral view. All the vessels are branches of the internal and external carotid arteries. *B.* Vertex view, showing the five pairs of arteries supplying the scalp. There is an extensive interconnecting network of vessels across the top of the head.

The major vessel entering laterally is the superficial temporal artery, one of the two terminal branches of the external carotid. The superficial temporal is the largest artery supplying the scalp and is the most useful for anastomosis in scalp replantation. This artery passes over the zygoma anterior to the tragus. At approximately the level of the superior pole of the ear, the artery divides into an anterior (frontal) branch and a posterior (parietal) branch. The frontal branch joins with branches of the supraorbital artery, and the parietal branch anastomoses freely with the posterior auricular and occipital arteries.

The posterior portion of the scalp is supplied by two branches of the external carotid artery: the posterior auricular artery and the occipital artery. The posterior auricular artery is a small branch of the external carotid which passes cephalically and posteriorly behind the ear over the mastoid process. The occipital artery is larger and enters the scalp posteriorly on each side at approximately the superior nuchal line.

After entering the scalp, the arteries form an extensive interconnecting network of vessels across the most cephalic portion of the scalp (Fig. 198-2B). The vessels are located in the deep portion of the fibrofatty layer of the scalp just above the galea. It is convenient therefore to think of the scalp as having an axial pattern. Because of this fact, large scalp flaps can be developed without a prior delay procedure. In designing scalp flaps, however, one should attempt to base the flaps laterally and to include the major vessels where possible (Figs. 198-3 and 198-4). The use of a Doppler device is helpful here.

Nerve Supply

Sensation of the scalp is supplied by branches of the fifth cranial nerve anteriorly and by branches of dorsal rami of cervical nerves posteriorly. Anteriorly, the major cutaneous

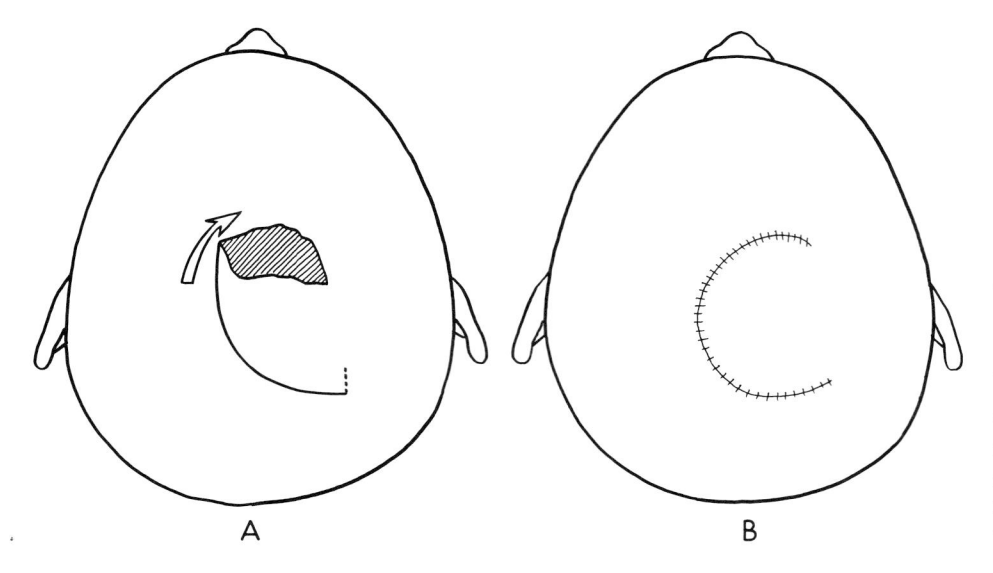

Figure 198-3 A simple rotation flap. *A.* Many defects in the scalp which are too large for primary approximation can be closed by a simple rotation flap. The dotted line indicates a back cut which may sometimes be necessary. *B.* If the rotation flap is large enough, the defect can be closed without using a skin graft.

nerves are the supraorbital and supratrochlear nerves, which are branches of the ophthalmic division of the fifth cranial nerve. These accompany the arteries of the same name and supply the scalp as far posteriorly as a line drawn across the top of the head from one ear to the other. Posterior to this line, the scalp is supplied by the greater and lesser occipital nerves and a portion of the greater auricular nerve, all branches of the dorsal rami of C2 through C4. The parietal area on both sides is supplied by the zygomaticotemporal nerve (a branch of the maxillary division of the fifth cranial nerve) and the auriculotemporal nerve (a branch of the mandibular division of the fifth cranial nerve).

Lymphatics

The lymphatic drainage of the scalp, in general, parallels the neurovascular supply. The lower portion of the forehead drains through the face into the submandibular nodes. The upper frontal and parietal areas drain into the superficial parotid group of nodes which are located superficial to the parotid gland, just in front of the tragus. Both the submandibular and superficial parotid nodes drain to the deep cervical nodes. The coronal and occipital portions of the scalp drain to the retroauricular nodes and then to the superficial cervical nodes. Thus it can be seen that the anterior portion of the scalp drains to the deep cervical nodes and the posterior part of the scalp drains to the superficial cervical nodes. The watershed runs generally along a line which passes from the superior pole of one ear to the other.

Examination and Primary Care of Scalp Injuries

A consideration of the basic principles of trauma care is rarely more important than in the examination and treatment of scalp injuries. Injuries sufficient to damage the scalp may also damage the underlying skull. Injuries to the scalp

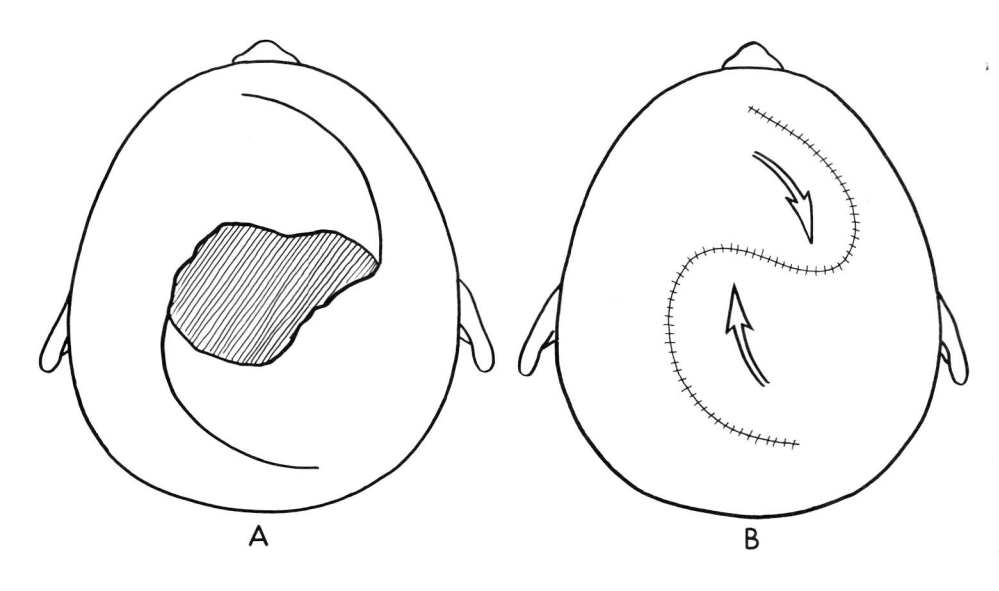

Figure 198-4 Larger defects (*A*) can be closed using multiple rotation flaps (*B*). The base of each flap should include major arteries if possible.

are usually obvious and spectacular injuries, but it should be kept firmly in mind that they may not be the most lethal injuries. A complete examination of the whole patient is mandatory since life-threatening, but perhaps less obvious, injuries of the chest or abdomen take precedence over scalp lacerations. As with any trauma to the head and neck, attention should be given to the possibility of cervical spine injuries. If there is any question of injury to this area, a cross-table lateral x-ray film of the cervical spine should be obtained before the patient is moved.

All examinations of scalp wounds should be performed using sterile technique. Many times an underlying skull fracture can be palpated in the depths of a scalp laceration.

Because of the rich blood supply to the scalp, there may be copious bleeding. In the absence of an underlying skull fracture, the best method to control scalp bleeding is pressure directly over the wound. The pressure should be firm and continuous, and one should resist the temptation to keep dabbing at the wound. Because of the tendency for scalp wounds to gape, many irregular lacerations give the initial impression that tissue has been lost. However, after cleaning and sorting out the jigsaw puzzle, one frequently finds that most of the tissue is present. Most scalp injuries can be dealt with immediately, but it is possible to delay closure of scalp wounds for up to 24 h if necessary if the patient is in poor condition or if other more life-threatening injuries are present.[4]

Lacerations

Lacerations of the scalp can take many forms. They may be small and linear, which can make them difficult to detect beneath matted, blood-soaked hair, or they may be large and stellate, giving the often erroneous impression that tissue is missing. Because of the amount of tension in the galea, wounds which include this layer tend to gape considerably. This tendency of the galea to retract offers a form of protection, however. Since the main blood vessels are located in the subcutaneous fascia, they do not contract. If the galea is lacerated, however, the contraction of this layer will cause retraction of the vessels also. Thus superficial lacerations with the galea intact may bleed more profusely than deep lacerations with the galea cut.

The best technique for stopping bleeding in scalp lacerations is circumferential pressure of the surrounding scalp against the skull. One should always make sure that no underlying skull fracture is present. In very large and gaping wounds, another useful technique is to place clamps on the galea and draw this back over the dermis, thereby compressing the vessels.

Most simple lacerations can be closed under local anesthesia. Scalp lacerations should be closed in two layers. The first layer approximates the galea and should be done with an absorbable suture such as one of polyglycolic acid. The galea is the strongest layer of the scalp and should always be repaired if possible. It is unnecessary to place other stitches in the subcutaneous fascia. The skin is then closed with monofilament nylon suture. Interrupted or running sutures may be used, and one should take fairly healthy bits of tissue on each side of the wound. Varying the depth of the stitch from one side of the wound to the other can help make the skin edges come together evenly.

In the case of extensive and stellate lacerations, or in very young children, it is necessary to use general anesthesia in the operating room. Because of the rich blood supply, extensive debridement is both unnecessary and unwise, but all obviously devitalized tissue should be removed. Following closure, a compression dressing is helpful, particularly if there has been undermining of the subgaleal space, since subgaleal hematomas may take weeks to resorb. Drains beneath the galea are rarely necessary. Sutures should remain in place 7 to 10 days.

Avulsions

Avulsions of the scalp usually occur in the loose areolar tissue between the galea and pericranium. Most scalp avulsions occur when a portion of hair is pulled at a tangential angle (Fig. 198-5). If hair is pulled perpendicularly away from the skull, this may result in avulsion of hair only.

The treatment of scalp avulsions depends in large part on the amount of scalp avulsed. If the defect is small, it can be repaired using either single or multiple rotation flaps (Figs. 198-3 and 198-4). Many times the wounds can be closed without leaving a donor defect which requires grafting. When constructing either single or multiple flaps in the scalp, additional length can be obtained by carefully incising the galea with parallel cuts on the underside of the flap and allowing the flap to expand like an accordion. Extreme care should be taken when performing this maneuver, since the blood vessels are located just above the galea.

If the defect is too large for multiple rotation flaps, and the avulsed segment too badly damaged for replantation, a skin graft should be applied if the pericranium is intact. This will provide wound coverage and prevent desiccation and infection of the tissues and will allow more definitive reconstruction at a later date. Split-thickness skin grafts take readily on pericranium, due to its excellent blood supply. Skin grafts may be harvested from any suitable donor site, such as the anterior thigh. However, with scalp avulsions that are too large for closure with local scalp tissue, every attempt should be made to replant the avulsed scalp using microvascular surgical techniques.

Replantation of an Avulsed Scalp

Total avulsion of the scalp has declined in frequency since the closure of the western frontier, but the injury still occurs as a result of industrial or other types of accidents. Before the age of microvascular surgery, many scalp avulsions were treated by simply replacing the scalp as a free graft. The success rate with this form of treatment was dismally low, with perhaps only one successful case having been reported without the use of vascular anastomoses.[6] The first reported successful replantation of a scalp using microvascular anastomoses was reported in 1976.[8] Since then, there have been

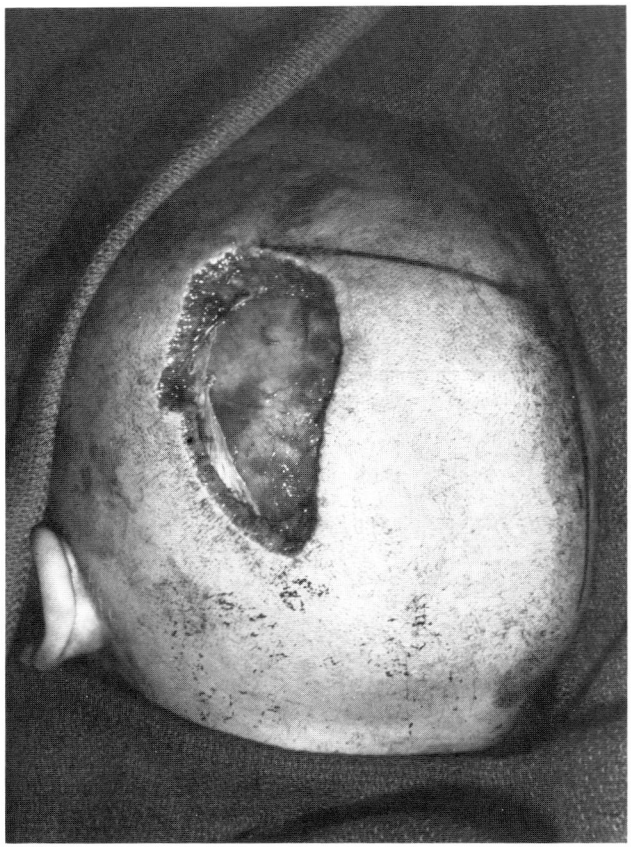

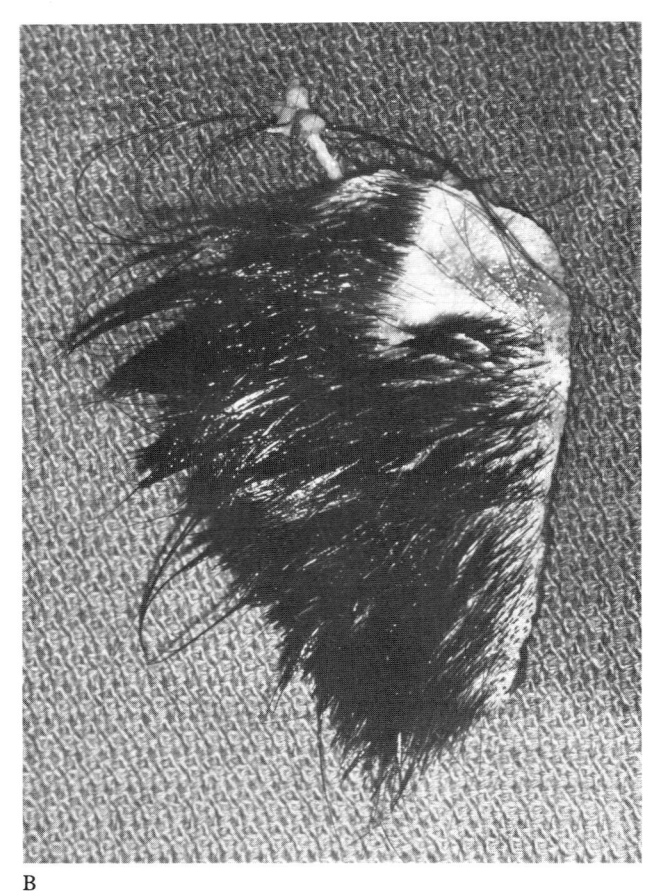

Figure 198-5 Avulsion of a portion of the scalp after the hair was caught in machinery. *A.* A rotation flap for closure has been outlined. *B.* The avulsed portion of scalp. The hair was pulled tangentially. If the pull had been perpendicular, this would have resulted in avulsion of the hair only.

some 10 reported cases of microvascular replantation of the scalp which have been successful.[1] The percentage of scalp loss has varied from 20 to 100 percent, with only three cases of successful replantation of a greater than 90 percent avulsion.

Despite the difficulties inherent in doing scalp replantations, it should now be considered the procedure of choice with significant scalp avulsions, since the alternatives are much less satisfactory, both physiologically and aesthetically. The principles and technique of scalp replantation can be best illustrated by a representative case.

Figure 198-6 shows a previously unreported case of total avulsion of the scalp and a portion of the right ear. The patient worked near machinery which rotated at high speed. She had long hair, which she kept in a ponytail. The ponytail became caught in the rotating machinery, resulting in total avulsion of the scalp from the eyebrows to the occipital area. The scalp was packed with ice and transported with the patient to the hospital, where she arrived approximately 4 h after the injury. While the patient was being resuscitated in the emergency department, the avulsed scalp was immediately transferred to the operating room. The scalp was first shaved and cleansed on an ice table. The superficial temporal vessels on each side were dissected out until normal vessel was found.

At the completion of this preparation, the patient had arrived in the operating room and was anesthetized. The proximal superficial temporal vessels were then dissected out on both sides and the scalp tacked in place with several stay sutures. Although in many cases of digital replantation it is advisable to repair the veins first, in most scalp avulsions, it is advisable to repair the artery first, due to the long ischemia time. In this case, the superficial temporal artery on the side of the avulsed ear was repaired first. Following this repair, the scalp immediately became pink, as did the avulsed ear. A demonstration that a single good artery can support the whole scalp was seen from the fact that after successful completion of the first arterial anastomosis, oxygenated blood and venous blood were seen coming from the opposite superficial temporal artery and vein. In this case, both superficial temporal arteries and veins were repaired. A vein graft was necessary for the left artery. No anticoagulants were used preoperatively or intraoperatively, but dextran, aspirin, and dipyridamole were given postoperatively. Early postoperative results are shown in Figs. 198-7 and 198-8.

Scalp Injuries

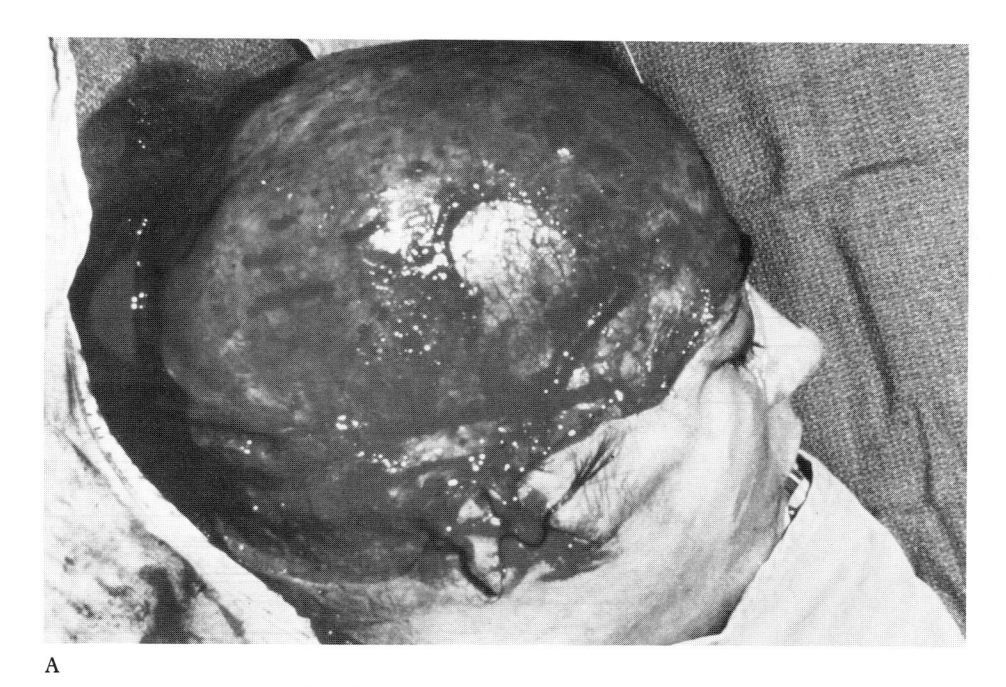

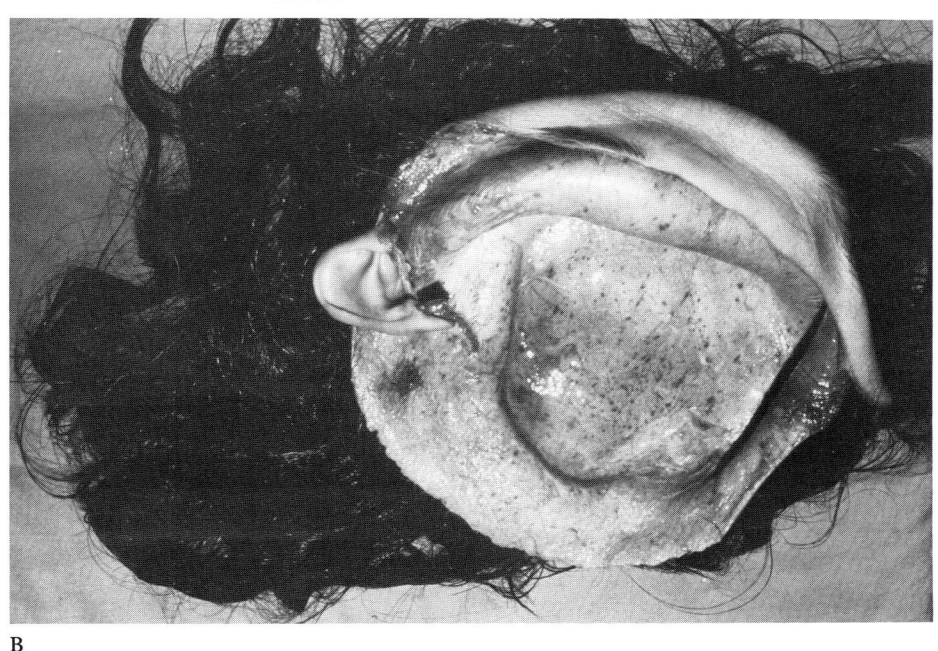

Figure 198-6 Total avulsion of the scalp and right ear from the eyebrows to the nuchal line. *A.* Note that the pericranium is intact. *B.* The avulsed scalp. The right ear and right eyebrow can be clearly seen.

A question that arises in scalp avulsions is whether one should attempt to repair the nerves. It is probably better not to do this, because the dissection necessary to isolate the nerves may put the already completed anastomoses at risk. After 1 year (Fig. 198-9) this patient had recovery of sensation to all areas except for a small spot on the very superior portion of the scalp.

In cases of extensive scalp avulsion in which the pericranium has also been avulsed and in which a scalp replantation is impossible, one must resort to other measures. Obviously a skin graft will not take on bare bone. Several techniques have stood the test of time for promoting the formation of granulation tissue which will accept a skin graft. One is to make multiple drill holes through the outer table of the skull into the diploic space (Fig. 198-10*A*). This will result in the development of granulation tissue, but the process may take several weeks or months. Another technique is to remove the outer table of the skull using an osteotome (Fig. 198-10*B*). In this case a skin graft may be applied immediately; however, hematomas are more common after immediate application of the graft, and it is usually advisable to wait several days until granulation tissue has formed.

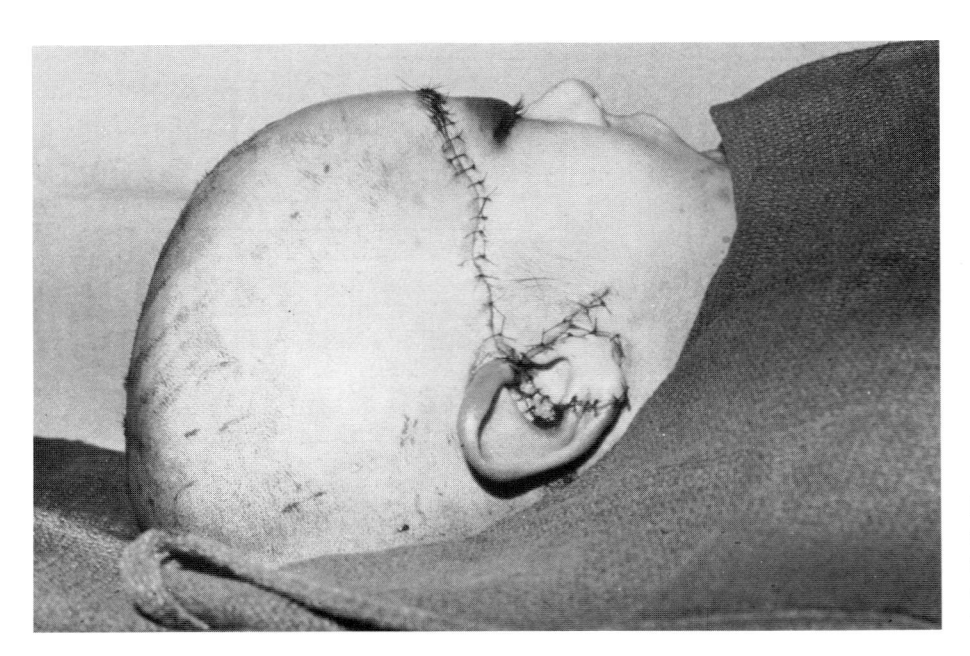

Figure 198-7 Immediately after operation the entire scalp and right ear are viable. Both superficial temporal vessels were anastomosed. ✓

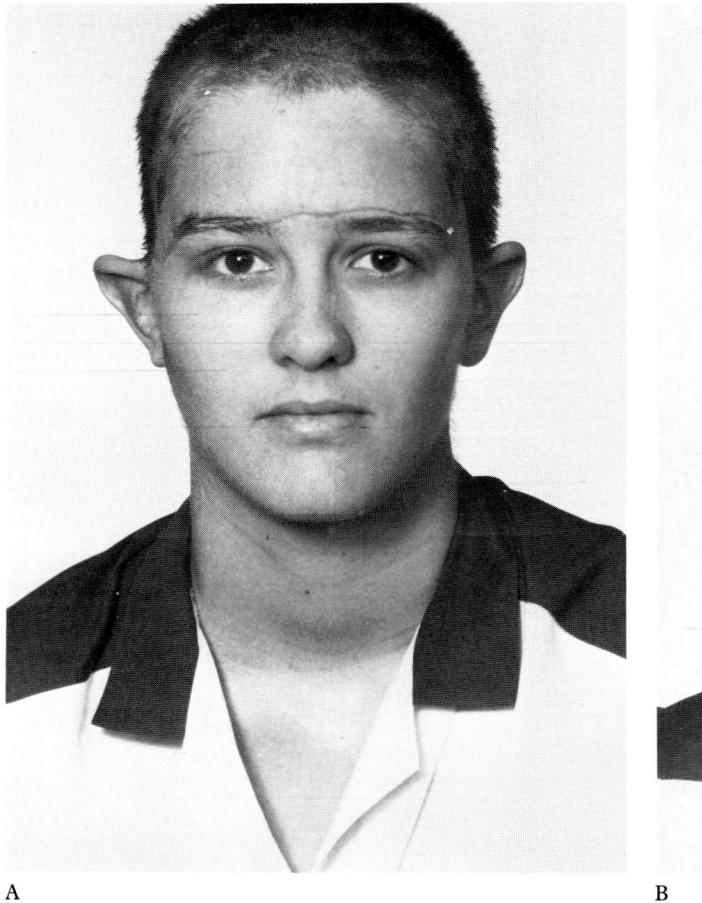

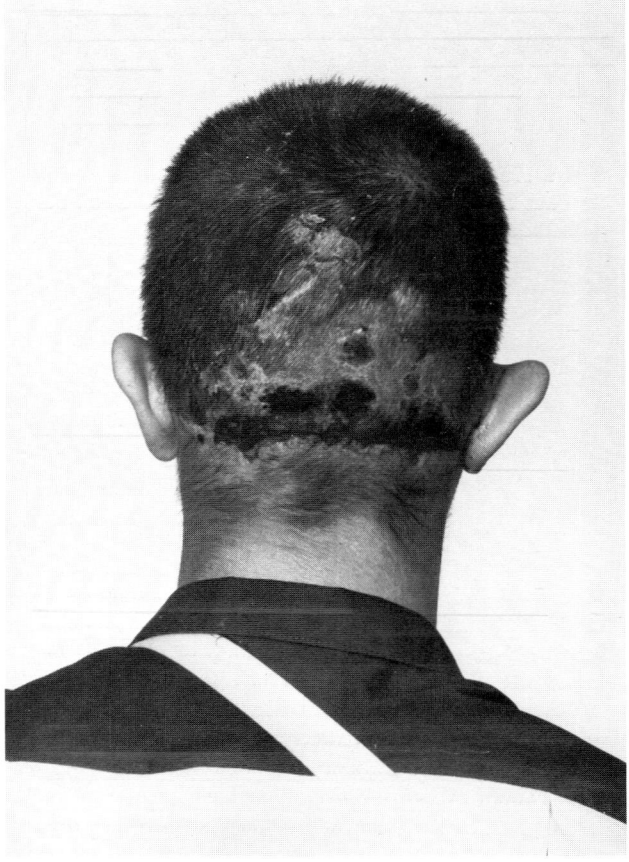

Figure 198-8 *A.* The patient 1 month after scalp replantation. The hair is already beginning to grow. *B.* A small amount of necrosis developed at the most posterior portion of the replanted scalp. This is because this portion of scalp was tangentially lacerated and is farthest from the blood supply.

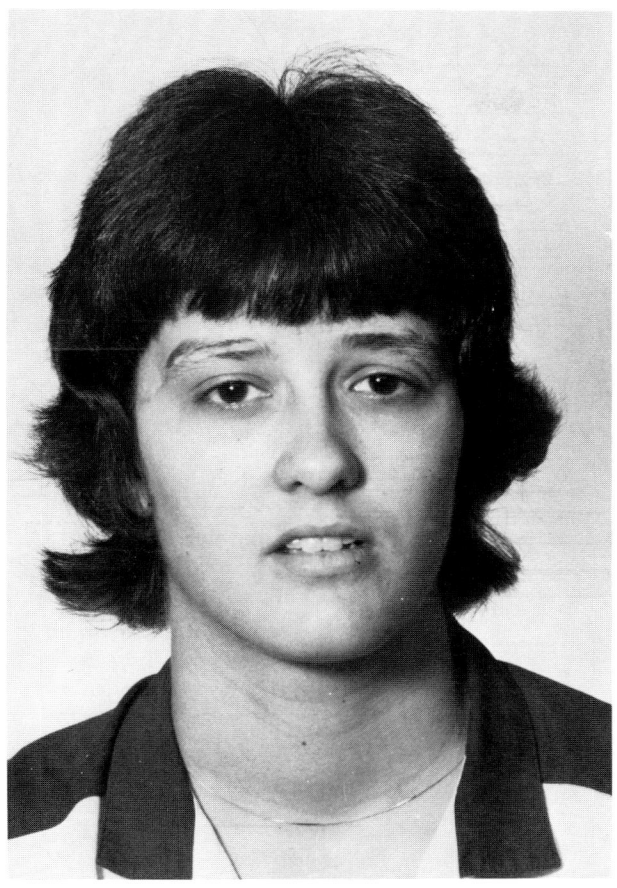

Figure 198-9 One year following the operation, the patient has luxuriant hair growth, and sensation in all parts of the scalp except the most superior portion.

Because of the length of time required for granulation tissue to develop and also because of the long-term instability of a split-thickness skin graft on the skull, the preferred technique now is placement of a distant flap of skin and subcutaneous tissue, with or without muscle. Recent developments in musculocutaneous flaps and in microvascular surgery have made it unnecessary to do multiple-staged pedicle flap techniques.

Some scalp defects can be reached easily by musculocutaneous flaps such as a latissimus dorsi flap or a trapezius flap. However the safe arc of rotation of most musculocutaneous flaps reaches to a point approximately at the level of the upper pole of the ear. Defects in the central superior portion of the scalp are probably best handled by a microvascular free tissue transfer. A number of donor sites are available which will provide durable functional skin cover for this area without excessive bulk.

The patient shown in Fig. 198-11 sustained deep thermal burns to the superior portion of the scalp. A portion of the wound was of partial thickness and healed in the usual fashion; however, the central portion of the wound was of full thickness, including pericranium. An attempt was made to stimulate the development of granulation tissue by removing the outer table of the skull; over a 4-week period, this resulted in only spotty development of granulations. The area was then resurfaced using a free scapular flap based on the circumflex scapular vessels which were anastomosed to the superficial temporal vessels (Fig. 198-11B). Other potential free flaps for this situation are the groin flap and the dorsalis pedis flap. The groin flap is hampered by having a short pedicle which frequently requires a vein graft, and the dorsalis pedis flap is a difficult flap to dissect and has considerable donor site morbidity. In addition, any free flap requires special techniques which may not be available in most hospitals.

Injuries by Physical and Chemical Agents

Thermal Burns

Because of its exposed and prominent position, the scalp is frequently injured by physical and chemical agents. Thermal injury to the scalp may occur alone or, perhaps more frequently, in conjunction with burns elsewhere. For this reason, the initial resuscitation involves close attention to fluid and electrolyte balance as well as wound care. The reader is referred to standard works on the treatment of burns. The scalp represents only about 4 percent of the total body surface area in adults (slightly greater in children), and for this reason isolated burns of the scalp do not require a great deal of attention to systemic effects.

The scalp has thick skin with a remarkable capacity to regenerate epithelium. This is due to the presence of many hair follicles and other epithelial adnexal structures. For these reasons, burns which would be full thickness in other parts of the body will eventually re-epithelialize in the scalp.

The treatment of scalp burns should, therefore, be conservative. Burn wounds may be covered with topical antibiotic agents such as silver sulfadiazine or povidone-iodine, but these dressings are frequently messy and difficult to keep in place. Another alternative is exposure. The wounds are cleansed initially, with removal of any devitalized debris. They are allowed to dry and are protected until re-epithelialization takes place.

Full-thickness burns of the scalp, including the pericranium, such as sustained by the patient shown in Fig. 198-11, are unusual. In these situations, although some areas may re-epithelialize, one frequently has to resort to one of the techniques described earlier for repair.

Electrical Burns

Electrical burns of the scalp occur when a person's head comes into contact with high tension wires, and usually involve several thousand volts of electricity. Most authors consider the damage to be the result of heat generated by the resistance of the tissues to the passage of the electric current. The amount of heat generated for a given current depends on the resistance of the specific tissue (Joule's law). Skin and bone, both present in large quantity in the head, have a higher resistance than other tissues. Resistance of the skin is further influenced by thickness, moisture, and the amount

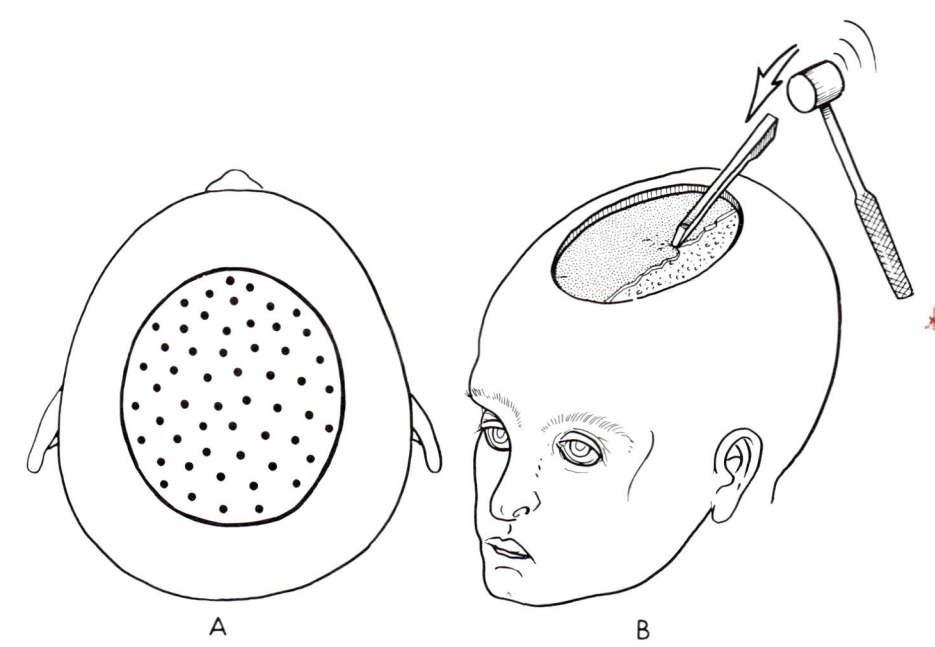

Figure 198-10 Methods of promoting granulation tissue on bare skull. *A.* The method of using multiple drill holes into the diploic space. The holes should be approximately 1 to 2 mm in diameter and should be no further than 1 cm apart. *B.* The method of removing the outer table of the skull. The immediate or delayed application of a skin graft may be done.

of vessels or nerves present. The injury may be further compounded by the phenomenon of "arcing," in which a spark is generated between the wire and the contact point. It should also be kept in mind that damage is also produced elsewhere in the body at the exit point, although usually of lesser degree due to dissipation of the current. Damage to respiratory centers and the heart must also be anticipated and respiration and cardiovascular functions supported if necessary.

The treatment of electrical burns of the scalp is based on the principle of removal of devitalized tissue and replacement as necessary to provide durable skin coverage and underlying bony support. The characteristic cross-sectional shape of the devitalized area has been well described.[9] The lesion is usually crescent- or saucer-shaped, with the deeper burn toward the center and becoming more superficial toward the periphery. High-tension electrical burns of the scalp are always of full thickness, extending to and including bone.

The traditional treatment has been to debride the dead scalp and cranium and then await sequestration of bone. If the diploe was affected, a full-thickness section of the skull was removed. Occasionally, only the outer table required removal, with subsequent granulation of the underlying diploe. This sequence of debridement, sequestration, sequestrectomy, and repair can take many weeks or months, with the constant danger of infection of the underlying dura.

More recently, several authors have advocated a more radical approach, which may give improved results.[7,10] They have suggested thorough debridement of devitalized scalp and pericranium followed by immediate flap coverage of the underlying bone, regardless of its apparent nonviability. The rationale is that although the bone may be dead, it will still function as a perfectly shaped "in-situ" bone graft. Coverage can be obtained by local scalp flaps or by distant flaps. Follow-up by x-ray studies and bone biopsy have shown regeneration of normal bony architecture, thus obviating the need for future cranioplasty.

Chemical Burns

Injuries of the scalp by chemical agents may occur intentionally as in an assault, or much more frequently as an accident, particularly in children. Lye burns are more common than acid burns. Several characteristics of chemical burns make them different from other types of burns. Damage to tissues in chemical burns is due to the action of free hydroxide or hydrogen ions in the tissues. Once these compounds come in contact with the skin, damage will continue until the agent is removed or neutralized by combining with ions in the tissues. It has been shown that irreversible cellular changes will take place if the pH is below 2.5 or above 11.5.[5] The ability to withstand this wide range of pH is due to the buffering effect present in normal tissues.

In general, the effects of different chemicals on the skin are determined by (1) concentration, (2) duration of contact, (3) penetrability of the compound, (4) quantity, and (5) manner of action.[2] In addition, especially in the case of lye burns, there is a latent period before the damage begins to be apparent. On the basis of these factors, the rationale for treatment is readily apparent. The only factor which can be influenced by the action of a physician is the duration of contact. One should therefore institute immediate, copious, and continuous irrigation of chemical burns with sterile water. Following this, an attempt can be made to neutralize the offending agent. For lye burns, dilute acetic acid can be used, and for acid burns, a dilute sodium bicarbonate solution can be used. It is important to remember that one should not attempt to neutralize the agent before thorough irrigation with water, since the neutralization reaction may cause further damage from the heat produced.

Scalp Injuries

Figure 198-11 Thermal burns of the scalp. *A.* The central superior portion of the burn included the pericranium. After removing the outer table of the skull, only spotty granulation tissue developed over a 3-week period. *B.* The defect was repaired using a vascularized scapular cutaneous flap. The flap was anastomosed to the superficial temporal vessels.

The depth of damage is sometimes difficult to determine in chemical burns, and for this reason debridement should be conservative. When the damaged area is well demarcated, however, it can be excised and a skin graft applied.

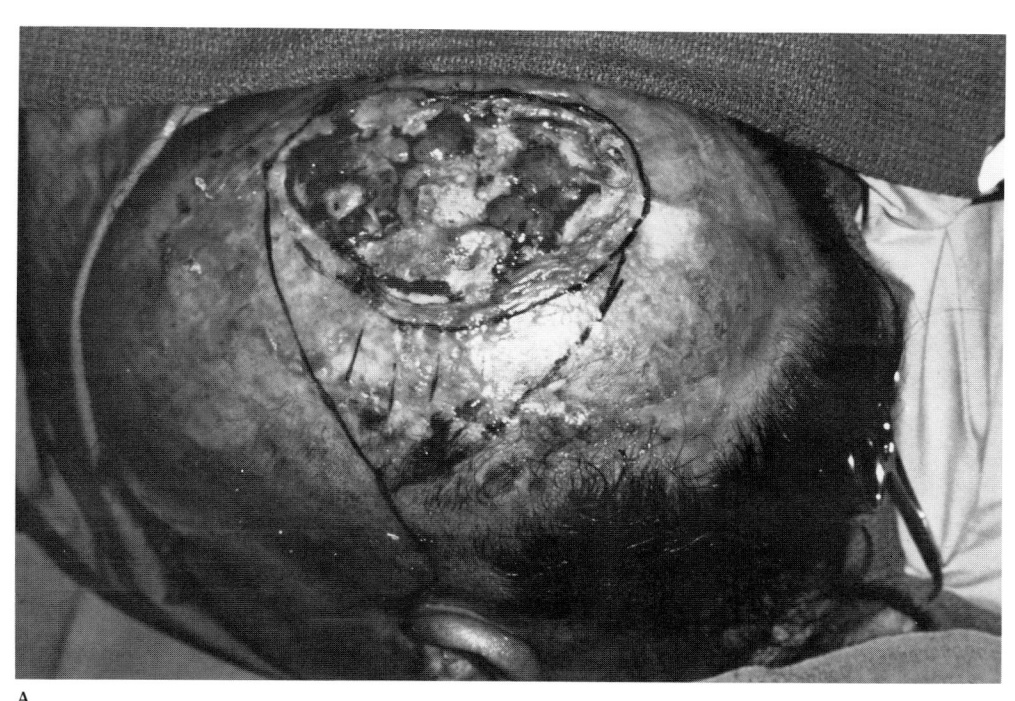

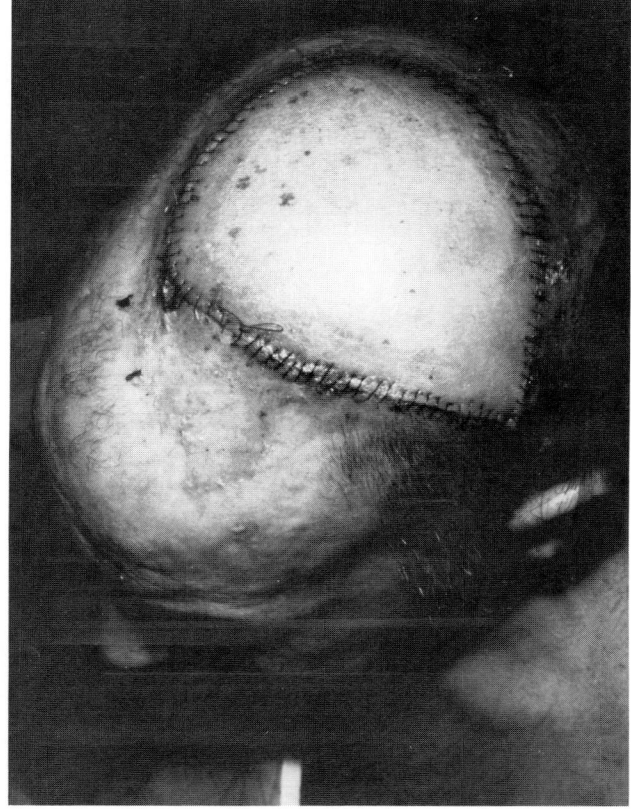

Radiation Injuries

Radiation burns usually occur as a result of accidental overexposure due to lack of filtration, or due to intentional or unintentional overlapping of fields. The result may be both an acute and chronic radiodermatitis. Acute radiodermatitis is characterized by initial erythema and edema of the skin, with blanching in the areas of greatest exposure. This may last up to 48 h and then subside rapidly. During this period of time the lesions are exquisitely painful. This may be followed by a period of several days in which symptoms and signs disappear, but after approximately 1 week, a secondary erythema begins to develop which may be complicated by extravasation of blood into the erythematous areas. This may progress to blisters with necrosis and ulceration of the underlying skin.[3] These ulcers are very difficult to heal due to radiation-induced endarteritis in the adjacent skin. The usual treatment for acute radiation ulcerations of the skin is excision and grafting, but this should be delayed until final demarcation has taken place.

References

1. Alpert BS, Buncke HJ, Mathes SJ: Surgical treatment of the totally avulsed scalp. Clin Plast Surg 9:145–159. 1982
2. Bromberg BE, Song IC, Walden RH: Hydrotherapy of chemical burns. Plast Reconstr Surg 35:85–95, 1965.
3. Cairns RJ, Champion RH, Wilkinson DS: Cutaneous reactions to physical agents, in Rook A, Wilkinson DS, Ebling FJG (eds): *Textbook of Dermatology*, 1st ed. Philadelphia, Davis, 1968, pp 323–361.
4. Dingman RO, Argenta LC: The surgical repair of traumatic defects of the scalp. Clin Plast Surg 9:131–144, 1982.
5. Friedenwald JS, Hughes WF Jr, Herrmann H: Acid-base tolerance of the cornea. Arch Ophthalmol 31:279–283, 1944.
6. Lu MM: Successful replacement of avulsed scalp: Case report. Reconstr Surg 43: 231–234, 1969.
7. Luce EA, Hoopes JE: Electrical burn of the scalp and skull: Case report. Plast Reconstr Surg 54: 359–363, 1974.
8. Miller GDH, Anstee EJ, Snell JA: Successful replantation of an avulsed scalp by microvascular anastomoses. Plast Reconstr Surg 58:133–136, 1976.
9. Stuckey JG Jr: The surgical management of massive electrical burns of the scalp. Plast Reconstr Surg 32: 538–543, 1963.
10. Worthen EF: Regeneration of the skull following a deep electrical burn. Plast Reconstr Surg 48:1–4, 1971.

199
Cephalhematoma and Subgaleal Hematoma

Derek A. Bruce
Luis Schut
Leslie N. Sutton

A cephalhematoma is a collection of blood under the periosteum of a skull bone. This lesion is limited by the pericranial attachments of the edges of the sutures and, therefore, does not cross suture lines. The mass is immobile, but the scalp can often be moved freely over the mass. Cephalhematomas occur most frequently in the neonatal period and are rare at other times of life. Usually, there is no associated skull fracture,[1] and the mechanism of formation of the cephalhematoma is unclear. It may be that prolonged or sudden compression of the skull results in sudden inward movement, displacing the bone away from the periosteum, or that some shearing force is set up between the periosteum and skull bone during delivery. In infancy, there are no real tables to the skull, and thus, when the periosteum is stripped from the underlying bone, hemorrhage occurs.

A subgaleal hematoma is a collection of blood in the space between the pericranium and the aponeurotic galeal layer of the scalp (external to the bones of the calvarium are five layers: skin, subcutaneous tissue, galea aponeurotica, loose connective tissue, and pericranium). Subgaleal hematomas can occur at any age but are particularly common after head trauma in the infant and young child (0 to 5 years of age). Typically, the lesion is unassociated with bony trauma, but in children under 1 year of age there is frequently a linear skull fracture. The fracture may be quite extensive in the child less than 1 year old, and may cross suture lines. Because the spread of this hematoma is uninhibited by the pericranial attachments, a soft, fluctuant mass can spread markedly, and frequently it will spread across the midline.

Cephalhematoma is almost exclusively seen in the newborn period. The presentation is of a firm, localized mass deep to the scalp, most frequently in the parietal region and rarely ever frontal. Usually, the appearance of the skin is normal unless forceps have been used. This lesion is uncommon in premature infants. The mass is initially firm, and the scalp can frequently be moved freely over the mass. This lesion is limited by the attachment of the suture lines, and therefore, a diagnosis is easily made. X-rays films of the skull are usually normal except for evidence of soft tissue swelling. There is rarely any intracranial injury. The acute treatment of this lesion is to leave it alone. Tapping or draining is contraindicated because of the risk of secondary infection and the fact that removal of the blood may lead to anemia in the child. More than 80 percent of these lesions become increasingly fluctuant with time and gradually resolve over 2 to 3 weeks. The only complication of this lesion is the development of a calcified cephalhematoma. This is apparent within the first few weeks of life when the lesion, instead of becoming smaller and softer, remains firm and large. The radiographic appearance of a calcified cephalhematoma is classical (Fig. 199-1). Because of the cosmetic disfiguration, these lesions require surgical removal. There is a plane between the outer table of the cranium and the calcified mass, and thus it is not necessary to open the calvarium. At surgery, frequently, the center of the mass is found to be a liquid hematoma or organized clot. It is suggested that, if the cephalhematoma has not disappeared within 6 weeks after birth, skull films be obtained. If the hematoma has become calcified, surgery is indicated.

A subgaleal hematoma rarely presents a diagnostic problem. Occasionally, a baby less than 1 year of age is seen a week or more following minor trauma with findings of a large fluctuant mass extending over much of the skull. The fluid is readily ballottable, and the parents will state that the lesion was definitely not present in the first few days following injury. Frequently, x-ray films reveal a linear fracture, and the diagnosis of cerebrospinal fluid leakage into the subgaleal space has often been made. This is never correct, and the true diagnosis is a subgaleal hematoma. A careful history will confirm the presence of a localized hematoma in the first few days after trauma. As the hematoma liquefies, it spreads in the subgaleal space, and the appearance can be very dramatic. In children under 1 year of age, blood loss into the trapped space can occasionally be severe enough to produce anemia, and transfusion is sometimes required. There is no indication to tap these collections because of the high risk of infection. The treatment is to reassure the parents that the mass will resolve and, if the collection is large, to obtain serial hemoglobin and hematocrit determinations. If the child is seen at the time of minor trauma, it is advisable to inform the parents that a soft, fluctuant mass may appear over the subsequent few days. This will markedly diminish parental concern and prevent the doctor's being forced into unnecessary treatment.

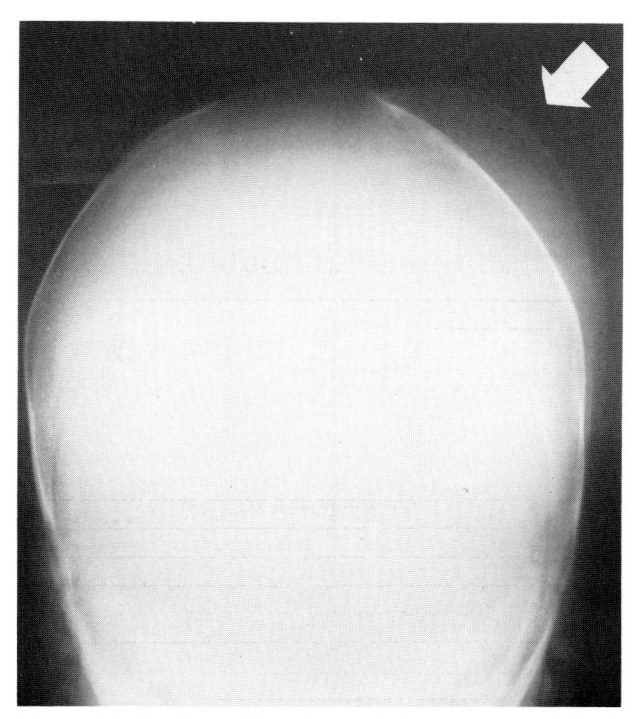

Figure 199-1 X-ray film of the skull showing a calcified cephalhematoma (*arrow*) in an 8-week-old male infant.

Reference

1. Kendall N, Woloshin H: Cephalohematoma: Associated with fracture of the skull. J Pediatr 41:125–132, 1952.

200
Skull Fractures
L. M. Thomas

Skull fractures most commonly result from impact injuries, although crushing forces can cause the bones of the skull to fracture. Impact may be investigated with a force transducer recording the event in terms of force as a function of time, or impulse. Many variables contribute to the shape of the impulse; the more obvious include the relative masses of the head and the impacting object, the area of impact, and the elastic or viscoelastic properties of the skull and the object. The impulse may deform or accelerate the head, or both, depending upon its shape. In order to produce a fracture, the force must rise to a level of 900 to 1700 lb in 0.001 s or less. If the circumstances of the impact are such to cause the force level to rise at a slower rate, the fracture level will not be reached and the energy will be dissipated by accelerating the head. The basic mechanical engineering aspects of skull fractures were elucidated thoroughly by Gurdjian and Lissner in the 1940s and 1950s at our institution.[3]

The skull is for practical purposes a closed ellipsoid. It may be divided into the cranium, or vault, and the base. It averages 2 to 6 mm in thickness, although areas of stress concentration, the buttresses, may be considerably thicker. The bones of the vault are composed of solid inner and outer tables separated by cancellous bone called the diploe.

Fractures of the skull may be classified as linear or depressed, and either of these may be further classified as open or closed depending upon whether there is an overlying scalp laceration or extension of the fracture into the area of the air-bearing sinuses.

Linear Fractures

Linear fractures result from elastic deformation of the skull[3] and constitute 80 percent of skull fractures. When the skull receives a blow of moderate energy and velocity, the area receiving the blow bends inward. A simultaneous outbending occurs at a point distant from the impact. The fracture is initiated in the outbent area or areas, when it or they fail in tension. The fracture extends toward the impact site and away from it toward the base.

The prognostic significance of a closed linear fracture is as an index of the severity of the blow. A fracture traversing the middle meningeal groove should alert the surgeon to the potential for an epidural hematoma. However, closed linear fractures require no specific treatment.

Diastatic fractures are those fractures that result in a separation at a suture line, usually the lambdoid or coronal suture, and are more common in infants. Fractures with marked separation are also referred to as diastatic and likewise are more common in the infant, undoubtedly because of the incomplete calcification and lack of tensile strength of the bones of the calvarium. As the child reaches the age of 2 to 3 years, the adult pattern of linear skull fracture is more likely.

Open linear fractures deserve a careful inspection for the presence of foreign material but ordinarily will require only soft tissue debridement and closure. If a linear fracture extends into an air-bearing sinus such as the frontal sinus, no specific treatment is required although it is technically an open fracture. Antibiotics should not be given prophylactically. The presence of a linear fracture extending into the sinus should alert the observer to the possibility of a more serious fracture of the posterior wall of the sinus. Tomograms of the area may be required.

Depressed Skull Fractures

Depressed skull fractures result from an energy concentration sufficient to cause local failure of the bone. They may be divided into *perforating fractures*, resulting from a small mass such as a bullet moving at a high velocity; *penetrating fractures*, resulting from moderately high velocity impacts as from a shell fragment; and the more common *depressed fractures* with comminuted fragments, resulting from a slower-moving object of high kinetic energy such as a hammer or baseball bat. By definition, a fracture is depressed if a fragment is depressed to the thickness of the skull. A depressed fracture may not be clearly defined by standard x-ray films of the skull. If it is suspected by the presence of a bony double density or a circular fracture line, tangential views should be obtained. Depressed fractures may be either open or closed; open depressed fractures are more common.

Several features of depressed skull fractures must be understood to gain insight into the rationale of management:

1. The fracture is of greater area on the inner table.
2. There are commonly several fragments that may be tipped or twisted.
3. There is frequent tearing of the underlying dura or brain.
4. The static view at the time of the x-ray examination does not represent the depth to which the fragments penetrated at the time of impact.

Depressed fractures may produce neurological deficit as the result of cortical damage occurring at the time of impact. The same cortical injury may result in the formation of an epileptogenic focus.[10] Traditionally, elevation of depressed fractures has been recommended to alleviate neurological deficit and to reduce the incidence of post-traumatic epilepsy. Jennett has shown that the incidence of post-traumatic epilepsy is not decreased by fracture elevation.[5] Likewise, neurological deficits do not seem to be reversed by fracture elevation.

With these features in mind, a practical list of surgical indications in the treatment of a depressed skull fracture can be developed. The principal indication for the operative management of a closed depressed fracture is cosmetic. Since 50 percent of depressed fractures occur in the frontal area, cosmetic indications for surgery are often encountered. The presence of an increasing neurological deficit or radiographic evidence of an intracranial hematoma are obvious surgical indications, no different here than in other forms of head injury. The presence of deeply embedded bony fragments may require debridement.

The main indication for bony elevation in open depressed skull fracture is to prevent infection by the careful debridement of contaminated and necrotic tissue and the removal of foreign material. Debridement of necrotic brain and hematomas and dural repair are also important. Such early operative cleansing will do much to reduce both neurological deficit and post-traumatic epilepsy, both of which are greatly increased by infection or hematoma formation.[6,7,10]

Closed depressed fractures should be elevated through a cosmetically acceptable incision. Either an S-shaped curvilinear incision or a horseshoe flap may be utilized. Either incision must be planned to allow ample exposure, as the fracture, particularly of the inner table, is ordinarily larger than anticipated. Plans to allow extension of the incision must be incorporated in the original preparation and draping.

Open depressed fractures require debridement of the skin edges, and here the S incision is most effective. The excision of contaminated tissue should include the pericranium. As with the closed fracture, ample exposure is mandatory.

Several rules should be applied in the surgical management of depressed fractures; additional safeguards are needed in selected circumstances. Depressed fragments must not be twisted or levered as the deep edges may be sharp and will damage the cortex. It is preferable to begin with a trephine opening in normal bone adjacent to the depression. Normal dura can be visualized and the fragments removed carefully, using rongeurs. After the fragments have been removed, the dura should be inspected. If the dura is bulging or discolored, even though intact, it is advisable to incise it and inspect the underlying brain. Necrotic areas and blood clots should be debrided carefully. After meticulous hemostasis, the dura should be carefully and completely closed. When the dura has been torn by the depressed fracture, it should be carefully debrided. Again, an adequate dural closure is necessary, and a graft of pericranium, temporal fascia, or some similar tissue should be used if necessary. A dural substitute is not adequate and should not be used.

There is no consensus about the use of the depressed bone fragments for cranial repair. If the wound is older than 24-h or is obviously grossly contaminated, the fragments should be discarded. If the wound is fresh and reasonably clean, the fragments may be used to construct a cranioplasty, being held together with nonmetallic sutures if needed.[6] Acrylic cranioplasty is not advisable at the time of debridement. If the bone fragments are not replaced, elective cranioplasty may be planned in 3 to 4 months.

Skull Fractures

The incidence of late post-traumatic epilepsy is greatly increased if the dura is lacerated, if there is a greater than 24-h post-traumatic amnesia, or if one or more seizures occur in the first week. Prophylactic anticonvulsive therapy is reasonable if any one of these risk factors is present.

Dural Venous Sinus Injuries

Depressed skull fractures that are situated over major dural venous sinuses such as the sagittal and transverse sinuses pose a special problem. A bony fragment may have torn into the sinus, and when the fragment is removed, catastrophic bleeding may occur. Adequate precautions must be taken. Operation should not commence until the surgical team is prepared to deal with massive hemorrhage. The principle of wide exposure is essential. Access to the sinus must be obtained to ensure proximal and distal control before the fragments are manipulated.

A tear in the sagittal sinus may be ligated in the anterior one-third without expectation of difficulty from venous stasis. Ligation of the middle one-third is questionable; the posterior one-third should not be ligated. The sinus tear may be simply sutured, may need oversewing with muscle stamps or Gelfoam (absorbable gelatin sponge; The Upjohn Company, Kalamazoo, Mich.), or may need a patch graft of dura mater or vein. Large lacerations may require closure over a shunt, which will allow a more leisurely repair.[8]

The results of transverse sinus ligation are more difficult to predict because of the normal anatomical variations at the torcular. Preoperative angiography is helpful.

If the depressed fracture overlying a venous sinus is closed and does not present with a mass effect or a major cosmetic problem, it should not be elevated unless unexplained intracranial hypertension develops. This may be the result of sinus occlusion, which should be confirmed by angiography before repair is undertaken.

Depressed Fractures Involving the Frontal Sinus

One-half of depressed fractures occur in the frontal area; many of these may involve the frontal sinus. Unconsciousness and focal neurological deficits are not common with fractures of the frontal sinus. However, considerable dural and cerebral involvement may be present. The thin cribriform plate is often shattered, and both frontal poles may be injured. The immediate mortality rate is low; complications are more apt to occur and include cerebrospinal fluid rhinorrhea, pneumocephalus, meningitis, and brain abscess.

Operative treatment of depressed fractures of the frontal sinus should be undertaken as soon as the patient's condition permits. An adequate exposure must be obtained. The comminuted bone fragments should be removed from the anterior wall of the sinus, and the mucous membrane completely excised. The posterior wall must be inspected and, if fractured, should be excised to expose the dura. Sufficient bone should be removed to repair the dura. Usually dural tears in the cribriform plate area can be repaired by an extradural approach.[11]

Basilar Skull Fractures

Basilar skull fractures are most commonly an extension of fractures of the vault.[4] They may occur separately as a result of stress concentration occurring among the many perforating foramina or from indirect force such as the lower jaw or vertebral column impacting against the condyloid processes or occipital condyles, respectively. The usual locations are the petrous portion of the temporal bone, the orbital surface of the frontal bone, and the basiocciput.[9] These fractures are difficult to diagnose by ordinary x-ray examination and frequently are inferred because of clinical signs such as cerebrospinal fluid otorrhea or rhinorrhea, hemotympanum, ecchymosis over the mastoid process (Battle's sign), periorbital ecchymoses (raccoon eyes), or deficits in cranial nerves that exit through the base. Anosmia may occur in fractures of the frontal base, as may carotid-cavernous fistula. Carotid-cavernous fistula may also occur with basilar fractures involving the middle fossa. Middle fossa fractures may be suspected to involve the sella turcica if an air-fluid level is seen in the sphenoid sinus on a brow-up lateral x-ray film. Recognition is important, as acute or delayed endocrine disturbances may occur.

Two types of fracture of the petrous bone are recognized, longitudinal and transverse, the terms referring to the long axis of the petrous pyramid. The more common longitudinal fracture usually begins in the squamosal part of the temporal bone from a lateral blow to the head. The fracture extends medially and downward to deform the external canal or tear the tympanic membrane, either of which will result in bleeding from the ear. More severe longitudinal fractures may involve the middle ear and disrupt the ossicular chain. The facial nerve may be involved in its horizontal or middle ear course. The dura may be torn, and cerebrospinal fluid will escape to the middle ear and thence through the torn tympanic membrane to the external auditory canal. If the tympanic membrane is intact, the fluid may escape through the eustachian tube to the nasopharynx.

Transverse fractures commonly result from occipital or occipitomastoid blows. The blows required to produce this fracture are more severe and result in higher early mortality. Medial transverse fractures disrupt the internal auditory canal and cochlea, injuring both seventh and eighth cranial nerves in the internal auditory canal. Lateral fractures disrupt both the vestibular and cochlear components of the labyrinthine capsule and may injure the facial nerve in its horizontal middle ear course. Transverse fractures seldom cause cerebrospinal fluid otorrhea.

Diagnosis in Petrous Bone Fracture

Neuro-otologic examination of a patient with a suspected basilar fracture should include an evaluation of bleeding from the ear, hemotympanum, cerebrospinal fluid otorrhea, ecchymosis of the mastoid area, facial paralysis, dizziness or vertigo, nystagmus, tinnitus, and hearing impairment. Bleeding from the ear following head trauma ordinarily signifies a basilar skull fracture. Occasionally blood may run into the ear from external lacerations. It is best to defer cleansing the external canal to reduce potential infection; if localization of the bleeding point is essential, careful cleansing using sterile technique may be accomplished.

Facial paralysis is seen in approximately 50 percent of patients with transverse fractures and 20 percent of patients with longitudinal fractures. Facial paralysis can be characterized as follows: complete or incomplete; immediate or delayed; due to neurapraxia or axonotmesis; due to injury proximal or distal to the geniculate ganglion.

The prognosis in incomplete paralysis (paresis) is excellent. A delayed onset has a more favorable prognosis than an immediate paralysis. An electrical nerve stimulator may be used to determine axonal degeneration. The stimulator is placed over the facial nerve trunk as it exits from the stylomastoid foramen. A normal nerve will respond to between 3 and 7 mA of current. If the paralyzed side has a substantially higher threshold or develops such, an assumption of axonal degeneration can be made. This can be confirmed by electromyography, but there is a 10- to 14-day latency before fibrillation potentials appear.

Localization of the injury in relation to the geniculate ganglion is important in planning surgical approaches. The presence or absence of lacrimation, mediated by the greater superficial petrosal nerve, is easily detected by placing a narrow strip of filter paper in the conjunctival sac of each eye and comparing the wetting of the papers over 5 min (Schirmer test).

Vertiginous dizziness is due to a vestibular disorder and is associated with nystagmus. If the vestibular nerve or vestibular labyrinth is damaged, as with a transverse fracture, immediate vertigo occurs and will subside in 3 to 4 weeks. Thereafter, there will be little or no response to caloric testing in the involved ear. Longitudinal fractures less frequently result in serious or persistent vestibular damage.

Tinnitus due to inner ear or acoustic nerve damage usually has a constant buzzing or ringing characteristic, in contrast to the low-pitched pulsatile tinnitus of vascular origin. Hearing impairment almost always occurs in temporal bone fracture. The loss may be conductive or sensorineural, but is usually a combination of the two. Early tuning fork tests of hearing lateralization (Weber test) and bone conduction compared with air conduction (Rinne test) may suffice, but should be followed by audiometry.

Treatment of Injuries Associated with Temporal Bone Fracture

If a patient has complete facial paralysis of immediate onset coincident with the temporal bone fracture, the facial nerve should be explored.[2] Partial or delayed paresis should be observed, as recovery is the rule. If electrical signs of axonal degeneration develop, exploration is worthwhile. Exploration of the distal nerve (lacrimation intact) is carried out through a standard mastoid approach; proximal lesions may be approached through the middle fossa or by a translabyrinthine route. Bony decompression may suffice, but nerve grafting may be required if the nerve has been severed.

Cochlear and vestibular injuries respond poorly to any known treatment. Vestibular depressant drugs may be of limited benefit.

References

1. Bakay L, Glasauer FE: *Head Injury*. Boston, Little, Brown, 1980, pp 72–73.
2. Becker DP, Miller JD, Young HF, Selhorst JB, Kishore PRS, Greenberg RP, Rosner MJ, Ward JD: Diagnosis and treatment of head injury in adults, in Youmans JR (ed): *Neurological Surgery*, 2d ed. Philadelphia, Saunders, 1982, pp 1938–2083.
3. Gurdjian ES, Lissner HR: Deformations of the skull in head injury studied by the "stresscoat" technique: Quantitative determinations. Surg Gynecol Obstet 83:219–233, 1946.
4. Gurdjian ES, Webster JE: *Head Injuries: Mechanisms, Diagnosis, and Management*. Boston, Little, Brown, 1958, p 76, p 211.
5. Jennett B: *Epilepsy after Non-Missile Head Injuries*, 2d ed. London, Heinemann, 1975, p 179.
6. Jennett B, Miller JD: Infection after depressed fracture of skull: Implications for management of nonmissile injuries. J Neurosurg 36:333–339, 1972.
7. Jennett B, Miller JD, Braakman R: Epilepsy after nonmissile depressed skull fracture. J Neurosurg 41:208–216, 1974.
8. Kapp JP, Gielchinsky I, Deardourff SL: Operative techniques for management of lesions involving the dural venous sinuses. Surg Neurol 7:339–342, 1977.
9. McLaurin RL, McLennan JE: Diagnosis and treatment of head injury in children, in Youmans JR (ed): *Neurological Surgery*, 2d ed. Philadelphia, Saunders, 1982, pp 2084–2136.
10. Miller JD, Jennett WB: Complications of depressed skull fracture. Lancet 2:991–995, 1968.
11. Thomas LM, Hodgson VR, Gurdjian ES: Skull fracture and management of open head injury, in Youmans JR (ed): *Neurological Surgery*. Philadelphia, Saunders, 1973, pp 969–977.

201
Growing Skull Fractures of Childhood

Timothy B. Scarff
Michael Fine

Linear or nonlinear calvarial fractures that enlarge with time are termed "growing" skull fractures. A pulsatile mass of encysted fluid (or, less commonly, brain tissue) usually protrudes through the cranial defect (Fig. 201-1). Growing skull fractures occur only in young children and have also been called *leptomeningeal cysts* because of the associated cystic masses. These rare fractures were first described clinically in 1816, pathologically in 1856, and radiologically in 1937; they were extensively reviewed by Lende and Erickson in 1961.[2]

Pathogenesis

Not all of the factors involved in the formation of growing skull fractures are known. Rupture of the dura and arachnoid underlying the original fracture must occur, producing a subgaleal fluid pocket that may or may not be clinically evident. The concurrence of immature membranous bone or rapidly growing brain is necessary, as these fractures do not occur in adults. Coincidentally, increased intracranial pressure or excessive original width of the fracture line are not factors directly responsible for the development of growing fractures. Growing fractures are not seen in other bones of the body, or in other than preteen children; 90 percent occur in children under 3 years of age. Underlying brain destruction, a ventriculosubarachnoid fistula, or the development of low-grade hydrocephalus may be present but have not been proved causative.[2] Despite breaching of the arachnoid and nonwatertight dural closures, growing "fractures" apparently never occur in patients who have had a craniotomy, whatever the age.

Dense arachnoidal loculations and brain with cystic degeneration often protrude into or underlie the growing fracture. These cavities are usually not in free communication with the subarachnoid space and may be a result of the original injury rather than a cause or result of fracture growth.[2,5,6]

Early authors recognized the invariable presence of dural lacerations in growing skull fractures, and thought that pulsations of intact arachnoid produced the fracture enlargement.[6] Goldstein et al. developed an animal model in puppies that reproduced some of the features of the clinical entity.[1] They produced 1-mm-wide craniotomy lines and lacerated the underlying dura in the experimental portions of the craniotomy. Varieties of dural-pericranial pouches were created within the craniotomy lines. They concluded that arachnoidal rupture and free communication of subarachnoid fluid with the pouch was an essential precondition for fracture growth. Interestingly, they noted that interposition of fibrous tissue in the fracture line prevented healing of even nongrowing fractures. Their results were not dramatic, however, with only 7 of 55 animals having a fracture diastasis of 3 mm of more. In the group with the subarachnoid space opened, the average fracture width was 2.1 mm; in the group with an intact arachnoid, the fracture width averaged 1.5 mm; and in the control group, fracture lines averaged 0.6 mm in width. Animals were observed an average of 45 days (4 to 140 days), sufficiently long for the largest of the growing fractures (7.5 mm wide) to be documented. None showed the cystic encephalomalacia and other changes so commonly seen with growing fractures in humans.

Stein and Tenner performed angiography on six children with growing skull fractures, from 10 days to 3 years following the initial trauma.[5] They documented cerebral herniation through the fractures in all, and thought that herniation (and subsequent tissue necrosis) may be a prerequisite for growing fractures in humans. Their theory would correlate clinically with the very frequent occurrence of cerebral atrophy, retardation, hemiparesis, and seizures, and would also explain the operative findings of cystic encephalomalacia.

Clinical Features

Growing skull fractures are rare lesions, complicating 0.6 percent of skull fractures in one large series.[3] They occur following cranial injuries at birth or up to 7 or 8 years of age. Typically months to years after an injury a pulsatile cranial defect is noted over a convexity. The history usually discloses a significant cranial injury, often with a subgaleal fluid collection. Alternatively, the original insult may have been sufficiently minor that no x-ray films were taken. Older infants and children are apt to experience post-traumatic paresis or a seizure disorder, but younger infants may be normal or have only a mildly hypotrophic extremity. The

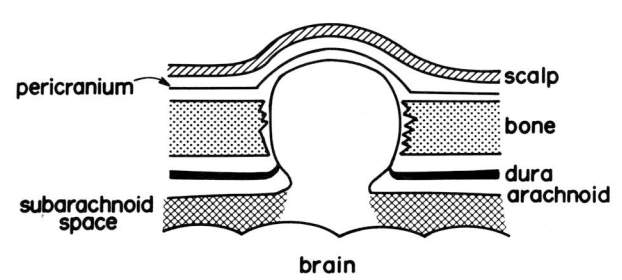

Figure 201-1 Basic conditions common to all growing fractures. The cystic pouch extending through the fracture is probably a residuum of cerebral herniation.

1627

hemiparesis is generally not progressive, but seizures may be resistant to medical management. Low-grade (post-traumatic) hydrocephalus or a mildly hyptertensive porencephaly may be present, and may possibly contribute to poor seizure control or hemiparesis.

Radiological Features

X-ray films of the skull obtained at the time of the initial injury usually show a linear, horizontal, often quite diastatic, frontoparietal or parieto-occipital fracture (Fig. 201-2). Less commonly, the fracture may be depressed, stellate, or involve both sides of the head. With the development of a growing fracture, the fracture line widens slowly. As years go by, plain films show an irregular enlarging defect of both tables, which may measure as much as 10 cm on a side. The edges are sclerotic and scalloped, and may be everted (Fig. 201-3). Adjacent bone may show pressure indentation from arachnoidal or parenchymal cysts that do not communicate with the subarachnoid space. Ventriculography or CT scanning usually shows enlargement of the ipsilateral ventricle with a shift to that side. A CT scan may show multicystic encephalomalacia or arachnoidal loculations in the area of the defect. Rarely, ventricular enlargement and cysts produce shifts away from the fracture site.

Management

Early and aggressive surgical treatment of growing skull fractures is generally advocated.[2,4-6] Operation is designed to accomplish four goals: (1) to debride and remove necrotic brain; (2) to communicate subarachnoid loculations; (3) to reconstruct the leptomeninges; and (4) to cover the cranial defect. Debridement is performed widely, enlarging the bony defect as necessary and breaking down loculations at

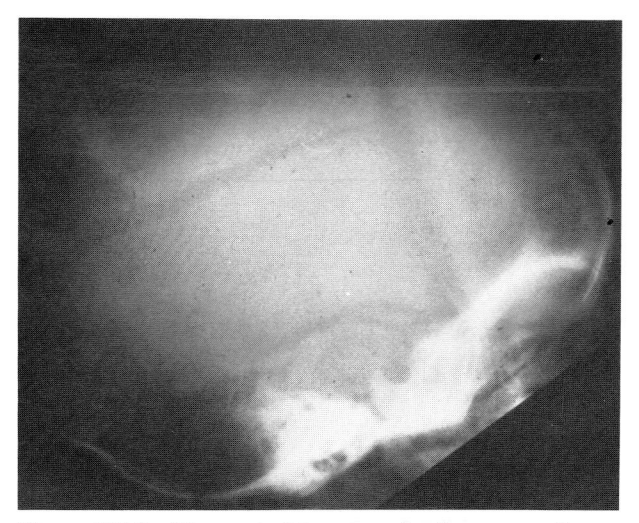

Figure 201-2 The typical location of a linear, usually parietal, fracture in an infant that can lead to a growing fracture.

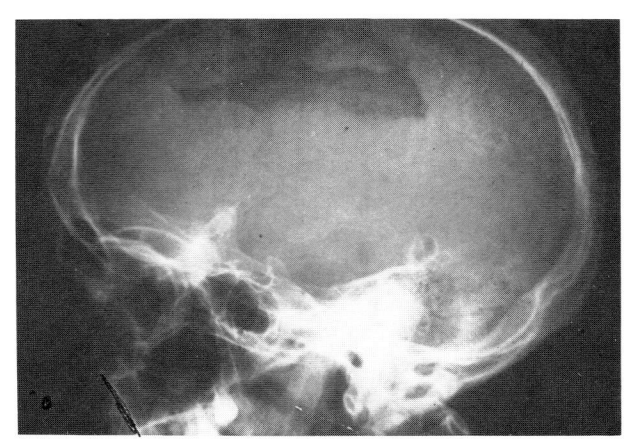

Figure 201-3 A growing parietal skull fracture. Note the eroded and scalloped bone edges.

the same time. Dural repair is accomplished by means of a temporalis or fascia lata graft, again enlarging the bony defect as necessary to secure normal dura. The cranioplasty is generally performed with acrylic and is more easily accomplished if the defect is small.

Ramamurthi et al. have advocated nonsurgical treatment of growing skull fractures.[3] They note that a pre-existing hemiparesis is unlikely to be improved with operation, but agree that epilepsy is better controlled. However, in their own case material, two of four patients apparently had a progressive hemiparesis during the active growth of the fracture.

Very early surgical intervention (10 days after injury) both for cerebral herniation and widely diastatic fractures has been recommended.[4,5] However, Sekhar and Scarff have documented a phenomenon of "pseudogrowth" of fractures in very young infants. Skull films taken up to 6 weeks after injury may show true widening of the fracture, but these fractures may heal normally in several more weeks.[4] X-ray evidence of true fracture growth would be present between 3 and 6 months following injury.

Improvement of hemiparesis has not been frequently reported, but many authors describe marked amelioration of seizures. Early correction of documented growing fractures carries an acceptable surgical risk, is technically easier, provides better cosmetic results, and may prevent progressive encephalomalacia.

References

1. Goldstein F, Sakoda T, Kepes JJ, Davidson K, Brackett CE: Enlarging skull fractures: An experimental study. J Neurosurg 27:541–550, 1967.
2. Lende RA, Erickson TC: Growing skull fractures of childhood. J Neurosurg 18:479–489, 1961.
3. Ramamurthi B, Kalyanaraman S: Rationale for surgery in growing fractures of the skull. J Neurosurg 32:427–430, 1970.
4. Sekhar LN, Scarff TB: Pseudogrowth in skull fractures of childhood. Neurosurgery. 6:285–289, 1980.
5. Stein BM, Tenner MS: Enlargement of skull fracture in childhood due to cerebral herniation. Arch Neurol 26:137–143, 1972.
6. Taveras JM, Ransohoff J: Leptomeningeal cysts of the brain following trauma with erosion of the skull: A study of seven cases treated by surgery. J Neurosurg 10:233–241, 1953.

202
Facial Fractures

Ronald Riefkohl
Gregory S. Georgiade
Nicholas G. Georgiade

Fractures of the facial skeleton consequent to violent accidents may cause tragic facial deformities in addition to significant disruption of vital physiological processes. It is imperative that the physician treating these facial fractures understands the anatomy, pathology, and surgery of the head and neck and has had extensive training in the management of trauma victims.

Etiology and Incidence

The most common causes of facial fractures are high-speed motor vehicle accidents, assaults, and sporting injuries.[1,5,9] Usually motor vehicle accidents account for 40 to 50 percent of all fractures, and assaults account for another one-third. In 70 to 80 percent of the patients with midfacial fractures, the cause of injury is a high-speed motor vehicle accident.[1] The mandible is the bone most commonly fractured.[5] Next in frequency is the zygomaticomaxillary complex, then the nasoethmoid complex, and finally, the maxilla.

Emergency Room Management

The first consideration is the assurance of a patent airway. The oropharynx should be cleared of fragments of teeth, blood clots, dentures, and other foreign bodies. Anterior mandibular fractures may be associated with airway obstruction caused by the tongue falling into the pharynx because of lost anterior fixation.[5] Treatment is forward traction of the tongue with either a heavy stitch or a towel clamp. Emergency tracheal intubation may be necessary in some patients. It is futile to attempt orotracheal intubation in the presence of bleeding intraoral lacerations, and nasotracheal intubation will be difficult in the presence of midface fractures. A tracheostomy is often the safest and quickest means of establishing an airway, but it should be executed under optimum conditions. Early tracheostomy is also preferable for patients with multiple extensive facial fractures, fractures associated with a severe intracranial injury, and fractures that will require both nasal packing and intermaxillary fixation.

After an airway is secured, hemorrhage from wounds of the face, scalp, and mouth is stopped, if possible by simple pressure, but larger vessels may be temporarily suture-ligated until definitive operative exploration of the wound is made. A considerable volume of blood may be swallowed and thus be unaccounted for in the estimation of the patient's blood loss.

After the patient's condition is stabilized, a careful neurological examination is completed; then the chest, abdomen, and extremities are evaluated. Lastly, the facial injuries and the head and neck are examined.

In the emergency room, preliminary facial roentgenograms are obtained to confirm the clinical impression of facial fracture. In addition, views of the skull, cervical spine, and chest are essential. In many instances, high-quality films and other sophisticated studies, such as plain or computed tomography,[4] are necessary to accurately define the extent of injury.

Many patients with facial fractures, especially those caused by great violence, have other associated injuries that may be life-threatening. The incidence of associated injuries depends on the nature of the causative factors, with a higher incidence of associated injuries occurring in victims of high-speed accidents.[9,14]

Some of the major concomitant injuries that are frequently associated with facial fractures include pneumothorax, hemothorax, adult respiratory distress syndrome, basilar skull fracture, intra-abdominal injuries, cervical spine fractures, genitourinary injuries, and extremity fractures.[5]

Specialty consultations should be obtained while the patient is in the emergency room so that other injuries are managed immediately. Life-threatening injuries have treatment precedence over facial fractures, although occasionally temporary measures are required to facilitate later definitive fracture treatment. It is preferable if the patient is managed by a physician who is able to assess the overall situation and orchestrate the modalities and timing of treatment of multiple injuries, as well as recognize early symptoms and signs of further complications.

Facial fractures should be treated early. However, treatment may be delayed if the patient's condition is unstable. Furthermore, facial fractures should not be treated until complete radiological evaluation, which may include tomography, has been accomplished. Treatment should also be deferred if there is marked soft tissue edema, or if special splints are necessary for proper management. On the other hand, the possibility of infection increases proportionally with the time interval between the injury and the time of treatment.[5] If definitive treatment of jaw fractures must be deferred, it may be necessary to implement temporary fixation by application of dental arch bars. Leakage of cerebrospinal fluid is not a contraindication to early surgery, but it should be thoroughly evaluated prior to undertaking fracture reduction.[5]

After the clinical and radiological evaluation, photographs are obtained and soft tissue wounds are managed appropriately. Tetanus prophylaxis should be resolved, and prophylactic antibiotics should be administered if there are open fractures or if there is severe contamination of the wound.

General Principles of Treatment

The method selected to manage the injury should be the simplest and most direct. Basic operative principles include exposure of the fractures through existing lacerations or esthetically placed incisions, wound irrigation and debridement, gentle handling of tissues, perfect hemostasis, aspiration of blood and other debris from sinus cavities, obliteration of dead space by accurate layered wound closure, and accurate operative reduction and internal fixation of fractures. An adequate airway is critical postoperatively, as the surgical trauma will compound the edema from the initial injury.

Patients who have a tracheostomy are unable to communicate except by writing; thus they should be provided with pen and paper. Early ambulation prevents thrombophlebitis and pulmonary embolism and improves patient morale. Soft tissue wounds are kept clean by daily care.

If intermaxillary fixation is necessary, initial postoperative feedings are administered through a nasogastric tube, and after several days feedings may be in the form of a blenderized oral diet. Oral hygiene is maintained with a dilute peroxide mixture or commercial mouthwash. Wire cutters or strong scissors are taped to the bed for immediate use in case the intermaxillary fixation must be released temporarily. The gums and buccal mucosa may become irritated from wires or arch bars; if irritation develops, wax is applied to the arch bars and wires.

Specific Fractures

Zygomatic Fractures

The prominence and architecture of the zygoma render it highly susceptible to fracture. A zygomatic fracture is the most common facial fracture in many series, but isolated fractures of the zygoma are not common.[1,5,13,17]

The zygomatic bone is a strong buttress between the maxilla and the cranium. The articulations with the maxilla and frontal bone are broad and strong, but the articulations with the sphenoid and temporal bones are thin and weak. The zygomatic bone forms a portion of the lateral wall and floor of the orbit, and in a few individuals may form the lateral superior wall of the maxillary sinus.[5] Although fractures through the bone may occur, most fractures disrupt the articulations with adjacent bones (Fig. 202-1).

There are numerous classification schemes for zygomatic fractures,[10] but a simple system based on displacement and stability of the zygoma is most applicable for treatment planning.[12]

Clinical findings depend upon when the patient is first seen. If the patient is seen immediately after injury when there is minimal edema, there may be flattening of the malar eminence, bony irregularities, abnormal motion, crepitation, and anesthesia of the cheek. If seen later, periorbital edema and ecchymosis and subconjunctival hemorrhage may be the only obvious findings. With posterior and downward displacement of the zygoma, the lateral canthus, the lower eyelid, and the globe are also displaced inferiorly. The fracture through the orbital floor will tear the maxillary sinus mucosa and may result in epistaxis. There may be trismus because of impingement of the mandibular coronoid process against the posteriorly displaced zygoma, or because of medial displacement of the zygomatic arch with impingement of the fragments against the temporalis muscle and coronoid process. Anesthesia in the distribution of the infraorbital nerve is probably the most common finding and is only rarely absent. Diplopia may also be present.

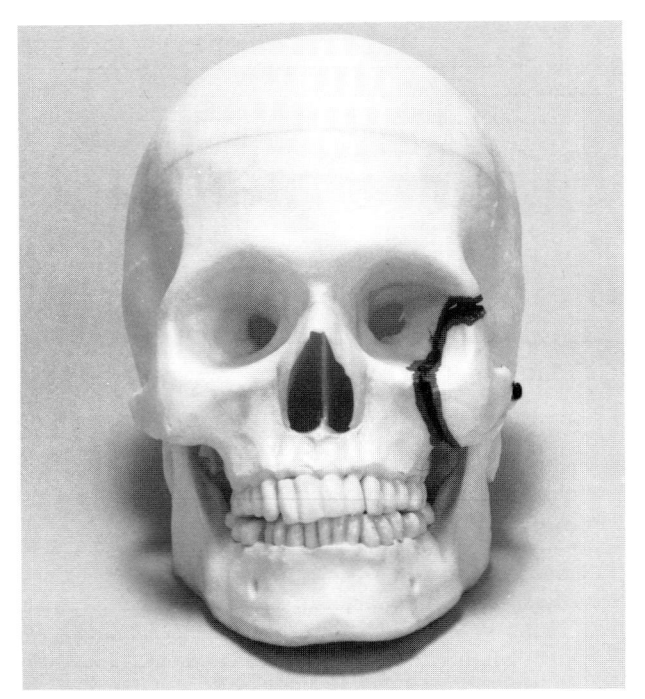

Figure 202-1 Zygomatic bone fracture. The most common site for fracture is at the articulations with adjacent bones.

The Water's view roentgenogram best demonstrates the fracture and the degree of zygomatic displacement, but the submentovertex view is necessary to visualize a fracture of the zygomatic arch. Commonly seen is opacification of the maxillary sinus, and in nondisplaced fractures, this may be the only radiographic finding.

After the patient has been stabilized satisfactorily and an ophthalmologist has evaluated the eye, treatment may be instituted. Nondisplaced and minimally displaced fractures do not require treatment; however, many fractures are actually displaced more than is evident from clinical and radiographic examination. Displaced fractures may be treated by closed reduction, but because there is a high incidence of redisplacement, displaced zygomatic fractures should be reduced and internally ligated. Old, impacted fractures may require considerable force for reduction because of organization and fibrous union. If treated within 6 weeks, however, the bones may still be repositioned. If there is unstable posterior displacement of the zygoma, which will cause later deformity, a 0.045 Kirschner pin may be driven across the face, engaging the opposite zygomatic bone. The K pin is then removed under local anesthesia in 4 to 6 weeks. This technique may be underutilized at present, since a recent review indicated that malunion was found in one-third of the patients treated with transosseous wires alone.[13]

Unstable, multiple fractures of the zygomatic arch are difficult to manage. The fragments may be skewered by a small K pin, or held in place by Penrose drain packing, or the fragments may be exposed and wired directly through appropriately placed incisions to avoid the branches of the facial nerve.[5]

If the orbital floor is extensively comminuted, it must be reconstructed by autogenous tissue or by an artificial implant. Packing placed in the maxillary sinus must be removed in 7 to 10 days and, therefore, does not provide permanent stabilization of the orbital floor.[5]

The most common complication of zygomatic fractures is persistent infraorbital nerve anesthesia. In the majority of cases, this gradually resolves over a 6- to 12-month period, but if there is no recovery, or if annoying dysethesia and anesthesia are present, then the infraorbital nerve should be explored. Other common complications include malunion with facial deformity, diplopia, and enophthalmos. Ocular complications include blindness, extraocular muscle dysfunction, and permanent diplopia. Nonunion and infection are rare. Chronic maxillary sinusitis may occur, particularly if sinus packing was a component of treatment. Fibro-osseous ankylosis involving the coronoid process is also rare.

Orbital Fractures

After sufficient trauma in the vicinity of the orbit to cause a fracture, a complete ophthalmologic evaluation is necessary prior to manipulation of the fractured bones.

Orbital fractures are classified as pure or impure blow-out fractures, and orbital fractures associated with concomitant maxillary, zygomatic, or naso-orbital fractures.[2,5] A pure blow-out fracture involves the orbital floor exclusively, whereas an impure blow-out fracture involves the orbital floor and the inferior orbital rim. The basis of this classification is the contention that a blow-out fracture is a distinct injury having a specific pathophysiology and clinical presentation. The blow-out fracture supposedly is caused by an impact to the globe that in turn transmits the force by hydraulic pressure to the orbital floor, causing a fracture.[5] This mechanism may be incorrect, since the inferior orbital rim may bend as much as 1 cm without fracturing, yet buckling and fracturing of the orbital floor results.[5]

The most common clinical finding in a blow-out fracture is diplopia. It may be present on admission but absent the following day or several days later. Diplopia, a result of deviation of the visual axis, may be caused by entrapment of soft tissues, such as the inferior rectus or inferior oblique muscle, in the fracture line.[5] However, since the orbital fat surrounding the globe and extraocular muscles has an intricate fibrous system that apparently has an important role in movements of the globe and gliding of the extraocular muscles,[11] incarceration of orbital fat rather than muscle may be the cause of diplopia. Diplopia may also be caused by downward displacement of the globe, although the binocular fusion mechanism easily compensates for globe displacement.[11] Injury to the motor nerves to the inferior oblique or inferior rectus muscle may also result in diplopia. Additional possible causes are injury to other cranial nerves or extraocular muscles, or disruption of muscle attachments. Edema and hemorrhage within the muscles may also play a role.

Enophthalmos, a common finding with blow-out fractures, may be difficult to recognize clinically and is seldom noticed by the patient. It is significant when there is greater than a 2-mm discrepancy in the cornea to lateral orbital rim distance compared with the normal side, and is disfiguring when this discrepancy is greater than 5 mm.[5] The precise cause of enophthalmos is unclear, but is probably related to enlargement of the orbital cavity and escape of orbital fat through the fracture. Progressive late enophthalmos is probably due to orbital fat necrosis, resolution of edema and hematoma, and a low-grade inflammatory process. Enophthalmos results in a pseudoptosis of the upper eyelid, a deepening of the superior tarsal fold, and a shortening of the horizontal dimension of the palpebral fissure.

Other possible clinical findings with a blow-out fracture are subconjunctival hemorrhage, bleeding from the lacrimal canaliculus, periorbital ecchymosis, and anesthesia of the infraorbital nerve. With impure blow-out fractures, there may be a palpable bone irregularity, abnormal motion, soft tissue crepitation, and bone tenderness.

Radiographic opacification of the maxillary sinus without other signs of injury is not reliable evidence of a blow-out fracture.

The presence of diplopia is important to management decisions. However, many patients with diplopia immediately after injury, if not treated, will experience spontaneous resolution of the diplopia.[6,16] Thus, diplopia alone is not necessarily an indication for surgery. Patients with diplopia alone should be treated by observation. If diplopia is still present after 2 weeks, then orbital exploration is indicated. A limitation of forced rotation of the eyeball (positive forced duction test), particularly if associated with significant enophthalmos or radiological evidence of a large defect in the orbital floor, is a definite indication for operation.

Treatment principles of blow-out fractures include release of entrapped structures, replacement of escaped orbital fat into the orbital cavity, and restoration of the orbital cavity to its former size and shape.[5] Surgery may be postponed until the edema resolves, provided that this does not extend beyond 7 days.

The orbital floor is usually exposed through a short incision through the lower eyelid, but many surgeons prefer a transconjunctival approach despite the reduced exposure.[5] Perhaps a transconjunctival incision is preferable for individuals with a tendency for hypertrophic scars or keloids. After exposing the inferior orbital rim, the periosteum is incised and elevated and the entire fracture and adjacent undamaged bone are exposed. Large angulated fragments are repositioned, and if the orbital floor defect is sizable, the floor must be reconstituted with either autogenous cartilage or bone, or with an artificial implant. After release of entrapped structures, there should be free rotation of the globe demonstrated by the forced duction test.

In many instances there is an associated blow-out fracture of the medial orbital wall, and perhaps this is the cause of late enophthalmos. Medial wall fractures are suspected if there is radiographic evidence of air within the orbit, clouding of the ethmoid sinus, or displacement of the medial orbital wall. Fractures through the lateral orbital wall and roof of the orbit are rare and usually are associated with more severe injuries.[5] These fractures require evaluation by routine or computed tomography. Fractures involving extensive bone disruption are treated by placing an implant over the defect.

Clinical findings of orbital fractures associated with high maxillary, naso-orbital, or zygomatic fractures are similar to those of the blow-out fracture, except that the forced duction test is usually negative.[5] Treatment is similar to the treatment of the blow-out fracture.

Orbital floor fractures may be complicated by late structural deformities subsequent to malunion or nonunion. Artificial implants may become infected and extrude, may cause extraocular muscle dysfunction, or rarely may compress the optic nerve.[5] Bone graft implants may resorb, resulting in enophthalmos. There may be permanent damage to the extraocular muscles and, consequently, muscle imbalance that requires subsequent corrective surgery. Enophthalmos and its sequelae are unfortunately common after orbital fractures. Ocular complications have been reported in 15 to 30 percent of orbital fractures, with loss of vision the most severe problem.[9,14] If the patient arrives in the emergency room with loss of vision, then routine or computed tomography should be done immediately to determine if optic nerve or orbital exploration is indicated.[4] Blepharoptosis due to injury to the levator muscle or its innervation is uncommon. Vertical shortening of the lower eyelid occurs with severely displaced inferior orbital rim fractures and results in disfiguring scleral show, ectropion, or entropion.

The superior orbital fissure syndrome is associated with severe orbital, naso-orbital, or zygomatic fractures. The fracture extends through the superior orbital fissure and can involve the optic foramen. This causes interference with the function of cranial nerves III, IV, V_1, and VI because of bleeding into the orbital muscle cone space between the intermuscular membrane and Tenon's capsule, which results in compression of the nerves against the margins of the superior orbital fissure. The syndrome consists of ophthalmoplegia, blepharoptosis, and anesthesia of the cornea and skin in the distribution of the supratrochlear and supraorbital nerves. If there is a parasympathetic block, there will be a fixed, dilated pupil. Because of paralysis of the motor nerves, the eye does not move and is proptotic. The maxillary division of the trigeminal nerve may also be involved if the fracture extends through the foramen rotundum. The syndrome may be complete, but in most instances is partial. There is also an orbital apex syndrome, which consists of the superior orbital fissure syndrome plus blindness due to impingement of the optic nerve by bone fragments. Treatment consists of exploration and decompression of the hematoma and replacement or removal of bone fragments.[5]

Naso-Orbital Fractures

With a naso-orbital fracture, the nasal bones are forced back into the interorbital space, which is formed by the ethmoid sinuses, the superior and middle turbinates, and the perpendicular plate of the ethmoid bone.[3] The thin and fragile medial orbital walls may comminute extensively, and fragments of the roof of the interorbital space may enter the anterior cranial fossa, either at the cribriform plate or at the roof of the ethmoid sinuses. Laceration of the dura or olfactory nerve sheath, perforation of the brain, or necrosis of brain tissue may occur in serious injuries.[3] The levator palpebrae muscle, the medial canthal ligament, the lacrimal sac, or the lacrimal canaliculus may also be injured.

Clinical findings may include flattening and shortening of the nose, edema and distortion of the medial canthal region, ecchymosis and edema of the eyelids, subconjunctival hemorrhage, epistaxis, traumatic telecanthus, crepitation, and possibly CSF rhinorrhea. Plain roentgenograms are deceiving since abnormalities may be missed. Plain or computed tomography is necessary to precisely define the full extent of the fracture.[3]

Treatment of naso-orbital injuries should be delayed until a thorough evaluation is completed and extensive edema has subsided. CSF rhinorrhea is not a contraindication to surgery, and in many instances will cease after reduction of the fracture.[3]

Although it is possible to expose these fractures through a coronal incision, a transverse nasal incision plus bilateral medial canthal incisions heal with fairly inconspicuous scars and provide excellent direct exposure.[3] The medial canthal ligaments must be identified and reattached with transnasal wires, although occasionally primary bone grafts may be necessary to properly secure the canthi.[3] Also, a primary bone graft may be incorporated to restore the nasal dorsum.

Complications of naso-orbital fractures include structural deformities if treatment was delayed, medial canthal displacement, nasal saddle deformity, ocular complications, lacrimal system injuries (such as canalicular interruption, mucocele, and inflammatory conditions involving the lacrimal sac), blepharoptosis subsequent to loss of function of the levator muscle, and CSF rhinorrhea with recurrent meningitis.[3]

Supraorbital and Frontal Sinus Fractures

The paired frontal sinuses within the frontal bone are formed by the frontal bone and supraorbital rims. The posterior wall of the sinus is thin, yet it rarely is fractured.[15] These fractures may occur independently, but ordinarily they are associated with naso-orbital fractures or other serious facial fractures.

The clinical diagnosis is based on the findings of edema, tenderness, ecchymosis, deformity, crepitation, and abnormal motion. There may be anesthesia of the forehead because of injury to the supratrochlear and supraorbital nerves, or the trochlea of the superior oblique muscle may be injured, resulting in diplopia. There may also be CSF rhinorrhea.

Roentgenograms often fail to delineate the posterior wall of the sinus, but intracranial aerocele is pathognomonic for a posterior wall fracture and dural tear.[15]

Treatment nearly always consists of operative reduction and internal fixation, but it is advisable to observe the patient's neurological signs for 48 to 72 h prior to the operation.[5] A coronal incision is preferred for fracture exposure or to provide access for an intracranial procedure, if necessary. For extensive injury with severe comminution, the bone fragments and all sinus mucosa are removed and bone chips are packed into the frontonasal duct. The forehead defect may be reconstructed later. Treatment of a unilateral fracture should include resection of the intersinusoidal septum to ensure drainage. Less serious fractures are elevated and ligated with fine stainless steel wires. Various means of maintaining elevation of unstable fragments are available, such as a halo frame, a plaster head cap with outriggers, or a small Foley or Fogarty balloon catheter placed into the sinus. Isolated injuries to the nasofrontal duct are treated by either direct repair and the insertion of a temporary obturator, or by a Lynch-type frontoethmoidectomy.[15] Posterior table fractures, if nondisplaced, require no treatment, but if displaced and associated with anterior wall injury, then sinus ablation and secondary cranioplasty are indicated.

Untreated anterior frontal wall fractures may result in deformity or nasofrontal duct obstruction with subsequent acute and chronic sinusitis, mucocele, pyocele, and intracranial or orbital infection. Another possible complication is acute and chronic sinusitis. Patients should be followed carefully for evidence of persistent sinus fluid, suggesting nasofrontal duct obstruction.

Nasal Fractures

Nasal fractures usually occur at the junction of the thick with the thin section of the nasal bone and are rare in the upper, thick section except when associated with naso-orbital, Le Fort II, or Le Fort III fractures.[5]

Nasal fractures are classified into unilateral fracture with or without displacement, bilateral fracture with fracture of the septum, and the open book fracture with severe comminution.[5,7] There may be concomitant injury to the nasolacrimal system, the perpendicular plate of the ethmoid bone, the ethmoid sinus, the cribriform plate, and the orbital plate of the frontal bone. The margins of the pyriform aperture may also be involved. Nasal fractures rarely occur without injury to the cartilaginous septum; however, septal injuries are easy to miss, particularly in children.

Clinical findings may include edema and tenderness, deformity, periorbital ecchymosis and edema, subconjunctival hemorrhage, nasal obstruction and epistaxis, mobility, and crepitation. Intranasal evaluation is facilitated by the application of a vasoconstrictor agent to the mucosa. Standard facial roentgenograms may not reveal the nasal fracture; soft tissue technique or xeroradiograms are preferable.

Nasal fractures are treated by closed reduction, either immediately after injury, if edema is not marked, or a week to 10 days afterward, when edema has subsided. An Asche forceps is used to elevate and manipulate the fragments into position. Telescoping of the septum may require open reduction; for unstable septal fractures, intranasal silicone splints are necessary until fixation occurs. The nasal cavities are packed with medicated gauze, and an external plaster splint is placed on the nose for 7 days. Rarely, a nasal fracture requires open reduction, but probably this should be undertaken as an elective procedure later.

Complications of nasal fractures include hematoma of the septum and its possible sequelae, infection, synechiae between the septum and turbinates, nasal obstruction, malunion and deformity, and nonunion.

Maxillary Fractures

The architectural arrangement of the maxilla is in the form of a bone mass capable of resisting considerable violence. Most maxillary fractures are caused by direct impact, although some occur by forces transmitted through the mandible. Muscular contraction has a minimal effect on displacement of maxillary fragments, but in the Le Fort II and III fractures, mastication may have a small role.[5]

Le Fort's experimental work with cadavers evolved into the classification of maxillary fractures into alveolar fractures; transverse fractures (Le Fort I), in which the fracture line crosses the pterygoid plates and maxilla just above the apices of the teeth (Fig. 202-2); pyramidal fractures (Le Fort II), in which the transverse fracture line extends obliquely upward across the inferior orbital rim and orbital floor to the medial orbital wall and then across the nasofrontal suture (Fig. 202-3); craniofacial dysfunction fractures (Le Fort III), in which the fracture involves the zygomatic arches, the zygomaticofrontal suture line, the nasofrontal suture line, the pterygoid plates, and the orbital floors, thus separating the entire maxilla from its cranial attachment (Fig. 202-4); and finally, vertical fractures, which occur just off the midline and are associated with other fractures of the maxilla. Le Fort II fractures are the most common and Le Fort III are the least common type of maxillary fracture.[5] The most common cause of maxillary fractures is the automotive

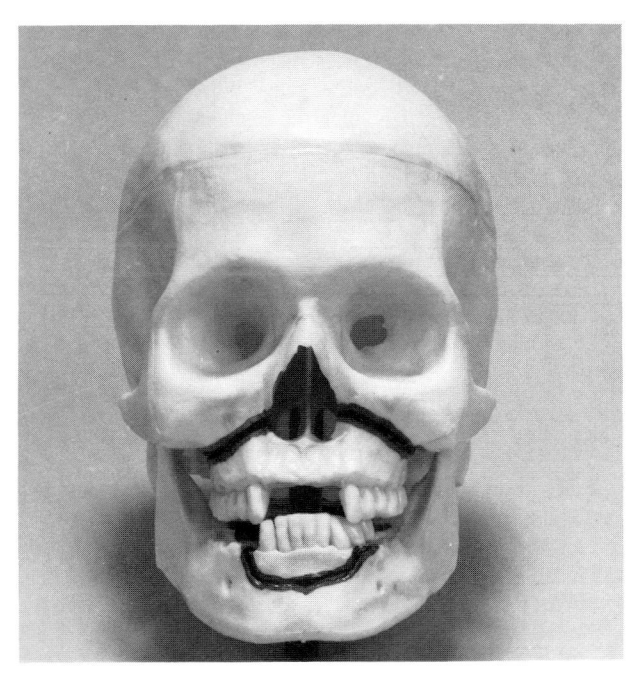

Figure 202-2 Le Fort I (transverse) maxillary fracture. The model also depicts an alveolar fracture of the mandible.

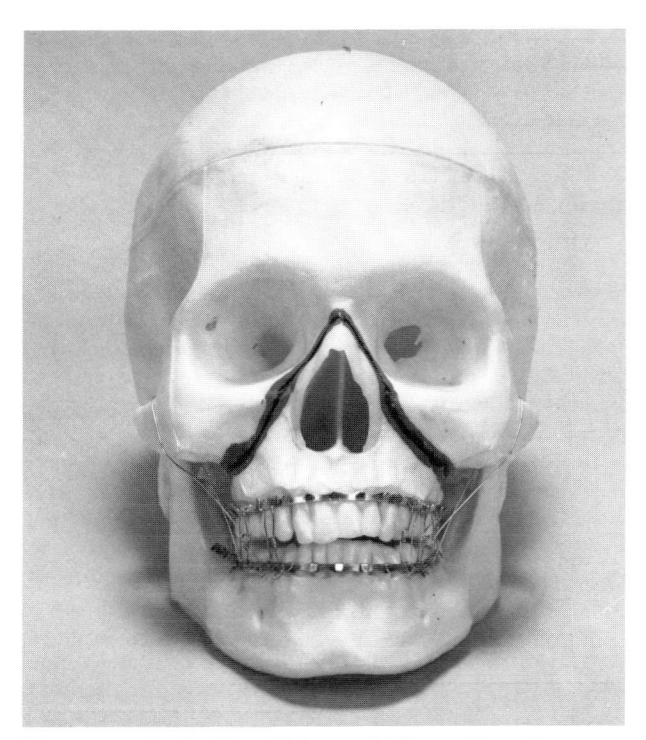

Figure 202-3 Le Fort II (pyramidal) maxillary fracture. Arch bars have been ligated to the teeth and to one another. Note the two suspension wires looped around the zygomatic arches and secured to the mandibular arch bar.

"guest passenger" injury, in which the individual is thrown forward during a collision and strikes the middle third of the face.[5] The consequent fracture depends on the direction and level of the impact. In many patients, multiple maxillary fractures occur concomitantly; this is especially common with the more serious injuries. Also, most patients with a fractured maxilla have another facial bone fracture.

Clinical findings may include epistaxis, periorbital ecchymosis, subconjunctival hemorrhage, facial edema, malocclusion often associated with an anterior open bite, submucosal hemorrhage or mucosal lacerations, a "dish-face" or "donkey-face" appearance, palpable bony irregularities, abnormal mobility unless the segments are impacted, crepitation, and CSF rhinorrhea. With Le Fort II and III fractures, the cribriform plate may be injured, and thus the nasal cavities should not be packed. With high Le Fort fractures there may be damage to the ethmoid bones, the nasal septum, and the lacrimal area, resulting in traumatic telecanthus. The nasolacrimal apparatus and cribriform plate are also frequently injured.

Radiographic evidence of maxillary fracture may be minimal, and in many instances, changes are absent entirely. There may be clouding of the maxillary or ethmoid sinuses, and in the Le Fort II and III types the fractures of the orbits and nasal bridge may be visible. The best radiographic view is the Water's view, but occlusal films, plain or computed tomography, or pantomography x-ray films may be necessary to further define the fracture.

Proper reduction and fixation of jaw fractures depends upon the restoration and maintenance of occlusion for a period of time. The maxillary and mandibular first molars are the guides for determining the correct establishment of normal occlusion,[5] but the abraded surfaces on occlusal and incisal areas of the teeth serve as useful landmarks. Fracture realignment will not be possible unless accurate occlusion is first restored.

Arch bars are ligated to all teeth, but traction should not be applied to the incisor region because the conical shape of these teeth and their roots may result in loosening. If traction in the anterior region is necessary, a circumferential mandibular wire and a maxillary suspension wire to the anterior nasal spine or pyriform aperture will provide the required stability.

The timing of treatment will depend on the extent of injury, but if definitive treatment is deferred, it may be appropriate to apply an arch bar for temporary stabilization, particularly if there are alveolar or vertical fractures. Isolated alveolar fractures are managed by application of an arch bar or by simple ligation of teeth on the fracture fragment to adjacent teeth.[5] A few weeks of intermaxillary fixation may be necessary if good occlusion is not achieved with simple arch bar application.

Le Fort I fractures, provided there are sufficient teeth, are treated by application of arch bars and intermaxillary fixation.[5] Maxillary suspension to solid bone above the line of fracture is also necessary. Secure fixation may be obtained by permanent wires to either the pyriform aperture or inferior orbital rims, or by temporary external suspension wires secured to the zygomatic arches or zygomatic processes of

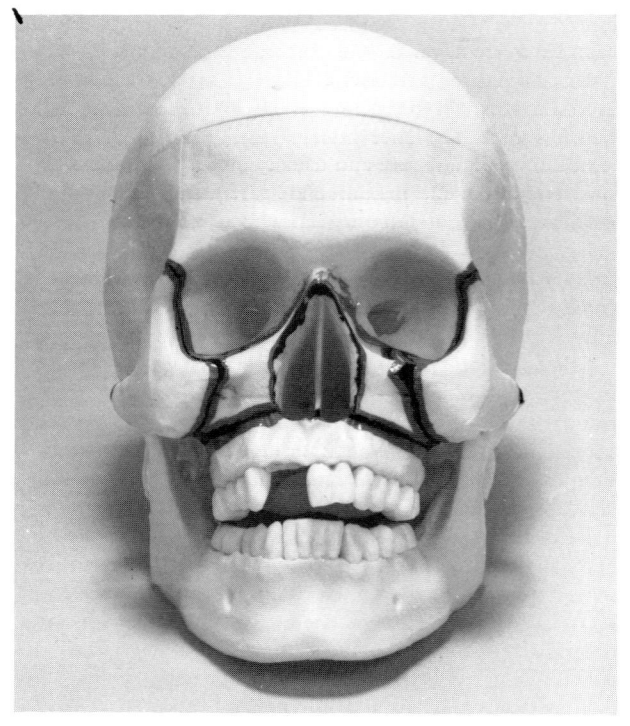

Figure 202-4 The model demonstrates a combination of Le Fort fractures. There are Le Fort I, II, and III fractures. The Le Fort III lines extend across the zygomaticofrontal suture, then across the lateral orbital wall to the pterygomaxillary suture which is disrupted.

the frontal bone. Temporary suspension wires should be ligated to the mandibular arch bar. Rarely, an external suspension device such as a halo frame is necessary.

Le Fort II and III fractures are approached in a similar manner, but in these more complex fractures it is best to internally ligate the fracture fragments at the infraorbital rims, the nasofrontal region, and the zygomaticofrontal region. As with the Le Fort I fracture, suspension to solid bone above combined with intermaxillary fixation is necessary. Suspension wires and intermaxillary fixation are usually left in place for 6 to 8 weeks.

Fractures of the edentulous maxilla are definitely uncommon unless associated with extensive fractures of the middle third of the face.[5] The absence of teeth prevents transmission of forces to the maxilla, and if the patient is wearing dentures they usually absorb most of the violence. When an edentulous maxilla fractures, there is usually minimal displacement. Treatment is unnecessary since the maxillary-mandibular relationship may be adjusted 4 to 6 weeks later by fabrication of new dentures. When there is significant displacement, however, the fracture fragments should be operatively reduced and immobilized by internal wires; prefabricated dentures are secured and suspended above to solid bone as with other maxillary fractures.

When the anterior maxillary wall is crushed into multiple small fragments resulting in deformity, treatment is by packing of the maxillary sinus through a Caldwell approach and delivery of the packing through a nasal antrostomy. The packing is removed in 10 days.

Complications of maxillary fractures are rare. Profuse hemorrhage may be treated by direct ligature or packing. Uncontrolled bleeding from the internal maxillary artery is managed by removal of the posterior wall of the maxilla through a Caldwell approach and direct ligation of the vessel. Nasal airway obstruction is common with maxillary fractures, especially once intermaxillary fixation is implemented. Infection is rare and usually involves the maxillary sinus. Nonunion and malunion are rare unless there is considerable destruction of bone. Extraocular muscle imbalance is also a possibility if the fractures transgress the orbits.

Mandibular Fractures

Although the mandible is a strong bone, there are inherent areas of weakness in the region of the mental foramina, the condylar necks, and at the angles where the bodies join the rami. With resorption of alveolar bone consequent to loss of teeth, the mandible thins and is more prone to fracture.[5] The most common site for mandibular fracture is the angle, accounting for 30 percent of fractures. Next in frequency is the body (27 percent) followed by the condyle (20 percent). The least common location for fracture is the coronoid process.[8] About 60 percent of patients with a mandibular fracture have other mandibular fractures; 80 percent have two fractures, 50 percent have three fractures, 4 percent have four fractures, and 3 percent have more than four fractures. In 95 percent of the patients with multiple mandibular fractures, the fractures occur in separate areas of the mandible.[8]

Mandibular fractures may be classified on the basis of fracture direction and displacement.[5] Another useful classification is based on the presence or absence of serviceable teeth in the fracture segments, since this is so critical for treatment.[5] With a class I fracture, there are teeth on both sides of the fracture, with a class II fracture there are teeth on only one side of the fracture, and with a class III fracture, there are no teeth at all.

Clinical findings with mandibular fractures may include pain with motion, tenderness, soft tissue edema, subcutaneous or submucosal hematoma, deformity, malocclusion, abnormal mobility, and crepitation. Deviation of the chin when the mouth is opened suggests a fracture of the condyle. The mandible deviates toward the side of the fracture, and there will also be premature occlusion on the same side plus an open bite on the opposite side. There may also be tenderness of the temporomandibular joint. If there are bilateral condylar fractures, there is a bilateral open bite with occlusion only on the posterior teeth. The patient also complains of pain with attempts to open the mouth, but the mandible does not deviate.

Posteroanterior and lateral roentgenograms of the mandible may reveal a fracture, but pantomography x-ray films are more informative. Fractures involving the condyle may require tomography for precise delineation, and occlusal dental views are necessary to visualize small alveolar fractures.

The factors influencing displacement of fracture segments include the site of the fracture, the direction and angulation of the fracture, the presence or absence of teeth adjacent to the fracture, the direction of pull of muscles attached to the fragments, and the direction and intensity of the impact.[5] The muscles attaching to the mandibular fragments are mainly responsible for displacement. The strong posterior group of muscles pulls the jaw up, forward, and medially, and the weak anterior group depresses the jaw. A fracture may be favorable or unfavorable depending on both the orientation and the bevel of the fracture (Fig. 202-5). Muscle action on the two fragments either distracts or impacts the fragments.

Treatment of mandibular fractures is based on the type of fracture, its location, and whether it is favorable or unfavorable. When teeth are in the mandibular fracture line, they should be extracted if there is extreme mobility, fracture of the root of the tooth, or pre-existing apical disease.

A class I fracture is treated with intermaxillary fixation provided the fracture is favorable. However, if the fracture is unfavorable, operative reduction and internal fixation are necessary. With proper open reduction and internal fixation the teeth usually assume good alignment and interdigitation, but occasionally good interdigitation is not achieved with initial reduction and several days of rubber band traction are necessary to bring about normal occlusion. After normal occlusion is achieved, the rubber bands are removed and stainless steel wires are applied.

Class II fractures are treated in a similar manner, but in general, operative reduction and internal fixation are usually necessary.[5] External pins or internal plates may be necessary, particularly for comminuted fractures in the region of the angle. These latter techniques have the disadvantage of greater periosteal dissection and also risk damage to teeth from drilling holes through bone.

Class III fractures of the mandible usually occur in areas

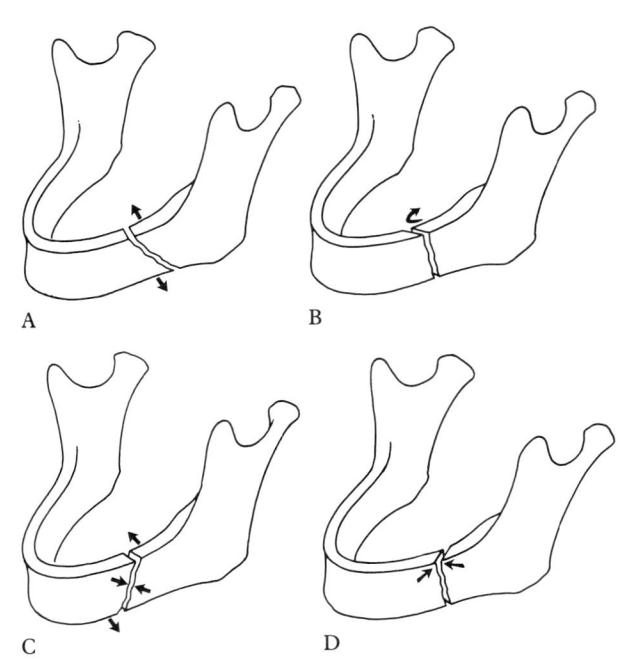

Figure 202-5 The effects of mandibular fracture orientation on fragment displacement. *A.* The posterior fragment will be displaced cephalad and the anterior fragment caudad by muscle contraction. *B.* The bevel of a vertical fracture may permit medial displacement of the posterior fragment because of muscle contraction. *C, D.* In these fractures, muscle contraction impacts the fracture fragments.

of the bone where atrophy is most marked. Because of the redundant soft tissue overlying the mandible, these fractures are rarely compound. In general, these fractures require an intraoral appliance even if there is minimal or absent displacement.[5]

Direct circumferential wiring of the fragments if the fracture is sufficiently oblique may suffice, but transosseous wiring is more reliable. The fracture may be exposed through either intraoral or extraoral incisions. Wire ligatures may require removal later if there is mucosal irritation caused by a denture.

Fractures of the mandibular condyle usually occur by indirect trauma as the condyle is protected by the overlying zygomatic arch. The fracture may occur either above or below the insertion of the lateral pterygoid muscle on the condylar neck. If the fracture is above the insertion, then the fracture is intra-articular. However, if the fracture is below the insertion, then the lateral pterygoid muscle will distract the proximal fragment anteriorly and medially. The proximal fragment may be minimally displaced or, rarely, completely dislocated out of the joint capsule. Usually the proximal fragment gradually returns to its normal position, but there may be some absorption and remodeling after fracture healing. Ordinarily, intermaxillary fixation alone is adequate treatment.[5] Direct reduction is necessary if dental occlusion cannot be reproduced, if there is an alteration in the vertical dimension of the face, or if the dislocation of the fragment will hinder primary osseous healing.[8] If the proximal fragment is displaced more than 90 degrees, particularly in chil-

dren and edentulous patients, open reduction and internal fixation is indicated through either a preauricular or a Risdon incision.[5]

Mandibular fractures may be complicated by infection, which is minimized by wound debridement, accurate fixation, and the intravenous administration of antibiotics. Avascular necrosis, osteitis, and osteomyelitis are rare. However, ankylosis of the temporomandibular joint, nonunion, malunion, delayed union, anesthesia in the distribution of the inferior alveolar nerve, facial deformity, and malocclusion may occur.

Multiple Complex Fractures

Multiple facial fractures are usually a result of high-speed vehicular accidents. Serious life-threatening associated injuries are common, and the treatment of facial fractures has a low priority in the overall management of the patient.

Initial radiographic evaluation is usually not possible

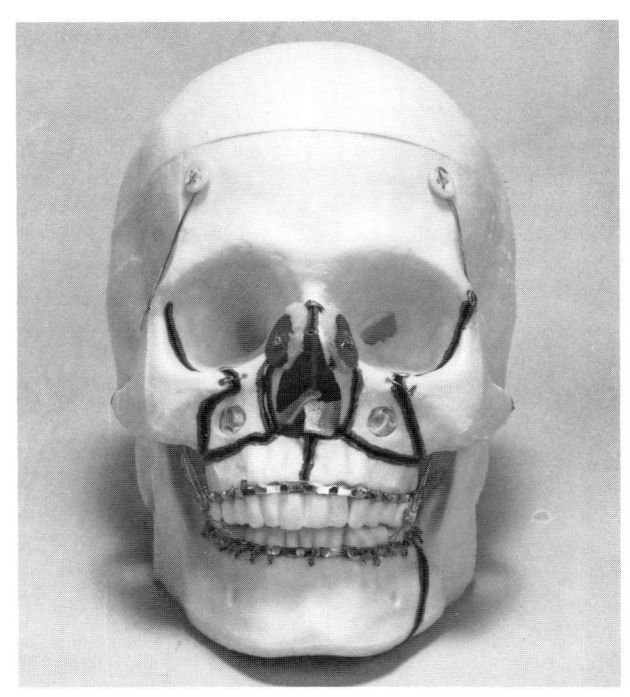

Figure 202-6 This model illustrates the repair of multiple facial fractures. The mandibular fracture is favorably oriented, and thus internal ligation is unnecessary. Arch bars have been applied to the teeth, and the inferior orbital rims and zygomaticofrontal sutures are internally ligated. Transnasal wires are secured over padded lead plates to support the naso-orbital fracture. Two suspension wires pass from the mandibular arch bar and behind the body of the zygoma to holes just above the zygomaticofrontal sutures. "Pull-out" wires are looped around the suspension wires, then passed subcutaneously upward to pierce the skin high on the forehead. These pull-out wires are tied over plastic buttons, and when the intermaxillary fixation is released, these wires are used to retrieve the two maxillary suspension wires.

because of the nature of the associated injuries, but after the patient is stabilized and other concomitant injuries are managed, a proper and thorough evaluation may be undertaken. The optimal time for fracture treatment is within the first 6 h, before massive edema develops, but this may not be practical when there are other injuries.

The most important principle of treatment of multiple facial fractures is direct operative reduction and internal fixation, combined with external suspension if instability is present (Fig. 202-6). Unstable mandibular fractures are first operatively reduced and internally ligated, and arch bars are applied to the teeth. Next, the orbital floors are explored and displaced fractures involving the infraorbital rim are ligated. Incisions in the lateral eyebrow provide access to the zygomaticofrontal region to secure fractures there and to attach maxillary suspension wires. Fractures of the naso-orbital region are then exposed, reduced, and internally ligated, and displaced medial canthi are reattached. Maxillary suspension wires and the arch bars are finally ligated.

References

1. Barclay TL: Four hundred malar-zygomatic fractures, in Wallace AB (ed): *Transactions of the International Society of Plastic Surgery, Second Congress.* Edinburgh, Livingstone, 1960, pp 259–265.
2. Converse JM, Smith B, Wood-Smith D: Orbital and nasoorbital fractures, in Converse JM (ed): *Reconstructive Plastic Surgery.* Philadelphia, Saunders, 1977, pp 748–793.
3. Cruse CW, Blevins PK, Luce EA: Naso-ethmoid-orbital fractures. J Trauma 20:551–556, 1980.
4. Daffner RH, Gehweiler JA, Osborne DR, Roberts L: Computed tomography in the evaluation of severe facial trauma. In press.
5. Dingman RO, Converse JM: The clinical management of facial injuries and fractures of the facial bones, in Converse JM (ed): *Reconstructive Plastic Surgery,* 2d ed. Philadelphia, Saunders, 1977, pp 599–747.
6. Emery JM, von Noorden GK, Schlernitzauer DA: Orbital floor fractures: Long term follow-up of cases with and without surgical repair. Trans Am Acad Ophthalmol Otolaryngol 75:802–812, 1971.
7. Harrison DH: Nasal injuries: Their pathogenesis and treatment. Br J Plast Surg 32: 57–64, 1979.
8. James RB, Fredrickson C, Kent NJ: Prospective study of mandibular fractures. J Oral Surg 39:275–281, 1981.
9. Jurkiewicz MJ, Nickell WB: Fractures of the skeleton of the face. J Trauma 11:947–958, 1971.
10. Knight JS, North JF: The classification of malar fractures: An analysis of displacement as a guide to treatment. Br J Plast Surg 13:325–339, 1961.
11. Koornneef, L: Current concepts on the management of orbital blow-out fractures. Ann Plast Surg 9:185–200, 1982.
12. Larsen OD, Thomsen M: Zygomatic fractures: I. A simplified classification for practical use. Scand J Plast Reconstr Surg 12:55–58, 1978.
13. Larsen OD, Thomsen M: Zygomatic fractures: II. A follow-up study of 137 patients. Scand J Plast Reconstr Surg 12:59–63, 1978.
14. McCoy FJ, Chandler RA, Magnan CG Jr, Moore JR, Siemsen G: An analysis of facial fractures and their complications. Plast Reconstr Surg 29:381–391, 1962.
15. Newman MH, Travis LW: Frontal sinus fractures. Laryngoscope 83:1281–1292, 1973.
16. Putterman AM, Stevens T, Urist MJ: Nonsurgical management of blow-out fractures of the orbital floor. Am J Ophthalmol 77:232–239, 1974.
17. Tempest MN: The surgical management of displaced fractures of the malar bone and zygomatic arch: A review of 275 consecutive cases, in Wallace AB (ed): *Transactions of the International Society of Plastic Surgery, Second Congress.* Edinburgh, Livingstone, 1960, p 259.

203
Cerebrospinal Fluid Fistula
Ayub Khan Ommaya

Management of cerebrospinal fluid (CSF) leakage from the nose or ear demands a clear understanding of the etiology and pathogenesis of such dural fistulas. The majority of such leaks occur through the base of the skull, a fact undoubtedly related to the particular anatomy of the area and the inexorable force of gravity. The fundamental cause of CSF leakage is a meningeal fistula caused by a number of factors that will be discussed below. It should also be emphasized, however, that a second critical factor is impaired tissue repair, which may be due to lack of proper closure, inadequate support of weak healing tissues, and poor healing of tissues due to infection, metabolic disorders, or other chronic diseases. Leakage is facilitated when the intracranial pressure (ICP) is elevated from any cause.

Although traumatic leakage of CSF is overwhelmingly more common, the first published case of CSF rhinorrhea was of a nontraumatic "high-pressure" type due to hydrocephalus.[42] This report by Miller in 1826 was followed by that of King in 1834,[32] and of Thomson in 1899 on so-called spontaneous rhinorrhea.[57] Neurosurgical treatment of such dural fistulas began much later with the work of Grant[24] and Dandy.[12] Three cases of traumatic leakage treated surgically were reported in 1927 by Cushing.[11] The first series of cases treated by a transcranial extradural repair using fascia lata was published by Cairns in 1937.[7] The transnasal approach to this problem was limited to cauterization until 1948, when Dohlman described a transnasal (transethmoidal) approach that could seal off leaks through the cribriform plate with a septal and middle turbinate flap.[16] The intradural repair technique that is currently the most widely used method was first used by Taylor, as reported by Eden in 1941.[19]

Classification

We previously published an etiologic classification developed some years ago that has been generally accepted (Fig. 203-1).[46,48,54] The categories shown are for didactic purposes and are certainly not mutually exclusive insofar as the mechanism of leakage is concerned. Certain cases of delayed-onset traumatic CSF rhinorrhea have symptoms and signs identical to those of nontraumatic cases, and the actual precipitating cause of the leak may be identical. Voena has described such cases in which a congenital anomaly was found.[60] Analogously, the onset of nontraumatic CSF rhinorrhea in certain cases of pituitary tumor not subjected to surgery but treated with x-irradiation suggests atrophy of tissues as a common etiologic factor with delayed-onset traumatic leaks. However, the mode of onset, complications, and role of raised ICP in the traumatic and nontraumatic groups are significantly different. Nontraumatic leaks are much less common, are insidious in onset, and may persist for years. In the majority of traumatic cases (>50 percent) rhinorrhea stops within 1 week and in most within 6 months. The flow of CSF is greater in the nontraumatic type, the side affected is not constant, aeroceles rarely develop intracranially, and anosmia, found in 78 percent of traumatic cases, is rare. Headache is common in nontraumatic cases. Traumatic CSF leaks bear no relationship to age or sex, whereas the nontraumatic variety affects adults mainly over 30 and females twice as often as males. Meningitis, the main danger in traumatic cases, is much less common in the nontraumatic variety. These and other contrasts between the two major subdivisions of dural fistula are given in Table 203-1.

There is a certain degree of semantic confusion in the literature concerning the nasal leakage of CSF when trauma is not the cause. The term *spontaneous CSF rhinorrhea* has been used more or less consistently to describe such cases since the monograph by St. Clair Thomson in 1899.[57] Further subdivision of this category into *primary spontaneous* (or *idiopathic*) *rhinorrhea* when no precipitating cause could be found and *secondary spontaneous rhinorrhea* when a cause, usually a tumor, was discovered clearly reveal the nosological inadequacy of such a term as *spontaneous* CSF rhinorrhea, which indicates neither the pathogenesis nor the natural history of the disease. The word *spontaneous* means "arising from natural impulse, without external stimulant, or having a self-contained cause or origin, or arising from or entirely determined by the internal operative or directive forces of the organism" (*Shorter Oxford English Dictionary*, 1962). Careful study of the natural history of patients suffering from nontraumatic CSF leaks reveals no actual case that can fit such a definition—that is, in being truly "spontaneous"—hence our preference for the more general term, *nontraumatic CSF rhinorrhea*. This category may then be subdivided etiologically as shown in Fig. 203-1.

A very important subdivision of the nontraumatic group is into *high-pressure* and *normal-pressure* categories. In the high-pressure category the leakage of cerebrospinal fluid is usually acting as a safety valve, closure of which may worsen the patient's condition if the causative lesion is not treated.

Diagnosis

Identification of CSF as the leaking fluid usually must precede demonstration of the cause as well as localization of the fistula itself. Biochemical tests on the collected fluid must show values for sugar of more than 30 mg/dl to be conclu-

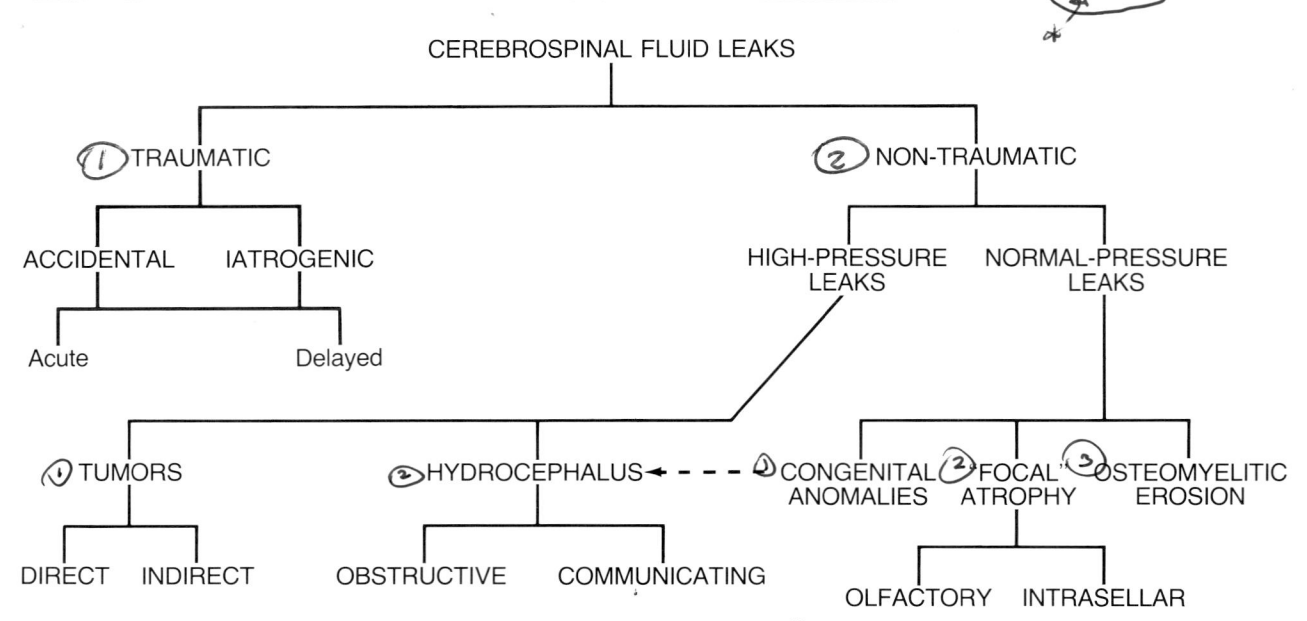

Figure 203-1 Classification of CSF leaks. (Redrawn from Ommaya et al.[48])

TABLE 203-1 Features of Traumatic and Nontraumatic CSF Leakage

Traumatic	Nontraumatic
Incidence	
Approximately 2% of unselected head injuries, relatively common condition	Rare condition; only 82 cases cited in literature
Age and Sex	
Irrespective of age, sex	Usually in mature adults (over 28); average age 43; females predominate (2:1)
Onset	
Usually within 48 h of trauma; occasionally after a few weeks; rarely after months; longest interval reported is 4½ years; onset is always abrupt	Insidious, often mistaken for allergic rhinitis; later becomes profuse flow; in a few cases, after bout of headache, sneezing
Duration of Leakage	
Over 70 percent ease within 1 week, 20–30% may continue for months; it is very unusual for flow to persist for years; nearly all stop within 6 months; recurrent leakage is very rare	Untreated leak may persist for years; in about one-third of cases spontaneous arrest occurs; flow is characteristically intermittent; recurrent leak after long stoppage is common
Amount of Leakage	
From few drops to few ounces daily; profuse leakage extremely unusual	Usually profuse flow; varies from few ounces to over 30 oz daily
Laterality	
Usually unilateral, and this often indicates side of fistula, but side of fracture is better index	Variable; bears no relation to side of fistula
Aerocele and Intracranial Air	
Found in about 20% of cases	Unusual
Anosmia	
Present in 78% of cases	Sense of smell usually preserved
Headache	
Relatively uncommon; in about 10% of cases, usually when marked aerocele or profuse flow is present; this headache is not relieved by flow	Fairly common; characteristically, cessation of flow associated with headache, then relieved by onset of flow, particularly seen in the high-pressure category
Risk of Infection	
High, from 25% to 50% of untreated cases	Lower when factor of longer duration is taken into consideration; appears to be especially true of those cases due to intracranial tumors, that is, high-pressure leaks

SOURCE: Modified from Ommaya et al.[48]

sive. It should be noted, however, that although a test with a Dextrostix reagent strip (Ames Division, Miles Laboratories, Inc., Elkhart, Ind.) has a 45 to 75 percent chance of positive results with normal nasal secretions, a negative test is often very useful, particularly in traumatic cases with serosanguinous leaks.[22] Positive identification of CSF necessitates introduction of suitable tracers into the CSF cavities and their recovery in the nasal discharge and is combined with the methods of fistula localization considered below.[39]

Over half of the cases with nontraumatic rhinorrhea are high-pressure leaks due to tumors, and the diagnostic approach to such patients should therefore be the same as that for patients with epilepsy of late onset, i.e., to vigorously pursue the possibility of a space-occupying lesion with the added proviso that the fistula must also be localized.

The precise localization of the leakage is often a difficult and challenging problem. Possible leaking sites may be numerous and may occur in the anterior, middle, and posterior fossae. Most frequently the CSF reaches the nasal cavity through the frontal sinus, the lamina cribrosa, the sphenoidal roof, or the petrous bone via the middle ear and the eustachian tube. Lateralization of the leak according to nostril side is not reliable.

Table 203-2 summarizes the techniques available for localization and lateralization of CSF fistulas. These include the use of dyes, fluorescent substances, radioactive tracers, and radiographic techniques.[3] Dyes (methylene blue, phenolsulfonphthalein, indigo carmine) have been introduced before or during surgery within the subarachnoidal spaces or intranasally for visual localization of the fistula. Fluorescein has also been used. However, most of these dyes, and particularly methylene blue, can cause significant morbidity.[63] In 1956, the use of radioactive sodium (^{24}Na) injected into the cisterna magna and detected by cotton pledgets distributed against the walls and roof of the nose and nasopharynx and the openings of the eustachian tubes was reported by Crow et al.[10] Similar isotope-counting techniques have been reported employing radioiodinated serum albumin (RISA). Isotope cisternography was introduced by our group at the National Institutes of Health and has been used successfully to visualize the fistula in many cases of traumatic and nontraumatic CSF rhinorrhea.[13,15,48] In 1972, a review of the use of isotopes in the assessment of CSF pathways was published by Holman and Davis.[26]

Plain roentgenograms may demonstrate air-fluid levels within the sphenoid sinus as well as reveal an enlarged sella turcica, and tomography may demonstrate suspicious bone defects. Pneumoencephalography has also been used to show a dilated intrasellar subarachnoid pocket, which, by acting as a tense, pulsating cyst, may be responsible for a rupture in the sellar floor.[6,20] The use of a pneumoencephalogram to decide between such a cyst and a pituitary adenoma has now been completely replaced by CT scanning. Subdural pneumography may be useful in traumatic cases with leaks through the anterior cranial fossa. Various attempts have been made to localize a CSF fistula by Pantopaque or metrizamide injected into the subarachnoid space,[52] into the ventricular system, into a pneumocephalic cavity, or intranasally.[55] After the injection of such media the passage of the opaque material is observed with fluoroscopy and radiography. The use of less irritating water-soluble positive contrast media such as metrizamide combined with CT scanning and suitable image reconstruction can often be extremely useful in pinpointing leak locations. However, despite the foregoing, it should be noted that the dictum of Dandy that visualization of the fistula may on occasion be impossible is still true today.

TABLE 203-2 Diagnostic Procedures for CSF Fistula Localization

Modality	Agent	Comment
A. Dyes	1. PSP 2. Indigo carmine	Dyes are not recommended unless radioisotopes are not available
B. Photoluminescence	Fluorescein	As for A
C. Radiography with x-ray films and computed tomography	1. Conventional films of skull base 2. Tomography (pluridirectional) 3. Pneumoencephalography 4. Subdural pneumography (with tomography) 5. Positive contrast radiography	All are useful procedures. Provisos are: 1. Must show paranasal sinuses 2. Is particularly of value in traumatic leaks and in high-pressure nontraumatic leaks 3. Useful mainly for anterior leaks communicating with ventricles 4. Applicable only to frontal traumatic leaks 5. Especially of value in posterior and middle fossa leaks using metrizamide CT cisternography
D. Radioisotopic assessment	1. ^{99m}Tc-labeled albumin 2. Chelated ^{169}Yb-labeled diphosphothiamine	Fistula track only seen if leak is profuse and track large; accumulation of nuclide in sinus also helps localization; AP views are essential
E. Surgical methods	Retrograde air insufflation via nasopharynx while surgeon looks for bubbles intracranially	Carries risk of introducing infection and is therefore not recommended

Traumatic CSF Leaks

Diagnosis of Traumatic Leaks

CSF leaks after trauma produce the risk for meningitis that may on occasion be fulminant in onset. Lewin has reported one patient with a fracture involving the frontal sinus, who died within 36 h after CSF rhinorrhea following head injury.[35] Pyogenic meningitis developed and the patient died in spite of antibiotics started within a few hours of the injury. Wehrle et al. reported a 21 percent incidence of meningitis after traumatic CSF leaks.[62] Lewin noted that in two-thirds of the patients in his extensive series leaks started within 48 h of the trauma while in the majority of the remainder delayed leaks occurred up to 3 months after head injury. In a few cases the onset was delayed by many months or even years, the longest delay being 9 years in this series. The longest published delayed onset of CSF rhinorrhea was 14 years.[36] Spontaneous closure of such fistulas occurs by adhesions or herniations of brain into bony crevices or by granulation tissue resulting from local meningitis. The quality of closure is thus often inadequate, and the risk of meningitis may remain in some cases of spontaneous closure. It is imperative, therefore, to search for evidence of CSF leakage in all patients with head injury, particularly those with fractures of the skull base. Specific fracture patterns that should be looked for are a fracture that passes through the frontal or ethmoidal sinuses or the common middle fossa fracture that passes parallel to the long axis of the petrous bone. The latter type of fracture almost always involves the middle ear, and if the tympanic membrane is torn, CSF otorrhea is evident. If the tympanic membrane is not torn, fluid will be visible through it in the middle ear. Transverse temporal bone fractures pass at right angles to the petrous pyramid and thus damage the membranous labyrinth but rarely tear the tympanic membrane. Meningitis is usually of delayed onset in such cases. Many cases of meningitis may be due to an undiagnosed transverse temporal fracture, the healing of endochondral bone being notoriously poor. An episode of otitis media at any time following such a fracture is capable of causing meningitis because of the communication between middle ear and subarachnoid space.[30]

In acute traumatic leaks, the CSF invariably is bloody initially and then becomes clear. Delayed leaks may present with a fairly sudden copious gush or as an attack of meningitis without an obvious leak. The rate and constancy of the leakage are probably key factors in determining the onset of meningitis. Copious, continuous leakage is probably less likely to be associated with meningitis than is a scanty, "stop and go" type of leak.

The overall incidence of CSF leaks in head-injured patients varies between 0.25 to 0.5 percent. In Lewin's series of 100 unselected patients with head injury, 7 percent had basal skull fractures, of which one-third, or 2 percent, of the total had CSF leaks.[35] One-quarter of these patients (i.e., 0.5 percent of the total) developed meningitis. MacGee and associates reported a lower incidence of 0.25 percent in their series.[37]

In addition to the clinical search for evidence of a CSF leak or meningitis, the skull films should also be carefully examined for the presence of fluid levels in the sinuses[48] and for the presence of intracranial air. In Lewin's series, air was present intracranially in one-third of the patients with CSF leakage.[35] Marc and Schecter have described a pneumoencephalographic technique by which positioning the patient with a leak can create an air-fluid level in the sphenoid sinus if that is the site of the fistula.[38] A similar maneuver can also be used prior to CT scanning. Other clinical evidence may also alert one to the possibility of a fractured sinus and thus the risk of CSF leak and meningitis. Thus, CSF escaping via the ethmoidal sinuses may collect in the periorbital tissues to cause local edema. In 50 percent of patients with fractures involving the sphenoid sinus, nearby structures are damaged and form the presenting neurological deficit, e.g., visual defects due to chiasmatic injury and evidence of trauma to the hypothalamus or internal carotid artery. However, one-third of patients with fractures involving the paranasal sinuses but with no obvious leak will be found to have no dural tear on intracranial exploration of the sinus fracture.

Although gamma scintigraphic display of the CSF fistula is eminently desirable, there is still a place for the simpler method of Crow et al., particularly when plain x-ray films show a fracture passing through the cribriform plate and a gamma camera is not available.[10,29] A quantitative variant of this technique using chelated ^{111}In-labeled DTPA has also been published.[45] Results of a detailed analysis of the use of isotope cisternography in CSF rhinorrhea by Oberson[45] are summarized in Table 203-3. There were a total of 71 patients referred with a clinical suspicion of CSF rhinorrhea. The necessity for persistance and care in the use of this method is illustrated by the fact that of 29 definite leaks displayed, the majority (i.e., 7 of 11 large and 10 of 18 small fistulas) were seen only on the 24-h scan. A basal cisternal pouch was not thought to be diagnostic unless it was retained on the 24-h scan. Lateralization of the leak, a key need for the surgeon, was possible in only one-third of cases, an experience in keeping with our own.[14] Measurable isotope contamination of the nasopharynx was variable and did not correspond to the side of the fistula in 10 percent of cases. The 34 patients who had negative radioisotope signs in spite of a clinical suspicion of CSF rhinorrhea or otorrhea had no subsequent evidence of a leak in their clinical course, and none developed meningitis. All patients with a positive scan had radioactive handkerchiefs. Washing of the nostrils with physiological water demonstrated contamination of the mucosa in eight cases of CSF fistula without evidence of rhinorrhea. In cases where the handkerchiefs were equivocal, radioactivity in the saliva was compared with the activity of the rinsing water. The test is considered positive only if the radioactivity of the handkerchief is greater than that of the saliva. The saliva is always somewhat radioactive because the resorption of radioiodine varies from one solution to another depending on the stability of the preparation. Alazraki and associates have recommended the use of 10 percent dextrose in water as a vehicle for the radioisotope in order to provide a hyperbaric medium, which apparently results in fewer scan failures, higher count efficiency, and decreased radiation exposure.[2]

In difficult cases where the side and site of the fistula are not obvious, and particularly in cases of CSF otorrhea where it is not clear whether the leak is via the middle fossa or posterior fossa, positive contrast myeloencephalography and ventriculography are recommended.[17] Special care must be taken to use small amounts of the contrast medium and careful x-ray techniques. The risk of meningeal inflammation must always be kept in mind. (This caveat is true for all methods used to display the fistulous tract using chemical substances.)

Iatrogenic Traumatic Fistulae

CSF leakage through the nose after pituitary surgery and through the ear after surgery in the cerebellopontine angle had been much more common in the past. With the introduction of the surgical microscope and the enormous facilitation of technique, this complication has been markedly reduced. In recent series, CSF leakage has been reported in only 5 to 10 percent of cases of acoustic neuroma[28,64] and in 3 to 6 percent of patients undergoing microneurosurgical pituitary surgery.[9,59] The routine use of fat grafts and fascial and muscle stamps to close any fistula created at the time of surgery has significantly reduced the incidence of this complication in contemporary practice.

Treatment of Traumatic Leaks

The surgical approach to traumatic leaks ranges from the vigorous one of Cairns[7,8] and Lewin,[35] who recommended exploration and repair of all leaks as soon as the patient is fit for surgery, to the more moderate approach of waiting to see if spontaneous arrest will occur. Apart from the special case of fractures involving the frontal sinus, which have a high risk of meningitis, the data are inadequate to justify immediate repair of dural fistulas caused by trauma. Five areas of controversy that do require further discussion are as follows:

1. **Duration of conservative management before surgery** Most leaks stop spontaneously, and a significant number do not develop complications. Moreover, no surgical repair guarantees closure of all possible leaks. It is reasonable, therefore, to wait for the general condition of the patient to stabilize after the head injury. During the first week to 2 weeks, an indication for surgery is: (1) no

TABLE 203-3 Radioisotope Signs and Incidence in CSF Rhinorrhea*

Sign	No. of Cases	Time of Positive Scan (No. of Cases)	
		On First Day	On Second Day
No visible fistula	34	0	0
Large fistula	11	4	11
Small fistula	18	6	16
Basal cisternal pouch	22	13	20
Rhinopharyngeal contamination	19	6	17
Radioactive handkerchiefs	29	15	29
Rinsings from nostrils	8	–	8

*Summarized from Oberson.[45]

decrease in the rate of CSF flow over 6 to 8 days, (2) an initial decrease of flow followed by continuation of flow for more than 10 to 12 days, (3) the presence of intracranial air on x-ray examination, (4) meningitis (surgery to follow medical control and recovery from meningitis), or (5) a special circumstance, e.g., a very extensive skull fracture involving the sinuses, especially frontal, or, in the course of surgery for a compound skull fracture, discovery of a dural tear.

2. **Antibiotics** Nose and throat cultures should be taken immediately, and all patients should be placed on antibiotics immediately thereafter. The antibiotics should be changed according to the culture results as they are discovered. Postoperative antibiotics are required only for 3 to 5 days. Broad-spectrum antibiotics are not recommended, and all cultures must be repeated at 48-h intervals in the first week.

3. **Timing of sinus repair** It is not necessary that sinus repair should precede the fistula repair. Cairns showed that sinusitis rarely follows sinus injury, whereas meningitis is a real risk.[7,8] The only exception to this advice is in the case of mastoid sinus injuries. Repair of the mastoid sinuses should precede closure of a related CSF fistula.

4. **CSF drainage** This should not be used because of the high risk of reversing the flow gradient and inducing infection.

5. **Timing of reduction of facial fractures in association with CSF rhinorrhea** Collins has reviewed 19 patients of this type and recommends early reduction (within 48 h) of the facial fractures to avoid poor primary healing of the fracture as well as the risk of meningitis. This author also emphasizes the increased difficulty of reducing partly healed fractures and the supportive advantage of a reconstituted bony support structure at the time of surgical closure of the CSF fistula.

Conservative management while waiting for the decision about operation should consist of total bed rest, 15 to 20 degree elevation of the head to decrease ventricular pressure, cultures of the nose and throat, and penicillin, 1 to 2 million units per day. In children, ampicillin is of value because of the risk of *Haemophilus influenzae* infection. Traumatic otorrhea stops spontaneously more frequently than traumatic rhinorrhea and, if persistent, is suggestive of raised intracranial pressure.

Nontraumatic CSF Leaks

Diagnosis of Nontraumatic Leaks

The clinical presentation of nontraumatic leaks is clearly different as indicated earlier and as summarized in Table 203-1. Patients may present either with a leak as part of a neurological picture of a space-occupying lesion (i.e., a high-pressure leak), as a simple "leaky nose" often mistaken to be a "rhinitis," or as recurrent meningitis without an obvious leak. The flow of CSF is usually more copious than with a traumatic leak and is often heavier on arising in the morning.

This type of CSF leakage seldom stops spontaneously, and thus the first aim in diagnosis is to determine whether a high-pressure or normal-pressure type of mechanism is causative. Our experience with 19 cases of nontraumatic leaks in these two major subcategories is summarized in Tables 203-4 and 203-5.

Each of the etiologic factors in the two categories will now be reviewed in turn. Leakage caused by tumors is subdivided in our classification into *direct* and *indirect* types. This indicates the two ways in which the fistula may be created by the tumor—that is, either directly by tumor eroding the meninges and bone (cases 9 to 15 in Table 203-5) or indirectly via high intracranial pressure causing erosion of anatomically fragile areas of the skull base (cases 16, 17, and 18 in Table 203-5). It is significant that in all three of these indirect rhinorrheas the fistula was in the cribriform plate, an indication of the fragility of this area. Previous reports on tumor-induced CSF rhinorrhea[23,50,56] have emphasized that pituitary tumors are the commonest lesions, and in our series of 10 patients with high-pressure leaks there were four such cases (cases 9, 13, 14, and 15 in Table 203-5). It should be stressed that CSF rhinorrhea is an extremely rare complication of such tumors.

Congenital anomalies and hydrocephalus are much less common than tumors in causing CSF rhinorrhea. The earliest report was by Miller, in which the hydrocephalus was the communicating type.[42] Occasionally hydrocephalus is associated with a congenital anomaly as the cause of a *high-pressure* CSF leak, and such an association has been reported with Crouzon's disease and Albers-Schoenberg disease (osteopetrosis). In the majority of cases, however, congenital anomalies are etiologically more important for *normal-pressure* leaks. Here nasal encephalocele is the usual lesion discovered (case 4 in Table 203-5), and such patients are the usual examples of normal pressure leaks occurring in childhood.

Congenital anomalies may also play a role in the next category of our classification, namely "focal atrophy." We first proposed this speculative idea in 1968, suggesting that the normal contents of the cribriform plate or sella turcica areas are reduced in bulk. This atrophy may be due to ischemia, and the empty space thus created is filled with an arachnoidal pouch. This pouch, which is simply an extension of the normal CSF space, e.g., the intrasellar cistern, enables the normal CSF pressure pulse to exert a focal and continually erosive effect analogous to the creation of cranial vault excavations by the arachnoidal granulations. This concept of focal atrophy was developed to explain the mechanism of CSF rhinorrhea in three of our patients with sellar leaks (cases 2, 7, and 8 in Table 203-4). It may also be invoked to explain normal-pressure CSF leaks from any site in adults. In this it agrees quite well with the hypothesis advanced by O'Connell.[47] He described in two patients a combination of an excavated lamina cribrosa plus a shrunken olfactory bulb, enabling the development of a pulsating pocket of CSF over the fistula. In our series, case 1 in Table 203-4 appeared to have a similar lesion. A recent report by Front and Penning described three cases of recurrent meningitis without obvious rhinorrhea in whom a pouch of arachnoid bulged through the floor of the anterior cranial fossa into the nasal cavity.[21]

TABLE 203-4 Summary of Case Material, Normal-Pressure Leaks

Case No.	Age	Lesion*	Surgery for Lesion	Surgery for Rhinorrhea	Result Lesion	Result Rhinorrhea	Follow-up Results
1	54	Hole in cribriform plate with arachnoid hernia	Yes	Yes (same operation)	Recurred	Recurred	Leak persists minimally 10 yr after surgery with no attacks of meningitis.
2	58	Arachnoid hernia into enlarged "empty sella"	Yes	Yes (same operation)	Cured	Cured	No further leak 6 yr after surgery; patient well.
3	32	Hole in cribriform plate with meningeal hernia	Yes	Yes (same operation)	Cured	Cured	No further leak 25 yr after surgery; patient well.
4	4	Nasal encephalocele	Yes	Yes (same operation)	Cured	Cured	No further leak 16 yr after surgery; patient well.
5	24	Hole in cribiform plate with brain and meningeal hernia	Yes	Yes (same operation)	Cured	Cured	No further leak 16 yr after surgery; patient well.
6	52	Hole in anterior cranial fossa with meningeal hernia	Yes	Yes (5 operations)	Recurred	Recurred	Leak persisted until death 11 yr after first operation; autopsy confirmed congenital hole; no evidence of tumor.
7	50	Hole in front of sella turcica	Yes	Yes (same operation)	Cured	Cured	No further leak 6 yr after surgery; patient well.
8	48	Hole in floor of sella with arachnoid hernia into sella	Yes	Yes (same operation)	Cured	Cured	No further leak 6 yr after surgery; patient well.
9	43	Hole in posterior aspect of sella floor in patient diagnosed as having "pituitary tumor" but having an empty sella with 3 yr of scanty CSF leak	No	Yes	Unchanged	Cured	No further leak at 1 yr after surgery.

*Analysis of 50 cases of normal-pressure nontraumatic leaks suggest an equal probability for the site of the fistula to be either in the cribriform zone or in the floor of the sella and through the sphenoid sinus.

Recently Leclercq et al. reviewed the "empty sella" syndrome and presented arguments indicating that a more suitable name for this example of focal atrophy would be *intrasellar arachnoidocele*.[34] They argued that the sella is filled with a fluid pouch of arachnoid overlying a normal though shrunken pituitary gland. The syndrome is relatively benign, as noted earlier by others.[5,18,25,31,41] These authors would reserve the term *empty sella* for the sella "emptied" by surgery.

Drolet et al. reported one additional case of empty sella with a CSF leak that illustrates important points in the diagnosis and treatment of such lesions.[18] Because of the posterolateral position of the fistula, it required three operations to stop the leak. The third successful operation, which approached the fistula via the transnasal trans-sphenoidal route, was the only one that could truly disclose the site of the fistula. Our most recent case in this category is given as case 9 in Table 203-4.

The anatomy of the sphenoid bone in relation to CSF leaks has been carefully studied by A.C. Hooper.[27] In 138 adult sphenoids, 27 defects were found that could become potential sites for fistulas associated with CSF rhinorrhea. Fourteen holes were located at the site of the superior opening of the transient lateral craniopharyngeal canal. The remaining 13 were along the pathway of the internal carotid artery. Hooper concluded that the gross and microscopic appearances of these defects were consistent with their production by a process of focal atrophy as suggested by us in 1968.

Minor degrees of congenital meningeal and meningocerebral hernia can also act as actual or potential pathways in the anterior skull base and present in adult life with CSF rhinorrhea, for example, cases 3, 5, and 6 in Table 203-4. The majority of case reports of "primary spontaneous" rhinorrhea are explicable by this etiology. The genesis of such a leak, aside from the role of focal atrophy, is probably related to the attainment of the maximal CSF pressure in adults, which is almost three times that of infants, as well as in association with factors such as sneezing, coughing, or other causes of normal fluctuations in CSF pressure.[47]

TABLE 203-5 Summary of Case Material, High-Pressure Leaks

Case No.	Lesion*	Surgery for Lesion	Surgery for Rhinorrhea	Result Lesion	Result Rhinorrhea	Follow-up Results
10	Pituitary adenoma; leak via sella floor	Yes (1)†	Yes (2)	Cured	Recurred	Leak persists 6 yr. after surgery; on replacement therapy and penicillin.
11	Acoustic neurinoma; leak via eustachian tube?	Yes (1)	No	Cured	Cured	No leak for 6 yr.
12	Acoustic neurinoma; leak via eustachian tube?	Yes (2)	No	Cured	Cured	No leak for 9 yr.
13	Nasopharyngeal carcinoma	Yes (1)	No	Persisted	Stopped	Died after 1 yr; no autopsy.
14	Pituitary adenoma	Yes (1) +DXr‡	No	Persists	Stopped	No leak 5 yr later.
15	Pituitary tumor	No DXr only	No	?Cured	Persists	Minimal leak persists; patient refuses surgery; 6 yr.
16	Pituitary adenocarcinoma; leak via sellar floor	Yes (2) +DXr	Yes	?Cured	Cured	Massive tumor regressed after radiation; no tumor recurrence for 3 yr, leak arrested.
17	Third ventricle tumor; leak in cribriform plate	No	Yes (shunt)	Persists	Cured	No leak for 11 yr.
18	Cerebellar glioma; leak via cribriform plate	Yes (3)	Yes (1)	?Cured	Cured	No leak or tumor recurrence for 6 yr.
19	Cerebellar glioma; leak via cribriform plate	Yes (3)	Yes (2)	?Cured	Persisted	Died after second leak surgery from pulmonary embolism

*Analysis of 50 cases of high-pressure leaks suggest the following distribution for sites of fistulas: cribriform zone = 75%, sellar floor = 21%, and via the eustachian tube = 4%. This distribution did *not* correspond to the sites of tumors, most of which were pituitary lesions.
†Numbers in parentheses refer to number of operations
‡DXr = Deep x-ray therapy

The final etiologic category is of osteomyelitic erosion. This is a very rare cause,[43] and we have not had a single patient with this condition.

Nontraumatic Otorrhea

CSF fistulas of the temporal bone without preceding trauma are rare. They usually present as otorrhea, but just like the traumatic fistulas, they may present as rhinorrhea via the eustachian tube. Otorrhea is often unrecognized, especially if the tympanic membrane is intact, as in the case reported by Kramer et al. in which a congenital defect in the temporal bone led to occult otorrhea that simulated serous otitis media.[33] Tomography showed the bony defect clearly.

Treatment of Nontraumatic Leaks

The treatment of nontraumatic CSF leaks is primarily surgical, although nonsurgical measures have resulted in successful management of such patients on rare occasions. The principles of treatment of both traumatic and nontraumatic leaks is summarized in Table 203-6.

Remission of leakage, rarely permanent, may follow lumbar puncture, meningitis, or dye injection. It has been reported that long-term medical management with antibiotics is possible,[4] but with the increasing number of resistant organisms, this conservative therapy becomes hard to justify. Repeated lumbar punctures have been tried and recommended, but this may now be considered an obsolete method and, as indicated above, liable to precipitate meningitis. Instillation of substances such as silver nitrate nasally to promote closure of the fistula from below has not been routinely successful, but a recent cure of a case of CSF rhinorrhea has been reported following the application of methyl 2-cyanoacrylate to the roof of the ethmoid sinus.[23] It is often recommended that following the identification of CSF in a rhinorrhea, expectant treatment—including nursing in a semi-Fowler position and discouragement of nose blowing, sneezing, and straining—and antibiotic administration be tried for 6 to 8 weeks before surgery is considered.

TABLE 203-6 Summary of Principles of Treatment of CSF Leaks

Traumatic Rhinorrhea[35]
1. Intradural surgical repair of the dural laceration is recommended for *all* cases of proven CSF rhinorrhea as prophylaxis against infection.
2. Surgery should be performed 10–14 days after trauma for *acute* leaks and as soon as possible after the onset of delayed CSF rhinorrhea.
3. Conservative management is reserved for older and poor risk patients only.

Nontraumatic Rhinorrhea[48]
1. *High-pressure leaks* Treat the cause, e.g., remove a tumor or perform CSF shunt surgery for hydrocephalus. Only if the leak persists after the cause is treated should the fistula be localized and surgically closed.
2. *Normal-pressure leaks* The fistula will be found either in the anterior fossa (usually via the cribiform area) or in the middle fossa (usually via the sellar or parasellar area and sphenoid sinus). Localize and close either by an intradural or trans-sphenoidal method.

While it is true that the majority of cases of CSF rhinorrhea, particularly the traumatic variety, will stop leaking, it would be risky to suggest that this conservative therapy be adopted routinely. Indeed, the occurrence of repeated attacks of meningitis after spontaneous closure of such fistulas, even in the absence of obvious leakage of fluid,[53] would support a more active approach to some of these patients. Thus, in nontraumatic CSF rhinorrhea, a conservative attitude is probably justifiable only in those patients with high-pressure leaks in whom the causal lesion cannot be removed. This was the initial management of our case 15 in Table 203-5. However, after apparently complete regression of her adenocarcinoma following deep x-ray therapy, her fistula was closed intracranially to prevent recurrent meningitis.

In normal-pressure leaks, surgical repair of the fistula is usually easy and is to be recommended as soon as the diagnosis is established. A cautionary note should be made regarding anesthesia for such surgery. Positive pressure respiration at induction must be carefully avoided to protect against the risk of infection. Thus, tracheal intubation while the patient is awake is recommended.

The use of synthetic adhesives has been reviewed by VanderArk et al. and should be considered in the difficult case not responding to the more routine methods described above.[58] Nystrom[44] and Probst and Rahn[49] have used a combination of an adhesive (Biobond) and fascia to achieve good results.

Surgical Techniques for Fistula Closure

The techniques for fistula closure may be considered briefly under two headings: first, the extracranial, usually transnasal, approach, and, secondly, the intracranial approach. An extracranial, extranasal approach to fistulas through the frontal and ethmoidal sinuses has been recently recommended by Aboulker et al.[1] Mennig has described a transethmoidal trans-sphenoidal approach to repair a fistula through the floor of the sella turcica that was successful after an intracranial attempt at closing the leak had failed.[40] A recent review of such extracranial techniques may be found in a paper by Vrabec and Hallberg.[61] In my opinion, such extracranial techniques should be reserved for sellar and parasellar leaks in the carefully selected patient in whom the etiology of the leak has been clearly understood and the fistula tract demonstrated and in whom the intracranial methods cannot be undertaken for definite reasons. The rationale for this opinion is that CSF rhinorrhea is not simply a matter of closure of the bony defect but, more importantly, necessitates repair of the meningeal defects. Such meningeal repairs are best conducted after adequate inspection intradurally, and rhinological procedures seldom provide an adequate view within the dura mater except for the lower part of the sella turcica as exposed through the sphenoid sinus. Therefore, leaks through the sella turcica and sphenoid sinus are best approached via the microneurosurgical trans-spenoidal route. In one case we were able to stop a trans-sphenoidal leak using tantalum-impregnated methacrylate after three prior craniotomies had failed to stop the flow. Use of intraoperative fluoroscopy while injecting the opacified semiliquid methacrylate transnasally enabled complete and solid filling of the sphenoid sinus after polymerization had occurred.

Intracranial procedures have been adequately described by Dandy,[12] and only a few comments are necessary. The crucial factor in adequate surgical treatment is closure of the meningeal defect. This is often quite small in nontraumatic leaks and easy to overlook. Some neurosurgeons have resorted to filling the craniotomy site with saline, and with the help of the anesthesiologist they obtain a visual demonstration of the hole by forcing air from the nasopharynx into the exposure area, where the escape of bubbles may be seen.[51] However, with accurate preoperative diagnosis, this maneuver with its attendant risk of sepsis may be avoided. After demonstration of the meningeal defect, the patient's own fascia lata, pericranium, muscle, or strips of fat may be used to provide the intradural repair, with fascia lata plus fat grafts being most satisfactory. It is not essential to strip the dura and to seal bony defects exposed with bone wax, acrylic cements, or other substances. This is necessary only where the bony defect is large enough to necessitate support of the intradural graft. In such cases, methyl methacrylate is a satisfactory caulking material.

The intracranial, intradural approach is recommended for most traumatic and nontraumatic cerebrospinal fistulas, with careful "patching" of the fistula site, preferably using the patient's own fat with or without fascia lata as free grafts. Sealing of subjacent bony defects is required only when the hole is of significant size—for example, greater than 2 mm in diameter. In high-pressure leaks, removal or bypass of the tumor or obstruction should always precede repair of the fistula, which should be carried out only where it is positively established that the "safety valve" function of the CSF leakage is no longer required. In normal-pressure leaks, obliteration of the arachnoid hernia should accompany careful intradural repair of the fistula.

References

1. Aboulker P, Le Beau J, Sterkers JM, Elbaz P: Traitement des fistules méningées ethmoïdo-frontales: A propos de 15 cas opérés avec succès par voie exocrânienne. Ann Otolaryngol Chir Cervicofac 83:27–32, 1966.
2. Alazraki NP, Halpern SE, Ashburn WL, Coel M: Hyberbaric cisternography: Experience in humans. J Nucl Med 14:226–229, 1973.
3. Allen MB Jr, El Gammal T, Ihnen M, Cowan MA: Fistula detection in cerebrospinal fluid leakage. J Neurol Neurosurg Psychiatry 35:664–668, 1972.
4. Anderson WM, Schwarz GA, Gammon GD: Chronic spontaneous cerebrospinal rhinorrhea. Arch Intern Med 107:723–731, 1961.
5. Bernasconi V, Giovanelli MA, Papo I: Primary empty sella. J Neurosurg 36:157–161, 1972.
6. Busch W: Die Morphologie der Sella turcica und ihre Beziehungen zur Hypophyse. Virchows Arch [Pathol Anat] 320:437–458, 1951.
7. Cairns H: Injuries of the frontal and ethmoidal sinuses with special reference to cerebrospinal fluid rhinorrhoea and aeroceles. J Laryngol Otol 52:589–623, 1937.
8. Cairns H: Discussion on injuries of the frontal and ethmoidal sinuses. Proc R Soc Med 35:809–810, 1942.

9. Ciric IS, Tarkington J: Transsphenoidal microsurgery. Surg Neurol 2:207–212, 1974.
10. Crow HJ, Keogh C, Northfield DWC: The localisation of cerebrospinal-fluid fistulae. Lancet 2:325–327, 1956.
11. Cushing H: Experiences with orbito-ethmoidal osteomata having intracranial complications. Surg Gynecol Obstet 44:721–742, 1927.
12. Dandy WE: Pneumocephalus (intracranial pneumatocele or aerocele). Arch Surg 12:949–982, 1926.
13. Di Chiro G, Grove AS Jr: Evaluation of surgical and spontaneous cerebrospinal fluid shunts by isotope scanning. J Neurosurg 24:743–748, 1966.
14. Di Chiro G, Ommaya AK, Ashburn W, Briner WH: Isotope cisternography in the diagnosis and follow-up of cerebrospinal fluid rhinorrhea. J Neurosurg 28:522–529, 1968.
15. Di Chiro G, Reames PM, Matthews WB Jr: RISA-ventriculography and RISA-cisternography. Neurology (Minneap) 14:185–191, 1964.
16. Dohlman G: Spontaneous cerebrospinal rhinorrhea: Case operated by rhinologic methods. Act Otolaryngol [Suppl] (Stockh) 67:20–23, 1948.
17. Doron Y, Simon J, Peyser E: Positive contrast myeloencephalography for visualization of cerebrospinal fluid fistula. Neuroradiology 3:228–230, 1972.
18. Drolet M, Bouche B, Bélanger C: Syndrome de la grosse selle turcique vide et de la rhinorrhée du liquide céphalo-rachidien. Can Med Assoc J 107:1199–1202, 1972.
19. Eden K: Traumatic cerebrospinal rhinorrhoea: Repair of the fistula by a transfrontal intradural operation. Br J Surg 29:299–303, 1941.
20. Engels EP: Roentgenographic demonstration of a hypophysial subarachnoid space. AJR 80:1001–1004, 1958.
21. Front D, Penning L: Occult spontaneous cerebrospinal fluid rhinorrhea diagnosed by isotope cisternography. Neuroradiology 2:167–169, 1971.
22. Gadeholt H: The reaction of glucose-oxidase test paper in normal nasal secretion. Acta Otolaryngol (Stockh) 58:271–272, 1964.
23. Gotham JE, Meyer JS, Gilroy J, Bauer RB: Observations on cerebrospinal fluid rhinorrhea and pneumocephalus. Ann Otol Rhinol Laryngol 74:215–233, 1965.
24. Grant FC: Intracranial aerocele following fracture of the skull: Report of a case with review of the literature. Surg Gynecol Obstet 36:251–255, 1923.
25. Hodgson SF, Randall RV, Holman CB, MacCarty CS: Empty sella syndrome. Med Clin North Am 56:897–907, 1972.
26. Holman BL, Davis DO: Radioisotopic assessment of cerebrospinal fluid pathways. Prog Nucl Med 1:359–375, 1972.
27. Hooper AC: Sphenoidal defects—a possible cause of cerebrospinal fluid rhinorrhoea. J Neurol Neurosurg Psychiatry 34:739–742, 1971.
28. House WF, Hitselberger WE: Surgical complications of acoustic tumor surgery. Arch Otolaryngol 88:659–667, 1968.
29. Jacobson I, Maran AG: Localization of cerebrospinal fluid rhinorrhea. Arch Otolaryngol 93:79–80, 1971.
30. Jones HM: The problem of recurrent meningitis. J R Soc Med 67:1141–1147, 1974.
31. Keravel Y: Contribution au diagnostic et au traitement chirurgical de la selle turcique "vide." Thèse de Doctorat en Médecine, Paris, 1973.
32. King D: Report to Westminster Medical Society. London Med Surg J 4:823–825, 1834.
33. Kramer SA, Yanagisawa E, Smith HW: Spontaneous cerebrospinal fluid otorrhea simulating serous otitis media. Laryngoscope 81:1083–1089, 1971.
34. Leclercq TA, Hardy J, Vezina JL, Mercky F: Intrasellar arachnoidocele and the so-called empty sella syndrome. Surg Neurol 2:295–299, 1974.
35. Lewin W: Cerebrospinal fluid rhinorrhea in nonmissile head injuries. Clin Neurosurg 12: 237–252, 1966.
36. Linell EA, Robinson WL: Head injuries and meningitis. J Neurol Neurosurg Psychiatry 4:23–31, 1941.
37. MacGee EE, Cauthen JC, Brackett CE: Meningitis following acute traumatic cerebrospinal fluid fistula. J Neurosurg 33:312–316, 1970.
38. Marc JA, Schecter MD: The significance of fluid-gas displacement in the sphenoid sinus in post-traumatic cerebrospinal fluid rhinorrhea. Radiology 108:603–606, 1973.
39. McKusick KA, Malmud LS, Lordela PA, Wagner HN Jr: Radionuclide cisternography: Normal values for nasal secretion of intrathecally injected ^{111}In-DTPA. J Nucl Med 14:933–934, 1973.
40. Mennig H: Heilung einer schwierigen Liquorfistel durch rhinochirugisches Vorgehen. Laryngol Rhinol Otol (Stuttg) 43:412–419, 1964.
41. Metzger J, Helias A, Messimy R, Fischgold H: Nouveaux cas de selles turciques dites vides avec signes neuro-ophtalmologiques ou rhinorrhée. Rev Neurol (Paris) 123:435–442, 1970.
42. Miller C: Case of hydrocephalus chronicus, with some unusual symptoms and appearances on dissection. Trans Med Chir Soc Edinb 2:243–248, 1826.
43. Nori A, Carteri A: Rinoliquorrea: Trattamento e risultati a distanza. Chir Ital 16:161–165, 1964.
44. Nystrom SHM: On the use of Biobond in the treatment of cerebrospinal rhinorrhea and frontobasal fistula. Int Surg 54:332–340, 1970.
45. Oberson R: Radioisotopic diagnosis of rhinorrhea. Radiol Clin Biol 41:28–35, 1972.
46. Obrador S: Primary non-traumatic spontaneous cerebro-spinal fluid rhinorrhea with normal cerebro-spinal fluid pressure. Schweiz Arch Neurol Neurochir Psychiatr 111:369–376, 1972.
47. O'Connell JEA: Primary spontaneous cerebrospinal fluid rhinorrhea. J Neurol Neurosurg Psychiatry 27:241–246, 1964.
48. Ommaya AK, Di Chiro G, Baldwin M, Pennybacker JB: Non-traumatic cerebrospinal fluid rhinorrhea. J Neurol Neurosurg Psychiatry 31:214–225, 1968.
49. Probst C, Rahn BA: La fermeture plastique des fistules frontobasales au moyen de Biobond-Tabotamp: Expériences cliniques et expérimentales. Neurochirurgie 18:203–212, 1972.
50. Raskin R: Cerebrospinal fluid rhinorrhea and otorrhea: Diagnosis and treatment in 35 cases. Int Surg 43:141–154, 1965.
51. Ray BS, Bergland R: Cerebrospinal fluid fistula: Clinical aspects, techniques of localization, and methods of closure. J Neurosurg 30:399–405, 1969.
52. Rockett FX, Wittenborg MH, Shillito J Jr, Matson DD: Pantopaque visualization of a congenital dural defect of the internal auditory meatus causing rhinorrhea; Report of a case. AJR 91:640–646, 1964.
53. Schneider RC, Thompson JM: Chronic and delayed traumatic cerebrospinal rhinorrhea as a source of recurrent attacks of meningitis. Ann Surg 145:517–529, 1957.
54. Spetzler RF, Wilson CB: Dural fistulae and their repair, in Youmans JR (ed): *Neurological Surgery*, 2d ed. Philadelphia, Saunders, 1982, pp 2209–2227.
55. Teng P, Edalatpour N: Cerebrospinal fluid rhinorrhea with demonstration of cranionasal fistula with Pantopaque. Radiology 81:802–806, 1963.
56. Teng P, Papatheodorou C: Cerebrospinal rhinorrhea and otorrhea. Arch Otolaryngol 82:56–61, 1965.
57. Thomson St C: *The Cerebrospinal Fluid; Its Spontaneous Escape from the Nose*. London, Cassell, 1899.
58. VanderArk GD, Pitkethly DT, Ducker TB, Kempe LG: Repair of cerebrospinal fluid fistulas using a tissue adhesive. J Neurosurg 33:151–155, 1970.

59. VanGilder JC, Goldenberg IS: Hypophysectomy in metastatic breast cancer. Arch Surg 110:293–295, 1975.
60. Voena G: Considerazioni su un caso di grave cranio-rino-liquorrea da persistenza del canale basi-occipitale. Arch Ital Otol 70:212–222, 1959.
61. Vrabec DP, Hallberg OE: Cerebrospinal fluid rhinorrhea. Arch Otolaryngol 80:218–229, 1964.
62. Wehrle PF, Mathies AW Jr, Leedom JM: Management of bacterial meningitis. Clin Neurosurg 14:72–85, 1967.
63. Wolman L: The neuropathological effects resulting from the intrathecal injection of chemical substances. Paraplegia 4:97–115, 1966.
64. Yasargil MG, Fox JL: The microsurgical approach to acoustic neurinomas. Surg Neurol 2:393–398, 1974.

204
Cranial Defects and Cranioplasty
Donald J. Prolo

The cranium is the province of the neurosurgeon, who must respect and be knowledgeable of its unique biological nature no less than that of the brain itself. Craniotomy for various cerebral lesions requires safe passage to and from cephalic areas with eventual restoration of conformity of the head. The temporary exteriorization of sections of the skull, either free or hinged on a muscle pedicle, in every craniotomy is followed by a form of fresh autogeneic (formerly autogenous) cranioplasty. Discontinuity defects of the cranium for which there is no replaceable skull section have engaged the ingenuity of surgeons from antiquity to the present. The problem of reconstructing the smooth symmetrical and rounded contours of the skull is complex, the moment for accomplishing this is often fleeting, and the diversity of methods advanced through the years testifies to the unsolved nature of this Sisyphean task.

Brief Historical Review

Operations on the cranium long antedated procedures on the brain.[46] Primitive races trephined by scraping away bone until dura was exposed. Coconut shells were used by South Sea Islanders to repair the defect. Petronius in 1565 used a gold plate to repair cleft palates—the first use of an alloplastic material to repair a defect. J. van Meekren is credited with the first bone graft in history when in 1670 he used canine bone to repair a skull defect in a Russian; however, he removed the implant under threat of excommunication by the church. Merrem in 1810 transplanted bone in dogs, and in 1821 P. von Walther performed the first human autogeneic bone graft. The work of Ollier in 1859 established the importance of periosteum in bone regeneration. Macewen in 1873 reimplanted calvarial bone fragments after treating them with bichloride of mercury, and in 1878 he was the first to transplant a human bone allograft.[9]

In 1889 Senn wrote on the repair of cranial defects with antiseptic decalcified bone. In that same year Seydel transplanted an autograft of tibia with attached periosteum to repair a parietal defect. Müller and König in 1890 independently advocated a flap of scalp periosteum and outer skull table to be swung over a skull defect. Bunge (1903) first used fresh osteoperiosteal homograft (allograft) skull. The work of Sicard, Dambrin, and Roger from 1917 to 1919 introduced cadaver skull in cranioplasty. The transplantation of fresh autogeneic bone in cranioplasty followed the initial work of Kappis (1915) with whole ribs, Brown (1917) with split ribs, and Mauclaire (1914) with ilium.[18,46,61] The histological sequence of autogeneic bone transplant repair was first fully documented by Axhausen in 1907, who described the process of invasion of blood vessels along pre-existing channels followed by dynamic reconstructive processes of resorption and appositional new bone formation (*schleichender Ersatz*, translated "creeping substitution").[9]

Alloplastic repair of cranial defects has followed the availability of various plastics and metals throughout this past century. Celluloid, used by Fraenkel in 1890, had an extensive trial but later was abandoned because of cellular reactions and biodegradative processes in tissue.[18,46,61] Aluminum, one of the first metals used by Booth and Curtis in 1893, was soon followed by gold, utilized successfully by Gersten (1895) and more extensively tried by Estor (1916). Subsequently many metals have had clinical trials, including vitallium alloy (cobalt, chromium, and molybdenum) used by Geib (1941), tantalum by Pudenz and Odom (1942) and Fulcher (1943), stainless steel mesh by Boldrey (1944), stainless steel by Scott, Wycis, and Murtagh (1956), titanium by Simpson (1965) and Gordon and Blair (1974).[6,53] Seven decades after its introduction, Black (1978) returned to the use of aluminum because of its malleability, radiolucency, and low tissue reactivity.[5]

Acrylic resins became available as industrial materials in 1937. Under trade names of Vitacrilic, Lucite, Plexiglas, Crystallite, or Cranioplastic, methyl methacrylate was introduced to human cranioplasty by Zander in October 1940.[61] A one-stage acrylic method described by Spence (1954) is now the most widely used method.[50] Galicich and Hovind in 1967 found that incorporating stainless steel mesh within the methyl methacrylate rendered it less brittle.[15] More recently Habal et al. have reconstructed cranial defects with an alloplastic tray of polyurethane terephthalate (cured Dacron-urethrane composite) filled with autogeneic cancellous bone.[22] Polyethylene, introduced by Alexander and Dillard in 1950, has never achieved broad usage because of difficulties in obtaining a pure form.[29,53] Softness of Silastic rubber has militated against its general use since it was first employed for cranioplasty by Courtemanche and Thompson in 1968.[11]

Over this past century the plethora of methods tried and later abandoned for various reasons has paralleled the increasing need for a suitable implant. The incidence of trauma through wars and vehicular accidents and multiplying neurosurgical procedures have provided an experimental base upon which principles of cranioplasty have evolved.

Causes of Skull Defects; Indications for and Timing of Cranioplasty

Skull defects most commonly result from trauma. Contaminated compound depressed skull fractures among civilians and penetrating head injuries among military personnel are the most frequent causes. More recently, a defect resulting from a growing skull fracture has been found in children usually under 3 years of age with an antecedent (usually parietal) skull fracture within 4 to 6 months, and associated with a dural tear, cerebral herniation, and ventricular dilatation and porencephaly.[20,30]

Skull defects also arise from excision of tumors (osteomas, hemangiomas, meningiomas, eosinophilic granulomas, epidermoids, metastatic tumors, fibrous dysplasia), from infections (osteomyelitis, infected skull flaps), from aseptic necrosis of skull flaps, from radionecrosis and electrical burns of the skull, and from congenital absence of portions of the skull (encephaloceles, large parietal foramina, and other anomalies of the obelion). Cerebral swelling from brain tumors, trauma, infections, and lead intoxication at times requires external decompression and thereby results in a skull defect.

Defects larger than 2 to 3 cm over the cerebral convexity and all defects in the glabrous frontal areas are universally repaired. Exceptions to this general rule include deficient skull under temporal or occipital muscles or calvarial discontinuity in the elderly or mentally encumbered. If cerebral seizures occur among these latter patients, a cranioplasty should be done to protect the brain.

Among the possible indications for cranioplasty, the two commonly accepted ones address issues of cerebral protection and appearance. These two indications also partially delimit materials used to restore the integrity of the cranium. Although the relief of wound discomfort and seizures was once thought to follow cranioplasty, this does not seem to be the case. Neither is the "syndrome of the trephined," consisting of headaches, dizziness, intolerance of vibration and noise, irritability, fatigability, loss of motivation and concentration, depression and anxiety, universally accepted as an indication to reconstruct the skull.[19,59] This last constellation of symptoms is regaining some credibility from recent reports that describe the effects of direct atmospheric pressure on the brain.[14,52] Both ventricular migration toward a small defect with a corresponding ipsilateral midline shift and contralateral shift of central structures under a large defect have been reported.[30,51,52] Associated with this anatomical displacement of brain has been contralateral hemiplegia,[52] increased intracranial pressure, hemispheric collapse,[51] and cerebrospinal hydrodynamic changes[14] in patients with large cranial defects. In these large defects with anatomical displacement of cerebral structures, the return of the patient to normal after cranioplasty was noted in each of the above reports.

Four persuasive indications for cranioplasty, therefore, are restoration of cerebral protection, physical appearance, and intracranial pressure relationships and the provision of an intact vault for the normal growth and development of cephalic structures in the young. Evidence supportive of the organic basis of the syndrome of the trephined is the improvement in symptoms following cranioplasty with the reversion of intracranial pressure relationships to normal. Convulsive disorders and wound tenderness are unlikely to benefit from cranioplasty.

Contraindications to cranioplasty include the presence of hydrocephalus, cerebral swelling, infection, a compound wound, contiguous functional paranasal sinuses (as indicated by air within a sinus on x-ray), and thin, scarred, or devitalized scalp. Children under 6 years of age will frequently regenerate skull, provided that the dura is intact and not grafted. At least 1 year after craniectomy should elapse before considering a cranioplasty in children.

The timing of cranioplasty is critical to avoid infection developing in devitalized autografts or about alloplastic substances. It is generally accepted that cranioplasty should be delayed 3 to 6 months after compound wounds and at least 1 year after a wound infection. The report of Rish et al. in 1979 based on 491 cranioplasties performed by numerous neurosurgeons clearly established the desirability of waiting 1 year after penetrating or compound cranial injuries.[47] The use of stainless steel mesh and antibiotics by Koslow and Ransohoff suggests an alternative method in rare and exceptional circumstances.[32]

Attributes of Ideal Cranioplastic Material

Most will agree that no alloplastic plate will ever exceed in quality the properties of viable full-thickness autogeneic skull. That such tissue is quantitatively unavailable explains the search for an acceptable, albeit imperfect, substitute. An ideal material would be (1) viable and thereby capable of growth and resistant to infection, (2) radiolucent, (3) thermally nonconductive with a coefficient of expansion identical with that of the surrounding skull, (4) nonionizing and noncorrosive, (5) stable (durable, nonbiodegradable), (6) inert (nonreactive, nonantigenic, nonsensitizing, noncarcinogenic), (7) esthetically pleasing, (8) protective with equivalent biomechanical properties compared with the skull, (9) malleable and easily contoured, (10) inexpensive, (11) readily available, and (12) sterilizable.[13] For various reasons no present material satisfies all of these criteria.

Autogeneic bone (rib, ilium) removed from its blood supply slowly becomes viable and capable of growth and resistant to infection. The frequently unsatisfactory esthetic result (up to 50 percent),[31] the necessity to harvest and thereby violate another area of the body, and the tendency for the cranioplasty to resorb with compromised biomechanical properties are all disadvantages in the use of autogeneic rib or ilium.

Metals are strong, can be sterilized, and do not require a second operation. However, they more often become infected, they indent, they conduct cold and heat, they ionize and corrode, they are difficult to shape, and they usually are radiopaque.

Acrylic resins provide favorable properties, including strength, esthetic qualities, inertness, availability, thermal nonconductivity, and ease of application. The plate remains a foreign body, however, with attendant risks of infection, brittleness, and stationary size. With a pore size of 50 μm, bacteria may colonize within the plate.[21] Methyl methacrylate is well tolerated both for cranioplasty and aneuroplasty,[7,8,23] but macrophages aggregate around implants and methyl methacrylate particles have been found in the liver.[21] No report of carcinoma or sarcoma has followed the use of any plastic, including polyethylene in humans, despite the reports in rats.[40]

Technique of Cranioplasty with Methyl Methacrylate

The use of methyl methacrylate has been widespread since Spence described the one-stage method in 1954.[50] The brittleness of this material resulted in reports of fractures,[26,27] leading Galicich and Hovind to recommend embedding wire mesh within the plate during the autopolymerization process.[15] Lake et al. confirmed the more favorable mechanical properties of methyl methacrylate strengthened by coarse wire mesh.[33] The plate should be at least 5 mm thick, except over temporal regions or in a child's skull (Figs. 204-1 and 204-2).

Preparation of the Patient

Because acrylic is a foreign body, some neurosurgeons will deliver preoperative antibiotics active against *Staphylococcus* species, and continue them for 48 h postoperatively. All the hair over the scalp is clipped on the ward, and the scalp is scrubbed with disinfectant soap several times. After the induction of general anesthesia the entire head is shaved and then positioned with the plane of the skull defect horizontal in order to facilitate molding of the congealing plastic later (Fig. 204-1).

Preparation of the Wound

Scalp flaps must be designed to lie outside of the defect, behind the hairline, never parallel to previous wounds and scars, and with a broad base to accommodate the vascular supply to the area of skin within the flap. If an incision is made through the old scar, one must exercise great care to avoid incising the dura. The entire scalp flap is elevated cautiously to avoid penetrating the dura in areas where it is adherent to the scalp. Emphasis must be placed on maintaining the full thickness of the scalp, especially where it will overlie the acrylic plate. The temporalis muscle is reflected off the dura. The pericranium surrounding the cranial defect should be incised and the margins of the defect demarcated by removing soft tissue down to the dura with a curette. A 3- to 5-mm ledge is then drilled along the entire circumference of the defect to the diploe with a high-speed burr. This allows the edges of the acrylic plate to be recessed and provides a smooth contour and firm fixation. At least four drill holes are placed through the skull around the circumference of the defect for securing the plate.

Preparation and Positioning of the Acrylic Plate

Strips of bulk cotton soaked in saline and of variable thickness are laid over the dura within the defect to establish the desired contour over which the plate will be molded. This material also further protects the brain from thermal or chemical injury from the acrylic plate.[2,16,36] Methylene blue or another marker is used to outline the edges of the defect along the ledge. A sheet of paper is then placed over the defect, and the outline of the defect is transposed onto the paper. This pattern is superimposed onto coarse 20- or 24-gauge foundation stainless steel wire mesh, and an appropriate configuration of wire mesh is prepared. The wire mesh is then contoured over the bulk cotton in the defect. Thin radial sectors may be cut into the mesh to help in bending the coarse wire mesh. The wire mesh must be coarse enough to permit penetration by the methyl methacrylate. A clamp is used to open up holes in the wire at 2-cm intervals.

A sheet of polyethylene folded along one edge is laid over the defect. In between the two layers of the sheet, the contoured wire mesh is positioned. Liquid monomer (the catalyst) is then added to the powdered methacrylate polymer. This mixture is continuously stirred until its consistency is doughy (soft putty), at which time it is poured over the wire mesh in between the layers of polyethylene sheet. Enough methyl methacrylate is mixed to form a plate at least 5 mm thick for the adult skull. The surgeon, assistant surgeon, and nurse then firmly press with their fingers along the edges of the defect to establish the boundaries of the plate. Intermittent molding of the plate will smooth out irregularities and promote equal thickness. Because this autopolymerization process is exothermic, cold saline should be irrigated over the plate while it hardens.[16,37] Studies have shown the subdural temperatures to rise very little.

When the plate solidifies enough to hold its shape, it is removed from its position over the defect at a time when the exothermic process peaks. The plate is then trimmed, and irregularities are removed with a drill. In the areas of the previously placed holes in the wire mesh, the drill is used to create 3- to 5-mm openings in the plate. This allows egress of epidural fluid and fibrosis to occur through the plate, with the scalp eventually becoming adherent to it. Smaller drill holes are placed at four points along the edges of the plate opposite holes in the skull in order to secure the plate in position with 28-gauge stainless steel wire. The high-speed drill is then further used to remove any excrescences over the plate. Bulk cotton overlying the dura is removed before copious saline irrigation purges the wound of debris. The temporalis muscle, galea, and skin are closed in layers.

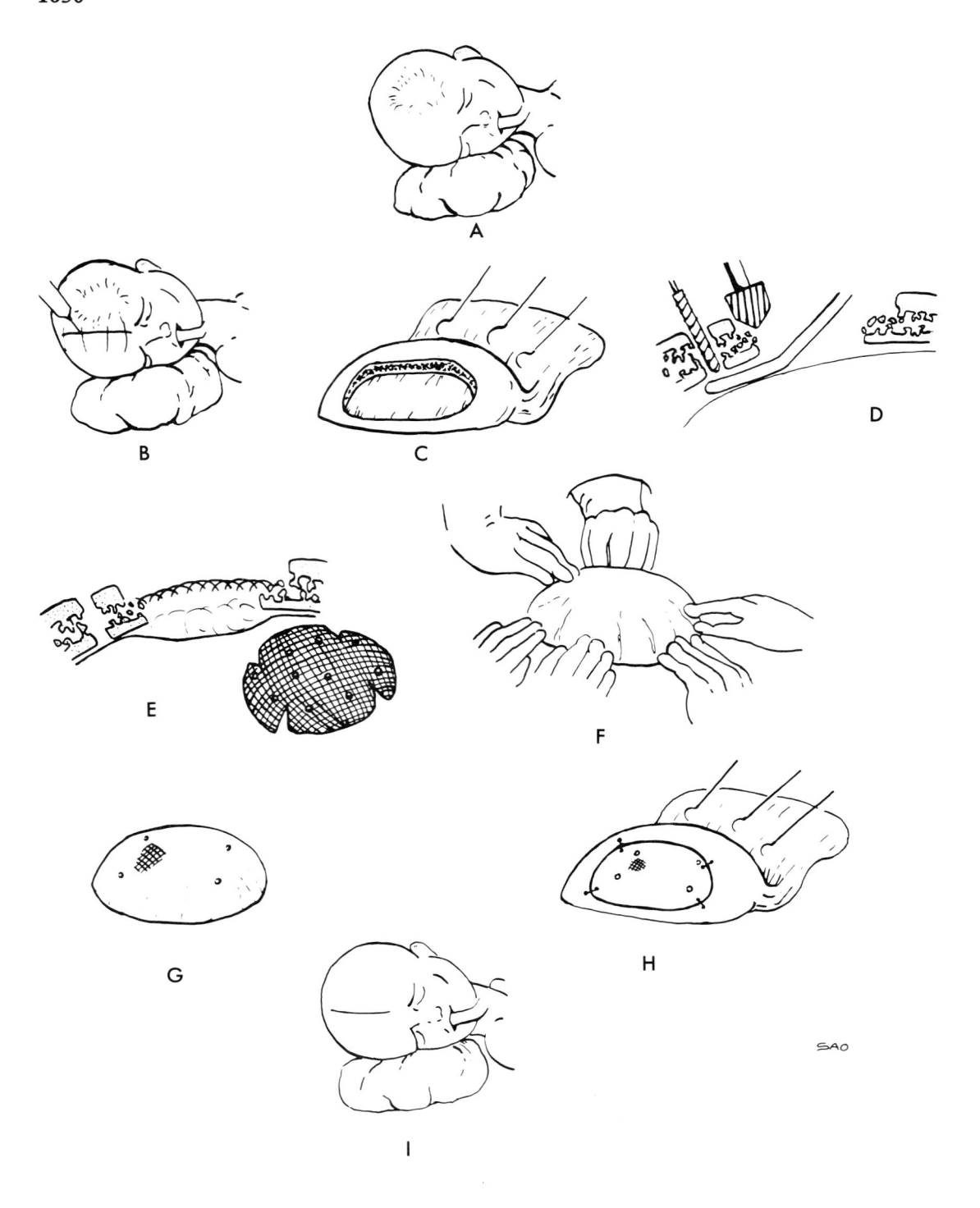

The postoperative roentgenographic appearance of such a plate demonstrates the wire mesh separated by a margin of acrylic from the edge of the skull defect (Fig. 204-2A and B). The contour of such a plate should follow that of the brain. Otherwise, in striving for perfect symmetry of the skull, one risks excessive pressure on the brain. Stainless steel wire mesh embedded within the acrylic plate imposes minimal artifact on the computed tomogram (Fig. 204-2C).

As an alternative to direct formation of an acrylic plate, some neurosurgeons prefer the prefabrication of such an implant by impression techniques in order to ensure a good cosmetic result and reduce operating time. Maniscalco and Garcia-Bengochea,[36] Jordan et al.,[28] and Cooper et al.[10] have described such procedures, which require the services of a

Figure 204-1 Methyl methacrylate cranioplasty. Acrylic cranioplasty lends itself to all regions of the skull except in areas of infection or in direct contiguity with functional paranasal sinuses. *A.* At operation, the head is positioned with the plane of the defect horizontal to facilitate later molding of the hardening plastic. *B.* The scalp incision is outlined on the skin outside the area of the defect and is infiltrated with a local anesthetic containing adrenalin. *C.* The margins of the defect are defined with removal of soft tissue down to the dura; penetration of this protective membrane is avoided. *D.* With a drill, a 5-mm ledge is carved around the defect. At least four holes are placed around the defect. *E.* Bulk cotton is placed over the dura to approximate the normal cranial contour. Methylene blue is traced over the ledge. This outline is then transferred onto paper spread over the defect. A paper pattern of the defect is then placed over 20-gauge stainless steel wire mesh, and the wire mesh is cut in the shape of the defect. Sectors are cut out of the wire mesh to facilitate bending it, and 5-mm holes are opened up in the mesh with a small clamp. *F.* Enough acrylic monomer and polymer are mixed to provide for a 5-mm thick plate. The wire mesh and acrylic of doughy consistency are placed within a folded plastic sheet that is positioned over the defect. At least three pairs of hands are positioned around the defect to fashion a plate of desired shape and thickness. *G.* Excrescences are removed with a burr, and holes are drilled around the edges of the plate to secure it to the skull and through the interior of the plate to allow for the escape of extradural fluid and penetration of binding fibroblasts. *H.* The plate is secured with 28-gauge stainless steel wire, and the wound is closed (*I*).

dental prosthetics laboratory. If the patient's own bone flap or that of another patient of identical cranial contour is available for use as a model, a plate may be prefabricated without estimating margins of the defect through the intact scalp.[4] Asimacopoulos et al. reported forming an impression and thereafter a plate of methyl methacrylate during the operative procedure to improve the cosmetic appearance and strength of the implant.[2] The prefabrication techniques are most applicable for very large hemicraniectomy defects, where irregularities and low stress points in the plate may be eliminated.[10,28,29,36]

Methyl methacrylate is available commercially (Cranioplastic; Codman & Shurtleff, Inc., Randolph, Mass.). Although aluminum wire mesh has the most favorable combination of strength, malleability, and radiolucency, the Food and Drug Administration has not approved its use. Most vendors now have stopped supplying stainless steel wire mesh, but implantable-grade stainless steel wire mesh of various gauges is available from Melrath Gasket, Philadelphia, Pa.

Technique of Autogeneic Bone Cranioplasty

Despite the universal popularity of cranioplasty with methyl methacrylate, there are indications for autogeneic bone grafting of skull defects.[31,34,35,38] In children undergoing active growth of brain and skull, autogeneic bone grafting is obviously advantageous because of the capacity of the bone to respond to developmental forces pari passu with surrounding skull. It has been shown further that viable bone is more resistant to infection. When an alloplastic plate must be removed in an adult because of infection, fracture, or hypersensitivity, then consideration must be given to the use of autogeneic rib or ilium. Although Kappis in 1915 used whole rib, it was Brown in 1917 who suggested splitting the rib to obtain greater volume of the bone and to more easily contour the autograft. Credit must be given to Longacre for emphasizing the clinical utility of autogeneic rib and providing a scientific base through studies in the monkey.[35] He emphasized the unique osteogenic proliferative capacity of transplanted rib, the large reservoir of autogeneic ribs within the body, and its regenerative character. If its thoracic periosteal bed is preserved, rib regenerates within 5 weeks in the young child, and if necessary may be used again for transplantation. McClintock and Dingman reported the successful use of iliac bone for cranioplasty in 1951 even before the studies of Longacre.[53]

Two operative fields are necessary for autogeneic bone cranioplasty (Fig. 204-3). The source of autogeneic bone for smaller defects may be the iliac crest. For larger defects rib grafts should be employed. Incisions for rib grafts are made to take some alternate combination of ribs (e.g., ribs 4 and 6). The thoracic incision is curved posteriorly to allow exposure of more ribs. An incision is made through the periosteum overlying the rib, and as much rib as possible is removed from the transverse process to the costal cartilage.

An estimate of the total length of rib needed is determined by the formula $L = A/W \times 2$, where L is the length of the rib required in centimeters, A is the surface area of the defect in square centimeters, and W is the average width of the rib in centimeters.[38] Ribs are cut 4 mm longer than the defect. The costal periosteum is then closed with no. 000 catgut suture. If the pleural cavity is entered, closure should be effected at the time of a Valsalva maneuver. The chest wall is then closed.

The cranial wound is prepared in the same manner described above for alloplastic cranioplasty. In this case, however, the eburnated margins of the defect must be curetted and rid of fibrous tissue back to bleeding bone. The high-speed drill may destroy cells by heat production. It and the use of bone wax should be avoided. Either a 1-cm ledge is created along the edge of the defect on which to inlay the rib or a groove may be tunneled between the inner and outer tables of the skull to position the tapered ends of the ribs. The ribs are split with osteotomes and contoured with strong clamps or bone benders to provide a suitable cosmetic result. It is extremely important that the sections of rib be firmly secured to the exposed corticocancellous bone at the margins of the defect. Contact compression forces at the junction between autograft and host skull ultimately deter-

A

B

C

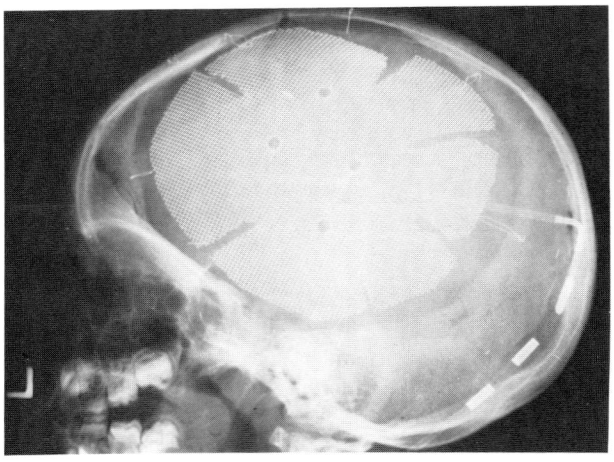

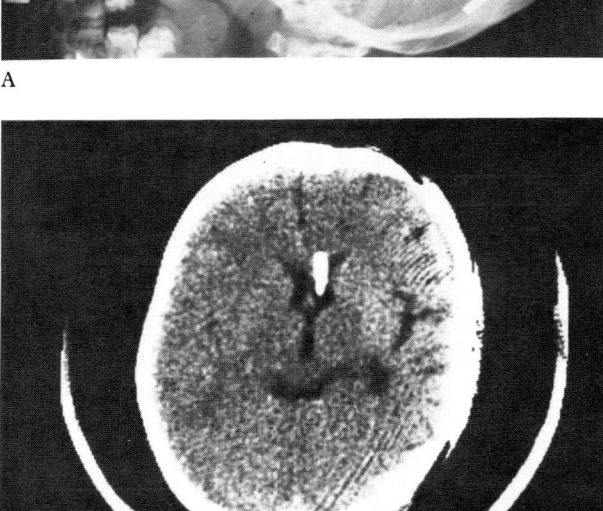

mine whether the grafts will become viable or subsequently will resorb. The inlaid ribs are then secured at either end with 28-gauge stainless steel wire. Adjacent ribs have either the cortical or the medullary surface facing the dura. Adjacent ribs must be closely approximated to one another to stimulate osseous rather than fibrous union. Wiring adjacent ribs together in the manner of a chain-linked fence has even been suggested.[38] The wound is closed in layers as described above, and a mild compressive dressing is applied.

Complications and Results

Complications from cranioplasty may be divided between those characteristic of the operative procedure in general and those more related to the type of implant used. The risks for life in a patient with marginal cardiopulmonary reserve who is bedridden or sedentary are extraordinary when considering a procedure designed for cerebral protection and appearance. If a large prefabricated plate does not fol-

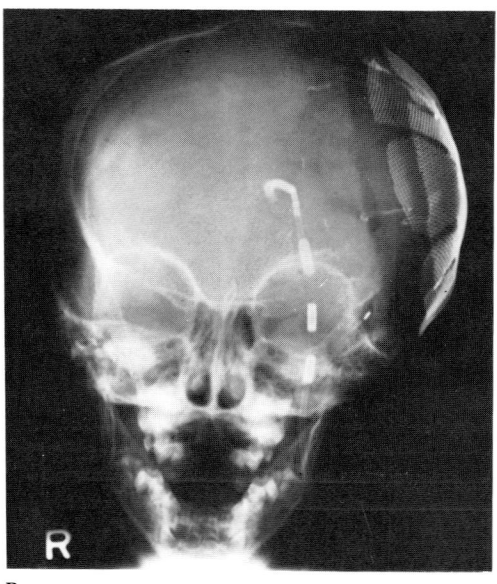

Figure 204-2 A 2-year-old patient with a cranioplasty. *A.* A lateral skull film shows the methyl methacrylate-stainless steel wire mesh plate. The wire mesh does not reach the margins of the defect and is surrounded by and embedded within a 5-mm-thick acrylic plate. A diversionary shunt performed 9 months previously for communicating hydrocephalus is seen. *B.* An anteroposterior skull film also shows the acrylic-mesh cranioplasty. A rim of acrylic surrounds the mesh. The child's head is asymmetrical from hydrocephalus and disturbed cranial growth after a severe injury with cerebral swelling and an acute subdural hematoma. *C.* A CT scan shows brain reaching the inner portion of the acrylic-mesh plate, some artifact from the wire mesh, and evidence of treated communicating hydrocephalus.

Figure 204-3 Autogeneic rib cranioplasty. *A.* This cranioplasty is indicated in defects previously infected or contiguous with paranasal sinuses and is used by some neurosurgeons in children. *B.* The scalp incision is made behind the hairline and never directly over the defect. *C.* The skull defect is exposed, with removal of all soft tissue from the margins of the defect to the dura. A curette is used to fashion a ledge (*D*) or a groove (*G*) for inlaying the tapered ends of the rib. *E.* Alternate ribs are removed and are split with an osteotome (*F*) after a groove is made along one edge. *H.* Split-thickness ribs are placed across the defect with alternate medullary or cortical surfaces facing the dura. The ribs are stabilized in position with 28-gauge stainless steel wire at each end and also across the middle with interlocking wire to hold the ribs in tight contact and thus stimulate bony union.

Cranial Defects and Cranioplasty

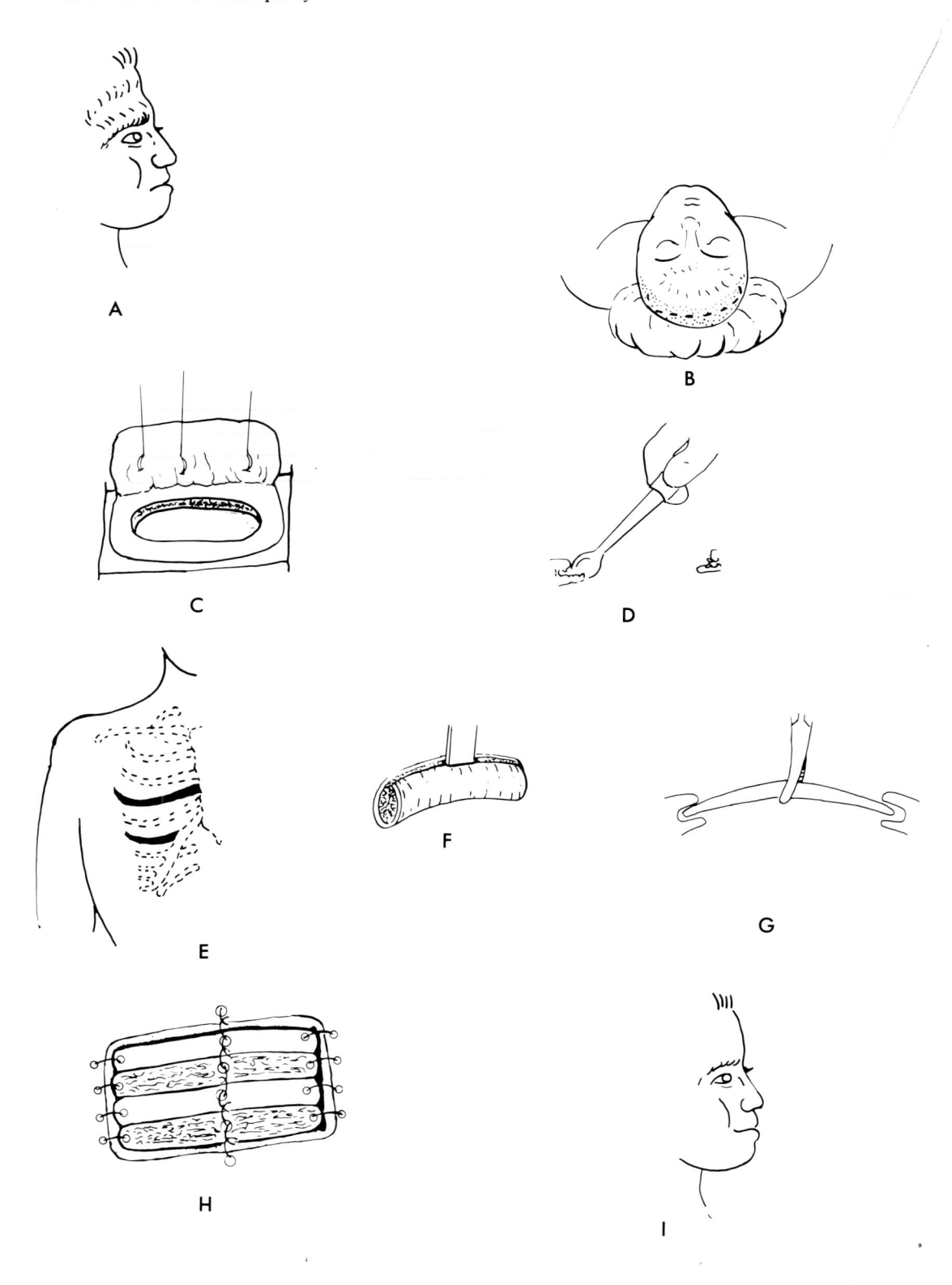

low the cranial contours, compression of the underlying brain and internal herniation may result and death may occur. Infection in a plate with subsequent meningitis or cerebral abscess formation may lead to permanent morbidity or even death. A frequent instructive comment by all authors is the need to obliterate contiguous paranasal sinuses months before implanting any plate. Otherwise the alloplastic material or devitalized autogeneic bone are subject to external microbial colonization.[23]

Metallic and plastic plates are foreign bodies that become encapsulated by host tissue. Sinus tracts between plate and skin, granulomas, and pneumatoceles have been reported.[53] Plates may loosen and erode the skin. Acrylic plates, especially brittle unless they are fortified with stainless steel mesh, may fracture and injure the underlying brain or protrude through the skin. Infection remains the predominant concern for all foreign bodies, and if infection does occur, these foreign bodies must be removed. Autogeneic bone grafts are initially nonviable and therefore are subject to infection. These grafts later may resorb or lead to cosmetically undesirable ridges.

The mortality rate for cranioplasty is very low. Even before the modern era, Grant and Norcross reported a mortality rate of 0.73 percent among 1385 reported cases.[18] Whereas complications of cranioplasty with tantalum were relatively frequent,[60] a much more favorable experience with methyl methacrylate has been apparent. Infection rates usually range between 1 and 8 percent,[23,47,54,63] with an inexplicably high rate of 12 percent in one report.[41] Hammon and Kempe reported 1 percent infection, 2 percent morbidity, and no mortality among 417 cranioplasties.[23] The most comprehensive survey consisted of 491 cranioplasties performed by many surgeons and was published by Rish et al. in 1979.[47] Their mortality rate of 0.2 percent with total morbidity of 5.5 percent (infection rate of 3.7 percent, plate loss 3.1 percent) is likely representative of the results achievable in the community practice of neurosurgery.

Through the past 40 years of usage there have been no reports of malignancy associated with implanting acrylic resin, and the plastic is well tolerated by the adjoining tissue.[7,8] In general the cosmetic result with methyl methacrylate is favorable, although large plates may give the head a flattened appearance, and wire mesh must be imbedded to prevent fracture of these brittle prostheses.

Autogeneic bone is preferred by many, especially in children and generally in areas of previous infections or adjacent to sinuses.[18,31,34,35,41,48] Among 55 cranioplasties with autogeneic bone (46 rib cranioplasties, 9 ilium cranioplasties), Körloff et al. in 1973 reported 1 infection.[31] The cosmetic result was satisfactory in only 50 percent of these cases, however. Petty (1974) reported no infections in 19 rib cranioplasties and only 1 case of resorption.[41] Leivy and Tovi (1970) reported no complications among 9 patients (7 cranioplasties with rib, 2 with ilium).[34] Including the use of osteoperiosteal grafts of skull, Grant and Norcross (1939) reported an infection rate of 5.1 percent among 89 cases (75 osteoperiosteal grafts, 7 rib grafts, etc.). They recommended use of the seventh and ninth ribs for defects larger than 6 × 6 cm.[18] Santoni-Rugiu (1969) transplanted 12 osteoperiosteal grafts from adjacent cranium without complications.[48]

General disinclination to use autogeneic bone among many neurosurgeons results from the need for two operative fields, more operative time, difficulty sculpturing the autograft, some tendency for the grafts to resorb, donor wound complications (pain, pneumothorax), and the frequently unacceptable cosmetic result.

Preservation and Delayed Reimplantation of Skull Flaps

Sections of cranium are often exteriorized for various periods of time with the prospect of delayed reimplantation. Treatment of skull after removal determines in large part its natural history after replacement. Odom et al. (1952)[39] and Abbott (1953)[1] reported success with delayed cranioplasty after freezing the autograft. Hancock (1963) cautioned against autoclaving exteriorized skull because of the high rate of aseptic necrosis and infection with these replaced frozen autografts.[24] Fresh bone separated from its blood supply dies, with the exception of some periosteal, endosteal, and medullary cells and osteocytes within 0.2 mm of cortical bone surfaces. Frozen bone is entirely devitalized. The reorganization of a dead bone plate requires revascularization followed by resorption of dead bone trabeculae and cortex, then finally appositional new bone formation.[42] After bone is frozen, there is impaired coupling of new bone formation to follow the initial resorptive phase.

At this time the only generally accepted method of preserving cranium is by freezing to −70°C or freeze-drying after aseptic removal from the skull. The extent of resorption within these frozen plates is considerable in many and is not reduced even by augmentation with fresh corticocancellous bone. Some of these frozen plates must be removed later and an acrylic cranioplasty performed if resorptive processes leave a thin, unprotective, and cosmetically undesirable plate. The length of time the cranial flap is frozen has no bearing on the outcome; neither does sterilization with ethylene oxide adversely affect the biological events in the replaced plate.[43] Despite this tendency toward resorption, restoration of skull with frozen autogeneic skull is generally successful, except in individuals under 13.[24] In younger people with a very thin cranium, resorption reduces the replaced plate to only a small remnant.

In an effort to prevent resorption of an externalized plate, many clinicians have tried novel approaches for cranial bone preservation. Kreider (1920) and more recently Häuptli and Segantini (1980) have implanted the skull section subcutaneously in the abdomen.[25,46] This technique would likely maintain viability of some superficial cells and perhaps some matrix proteins. Yamada et al. advocated coating the exteriorized bone graft with acrylic resin to reduce resorption, but report an infection rate of 11 percent.[62]

Skull that is contaminated may never be boiled or autoclaved without denaturation of the essential bone proteins (and resultant nearly universal resorption). Cold-cycle ethylene oxide may be used to sterilize skull provided residues are desorbed by lyophilization or prolonged aeration over at least 5 days at room temperature.[44]

The fresh autograft of skull remains the best graft. No preservative method for bone yet equals the osteogenic capacity of a fresh autograft.[43] That such a graft is unavailable accounts for the search for a suitable alternative.

Prospects for the Future

Calvarial bone has the lowest regenerative capacity of any bone within the body. This characteristic led Barth (1893–1898) to conclude in error that all fresh transplanted bone dies and must be replaced by surrounding tissues.[9] It is known that fractures of the cranial base (of chondral origin) heal faster than those over the convexity (of membranous origin).[35]

In an elegant series of experiments in growing rabbits,

Uddströmer (1978) demonstrated the inherent deficiency of periosteum from skull to form bone.[55,56] Isolated periosteum of tibia over tibial defects had seven times the potency for osteogenesis compared with skull periosteum placed over skull defects. Tibial periosteum transplanted over skull defects reproduced calvarial-like bone, and skull periosteum placed over tibial defects increased its osteogenic capacity fivefold. It may be concluded that environmental functional demands influence the type of bone formation and final structure, but there are intrinsic differences between long and membranous bone periosteum in the amount of bone formed.

It is possible that in the adult skull, the diminished functional demands and stresses (Wolff's law) result in the predominance of resorption over appositional new bone formation in the implant. There are further biological differences in the proliferative capacities of living periosteum derived from bone of cartilaginous versus that of membranous origin. Bone modified by physical (boiling, freezing, irradiation) and chemical treatments further must lose structural proteins, which ordinarily enhance new bone formation at the recipient site.

Bone is one of the few organs in the body that retains the primordial capacity to induce regeneration of lost parts. A bone morphogenetic hydrophobic glycoprotein of low molecular weight has been characterized.[58] This "bone morphogenetic protein" induces cell differentiation in perivascular mesenchymal and other undifferentiated cells. More recently a human skeletal growth factor isolated from demineralized adult human bone matrix has been shown to increase the proliferation rate of embryonic chick bone cells in culture.[12] This mitogen putatively released from resorbing bone is postulated to couple bone resorption to formation by interacting locally and selectively with osteoblastic progenitor cells, thereby regulating the amount of bone formed.

Senn in 1889 reported demineralized bovine bone to have some osteogenic capacity. More recently Shehadi (1970) and Bakamjian and Leonard (1977) reported the osteogenic capacity of even undemineralized bone powder.[3,49] Experimental and clinical studies confirm the well-established findings of Urist, Reddi, and others that demineralized bone is osteogenic.[17,45,57]

In the future, research will be directed at characterizing and preserving osteogenic factors in bone and maximizing conditions at the bone graft site that promote appositional new bone formation. An implant of human bone for cranioplasty at once conveying immediate protection to the brain, reconstructing symmetrical contours for the head, and capable of undergoing revitalization with prospects for evolutionary viability is the goal for the future.

References

1. Abbott KH: Use of frozen cranial bone flaps for autogenous and homologous grafts in cranioplasty and spinal interbody fusion. J Neurosurg 10:380–388, 1953.
2. Asimacopoulos TJ, Papadakis N, Mark VH: A new method of cranioplasty: Technical note. J Neurosurg 47:790–792, 1977.
3. Bakamjian VY, Leonard AG: Bone dust cranioplasty: Case report. Plast Reconstr Surg 60:784–788, 1977.
4. Bernstein TW, Stewart WA, Andrews EE: Cranioplasty: Utilization of bank bone flaps to prepare acrylic cranioplasties: A technical note. J Trauma 12:133–134, 1972.
5. Black SPW: Reconstruction of the supraorbital ridge using aluminum. Surg Neurol 9:121–128, 1978.
6. Blair GAS, Fannin TF, Gordon DS: Titanium-strip cranioplasty. Br Med J 2:907–908, 1976.
7. Cabanela ME, Coventry MB, MacCarty CS, Miller WE: The fate of patients with methyl methacrylate cranioplasty. J Bone Joint Surg [Am] 54A:278–281, 1972.
8. Charnley J: The reaction of bone to self-curing acrylic cement: A long-term histological study in man. J Bone Joint Surg [Br] 52B:340–353, 1970.
9. Chase SW, Herndon CH: The fate of autogenous and homogenous bone grafts: A historical review. J Bone Joint Surg [Am] 37A:809–841, 1955.
10. Cooper PR, Schechter B, Jacobs GB, Rubin RC, Wille RL: A pre-formed methyl methacrylate cranioplasty. Surg Neurol 8:219–221, 1977.
11. Courtemanche AD, Thompson GB: Silastic cranioplasty following craniofacial injuries. Plast Reconstr Surg 41:165–170, 1968.
12. Farley JR, Baylink DJ: Purification of a skeletal growth factor from human bone. Biochemistry 21:3502-3507, 1982.
13. Firtell DN, Grisius RJ: Cranioplasty of the difficult frontal region. J Prosthet Dent 46:425–429, 1981.
14. Fodstad H, Ekstedt J, Fridén H: CSF hydrodynamic studies before and after cranioplasty. Acta Neurochir (Wien) [Suppl] 28:514–518, 1979.
15. Galicich JH, Hovind KH: Stainless steel mesh-acrylic cranioplasty: Technical note. J Neurosurg 27:376–378, 1967.
16. Genest AS: Cranioplasty made easier. Surg Neurol 10:255–257, 1978.
17. Glowacki J, Kaban LB, Murray JE, Folkman J, Mulliken JB: Application of the biological principle of induced osteogenesis for craniofacial defects. Lancet 1:959–963, 1981.
18. Grant FC, Norcross NC: Repair of cranial defects by cranioplasty. Ann Surg 110:488–512, 1939.
19. Grantham EG, Landis HP: Cranioplasty and the post-traumatic syndrome. J Neurosurg 5:19–22, 1948.
20. Haar FL: Complication of linear skull fracture in young children. Am J Dis Child 129:1197–1200, 1975.
21. Habal MB: Current status of biomaterial's clinical applications in plastic and reconstructive surgery. Biomater Med Devices Artif Organs 7:229–241, 1979.
22. Habal MB, Leake DL, Maniscalco JE: A new method for reconstruction of major defects in the cranial vault. Surg Neurol 6:137–138, 1976.
23. Hammon WM, Kempe LG: Methyl methacrylate cranioplasty: 13 years experience with 417 patients. Acta Neurochir (Wien) 25:69–77, 1971.
24. Hancock DO: The fate of replaced bone flaps. J Neurosurg 20:983–984, 1963.
25. Häuptli J, Segantini P: Neue Aufbewahrungsart von Schädelkalottenstücken nach dekompressiver Kraniotomie. Helv Chir Acta 47:121–124, 1980.
26. Henry HM, Guerrero C, Moody RA: Cerebrospinal fluid fistula from fractured acrylic cranioplasty plate. J Neurosurg 45:227–228, 1976.
27. Jackson IJ, Hoffmann GT: Depressed comminuted fracture of a plastic cranioplasty. J Neurosurg 13:116–117, 1956.
28. Jordan RD, White JT, Schupper N: Technique for cranioplasty prosthesis fabrication. J Prosthet Dent 40:230–233, 1978.
29. Karvounis PC, Chiu J, Sabin H: The use of prefabricated polyethylene plate for cranioplasty. J Trauma 10:249–254, 1970.
30. Kingsley D, Till K, Hoare R: Growing fractures of the skull. J Neurol Neurosurg Psychiatry 41:312–318, 1978.

31. Körlof B, Nylén B, Rietz K: Bone grafting of skull defects: A report on 55 cases. Plast Reconstr Surg 52:378–383, 1973.
32. Koslow M, Ransohoff J: Primary wire mesh cranioplasty in flap infections. Neurosurgery 4:290–291, 1979.
33. Lake PA, Morin MA, Pitts FW: Radiolucent prosthesis of mesh-reinforced acrylic: Technical note. J Neurosurg 32:597–602, 1970.
34. Leivy DM, Tovi D: Autogenous bone cranioplasty. Acta Chir Scand 136:385–387, 1970.
35. Longacre JJ: Deformities of the forehead, scalp and cranium, in Converse JM (ed): *Reconstructive Plastic Surgery*, vol 2. Philadelphia, Saunders, 1964, pp 564–597.
36. Maniscalco JE, Garcia-Bengochea F: Cranioplasty: A method of prefabricating alloplastic plates. Surg Neurol 2:339–341, 1974.
37. McComb JG, Heiden J, Weiss MH: Cortical damage from methyl methacrylate cranioplasty. Neurosurgery 3:233, 1978.
38. Munro IR, Guyuron B: Split-rib cranioplasty. Ann Plast Surg 7:341–346, 1981.
39. Odom GL, Woodhall B, Wrenn FR Jr: The use of refrigerated autogenous bone flaps for cranioplasty. J Neurosurg 9:606–610, 1952.
40. Olson NR, Newman MH: Acrylic frontal cranioplasty. Arch Otolaryngol 89:774–777, 1969.
41. Petty PG: Cranioplasty: A follow-up study. Med J Aust 2:806–808, 1974.
42. Prolo, DJ, Burres KP, McLaughlin WT, Christensen AH: Autogenous skull cranioplasty: Fresh and preserved (frozen), with consideration of the cellular response. Neurosurgery 4:18–29, 1979.
43. Prolo DJ, Pedrotti PW, Burres KP, Oklund S: Superior osteogenesis in transplanted allogeneic canine skull following chemical sterilization. Clin Orthop 168:230–242, 1982.
44. Prolo DJ, Pedrotti PW, White DH: Ethylene oxide sterilization of bone, dura mater, and fascia lata for human transplantation. Neurosurgery 6:529–539, 1980.
45. Reddi AH, Huggins C: Biochemical sequences in the transformation of normal fibroblasts in adolescent rats. Proc Natl Acad Sci USA 69:1601–1605, 1972.
46. Reeves DL: *Cranioplasty.* Springfield, Ill., Charles C Thomas, 1950.
47. Rish BL, Dillon JD, Meirowsky AM, Caveness WF, Mohr JP, Kistler JP, Weiss GH: Cranioplasty: A review of 1030 cases of penetrating head injury. Neurosurgery 4:381–385, 1979.
48. Santoni-Rugiu P: Repair of skull defects by outer table osteoperiosteal free grafts. Plast Reconstr Surg 43:157–161, 1969.
49. Shehadi SI: Skull reconstruction with bone dust. Br J Plast Surg 23: 227–237, 1970.
50. Spence WT: Form-fitting plastic cranioplasty. J Neurosurg 11:219–225, 1954.
51. Stula D, Müller HR: Schädeldachplastic nach grossen dekompressiven Kraniotonien mit Massenverschieburg; CT Analyse. Neurochirurgia (Stuttg) 23:41–46, 1980.
52. Tabaddor K, LaMorgese J: Complication of a large cranial defect: Case report. J Neurosurg 44:506–508, 1976.
53. Timmons RL: Cranial defects and their repair, in Youmans JR (ed): *Neurological Surgery: A Comprehensive Reference Guide to the Diagnosis and Management of Neurosurgical Problems*, 2d ed. Philadelphia, Saunders, 1982, pp 2228–2250.
54. Tysvaer AT, Hovind KH: Stainless steel mesh-acrylic cranioplasty. J Trauma 17:231–233, 1977.
55. Uddströmer L: The osteogenic capacity of tubular and membranous bone periosteum: A qualitative and quantitative experimental study in growing rabbits. Scand J Plast Reconstr Surg 12:195–205, 1978.
56. Uddströmer L, Ritsilä V: Osteogenic capacity of periosteal grafts: A qualititative and quantitative study of membranous and tubular bone periosteum in young rabbits. Scand J Plast Reconstr Surg 12:207–214, 1978.
57. Urist MR: Surface-decalcified allogeneic bone (SDAB) implants: A preliminary report of 10 cases and 25 comparable operations with undecalcified lyophilized bone implants. Clin Orthop 56:37–50, 1968.
58. Urist MR, Lietze A, Mizutani H, Takagi K, Triffitt JT, Amstutz J, DeLange R, Termine J, Finerman GAM: A bovine low molecular weight bone morphogenetic protein (BMP) fraction. Clin Orthop 162:219–232, 1982.
59. Walker AE, Erculei F: The late results of cranioplasty. Arch Neurol 9:105–110, 1963.
60. White JC: Late complications following cranioplasty with alloplastic plates. Ann Surg 128:743–755, 1948.
61. Woolf JI, Walker AE: Cranioplasty: Collective review. Int Abst Surg 81:1–23, 1945.
62. Yamada H, Sakai N, Takada M, Ando T, Kagawa Y: Cranioplasty utilizing a preserved autogenous bone flap coated with acrylic resin. Acta Neurochir (Wien) 52:273–280, 1980.
63. Zotti G, De Vito R: Cranioplastica con resina acrilica: Considerazioni su 139 casi. Minerva Med 62:3760–3769, 1971.

205
Traumatic Intracranial Hematomas

Paul R. Cooper

Impact injury to the head has the potential for producing a variety of hemorrhagic lesions within the substance of the brain and in the epidural and subdural space. Although it is useful to think of these lesions as distinct clinical entities, it must be realized that more often than not two or more types of hemorrhagic lesion coexist or are associated with diffuse brain injuries of a nonhemorrhagic nature. Moreover, because the brain reacts in similar fashion to a variety of traumatic lesions, the clinical appearance of each of these lesions tends to be less distinct than might be assumed from a textbook discussion.

Acute Subdural Hematoma

It is convenient to divide subdural hematoma (SDH) into acute lesions, which present within 48 to 72 h of injury, subacute hematomas, which are manifest between 3 and 20 days, and chronic hematomas, which produce symptoms from 3 weeks to several months after injury.

Pathogenesis

Acute SDH occurs in approximately 10 to 15 percent of patients with severe head injury. Injury from high-speed impact causes the brain to accelerate within the skull and results in tearing of veins that traverse the space between the cortical surface and the dural venous sinuses. Subdural hemorrhages also result from injury to the surface of the brain with bleeding from cortical vessels into the subdural space.

The impact that produces an acute SDH may also cause severe parenchymal injury, which can have a greater influence on the patient's outcome and prognosis than the presence of the hematoma in the subdural space. The presence of these parenchymal injuries explains, in large part, why the morbidity and mortality for acute SDH is so much worse than those seen with acute epidural hematoma.

Clinical Findings; Diagnosis

The patient's clinical findings are related to the size and rapidity of growth of the SDH and the severity of impact injury to the brain. Patients who are rendered immediately unconscious with decerebrate posturing at the time of injury may be assumed to have sustained diffuse (and perhaps irreversible) injury to the cerebral parenchyma. Recovery often does not take place no matter how rapidly the hematoma is removed or intracranial pressure (ICP) controlled.

In patients with less severe injuries, the temporal sequence of changes in the level of consciousness is determined by the magnitude of the impact injury and the rapidity of hematoma accumulation. Those patients with relatively minor injuries may lose consciousness only briefly, or not at all, at the time of impact. However, with expansion of the hematoma, consciousness is gradually lost in the early post-traumatic period.

An altered level of consciousness, pupillary inequality, and motor deficit are frequently noted signs in patients with acute SDH (Table 205-1). These signs are seen with other expanding intracranial mass lesions and are not pathognomonic for SDH. However, regardless of the type of mass, these signs may provide information as to the side of the lesion: mass lesions will usually be found ipsilateral to the side of the pupillary dilatation and contralateral to the side of the motor deficit. Contralateral (falsely localizing) pupillary dilatation may be seen as a result of direct trauma to the globe, oculomotor or optic nerve injury, or direct midbrain trauma. Ipsilateral (falsely localizing) motor deficit is not uncommon and results from cerebral parenchymal injury on the side opposite the SDH or from compression of the contralateral cerebral peduncle against the tentorial edge.[15]

Specialized Diagnostic Examinations

Skull roentgenograms are commonly obtained in patients with head injury who also have focal neurological deficit or a depressed level of consciousness, in a search for a linear skull fracture. However, the presence of a linear skull fracture does not reliably predict the presence or the site of an intracranial hematoma. Although skull films may be used to assess a pineal shift, emergency room skull films are often of poor quality and a pineal shift is identified less than 20 percent of the time in patients with acute SDH.[17,18] For the obtunded patient suspected of having an SDH or other intracranial hematoma, skull films delay the diagnostic evaluation, provide little information that will enable the neurosurgeon to make therapeutic decisions, and are unnecessary

TABLE 205-1 Frequency of Various Signs in Patients with Acute Subdural Hematoma*

Sign	Patients, %
Anisocoria	47
Papilledema	16
Cranial nerve VI palsy	5
Hemiparesis	47

*As compiled from a number of large series in the literature.

except to evaluate a depressed skull fracture or localize the site of a cerebrospinal fluid fistula.

The preferred diagnostic procedure for patients suspected of having an acute SDH is the CT scan, as it is rapid, visualizes the entire intracranial compartment, and can reliably distinguish the density and thus the nature of intra- and extra-axial mass lesions (Fig. 205-1). If a CT scanner is not available, carotid angiography is an acceptable alternative means of diagnosis.

Treatment

Patients who are admitted with a depressed level of consciousness and a suspected intracranial mass should be assumed to have an increase in ICP. Medical treatment to lower elevated ICP should begin after the initial evaluation and is discussed elsewhere in this volume. The definitive treatment of acute SDH consists of operative removal using a large craniotomy centered over the maximum thickness of the hematoma.[7,29] Wide exposure provided by craniotomy allows complete removal of solid clot and visualization and control of the source of hemorrhage. When present, contused brain is resected and intraparenchymal hematomas are evacuated. We leave a drain in the subdural space, close the dura around the drain, and wire the bone flap in place. In the postoperative period the ICP is monitored; a CT scan is obtained within 24 h of operation and again 2 days later, even if the patient is apparently doing well, to rule out the presence of recurrent extra-axial hematoma or delayed parenchymal bleeding.

Burr holes or trephines have been used in the past for the treatment of acute SDH. For the rapidly deteriorating patient with clear signs of focality, emergency burr holes are useful to diagnose the presence of an acute SDH and to evacuate enough hematoma to stabilize the patient's neurological condition or to reverse signs of herniation. However, burr holes or small trephine openings are inadequate for the definitive treatment of acute SDH as visualization of the hematoma is limited and total evacuation of a solid hematoma cannot be accomplished through small openings.[13]

Large decompressive craniectomies have been proposed as a means of improving mortality from acute SDH by providing for external decompression of a swollen brain.[24] Decompression does reduce ICP and beneficially affects intracranial compliance, but outcome has not been improved by this procedure. The failure to improve morbidity is probably a result of the severe parenchymal injury sustained by many patients with acute SDH that cannot be reversed by decompression. Moreover, there is experimental evidence that decompression may increase edema formation and result in strangulation of cortical vessels at the edges of the craniectomy and produce cerebral infarction.[5]

Complications

As many as one-half of patients will have elevations of ICP following operation.[20] CT scanning will clarify the cause of these elevations and distinguish those patients who need reoperation from those whose ICP should be managed medically. The commonest cause of elevation of ICP in the postoperative period is cerebral swelling and results from brain compression by the SDH and direct parenchymal injury sustained at the time of trauma. The edema is often diffuse and generally is not amenable to operative treatment. Therapy consists of control of ICP using medical means.

Recurrent or residual hematoma is not an uncommon complication. If the hematoma is small and the ICP not elevated, operative removal may not be necessary, although the patient may eventually develop a chronic SDH with cerebral compression. Large hematomas or those associated with ICP elevations should be removed. Delayed intracerebral hemorrhage may occur into areas of brain that have sustained shearing or loci with minor contusions on the initial CT scan. This complication is more frequent than had been suspected in the past but is readily identified by frequent CT scanning in the postoperative period. Seizures occur in over one-third of patients, and anticonvulsant medication should be given prophylactically to all patients and continued for at least 1 year following operation.

Outcome

The outcome from acute SDH has been generally unsatisfactory. The majority of series in the literature report a mortality of over 50 percent, and none records a mortality of less

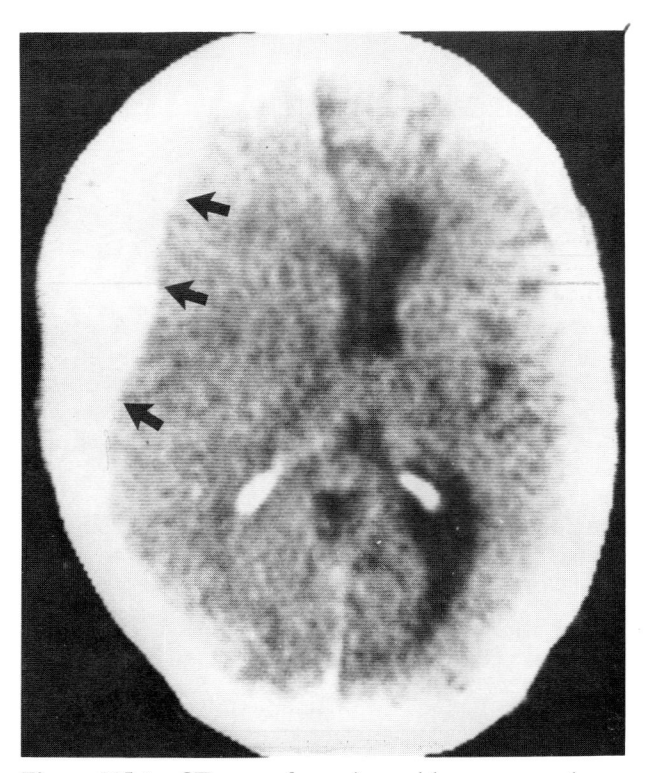

Figure 205-1 CT scan of a patient with an acute subdural hematoma (*arrows*). Although the density appears similar to that of bone, when the windows on the CT scanner were changed, it clearly showed a hematoma between the skull and the brain. Note also the compression and shift of the lateral ventricles.

than 35 percent. Of those patients who do survive, most do not return to normal functioning and a significant number have disabilities that render them dependent.

For the individual patient, however, there are factors that affect outcome in either a beneficial or detrimental way. McKissock et al. found that mortality in patients under age 40 was 20 percent, whereas those over that age had a 65 percent mortality.[17] Others have found that mortality changes after the age of 50 or 60.[29] Patients who are conscious at the time of operation have a mortality of 9 percent, whereas unconscious patients have a 40 to 65 percent mortality.[13] Recently Seelig et al. have shown that prompt operation has an important bearing on outcome; patients with functional survival had an operation within 170 min of their injury, and those who died had an operation on the average 390 min from trauma.[25] Associated brain injury also influences outcome; acute SDH without evidence of parenchymal injury is associated with a mortality of 22 percent, but those patients with concurrent brain injury have a mortality between 30 and 64 percent.[13]

Subacute and Chronic Subdural Hematoma

SDH developing between 3 days and 3 weeks after head injury are termed *subacute*, and those that are manifest longer than 3 weeks after injury are defined as *chronic*. There has been little written about subacute SDH, and for all practical purposes those hematomas that produce symptoms within the first week clinically resemble acute SDH and those that are manifest from 1 to 3 weeks after injury are much like chronic SDH.

The incidence of chronic SDH is 1 to 2 per 100,000 people per year.[8] The majority of patients are 50 years of age or older. Between one-quarter and one-half have no history of head injury, and in those with a history of trauma the injury is often a mild one. A significant proportion of patients are predisposed to SDH because of chronic alcoholism, epilepsy, or coagulopathies.

Pathogenesis

Small amounts of hemorrhage into the subdural space or larger hematomas in patients with brain atrophy may fail to produce symptoms. Within 1 week the hematoma is covered by an outer membrane beneath the dura, and by 3 weeks an inner membrane forms between the hematoma and the arachnoid surface over the brain, thus completely enclosing the hematoma. During this period the hematoma liquefies and becomes progressively more hypodense on the CT scan. In the next weeks, in some patients the hematoma gradually enlarges and in others there is gradual resorption of the liquefied blood.

It has been postulated that a chronic SDH enlarges because the capsule acts as an osmotic membrane with cerebrospinal fluid diffusing into the hematoma and increasing the volume contained within the capsule. Zollinger and Gross suggested that the flow across the membrane occurs as a result of an increase in osmotic pressure from a breakdown of hemoglobin molecules.[34]

These theories have now been discredited with the documentation that the osmolality of the hematoma does not change with time.[31] Moreover, the albumin/gamma globulin and albumin/total protein ratios in the hematoma are higher than in serum. It is likely that albumin diffuses across the hematoma membrane and that the hematoma also enlarges from recurrent hemorrhage into its surrounding membranes.[11]

There is considerable angiographic and CT evidence that some hematomas regress in size and do not need surgical treatment. It is likely that there is a balance between hematoma production and resorption; when resorption exceeds production, the hematoma will shrink, and conversely when production exceeds resorption, the hematoma will enlarge.

Symptoms and Signs

The symptoms and signs of chronic SDH are variable and are not pathognomonic. In the elderly patient the insidious onset of symptoms is sometimes interpreted as dementia. In other patients the onset of a motor deficit is confused with a cerebrovascular accident, transient ischemic attacks, or a brain tumor. Common signs are listed in Table 205-2.

Diagnostic Evaluation

The diagnostic procedure of choice for the evaluation of a chronic SDH is the CT scan. In the first week after injury a chronic SDH appears hyperdense in relation to brain, and in the next 2 weeks most hematomas will appear isodense (although some will appear hyperdense or hypodense). After 3 weeks the vast majority will be hypodense and will assume a lenticular appearance (Fig. 205-2). Nevertheless, because recurrent bleeding frequently occurs from the vascular hematoma membranes, chronic SDH can appear as an admixture of hypo- and hyperdense material.

With older and less sophisticated CT scans, isodense hematomas were not always readily distinguished from the cerebral parenchyma. The shift of midline structures was often mistakenly attributed to cerebral swelling or even a neoplastic process. Bilateral isodense SDHs were even more likely to result in misdiagnosis because a midline shift was not present. Most of the newer CT scanners show the interface between cortical gray matter and the underlying white matter quite well. When the interface is seen well away from

TABLE 205-2 Frequency of Various Signs in Patients with Chronic Subdural Hematoma*

Sign	Patients, %
Hemiparesis	45
Papilledema	24
Hemianopsia	7
Cranial nerve III abnormality	11
Impaired consciousness	53

*Mean calculated from several large series in the literature.

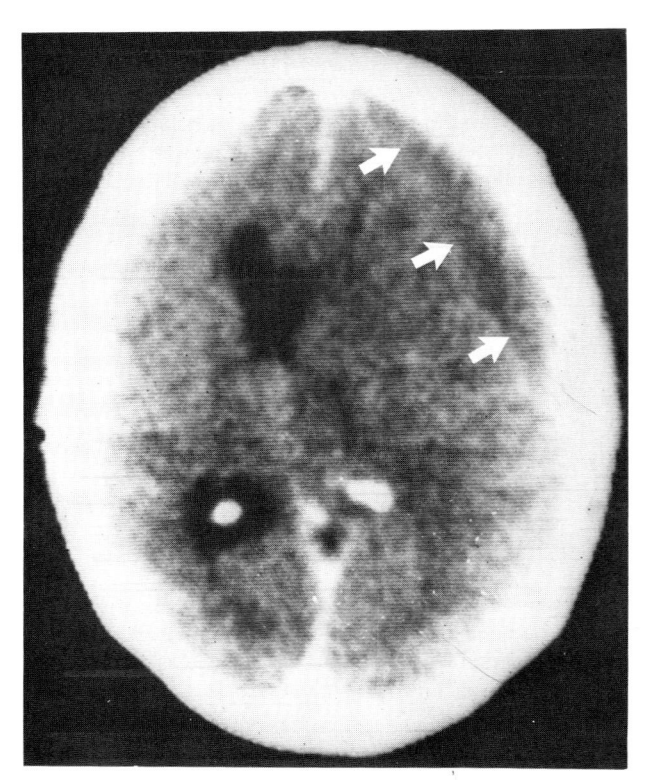

Figure 205-2 This CT scan shows a hypodense extraparenchymal lesion characteristic of a chronic subdural hematoma (*arrows*). The shift of the ventricular system is considerable, and multiple other CT cuts also showed the chronic hematoma.

the inner table, a chronic SDH should be suspected. If there is remaining uncertainty, contrast material (300 ml of 30% diatrizoate meglumine) injected intravenously will cause the membranes of an otherwise isodense hematoma to opacify.

Cerebral angiography was formerly the primary modality for the diagnosis of chronic SDH; the hematoma appears as an avascular space between the brain and skull at the frontal or occipital poles. Between 15 and 20 percent of chronic SDHs are bilateral, so bilateral carotid injections must be performed in all patients.

Treatment

Chronic SDH has been managed by both medical and surgical means. Proponents of medical management have used combinations of bed rest, osmotic diuretics, and corticosteroids in selected patients who had minimal neurological signs.[2,27] Unfortunately, medical treatment is unsuccessful in a considerable number of patients[2] and entails the risks of prolonged immobilization and the administration of corticosteroids and potent diuretics; sudden neurological deterioration is not uncommon.

Prevailing opinion today overwhelmingly supports the operative treatment of these lesions. Evacuation of a chronic SDH has been achieved with the use of craniotomy, burr holes, or with twist drill aspiration. Putnam and Cushing advocated craniotomy because of the exposure it provided for treatment of the solid components of the SDH.[23] Others have employed craniotomy to enable removal of the membranes surrounding the hematoma. There is no evidence that craniotomy is necessary for the adequate treatment of chronic SDH. These hematomas are liquid, and removal may be accomplished without a craniotomy. Similarly, removal of membranes is unnecessary and has no advantage over simple hematoma evacuation.

The most frequently employed treatment of chronic SDH has been evacuation using burr holes at the site of maximum hematoma thickness. A single burr hole is usually sufficient, although two burr holes are sometimes helpful. In the postoperative period a catheter is left in the subdural space for 24 h to remove any residual hematoma using gravity drainage or gentle suction.

Twist drill craniostomy performed at the bedside using local anesthesia is also an effective treatment for most hypodense or isodense chronic SDHs.[28] A twist drill hole is made at a 45 degree angle to the skull, and a Scott cannula or small pediatric feeding tube is passed into the subdural space and connected to a closed sterile collection system. Because rapid evacuation of a chronic SDH by craniotomy or other means can cause brain shift, neurological deterioration, or brain stem hemorrhages,[17] we initially place the drainage bag at or slightly below the patient's head and gradually lower the bag over a period of hours to facilitate slow drainage. After 24 h the subdural drain is removed and the patient is allowed out of bed.

Occasionally when the CT scan shows a loculated hematoma, two twist drill drains must be inserted. Twist drill drainage will not work if the hematoma has a significant solid component. When the CT scan shows a hyperdense collection, the solid hematoma should be evacuated using a burr hole or a small trephine opening.

Complications

The frequent use of the CT scan to follow the postoperative progress of patients with a chronic SDH shows that residual hematoma is quite common regardless of the operative technique used. In spite of this, removal of most of the hematoma will generally result in alleviation of symptoms, and the residual hematoma will gradually resorb over a period of weeks.

True reaccumulation of the hematoma is reported to occur as often as 45 percent of the time in some series and probably results from bleeding from the vascular outer membrane. The possibility that reaccumulation has occurred should be considered in all patients who deteriorate or who do not improve after operation. When this is suspected, a CT scan should be obtained, and if reaccumulation has occurred, the CT scan will show a hematoma that is hyperdense or of mixed density.

When bilateral hematomas exist, it is essential that both be evacuated. If only one is removed, the remaining hematoma can cause a rapid shift of midline structures with resultant neurological deterioration.

Infectious complications include subdural empyema, brain abscess, and meningitis. These are uncommon and occur in less than 1 percent of patients. Seizures are reported in about 10 percent of cases, and all patients with a chronic

SDH should be treated prophylactically with anticonvulsant medication.

Results of Treatment

The mortality following treatment of a chronic SDH is less than 10 percent in most large series, and about 75 percent of patients are able to resume normal functioning. Outcome correlates most closely with the patient's neurological state at the time of treatment; McKissock et al. reported a 13 percent mortality in patients who were comatose or stuporous at the time of operation and a 5 percent mortality in patients who were alert or drowsy.[17]

Subdural Hygroma

Collections of clear, xanthochromic, or slightly bloody fluid in the subdural space following head injury are termed *subdural hygromas*. Hygromas probably form as a result of a tear in the arachnoid with the escape of cerebrospinal fluid into the subdural space.[9,26,29] Enlargement occurs as cerebrospinal fluid becomes trapped in the subdural space.

Subdural hygromas represent about 10 percent of all traumatic intracranial mass lesions. The severity of the precipitating head injury varies from very minor to severe, and the reported age of patients ranges from infancy to the seventies. Subdural hygromas are frequently seen in association with other injuries to the cerebral parenchyma, and the time after injury that the hygroma is discovered depends, in large part, on the nature of the underlying brain injury. Many patients are asymptomatic, but depression of the level of consciousness and a focal motor deficit are common manifestations.

The CT scan shows a crescentic extra-axial collection with a density similar to that of cerebrospinal fluid (Fig. 205-3). The collections are bilateral in more than half of patients, but even when unilateral the midline shift is often small or absent and serves to distinguish hygromas from chronic SDHs. Unlike the chronic SDH, there are no membranes and there is no enhancement with intravenous contrast injection. In patients who are asymptomatic, treatment is not necessary. In symptomatic patients therapy consists of burr hole or twist drill drainage. In patients with coexisting parenchymal lesions, a craniotomy may be necessary. Because of the nature of the lesion, recurrence is frequent. Mortality ranges from 12 to 25 percent and is highest in those patients with severe parenchymal injuries.

Extradural Hematoma

Epidemiology

Extradural hematoma (EDH), a collection of blood between the inner table of the skull and the dura, is an infrequent sequel of head injury and occurs in less than 2 percent of patients admitted with craniocerebral trauma.[12] The age distribution of patients with EDH is generally similar to that

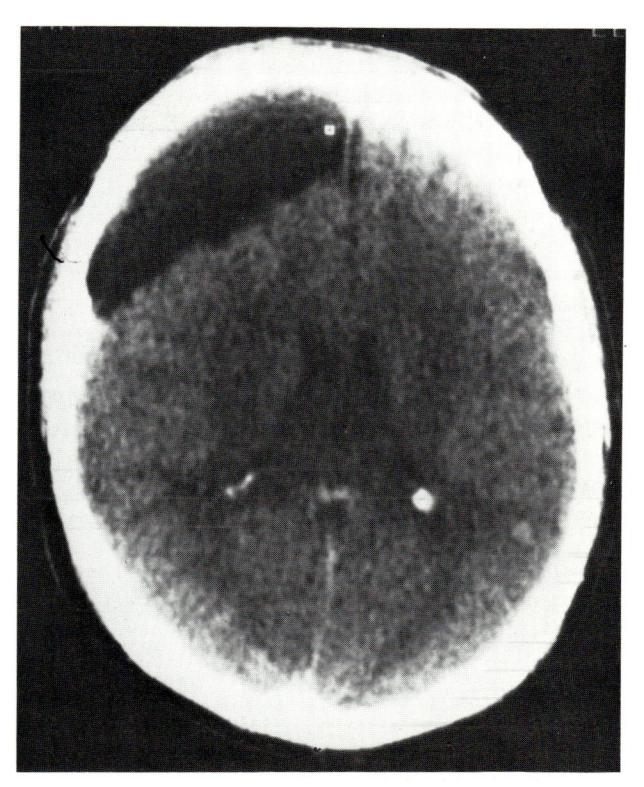

Figure 205-3 This CT scan shows a frontal subdural hygroma. The lesion density is the same as that of cerebrospinal fluid. There is no ventricular shift and only slight effacement of the frontal horn of the lateral ventricle. At operation (performed for severe headache), clear colorless fluid not enclosed by membranes was removed.

seen in patients with other types of head injury. However, it is rare in those over the age of 60 (probably as a result of the increased adherence of the dura to the inner table of the skull in the elderly) and in children in the first 2 years of life.

Pathogenesis

Impact to the skull causes inbending and stripping of the dura mater from the inner table. The skull is usually (although not invariably) fractured, and meningeal vessels are torn. Bleeding occurs into the region where the dura has been separated from the inner table of the skull, and the dura is further stripped by a confluent hematoma.

EDH results from injury to the middle meningeal artery or vein, diploic veins, or the dural venous sinuses. In over 50 percent of patients, the hematoma rises from the middle meningeal artery. In one-third the middle meningeal vein is the source of the hematoma, and in the remainder diploic veins or a torn dural venous sinus give rise to the hemorrhage. The hematoma is almost always unilateral, and the majority are found in the temporal region, although extension to adjacent frontal, parietal, and occipital areas is common. In adults a fracture is present 90 percent of the time, although in children fractures are less commonly found.

Associated intracranial injury occurs in a minority of patients, and in this sense EDH is quite different from an acute SDH where associated parenchymal injury is usual and has such a detrimental influence on outcome.

Clinical Manifestations

Patients with EDH present with one of five clinical courses:

1. Conscious throughout
2. Unconscious throughout
3. Initially conscious and subsequently unconscious
4. Initially unconscious and subsequently lucid
5. Initially unconscious followed by a lucid interval and then unconscious once again

The concept of a "lucid interval" has come to be associated with EDH; a transient loss of consciousness results from a concussive blow and is followed by a return of consciousness until the growing EDH results in unconsciousness once again. Although a lucid interval is sometimes seen in patients with EDH, it is less frequent than is commonly imagined and is the mode of presentation in less than one-third of patients reported in the literature. Moreover, a lucid interval is not pathognomonic for EDH, and other post-traumatic mass lesions can present in a similar fashion.

The rapidity of the appearance of symptoms and signs in patients with EDH is variable: one-third of patients come to the operating room within 12 h of injury and between 60 and 75 percent within 48 h. In the remaining patients the hematoma develops between 2 and 7 days following injury. Rarely patients may present after the first week; a lengthy interval from trauma to the time of clinical presentation is most commonly associated with hematomas originating from a laceration of the middle meningeal vein or a dural venous sinus.

The clinical signs associated with EDH depend on the rapidity of the growth of the hematoma and the presence of associated intradural lesions. Depression of the level of consciousness, hemiparesis, and pupillary dilatation are frequently seen with EDH but are not pathognomonic and are of little use in distinguishing EDH from other post-traumatic intracranial mass lesions.

Diagnosis

When an EDH is suspected, a CT scan should be performed; the hematoma will appear as a hyperdense, biconvex area between the skull and the brain (Fig. 205-4).

Treatment

The condition of most patients can be stabilized initially with diuretics and hyperventilation so that a CT scan can be obtained to confirm the diagnosis. Following the CT scan, an immediate craniotomy with evacuation of the hematoma is the treatment of choice. In the rapidly deteriorating patient with a suspected EDH, a CT scan is inappropriate, and a burr hole is placed ipsilateral to the side of pupillary dilatation and contralateral to the side of motor signs. After emergency hematoma evacuation, there is usually a rapid improvement in neurological signs and the patient is taken to the operating room where a craniotomy is made that is large enough to expose the site of bleeding and to visualize and remove the entire hematoma. In those patients who have not had a preoperative CT scan the dura should be opened to rule out an underlying acute SDH and a postoperative scan is obtained to identify any other occult intradural lesions.

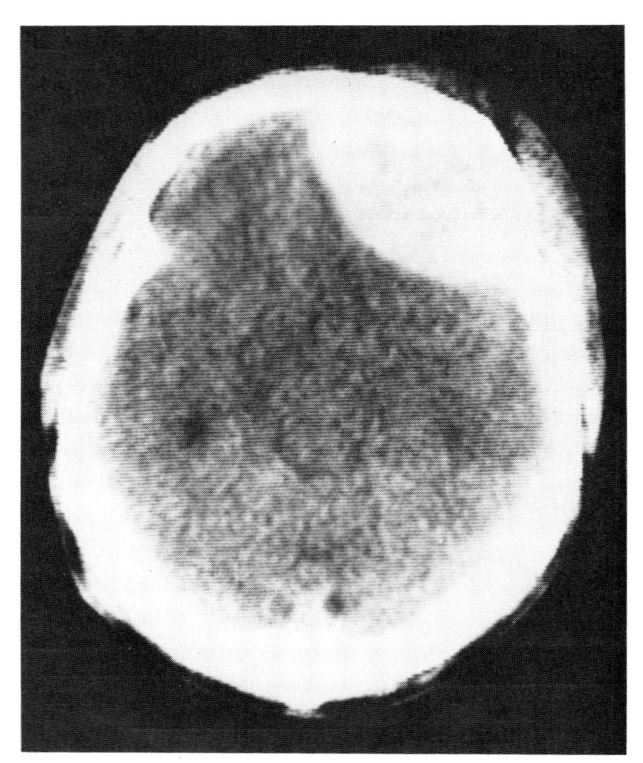

Figure 205-4 A CT scan showing a large hyperdense frontal epidural hematoma.

Complications

Delay in diagnosis and treatment is the most common preventable cause of morbidity and mortality. In one study the mean delay in evacuation of the hematoma in patients who made a good recovery was 2 h and in those who died was over 15 h.[19]

Although the placement of burr holes is an acceptable life-saving emergency procedure, burr holes are inadequate as the definitive treatment of EDH. Recurrent or residual hematoma may result from failure to gain full access to the hematoma, the lacerated meningeal vessel, or multiple small bleeders on the dura where it has been stripped off the inner table of the skull.

Outcome

Mortality following treatment of EDH varies from 15 to 43 percent.[12,21] Mortality is low (5 to 10 percent) in children and increases sharply in those over age 40 (35 to 50 percent). Associated intracranial lesions such as SDH, intracerebral hematoma, and cerebral contusion have a detrimental effect on outcome and result in a mortality rate four times greater than that seen in patients without such lesions. Patients who are alert or slightly lethargic at the time of operation should have virtually no mortality, while those who are unconscious with brain stem signs will have a mortality well over 50 percent.

Cerebral Contusion

Cerebral contusions consist of heterogeneous areas of hemorrhage, brain necrosis, and infarction. It is the most frequently seen lesion following head injury at autopsy and on CT scan. Cerebral contusions are usually multiple and are commonly associated with other intracranial hemorrhagic lesions.

Contusions occur in brain underlying the site of impact (coup lesions) although the largest and most serious contrecoup contusions are generally seen far from the site of impact at the frontal and temporal poles as a result of injury against the bony floor of the frontal and middle fossa as the brain accelerates within the skull. Contusion of the medial cerebral hemispheres or corpus callosum may occur as a result of acceleration of the brain against the falx cerebri. Small hemorrhagic lesions are also found in the deep white and gray matter and result from the shearing that occurs with rapid acceleration and deceleration of the brain.

Symptoms and Signs

The symptoms and signs produced by cerebral contusion will vary according to the size and location of the contusion and the type of associated lesions. Small contusions pose no threat to the patient's life, but when they occur in speech areas of the dominant hemisphere or in the motor cortex, permanent deficit can result. Large contusions or multiple ones involving both frontal and temporal lobes (the so-called tetrapolar injury) may produce elevations of ICP.

In the period following the injury, the contused areas become necrotic and heterogeneously hemorrhagic. Although the hemorrhage is eventually resorbed, the total mass effect may initially increase as a result of edema around the contused brain, with a rise in ICP, depression of the patient's level of consciousness, and the appearance or exacerbation of focal neurological deficits.

Diagnosis

The diagnosis of cerebral contusion is established by the CT scan; hemorrhagic contusions appear as small areas of increased density mixed with areas of decreased density characteristic of edema and necrotic brain (Fig. 205-5).

Treatment

Patients with small or deep lesions are managed nonoperatively. Patients with larger contusions and mass effect should have a craniotomy at the time of presentation. Although medical management of increased ICP has been used to avoid operation, patients with an apparently stable neurological status may suddenly herniate as long as 7 to 9 days following injury. For this reason large contusions are resected shortly after injury, minimizing the chances for subsequent neurological deterioration.

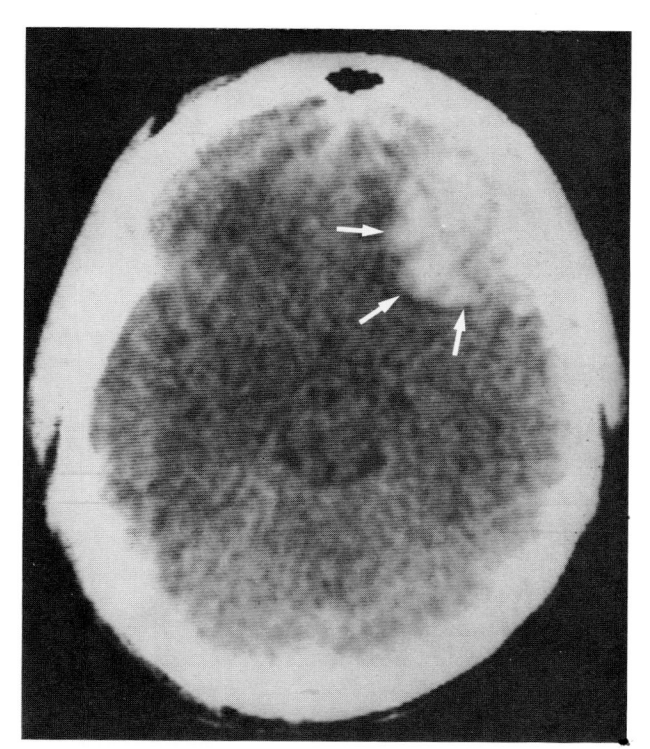

Figure 205-5 A CT scan showing a post-traumatic frontal intracerebral hematoma (*arrows*). The superficial location in the frontal or temporal area is characteristic of a traumatic hematoma.

Outcome

The mortality from cerebral contusion has been reported to be from 25 to 60 percent. Outcome is influenced by the same factors that are important for other mass lesions and that have been discussed in previous sections of this chapter.

Intracerebral Hematoma

Traumatic intracerebral hematomas are well-defined, homogeneous areas of hemorrhage that appear hyperdense on the CT scan. Before the use of the CT scan, the incidence of traumatic intracerebral hematoma was reported as 0.6 percent.[14] However, CT scan visualization of intracranial hematomas occurs as frequently as 12 percent of the time.[33]

Pathogenesis

The cause of intracerebral hematoma is similar to that which produces contrecoup contusions as the brain is propelled forward in the cranium. Confluent hemorrhages resulting from trauma are found in the same locations as cerebral contusions: the frontal and temporal lobes account for 80 to 90 percent of total hemorrhages. Hemorrhages may also be found in the corpus callosum, brain stem, and deep gray matter as a result of shearing injury. Multiple hemorrhages are seen in 20 percent of patients, and 60 percent of intracerebral hemorrhages are associated with extracerebral hematomas.[3,6] CT evaluation of patients with acute head injury has revealed that intraventricular hemorrhages are not uncommon and can be seen in the absence of CT-demonstrable parenchymal injury.

Symptoms and Signs

The injury that results in intracerebral hemorrhage is generally severe, and over one-half of all patients lose consciousness as a direct result of the impact. The subsequent level of consciousness is determined by the severity of the impact injury and the growth of the intracerebral hematoma or of coexisting extracerebral hematomas.

The symptoms and signs of intracerebral hematoma are not pathognomonic, and this entity cannot be reliably distinguished from other intracranial mass lesions on clinical grounds alone. The fact that these lesions so frequently coexist with extracerebral collections makes their diagnosis even more difficult. The neurological findings depend on the location and size of the hematoma. Enlargement of the hematoma or surrounding edema appearing in the days following injury may produce additional mass effect with deterioration of consciousness and an increase in neurological deficit.

Diagnosis

The CT scan is the favored diagnostic procedure for the detection of intracerebral hematomas and will reliably distinguish mass effect caused by parenchymal hematomas from edema or cerebral contusions, a distinction that cannot be made by angiography (Fig. 205-6).

Treatment

Patients with a large intracerebral hematoma with a midline shift, altered consciousness, and a focal deficit require operative evacuation of the hematoma. We fashion a large craniotomy centered over the site of the hematoma (which facilitates complete hematoma removal), resect adjacent injured brain, and evacuate extraparenchymal hematomas. Patients whose hematomas are small (whether or not a neurological deficit is present) usually do not need an operation. Similarly, patients with hemorrhages involving the deep white matter or basal ganglia are not operative candidates.

Teasdale et al. report that when the initial ICP is greater than 20 mmHg, most patients will need an operation.[30] Patients who are initially not considered operative candidates should have ICP monitoring if indicated and serial CT scans every 2 to 4 days for the first week or 10 days following injury. Operation is indicated if the ICP cannot be controlled by medical means or if there is an increasing mass effect from hematoma growth or edema. Temporal lobe hematomas are an especially dangerous entity because of their proximity to the incisura and midbrain. In spite of an ICP that is often surprisingly low, and minimal midline shift on a CT scan, rapid neurological deterioration with little or no warning is a frequent occurrence. For this reason we have been aggressive in treating these lesions with early operation and hematoma removal.

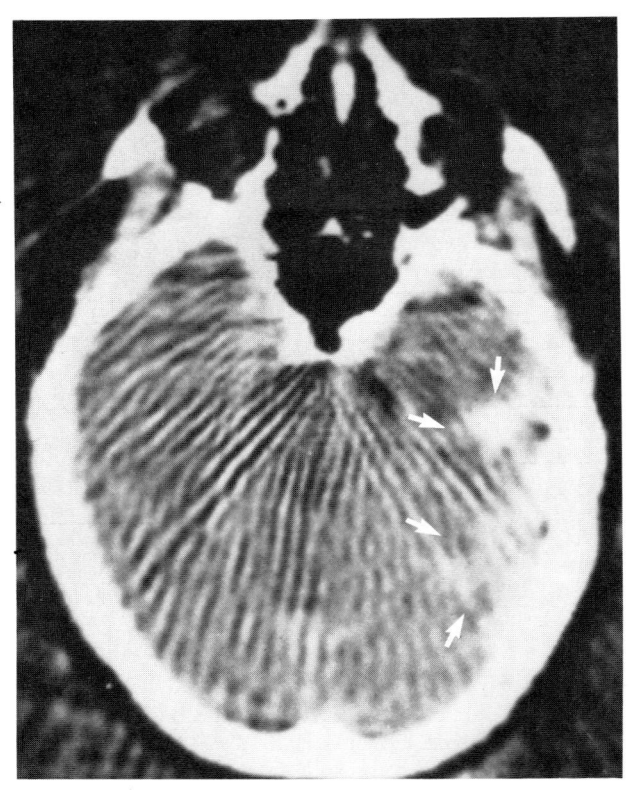

Figure 205-6 This CT scan shows multiple small contusions (*arrows*). The superficial location in the temporal area is common. This scan was performed shortly after injury, and subsequent scans showed areas of edema around the lesions.

Outcome

Mortality from 25 percent[14] to 72 percent[3] has been reported and is dependent to a large degree on the patient's neurological status at the time of operation: patients who were conscious at operation had a mortality of 6 percent, whereas those who were unconscious had a mortality of 45 percent.

Mass Lesions of the Posterior Fossa

Posterior fossa structures are remarkably well protected from injury; traumatically induced hemorrhagic lesions are unusual and represent less than 5 percent of all intracranial traumatic lesions. EDH is the commonest lesion seen, followed by SDH and intracerebellar hematoma.

Epidural Hematoma of the Posterior Fossa

The time of onset of neurological signs in patients with EDH of the posterior fossa is variable: about 40 percent of patients will become symptomatic in the first 24 h, just over 50 percent in the next 6 days, and a small percentage after 1 week.

Headache and stiff neck are common.[10,32] Cranial nerve deficits are sometimes present. Cerebellar signs are seen in less than one-half of all patients and are uncommon in those with a rapid course. Corticospinal tract findings may result from coexisting supratentorial injury or extension of the hematoma superiorly to overlie the occipital lobe. Later in the patient's course, corticospinal tract signs result from medullary compression and are associated with a depressed level of consciousness.

Because EDH of the posterior fossa is rare and coexisting supratentorial injury is often present, the diagnosis is often not suspected. Posterior fossa EDH or some other infratentorial mass should be considered when a depressed level of consciousness without localizing signs follows occipital trauma.

The CT scan will rapidly and accurately establish the diagnosis of posterior fossa EDH. In all head-injured patients, and particularly those with altered consciousness with few localizing signs, the posterior fossa should be scanned. In the past, ventriculography and angiography have been used for evaluation of suspected lesions. They have been superseded by the CT scan and are indicated only when the CT scanner is unavailable.

Treatment of these lesions is operative. Posterior fossa epidural hematomas usually arise from a tear in the dural venous sinuses underlying a skull fracture. Therefore a craniectomy is performed where the skull fracture crosses the torcular, transverse sinus, or sigmoid sinus. The craniectomy is enlarged superiorly, if needed, for visualization of a hematoma above the transverse sinus compressing the occipital lobe.

Outcome is most closely related to the patient's level of consciousness at the time of operation, and mortality is reported to range from 37 to 69 percent.[1,16]

Subdural Hematoma of the Posterior Fossa

Posterior fossa SDH composes less than 1 percent of the total number of SDHs reported. Bleeding from torn bridging veins over the cerebellum, injury to the dural venous sinuses, or hemorrhage from cerebellar contusions is the usual source of SDH.

Disturbance of consciousness, headache, and vomiting are common. Cranial nerve palsies, nuchal rigidity, and cerebellar signs are each seen in less than one-half of patients. The clinical course is variable, and symptoms and signs may appear immediately after injury or after an interval of over 24 h.

Treatment is similar to that described for posterior fossa EDH. After removal of an SDH, a careful search must be made for the injured vessels giving rise to the hematoma and hemostasis obtained to prevent recurrence. Mortality is reported to be in the range of 50 percent.[4]

Traumatic Intracerebellar Hematoma

Traumatic intracerebellar hematomas are unusual lesions that originate from direct blows to the suboccipital area. A fracture is frequently present.[32] Posterior fossa SDH is a frequent co-existing lesion. Symptoms and signs are indistinguishable from those produced by extra-axial posterior fossa lesions. Operative treatment consists of removal of the hematoma and adjacent contused cerebellum. Associated supratentorial contrecoup contusions and hematomas are frequently found, and attention is first directed to the lesion that is felt to be the most clinically significant. Mortality is high, and survivors are often left with significant neurological impairment.[22]

References

1. Beller AJ, Peyser E: Extradural cerebellar hematoma: Report of three cases with review of the literature. J Neurosurg 9:291–298, 1952.
2. Bender MB, Christoff N: Nonsurgical treatment of subdural hematomas. Arch Neurol 31:73–79, 1974.
3. Browder J, Turney MF: Intracerebral hemorrhage of traumatic origin: Its surgical treatment. NY State J Med 42:2230–2235, 1942.
4. Ciembroniewicz JE: Subdural hematoma of the posterior fossa: Review of the literature with addition of 3 cases. J Neurosurg 22:465–473, 1965.
5. Cooper PR, Hagler H, Clark WK, Barnett P: Enhancement of experimental cerebral edema after decompressive craniectomy: Implications for the management of severe head injuries. Neurosurgery 4:296–300, 1979.
6. Dublin AB, French BN, Rennick JM: Computed tomography in head trauma. Radiology 122:365–369, 1977.
7. Fell DA, Fitzgerald S, Moiel RH, Caram P: Acute subdural hematomas: Review of 144 cases. J Neurosurg 42:37–42, 1975.
8. Fogelholm R, Waltimo O: Epidemiology of chronic subdural haematoma. Acta Neurochir (Wien) 32:247–250, 1975.
9. Hoff J, Bates E, Barnes B, Glickman M, Margolis T: Traumatic subdural hygroma. J Trauma 13:870–876, 1973.
10. Hooper RS: Extradural haemorrhages of the posterior fossa. Br J Surg 42:19–26, 1954.
11. Ito H, Komai T, Yamamoto S: Fibrinolytic enzyme in the lining walls of chronic subdural hematoma. J Neurosurg 48:197–200, 1978.
12. Jamieson KG, Yelland JDN: Extradural hematoma: Report of 167 cases. J Neurosurg 29:13–23, 1968.
13. Jamieson KG, Yelland JDN: Surgically treated traumatic subdural hematomas. J Neurosurg 37:137–149, 1972.
14. Jamieson KG, Yelland JDN: Traumatic intracerebral hematoma: Report of 63 surgically treated cases. J Neurosurg 37:528–532, 1972.
15. Kernohan JW, Woltman HW: Incisura of the crus due to contralateral brain tumor. Arch Neurol Psychiatry, 21:274–287, 1929.
16. Kosary IZ, Goldhammer Y, Lerner MA: Acute extradural hematoma of the posterior fossa. J Neurosurg 24:1007–1012, 1966.
17. McKissock W, Richardson A, Bloom WH: Subdural haematoma: A review of 389 cases. Lancet 1:1365–1369, 1960.
18. McLaurin RL, Tutor FH: Acute subdural hematoma: Review of 90 cases. J Neurosurg 18:61–67, 1961.
19. Mendelow AD, Karmi MZ, Paul KS, Fuller GAG, Gillingham FJ: Extradural haematoma: Effect of delayed treatment. Br Med J 1:1240–1242, 1979.

20. Miller JD, Becker DP, Ward JD, Sullivan HG, Adams WE, Rosner MJ: Significance of intracranial hypertension in severe head injury. J Neurosurg 47:503–516, 1977.
21. Phonprasert C, Suwanwela C, Hongsaprabhas C, Prichayudh P, O'Charoen S: Extradural hematoma: Analysis of 138 cases. J Trauma 20:679–683, 1980.
22. Pozzati E, Grossi C, Padovani R: Traumatic intracerebellar hematomas. J Neurosurg 56:691–694, 1982.
23. Putnam TJ, Cushing H: Chronic subdural hematoma: Its pathology, its relation to pachymeningitis hemorrhagica and its surgical treatment. Arch Surg 11:329–393, 1925.
24. Ransohoff J, Benjamin MV, Gage L Jr, Epstein F: Hemicraniectomy in the management of acute subdural hematoma. J Neurosurg 34:70–76, 1971.
25. Seelig JM, Becker DP, Miller JD, Greenberg RP, Ward JD, Choi SC: Traumatic acute subdural hematoma: Major mortality reduction in comatose patients treated within four hours. N Engl J Med 304:1511–1518, 1981.
26. Stone JL, Lang RGR, Sugar O, Moody RA: Traumatic subdural hygroma. Neurosurgery 8:542–550, 1981.
27. Suzuki J, Takaku A: Nonsurgical treatment of chronic subdural hematoma. J Neurosurg 33:548–553, 1970.
28. Tabaddor K, Shulman K: Definitive treatment of chronic subdural hematoma by twist-drill craniostomy and closed-system drainage. J Neurosurg 46:220–226, 1977.
29. Talalla A, Morin MA: Acute traumatic subdural hematoma: A review of one hundred consecutive cases. J Trauma 11:771–777, 1971.
30. Teasdale G, Galbraith S, Jennett B: Operate or observe? ICP and the management of the 'silent' traumatic intracranial haematoma, in Shulman K, Marmarou A, Miller JD, Becker DP, Hochwald GM, Brock M (eds): *Intracranial Pressure IV*. Berlin, Springer-Verlag, 1980, pp 36–38.
31. Weir BKA: The osmolality of subdural hematoma fluid. J Neurosurg 34:528–533, 1971.
32. Wright RL: Traumatic hematomas of the posterior cranial fossa. J Neurosurg 25:402–409, 1966.
33. Zimmerman RA, Bilaniuk LT, Gennarelli T, Bruce D, Dolinskas C, Uzzell B: Cranial computed tomography in diagnosis and management of acute head trauma. AJR 131:27–34, 1978.
34. Zollinger R, Gross RE: Traumatic subdural hematoma: An explanation of the late onset of pressure symptoms. JAMA 103:245–249, 1934.

206
Delayed and Recurrent Intracranial Hematomas and Post-Traumatic Coagulopathies

Michael E. Miner

Patients with acute traumatic intracranial hematomas require prompt surgical decisions and frequently an emergency craniotomy. It is not widely appreciated that delayed intracerebral hematomas occur in up to 7 percent of patients with severe head injuries.[8] A smaller but significant number of patients who have had early emergency craniotomy for evacuation of an extracerebral hematoma develop recurrent intracranial hematomas within the first 10 days after their initial surgical treatment.[19] Thus, the incidence of delayed or recurrent traumatic intracerebral hematomas is significant, but, fortunately, both types of hematoma are relatively easily diagnosed by CT scan. However, the diagnosis of delayed and recurrent post-traumatic intracranial hematomas does require a high index of clinical suspicion, an understanding of the clinical features and CT findings, and, most importantly, an understanding of the pathophysiology of these lesions.

Clinical Features and CT Findings

The neurological abnormalities associated with delayed or recurrent intracranial hematomas that occur within the first week after severe head injury may be difficult to distinguish from those due to brain edema. A deteriorating state of consciousness, a newly developed third nerve palsy, or a rise in intracranial pressure does not differentiate which intracranial compartment has increased in volume. Laboratory evaluations also do not distinguish the cause, even though blood clotting abnormalities are more frequently associated with new brain destruction from hematoma than from brain swelling.

CT is currently the test of choice for diagnosing delayed or recurrent intracranial hematomas.[4] Delayed intracerebral hematomas are nearly always lobar, are frequently multiple, and often occur in areas of previously demonstrated cerebral contusion.[5,8] However, delayed intracerebral hematomas can occasionally be demonstrated even after an initially totally normal CT scan.[19] Small areas of contusion, best appreciated on the contrast-enhanced CT scan, frequently evolve into delayed parenchymal hemorrhages. We routinely rescan any patient with an area of traumatic brain contusion greater than 1 cm in diameter within 3 to 5 days after injury. Because delayed hematomas may be quite insidious, we rescan all patients with extra-axial hematomas in 3 to 5 days after injury regardless of their clinical recovery.

Delayed epidural and subdural hematomas occur in approximately equal proportions to delayed intracerebral hematomas.[19] The clinical signs are frequently insidious. This has prompted our policy of late CT scans on all severely head-injured patients who do not return to normal.

Pathophysiology

Over the past decade, it has become increasingly apparent that severe brain injury results in pathological changes in multiple organ systems. Accordingly, the best treatment for the head-injured person requires emphasis on the treatment of these other organ systems as well as the brain. A number of reports have noted that brain injury can result in abnormalities of blood coagulation. These coagulation changes themselves may also be the cause of cerebral hemorrhage or infarction, resulting in a self-perpetuating, ever-worsening course with a predictable outcome.[15] Neurosurgeons must be aware that head trauma can result in coagulopathies that can be successfully treated and must be able to recognize when and how to initiate treatment. To do this, a basic understanding of normal hemostasis and the required screening coagulation studies is essential.

Normal Coagulation

Normal hemostasis results from a complex series of reactions that are still incompletely understood. Platelets aggregate at the site of hemorrhage and serve to mechanically occlude the vessel. Serotonin and other vasoactive peptides are also released by platelets, resulting in a local vasoconstriction. Two fundamental clotting pathways are well described: the tissue-activated, or extrinsic, pathway and the plasma-originated, or intrinsic, pathway. The extrinsic pathway, initiated by tissue thromboplastin, requires calcium ions and plasma factor VII, which ultimately results in activated factor X, the Stuart factor. There are high concentrations of thromboplastin in the intima of small vessels throughout the body, but the brain has exceedingly high thromboplastin activity.[1,21,24]

The intrinsic pathway does not require thromboplastin but rather coagulation factors normally present in plasma (plasma factors IX and VIII), calcium ions and platelet phospholipid. This pathway results from a cascade of clotting enzymes converting precursors to activated forms that catalyze the next reaction.[12] Ultimately, both the intrinsic and the extrinsic pathways generate activated factor X, the Stuart factor. Although both pathways are complex, it is striking that a fibrin clot can be produced in a matter of seconds by the extrinsic pathway but requires several minutes to form by the intrinsic pathway. This time difference may be related to the normal function of the two pathways. A final common pathway, originating from activated Stuart factor, catalyzes the conversion of prothrombin to thrombin, which in turn catalyzes the conversion of fibrinogen to fibrin. Fibrin monomers can self-polymerize to yield a durable vascular occlusion and thus hemostasis.

Intravascular coagulation is a normal process that is constantly occurring throughout all organs. Similarly, fibrinolysis is constantly occurring as a normal process. Although the control of this homeostatic mechanism is incompletely understood, it is amazingly accurate. Plasminogen activator substance, present in blood and many body tissues, converts plasminogen to plasmin, which functions to dissolve fibrin clots. Fibrin clots are thus split or degraded to smaller molecules (fibrin split products or degradation products) that are themselves antihemostatic in that they inhibit the polymerization of fibrin monomers.

Although the foregoing is a brief overview of normal hemostasis, it allows the screening tests for blood clotting and fibrinolysis to be defined. Platelet quantification is important because platelet aggregation is the initial step in hemostasis. Furthermore, platelets are critical to the intrinsic clotting pathway. The prothrombin time primarily screens for abnormalities in the extrinsic pathway, whereas a normal activated partial thromboplastin time (APTT) reflects the integrity of the intrinsic clotting pathway. However, even minor abnormalities of these clotting tests may indicate major hemostatic abnormalities. The prothrombin time and the APPT do not become prolonged until one or more of the clotting factors decreases to 20 to 30 percent of normal. Fibrinogen quantification provides information about the integrity of the final common pathway to hemostasis. The level of fibrin split products reflects the magnitude of fibrinolytic activity.

Screening tests are arbitrary. Therefore, there may be good justification to utilize a wide variety of screening tests to determine the integrity of the clotting and fibrinolysis systems. However, we have found that the results of platelet, fibrinogen, and fibrin split product quantification together with the prothrombin time and APTT provide the neurosurgeon with sufficient data to make therapeutic decisions in the management of patients with acute head injuries. These test results also allow our hematology colleagues information about where to focus their attention when more specific tests are required.

Disseminated Intravascular Coagulation and Fibrinolysis Syndrome

Disseminated intravascular coagulation and fibrinolysis (DICF) is an abnormal hemostatic syndrome that results from a pathological activation of the blood-clotting enzymes. Either the intrinsic or the extrinsic clotting enzymes, or both, may initiate the process, but the net result is abnormal intravascular clotting with simultaneous consumption of clotting factors. This consumption of clotting factors is coupled with a diffuse intravascular lysis of clots, which, at its end stage, results in impaired hemostasis and spontaneous hemorrhages. Either the coagulation or the fibrinolytic component may predominate, but usually both components are evident in the laboratory evaluation. The laboratory evidence of DICF may be present even when there is no clinically recognizable disorder.[11] DICF may be precipitated by a variety of disorders, but it is always a secondary event triggered by another process.[14,16]

Relationship between DICF and Head Injury

Several reports have discussed the association between severe brain injury and clinically obvious bleeding abnormalities.[3,6,7,10,18,19,20,23] The vast majority of patients have died after a short period of observation. However, Goodnight et al. observed one patient with "massive blunt trauma" and two with gunshot wounds to the brain who survived in spite of laboratory evidence of DICF.[7] On the other hand, Preston et al. reported two patients with relatively trivial head injuries who developed DICF.[18] Several authors have observed that severe coagulopathies associated with brain injury result in microthrombi in multiple organs, including the brain, lungs, and kidneys,[3,18,25] whereas others have found no such microthrombi.[10,13] The contribution of DICF to intraoperative bleeding has been reported and is a very real phenomenon to the trauma surgeon.[7] Recently, DICF has been directly and causally related to delayed and recurrent intracranial hematomas.[9]

van der Sande et al. found that coagulation studies drawn within 24 h of the time of injury were abnormal in 64 percent of patients with severe head injuries,[23] which closely compares with the 56 percent that Pondaag found in a similar group of patients.[17] We have observed that 90 percent of all of our severely brain-injured patients have one or more hemostatic abnormalities if the patient is screened within 2 h of injury. It is also of note that over half of our patients with mild head injuries have one or more hemostatic abnormalities. Thus, it would appear that hemostatic abnormalities are common after brain injury, are more frequent after severe injury, and will be found most often if the patient is evaluated soon after injury.

In our experience, the fibrin split product level is the most frequently abnormal of the screening tests, being elevated in over two-thirds of all head-injured patients upon admission. van der Sande et al. concluded that fibrin split product elevations reflect the amount of brain tissue damage.[22,23] In general we would agree, but we have evaluated several patients with mild head injuries who had extreme but transient elevations of the fibrin split products. Fibrinogen levels were decreased in over 40 percent of our patients. The frequent elevation of fibrin split products and decrease in fibrinogen levels serve to emphasize that fibrinolysis is a very real phenomenon in head-injured patients. Although the clotting screening tests indicate that abnormalities of the thromboplastin-activated extrinsic clotting system occur more frequently than abnormalities of the intrinsic system, abnormalities of both systems are common and both systems can be abnormal at the same time in a single patient. Abnormal platelet counts are relatively uncommon but were present in over 5 percent of our severely head-injured patients. Our experience indicates that the frequency of hemostatic abnormalities is directly related to the severity of the neurological deficits on admission and that patients who would be predicted to have more cell destruction (i.e., patients with gunshot wounds and depressed skull fractures) have a greater incidence of hemostatic abnormalities than patients with less brain tissue destruction.

The disseminated intravascular coagulation and fibrinolysis syndrome is difficult to define from the results of clotting studies because relatively minor abnormalities of the clotting tests may indicate major hemostatic abnormalities. Indeed, the PT and APTT values do not become prolonged until one or more of the clotting factors decreases to 20 to 30 percent of normal. The laboratory diagnosis of DICF may be rather liberal and only require the demonstration of fibrin split products in the serum or decreased levels of fibrinogen or numbers of platelets.[9] On the other hand, others have defined DICF as a fibrinogen level below 130 μg/dl and fibrin split products greater than 40 μg/ml.[17] If either of these sets of criteria is used, 70 to 85 percent of our severely injured patients would have DICF. However, by requiring abnormalities in multiple (three or more) major hemostatic screening studies, we developed a somewhat more restrictive definition of DICF to ensure that a clotting disorder unequivocally existed and that it was severe. Even so, nearly half of our severely injured patients had DICF when initially evaluated.

Both abnormalities of individual clotting tests and "full-blown" DICF correlated with the severity and pathology of the brain injury. This implies not only that the incidence of clotting abnormalities is related to the amount of brain tissue destruction, but also that the severity of the coagulopathy is related to the severity of the injury. However, it is equally clear that the absence of demonstrable tissue destruction does not rule out DICF.

It is surprising that whereas we found that over 40 percent of severely brain-injured patients had DICF when first evaluated, this has not been a generally recognized phenomenon.[17] This may be because DICF following brain injury is either a transient phenomenon or has such a high mortality rate associated with it that most patients with severe head injuries and DICF do not survive to reach medical facilities. Case reports of DICF following head injury are generally from patients evaluated very soon after their injury, and all of our patients were initially evaluated less than 2 h after their injury. The relationship between DICF and morbidity and mortality after head injury is impressive. van der Sande et al. compared CT scans, neurological status, and coagulation studies on hospital admission and found that coagulation studies were more sensitive than CT scanning to demonstrate brain contusion.[23] In our studies, the presence of DICF increased mortality by a factor of three to six times, dependent on the pathology and severity of the injury.[15] However, the cause of death is not obvious in all cases. Many patients died after their clotting studies had returned to normal, and their autopsy studies generally did not indicate massive hemorrhage or intravascular clots. It is likely that the influence on mortality is due to diffuse microvascular fibrin deposits that plug small vessels and result in increased brain damage and multiple organ failure. Thus, DICF following brain injury may be life-threatening, may occur without overwhelming brain injury, may affect multiple organs, and may affect long-term recovery.

A Treatment Regimen for Delayed and Recurrent Intracerebral Hematomas and Post-Traumatic Coagulopathies

At the current time, we obtain coagulation screening tests on admission on all patients with diffuse brain injuries who are not following commands, as well as on all of those who have penetrating brain injuries or intracranial hematomas. Fresh frozen plasma is used as an initial resuscitation fluid if the prothrombin time or the activated partial thromboplastin time is increased or the fibrinogen level is less than 130 mg/dl. Platelet packs are given if the platelet count is less than 100,000 per cubic millimeter. If possible, we delay operation until the coagulation studies normalize. However, abnormal fibrin split product or fibrinogen levels are not seen as a contraindication to surgery but are treated with fresh frozen plasma as preparations are being made for surgery. If the clotting studies are abnormal, we use a hollow screw in the subarachnoid space to monitor intracranial pressure rather than a ventriculostomy.

An increase in intracranial pressure, a decrease in the state of consciousness, or the development of a focal or lateralizing finding prompts repeat CT scanning. Also, patients who have had cerebral contusions or hematomas visualized on their initial CT scan are routinely rescanned on the third to fifth day after injury. If a recurrent or delayed intracerebral hematoma is identified, repeat coagulation studies are performed and the same hematologic resuscitation is used as that used on admission. Surgical decisions and timing are based on the patient's clinical status, the CT scan, and the coagulation studies. We, of course, do not delay operating on life-threatening surgical lesions.[2] However, the correction of hemostatic abnormalities is just as important as the correction of a low hemoglobin or arterial oxygen tension. We have found that this policy decreases blood loss during operation, decreases morbidity, and, ultimately, saves lives.

References

1. Astrup T: Assay and content of tissue thromboplastin in different organs. Thromb Haemost 14:401–416, 1965.
2. Becker DP, Miller JD, Ward JD, Greenberg RP, Young HF, Sakalas R: The outcome from severe head injury with early diagnosis and intensive management. J Neurosurg 47:491–502, 1977.
3. Clark JA, Finelli RE, Netsky MG: Disseminated intravascular coagulation following cranial trauma: Case report. J Neurosurg 52:266–269, 1980.
4. Clifton GL, Grossman RG, Makela ME, Miner ME, Handel S, Sadhu V: Neurological course and correlated computerized tomography findings after severe closed head injury. J Neurosurg 52:611–624, 1980.
5. Diaz FG, Yock DH Jr, Larson D, Rockswald GL: Early diagnosis of delayed posttraumatic intracerebral hematomas. J Neurosurg 50:217–223, 1979.
6. Drayer BP, Poser CM: Disseminated intravascular coagulation and head trauma—two case studies. JAMA 231:174–175, 1975.
7. Goodnight SH, Kenoyer G, Rapaport SI, Patch MJ, Lee JA, Kurze T: Defibrination after brain tissue destruction: A serious complication of head injury. N Engl J Med 290:1043–1047, 1974.
8. Gudemann SK, Kishore PRS, Miller JD, Girevendulis AK, Lipper MH, Becker DP: The genesis and significance of delayed traumatic intracerebral hematoma. Neurosurgery 5:309–313, 1979.
9. Kaufman HH, Moake JL, Olson JD, Miner ME, duCret RP, Pruessner JL, Gildenberg PL: Delayed and recurrent intracranial hematomas related to disseminated intravascular clotting and fibrinolysis in head injury. Neurosurgery 7:445–450, 1980.
10. Keimowitz RM, Annis BL: Disseminated intravascular coagulation associated with massive brain injury. J Neurosurg 39:178–180, 1973.
11. Kim H, Suzuki M, Lie JT, Titus JL: Clinically unsuspected disseminated intravascular coagulation (DIC): An autopsy survey. Am J Clin Pathol 66:31–39, 1976.
12. Macfarlane RG: An enzyme cascade in the blood clotting mechanism and its function as a biochemical amplifier. Nature 202:498–499, 1964.
13. McGauley JL, Miller CA, Penner JA: Diagnosis and treatment of diffuse intravascular coagulation following cerebral trauma: Case report. J Neurosurg 43:374–376, 1975.
14. McKay DG, Latour JG, Parrish MH: Activation of Hageman Factor by α-adrenergic stimulation. Thromb Haemost 23:417–422, 1970.
15. Miner ME, Kaufman HK, Graham SH, Haar FH, Gildenberg PL: Disseminated intravascular coagulation, a fibrinolytic syndrome following head injury in children: Frequency and prognostic implications. J Pediatr 100:687–681, 1982.
16. Peck SD: Disseminated intravascular coagulation: How often have you missed it? Rocky Mt Med J 67:25–31, 1970.
17. Pondaag W: Disseminated intravascular coagulation related to outcome in head injury. Acta Neurochir (Wien) [Suppl] 28:98–102, 1979.
18. Preston FE, Malia RG, Sworn MJ, Timperley WR, Blackburn EK: Disseminated intravascular coagulation as a consequence of cerebral damage. J Neurol Neurosurg Psychiatry 37:241–248, 1974.
19. Pretorius ME, Kaufman HH: Rapid onset of delayed traumatic intracerebral haematoma with diffuse intravascular coagulation and fibrinolysis. Acta Neurochir (Wien) 65:103–109, 1982.
20. Strinchini A, Baudo F, Nosari AM, Panzocchi G, deCataldo F: Defibrination and head injury. Lancet 2:957, 1974.
21. Tovi D: Fibrinolytic activity of human brain: A histochemical study. Acta Neurol Scand 49:152–162, 1973.
22. van der Sande JJ, Emeis JJ, Lindeman J: Intravascular coagulation: A common phenomenon in minor experimental head injury. J Neurosurg 54:21–25, 1981.
23. van der Sande JJ, Veltkamp JJ, Boekhout-Mussert RJ, Vielvoye GJ: Hemostasis and computerized tomography in head injury: Their relationship to clinical features. J Neurosurg 55:718–724, 1981.
24. Vecht CJ, Sibinga CTS, Minderhoud JM: Disseminated intravascular coagulation and head injury. J Neurol Neurosurg Psychiatry 38:567–571, 1975.
25. Watts C: Disseminated intravascular coagulation. Surg Neurol 8:258–262, 1977.

207
Penetrating Wounds of the Head

Griffith R. Harsh, III
Griffith R. Harsh, IV

Missile injuries to the head account for the majority of penetrating wounds of the brain and are responsible for a significant number of deaths whether in times of war or peace. Baker et al. reported that in 1976 there were 100,761 Americans under 45 years of age who died as a result of trauma, yielding a death rate from injury of 46.9 per 100,000 persons.[1] According to their 1977 statistics from San Francisco, 50 percent of trauma deaths resulted from brain injury and 35 percent of those (brain injury deaths) from gunshot wounds to the head. Combining these figures reveals a national death rate (under age 45) from gunshot wounds to the head of 8.2 per 100,000 persons. Assuming the commonly reported mortality figure for civilian gunshot wounds to the head of 30 percent to 40 percent (35 percent) to be representative, the estimated annual incidence of gunshot wounds of the head is approximately 23.4 per 100,000 persons under age 45.

The neurosurgical management of all penetrating head wounds derives from the same fundamental concepts whether the penetration involves the scalp alone or the skull, dura, and brain, and whether the penetration is unilateral or bilateral. The intent of treatment in such penetrating wounds is to increase the incidence and quality of survival by prevention of early or late infection, by control and relief of increased intracranial pressure, and by reduction of secondary damage to the affected brain tissue.

Discussion in this chapter will focus on wounds penetrating the dura and brain produced by power-driven missiles (bullets or shell fragments). Other piercing injuries of course may be caused by such sharp objects as nails, sticks, pencils, pens, screwdrivers, hatchets, pointed toys, and rocks. Injuries caused by these objects evoke similar therapeutic considerations but are modified primarily by a general absence of significant impact force and its deleterious secondary consequences.

Much of the extant literature[7,9-12,21,22,24] referable to penetrating head wounds analyzes military experiences, but numbers of more recent writings deal with data extracted from civilian occurrences[14,16,18,20,23] and animal experimentation.[5,6,19] These diverse origins have occasionally led to an unfortunate and possibly irrelevant dichotomy in therapeutic considerations. Variations in patient populations from military to civilian practice (that is, patient age, missile origin, and high- versus low-impact velocity as well as time lag from wounding to definitive care) undoubtedly exist and may influence patient selection and outcome. However, they do not alter the basic therapeutic surgical tenets of thorough debridement with removal of all accessible bone or metallic fragments, hematoma evacuation and hemostasis followed by meticulous wound closure to re-establish impermeable barriers between the brain and the external environment, and the control of increased intracranial pressure.

Ballistic Considerations

Missiles damage tissues by transmitting energy in excess of the tissue's capacity to absorb or dissipate it. Anatomical and/or functional disruption of the tissue results. The energy released by a missile in its course through a tissue is a function of the change in kinetic energy experienced by the missile during the traverse of the tissue and is generally expressed by the formula $E = \frac{1}{2}m(V_i^2 - V_r^2)$ where m represents the mass of the missile; V_i, the impact velocity; and V_r, the residual velocity.[3]

The squaring of the velocity variables in this equation indicates the overwhelming importance of velocity in this energy transfer and, consequently, in the capacity of a missile to effect tissue disruption. Diminution of velocity of a missile as it passes through or stops within a tissue and, therefore, its energy release and destructive power are proportional to the retardation the missile experiences. As described by Hopkinson and Marshall, the damage inflicted by a missile then depends on the mass, velocity, and depth of penetration of the missile, modified by retardation to the missile, which is a reflection of missile shape, tissue density, and tissue composition.[15]

In most ballistic studies, the independent variable emphasized is velocity. Most modern rifles have muzzle velocities that exceed 750 m/s. The muzzle velocity of most handguns is less than 250 m/s. The velocity value relevant to head injury, however, is impact velocity, not muzzle velocity. Hammon has estimated that an impact velocity of at least 100 m/s is required to effect the explosive type of intracranial damage that often separates fatal head injuries from less severe ones.[12,13] Thus, the speed of sound (approximately 320 m/s) is a reasonable, though admittedly arbitrary, point of separation between high-velocity missiles and those of low velocity. This division on the basis of impact velocity corresponds roughly to the ballistics experts' distinction between missiles of high muzzle velocity (muzzle velocity greater than 750 m/s) occurring most commonly as military bullets or shrapnel fragments and missiles of low muzzle velocity (muzzle velocity less than 250 m/s) that are usually fired from civilian handguns. Excessive generalization from the tendency of military missiles to be of high-impact velocity and those of civilian missiles to be of low-impact velocity has contributed to unnecessarily dogmatic arguments between neurosurgeons with predominantly military experience and those in civilian practice regarding the aggressiveness of surgical approach. Certainly high-velocity-missile injuries are encountered in civilian practice (e.g., hunting rifle accidents) just as low-velocity-missile injuries are seen in military experience (e.g., wounds by a fragment from a distant grenade).

Pathophysiology

The impact of a missile to the head causes immediate tissue displacement and disruption that is soon followed by secondary alterations in the physiological parameters of the brain. Tissue disruption occurs at three anatomical levels:

1. Superficial soft tissue of the scalp is torn by the missile itself and, if the weapon is sufficiently close, by the pressure waves of gas combustion. Beyond the air-tissue interface, the gaseous pressure waves of weapon firing are of little significance.[18] Lacerated soft tissue carried intracranially by the force of the missile may act as a vehicle for inward transport of bacteria.
2. Bone is comminutedly fractured, and depressed edges may damage immediately subjacent vascular or cortical structures. In-driven fragments may act as secondary missiles.
3. Dura is perforated. Cerebral parenchyma is displaced by the missile and bone fragments and disrupted both along the missile path and at distant sites within the cranium by emanating shock waves and contrecoup injury.

The missile itself continues a path, determined by its velocity, angle of incidence, deformation, yaw, and structures encountered, that often extends at least to the inner table of the contralateral cranium. Then it may ricochet to form a second traverse, burst into smaller fragments, or become lodged in contralateral superficial structures, or it may penetrate the skull and scalp, completing a through-and-through perforating wound.[7]

As described by Hopkinson and Marshall, energy transfer from missile to tissue can cause tissue damage by three different mechanisms.[15] The prominence of each mechanism depends on the missile velocity. Missiles of low-impact velocity (less than 320 m/s) damage encountered tissue primarily by laceration and maceration. As the missile penetrates, tissues are torn apart and separate little more than the diameter of the missile. Pathologically evident damage is local only. At higher missile velocities, beginning at 100 m/s but becoming of truly significant consequence above 320 m/s, two other mechanisms, shock waves and temporary cavitation, are more destructive than the laceration caused by the missile itself.

Shock waves traveling in excess of the speed of sound in the tissue radiate from in front of the advancing missile. They are exceedingly brief (15 to 20 μs) and, in missiles of high velocities, may involve exceptionally high pressure fluctuations (1000 lb/in^2).[15] Even with missiles of lower velocities, shock waves of less magnitude may, by summation of their own reflected predecessors, grow into pressure pulses of significant amplitude and cause disruption of neural tissue structures and function at considerable distances from the missile trajectory.

In the case of missiles of highest velocity, most of the tissue damage results from temporary cavitation. As a high-velocity missile traverses the brain, a temporary conical cavity is formed as tissue in the region is pushed centrifugally from the surface of the missile. The diameter of this cavity is proportional to the change of the missile's kinetic energy along its path and may exceed that of the missile by 30-fold.[4] This cavity lasts only for 10 to 20 ms before its collapse, but as shown in the experiments of Hopkinson and Marshall it pulsates for 5 to 6 cycles of successively diminishing amplitude before subsiding to a permanent cavity.[15] During the formation of the temporary cavity, pressure within it may fall below atmospheric pressure, creating a pressure gradient such that surface debris may be drawn into the wound, spreading contamination along the missile tract. Tissues displaced secondary to the formation of the cavity may be damaged by the blast effect emanating from the bullet or by compression against distant unyielding dural and bony surfaces.

The shapes of both temporary and permanent cavities are modifications of a basic conical form with the base of the cone proximal and its apex distal. Variations from conicity result from yaw or missile irregularity yielding increased tissue damage due to an enhanced rate of missile slowing, and, consequently, of energy transfer. That exit wounds are frequently larger than wounds of entrance may be explained by increased missile deformation, yaw, and energy emission. Immediate hemorrhage from lacerated blood vessels may fill the permanent cavity and further intensify the existing mutilation (Fig. 207-1).

In summary, tissue damage from missiles of all velocities involves formation of a track of macerated tissue about the missile path. In addition, with medium- and perhaps even low-velocity injuries, summation of shock waves may cause physiological disruption at distant sites. As suggested by Kirkpatrick and Di Maio,[18] the studies of Sullivan et al.[25] lend credence to the postulation of brain stem injury through such a mechanism. Finally, at higher velocities, formation of a temporary cavity may be of such explosive character that the skull bursts.

The damage created instantaneously by the missile is soon compounded by a series of secondary changes that occur over minutes or hours. The first change, demonstrated in the elegant studies of Crockard et al.,[6] consists of a rise of intracranial pressure within 5 min to a peak as high as 100 torr. Missiles of higher impact velocity elicit a faster rise to a higher peak intracranial pressure than those of lower velocity. In their model, this ICP rise is associated with various cardiovascular changes. A fall in cardiac output and an immediate rise, followed by a rapid decline, in mean arterial pressure occurs. There is an early drop in cerebrovascular resistance (CVR) leading to an increase in cerebral blood volume (CBV) and further increase in intracranial pressure. Crockard et al. hypothesized the early formation of edema due to blood-brain barrier breakdown in the face of increased venous-capillary pressure consequent to the fall in cerebrovascular resistance.[6]

Subsequently, concomitant with sustained depression of cardiac output and blood pressure, there occurs a rise of CVR to high levels. In conjunction with ICP elevation, this causes decreased cerebral perfusion pressure (CPP), cerebral blood flow (CBF), and cerebral metabolic rate of oxygen, and indicates disruption of cerebrovascular autoregulation. After injuries of low velocity (90 m/s to exposed brain in their study), these changes may regress. At higher velocities

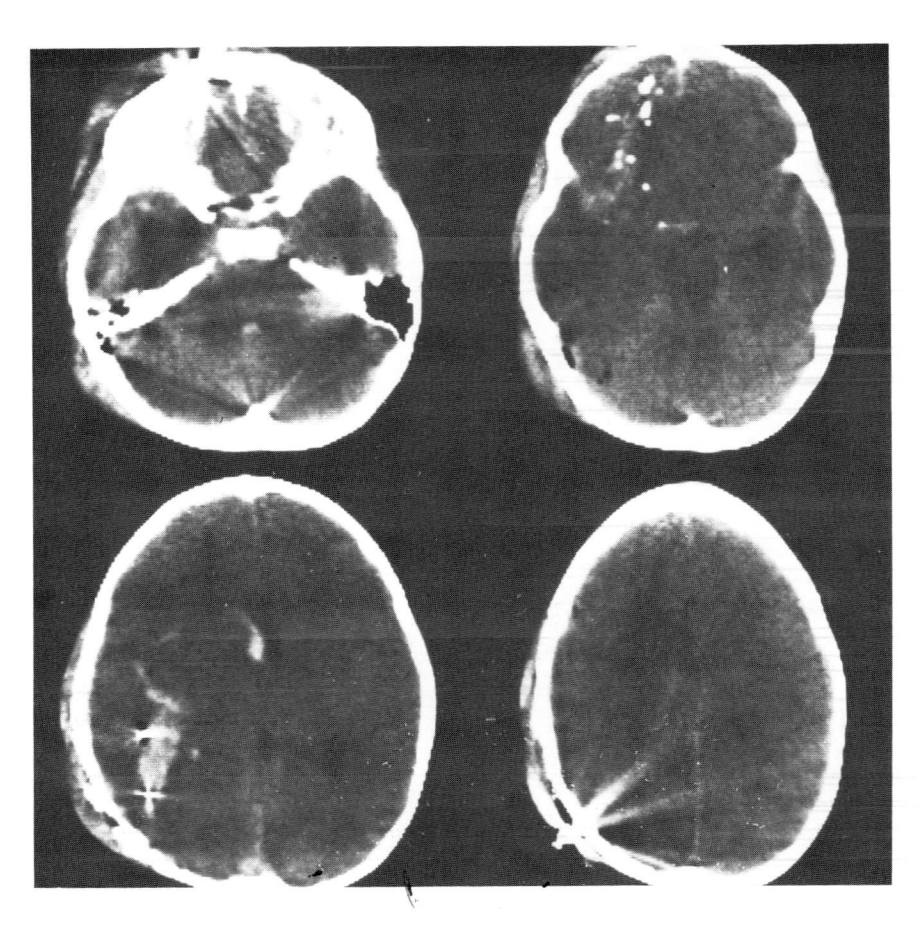

Figure 207-1 CT scans showing penetrating missile track, right supraorbital to right occipital area. Note fragments in the track, the distal permanent cavity distended by hemorrhage, and subependymal blood in the right lateral ventricle.

they persist until death from sustained inadequate perfusion intervenes. Cardiovascular suppression and disturbance of autoregulation may result from indirect brain stem injury due to the summation of initially low-amplitude shock waves in the posterior fossa.

Intracranial hemorrhage may contribute to additional intracranial hypertension. This may range from the mass collections of intracranial hematomas caused by disruption of larger vessels to contusion and extravasation either along the missile path or at brain surfaces displaced against rigid structures. The reported incidence of hematoma causing significant shift in civilian penetrating injuries ranges from 10 percent to 50 percent.[16] Traumatic aneurysms may result in later subarachnoid or intraparenchymal hemorrhage. Compression of adjacent tissue by an expanding blood collection may result in further mass effect by inducing surrounding vasogenic edema. Additional increase in intracranial pressure and various herniation syndromes and inadequate cerebral perfusion may result (Fig. 207-2).

Presentation

Presentation of a patient following missile injury to the brain is highly variable. Nearly all combinations of external signs of trauma and neurological deficit occur. Externally, wounds may be discrete with little soft tissue disruption (e.g., in orbital-facial injuries the entrance site may be covert) or they may involve extensive skin and muscle destruction. Bleeding may be sufficiently profuse to produce hypovolemic shock or may be minimal. Bone fracture may be almost linear, but most often it is comminuted, displaced, and accompanied by inward carriage of fragments and debris.

In both military and civilian settings, injuries to other parts of the body are common. From Vietnam, Hammon reported an incidence of 9.65 percent for chest injuries, 11.02 percent for abdominal injuries, 17.69 percent for facial injuries, and 2.06 percent for extremity injuries requiring amputation in patients with penetrating head wounds.[12]

Neurologically any combination of alteration of consciousness and focal deficit may be seen. Some degree of agitation or depression of awareness is usually found. Consciousness may or may not be lost in penetrating brain injury, though its presence should never be taken as a guarantee against sudden severe neurological deterioration. Focal deficits may be absent, indicating missile traverse of noneloquent brain, or they may be multiple and profound, usually reflecting cortical damage at the sites of entry, ricochet, or exit. Loss of brain stem reflexes may be only transient. When their appearance is progressive, particularly in sequences characteristic of herniation syndromes, progressive enlargement of an intracranial mass is suspected.

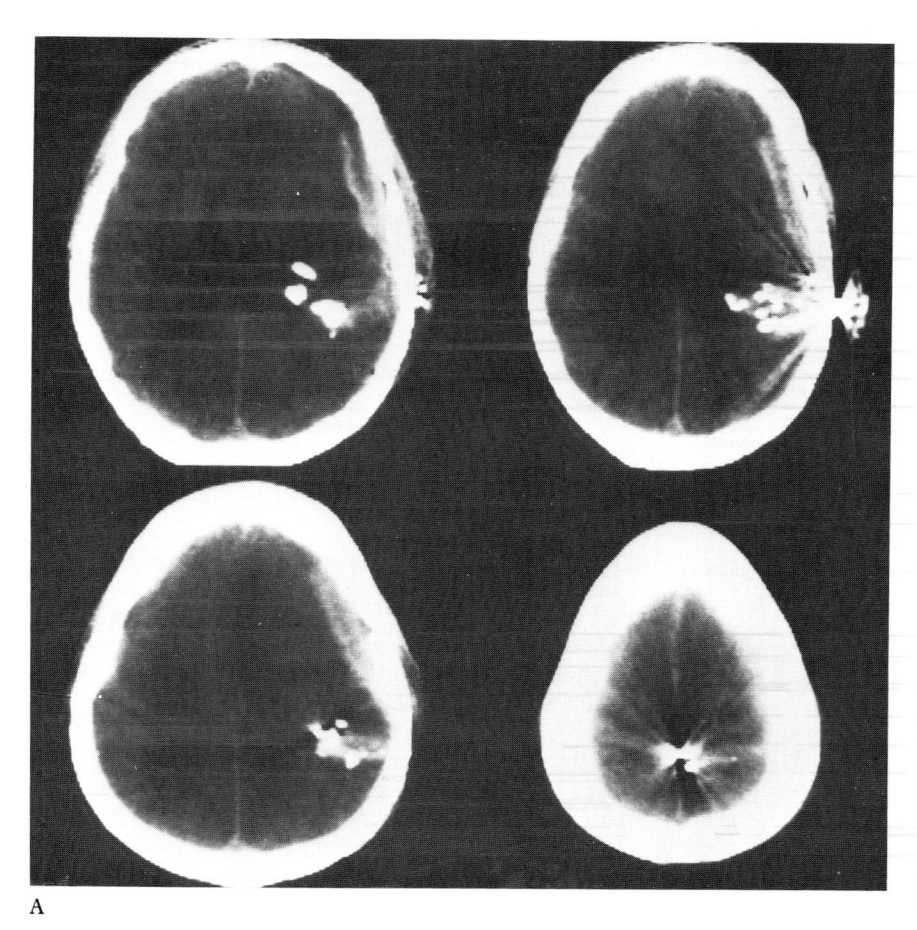

Figure 207-2 Left parietal missile injury. *A.* On the CT scans, note the extra- and intracranial fragments, subdural hematoma, track hemorrhage, left hemisphere swelling, and ventricular shift to the right, details not delineated by the accompanying plain x-ray films of the skull (*B, C*).

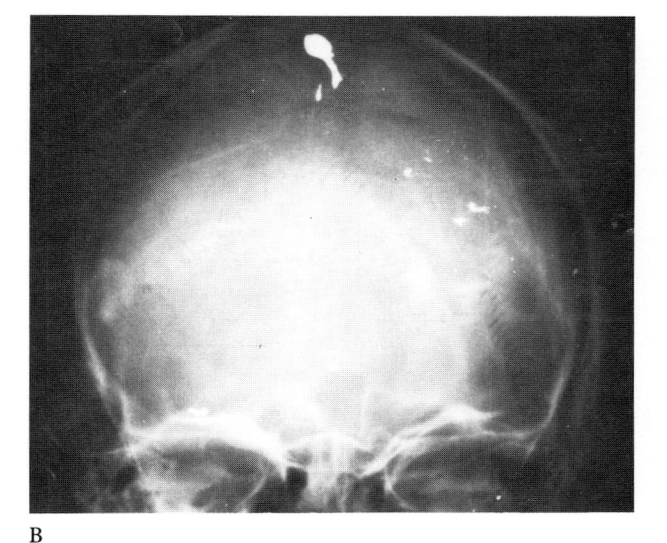

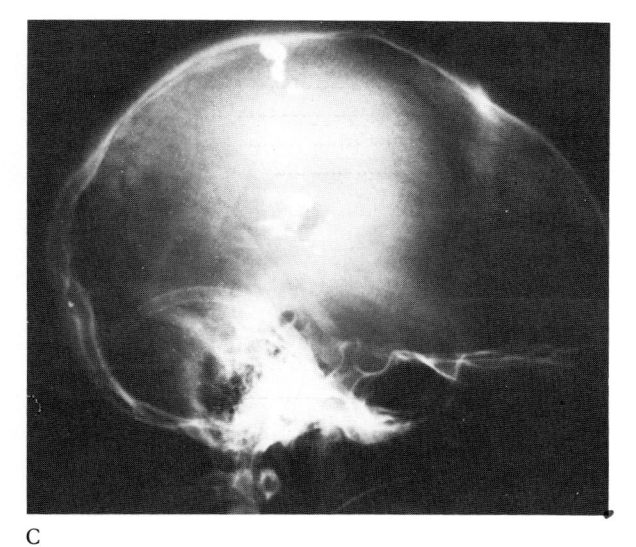

Primary Care

Proper care of a patient with a gunshot wound of the head first involves any necessary cardiopulmonary resuscitation. Endotracheal intubation is indicated in patients with stupor or a compromised airway. Significant bleeding from the scalp or other associated wounds should be controlled immediately. Cardiovascular compromise from volume loss, arrhythmia, or failure is corrected as rapidly as possible. The usual precautions for spine injury are observed. A search for abdominal, thoracic, or extremity injuries is made, and their appropriate treatment instituted or planned. In cases of multiple injury, first priority is given to the most life-threatening situation, and occasionally simultaneous laparotomy or thoracotomy and craniotomy are necessary.

Complete shaving of the head facilitates the search of small or cryptic wounds of entrance or exit. Open wounds exuding cerebrum or CSF should be bandaged appropriately. Neurological assessment should be as thorough as time permits, although the appearance of rapid deterioration with signs of progressive herniation requires immediate surgical intervention.

Anteroposterior and lateral x-ray films of the skull may be a sufficient guide for localization of entrance and exit wounds as well as intracranial bone and metallic fragments. Location of the latter may be an inaccurate indicator of the missile's true course as the missile may undergo tumbling or it may ricochet. If available, a CT scan should be obtained, as it provides the most definitive localization of track or other intracranial hematomas. Depending on the CT slice intervals, bone or metallic fragments and their potential relations to the ventricle may be discretely delineated (Fig. 207-3). Arteriography, formerly suggested for mass localization, is seldom indicated acutely, although it may be helpful in the evaluation of late sequelae such as a traumatic aneurysm or a carotid-cavernous fistula.

During such initial assessment and management, a decision regarding further treatment is made. It is at this point that the judgment of the surgeon is most severely taxed. Most would agree that the comatose, unresponsive patient with fixed dilated pupils and absence of an intracranial hematoma as proved by CT scan is not a candidate for immediate surgery. Similarly, most concur that the initially intact but subsequently deteriorating patient with a gunshot wound of the head requires immediate craniotomy. Between these extremes lie the problems. Categorical or protocol decisions would seem inappropriate. The surgeon at hand must individualize the decision, remembering that the relief of increased intracranial pressure and control of hemorrhage may be the only indication for immediate operation, but that prevention of infection and morbidity reduction mandate wound repair as soon as possible in any potentially salvageable individual.

Medical Therapy

Preoperative or intraoperative medical therapy consists of various measures to control intracranial pressure and to prevent seizures, infection, and gastrointestinal hemorrhage. Elevated intracranial pressure should be assumed in all cases that present with a depressed level of consciousness and should be treated empirically with hypocarbia and hyperosmotics. A preoperative dose of mannitol, 1 g/kg IV, is standard. Corticosteroids, usually dexamethasone (10 mg IV followed by 4 mg IV q 6 h), are commonly given, although there is no conclusive evidence of their efficacy. The high

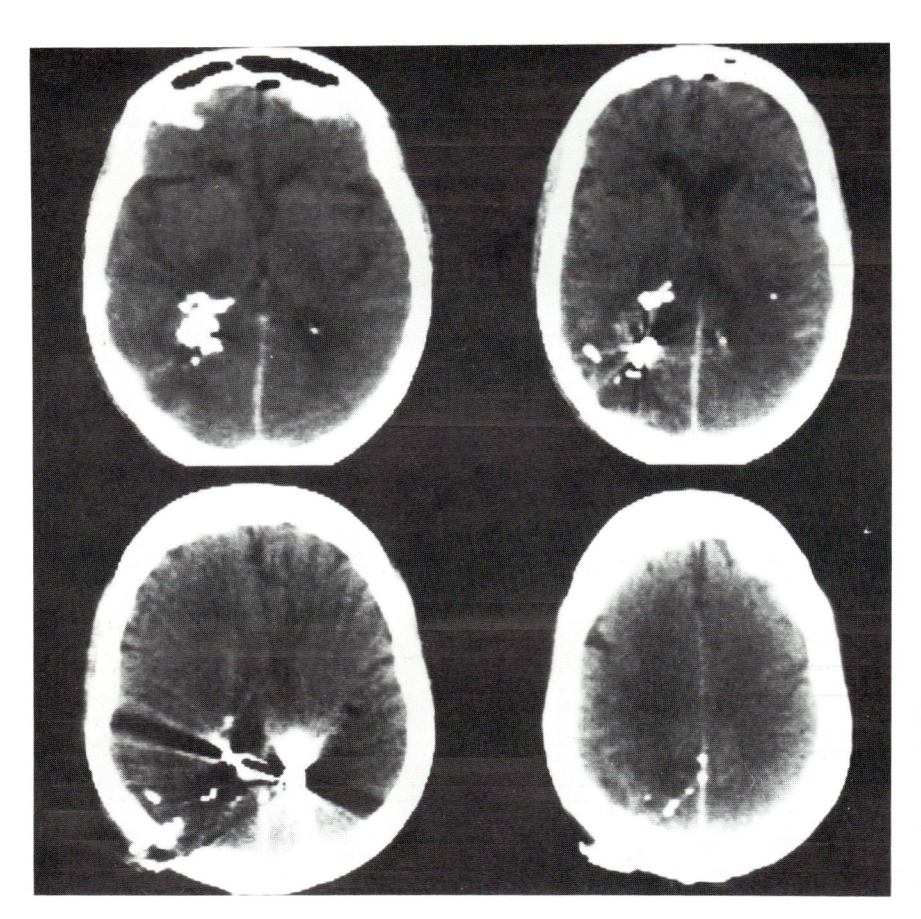

Figure 207-3 CT scans disclosing a right parietal to left parietal (transfalcine) penetrating wound. Note fragments in or adjacent to the ventricular trigone, interhemispheric blood, and proximity of the distal fragment to the falx.

incidence of late post-traumatic seizures complicating penetrating head wounds suggests the routine use of anticonvulsants, but recent studies question their efficacy as prophylaxis.[2,26,27]

Although no controlled prospective double-blind trials establishing their efficacy in preventing meningitis, abscess formation, and wound infection in missile wounds exist, and despite the possibility of selecting resistant organisms, prophylactic antibiotics are routinely used. Jennett and Teasdale[17] say there is no case for broad spectrum antibiotics in that organisms in traumatic meningitis are usually penicillin-sensitive, but the wide array of organisms cultured from wounds treated by Hagan[11] suggests the opposite. Currently the best broad spectrum coverage for non-nosocomially incurred wounds is probably nafcillin, chloramphenicol or moxalactam. Should infection arise, a change to organism-specific agents should immediately follow demonstration of sensitivity. In addition, tetanus toxoid should be administered routinely. In no case should antibiotic prophylaxis be considered adequate replacement for surgical treatment. Finally, insertion of a nasogastric tube for intermittent suction should be accompanied by antacid administration.

Surgical Treatment

Surgical intervention is directed toward the reduction of elevated intracranial pressure and the prevention of infection, seizures, and further loss of eloquent brain tissue. These can best be accomplished by removal of hematoma and meticulous hemostasis; thorough track cleansing with removal of debris, devitalized tissue, and bone and accessible missile fragments; and closure of the wound, creating impermeable barriers at dura, galea, and skin levels. The entire head is shaved and a thorough search for entrance and exit wounds is made. All of the scalp is prepared and draped in sterile fashion. The head is positioned to allow access first to entrance and then to exit wounds unless a distal intracranial hematoma evident on the preoperative CT scan mandates initial exit wound craniectomy.

The scalp wound should be totally excised, usually as an ellipse within a curvilinear incision. Dural exposure may be accomplished either through a bone flap incorporating the entrance defect with a central craniectomy circumferentially fashioned about the fracture or simply through a craniectomy of the penetration site centripetally effected from an adjacent burr hole. In either event, exposure should be large enough to allow access to tracts that may diverge from the perpendicular, to surrounding contusions, and to the full extent of extra-axial blood collections. Comminutedly fractured bone should be removed and discarded. Replacement of devitalized bone fragments, advocated by some in non-penetrating wounds, has no place in penetrating missile injuries of the brain. Dura is incised outwardly from the center of the penetration; devitalized dura is removed, but its debridement is minimized to facilitate closure. Dural sinus bleeding may be controlled by tamponade or oversewing.

The subdural space is inspected and any hematoma evacuated. The missile track through the parenchyma is then explored. All pulped, grossly contaminated tissue, regardless of anatomical area, is removed with gentle suction and irrigation. The track is followed deeply as resection of necrotic cerebrum, hematoma, and foreign debris is carried out in a circumferential pattern. Gentle palpation of the track with bayonet forceps, illumination with headlight or lighted retractors, and magnification with loupe may be helpful in a meticulous search for the removal of all accessible bone and metal fragments. Those removed, along with necrotic tissue, are routinely subjected to culture for microorganisms. Copious irrigation with bacitracin solution or saline is mandatory. Adequacy of resection is indicated by the ability of normal brain to maintain the resultant cavity. It is relaxed and pulsatile but usually does not collapse. Progressive protrusion or "swelling" of the brain might indicate deep or distant hematoma, which should be sought and evacuated.

Repeat subdural inspection is followed by dural closure that is often possible without grafting. If necessary, pericranium, temporal or occipital fascia, or fascia lata may be used as a dural graft. A watertight dural closure is crucial to the prevention of CSF leakage and the resultant risk of meningitis, to preclusion of extrusion of cerebral tissue (fungus formation), and to reduction of seizure incidence. A subdural or intraventricular catheter may be left in place for a short time to monitor pressure if swelling suggests its necessity. Closure of previously debrided soft tissue involves nonabsorbable suture in the galea and skin, or, if the wound is more than 36 h old, a single layer of stainless steel wire. Undermining or rotation flaps may be necessary to ensure tension-free, full-thickness coverage over the craniectomy.

Special Surgical Considerations

Tangential Wounds

Termed *gutter wounds* by Cushing[7], tangential wounds are those in which the missile delivers a glancing, nonpenetrating blow to the cranium. Such an injury may be associated with significant brain damage with or without visible bone involvement. If bone fragments are depressed or in-driven, usually at a right angle to the tangential missile path, they should be removed and the wound treated with the same diligence as any other penetrating wound. Even if there is no bone disruption or only a nondisplaced linear skull fracture, significant neurological injury may result from brain hematoma, laceration, or contusion underlying the point of tangential impact. Whether such an injury requires craniotomy and brain debridement remains somewhat controversial.[10] A hematoma of significant mass should be evacuated. Simple contusion should not be disturbed. The CT scan is of considerable help in arriving at an appropriate decision.

Opening of Intact Dura

Dura left intact by the injury should be opened at the time of operation if the neurological examination or CT scan, or a tense, protuberant, darkened appearance of the dura suggests an underlying mass.

Inferior Cranial Wounds

As pointed out by Dillon and Meirowsky[9], injuries from missiles that, in penetrating the orbit, maxillary region, sphenoid wing, or temporal bone, pierce the floor of the anterior or middle cranial fossa deserve special attention. The wound of entrance is frequently small and may go undetected. Such injuries have a high potential for infection, a common association with intracranial hemorrhage, and, consequently, a high mortality—27.9 percent opposed to 7.8 percent overall mortality for 1105 consecutive Korean war casualties with penetrating craniocerebral trauma. Their proximity to accessory air sinuses, basal intracranial vessels, and cranial nerves leads to a high incidence of such serious complications as pneumocephalus, cerebrospinal fluid otorhinorrhea, traumatic aneurysm, and arteriovenous fistula in addition to infection and hematoma. Direct disruption of brain stem structures is usually incompatible with life.

In this type of injury arteriography should precede operation. Craniotomy is the approach of choice in that exploration through a basally originating missile tract affords inadequate exposure. Meticulous debridement and irrigation are mandatory. Dural closure is essential and is best effected by intradural patch grafting. Primary suture is often not feasible, and extradural grafting has a high incidence of failure. Although avoidance of placement of foreign material is desirable, prevention of an inferior anterior cranial fossa encephalocele may necessitate wire mesh covering of the bony defect.

Perforation of Air Sinuses

When a missile has traversed an air sinus, bone fragments should be removed. Sinus mucosa must be totally exenterated, and the sinus ostium packed with fat or muscle. The cranial defect is then covered with pericranium or fascia. Dural closure must be watertight.

Removal of Fragments from Dural Sinuses

Bone fragments should be removed from dural venous sinuses. Adequate preparation includes obtaining whole blood for replacement of hemorrhage and securing both proximal and distal exposure of the involved sinus to allow its afferent and efferent control. After removal of the fragments, bleeding may be controlled with standard methods such as absorbable gelatin sponge, clips, or fascial patch graft if necessary. Temporary clamping of the sinus for primary repair or vein graft interposition while employing a bypass shunt may be feasible. Ligation of the sagittal sinus anterior to the coronal suture or of the nondominant transverse sinus is usually safe, but other sinus ligations are fraught with danger and should be avoided.

Retained Bone Fragments

Neurosurgeons disagree over the therapeutic implications of retained bone fragments. Those with predominantly military experience argue that postoperative demonstration of retained bone fragments indicates inadequate debridement and warrants immediate re-exploration. Those who have had primarily civilian practice suggest expectant management. Hammon states that re-exploration for retained bone fragments without exception reveals significant amounts of necrotic debris, and he unequivocally links clusters of bone fragments with high incidences of subsequent infection.[12] Hagan reported bacterial contamination, as proved by culture, of 56.4 percent of 62 patients with retained bone fragments at the time of re-exploration despite prophylactic antibiotics and the use of only aerobic cultures.[11]

Some argue that one can be more tolerant of retained bone fragments in civilian wounds because the contamination that occurs in such low-velocity injuries is often limited.[20,23] Most neurosurgeons, however, think that retained bone fragments that can be removed without increasing neurological dysfunction should be extracted whereas those more dangerously situated should be managed expectantly with frequent observation and scanning for abscess development.

The case is less strong for exploration for retrieval of retained metal fragments. Raimondi and Samuelson have argued that in low-velocity civilian wounds with limited tissue destruction, the value of extensive exploration in efforts to retrieve missile fragments is minimal and that they should be left.[23] Few would disagree with this premise as applied to fragment removal that might be associated with increased neurological deficit. However, in a military setting, Hagen found culture proven bacterial contamination of all removed metal fragments.[11]

In conclusion, removal of retained bone and metal fragments is highly desirable if this can be accomplished without increasing the neurological deficit. A longer interval between trauma and surgery warrants more aggressive initial debridement and attempted fragment removal. In addition, as emphasized by Small and Turner,[24] ventricular penetration mandates ventriculotomy for removal of all fragments, debris, and clot. Intraoperative ultrasound may be helpful in fragment localization. If additional neurological deficit is likely to be incurred by bone or metal fragment removal, they should be left undisturbed and the patient followed with CT scanning for abscess formation, late hemorrhage, or missile migration.

Wounds That Traverse the Midline

As pointed out by Meirowsky et al.,[22] special problems are posed by missile injuries that cross the midline. Although mortality in these cases was similar to that for all penetrating head injuries in Vietnam, there was a high incidence of infection, intracranial hematoma, and post-traumatic epilepsy. Should the missile cross the midline but not traverse the contralateral parenchyma, it may be removed from a position close to the dural reflection by incising the falx. If, on the other hand, the missile lies superficially on the contralateral side or if it is associated with a significant hematoma, a contralateral craniotomy should be performed. Should the ventricular system be penetrated by the missile, special care is necessary to assure thorough cleansing and removal of the mobile intraventricular fragments and debris.

Postoperative Care

Prevention of further injury to the brain during the postoperative period is crucial to the eventual outcome. This involves close neurological monitoring for signs of increased intracranial pressure or infection. An intracranial pressure monitor may be used if problems with pressure control are anticipated, but it should be removed as soon as possible given the contamination of the nearby wound. Intracranial hypertension should be investigated by an emergency CT scan and treated aggressively with mild sedation, perhaps paralysis, hypocapnia, hyperosmotic dehydrating agents, and, if indicated, a repeat operation. In addition, postoperative skull films or CT scans should always be obtained soon after surgery in search of retained bone fragments that may warrant early re-exploration. Prophylactic antibiotics are continued. Rigorous medical intensive care monitoring is essential for prevention of cardiac, pulmonary, or metabolic difficulties that might jeopardize brain recovery. Seizures require antiepileptic drugs.

Complications encountered in the early postoperative period include recurrent bleeding, uncontrolled intracranial hypertension, infection, CSF fistula, and retained fragments.[11] Recurrent bleeding mandates a repeat craniotomy, and infection requires obliteration of the source (repair of a continuing CSF fistula, removal of an abscess) and appropriate antibiotics.

Morbidity and Mortality

Brain damage resulting from missile penetration, or from consequences secondary to the penetration, determines the duration and quality of patient survival. The presenting neurological status is the best indicator of prognosis. Crockard tabulated the specific incidence of mortality as related to the initial level of consciousness, pupil reactivity, and blood pressure.[4] The mortality was 11.5 percent in awake, alert patients, 33.3 percent in lethargic patients, and 100 percent in unresponsive patients. Normal pupils were associated with a 34 percent mortality, and dilated pupils with a 96 percent mortality.

Factors significantly related to brain damage and its derivatives include missile nature and velocity, site of intracranial injury, and interval between injury and surgical intervention. Hammon reported an operative mortality of 7.64 percent from fragment wounds and 22.73 percent from gunshot wounds as compared with a 10 percent mortality from wounds resulting from handguns fired from distant range.[12] Multilobar injury is associated with higher mortality than unilobar damage. As expected, injury to the brain stem and diencephalon is more commonly fatal than that involving other areas.

The most frequent cause of death following a penetrating wound to the brain is either direct or indirect brain stem disruption. Other contributors to demise include massive cerebral destruction, infection, intracranial hemorrhage, seizures, and cardiopulmonary failure. Hammon claimed that operative complications, including hematoma and infection, were responsible for less than 5 percent of deaths and that associated injuries caused 9 percent of all perioperative fatalities.[12]

Results from penetrating missile wounds vary to some extent with the setting of the injury. Hubschmann et al. in their civilian practice reported a satisfactory outcome in 39 percent of cases in their series.[16] Fifty-four percent died, three-quarters of them without operation, and one-quarter after operation. Of their survivors, 71 percent were capable of self-care. Suicide attempts are associated with a high mortality—53.3 percent in Mississippi[20] and 90 percent in Finland.[14] Mortality from wartime wounds, on the other hand, has steadily declined as a result of improvement in technique, antibiotic therapy, and rapidity of evacuation. Cushing's application of the basic principles outlined above resulted in fall of mortality from 54.4 percent to 28.8 percent during World War I.[7] Small and Turner attained a 16.4 percent mortality rate during World War II.[24] Surgical mortality averaged 9.6 percent in both the Korean and Vietnam experiences.[11,13]

Conclusions

Whether penetrating brain wounds are sustained in military or civilian combat is of little consequence in management decisions. Wounding mechanisms are similar; differences occur in intensity of destructive force, reflecting variations in missile velocity and in the interval from trauma to treatment. The extremes of these variables are encountered in both military and civilian settings. The sound, well-established surgical principles of thorough scalp, bone, and brain debridement, with meticulous removal of bone and metal fragments that are accessible without producing an increased neurological deficit, and careful primary wound repair should be applied to both. Continued dedication to these principles, augmented by utilization of CT scanning and other new diagnostic techniques and by such increasingly effective therapeutic adjuncts as intracranial pressure and cardiorespiratory control, antibiotics, and anticonvulsants, is the "state of the art" requisite for the care of penetrating wounds of the head.

References

1. Baker CC, Oppenheimer L, Stephens B, Lewis FR, Trunkey DD: Epidemiology of trauma deaths. Am J Surg 140:144–148, 1980.
2. Caveness WF, Meirowsky AM, Rish BL, Mohr JP, Kistler JP, Dillon JD, Weiss GH: The nature of posttraumatic epilepsy. J Neurosurg 50:545–553, 1979.
3. Cooper PR: Gunshot wounds of the brain, in Cooper PR: *Head Injury.* Baltimore, Williams & Wilkins, 1982, pp 257–274.
4. Crockard HA: Bullet injuries of the brain. Ann Roy Coll Surg 55:111–123, 1974.
5. Crockard HA: Penetrating craniocerebral missile injuries. Int Anesthesiol Clin 17:307–326, 1979.
6. Crockard HA, Brown FD, Calica AB, Johns LM, Mullan S: Physiological consequences of experimental cerebral missile injury and use of data analysis to predict survival. J Neurosurg 46:784–794, 1977.
7. Cushing H: A study of a series of wounds involving the brain

and its enveloping structures. Br J Surg 5:558–684, 1918.
8. DeMuth WE Jr: Bullet velocity as applied to military rifle wounding capacity. J Trauma 9:27–38, 1969.
9. Dillon JD Jr, Meirowsky AM: Facio-orbito-cranial missile wounds. Surg Neurol 4:515–518, 1975.
10. Dodge PR, Meirowsky AM Tangential wounds of scalp and skull. J Neurosurg 9:472–483, 1952.
11. Hagan RD: Early complications following penetrating wounds of the brain. J Neurosurg 34:132–141, 1971.
12. Hammon WM: Analysis of 2187 consecutive penetrating wounds to the brain from Vietnam. J Neurosurg 34:127–131, 1971.
13. Hammon WM: Missile wounds, in Vinken PJ, Bruyn GW, Braakman R (eds): *Handbook of Clinical Neurology*, vol 23: *Injuries of the Brain and Skull*. Amsterdam, North-Holland Publishing Co, 1975, pp 505–526.
14. Hernesniemi J: Penetrating craniocerebral gunshot wounds in civilians. Acta Neurochir (Wien) 49:199–205, 1979.
15. Hopkinson DAW, Marshall TK: Firearm injuries. Br J Surg 54:344–353, 1967.
16. Hubschmann O, Shapiro K, Baden M, Shulman K: Craniocerebral gunshot injuries in civilian practice—prognostic criteria and surgical management: Experience with 82 cases. J Trauma 19:6–12, 1979.
17. Jennett B, Teasdale G: *Management of Head Injuries*. Philadelphia, Davis, 1981, pp 193–209.
18. Kirkpatrick JB, Di Maio V: Civilian gunshot wounds of the brain. J Neurosurg 49:185–198, 1978.
19. Levett JM, Johns LM, Replogle RL, Mullan S: Cardiovascular effects of experimental cerebral missile injury in primates. Surg Neurol 13:59–64, 1980.
20. Lillard PL: Five years experience with penetrating craniocerebral gunshot wounds. Surg Neurol 9:79–83, 1978.
21. Meirowsky AM: Secondary removal of retained bone fragments in missile wounds of the brain. J Neurosurg 57:617–621, 1982.
22. Meirowsky AM, Rish BL, Mohr JP, Caveness WF, Dillon JD, Kistler SP, Weiss GH: Definitive care of cerebral missile injuries crossing the midline. Milit Med 145:246–250, 1980.
23. Raimondi AJ, Samuelson GH: Craniocerebral gunshot wounds in civilian practice. J Neurosurg 32:647–653, 1970.
24. Small JM, Turner EA: A surgical experience of 1200 cases of penetrating brain wounds in battle, Europe, 1944–45. Br J Surg [War Surg Suppl] 1:62–74, 1947.
25. Sullivan HG, Martinez J, Becker DP, Miller JD, Griffith R, Wist AO: Fluid-percussion model of mechanical brain injury in the cat. J Neurosurg 45:520–534, 1976.
26. Young B, Rapp RP, Norton JA, Haack D, Tibbs PA, Bean JR: Failure of prophylactically administered phenytoin to prevent early posttraumatic seizures. J Neurosurg 58:231–235, 1983.
27. Young B, Rapp RP, Norton JA, Haack D, Tibbs PA, Bean JR: Failure of prophylactically administered phenytoin to prevent late posttraumatic seizures. J Neurosurg 58:236–241, 1983.

208
Vascular Lesions with Head Injury

Steven L. Giannotta
Jamshid Ahmadi

Trauma to cerebrovascular structures is a well-recognized concomitant of craniocerebral injury. Epidural hematoma and carotid-cavernous sinus fistula are two well-recognized sequelae of intracranial vascular disruption. Unfortunately, not all vascular injuries associated with head trauma are as readily identifiable nor are they associated with definite treatment guidelines. Symptoms and signs of major extra- or intracranial cerebrovascular injury such as carotid thrombosis may be delayed in onset or be totally unrecognized because of superimposed brain injury. The patient is at risk for further irreversible deterioration due to ischemia or emboli. Thus, early diagnosis of traumatic injury to major intra- or extracranial cerebrovascular structures is desirable if this admittedly small subset of head injuries is to be managed properly.

One of the most important advances in the diagnosis and management of head trauma made in the past 20 years is the advent of the computed tomography (CT) scanner. CT examination has become the definitive method of evaluating head-injured patients, essentially supplanting cerebral arteriography. Unhappily, arteriography still remains the definitive examination for documenting cerebrovascular lesions. Reliance on CT evaluation in head trauma may potentially decrease the number of occult vascular injuries identified. At our medical center, the number of cerebral angiographic examinations has fallen from approximately 900 per year to just over 200 per year since CT scanning has been available. The incidence of documented intracranial traumatic aneurysms over that period of time has fallen a proportional amount.[24] Since the majority of traumatic vascular injuries associated with head injury are not suspected prior to angiography, a high index of suspicion and a firm concept of the pathophysiology and presenting symptoms of vascular insufficiency associated with head trauma are needed.

In this chapter we will discuss a number of cerebrovascular lesions known to occur in association with head trauma. Although the list will by no means be exhaustive, a discussion of the presenting symptoms and signs, natural history, radiographic evaluation, pathology, and management may serve to emphasize the importance of early diagnosis and a high index of suspicion in the prevention of the "stroke after head injury" syndrome.

Extracranial Traumatic Arterial Lesions

Injury to the extracranial carotid and vertebral arteries is uncommon but certainly by no means rare. Well over 90 percent of the major arterial trauma in the neck is caused by penetrating wounds, especially from firearms.[31,48,52] Not surprisingly, our knowledge of the management of extracranial cerebrovascular injuries comes from reports from military actions in which the majority of injuries are penetrating.

In the setting of civilian head trauma, nonpenetrating traumatic lesions of the extracranial cerebral vasculature provide the most difficult diagnostic and management problems and will be the focus of this discussion.

Carotid Arterial Injuries

The incidence of extracranial carotid artery injuries in association with head trauma is generally unknown. In one series of 2000 head injuries, the carotid artery was found to be injured in 0.5 percent.[18] When one considers that more than 1.5 million head injuries occur in the United States each year, the problem assumes greater magnitude.[10] The mortality rate for a traumatic lesion of the carotid artery in the neck is between 20 and 40 percent.[26,30,45,64,66] This combined with the fact that the incidence of neurological deficit can be up to 80 percent in those who survive further underscores the importance of this entity.[52]

Presenting Symptoms and Signs

Because of the relatively low incidence of carotid artery injuries, a typical patient profile is difficult to construct. The majority of cases are subjects of isolated case presentations in the literature. Yamada et al., in a review of the literature, put together a series of 52 cases of blunt trauma to the carotid artery.[66] They found that 75 percent of the patients had some history of head injury prior to their presentation and 23 percent of these head injuries were severe. An important feature of this study was the fact that there was a significant delay in recognizing the vascular injury in 94 percent of the cases. A number of clinical features peculiar to traumatic lesions of the carotid artery may explain the reasons for this delay.

The most important symptoms of carotid arterial injury are those of cerebral ischemia. Following a traumatic incident, the patient may develop a hemiparesis or a hemisensory deficit with or without associated hemianopsia suggesting ischemia in the internal carotid territory.[43] Symptoms may be fleeting, as in transient ischemic attack (TIA), or more prolonged in their presentation, as in reversible ischemic neurological deficit (RIND). With severe ischemia, the neurological deficit worsens and eventually becomes permanent. Also, the level of consciousness may be affected, but frequently the neurological deficit is out of proportion to any reduction in the level of consciousness, in contradistinction to what would be expected solely as a result of the head injury.

Several factors may have a negative impact on the examiner's index of suspicion of an associated extracranial traumatic arterial lesion. Less than half of the patients in the series of Yamada et al. showed any sign of injury to the neck.[66] Those who did had only a bruise on the neck or at most an abrasion on the neck or forehead. Secondly, symptoms and signs of carotid territory insufficiency were delayed in their appearance. Less than 10 percent of the patients developed ischemic symptoms within 1 h of the time of the injury. Half of the patients remained asymptomatic for up to 10 h. Indeed, 17 percent of their cases were still asymptomatic with respect to the arterial injury at 24 h following the injury. The presence of associated injuries, especially traumatic brain injuries, can mask symptoms related to the arterial trauma. This is especially true in those cases where severe head injury accompanies the vascular lesions.

Other physical findings may herald the presence of an associated carotid injury in the setting of a traumatic brain injury. A number of patients will manifest a Horner's syndrome caused by injury to the sympathetic nerves surrounding the internal carotid artery. Also, the presence of a carotid bruit due to turbulence at the site of an unsuspected injury should cause one to further consider the possibility of an internal carotid lesion. The association of a fractured mandible with that of traumatic carotid injury has been underscored by a number of authors.[4,28,60] Although the mechanism is unclear, the presence of facial fractures, especially a mandible fracture, should alert one to the possibility of an underlying carotid injury.[4,59,60,63]

Mechanism of Injury

The cervical portion of the carotid artery can be injured in association with head trauma in several ways. The most common mechanism is that of direct blunt trauma to the neck. In this situation, the internal carotid artery just above the bifurcation seems to be the most vulnerable. It is theorized that the artery is rapidly compressed against the vertebral column, resulting in injury to the media or to the intima. As mentioned above, mandibular fractures may in some way be responsible for injuring the internal carotid artery above the bifurcation. A fracture fragment or bony spicule may compress the artery, causing disruption of one or more layers of the arterial wall. More likely the fracture simply identifies the patient most likely to have arterial trauma, much like a first rib fracture suggests a major injury to branches of the aortic arch.[49,60]

The internal carotid artery in its cervical portion can also be injured by stretching.[4] Boldrey et al. directed attention to this particular mechanism of injury.[7] Because the carotid is firmly rooted in the carotid canal at the base of the skull, a blow to the head or face that results in hyperextension and rotation can pull the internal carotid artery tightly against the lateral mass of either the C1 or C2 vertebra. Subsequent stretching or compression of the artery against the bony prominence causes intimal disruption and possibly hematoma formation in the media. This mechanism has been invoked to explain injuries that result in internal carotid artery dissections in the upper cervical portion. A number of young patients with high internal carotid dissections have been reported, suggesting that older people with more redundant elongated arteries may somehow be protected from this type of injury.[4,5,33,59]

Following an injury that results in disruption of the arterial intima, subsequent hemodynamic and thrombogenic events will determine the ultimate pathological injury. The fractured intima initially serves as a substrate for platelet deposition and thrombus formation. As this process proceeds, several different sequelae may occur. A concomitant mural hematoma may constrict the vessel lumen and predispose it to complete thrombosis. An ischemic infarction of the brain is the usual result. Prior to or in the absence of complete vessel occlusion, distal embolization of fragments from the growing thrombus may occur causing TIAs, seizures, or cerebral infarction.

Traumatically induced dissection of the internal carotid artery in the neck also occurs in association with head injury. As in thrombosis, the critical element is disruption of the intima. The rapid pulsatile blood column further elevates the intima and subintimal layers, occasionally over very long stretches of the vessel. This may proceed up to the carotid canal at the base of the skull. A long segment of severe stenosis may result in restriction of flow or serve as the site for the origination of cerebral emboli.[5,59]

Aneurysms may also result from injury of the carotid artery in association with head trauma. The majority of these lesions are found in association with traumatic dissection of the carotid artery. The arterial wall is thinned and weakened, and the pulsatile column of blood produces an aneurysm in association with an area of dissection. Turbulence may cause the aneurysm to enlarge and also provide for thrombus formation, which can subsequently go on to distal embolization. Patients may complain of a pulsatile neck mass, dysphagia, or noise in the neck that may radiate into the head. Also, lower cranial nerve palsies including hoarseness or weakness of the tongue may occur in association with large aneurysms of the carotid artery.[11,37,41,47,50]

Angiographic Signs

Thrombosis The typical picture of trauma-induced occlusion of the cervical internal carotid artery is abrupt blockage of flow of the contrast medium approximately 1 to 3 cm above the bifurcation of the common carotid artery in the neck. Regardless of the site of injury the entire cervical segment is usually occluded. Reconstitution of the intracranial portion of the internal carotid artery may occur from collateral circulation across the anterior or posterior communicating arteries or from the external carotid artery. Close scrutiny of intracranial vessels may show the presence of emboli or middle cerebral branch occlusions to suggest prior embolization. Occasionally retrograde flow in the upper cervical portion of the internal carotid artery is noted. This phenomenon, which is usually better appreciated on the later phases of the study, suggests that the internal carotid artery may be physiologically patent and that thromboendarterectomy may be a viable treatment alternative.

Dissection Although traumatic dissection can occur anywhere along the course of the internal carotid artery, it most frequently begins in the section of the artery adjacent to the C1 or C2 vertebra. An irregular narrowing of the contrast column over several centimeters is the typical angiographic picture. An intramural hematoma may almost totally occlude the artery, and thrombus formation may be apparent. The artery usually assumes its normal caliber in the region of the carotid canal at the base of the skull (Fig. 208-1). Branch occlusions or evidence of distal emboli may be seen in the intracranial vasculature.

Aneurysm Dissecting aneurysms may present as an irregular enlargement of the contrast column in association with segmental narrowing of the cervical internal carotid artery. These aneurysms tend to become more localized and saccular in nature. False aneurysms of the internal carotid not in association with dissection usually present as saccular expansions of the vessel with a small communication to the lumen (Fig. 208-2). Irregularities in the lumen may suggest the presence of thrombus material, again emphasizing the potential for these lesions to be a source of intracranial emboli.

Treatment

Successful management of trauma-induced extracranial carotid lesions will be influenced by three major factors: the type of injury as depicted by carotid angiography, the location of the injury along the course of the internal carotid artery, and the pre-existing severity of the neurological deficit. The rapidity with which the diagnosis is made will influence two of these factors, namely the type of angiographic injury (stenosis versus occlusion) and the amount of neurological deficit. Therefore, the key to successful management of these injuries is early diagnosis.

The treatment of patients with carotid thrombosis will

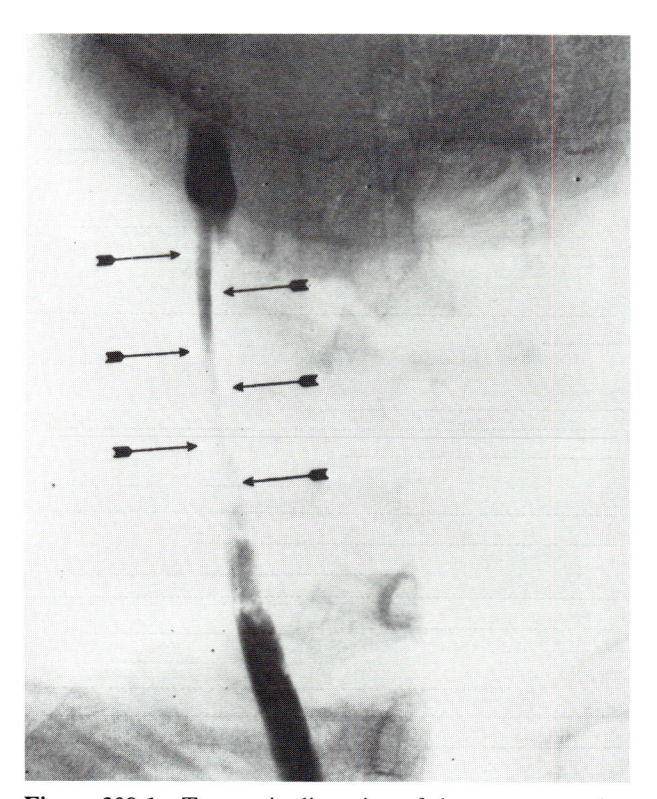

Figure 208-1 Traumatic dissection of the common and internal carotid arteries. Management included thromboendarterectomy and intimal repair.

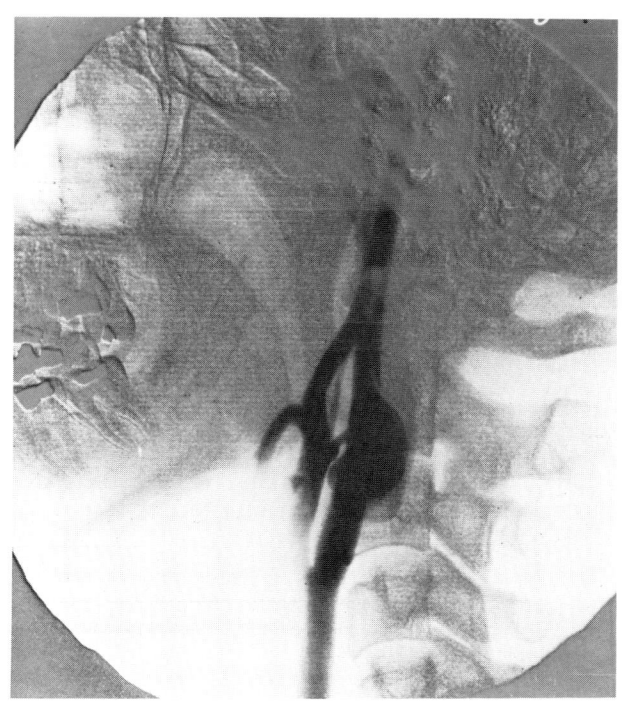

Figure 208-2 Traumatic aneurysm of the cervical internal carotid artery. Management included resection and autogenous vein grafting.

depend on the stage at which it is diagnosed. Those with a completed stroke of more than 12 h in duration or who present in coma will most likely prove refractory to any type of treatment. Patients with fluctuating neurological symptoms in the face of an acutely occluded internal carotid artery may benefit from urgent exploration and thromboendarterectomy. Extraction of the thrombus with repair of the detached intima has been successful in restoring flow in approximately half of the cases in which this has been attempted.[30,45,64] Furthermore, Yamada, Perry, Jernigan, Little, and others have reported dramatic reversal of ischemic neurological deficits following emergent thromboendarterectomy for traumatic cervical carotid occlusion.[28,33,45,66] Acute revascularization via an extracranial-intracranial (EC-IC) bypass is probably not indicated for an asymptomatic occlusion and is at best hazardous in the face of a moderate or severe deficit. In those patients with TIAs or RINDs where thromboendarterectomy has been unsuccessful, revascularization may be beneficial. Unfortunately there is little current information to support this concept.

An indication for a delayed attempt at thromboendarterectomy in a patient with a minimal neurological deficit may exist if the patient receives early anticoagulation therapy with heparin. In this situation a soft thrombus without significant organization may be found occluding the internal carotid artery. Extraction of the thrombus using Fogarty catheters may be possible with subsequent restoration of antegrade flow.

Prior to any thoughts of surgical therapy, the patient who presents with an occluded carotid artery with or without ischemic neurological deficits should be managed with attempts to increase cerebral perfusion. Hypotension resulting from associated injuries should be rapidly reversed with fluid therapy or pressor agents. In those few patients found to have a carotid occlusion in the absence of neurological symptoms, a high circulating intravascular volume should be maintained in order to obviate any potential hypotensive episodes in the first few days following the injury. Those patients who have a mild to moderate neurological deficit and who may or may not be candidates for surgical therapy may benefit by trial of induced hypervolemia or hypertension with close hemodynamic and neurological monitoring.[29,46] Patients who have severe neurological deficits are not candidates for surgery, and attempts to open the occluded carotid artery have usually ended in failure.

Specific guidelines for the treatment of traumatic carotid dissection are still a matter of anecdote because of the fact that the natural history of this entity has not been defined. Although a number of these cases have presented with neurological deficits presumably due to emboli, some have remained asymptomatic during follow-up. Stringer and Kelly presented six cases of traumatic dissection of the extracranial carotid artery, all of which were treated conservatively.[59] Those patients who were found to have angiographically demonstrable intracranial emboli were recommended for anticoagulation therapy with heparin. New and Momose and Sullivan et al. have reported cases in which the dissection has eventually resolved completely; however, other cases have been documented to result in pseudoaneurysm formation, complete thrombosis, or further embolization.[4,41,60] Several reports in the literature have suggested that if the dissection is surgically approachable, repair of the injured intima can be accomplished safely.[30,66] If, after antiplatelet or anticoagulant therapy, follow-up angiography demonstrates the progression of stenosis or evidence of thrombus formation, or if the patient's course suggests further ischemia, thromboendarterectomy or resection with grafting is warranted. Again, the type of therapy depends on the location of the lesion. In high lesions that are inaccessible, gradual carotid occlusion with or without EC-IC bypass grafting may be the best choice for reducing the possibility of distal embolization.[5]

The management of dissecting or false aneurysms is not without controversy. Authors have brought attention to the fact that these lesions can harbor thrombus material that can serve as a source of emboli.[11,47,50] Other potential complications such as hemorrhage, further enlargement, or compression of surrounding neurological structures are much less likely. If accessible, traumatic carotid aneurysms should be treated by aneurysmorrhaphy, resection and end-to-end anastomosis, or resection and reconstitution of the vessel using an interposition graft.[37,39,47] Inaccessibly high lesions of the internal carotid artery may also best be treated with EC-IC bypass grafting and gradual carotid occlusion in the neck. Those patients thought to be candidates for gradual occlusion of the internal carotid artery without a prior EC-IC bypass should be managed with a high circulating blood volume and induced hypertension as necessary to avoid an ischemic neurological deficit.[23]

The outcome will be governed by the severity of the initial neurological insult and to a lesser extent the physician's ability to obviate further neurological impairment.[30,31,52]

Although a number of patients have been reported whose neurological deficit has cleared following reconstitution of flow, the majority of neurological insults from carotid artery trauma are likely due to emboli. Therefore, reversal of neurological deficit will continue to be a rare event due to surgery alone.

Vertebral Artery Injuries

Injuries to the cervical portion of the vertebral artery occur infrequently. Rich and Spencer reported approximately 7000 war-related and civilian arterial injuries and could document only 15 cases of vertebral artery trauma.[48] The relatively deep position of the vertebral artery in the neck associated with its protection by the foramina transversaria tends to reduce its vulnerability to both blunt and penetrating injuries. Further, the relative redundancy of the vertebral system makes injuries to one vertebral artery less likely to cause ischemic cerebrovascular symptoms. Most instances of trauma to the cervical vertebral arteries are due to blunt injury, and are infrequently associated with concomitant head injury. Injuries have been reported in conjunction with cervical spine fracture, chiropractic manipulation, yoga exercises, and sporting injuries.[9,13,16,22,58] There are, however, a small number of reported injuries associated with mild head and neck trauma that can result in symptomatic injury to the cervical portion of the vertebral artery.[16,22] This usually results in thrombosis of one vertebral artery, occasionally with propagation of the thrombus into the intracranial portion. This may ultimately result in ischemic infarction in the cerebellum and brain stem, the diagnosis of which is made at autopsy or after irreversible ischemic neurological deficit has taken place. Meier et al. have reported that the liberal use of four-vessel angiography in patients suspected of having major vascular injury in the neck will increase the yield in documenting vertebral artery injuries.[39] Therefore, a discussion of the circumstances surrounding vertebral artery trauma as well as the related symptoms and signs is in order.

Symptoms and Signs

The majority of patients with vertebral artery injuries associated with head and neck trauma will present with the delayed onset of symptoms and signs of brain stem or cerebellar ischemia. Vertigo, blurred vision, ataxia, and dysarthria are common. In the setting of cervical vertebral artery trauma, neck ache, suboccipital pain, and headache are also frequent concomitants. The classical Wallenberg syndrome as a result of trauma to the vertebral artery is also known to occur following minor head and neck injury.[9,13,22,32] This results in a Horner's syndrome with decreased sensation to pain and temperature on the ipsilateral face and contralateral arm and leg in association with ataxia on the ipsilateral side. These symptoms may follow any traumatic incident that causes acute hyperextension or rotation of the cervical spine. Frequently the head injury is minor, and usually the patient will not be able to recall a period of unconsciousness. Neurological symptoms may be delayed as long as a month after the trauma but usually occur within 24 h. In some cases associated neck movements serve to exacerbate the symptoms of ischemia.[58] This situation should alert the treating physician to a potential vertebral artery injury.

Schneider and Schemm brought our attention to the occurrence of spinal cord ischemia from vertebral arterial insufficiency due to cervical trauma.[54] They theorized that traumatic vertebral artery occlusion may compromise blood flow to the anterior spinal artery, producing ischemia to the cervical portion of the spinal cord. The manifestations would include a typical central cord lesion with disproportionately more motor impairment of the upper than the lower extremities, bladder dysfunction, and varying degrees of sensory loss below the level of the lesion.

Outward signs of trauma to the head or neck may be lacking or simply exist in the form of bruises or abrasions. Neck pain, as noted in some patients with vertebral artery injuries, may be simply ascribed to bony or ligamentous injury to the spine. Therefore one must maintain a very high index of suspicion when dealing with patients with minor head and neck injury.

Mechanism of Injury

Injuries to the extracranial vertebral artery commonly occur in three places. The artery is susceptible to blunt or penetrating injury below or at its entrance into the foramen transversarium at C6. It is here that the artery, relatively free in the base of the neck, becomes fixed to the bony orifice of the foramen. This combined with the fact that the mobility of the cervical spine is greatest at the C5-6 joint makes the vertebral artery particularly vulnerable to hyperextension injuries. The vessel can be stretched at its entrance into the foramen, causing a mural hemorrhage or possibly an intimal disruption culminating ultimately in thrombosis or distal embolization. The artery is also susceptible to injuries at the atlantoaxial joint and the atlanto-occipital joint. In this region the spine has its greatest rotational mobility. Stretch injuries are liable to occur during rotation and extension because of the relative fixation of the artery at the atlanto-occipital membrane. Cadaver studies have shown that the vertebral artery can be occluded or narrowed when the head is rotated toward the opposite side.[62] This may occur even when movement is within physiological limits. Therefore it is not surprising that traumatically induced extension and rotation injures the vessel. The presence of congenital spinal abnormalities such as congenital subluxations or fusions tends to increase the mobility of the adjacent cervical spinal segments and increases the possibility of stretch injury to the vertebral artery.[58] Patients with these anomalies should be closely scrutinized for any delayed symptoms of cerebrovascular insufficiency.

Injuries to the cervical vertebral arteries most commonly result in thrombosis. However, intimal disruption, dissection, aneurysm formation, and fistula formation are also known to occur. Ischemia usually results from distal embolization but also may result from flow-restrictive lesions in dominant vertebral arteries.

Treatment

Little has been written about the management of acute vertebral artery injury because of the fact that the diagnosis is frequently delayed or is only made at the time of autopsy.

Scrutiny of the few cases that exist in the literature suggests that it is not unusual for a lucid interval to occur before episodes of vertebrobasilar ischemia. Thus a high index of suspicion and early and liberal use of angiography in suspected arterial lesions may provide for management alternatives.

As with carotid arterial injuries, treatment will depend on the location and nature of the lesion as well as any existing neurological deficit. Total occlusion of the vertebral artery may not lead to ischemic symptoms because of a patent vertebral artery on the other side. In this instance no further therapy is warranted. In those cases where vertebral thrombosis results in significant neurological symptoms, attempts at thrombus removal or thromboendarterectomy of the vertebral artery have usually been unsuccessful.[58] Supportive therapy with a trial of increased intravascular volume or mild hypertension may obviate some of the ischemic manifestations. Other injuries including traumatic narrowing, dissection, and mural hemorrhage with pseudoaneurysm formation are potential sources for distal embolization. In documented cases of embolization with mild or transient neurological deficits, anticoagulation with heparin is recommended with consideration given to repair of the vessel. If angiography documents that the injured vessel is the dominant vertebral, reconstruction or repair using suitable graft material or possibly ligation or balloon occlusion with concomitant EC-IC bypass grafting might be contemplated. In a situation where the nondominant vertebral artery is injured and is considered to be nonrepairable, a successful trial of balloon occlusion under local anesthesia may be followed by permanent occlusion. In the presence of a major cerebral infarction, revascularization or anticoagulation should only be attempted as a last resort.

In those patients in whom cervical subluxation or cervical spondylosis has caused or exacerbated vertebral arterial stenosis, decompression or fusion may be all that is necessary to avoid further trauma to the artery and obviate further ischemic episodes.[58] Follow-up angiography is strongly recommended in vertebral dissection and traumatic aneurysm formation. Evidence of increasing stenosis or enlargement of the aneurysm in those patients initially treated with conservative measures should prompt surgical intervention to avoid the potential for emboli or vertebrobasilar ischemia.

Intracranial Vascular Injuries

Disruption of intracranial vasculature is the rule rather than the exception with severe head injury. Subarachnoid hemorrhage due to loss of integrity of small pial vessels can be documented in the majority of fatal brain injuries. However, documentation of traumatic lesions to major branches of the circle of Willis or to dural venous sinuses is relatively uncommon in blunt head trauma. In a series of over 2000 head injuries from Scandinavia, injury to a major intracranial vessel as proved by angiography or at autopsy occurred in just over 3 percent of the cases.[18] A report from Canada surveyed 431 industrial head injuries; nine cases were found that demonstrated evidence of trauma-induced cerebral arterial occlusion.[6] A review of these types of injuries with discussion of presenting symptoms, mechanisms, and outcome should help to emphasize the difficulty in identifying and treating these patients.

Occlusion

The most common intracranial arterial structure to be occluded in blunt head injury is the internal carotid artery. Although the majority of injuries to the internal carotid occur in its cervical portion, injury at the base of the skull, within the carotid canal, or at its cavernous segment has been reported with some regularity.[1,3,38,67] Injuries to the carotid artery at the skull base occur usually in the setting of major head trauma. The patient is typically admitted comatose following an auto accident. Within 24 h the neurological condition deteriorates further, during which time evidence of a hemiparesis may emerge. In slightly less than one-third of intracranial carotid injuries, head trauma may be relatively mild.[1,67] In this situation the clinical syndrome mimics that of traumatically induced carotid occlusion in the neck.

Several important mechanisms are thought to be responsible for intracranial carotid thrombosis secondary to head trauma. Autopsies frequently demonstrate a fracture at the base of the skull that narrows the carotid canal. Fracture fragments may compress the vessel, causing irreversible injury and subsequent thrombosis. Pathological examination may reveal an intimal dissection, mural hematoma, aneurysm formation, or total disruption. In the absence of a fracture, stretching or torsion of the carotid artery as it exits from the carotid canal or the cavernous sinus is thought to be another cause of occlusion. Differential motion between the brain and skull during acute acceleration and deceleration can compress the arterial wall, setting in motion the thrombotic process. An equally important mechanism for intracranial thrombosis of the carotid artery involves emboli originating more proximally in the vessel secondary to an arterial injury in the neck. In a small number of cases, usually older individuals, traumatic disruption of atherosclerotic plaques may also cause distal embolization and possibly internal carotid occlusion.[5,25,36]

Radiographically, an abrupt, usually smooth obstruction or stenosis is noted near the skull base (Fig. 208-3). Frequently the occlusion will propagate to the next patent branch, namely the ophthalmic artery. Occlusion may, however, extend to the internal carotid bifurcation, resulting in cerebral infarction. Evidence of distal embolization including the absence of small branches of the middle cerebral artery or intraluminal filling defects may also be appreciated.[1,67]

Eighty-five percent of patients with traumatic internal carotid artery occlusion at the base of the skull or intracranially can be expected to die or suffer a severe neurological deficit.[1,36,67] The severity of head injury also governs the outcome. Aarabi and McQueen, reviewing reports of 21 cases, found that of 15 who suffered major brain trauma, 12 died.[1] There was only 1 death among the 6 patients who suffered minor head trauma. Management of intracranial thrombosis of the internal carotid artery remains a frustrating exercise. In those patients who have suffered a major ischemic neurological deficit, steroid administration and attempts to control the intracranial pressure may be of some

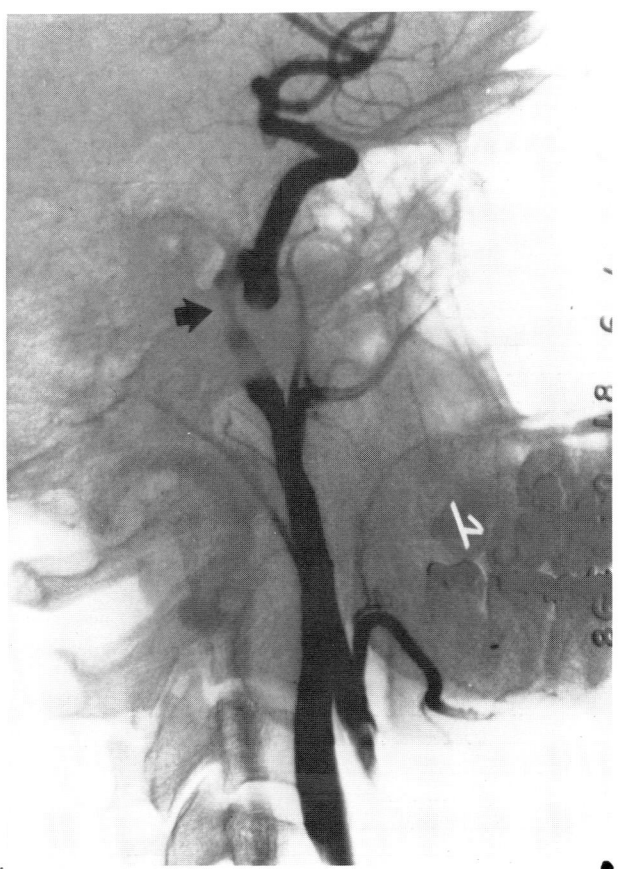

Figure 208-3 Narrowing of the internal carotid artery associated with a basilar skull fracture.

potential benefit. Barbiturate-induced coma has also been utilized in this setting with unspectacular results. Acute revascularization also seems an unlikely adjunct to the management of these cases since the diagnosis is usually delayed and cerebral infarction has already occurred. In those few instances where emboli are found to occur in the absence of a major infarction, anticoagulation may be attempted in order to obviate further neurological deficit.

Occlusion of other major intracranial vessels has also been documented subsequent to head trauma. Evidence of injury to cerebral cortical branches may be seen, especially in relation to calvarial fractures. Findings may include branch occlusion, segmental narrowing, traumatic aneurysm formation, or slow flow in the cortical surface veins. A sharp angulation of a damaged cortical branch (Z deformity) is suggestive of entrapment of the vessel within the fracture line.[53]

Dujovny et al. cataloged eight cases of traumatically induced middle cerebral artery thrombosis.[15] Five were caused by motor vehicle accidents, and the remaining three were caused by falls. Five of their patients demonstrated a lucid interval, which varied from 9 to 15 days. Either after the lucid interval or from the outset of the traumatic event, a contralateral hemiparesis or hemiplegia occurred. Four patients also demonstrated a homonymous hemianopsia. No obvious injury to the head was present on physical examination, and x-ray films of the skull revealed a linear skull fracture in only two patients. All patients had occlusion of the middle cerebral artery at its origin from the internal carotid bifurcation. One patient in their series died, and although the remainder suffered severe cerebral infarctions, four eventually became ambulatory. This report is in sharp distinction to others that suggest a 38 percent mortality rate for traumatically induced middle cerebral artery thrombosis.[25,27,34,51]

The mechanisms of middle cerebral artery thrombosis secondary to trauma are incompletely explained. The middle cerebral artery may become occluded indirectly secondary to injury to the internal carotid artery. In a report of three cases and a review of the literature, Hollin and colleagues suggested that one-third of the cases of traumatic middle cerebral artery occlusion were caused by emboli from injury to the internal carotid.[25] Alternatively, the middle cerebral artery may be compressed by extracerebral or intracerebral hematomas. A more likely mechanism for thrombosis of the middle cerebral artery is stretching due to acceleration or deceleration of the brain resulting from blunt head trauma. Others have theorized that the artery may directly impact against the sphenoid bone causing intimal dissection or a mural hematoma resulting in eventual occlusion.[34,55]

The management of traumatically induced middle cerebral occlusion remains empirical and supportive only. In the majority of those patients who survive and have follow-up angiography, the middle cerebral artery is again patent.[34]

Basilar artery occlusion has also been noted secondary to head trauma.[56,57] These patients invariably present with ischemic brain stem symptoms, and the majority of them do not survive. Basilar artery occlusion or stenosis can often be inferred from a carotid arteriogram that shows filling of the distal basilar artery through a posterior communicating artery. This observation should prompt complete examination of the vertebrobasilar circulation. Not infrequently the basilar artery may be occluded due to associated injury to one or both vertebral arteries, which then act as a source of emboli. Basilar occlusion may also be related to a fracture at the base of the skull across the clivus, which in some instances may serve to trap the artery within the fracture.[57] The majority of cases of basilar artery occlusion are documented at the time of autopsy; thus, no satisfactory treatment regimen has yet evolved.

Traumatic Aneurysms

Traumatically induced intracranial artery aneurysms are rare lesions. None of the intracranial aneurysms cataloged in the Cooperative Aneurysm Study was of traumatic origin. Parkinson and West collected five cases of traumatically induced intracranial aneurysm, adding to them six cases of traumatically induced fistula, and emphasized the fact that since angiography has been replaced by CT scanning in the evaluation of head injuries, these aneurysms are even more likely to escape attention.[44] Our own experience tends to confirm this. Since 1977, when we began to use the CT scanner in our department, the number of traumatic intracranial aneurysms documented by angiography has dropped dramatically.[24]

Our experience with traumatic intracranial aneurysms is based on over 30 cases since 1968. The majority of these were unsuspected and were found in conjunction with angiographic evaluation usually in an unconscious head trauma victim. The most common mode of presentation in symptomatic patients is that of delayed subarachnoid hemorrhage following a head injury. Typically a decrease in the level of consciousness to the point of coma heralds the subarachnoid hemorrhage. Further evaluation may reveal nuchal rigidity or complaints of a severe headache. Unless a high index of suspicion is maintained, the symptoms may be ascribed to an intracranial expanding process such as a hematoma or edema or possibly post-traumatic hydrocephalus. Other presenting symptoms include progressive deterioration following head trauma, most likely due to vasospasm following rupture of the aneurysm. Epistaxis or a delayed cranial nerve palsy following trauma may also give evidence of the presence of an internal carotid aneurysm near the skull base. Extracerebral hematomas following trivial head trauma and unexplained arterial bleeding during hematoma removal have all been reported as evidence of traumatically induced cerebral aneurysms.[2,8,21,24,44,53]

Blunt head trauma is responsible for the majority of these lesions. Up to 40 percent may be seen in the absence of a fracture on skull films.[8] Penetrating lesions including in-driven bone fragments and missiles of various genre such as radio antennas, umbrella tips, bullets, knives, and surgical instruments are responsible for a high proportion of these cases.

Theories regarding the mechanism of traumatic cerebral aneurysm formation abound. Blunt trauma can produce the vascular injury as a result of differential velocity of the brain and skull. The brain and its vessels impact against bony or connective tissue protuberances such as the falx, tentorium, or sphenoid wing. Traction injuries thought to be due to adhesions between cortical vessels and the underlying dura as described by Drake are also believed to be operative in producing traumatic tears of cortical arteries with subsequent aneurysm formation.[14] Trapping of the cortical vessel in a fracture site has also been reported as a mechanism for traumatic cerebral aneurysm formation.[53]

The majority of traumatic cerebral aneurysms are located on branches of the middle cerebral artery. The next most common site is the internal carotid artery as it enters the skull. The pericallosal artery, most likely because of its proximity to the falx, is another important site for the occurrence of traumatically induced aneurysms.

Angiographic hallmarks including delayed filling and emptying of the aneurysm, an irregular contour, the absence of a neck, and a peripheral location other than at a branching point tend to distinguish the traumatically induced aneurysm from that of the congenital atherosclerotic form.

A review of the literature shows that in those cases where no immediate surgical treatment was rendered, 40 percent of the aneurysms bled at some point after the diagnosis was made. Further, 21 percent were found to enlarge with follow-up cerebral angiography. This often occurred within 3 weeks of the trauma. A small number of aneurysms were noted to become either smaller or totally thrombosed on follow-up angiography.[2,8,21,24]

As with other types of intracranial aneurysm, management is directed toward avoiding recurrent hemorrhage. Fleischer et al. reported increased survival rates in those patients treated surgically.[21] Unfortunately, the amount of underlying brain injury may negatively affect the outcome in selected cases. Operative mortality now hovers around 16 percent. Conservative therapy in these lesions has produced a mortality of 41 percent.[24]

Arteriovenous Fistula

Arteriovenous fistulas secondary to head injury are not rare lesions. The most dramatic and therefore most well recognized is the carotid-cavernous sinus fistula. This lesion is discussed in more detail in another section of this text. The remainder of traumatic fistulas usually involve dural vessels and are found incidentally at the time of angiography.

An arteriovenous fistula fed by the middle meningeal artery can be found in 2 percent of head trauma victims.[19,20] Typically a fistulous communication develops between the meningeal artery and the accompanying veins, producing the so-called "tram track" sign (Fig. 208-4). However fistulas between the meningeal artery and diploic veins may also occur, usually in association with lacerations of the dura. These fistulas are almost always found in association with a fracture line. The fistula itself does not usually cause symptoms over and above those that result from the head injury. Thus they represent more of an arteriographic curiosity than a threat to the well-being of the patient. Spontaneous closure has been reported, but the natural history of these lesions is really unknown.

Traumatic dural AV fistulas usually do not produce symptoms. The few cases in the literature of symptomatic AV fistulas described headache, ophthalmologic complaints, and bruit developing in a delayed fashion from 30 days to 1

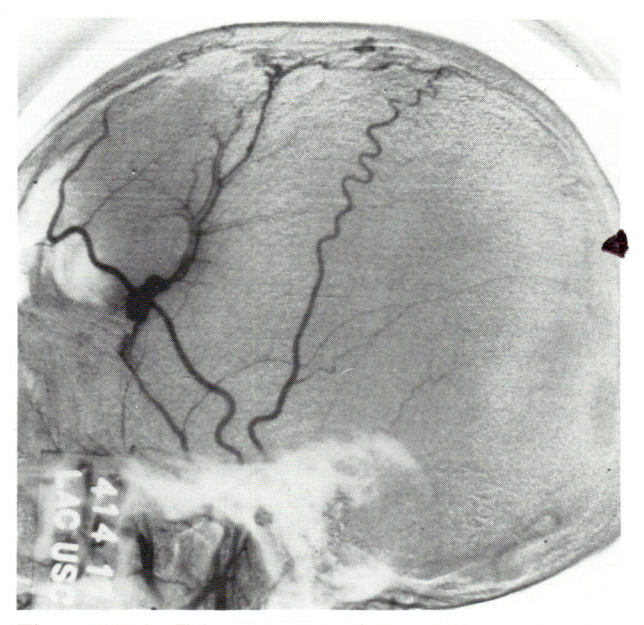

Figure 208-4 False aneurysm of the middle meningeal artery in association with an arteriovenous fistula. Note the "tram track" sign superior to the aneurysm.

year following the head injury.[12,20] In contradistinction, spontaneous dural AV fistulas have been known to present with subarachnoid hemorrhage, increased intracranial pressure, progressive neurological deficit, or hydrocephalus.[42]

An unusual case of traumatic AV fistula fed by cortical arteries was reported by Feldman et al.[19] Their case was unique in that cortical branches of the middle cerebral artery directly fed branches of the sagittal sinus. Eventually the sagittal sinus became completely arterialized and no longer served as a conduit for venous return. Treatment was eventually completed by totally excising the fistula, including most of the superior sagittal sinus.

Technology used in obliterating a carotid-cavernous fistula such as balloon occlusion or embolization is also used to obliterate fistulas in other areas. Parkinson and West reported six cases of traumatically induced AV fistula, five of which were directly approached and obliterated with contemporary surgical techniques; the sixth lesion was treated successfully by embolization with Gelfoam (absorbable gelatin sponge, The Upjohn Company, Kalamazoo, Mich.) by cannulating the left external carotid artery.

Vasospasm

Cerebral vasospasm, a common cause of ischemic symptoms following the rupture of a cerebral aneurysm, has also been implicated in the pathophysiology of head injury (Fig. 208-5). The reported incidence of angiographically demonstrable vascular narrowing following significant head trauma is between 5 and 50 percent.[65] Suwanwela and Suwanwela reviewed the angiograms of 350 patients with moderate head injuries and found narrowing of the internal carotid, middle cerebral, or anterior cerebral arteries in 5.1 percent.[61] Selecting only those cases with the most severe injuries increases the rate to 58 percent.[35]

Data from human as well as experimental cases suggest that the accumulation of blood in the subarachnoid space is in part responsible for the vascular narrowing.[17,38] McCullough et al. found a direct correlation between the magnitude of hemorrhage in the basal cisterns and the degree of narrowing on angiography.[38] Other mechanisms, such as associated brain or vascular damage, certainly contribute to this phenomenon.

Evidence linking angiographic constriction with neurological deficit is lacking. Miller and Gudeman studied the CT scans of 162 patients with severe head injury and found a 14 percent incidence of low-density lesions unassociated with hematomas or contusions.[40] Autopsy data on some of the fatal cases confirmed the suspicion that these were areas of ischemic damage. Unfortunately, because of the relative lack of angiographic data in these cases, vasospasm remains a possible but as yet unverified explanation for their findings. Until further research into this phenomenon is available, the contribution of vasospasm to cerebral ischemia following head injury will remain conjectural.

As CT scanning continues to supplant cerebral angiography as the sole method of evaluating head trauma patients, information about the exact frequency and influence on prognosis of major vascular injuries will remain scarce. Increasing vigilance on the part of the physician, with liberal use of angiography in high-risk patients or those who deteriorate inexplicably, may allow for better management alternatives.

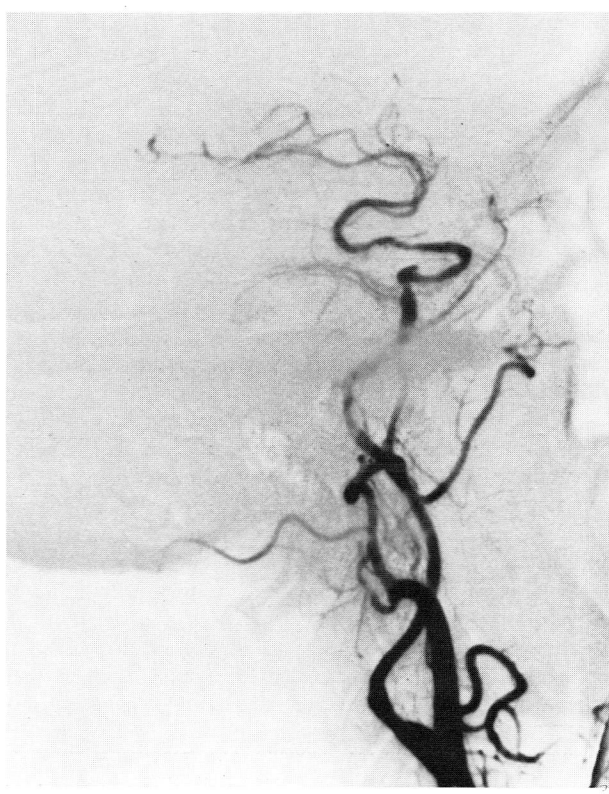

Figure 208-5 Spasm of the internal carotid artery and its branches associated with severe head injury and intracranial hemorrhage.

References

1. Aarabi B, McQueen JD: Traumatic internal carotid occlusion at the base of the skull. Surg Neurol 10:233–236, 1978.
2. Acosta C, Williams PE Jr, Clark K: Traumatic aneurysms of the cerebral vessels. J Neurosurg 36:531–536, 1972.
3. Ajir F, Tibbetts JC: Post-traumatic occlusion of the supraclinoid internal carotid artery. Neurosurgery 9:173–176, 1981.
4. Batzdorf U, Bentson JR, Machleder HI: Blunt trauma to the high cervical carotid artery. Neurosurgery 5:195–201, 1979.
5. Bergquist BJ, Boone SC, Whaley RA: Traumatic dissection of the internal carotid artery treated by ECIC anastomosis. Stroke 12:73–76, 1981.
6. Blau A, Richardson JC: Strokes and head injury. Can J Neurol Sci 5:263–266, 1978.
7. Boldrey E, Maass L, Miller E: The role of atlantoid compression in the etiology of internal carotid thrombosis. J Neurosurg 13:127–139, 1956.
8. Burton C, Velasco F, Dorman J: Traumatic aneurysm of a peripheral cerebral artery: Review and case report. J Neurosurg 28:468–474, 1968.
9. Carpenter S: Injury of neck as cause of vertebral artery thrombosis. J Neurosurg 18:849–853, 1961.
10. Caveness WF: Incidence of craniocerebral trauma in the United States in 1976 with trend from 1970 to 1975. Adv Neurol 22:1–3, 1979.
11. Countee RW, Vijayanathan T, Barrese C: Cervical carotid an-

eurysm presenting as recurrent cerebral ischemia with head turning. Stroke 10:144–147, 1979.
12. Dennery JM, Ignacio BS: Post-traumatic arteriovenous fistula between the external carotid arteries and the superior longitudinal sinus: Report of a case. Can J Surg 10:333–336, 1967.
13. Dragon R, Saranchak H, Lakin P, Strauch G: Blunt injuries to the carotid and vertebral arteries. Am J Surg 141:497–500, 1981.
14. Drake CG: Subdural hematoma from arterial rupture. J Neurosurg 18:597–601, 1961.
15. Dujovny M, Laha RK, Decastro S, Briani S: Post-traumatic middle cerebral artery thrombosis. J Trauma 19:775–779, 1979.
16. Easton JD, Sherman DG: Cervical manipulation and stroke. Stroke 8:594–597, 1977.
17. Echlin F: Spasm of basilar and vertebral arteries caused by experimental subarachnoid hemorrhage. J Neurosurg 23:1–11, 1965.
18. El Gindi S, Salama M, Tawfik E, Aboul Nasr H, El Nadi F: A review of 2,000 patients with craniocerebral injuries with regard to intracranial haematomas and other vascular complications. Acta Neurochir (Wien) 48:237–244, 1979.
19. Feldman RA, Hieshima G, Giannotta SL, Gade GF: Traumatic dural arteriovenous fistula supplied by scalp, meningeal, and cortical arteries: Case report. Neurosurgery 6:670–674, 1980.
20. Fincher EF: Arteriovenous fistula between the middle meningeal artery and the greater petrosal sinus: Case report. Ann Surg 133:886–888, 1951.
21. Fleischer AS, Patton JM, Tindall GT: Cerebral aneurysms of traumatic origin. Surg Neurol 4:233–239, 1975.
22. Fraser RAR, Zimbler SM: Hindbrain stroke in children caused by extracranial vertebral artery trauma. Stroke 6:153–159, 1975.
23. Giannotta SL, McGillicuddy JE, Kindt GW: Gradual carotid artery occlusion in the treatment of inaccessible internal carotid artery aneurysms. Neurosurgery 5:417–421, 1979.
24. Giannotta SL, Weiss MH: Pitfalls in the diagnosis of head injury. Clin Neurosurg 29:288–299, 1982.
25. Hollin SA, Sukoff MH, Silverstein A, Gross SW: Post-traumatic middle cerebral artery occlusion. J Neurosurg 25:526–535, 1966.
26. Houck WS, Jackson JR, Odom GL, Young WG: Occlusion of the internal carotid artery in the neck secondary to closed trauma to the head and neck. Ann Surg 159:219–221, 1964.
27. Jacques S, Shelden CH, Rogers DT Jr, Trippi AC: Posttraumatic bilateral middle cerebral artery occlusion: Case report. J Neurosurg 42:217–221, 1975.
28. Jernigan WR, Gardner WC: Carotid artery injuries due to closed cervical trauma. J Trauma 11:429–435, 1971.
29. Kindt G, McGillicuddy J, Giannotta S, Pritz M: The reversal of neurologic deficit in patients with acute cerebral ischemia by profound increases in intravascular volume. Acta Neurol Scand [Suppl] 72:468–469, 1979.
30. Krajewski LP, Hertzer NR: Blunt carotid artery trauma: Report of two cases and review of the literature. Ann Surg 191:341–346, 1980.
31. Ledgerwood AM, Mullins RJ, Lucas CE: Primary repair vs ligation for carotid artery injuries. Arch Surg 115:488–493, 1980.
32. Levy RL, Dugan TM, Bernat JL, Keating J: Lateral medullary syndrome after neck injury. Neurology (NY) 30:788–790, 1980.
33. Little JM, May J, Vanderfield GK, Lamond S: Traumatic thrombosis of the internal carotid artery. Lancet 2:926–930, 1969.
34. Loar CR, Chadduck WM, Nugent GR: Traumatic occlusion of the middle cerebral artery: Case report. J Neurosurg 39:753–756, 1973.

35. Macpherson P, Graham DI: Arterial spasm and slowing of the cerebral circulation in the ischaemia of head injury. J Neurol Neurosurg Psychiatry 36:1069–1072, 1973.
36. Mastaglia FL, Savas S, Kakulas BA: Intracranial thrombosis of the internal carotid artery after closed head injury. J Neurol Neurosurg Psychiatry 32:383–388, 1969.
37. McCollum CH, Wheeler WG, Noon GP, DeBakey ME: Aneurysms of the extracranial carotid artery: Twenty-one years' experience. Am J Surg 137:196–200, 1979.
38. McCullough D, Nelson KM, Ommaya AK: The acute effects of experimental head injury on the vertebrobasilar circulation: Angiographic observations. J Trauma 11:422–428, 1971.
39. Meier DE, Brink BE, Fry WJ: Vertebral artery trauma: Acute recognition and treatment. Arch Surg 116:236–239, 1981.
40. Miller JD, Gudeman SK: Cerebral vasospasm after head injury, in Wilkins RH (ed): *Cerebral Arterial Spasm: Proceedings of the Second International Workshop, Amsterdam, The Netherlands*. Baltimore, Williams & Wilkins, 1980, pp 476–479.
41. New PFJ, Momose KJ: Traumatic dissection of the internal carotid artery at the atlantoaxial level, secondary to nonpenetrating injury. Radiology 93:41–49, 1969.
42. Newton TH, Hoyt WF: Dural arteriovenous shunts in the region of the cavernous sinus. Neuroradiology 1:71–81, 1970.
43. Olafson RA, Christoferson LA: The syndrome of carotid occlusion following minor craniocerebral trauma. J Neurosurg 33:636–639, 1970.
44. Parkinson D, West M: Traumatic intracranial aneurysms. J Neurosurg 52:11–20, 1980.
45. Perry MO, Snyder WH, Thal ER: Carotid artery injuries caused by blunt trauma. Ann Surg 192:74–77, 1980.
46. Pritz MB, Giannotta SL, Kindt GW, McGillicuddy JE, Prager RL: Treatment of patients with neurological deficits associated with cerebral vasospasm by intravascular volume expansion. Neurosurgery 3:364–368, 1978.
47. Rhodes EL, Stanley JC, Hoffman GL, Cronenwett JL, Fry WJ: Aneurysms of extracranial carotid arteries. Arch Surg 111:339–343, 1976.
48. Rich NM, Spencer FC: *Vascular Trauma*. Philadelphia, Saunders, 1978.
49. Richardson JD, McElvein RB, Trinkle JK: First rib fracture: A hallmark of severe trauma. Ann Surg 181:251–254, 1975.
50. Rittenhouse EA, Radke HM, Sumner DS: Carotid artery aneurysms: Review of the literature and report of a case with rupture into the oropharynx. Arch Surg 105:786–789, 1972.
51. Roessmann U, Miller RT: Thrombosis of the middle cerebral artery associated with birth trauma. Neurology (NY) 30:889–892, 1980.
52. Rubio PA, Reul GA Jr, Beall AC Jr, Jordan GL Jr, DeBakey ME: Acute carotid artery injury: 25 years' experience. J Trauma 14:967–973, 1974.
53. Rumbaugh CL, Bergeron RT, Kurze T: Intracranial vascular damage associated with skull fractures: Radiographic aspects. Radiology 104:81–87, 1972.
54. Schneider RC, Schemm GW: Vertebral artery insufficiency in acute and chronic spinal trauma: With special reference to the syndrome of acute central cervical spinal cord injury. J Neurosurg 18:348–360, 1961.
55. Scott GE, Neuberger KT, Denst J: Dissecting aneurysms of intracranial arteries. Neurology (NY) 10:22–27, 1960.
56. Shaw C, Alvord EC Jr: Injury of the basilar artery associated with closed head trauma. J Neurol Neurosurg Psychiatry 35:247–257, 1972.
57. Sights WP Jr: Incarceration of the basilar artery in a fracture of the clivus: Case report. J Neurosurg 28:588–591, 1968.
58. Simeone FA, Goldberg HI: Thrombosis of the vertebral artery from hyperextension injury to the neck: Case report. J Neurosurg 29:540–544, 1968.
59. Stringer WL, Kelly DL Jr: Traumatic dissection of the extra-

60. Sullivan HG, Vines FS, Becker DP: Sequelae of indirect internal carotid injury. Radiology 109:91–98, 1973.
61. Suwanwela C, Suwanwela N: Intracranial arterial narrowing and spasm in acute head injury. J Neurosurg 36:314–323, 1972.
62. Toole JF, Tucker SH: Influence of head position upon cerebral circulation. Arch Neurol 2:616–623, 1960.
63. Towne JB, Neis DD, Smith JW: Thrombosis of the internal carotid artery following blunt cervical trauma. Arch Surg 104:565–568, 1972.
64. Unger SW, Tucker WS Jr, Mrdeza MA, Wellons HA Jr, Chandler JG: Carotid arterial trauma. Surgery 87:477–487, 1980.
65. Wilkins RH: Trauma-induced cerebral vasospasm, in Wilkins RH (ed): *Cerebral Arterial Spasm: Proceedings of the Second International Workshop, Amsterdam, The Netherlands.* Baltimore, Williams & Wilkins, 1980, pp 472–475.
66. Yamada S, Kindt GW, Youmans JR: Carotid artery occlusion due to nonpenetrating injury. J Trauma 7:333–342, 1967.
67. Yashon D, Johnson AB II, Jane JA: Bilateral internal carotid artery occlusion secondary to closed head injuries. J Neurol Neurosurg Psychiatry 27:547–552, 1964.

209

Sequelae of Head Injury

Byron Young

Post-Traumatic Epilepsy

Post-traumatic epilepsy is divided into two types. Early post-traumatic epilepsy is defined as one or more seizures occurring within 1 week of head injury without any other obvious causes. Late post-traumatic epilepsy refers to seizures occurring more than 1 week after head injury. Post-traumatic epilepsy is not an infrequent occurrence. An estimated 422,000 persons per year are hospitalized in the United States for head injury.[15] The incidence of early epilepsy in large head injury studies ranges from 2.5 to 7 percent.[1,14] Late seizures occurred in 7.1 percent of the patients in the retrospective study by Annegers et al. of a civilian population during the first year following head injury.[1] Five percent of Jennett's series of unselected head injuries admitted to the hospital developed late epilepsy.[14] Based on these data, between 8000 and 30,000 individuals annually in the United States have an early or late post-traumatic seizure.

Early Post-Traumatic Epilepsy

Risk and Characteristics of Early Epilepsy

The risk of early post-traumatic seizures is related to the type and severity of brain injury. Subdural and intracerebral hematomas are associated with a 30 to 36 percent incidence of early seizures.[13] Epidural hematomas, frontal and parietal depressed skull fractures, and brain injuries with focal neurological signs or post-traumatic amnesia longer than 24 h are associated with an early seizure incidence of 9 to 13 percent.[7,13,14] Combat missile wounds have an early seizure incidence of about 2 to 6 percent.[2,29] The incidence of early seizures following civilian missile wounds has not been established in any large series. Only 1 to 2 percent of patients with minor head injuries without neurological signs have an early seizure.[14]

Age also seems to be a factor determining the susceptibility to early seizures.[14] Early seizures occurred more frequently in children under 5 years of age in Jennett's series. Early seizures more often began in the first hour and by 24 h in children than in adults.

Slightly less than one-third of early seizures occur within an hour of injury, one-third occur during the next 24 h, and slightly more than one-third occur during the remaining days of the first week.[14] Rish and Caveness also reported that early post-traumatic seizures occur most frequently during the first 5 days following a combat head injury, with a peak incidence on the first day.[26]

Focal seizures account for about one-half of early seizures. The majority of focal early seizures are focal motor seizures. Focal seizures occur more frequently after missile injuries than after blunt injuries.[14]

A generalized seizure occurring within a few moments of injury is termed *immediate epilepsy* and is distinguished by most investigators from the *early seizures* that occur more than a few seconds after injury. An immediate seizure follows a mild injury, is an infrequent occurrence, and, unlike early seizures, does not predispose to subsequent seizures.[14]

Significance of Early Epilepsy

The primary significance of early epilepsy is as a predictor of an increased risk of developing late post-traumatic seizures. About 25 percent of patients with an early seizure have late seizures. This high frequency of late seizures following early seizures includes even mild injuries that would, in the absence of an early seizure, have only a slight risk for late seizures. The risk for late seizures is unaffected by the number or type of early seizures, except that early focal seizures in children do not increase the risk of late seizures.[14]

The occurrence of an early seizure complicates the management of head-injured patients. Depression of consciousness following a seizure hinders the evaluation of the patient's neurological condition. Costly CT scans may have to be repeated to rule out the possibility of a newly developed intracranial mass lesion. Occasionally secondary complications, such as aspiration pneumonitis, are caused by post-traumatic seizures. Eleven percent of all patients, and 22 percent of children under the age of 5, develop status epilepticus.[14] In a series of 116 patients who were able to talk following a head injury but who subsequently died, there were two children, only mildly injured, whose sole cause of death was poorly controlled epilepsy.[27]

Prophylaxis of Early Post-Traumatic Epilepsy

The question of whether early post-traumatic seizures can be prevented by the prophylactic administration of phenytoin has not been studied extensively. Rish and Caveness used a prophylactic regimen in Vietnam to attempt to prevent early post-traumatic seizures.[26] They showed no significant difference in the number of seizures in treated and untreated cases. The issue of post-traumatic seizure prophylaxis was not resolved in this study since the anticonvulsant regimen used in this combat situation could not have provided therapeutic blood levels during the first few days after injury. Moreover, this was not a randomized, placebo-controlled, or double-blind study. In our study, more than 78 percent of the patients had therapeutic levels of phenytoin throughout the first week.[36] We found no significant difference between the treated and untreated groups. Based on the results of these studies, we recommend that phenytoin be used only after an early seizure has occurred. Phenytoin should then be administered promptly by an intravenous route in an attempt to prevent during this acute phase the occurrence of additional seizures and secondary complications directly attributable to such seizures. Phenytoin plasma concentrations of 25 to 30 μg/ml are often necessary to control early seizures. Loading doses should be calculated to provide these high phenytoin blood levels. Intravenously administered phenobarbital should be added if phenytoin alone does not provide seizure control. The literature contains no firm guidelines regarding the duration of anticonvulsant therapy after an early seizure based on the results of well-designed studies. The rationale for continuing anticonvulsant drugs beyond the first week after injury is to prevent late post-traumatic epilepsy. Our policy is to administer phenytoin for 6 months to patients having an early seizure that is not followed by a late seizure. Every attempt is made to maintain phenytoin blood levels in the high therapeutic range of 15 to 20 μg/ml. Phenytoin is then discontinued unless an electroencephalogram shows localized spikes or spikes and waves.[9] If a late post-traumatic seizure occurs, we continue anticonvulsants for at least 1 year after the last seizure. The decision about continued therapy is then based upon the number of late seizures that have occurred and the electroencephalographic findings.

Late Post-Traumatic Epilepsy

Risk and Characteristics of Late Epilepsy

The incidence of late epilepsy depends upon the severity of the head injury. Traumatic intracranial hematomas have a very high incidence of post-traumatic seizures ranging from one-fifth of the patients with epidural hematomas to almost one-half of the patients with subdural or intracerebral hematomas.[13] The incidence after depressed skull fractures depends upon a wide range of factors and ranges from only 4 to 5 percent to over 60 percent. Other associated factors, such as focal signs, dural laceration, post-traumatic amnesia longer than 24 h, or an early seizure, greatly increase the incidence of late seizures in patients with depressed fractures. In the absence of these factors, the incidence of late epilepsy is below 10 percent.[14] About one-third of patients with combat missile wounds develop post-traumatic seizures.[8] Certain characteristics of the injury are important risk factors for subsequent seizures. The extent of focal damage, the association of focal damage and prolonged coma, and injuries adjacent to the central sulcus increase the late seizure incidence. In the Vietnam war head injury series, one-half of the patients having early seizures had late seizures. Severe head injuries are not the only injuries that have a high likelihood of late epilepsy. A patient with a mild injury, but having an early seizure, has a 25 percent chance of having late seizures. A mild injury alone, without significant loss of consciousness and no early epilepsy, is associated with only a 1 to 2 percent chance of late seizures. Jennett's series provides considerable data based on the features of the injury for the accurate calculation of the exact risk of the individual patient for late epilepsy.[14]

Caveness, Potter, and others have suggested that the individual's personal or constitutional makeup, such as genetic traits, may play an important role in his or her susceptibility to post-traumatic epilepsy.[8,21] The significance of these factors remains unestablished. Electroencephalography performed soon after head injury provides little reliable data to predict the risk of late seizures.[9] However, after a late seizure has occurred, focal EEG abnormalities suggest an increased risk of additional seizures.

The frequency of late seizures varies within a wide range. There may be only a single seizure or so many that no effort is made to keep count. According to Caveness et al., once post-traumatic epilepsy is established, there is little change in the attack frequency.[8] Caveness divided his Korean war series cases into three frequency patterns: 1 to 3 seizures, 4 to 30 seizures, and more than 30 seizures. Each of these groups comprised about one-third of the seizure patients. In his series, which was based on a 10-year follow-up, one-half of those patients having early seizures developed late seizures. There is a highly significant relationship between the frequency and duration of seizures. The greater the frequency of seizures, the greater the probability of persistence.

Mechanisms of Late Post-Traumatic Epilepsy

Surgical specimens removed to control post-traumatic epilepsy show neuronal and oligodendroglial loss, gliosis, and hemosiderosis. The epileptogenic focus is adjacent to the injury site. The hyperirritable epileptogenic focus may be caused by mechanical stress or long-standing localized ischemia.[12] Tower demonstrated that an epileptogenic focus has biochemical defects in acetylcholine, glutamic acid, and potassium metabolism.[31,32] Schmidt et al. attributed the burst of autonomous electrical activity in the epileptogenic focus to a dendritic depolarization and the difference in potential between the cell body and the dendritic network.[30] Westrum et al. proposed that the decreased synaptic endings or dendrites within the epileptogenic focus permit postsynaptic hypersensitivity.[33] Gliotic changes may also impair the glial control of acid-base balance and allow an excessive excitability of adjacent neurons.[19]

Post-traumatic epilepsy is characterized by a latency period between the time of the trauma and the appearance of the first seizure. The brain injury presumably sets into motion a series of biochemical, electrical, and structural changes that lead to the development of an epileptogenic focus.[22] The time for development of the epileptogenic focus in humans appears to be about 8 weeks. After this incubation phase, late seizures make their appearance. In Jennett's series, the seizure incidence during the first week after head injury is 30 times the incidence in any one of the seven subsequent weeks.[14]

Prophylaxis of Late Post-Traumatic Epilepsy

Many patients make an excellent recovery from head injuries but retain a significant disability because of post-traumatic seizures. Late post-traumatic epilepsy has considerably more severe medical, economic, social, and psychological consequences than early post-traumatic epilepsy. Late post-traumatic seizures greatly lessen the chance for gainful employment after rehabilitation.

A large body of experimental evidence suggests that anticonvulsant prophylaxis tends to prevent epilepsy induced by a variety of epileptogenic causes.[23,37] However, the evidence from clinical studies testing the efficacy of late post-traumatic seizure prophylaxis is conflicting. The rationale for prophylactic administration of anticonvulsant drugs is to prevent or arrest the progression of the development of the epileptogenic focus.

Hoff and Hoff randomized 100 World War II head-injured patients into two groups: one group received 200 mg of phenytoin daily, and the others were untreated controls. In the first 4 years of the study only 4 percent of those treated developed epilepsy, while 38 percent of the control group had convulsions.[11] In Birkmayer's follow-up report in 1951, 6 percent of the treated group had suffered seizures compared to 51 percent of the controls.[4]

Popek published a Czechoslovakian study in 1969.[20] The patients were given phenytoin (200 mg/day) and phenobarbital (30 mg/day) for 2 years and were followed for 5 years. The 73 adults in the study ranged in age from 16 to 32 years. None of the treated patients developed post-traumatic seizures. Twenty-one percent of the controls developed seizures. When a control patient had a seizure, he or she was switched to the treatment group. Popek reported that none of the controls developed further seizures after being switched to the treated group. In 1981 Zervit and Musil reported the long-term follow-up of Popek's study.[38] By this time, 87 percent of the patients had been followed for more than 5 years and 37 percent more than 10 years. In this study the phenytoin dosage was 160 to 240 mg/day and the phenobarbital dose was 30 to 60 mg/day. Of the treated group, 2.1 percent had had post-traumatic seizures; of the control group, 25 percent had had seizures.

The results of Popek and Zervit and Musil have been tested by a controlled prospective double-blind study.[18] Phenobarbital (60 mg/day) and phenytoin (200 mg/day) were given for 18 months. In a 3- to 6-year follow-up of 103 patients, there was no significant difference between the active drug and placebo groups. In general, the studies of Hoff and Hoff, Birkmayer, Popek, and Zervit and Musil were not randomized, double-blind, and placebo-controlled investigations, and their results have not been duplicated by well-controlled studies.

In the Vietnam war an anticonvulsant regimen was included in the routine postoperative orders.[8] Eighty-four percent of the men received anticonvulsants within 24 h of injury. Seventy-five percent of the men received phenytoin in doses of 300 to 400 mg/day. Twenty percent received phenytoin plus phenobarbital in doses of 96 mg/day, and an additional 3 percent received phenobarbital alone. No blood levels of the drugs were obtained. The study included 1030 cases. In 453 cases the medical records indicated that medication had continued through successive hospital admissions for periods ranging from 3 months to 9 years. In 524 cases the medication was interrupted at varying periods after injury, and 53 men had no anticonvulsant medication prescribed. This program demonstrated no benefit of continuous therapy over interrupted therapy, which included cases receiving no treatment.

In 1979 we suggested that phenytoin reduces the incidence of late post-traumatic seizures.[35] These conclusions were based on comparisons with other large clinical series published by 1979 rather than by randomized treated and control groups. The seizure rate of 6 percent during the first year after head injury in our series in which all patients received phenytoin is almost identical to the 7.1 percent rate reported by Annegers et al. in 1980 in an untreated cohort of severe head-injured patients. The retrospective analysis by Wohns and Wyler of 62 patients with severe head injury concluded that "prophylactically administered phenytoin is effective in reducing post-traumatic epilepsy."[34] However, this study was not randomized, placebo-controlled, or double-blinded.

Subsequently, the results of our randomized, double-blind, placebo-controlled study showed that the early initiation and continued administration of phenytoin does not lessen the occurrence of late post-traumatic epilepsy.[37] A goal of the study was to administer sufficient phenytoin to immediately achieve and then maintain the plasma phenytoin concentration between 10 and 20 μg/ml throughout the 18 months of the study. The success of this effort was assessed by frequent phenytoin assays during the first week following injury and every 2 to 3 days during the remaining period of hospitalization. Outpatient assays were planned for 1, 3, 6, 9, 12, 15, and 18 months after the injury. More frequent assays were carried out when the plasma phenytoin concentration was not within the desired range or when the patient's clinical condition required more frequent outpatient visits. Difficulties were encountered in obtaining a high rate of compliance to keep drug plasma levels in the high therapeutic range for a prolonged time. At 6 months over one-half the patients with known blood levels of phenytoin were compliant, but this represented only about one-fourth of the initial patients given phenytoin. Phenytoin plasma concentrations were determined on the next clinic visit after the occurrence of the first late seizure. No patient who had just had a seizure had a plasma concentration above 12 µg/ml. The finding that no patient with a phenytoin plasma concentration of 12 µg/ml or higher had a seizure raises the question of whether high therapeutic doses might lessen the occurrence of post-traumatic epilepsy.

These results give no support for the continued use of phenytoin to provide blood concentrations in the low therapeutic range for prophylaxis against late post-traumatic seizures. If phenytoin is used for late seizure prophylaxis, these results suggest that only doses providing high therapeutic blood levels that are proved to be consistently maintained by frequent phenytoin plasma assays can be justified. Whether this regimen would be effective remains unproved. The difficulties in obtaining a high rate of compliance to keep drug plasma levels in the high therapeutic range for a prolonged time in head-injured patients makes this a difficult goal to achieve. Post-traumatic epilepsy is a major public health problem deserving of a large cooperative trial to determine if phenytoin at higher blood levels or other currently available or newly developed drugs can prevent the occurrence of post-traumatic epilepsy. However, at this time no well-controlled study proves the efficacy of post-traumatic epilepsy prophylaxis.

Resection of the epileptogenic focus rarely is required to control post-traumatic seizures intractable to medical management. Late post-traumatic seizures tend to diminish with time, and surgery should not be done for at least 2 years after the injury. The general principles of the surgical treatment of post-traumatic epilepsy are the same as for other focal seizures, as detailed in another chapter. Rasmussen's classical report indicates that 40 percent of patients became seizure-free after surgery, 26 percent had a significant reduction in seizure frequency, and 35 percent had no or only a moderate reduction in seizure frequency.[23]

Postconcussion Syndrome

The postconcussion syndrome refers to a variety of symptoms, such as headache, dizziness, forgetfulness, anxiety, irritability, and impaired concentration, following minor head injury.[6,10,16] Characteristically, there are no, or a dearth of, neurological signs. There are widely differing opinions about the cause of the postconcussion syndrome. This etiological controversy and the dilemma for the physician faced with the treatment of an individual patient centers on whether the symptoms are a psychological consequence of a seemingly trivial head injury, are caused by structural damage associated with a minor head injury, or are caused by a combination of both factors.

Post-traumatic headaches are characterized by their variability.[6] The headaches range from mild to excruciatingly severe, steady to intermittent, throbbing to dull, burning to pressure-like, and generalized to localized. Common causative factors are change in posture, stress, fatigue, or effort. Temporary respite can usually be obtained by rest or simple analgesics. The characteristics of the headache do not seem to be related to the length of persistence of the headache after the injury. However, headaches lasting longer than 2 months are commonly accompanied by dizziness, anxiety, fatigability, and impaired concentration.

Post-traumatic dizziness is intermittent, each episode usually lasting a few minutes.[10] A change in posture commonly initiates the attack, but stress is occasionally also a precipitating factor. The severity and frequency of attacks are highly variable. The symptoms usually subside with recumbency with the eyes closed.

Brenner et al. studied 200 patients who were hospitalized for a minor head injury and who were followed for 6 months or more.[6] Sixty-nine percent of their patients complained of headache at some time after injury. Thirty-two percent of their total cases (slightly less than one-half of those with headaches) had headaches for more than 2 months. Prolonged headaches occurred more often in patients with neurotic symptoms prior to injury, occupational difficulties, pending litigation, immediate emotional reaction to the injury, and scalp laceration. Prolonged headaches occurred infrequently after very mild injury or recreational accidents.

Fifty-one percent of these patients had dizziness at some time after injury.[10] Thirty-four percent of the total group (70 percent of the patients with dizziness) had dizziness persisting after discharge from the hospital. Twenty-three percent of the total group had dizziness lasting for more than 2 months. About three-fourths of patients having dizziness had headaches. Likewise, a similar proportion of those with headaches had dizziness. Dizziness persisting longer than 2 months was associated with neurosis or nervousness prior to the injury, anxiety, fatigability, impaired memory after hospitalization, occupational difficulties, pending litigation, retrograde amnesia, postoperative amnesia, disorientation, and definite loss of consciousness. True vertigo was much less common than dizziness. Only 6 percent of the patients in this series had true vertigo at some time after injury, but vertigo tended to be more persistent than dizziness.

In the study of Rimel et al., minor head injury was defined as cranial trauma with loss of consciousness for 20 min or less and an admission Glasgow coma score of 13 or higher.[24] Three months after injury, 78 percent of their patients complained of persistent headache. A change in memory was noted by 59 percent of the patients. Fourteen percent reported difficulties with the activities of daily life. Only one-sixth of the patients had no complaints. Mild neuropsychological impairment was detected in the majority of patients tested 3 months following injury. One-third of the patients who were employed before the injury were not employed 3 months after injury.

Brenner et al. and Friedman et al. concluded that both physical and psychological factors are important in persistent post-traumatic headache and dizziness.[6,10] The symptoms lasting only a few days or weeks are often due to local scalp injury or subtle structural brain injury or dysfunction.

The management of most patients with symptoms following mild injury depends upon the duration, severity, and type of symptoms. Most patients need no treatment other than encouragement and the passage of a little time to resume work and the normal activities of daily life. When disabling symptoms persist for more than 2 or 3 months, continued encouragement by the treating neurosurgeon often must be supplemented by psychiatric evaluation and occupational rehabilitative programs. Evoked sensory potential testing, electroencephalography, computed tomography scanning of the brain, and neuropsychological testing may be helpful in separating psychiatric and structural factors contributing to persistent symptoms. Mild analgesics, medication for vertigo and dizziness, and antidepressant or antianxiety drugs may be helpful. Fortunately, the postconcussion syndrome almost always resolves with the passage of time. In some cases, cessation of symptoms occurs only after the settlement of litigation.

Intellectual Impairment

The Glasgow outcome scale is widely used to grade overall recovery and adjustment to daily life after head injury. Only a few studies have been published, however, that precisely quantify intellectual and psychological recovery after severe closed head injury. Levin et al. evaluated the neuropsychological recovery of patients with severe head injuries.[17] They classified the injury as severe when the initial Glasgow coma scale score was 8 or less. Of the 27 patients selected for their study, 10 made a good recovery, 12 were moderately disabled, and 5 were severely disabled. The study included only patients who could be tested, that is, who improved beyond a persistent vegetative state. The median follow-up exceeded a year, and minimum follow-up was 6 months. This study showed that patients attaining a good recovery level on the Glasgow outcome scale "recovered to within one standard deviation of the population mean (100) on both the verbal and performance scales of the WAIS, that is, no patient had an IQ below 85." Patients with a good recovery had median verbal IQ scores of 94 and performance scores of 100; moderately disabled patients had a median verbal IQ of 90 and a median performance IQ of 88; severely disabled patients had a median verbal IQ of 66 and a median performance IQ of 60. The verbal IQ was not statistically different between patients achieving a good outcome and those having a moderately disabled outcome, but the performance IQ was significantly lower in the latter patients.

In the study of Levin et al., impairment of long-term memory storage was defective in 10 percent of patients with a good recovery (only 1 patient of 10), in one-third of moderately disabled patients, and in all severely disabled patients. About one-third of the patients had a deficit in memory storage or retrieval. Speech deficits were confined to moderate and severely disabled patients. Writing impairment was confined to severely disabled patients.

The study of neuropsychiatric symptoms and signs by Levin et al. tested for disordered thinking, hostility-suspicion, withdrawal-retardation, and anxietal depression. Disorders in these areas were infrequent in patients with a good recovery, but behavioral disturbances were very common in moderately and severely disabled patients. Two-thirds of the patients had chronic disability. Only one-fifth returned to full-time employment. Levin et al. suggested that a characteristic pattern of neuropsychological and psychiatric deficits are responsible for the chronic disability seen after severe closed head injury. The characteristic pattern includes impairment in performance IQ, memory, and retrieval of names, and behavioral changes such as thinking disturbance and withdrawal-retardation. These sequelae were minimal in patients with a good recovery. Moderately disabled patients varied widely in neuropsychological impairments, and severely disabled patients uniformly had marked neurobehavioral disturbances.

In the study by Rimel et al. of moderate head injury, which was defined as a Glasgow coma scale score of 9 to 12 at 6 h after admission to the hospital, 93 percent of the patients had headaches and 90 percent had memory impairment at 3 months after injury.[25] Forty-two percent had multiple subjective problems. Although 38 percent were categorized as having a good recovery at 3 months, only 4 percent were asymptomatic and only 31 percent were employed. Only 69 percent of those employed before injury were at work 3 months after injury. The significant predictor of employment was not a premorbid factor, such as age, education, and socioeconomic status, but was the severity of injury. Twenty-one percent of the patients in this study were chronically unemployed, and 21 percent were unskilled laborers. Some alcohol was present in the blood of 73 percent of the patients, and 53 percent were intoxicated. Forty-two percent had had a previous head injury. Definite neuropsychological impairment was shown by the Halstead-Reitan neuropsychological test battery in these patients. The proportions of patients scoring beyond the standard cutoff scores for the normal range ranged from 34 percent to 66 percent.

The minimum time from injury to full recovery depends upon the severity of injury. In Becker's study of mild head injury, substantial recovery occurred by 11 weeks.[3] The study by Bond and Brooks of severe closed head injuries suggests that the major part of recovery occurs within 6 months.[5] Considerable individual variations in recovery rate do occur and are dependent upon age, neurological findings, and preinjury ability.[16] Rosenbaum et al. indicate that significant improvement in motor function, overall functional state, and (to a lesser extent) intellectual function can occur in some cases for as long as 3 years.[28]

Rehabilitation

Rehabilitation efforts should commence as soon as practical after head injury. The rehabilitation team should consist of a physiatrist, clinical psychologist, physical therapist, speech therapist, occupational therapist, and social worker. The neurosurgeon usually serves as a consultant but ideally should be an active participant in a rehabilitation program. Rounds and conference attendance by the neurosurgeon, even if only once a month, can improve the rehabilitation effort and provide an important educational service to other members of the rehabilitation team. A psychiatrist is also an essential consultant.

The importance of counseling the family cannot be overemphasized. Misunderstanding and outright refusal to accept the effects of the head injury on a loved one are frequent. Carefully informing the family about realistic recovery rates and probable eventual outcome enhances the relationship between the family and the injured individual and fosters confidence and respect for the personnel attempting rehabilitation.

Some programs accept for rehabilitation patients who are still unconscious, but most allow entry into their program only after a potential for retraining is established, such as verbal or performance IQ test scores of at least 80. Programs accepting comatose patients can aid the family in tracheostomy care, nasogastric tube feeding, bladder care, and coping with the emotional and economic effects of the head injury. Individuals with potential for retraining are entered into programs that are designed to permit re-employment, or at least an independent daily life. Cognitive retraining, vocational rehabilitation, and management of behavioral or family problems form the mainstay of the rehabilitation program.

The studies of Bond and Brooks show that verbal ability recovers faster than nonverbal skills, that the severity of injury is the significant determinant of outcome, that severely injured individuals reach their final level of outcome sooner than less injured persons, that older patients are left with greater disability than younger patients, and that psychosocial factors have an important influence upon recovery.[5]

References

1. Annegers JF, Grabow JD, Groover RV, Laws ER Jr, Elveback LR, Kurland LT: Seizures after head trauma: A population study. Neurology (NY) 30:683–689, 1980.
2. Ascroft PB: Traumatic epilepsy after gunshot wounds of the head. Br Med J 1:739–744, 1941.
3. Becker B: Intellectual changes after closed head injury. J Clin Psychol 31:307–309, 1975.
4. Birkmayer von W: Die Behandlung der traumatischen Epilepsie. Wien Klin Wochenschr 63:606–609, 1951.
5. Bond MR, Brooks DN: Understanding the process of recovery as a basis for the investigation of rehabilitation for the brain injured. Scan J Rehabil Med 8:127–133, 1976.
6. Brenner C, Friedman AP, Merritt HH, Denny-Brown DE: Post-traumatic headache. J Neurosurg 1:379–391, 1944.
7. Caveness WF, Liss HR: Incidence of post-traumatic epilepsy. Epilepsia 2:123–129, 1961.
8. Caveness WF, Meirowsky AM, Rish BL, Mohr JP, Kistler JP, Dillon JD, Weiss GH: The nature of posttraumatic epilepsy. J Neurosurg 50:545–553, 1979.
9. Courjon J: A longitudinal electro-clinical study of 80 cases of post-traumatic epilepsy observed from the time of the original trauma. Epilepsia 11:29–36, 1970.
10. Friedman AP, Brenner C, Denny-Brown D: Post-traumatic vertigo and dizziness. J Neurosurg 2:36–46, 1945.
11. Hoff von H, Hoff H: Fortschritte in der Behandlung der Epilepsie. Monatschr Psychiat Neurol 114:105–118, 1947.
12. Jasper HH: Physiopathological mechanisms of post-traumatic epilepsy. Epilepsia 11:73–80, 1970.
13. Jennett B: Epilepsy and acute traumatic intracranial hematoma. J Neurol Neurosurg Psychiatry 38:378–381, 1974.
14. Jennett B: *Epilepsy after Non-Missile Head Injuries*, 2d ed. Chicago, Year Book, 1975.
15. Kalsbeck WD, McLaurin RL, Harris BSH, Miller JD: The national head and spinal cord injury survey: Major findings. J Neurosurg 53:S19–S31, 1980.
16. Levin HS, Benton AL, Grossman RG: *Neurobehavioral Consequences of Closed Head Injury*. New York, Oxford University Press, 1982.
17. Levin HS, Grossman RG, Rose JE, Teasdale G: Long-term neuropsychological outcome of closed head injury. J Neurosurg 50:412–422, 1979.
18. Penry JK, White BG, Brackett CE: A controlled prospective study of the pharmacologic prophylaxis of posttraumatic epilepsy. Neurology (NY) 29:600–601, 1979 (abstr).
19. Pollen DA, Trachtenberg MC: Neuroglia: Gliosis and focal epilepsy. Science 167:1252–1253, 1970.
20. Popek K: Preventive treatment of post-traumatic epilepsy following severe brain injury. Cesk Neurol 35:169–174, 1972.
21. Potter JM: The personal factor in the maturation of epileptogenic brain scars: Review and hypothesis. J Neurol Neurosurg Psychiatry 41:265–271, 1978.
22. Rapport RL II, Ojemann GA: Prophylactically administered phenytoin: Effects on the development of chronic cobalt-induced epilepsy in the cat. Arch Neurol 32:539–548, 1975.
23. Rasmussen T: Surgical therapy of post-traumatic epilepsy, in Walker AE, Caveness WF, Critchley M (eds): *The Late Effects of Head Injury*. Springfield, Ill, Charles C Thomas, 1969, pp 277–305.
24. Rimel RW, Giordani B, Barth JT, Boll TJ, Jane JA: Disability caused by minor head injury. Neurosurgery 9:221–228, 1981.
25. Rimel RW, Giordani B, Barth JT, Jane JA: Moderate head injury: Completing the clinical spectrum of brain trauma. Neurosurgery 11:344–351, 1982.
26. Rish BL, Caveness WF: Relation of prophylactic medication to the occurrence of early seizures following craniocerebral trauma. J Neurosurg 38:155–158, 1973.
27. Rose J, Valtonen S, Jennett B: Avoidable factors contributing to death afer head injury. Br Med J 2:615–618, 1977.
28. Rosenbaum M, Lipsitz N, Abraham J, Najenson T: A description of an intensive treatment project for the rehabilitation of severely brain-injured soldiers. Scand J Rehabil Med 10:1–6, 1978.
29. Russell WR, Whitty CWN: Studies in traumatic epilepsy: I. Factors influencing the incidence of epilepsy after brain wounds. J Neurol Neurosurg Psychiatry 20:293–301, 1957.
30. Schmidt RP, Thomas LB, Ward AA Jr: The hyper-excitable neurone: Micro-electrode studies of chronic epileptic foci in monkey. J Neurophysiol 22:285–296, 1959.
31. Tower DB: *Neurochemistry of Epilepsy: Seizure Mechanisms and Their Management*. Springfield, Ill, Charles C Thomas, 1960.
32. Tower DB, Elliott KAC: Activity of acetycholine system in human epileptogenic focus. J Appl Physiol 4:669–676, 1952.
33. Westrum LE, White LE, Ward AA Jr: Morphology of the experimental epileptic focus. J Neurosurg 21:1033–1046, 1964.
34. Wohns RNW, Wyler AR: Prophylactic phenytoin in severe head injuries. J Neurosurg 51:507–509, 1979.
35. Young B, Rapp R, Brooks WH, Madauss W, Norton JA: Posttraumatic epilepsy prophylaxis. Epilepsia 20:671–681, 1979.
36. Young B, Rapp RP, Norton JA, Haack D, Tibbs PA, Bean JR: Failure of prophylactically administered phenytoin to prevent early posttraumatic seizures. J Neurosurg 58:231–235, 1983.
37. Young B, Rapp RP, Norton JA, Haack D, Tibbs PA, Bean JR: Failure of prophylactically administered phenytoin to prevent late posttraumatic seizures. J Neurosurg 58:236–241, 1983.
38. Zervit Z, Musil F: Prophylactic treatment of posttraumatic epilepsy: Results of a long-term follow-up in Czechoslovakia. Epilepsia 22:315–320, 1981.

SECTION B
Spinal Trauma

210
Experimental Spinal Cord Injury
Arthur I. Kobrine
Jerald J. Bernstein

Contemporary thinking regarding acute spinal cord injury began in 1908, with Allen's comprehensive clinicopathological description of acute spinal cord injury in humans. He documented essentially for the first time the development of a central hemorrhagic lesion in the injured segment of the spinal cord. This unique pathological response of the spinal cord to trauma has been redocumented many times through the years, and the experimental data have been appropriately amplified. Allen's next contribution to the problem of spinal cord injury was the development of a laboratory model to study the pathophysiology of experimental spinal cord injury.[2] This basic model of a reproducible and graded spinal cord injury produced by dropping known weights through a vented tube and ultimately striking the dural-covered thoracic spinal cord of a surgically prepared laboratory animal is still in use today, and in fact is still the basic model used to study this problem. By multiplying the weight in grams by the distance in centimeters, Allen characterized the different injuries by their gram-centimeter (g-cm) product. His original observations that a 450 g-cm injury caused permanent paraplegia is still accepted as reasonably accurate for larger mammals.

It is now thought, however, that more accurate and sensitive standardization of the injury is necessary. Several investigators have questioned whether dropping 40 g a distance of 10 cm will create the same injury as dropping 10 g a distance of 40 cm. It has recently been suggested that perhaps the momentum of injury is the single most important physical factor related to the severity of injury. Although the basic weight drop model is still in wide use, measurements of velocity, force, and impulse are now possible. These physical characteristics more accurately describe the injury than the previous g-cm designation.

Other models used recently have employed an inflatable cuff surrounding the spinal cord, an aneurysm clip compressing the spinal cord for a specified time, and an inflatable epidural balloon causing intermittent, progressive, or acute spinal cord compression. All of these models are attempts to approximate the clinical situation.

In the clinical setting a wide variety of injuries exist. For example, there are patients who are rendered immediately and permanently paraplegic in whom no fracture or subluxation can be demonstrated. To be sure, transient subluxation or "pinching" had to occur at the moment of injury, but not afterward. Another group of patients demonstrate a marked subluxation of the cervical spine at the time of examination. In this group there was spinal cord injury at impact plus a prolonged period of spinal cord compression and ischemia. A third group demonstrate a mild to moderate amount of subluxation with little or no neurological impairment. In these patients, the instantaneous percussion injury did not transpire, and what neurological dysfunction they do demonstrate was probably caused by compression and is potentially reversible. It will not be possible to understand the pathophysiology in these clinical situations until laboratory models are developed that closely approximate them.

Following severe experimental impact injury of the spinal cord, the animal is essentially rendered immediately paraplegic. At this time, there is an immediate abolition of the sensory evoked response (SER), a good indication of the inability of the long tracts in the spinal cord to conduct an action potential across the injured spinal cord segment. However, there is essentially no change in both the light and electron microscopic examination of the injured segment at this time (3 min after impact). As time after impact progresses to several hours, one can appreciate the development of a central hemorrhagic lesion, with electron microscopic confirmation of tears in the basement membrane and endothelial lining of capillaries and small venules. The progressive development of the central hemorrhagic lesion has been cited by several investigators as being the pathological substrate of the observed neural dysfunction. However, there is an inverse temporal relationship between the development of the central hemorrhagic lesion and the clinical course of the animal. Animals injured with a severe impact injury are rendered immediately paraplegic, at a time when there are essentially no pathological changes. In animals that receive an incomplete lesion, the neurological dysfunction is worse immediately after impact, and they improve with time. In this latter group of animals, the pathological central lesion progresses as the clinical course improves.

Perhaps part of the confusion lies in the apparently limited fashion in which the spinal cord responds pathologically to various insults. The blood supply to the spinal cord arrives via two posterior spinal arteries and one anterior spinal artery, which lie in the subarachnoid space along the length of the spinal cord. The central area of the spinal cord is supplied by an end artery, the anterior sulcal artery, thereby making the central area more vulnerable to vascular occlusion. The dorsal, lateral, and ventral white matter of the spinal cord, the areas surrounding the central area, are supplied by an anastomotic pial network that receives blood from both posterior spinal arteries as well as the anterior spinal artery. Generally speaking, the spinal cord pathologically responds to insults, either mechanical or vascular, in much the same way, namely the development of a central hemorrhagic infarction. It is entirely possible, however, that a direct correlation between pathological anatomy and pathophysiology is not possible, and that the unique biomechanical aspects of the spinal cord (i.e., a central region of cells, relatively loose neuropil, and rich capillary supply, surrounded by longitudinally situated bundles of myelinated axons with a relatively sparse vascular supply) makes the central region vulnerable to injury, whether vascular or mechanical, but not in a cause-and-effect relationship.

Concomitant with, or soon after, the development of the central hemorrhagic infarction, there is an apparent breakdown of the pentilaminar tight junctions of the capillary endothelium (blood-cord barrier) in the surrounding white matter, with an extravasation of protein-rich fluid into the extracellular space of the neural parenchyma. However, the exact cause of this edema formation and its possible relationship to the post-traumatic neural dysfunction is still poorly understood. We do not know if this edema is an epiphenomenon (i.e., caused by the physical trauma, either by direct rupture of the small vessels or damage to the blood cord barrier, and concurrent with, but not related to, the neural dysfunction) or, in fact, central to the development of the neural dysfunction. Agents that are known to combat cerebral edema, such as dexamethasone, have been shown to have a beneficial effect when used to treat experimental spinal cord injury. However, Lewin et al. do not believe that this effect is due to dexamethasone's antiedema properties.[24] With the evolution of edema, the internal milieu of the spinal cord parenchyma changes, and the extracellular space is filled with a high-protein fluid derived from plasma. It is thought by some that the electrical properties of protein molecules can interfere with the normal depolarization-repolarization cycle necessary for the normal functioning of nervous tissue. If, in fact, this can be demonstrated, then vigorous treatment of the edema may prove valuable.

In 1972, Osterholm reported a series of experiments concerning the potential role of catecholamines in the pathophysiology of spinal cord injury. He measured norepinephrine levels of the injured spinal cord segment after experimental impact injury and reported a marked increase in measured levels of norepinephrine. Next, he injected norepinephrine directly into the parenchyma of the spinal cords of animals and noted the evolution of a central hemorrhagic lesion, apparently indistinguishable from the central lesion caused by trauma, as well as the development of paraplegia in the injected, uninjured animals. Lastly, he pretreated a group of animals with α-methyltyrosine, a norepinephrine blocker, and after impact injury reported that the treated animals neither were paraplegic nor developed the usual central hemorrhagic lesion. These experiments led Osterholm to suggest a unified theory concerning the pathophysiological response to spinal cord injury.[26] He suggested that the impact injury was responsible for the release of norepinephrine from injured neurons in the central gray matter of the impacted spinal cord segment. He thought that the norepinephrine then caused a marked vasoconstriction in the central cord area, leading to the development of the central hemorrhagic lesion. He further reasoned that the norepinephrine diffused into the lateral white matter, causing a progressive spreading ischemia in the white matter of the injured segment as well as for some distance caudal and rostral to the injury site. He suggested that the catecholamine-mediated ischemia in the white matter was, therefore, the pathological substrate of the observed neurological dysfunction (i.e., the paraplegia that occurs after experimental impact injury).

Since Osterholm's original work, workers in at least five separate laboratories have attempted to reproduce these observations, with negative results.[11,15,18,25,28] No other investigator has been able to demonstrate an increased norepinephrine level in the injured spinal cord segment at the impact site.

In 1980, Osterholm's group repeated his previous experiments with refined laboratory methods and biochemical assays.[1] They demonstrated a net depression in local tissue norepinephrine after injury, with essentially no change in dopamine levels. They explained the contradiction between these new results and the previous findings on the basis of apparent artifact in the initial study presumably caused by the nonselective nature of the biochemical assay used in the first study. They suggested that the conflicting data from other laboratories are possibly explainable on the basis of different magnitudes of injury, forms of injury, and sample size.

Experimental data concerning spinal cord blood flow (SCBF) changes after injury have been generally less helpful in understanding the pathophysiology of the neural dysfunction than one might think. We measured local blood flow in the lateral white matter of monkeys injured severely enough with the weight drop method to cause permanent paraplegia, and demonstrated consistently increased flow values, a hyperperfusion.[20] Bingham et al. repeated the above experimental conditions using the [^{14}C]antipyrine technique, rather than our hydrogen clearance technique, and also demonstrated a significant hyperemia in the lateral white matter of the injured spinal cord segment.[10] Several other investigators have demonstrated a hyperemia after injury when the systemic arterial pressure was maintained at preinjury levels, suggesting that the injury abolishes autoregulation and that the blood flow then becomes blood pressure–dependent.[30] Tator has consistently demonstrated an ischemia in the lateral white matter following experimental injury. However, his laboratory model of injury is not concussive (weight drop) but compressive, either by inflatable cuffs or aneurysm clips. This injury is ischemic by definition.[29]

D'Angelo et al. performed a series of experiments that suggest that the development of the central hemorrhagic lesion has little relation to the observed neurological dysfunction.[14] In their study, they removed the central gray matter area of the thoracic spinal cord in normal cats using a microsurgical technique. Postoperatively, these cats ran, jumped, and hopped in a normal fashion. This is not surprising since it is well known that the central gray matter in the thoracic area has no effect on movement of either the forelimbs or hind limbs. The long tracts in the lateral white matter carry impulses for leg movement, and integrity of these tracts is necessary to preserve function. Following stabilization of these animals, they were returned to the experimental laboratory and the previously operated spinal cord segment was exposed and injured, using the weight drop technique. Postoperatively, all of the animals were paraplegic. Upon postmortem examination, none of the animals demonstrated a central hemorrhagic lesion. This suggested to D'Angelo et al. that the evolution of the central hemorrhagic lesion following injury may, in effect, be an epiphenomenon and not significant in the development of the observed neurological dysfunction.

Recently Rawe et al. demonstrated that the extent of the central hemorrhagic lesion is in large part related to systemic arterial pressure following injury.[27] They were able to demonstrate a marked reduction in the development of the central hemorrhagic lesion if the animals were pretreated with phenoxybenzamine, which lowered their postinjury blood pressure. These data partially confirm the work of Smith et al., who demonstrated a loss of autoregulation with experimental impact trauma.[30] Under these conditions, therefore, blood flow in the spinal cord would be blood pressure–dependent. If vessels in the central cord were injured by trauma, leakage through them would be dependent upon blood pressure. However, these animals remain paraplegic in spite of the relative absence of the central hemorrhagic lesion.

One can now understand the difficulty in assessing the proper role of blood flow changes in the observed neurological dysfunction that follows spinal cord injury. The relative role of ischemia, if it exists, and its relationship to the direct effects of physical injury on neural structures in the overall pathophysiology of experimental spinal cord injury are poorly understood.

It has been theorized that the impact injury results in a biomolecular injury to the axonal membrane, interfering with the membrane's selective permeability to various cations, thereby changing the resting membrane potential and, hence, making the membrane relatively nonexcitable and nonconductive.[19] Figure 210-1 is a diagrammatic representation of the factors responsible for the resting membrane potential. If there were no restriction to sodium conductance through the membrane, and complete restriction to potassium, then the resting potential (RP) would equal E_{Na} (+58 mV). Conversely, if the resting membrane were completely impermeable to sodium but freely permeable to potassium, the RP would equal the E_K (−75 mV). As can be seen, the normal RP does approximate the E_K. The difference between the RP and E_K is accounted for by the small "leak" of sodium through the membrane that is normally occurring at rest. Thus, because of the membrane's restrictiveness to sodium at rest, the resting membrane potential is almost exclusively dependent on the relative intra- and extracellular concentrations of potassium only, which are maintained by the Na-K–dependent ATPase system (sodium pump).

However, if the impact were to disrupt the membrane's biomolecular structure such that the membrane lost its ability to be impermeable to sodium at rest, the resulting RP would more approximate the E_{Na}, and under such conditions, the membrane would become relatively nonexcitable.[3] Clinically, one observes this phenomenon as paraplegia. Re-establishment of the preinjury molecular configuration of the membrane might occur following a less severe injury, accounting for the return of function in experimental traumatic transient paraplegia.

We performed a series of experiments to test Tarlov's hypothesis that most neurological dysfunction secondary to trauma results from mechanical injury to neural tissue rather than from ischemia.[21-23] In our experiments, neural integrity of the long tracts of the spinal cord was monitored with spinal evoked responses, and local spinal cord blood flow was simultaneously measured using the hydrogen clearance

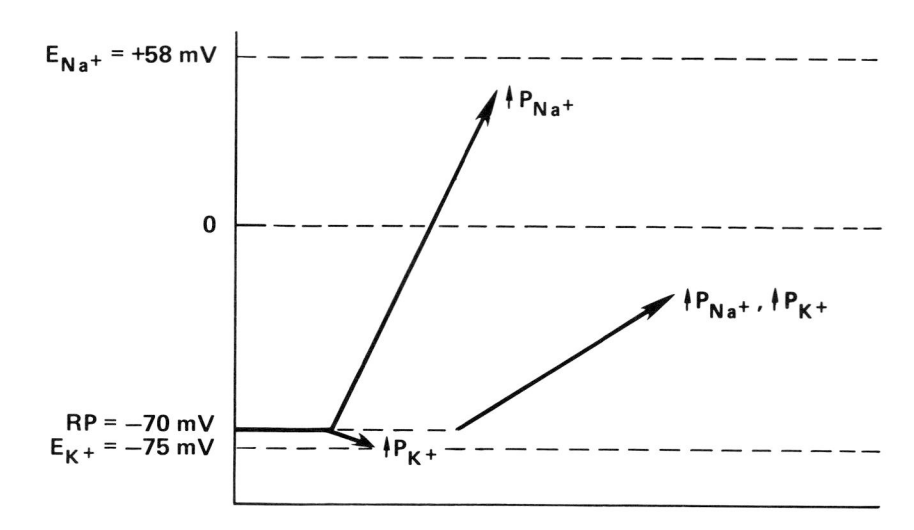

Figure 210-1 Diagrammatic representation of factors responsible for the resting membrane potential. See text for explanation.

Experimental Spinal Cord Injury

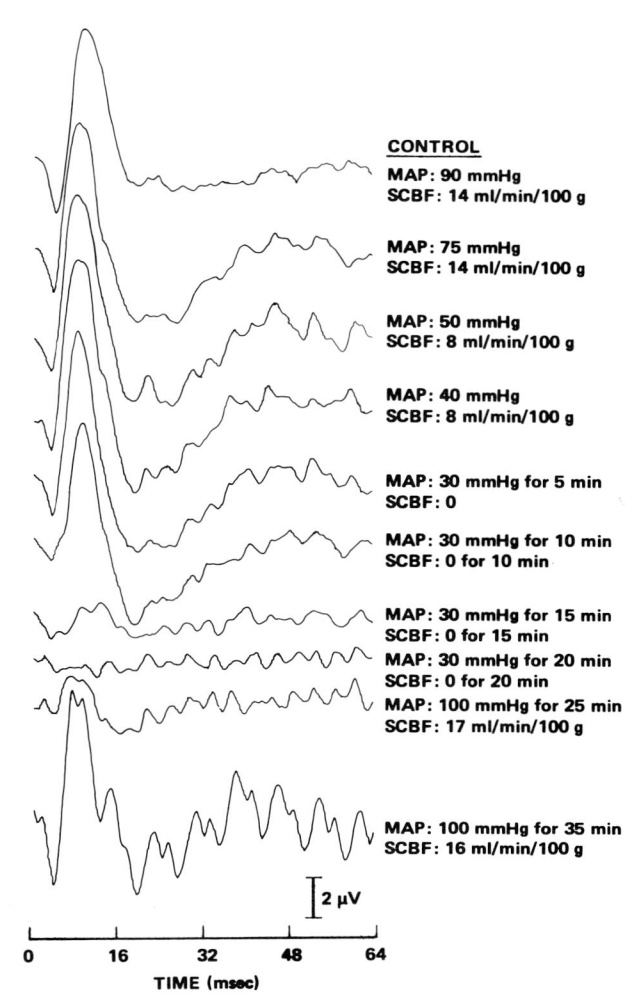

Figure 210-2 A series of SEPs from one animal from a progressive ischemia experiment. Note the loss of the SEP only after 20 min of absolute ischemia and the return of the SEP after reinstitution of the blood flow. MAP, mean arterial pressure; SCBF, spinal cord blood flow.

method (Figs. 210-2 to 210-4). This series of experiments demonstrated the following:

1. There was a relative insensitivity of long tract neural conduction (LTNC) to the effects of ischemia, with disappearance of the spinal evoked response (SER) only after 10 min or more of profound ischemia, essentially no change in the SER at spinal cord blood flow levels of approximately 25 percent normal (75 percent reduction), and complete return of the SER after a 5-min period of electrical silence (15 min of profound ischemia) upon reestablishment of the blood flow.
2. In the slow compression series the SER disappeared either concomitant with or several minutes after the development of essentially absolute ischemia. After a 5-min period of electrical silence, the balloon was deflated, and the SER returned in all animals within 1 h.[3] Acute balloon compression of the thoracic spinal cord for 15, 7, 5, 3, and 1 min caused immediate disappearance of the SER and complete focal ischemia of the compressed segment in all animals. Only the animals in the 1-min group demonstrated return of the SER.

It was thought that these results paralleled those of Tarlov.[32] In his experiments, blood flow was not measured; therefore, he could not document the degree of ischemia during compression. However, he demonstrated irreversibility of the injury in acute compression lasting longer than 1

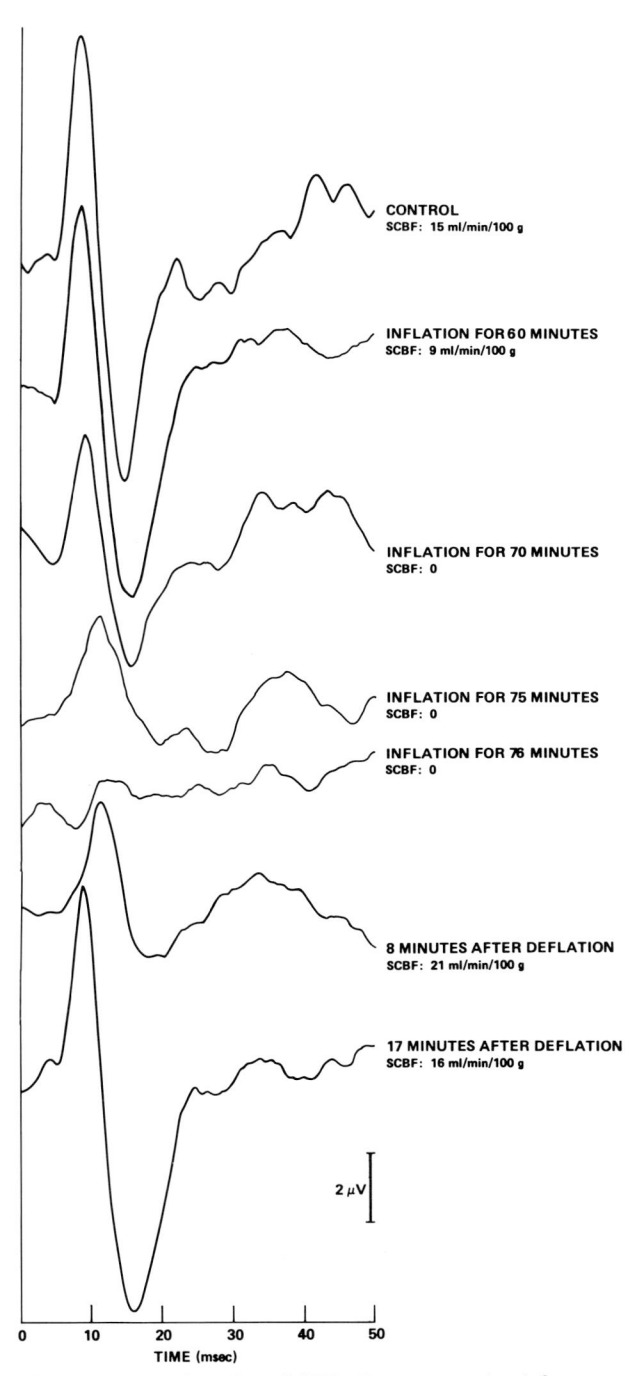

Figure 210-3 A series of SEPs from one animal from a slow compression experiment. Note that the blood flow falls to zero before the SEP disappears.

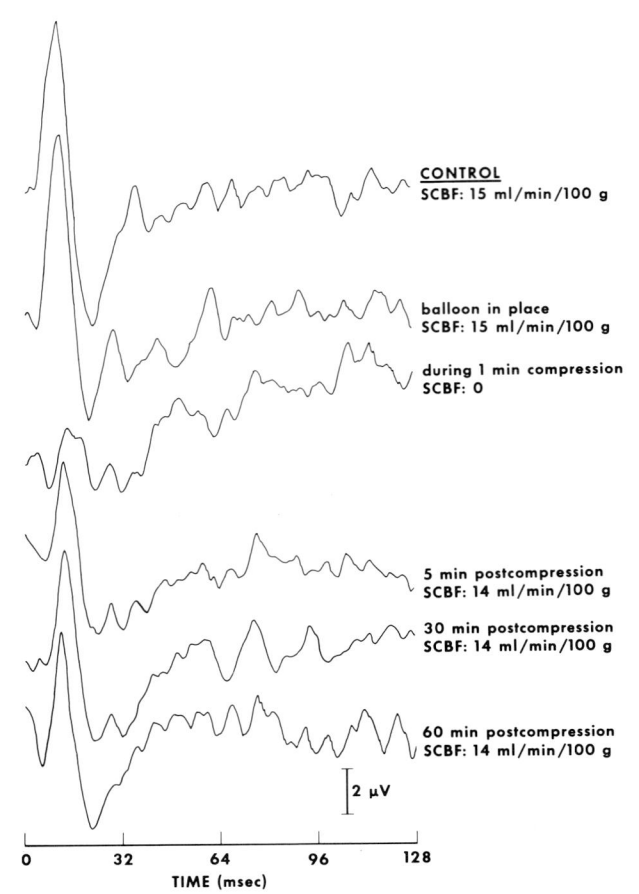

Figure 210-4 A series of SEPs from one animal from an acute compression experiment. Note the return of the SEP after 1 min of compression.

min and reversibility in slow compression when the SER was absent for up to 35 min. Tarlov concluded that mechanical deformation rather than ischemia accounted for the differences in observations between the two groups.

It has been suggested that two or more processes are at work, an immediate concussive injury that transiently "paralyzes" the neural membrane and should be reversible, and a subsequent progressive biochemical or metabolic injury, not yet understood, that is responsible for the long-term permanent neurological dysfunction. Hope that, in fact, two processes exist and that the second process is potentially reversible with treatment is the appropriate stimulus for continued research.

Demopoulous et al. have suggested a theory of pathophysiology based on free radical alteration of the membrane.[16] Their theory suggests that both regional ischemia and acute spinal cord injury are associated with distinct free radical pathology that affects the predominant membrane lipids in the traumatized zones. In their model of injury, the polyunsaturated fatty acids are selectively lost from the membrane phospholipids while saturated ones are not, because the unsaturated lipids are very susceptible to free radical damage. They suggest that the morphological damage seen after spinal cord injury could be the result of lipid peroxides, which are products of lipid free radical reactions,

inhibiting the synthesis of PGI_2, resulting in the initiation of an intravascular coagulation process.

Recently, enthusiasm has mounted concerning the use of opiate antagonists in the treatment of spinal cord injury. Flamm et al. reported an experiment in which naloxone-treated cats regained the ability to walk after a weight drop type of injury that caused permanent paraplegia in 9 of 10 control animals.[17] The possible mechanisms for this seemingly beneficial treatment are not understood at this time, and further experimental work as well as clinical studies are necessary. As the pathophysiology of the process is better understood and the anatomical substrate defined (e.g., membrane injury, metabolic insult, blood flow changes, etc.), perhaps a therapeutic regime could be developed to modify or reverse the concomitant neurological deficit.

Recent evidence has shown that there are regenerative responses after injury of the mammalian spinal cord.[4-9,12,13] These responses result in the growth of axonal sprouts as collateral branches of injured central nervous system axons or axonal sprouts of intact neurons in the area of lesions or degenerations (Fig. 210-5). The mechanism of inducing axonal sprouts has been partial denervation by a lesion in a given area of the brain or spinal cord.[4,13] In addition, sparing a dorsal root after rhizotomy rostrally and caudally and peripheral axotomy have been utilized. Axonal sprouting in the spinal cord results in the renewal of synapses in the central nervous system. This renewal is in the form of new axons, presynaptic terminals, and postsynaptic structures. Because of the limited regenerative capacity that has formerly been associated with injury of the spinal cord and brain, it is surprising to find such a response.

The actual regeneration or regrowth of axons from the tip of the severed axon is so limited that recent research in the area has not focused on this problem. However, oscillating synaptic renewal has been demonstrated in the mammalian

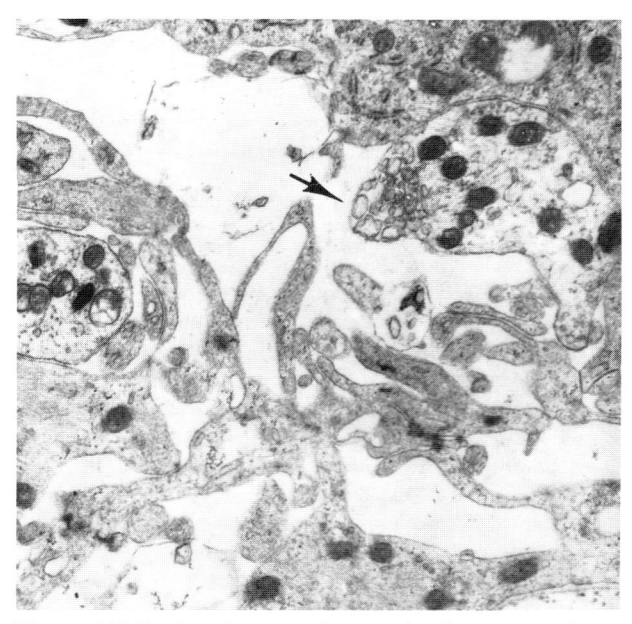

Figure 210-5 An electron micrograph of a regenerating axon in the hemisected spinal cord of the rat. A growth cone (*arrow*) is observed at the tip of the axon.

spinal cord. Following hemisection of the spinal cord, there is a cyclical renewal of synapses on neurons in layers IV, VII, and IX of the spinal cord.[4,6] This not only results in fluctuation of absolute numbers, but alteration in frequency of the types of terminals (based on morphology) in the synaptic complex. The numbers of terminals on spinal neurons rostral to the site of a spinal cord hemisection (T1-2) decreased at 10 to 20 days, increased at 30 days, and decreased at 45 and 60 days. From 60 to 90 days, the alteration in number of presynaptic terminals varied with the position of the postsynaptic neurons in the spinal cord. This phenomenon is interesting since axotomy of peripheral axons results in deafferentation of the central soma and dendrite of that neuron and axotomy of a peripheral nerve will result in a new synaptic pattern on the nerve cell body of origin.

Not only does the synaptic profile of the neuron soma change after axotomy of a peripheral nerve, but axotomy of the sciatic nerve results in cyclic degeneration and regeneration of dendrites over a 90-day period.[31] The dendrites in the rat spinal cord will degenerate and regenerate as much as 0.8 mm in a dendritic field. This appears to represent a mechanism for the formation of a new postsynaptic membrane. There is not only presynaptic, but postsynaptic renewal as well as subtle membrane shifts.

The consequences of spinal injury also affect the synaptology of the brain since a T13 dorsal column lesion results in an alteration of the absolute number of terminals in the relay nuclei up to and including the cortex. There is oscillating renewal in the number of terminals on nucleus gracilis neurons, the thalamus (ventralis pars lateralis), and the cortex. In essence, spinal cord injury results in alteration in brain synaptic morphology.[7]

If central nervous system axonal sprouts or regenerates could be induced to grow across the site of a lesion or contusion, would they form physiologically active synapses? When the cortical or deep cerebellar afferents to the red nucleus are lesioned, the remaining afferents to the affected neurons sprout. These sprouts are anatomically and physiologically demonstrable. Physiologically, the postsynaptic potential after intracellular recording from red nucleus neurons shifts in rise time and amplitude, demonstrating that the remaining afferents have shifted in position. The shift in position is to the membrane of red nucleus neurons which normally did not receive afferents from the cortex or deep cerebellar nuclei, but did so only after partial deafferentation of a given neuron. These data show that the new synapses are physiologically efficacious.

A new experimental approach to the problem of nonreplacement of central nervous system neurons is fetal grafting. In this process, fetal brain is placed in the brain of an adult mammal. This represents an attempt to make a viable substitute for nonfunctioning areas of brain, such as the substantia nigra in a patient with Parkinson's disease. There is an animal model that shows that rat fetal nigral implants are viable for long periods of time (10 months) in the rat caudate nucleus and result in suppression of motor deficits in substantia nigraectomized rats. In addition, spinal cord implants of early fetal spinal cord into adult rat spinal cord have had initial success. The neurons of the fetal implants distribute throughout the host spinal cord.[6]

These morphological regenerative responses have an underlying biochemical substrate. Although neurons do not divide in adult mammals, the structure as well as all components of the neurons are in a state of anabolic-catabolic balance. This results in the renewal of the structural and metabolic elements of the entire nervous system over time. Since the average half-life of a central nervous system protein is 15 days (with a wide range), there must be a turnover of the cellular membrane, organelles, and synaptic components. Neuronal presynaptic terminals receive their components for molecular renewal by transport in the axon (axoplasmic flow) and dendrite. The cytoskeleton of the axon is composed of, among other substances, tubulin, neurofilament triplet protein, and actin. These molecules are transported to the presynaptic terminal as neurotubules and neurofilaments. The tubules and filaments that constitute the axonal cytoskeleton are assembled at the rate of 1 to 4 mm/day in the soma and appear to be rate-limiting for the regeneration of peripheral nerves. Since this results in neurotubules and neurofilament anabolism with no catabolic process, it was postulated that production was balanced by the transport of a calcium-dependent protease enzyme that would disassemble the protein structure of the neurotubules and neurofilaments. Interestingly, an enzyme with these characteristics is found in axons. Alteration of the activity of the enzyme by local calcium concentration at the terminal could act as a growth-modulating process during development, growth, and regeneration. Mechanisms of modulation such as this model could be the method of catabolism of substances transported to the tip of axons (sprouts, regenerates, normals) by axoplasmic flow.

The mediation of synaptic renewal after trauma or as a natural process in the adult mammalian central nervous system must be initiated (or released) intracellularly, guided by intercellular recognition, and terminated with cellular adhesion. Factors that could produce this effect could originate from degeneration products, reactive neuroglia, adjacent axons, and/or the postsynaptic neuron.[6] These factors have been classified as trophic, tropic, antitropic, or antitrophic influences. A number of substances have been isolated that could enhance axon regeneration in the periphery, enhance central axonal sprouting, and produce directional growth of neurites in culture. These substances are often small diffusible peptides and appear to be released by degenerating nervous tissue, reactive neuroglia, and/or the pre- or postsynaptic complexes and neuron. Nerve growth factor has been shown to enhance the metabolism of cholaminergic neurons and results in neurite growth of the neuron. After initiation of the growth, the nerve fiber must be guided by internal and external cues to its site of termination. Many factors have been postulated, and most have some validity. The axon could be guided mechanically, by neurotropism, by chemical affinity, or by various combinations of these factors. The surface properties of the substrate along which the nerve fibers regenerate are critical and can form channels, or the substrate can have recognition molecules to which the membrane of the growing process orients. There are neurochemical and mechanical interactions between the growing neuronal process and the surface that it contacts (either neuronal or neuroglial). This interaction has been implicated as one of the factors responsible for the direction of growth. Glycoproteins have been shown to be active in the direction of growth as well as in cell adhesion and synapse formation during development. In adult mammals, glycoproteins are membrane surface components, but they are a minor component of the synaptic junction. During synaptic renewal, because of partial denervation of the hippocampus, the glycoproteins of the membrane surface are altered, suggesting an interlocking molecular recognition process.

These data show a relationship between the molecular structure (internal and external) and the neurochemical processes that result in the formation of organelles related to growth, guidance of the regenerating axon, and synapse formation in the regenerating central nervous system. These responses indicate that regeneration after injury to the human nervous system (such as paraplegia) should be possible and is amenable to further research in this area.

References

1. Alderman JL, Osterholm JL, D'Amore BR, Williams HD: Catecholamine alterations attending spinal cord injury: A re-analysis. Neurosurgery 6:412–417, 1980.
2. Allen AR: Surgery of experimental lesions of the spinal cord equivalent to crush injury of fracture dislocation of the spinal column: A preliminary report. JAMA 57:878–880, 1911.
3. Baker PF: The nerve axon. Sci Am 214(3):74–82, 1966.
4. Bernstein JJ, Bernstein ME: Neuronal alteration and reinnervation following axonal regeneration and sprouting in the mammalian spinal cord. Brain Behav Evol 8:135–161, 1973.
5. Bernstein JJ, Bernstein ME, Wells MR: Spinal cord regeneration and axonal sprouting in mammals, in Waxman SG (ed): *Physiology and Pathobiology of Axons*. New York, Raven Press, 1978, pp 407–420.
6. Bernstein JJ, Ganchrow D, Wells MR: Neurochemistry of synaptic renewal, in Flohr H, Precht W (eds): *Lesion-Induced Neuronal Plasticity in Sensorimotor Systems*. New York, Springer-Verlag, 1981, pp 75–86.
7. Bernstein JJ, Ganchrow D, Wells MR: Spinal cord injury results in alteration of brain microcircuitry, in Giuffrida-Stella AM, Haber B, Hashim G, Perez-Polo JR (eds): *Nervous System Regeneration*. New York, Alan L. Liss, 1983 (in press).
8. Bernstein JJ, Wells MR: Puromycin induction of transient regeneration in mammalian spinal cord, in McConnell PS, Boer GJ, Romijn HJ, van de Poll NE, Corner MA (eds): *Adaptive Capabilities of the Nervous System*. Amsterdam, Elsevier, North-Holland Biomedical Press, 1980, pp 21–38.
9. Bernstein JJ, Wells MR, Bernstein ME: Spinal cord regeneration: Synaptic renewal and neurochemistry, in Cotman CW (ed): *Neuronal Plasticity*. New York, Raven Press, 1978, pp 49–71.
10. Bingham WG, Goldman H, Friedman SJ, Murphy S, Yashon D, Hunt WE. Blood flow in normal and injured monkey spinal cord. J Neurosurg 43:162–171, 1975.
11. Bingham WG, Ruffolo R, Friedman SJ: Catecholamine levels in the injured spinal cord of monkeys. J Neurosurg 42:174–178, 1975.
12. Cotman CW: *Neuronal Plasticity*. New York, Raven Press, 1978.
13. Cotman CW, Nieto-Sampedro M, Harris EW: Synapse replacement in the nervous system of adult vertebrates. Physiol Rev 61:684–784, 1981.
14. D'Angelo CM, VanGilder JC, Taub A: Evoked cortical potentials in experimental spinal cord trauma. J Neurosurg 38:332–336, 1973.
15. de la Torre JC, Johnson CM, Harris LH, Kajihara K, Mullan S: Monoamine changes in experimental head and spinal cord trauma: Failure to confirm previous observations. Surg Neurol 2:5–11, 1974.
16. Demopoulous HB, Flamm ES, Pietronigro DD, Seligman ML: The free radical pathology and the microcirculation in the major central nervous system disorders. Acta Physiol Scand [Suppl] 492:91–119, 1980.
17. Flamm ES, Young W, Demopoulous HB, DeCrescito V, Tomasula JJ: Experimental spinal cord injury: Treatment with naloxone. Neurosurgery 10:227–231, 1982.
18. Hedeman LS, Shellenberger MK, Gordon JH: Studies in experimental spinal cord trauma. Part I: Alterations in catecholamine levels. J Neurosurg 40:37–43, 1974.
19. Kobrine AI: The neuronal theory of experimental traumatic spinal cord dysfunction. Surg Neurol 3:261–265, 1975.
20. Kobrine AI, Doyle TF, Martins AN: Local spinal cord blood flow in experimental traumatic myelopathy. J Neurosurg 42:144–150, 1974.
21. Kobrine AI, Evans DE, Rizzoli H: Correlation of spinal cord blood flow and function in experimental compression. Surg Neurol 10:54–59, 1978.
22. Kobrine AI, Evans DE, Rizzoli HV: The effect of ischemia on long-tract neural conduction in the spinal cord. J Neurosurg 50:639–644, 1979.
23. Kobrine AI, Evans DE, Rizzoli HV: Experimental acute balloon compression of the spinal cord. J Neurosurg 51:841–845, 1979.
24. Lewin MG, Hansebout RR, Pappius HM: Chemical characteristics of traumatic spinal cord edema in cats: Effect of steroids on potassium depletion. J Neurosurg 40:65–76, 1974.
25. Naftchi NE, Demeny M, DeCrescito V, Tomasula JJ, Flamm ES, Campbell JB: Biogenic amine concentrations in traumatized spinal cords of cats. J Neurosurg 40:52–57, 1974.
26. Osterholm JL: The pathophysiological response to spinal cord injury. J Neurosurg 40:3–34, 1974.
27. Rawe SE, D'Angelo CM, Collins WF Jr: The pressor response in experimental spinal cord trauma. Surg Forum 25:432–433, 1974.
28. Rawe SE, Roth RH, Boadle-Biber M, Collins WF: Norepinephrine levels in experimental spinal cord trauma: Part 1: Biochemical study of hemorrhagic necrosis. J Neurosurg 46:342–349, 1977.
29. Sandler AN, Tator CH: Review of the effect of spinal cord trauma on the vessels and blood flow in the spinal cord. J Neurosurg 45:638–646, 1976.
30. Smith AJK, McCreery DB, Bloedel JR, Chou S: Hypermia vasoparalysis and loss of autoregulation in the white matter following spinal cord injury. Presented at the Supplementary Session of the 26th Annual Meeting of the Congress of Neurological Surgeons, Point Clear, Alabama, October 31, 1976.
31. Standler NA and Bernstein JJ: Degeneration and regeneration of motoneuron dendrites after ventral root crush. Exp Neurol 75:600–615, 1982.
32. Tarlov IM: *Spinal Cord Compression: Mechanism of Paralysis and Treatment*. Springfield, Ill, Charles C Thomas, 1957.

211

High Cervical Spine Injuries

Richard C. Schneider

Traumatic lesions of the atlanto-occipital region and the upper cervical vertebrae with damage to the underlying cervicomedullary junction and high cervical spinal cord may cause unusual problems in diagnosis and treatment. However, with the development of improved plain x-ray views, computed tomography with and without metrizamide myelography, and perhaps cautious cineradiography in selected cases, the clinicians in the past decade have improved their diagnostic acumen, and more effective therapy for such lesions has evolved. Although many of the patients with such injuries succumb immediately, a surprising number survive with proper treatment. The reason is that there is proportionately more space for the spinal cord within its upper cervical spinal canal than in its lower one, so that a traumatic blow may avulse the laminar arches resulting in a decompression of the spinal cord in that region.

A review of the normal anatomical relationships enables one to better understand the mechanisms of injury and the factors involved in trauma to this area (Fig. 211-1). Anteriorly the anterior atlanto-occipital membrane joins with the anterior longitudinal ligament binding the clivus or basilar part of the occipital bone to the anterior ring of C1 and the odontoid and C2 vertebral body. The dens or odontoid process is held in close approximation to the anterior atlantal arch of the atlas by the alar ligaments, the transverse ligament, the cruciform membrane, and the tectorial membrane. The apical dental ligament that connects the clivus with the dens is rather weak and in most instances simply provides a small vessel to the bone. Although most of these ligaments are firm, they also permit considerable movement. To either side are the superior and inferior articular facets, and lateral to them are the foramina, which are traversed by the spinal nerves. In the cervical region the transverse processes are unusual for they have foramina transversaria, through which the vertebral arteries pass; these vessels then extend over the C1 laminae and enter the foramen magnum. The interspinous ligaments, the ligamentum flavum, and the capsular ligaments together with the anterior and posterior longitudinal ligaments help to stabilize the spine in this region.

Traumatic Atlanto-Occipital Dislocation

Atlanto-occipital dislocation is rather a rare injury, or at least one with which the patient frequently does not survive long enough to reach the hospital. Pang and Wilberger found only 13 documented reports of such cases in the world literature, with only 6 of these patients reported as surviving after admission to the hospital.[8] In 1966 when Gabrielsen and Maxwell reported their patient who had recovered (Fig. 211-2), they could find only two such patients in the literature with this lesion who had not succumbed; one of them was a child.[3]

Following trauma to the head the patient usually has a bout of unconsciousness, followed by disorientation with complete memory loss for the event and inability to verbalize, or acute respiratory arrest with death. Frequently there are abrasions on the chin, cheeks, or forehead, suggesting that there has been a hyperextension injury that permitted tearing of the strong ligaments, namely the transverse ligament, the tectorial and cruciform membranes, and the alar ligaments. If the abrasions are unilateral, it has been suggested that this indicates lateral flexion of the spine to the contralateral side.[8] The atlas itself is sustained in a central position by the anterior and posterior occipito-atlantal membranes and the anterior and posterior longitudinal ligaments. As a result, a blow to the chin with cervical hyperextension will result in slippage of the occiput backward on C1 when the ligaments rupture. The damage to the respiratory center in the medulla and a failure of the diaphragms to function as a result of cord and nerve damage most frequently result in cardiorespiratory cessation. The compression of the vertebral arteries laterally between the condyles and the laminae of C1 may also result in hypoxia and may cause brain stem infarction or hypoxia.

With roentgenographic diagnosis it is important to emphasize that the atlanto-occipital dislocation may not be visualized readily on some of the plain lateral cervical spine x-ray films and may be readily missed. It is frequently necessary to resort to tomography of this region to check on the relationship of the dens to the occipital condyles and possible abnormal separation between the condyles and superior articular facets. A suggestion has been made that with this lesion there is a lengthening of the normal distance (10 mm) between the basion of the skull and the tip of the dens, but this is not sufficiently accurate. A fluoroscopic check on the diaphragm should be made for paralysis of that structure. I have not had the opportunity to examine a patient with such a lesion with computed tomography. Although the use of vertebral arteriography has been reported, my experience with this procedure in high cervical cord injuries has included a respiratory arrest in one of these patients. I have therefore discontinued this practice.

The treatment of such cases is an emergency, for the patient's respirations may be impaired seriously. Blood gases should be drawn immediately. If there is any respiratory difficulty, intubation may be extremely difficult and dangerous. Gabrielsen and Maxwell noted in their case that with only a slight amount of traction the patient's cardiorespiratory function became compromised.[3] Therefore emergency

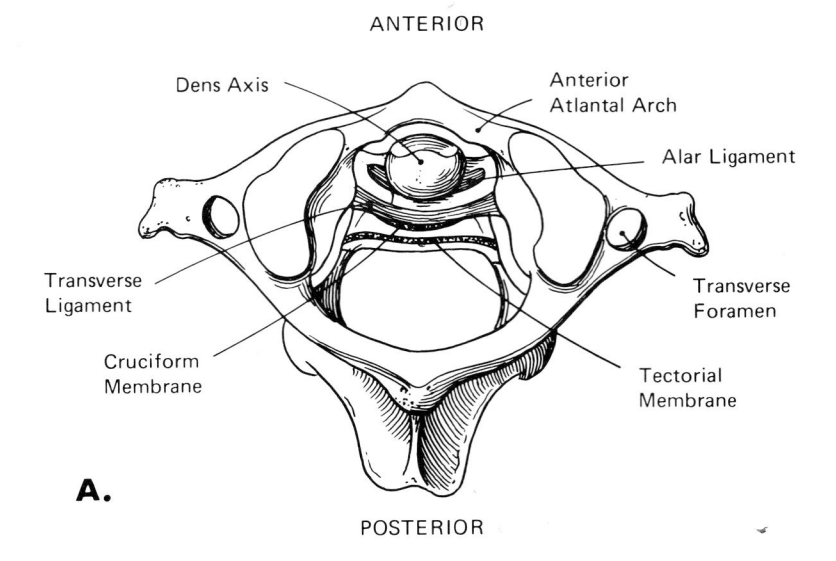

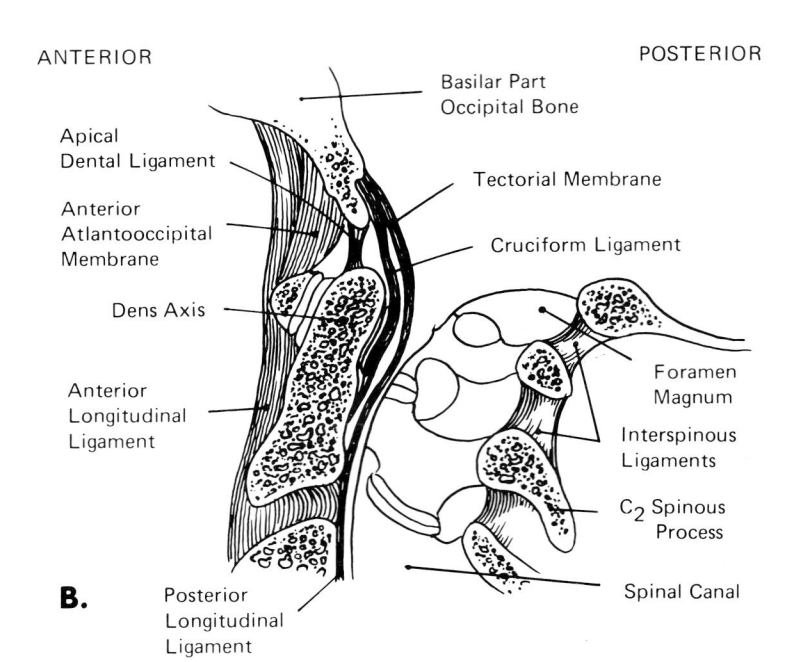

Figure 211-1 The normal anatomical relationships in the atlanto-occipital region. *A.* Superior view. *B.* Sagittal view.

tracheotomy with the least manipulation to the neck is often the procedure of choice. On several occasions the apparent head injury may call attention to the intracranial problem, causing the cervicomedullary junction lesion to be overlooked. After a suitable period of cardiorespiratory stabilization with immobilization on a frame in halo traction the patient's condition may become stabilized. After this point is reached, a posterior occipitoatlantoaxial fusion with the continued use of the halo traction and a body cast should be maintained, and this apparatus worn for a period of at least 12 weeks. Occasional checks should be made to ensure that the patient is maintained in proper alignment.

Jefferson's Fracture

In 1920 Jefferson published four cases of fracture of the atlas, which were initially regarded as rare fractures—no doubt because of the lack of suspicion that such a lesion existed and the major problems that occurred in detecting such a fracture prior to autopsy. Jefferson pinpointed bilateral fractures of the posterior arch of the atlas from a direct vertical blow to the head causing a "squeeze" of the atlas. This is the pattern most frequently recorded as the classical fracture, which bears his name (Fig. 211-3*A*). However,

High Cervical Spine Injuries

lateral mass, or fractures of the anterior and/or posterior arches and the vertebral body.[6] By far the most common lesions are the bilateral posterior arch fractures.

Jefferson described the mechanism as the head pressing firmly downward on the spinal column and the atlas being squeezed between the occipital condyles above and the axis below. As a result of the oblique position of the articular facets, the wedge-shaped lateral masses are displaced outward (Fig. 211-3B). The grooves for the vertebral artery are the sites where the arches of the atlas are weakest, and fractures occur at this site so that bursting fragments are displaced outward. With the widening of the spinal canal the cervicomedullary junction may remain unharmed, and the patient survives in some cases. Blows to the back of the head may also cause a classical posterior atlantal arch fracture or bony damage such as an odontoid fracture. With extreme flexion of the head and neck there may be associated and/or separate anterior arch fractures.

The symptoms and signs of nuchal rigidity and limitation of motion are present; the patient supports the forehead in the hands when looking downward, and on looking upward the patient supports the head with the hands posteriorly. Palpation in the pharynx may detect a protuberance, which is painful on pressure, in cases of fracture of the anterior arch. Dysphagia and thick speech occasionally may be associated with rotatory dislocation. Cervicomedullary and spinal cord injury are absent in 50 percent of the cases of atlantal fracture. The treatment is immobilization in halo traction for 12 weeks and then support with a cervical brace for 4 to

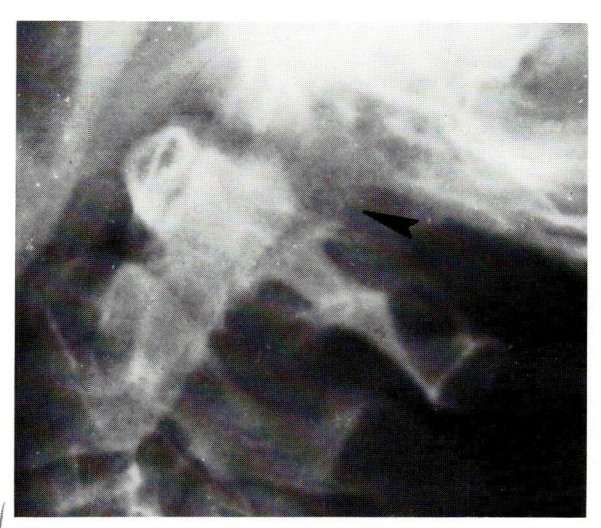

Figure 211-2 The complete atlanto-occipital separation (*arrowhead*) is readily noted on this lateral view from plain films of the cervical spine. (From Gabrielsen and Maxwell.[3])

during the next 4-year interval Jefferson searched the literature for all types of fractures of the atlas, finding 20 cases of isolated atlas fractures and 45 cases of fractures of the atlas complicated by fracture of the odontoid, compression of the

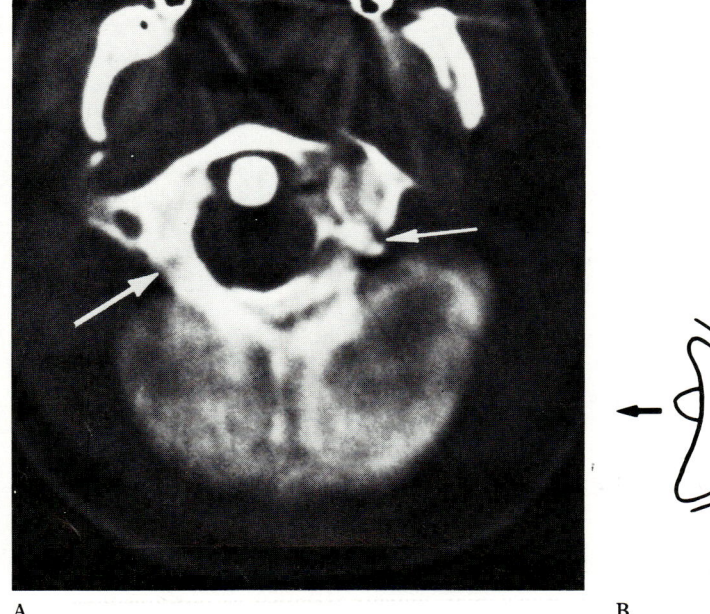

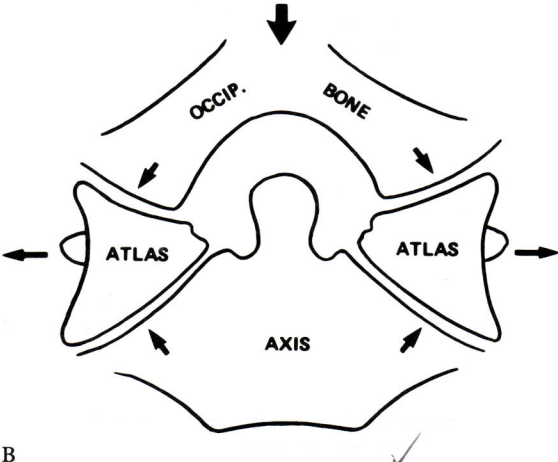

Figure 211-3 Jefferson fracture. *A.* This CT scan shows not only an asymmetrical Jefferson fracture with bilateral posterior arch fractures (*arrows*) but also extensive damage to the right articular facet. *B.* The mechanism of development of the Jefferson fracture of the atlas. The top arrow indicates the downward thrust of the occipital bone, transmitting its force through the occipital condyles against the arches of the atlas, driving them outward with a "bursting" effect.

Transaxial Cervicomedullary Injury

Almost 60 years have elapsed since Jefferson observed that "the vast majority of cervical injuries are produced by forces applied to the head and not directly to the neck."[6] To some extent his observations have remained unheeded. Thus far the bony changes that occur with a direct blow to the head and secondary damage to the atlas have been described. However there may be a deadly direct blow to the vertex *without* fracture of the skull or the cervical spine. After impact there is a rebounding of the brain with a direct transmission of force through the neural axis from the cerebral hemispheres into the brain stem and cervical spinal cord caudally to the level of the C2 segment, the site of the first dentate ligament attachment at the C2 level. This results in immediate cardiorespiratory paralysis and death due to petechial hemorrhages in the upper spinal cord (C2). The dynamic forces involved were witnessed in moving pictures of such a fatal football accident with subsequent postmortem support for this mechanism of injury (Fig. 211-4).[9] Gosch et al. provided experimental proof by simulated studies in the monkey on the impact track with the development of a similar lesion at the C2 level of the animal's spinal cord.[4]

Atlantoaxial Dislocation

Lesions of this type may fall primarily into three categories. They may be associated with (1) fractures of the odontoid process, (2) congenital deformities of the bones and ligaments, particularly the os odontoideum, and (3) tears of the supporting or restraining ligaments without any fracture but with disruption of the customary anatomical relationships.

Fractures of the Odontoid Process

It was stated in 1978 that there were over 500 cases of odontoid fracture reported in the literature; many more must have occurred in the interim.[11] The mechanisms of such injury may be acute blows to the face, the side or back of the head, or perhaps the traumatic traction use of the forceps at birth. The injuries in children appear to present a different problem than those in adult patients. It has been estimated by Sherk that fractures of the dens compose 75 percent of the cervical spine injuries in children, as contrasted with 10 percent to 15 percent in adults.[11] He has indicated that the skeletal attachment of the atlas and odontoid is only the cartilaginous plate between the ossification centers of the dens and axis. When these fractures of the dens occur through this region, it is between these two structures. After traction is applied by halo, the proper position is achieved, and maintenance is provided by a plaster jacket for 3 to 4 months, there is usually good healing in these youngsters.

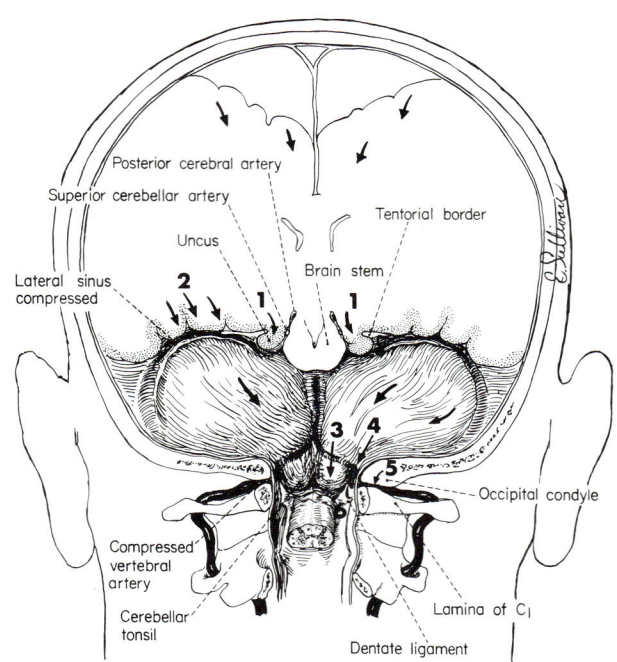

Figure 211-4 The dynamic mechanisms involved in the transaxial vertex impact injuries of Gosch et al.[4] The head strikes an object and the brain rebounds. It results in: (1) an acute tentorial pressure cone with uncal herniation with compression of the posterior cerebral artery, and possibly the superior cerebellar artery and brain stem; (2) obliteration of the subarachnoid space, bridging veins and lateral sinuses, blocking venous return and causing acute cerebral swelling; (3) an acute cerebellar pressure cone with compression of the medullary centers; (4) compression of the vertebral artery in the foramen magnum; and (5) occlusion of the vertebral arteries between the occipital condyles and C1 laminae. In addition, (6) the gradient of forces between the thrust of the freely moving cerebral hemispheres and the fixation of the cervical spinal cord by the first set of dentate ligaments results in central petechial hemorrhages at C2. This pathological lesion was first identified in a football player who sustained a vertex impact and had direct transmission of the force to the C2 level of the cord. It was confirmed by Gosch experimentally (From Schneider RC, Gosch HH, Norrell H, Jerva M, Combs LW, Smith RA: Vascular insufficiency and differential distortion of brain and cord caused by cervicomedullary football injuries. J Neurosurg 33:363–375, 1970.)

Fractures through the tip of the odontoid usually occur from disruption of the apical, transverse, and alar ligaments, and these heal satisfactorily in most instances with simple immobilization in a plaster jacket or halo for 3 or 4 months.

In contrast, when the fracture occurs at the base of the dens at the site of its union to the vertebral body in adults, there is disruption of the blood supply and often nonunion at this site. The impairment of the vascular supply to the dens is surprisingly complex.[5] The vertebral arteries provide an anterior and posterior ascending artery. This appears to arise at the level of C3 and passes both ventral and dorsal to

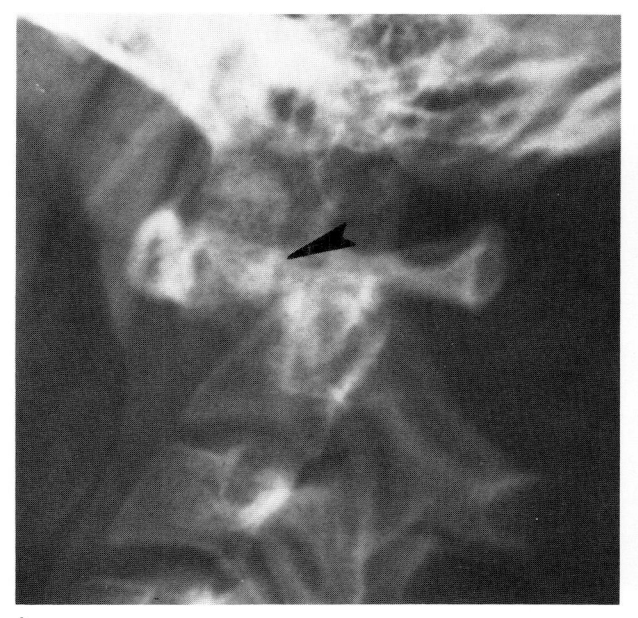

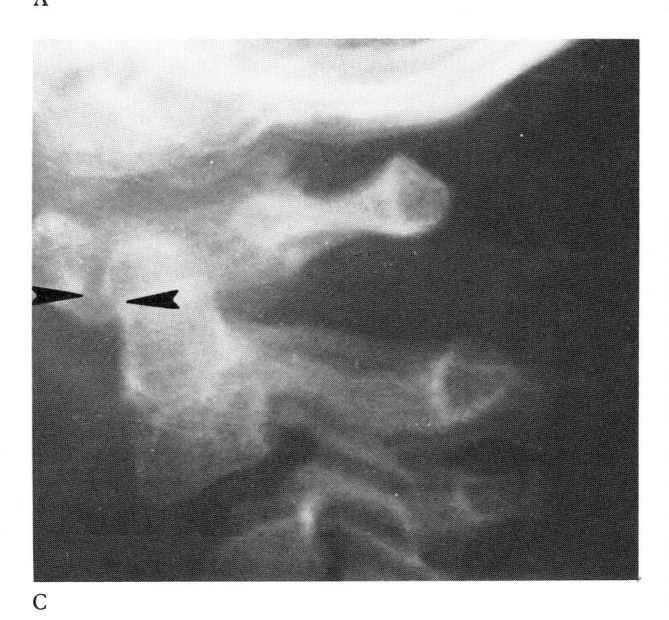

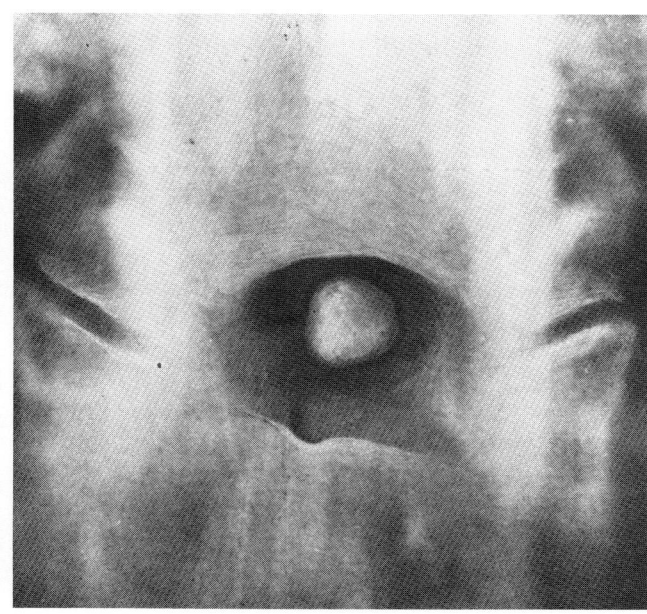

Figure 211-5 Atlantoaxial dislocations. *A*. Lateral view of the cervical spine demonstrating an anterior atlantoaxial dislocation secondary to a fracture of the odontoid (*arrowhead*) extending through the C2 vertebral body. *B*. A laminagram of an "open-mouth" view of the odontoid process revealed a completely separate apical ossicle, an os odontoideum, which in this case appeared to be posteriorly dislocated. (From Kline.[7]) *C*. The lateral cervical roentgenogram demonstrates the distance between the anterior ring of the first cervical vertebra and the odontoid process (*arrowheads*). Together with the widened distance between the C1 and C2 spinous processes it suggests tearing of the check ligaments at the atlantoaxial joint. (From Schneider RC: *Head and Neck Injuries in Football.* Baltimore, Williams & Wilkins, 1973.)

the body of the axis and the odontoid so that it forms an apical arcade of arteries in the region of the alar ligaments. From these vessels, branches enter the body of the axis and dens. Hensinger et al. have pointed out that lateral to the apex of the dens there are also ascending anterior arteries and an apical arcade of vessels that receive branches from the carotid arteries by way of the base of the skull and the alar ligaments.[5] They indicate that because of disruption of the blood supply and the fact that the dens is surrounded completely by synovial joint cavities, bony revascularization after fracture cannot readily occur from the branches of the vertebral artery at the C1 level. Fixation in such cases has been achieved by a bone graft with wiring of the C1 and C2 laminae in proper position posteriorly.

Finally, the third type of fracture to the base of the odontoid and into the C2 vertebral body is one that should heal with mere immobilization in a brace or possibly a cast for 3 or 4 months (Fig. 211-5*A*).

Congenital Anomalies of the Odontoid

Such anomalies are relatively rare. There are primarily three types of odontoid anomalies: complete absence, or aplasia; a partial failure of development, or hypoplasia, of the dens; and the os odontoideum, the most common maldevelopment of the three. Usually attention is called to these anomalies when some traumatic incident occurs. Hensinger et al.,[5] as

Os Odontoideum

This lesion occurs as a primitive articulation between the odontoid and the axis, leaving a large gap between the free ossicle and the axis (Fig. 211-5B).[2] This ossicle is rounded and oval and about half the size of the dens, and it is fixed solidly to the anterior ring of the atlas, moving in all directions with all motion. There is usually considerable instability, and Fielding has shown that cineradiography is invaluable in evaluating the pathological mechanisms in such lesions.

The patient with os odontoideum never suspects the dangerous existence in which he or she lives. Dr. Kline's patient (Fig. 211-5B) was a college student who barely touched her forehead to the roof on entering a car.[7] She became tetraplegic, apnoeic, and cyanotic. His quick clinical analysis of the condition of the patient with diaphragmatic breathing resulted in the application of traction and almost immediate recovery of function—thus saving her life. Stabilization by the wiring of the C1-2 laminae with insertion of a bone graft posteriorly is the procedure of choice.

Traumatic Tears of the Check Ligaments

Tears of the transverse and alar ligaments, as well as avulsion of the tectorial and cruciform membranes with severe hyperextension or forced flexion cervical injuries results more frequently in anterior atlantoaxial dislocations and less often in posterior ones. Occasionally this will occur in a patient who is at a fixed position in a motor vehicle which is struck from behind. The patients have soreness and neck

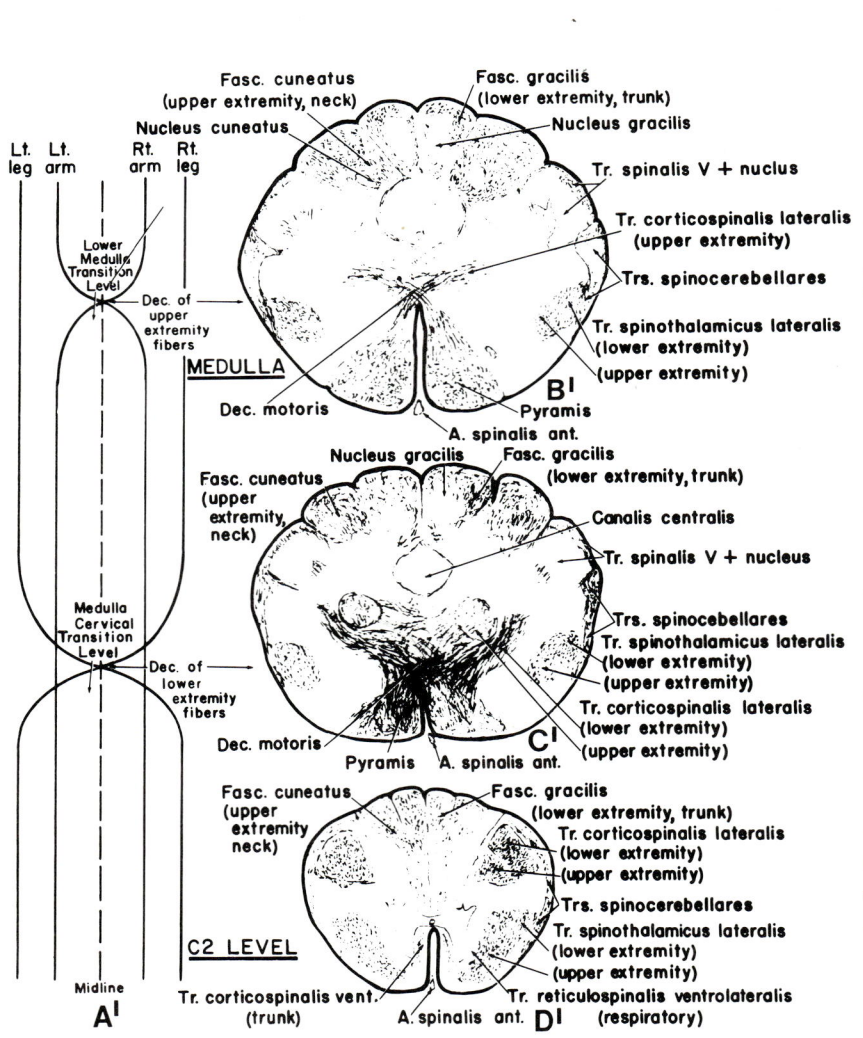

Figure 211-6 The neuroanatomical pathways concerned with brachial cruciate paralysis in cervicomedullary injuries. *A'*. This linear diagram depicts the relative positions of the components of the pyramidal tracts and their sites of decussation. The cross-sectional diagrams, *B'* to *D'*, show the relationships better. *B'*. At the medullary level the upper extremity fibers of the lateral corticospinal tracts are beginning to cross to the contralateral side. *C'*. At the level between the medulla and the C2 level of the cord, the upper extremity fibers decussate higher in the cervical cord and assume a more medial position in the lateral corticospinal tracts than fibers from the lower extremity. *D'*. More caudally, at the C2 level of the spinal cord, the decussation of the pyramidal tracts is completed: they have assumed their position in the posterolateral columns with the upper extremity fibers medially and the lower extremity fibers laterally. Note the relatively few uncrossed fibers of the ventral corticospinal tracts. With atlantoaxial dislocation the displaced odontoid may press medially under the medulla against the upper extremity decussation, causing motor weakness, while not impinging upon the uncrossed lower extremity fibers. This weakness in both upper extremities with good strength in the lower ones was designated by Bell[1] as brachial cruciate paralysis, thus mimicking the acute central cord injury syndrome.[8,11] (From Schneider RC: *Head and Neck Injuries in Football.* Baltimore, Williams & Wilkins, 1973.)

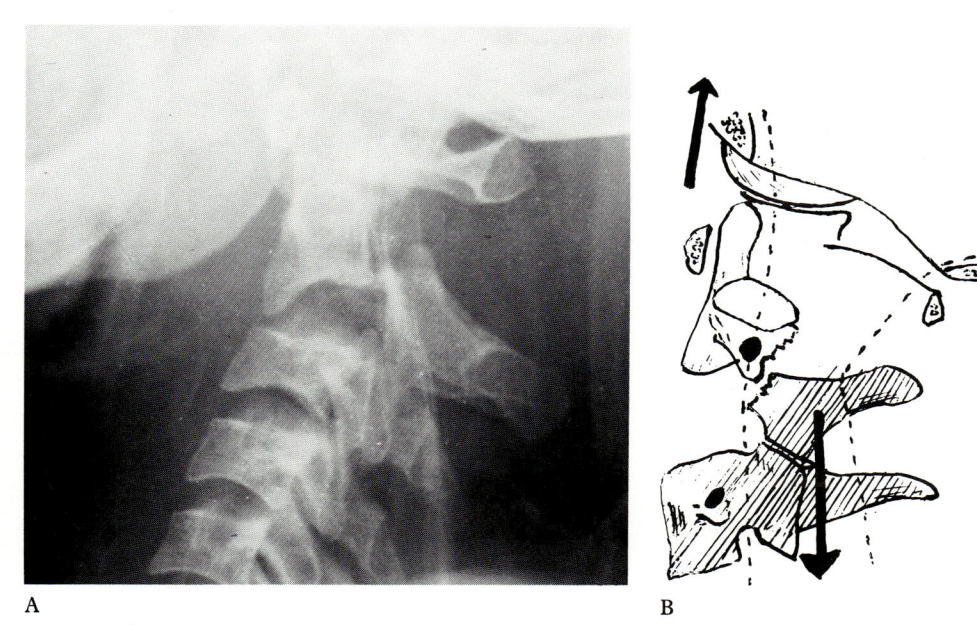

Figure 211-7 Hangman's fracture. *A*. The lateral radiographic view of the typical hangman's fracture. *B*. With a hangman's fracture there is an avulsion of the laminar arches of C2 and dislocation of the C2 vertebral body on C3. After fracture occurs, the forces will exert traction on the medulla and cord and compress the free space. (From Schneider et al.[10])

stiffness for a brief interval and then start to have pain in their shoulders. "Open-mouth" roentgenograms reveal an intact odontoid, but cautious lateral views in extension and flexion demonstrate the anterior ring of the atlas dislocating forward (Fig. 211-5C) or rarely a backward movement of the atlas posteriorly. These dislocations due to tears of the soft tissue ligaments will never heal spontaneously. Posterior fusion by bone graft and C1-2 laminal wiring is essential.

An important neurological discovery by Bell was his description of his "brachial cruciate paralysis syndrome."[1] With atlantoaxial dislocation, the dens may be pressed upward into the base of the medulla causing pressure on the pyramidal tracts in the midline with resulting paralysis of the upper extremities (Fig. 211-6). It is of importance because the condition mimics the acute central cervical cord injury syndrome. The neurological picture usually reverts to normal with simple traction that effects proper positioning, and then subsequent stabilization.

The Hangman's Fracture

This type of fracture is the avulsion of the laminar arches of C2 with some degree of dislocation of the C2 vertebral body on C3. The lesion was first described by Wood-Jones as the characteristic lesion resulting from judicial hanging performed by the platform drop technique.[12] In 1965, Schneider et al. reported eight such cases occurring in motor vehicle accident victims (Fig. 211-7A).[10] Two of these patients did not lose consciousness and recalled the details of the event. They had abrasions on their chins and/or faces and recalled "hanging" themselves on the steering wheel or the dashboard of the vehicle, respectively. The mechanism in these cases, and in most others, is a hyperextension injury. Occasionally this lesion has been reported in cervical flexion, but this is indeed rare. Professor A. J. E. Cave indicated that either in judicial hanging or in the motor vehicle accident the clivus of the skull and the C1 and C2 vertebral bodies move as a solitary unit avulsing the laminar arches (Fig. 211-7B).[10] In hanging, the weight of the body continues to pull downward and the body sways forward, cutting the vertebral arteries and destroying the cervicomedullary junction, with immediate death (Fig. 211-7B). In the case of the motor vehicle accident victim the weight of the body is supported after the initial blow without a further drop, so that the avulsed arches decompress the cervicomedullary junction and there usually is no neurological deficit. It is important to recognize these injuries, for these patients very seldom require surgical intervention and their lesion will heal with conservative therapy by merely placing the patient in a firm plastic cervical collar for a period of 10 weeks. Of our own patients only one out of a currently estimated 50 has been operated upon by an orthopedic surgeon, and at the time of operation the site of fracture dislocation was found to have already fused itself without instability.

In summary, lesions of the atlanto-occipital region and the upper cervical spine may be lethal, with immediate death, but an adequate understanding of the factors involved with a suspicion that such a lesion exists will often enable the proper diagnosis and recovery with a specific type of therapy.

References

1. Bell HS: Paralysis of both arms from injury of the upper portion of the pyramidal decussation: "Cruciate paralysis." J Neurosurg 33:376–380, 1970.
2. Dyck P: Os odontoideum in children: Neurological manifestations and surgical management. Neurosurgery 2:93–99, 1978.
3. Gabrielsen TO, Maxwell JA: Traumatic atlanto-occipital dislocation, with case report of a patient who survived. AJR 97:624–629, 1966.
4. Gosch HH, Gooding E, Schneider RC: Distortion and displacement of the brain in experimental head injuries. Surg Forum 20:425–426, 1969.
5. Hensinger RN, Fielding JW, Hawkins RJ: Congenital anomalies of the odontoid process. Orthop Clin North Am 9:901–912, 1978.
6. Jefferson G: Remarks on fractures of the first cervical vertebra: Founded on a portion of a Hunterian Lecture delivered at the Royal College of Surgeons of England, Feb 1924, in: *Selected Papers, Geoffrey Jefferson*. Springfield, Ill, Charles C Thomas, 1960, pp 213–231.
7. Kline DG: Atlanto-axial dislocation simulating a head injury: Hypoplasia of the odontoid: Case report. J Neurosurg 24:1013–1016, 1966.
8. Pang D, Wilberger JE Jr: Traumatic atlanto-occipital dislocation with survival; Case report and review. Neurosurgery 7:503–508, 1980.
9. Schneider RC, Crosby EC: Craniocerebral, cervicomedullary, and spinal injuries, in Schneider RC, Kahn EA, Crosby EC, Taren JA (eds): *Correlative Neurosurgery*, 3d ed. Springfield, Ill, Charles C Thomas, 1982, pp 1175–1300.
10. Schneider RC, Livingston KE, Cave AJE, Hamilton G: "Hangman's fracture" of the cervical spine. J Neurosurg 22:141–154, 1965.
11. Sherk HH: Fractures of the atlas and odontoid process. Orthop Clin North Am 9:973–984, 1978.
12. Wood-Jones F: The ideal lesion produced by judicial hanging. Lancet 1:53, 1913.

212
Mid- and Lower Cervical Spine Injuries
Martin H. Weiss

Serious injury to the cervical spinal cord is a problem of major public health proportions since the sequelae of such injuries are frequently devastating with respect to long-term disability for the patient and the demands on public resources generated by such disability. Our objective as physicians charged with the responsibility of caring for such individuals is to minimize the extent of spinal cord injury subsequent to cervical spine trauma while providing an environment for the cervical cord to recover maximally from existent damage.

At present our best available data indicate that the incidence of spinal column trauma throughout the country occurs at the rate of approximately 5 per 100,000 population. There will be approximately 5000 new cases of spinal cord injury throughout the United States per annum; of this group, approximately 10 percent of the spinal cord injuries (500 patients) will result in the genesis of a quadriplegic patient.

Spinal cord injury is most frequently a problem of the young adult male, occurring most commonly in the decade extending from age 16 to 25. The majority of spinal cord injuries occur as a consequence of road vehicular accidents; such accidents account for at least 50 percent of the spinal cord injuries seen throughout the country.[14] Various other contributing factors depend upon environmental and geographic considerations relative to the region of study. Interest has long focused on the significance of athletic participation as a cause of spine injury. Much focus has been directed toward contact sports as a precipitating cause; in fact, however, the occurrence of spinal cord injury subsequent to participation in football in the United States is rather insignificant when compared with other athletic activities.[6] Certainly, in the state of California, the greatest percentage of spinal cord injuries related to athletic participation occurs secondary to water sports (diving, surfing, and water skiing) and snow skiing participation. These activities account for more than 80 percent of the athletically related spinal cord injuries seen in California.[14,16] Interestingly, severe spinal cord injury is an uncommon occurrence in childhood, the frequency increasing directly with increasing age. When a cervical spine injury occurs in childhood, it is most commonly related to the upper cervical spine, almost all such injuries occurring between the levels of C1 and C4. Although utilization of seat belts in automobiles has contributed significantly to the reduction in mortality secondary to automobile accidents, an interesting observation has been made with respect to the occurrence of cervical spine injury secondary to the use of the lap-shoulder type of seat belts, which have contributed to the genesis of a small percentage of the overall number of spinal cord injuries. Certainly this occurrence pales in comparison to the protective effects of such seat belt utilization.

Cervical spinal cord injury appears to be a major contributing factor in acute death secondary to those traffic accidents resulting in severe head injuries. Approximately 20 percent of all fatal victims of traffic accidents have an associated severe cervical spinal cord injury that contributes significantly if not primarily to the mortality. Eighty percent of these lesions involve the articulations between the occiput, C1, and C2; only 20 percent involve the cervical spine below the level of the axis. Studies have shown that, in all auto injuries, cervical spine injuries occur with a frequency of 1 in 300 auto accidents requiring that the involved car be towed from the scene of the accident. If an occupant is ejected from the vehicle, the frequency of associated cervical spine injuries increases to 1 in 14. Interestingly, severe neck injuries are associated predominantly with impacts occurring at the front end or side; such injuries occur much less frequently with rear end impact.

The most common site of cervical vertebral body fracture is C5. Fracture-dislocation of the cervical spine occurs most commonly at the C5-6 interspace. As might well be expected, the incidence of neurological deficit in association with cervical spine injury is highest in those cases involving fracture-dislocation injuries. If one assesses the entire spinal column, 14 percent of fracture-dislocations are associated with significant neurological injury. However, 39 percent of cervical spine fractures are associated with significant neurological deficit, this being the highest incidence of neurological deficit related to spine injury. Indeed, when a cervical spine injury is associated with a fracture of the vertebral body and posterior elements, a 61 percent incidence of neurological deficit secondary to the injury is observed.[11,23] Multiple spinal fractures involving different anatomical sites occur in approximately 5 percent of cases;[4] such occurrences are obviously uncommon, but failure to recognize multiple levels of spine injury may result in devastating spinal cord damage at an unrecognized site of spinal injury.

Predisposing Factors

Undoubtedly the most important related factor with respect to the genesis of significant cervical spine injury is the concomitant occurrence of a serious head or trunk injury. Transmission of forces through the cranial vault to the cervical spine has been readily demonstrated; our general program of head-injury management requires that all patients rendered unconscious from a blow to the head should be considered a victim of an associated cervical spinal cord injury until proved otherwise. The high frequency of alcoholic intoxication associated with craniocerebral trauma is paralleled in cervical spinal cord injuries associated with traffic accidents. Not only does alcoholic intoxication contribute to the likelihood of becoming involved in such an accident but the potential chemical toxicity of ethanol on the traumatized spinal cord may increase the severity of the cord injury.

A number of underlying systemic medical diseases may also predispose one to the development of a spinal cord injury. Although rare, people with generalized seizure disorders or having electroconvulsive therapy have been reported to develop significant cervical spine injuries. Certainly unrecognized metastatic disease (both neoplastic and infectious) in the cervical spine renders an individual highly vulnerable to serious spinal cord injury subsequent to even trivial trauma. Of greatest consequence, however, is the existence of other underlying cervical spine diseases, either congenital or developmental. Three particular disorders that potentiate the occurrence of cervical spinal cord injury relate to the pre-existence of ankylosing spondylitis, degenerative spondylosis, or congenital fusion of cervical vertebrae. The first two of these are associated with a particularly high incidence of severe spinal cord injury related to trauma to the cervical spine; such injury most commonly occurs at the level of C5-7.[20,28,30]

Mechanisms

Biomechanical considerations of the various motion patterns that occur with respect to the cervical spine have been assessed in an attempt to understand the contribution of mechanical stresses to the development of specific spinal injuries. The cervical spine is subjected to varying forces of flexion, flexion-rotation, extension, and vertical compression or shear that result in damage to osseous, neural, and vascular components of the spine. Injury ensues when the head or neck is flexed, extended, or rotated on the trunk beyond physiological limits; the vertical application of force to the skull results in additional compressive forces that contribute to or may be the primary cause of an associated spinal cord injury.

Hyperflexion sprain is an entity that results from partial tearing of posterior ligamentous structures, including the interspinous ligaments that support the cervical spine. Although separation of the interspinous ligaments may be evident on stress x-rays in flexion, radiographic evaluation frequently demonstrates a normal spine. Pathological involvement of nerve roots or the spinal cord is rare under such circumstances; this entity may account for the syndrome of chronic neckache without neurological damage or radiographic evidence of acute spinal injury following trauma, which generally resolves with long-term immobilization.

The combination of forward flexion and rotation contributes to the development of *unilateral facet dislocation*. Under such circumstances one experiences tearing of the interspinous ligaments and the facet capsule on the involved side, resulting in forward displacement of the inferior facet at the level of the dislocation. In general, this results in less than a 50 percent anterior displacement between the involved vertebral bodies (most commonly C5 on C6, then C6 on C7 and C4 on C5). When the forces of distraction in flexion are greater, *bilateral dislocation and locking of facets* may occur. This phenomenon involves disruption of the interspinous ligaments as well as both facet capsules along with potential disruption of the posterior and anterior longitudinal ligaments that constrain the vertebral bodies. Under such circumstances, one frequently sees greater than 50 percent subluxation between the involved vertebral bodies; the loci of such lesions are similar to those of unilateral facet dislocation.

Under circumstances of unilateral facet dislocation, one frequently experiences entrapment and compression of a cervical nerve root with the potential for associated spinal cord injury at the level of subluxation. Such spinal cord injury is frequently of moderate extent resulting in an incomplete spinal cord lesion, although certainly not exclusively so. On the other hand, the extensive compromise of the spinal canal generated by bilateral facet dislocation frequently results in severe spinal cord injury of massive extent even though there have been scattered reports of *complete dislocation between vertebral bodies* in the absence of any neurological deficit.

The combination of hyperflexion combined with a compressive force applied to the anterior portion of the vertebral body results in a *wedge compression fracture*. Associated disruption of posterior ligamentous structures, evidenced by major separation of the spinous processes, results in instability of the cervical spine in association with such fractures. When major compressive forces are applied with the neck in flexion, the resulting vertical or axial loading stress results in the development of a *teardrop fracture*. This injury involves a comminuted fracture of the vertebral body in which the anterior-inferior vertebral fragment is triangular, giving rise to the name teardrop fracture. In such injuries, one frequently sees inferior portions of the vertebral body displaced posteriorly into the spinal canal, an injury that is frequently associated with major spinal cord damage. The extent of the traumatic myelopathy is generally thought to be dependent upon the amount of flexion at the time of the impact.

Although *hyperextension injuries* to the cervical spine formerly were considered uncommon, recent studies meticulously evaluating the mechanisms related to cervical spine injuries indicate that hyperextension injuries probably account for the majority of cervical spine injuries.[2,11] The most common mechanism underlying the severe spinal cord injury with a spine that appears normal radiographically seems to be that of hyperextension. Spinal cord injury secondary to hyperextension is a particularly frequent occurrence in patients who have underlying degenerative disease of the spine. In the presence of cervical spondylosis or ankylosing spondylitis, hyperextension of even a moderate degree may result in compression of the spinal cord between the posterior aspect of the vertebral body and the ligamentum flavum and lamina, resulting in severe spinal cord injury. In ankylosing spondylitis, a fracture may occur through an ankylosed disc space with resultant disruption of the anterior and posterior longitudinal ligaments, resulting in an unstable cervical spine injury. Such injuries are frequently associated with severe spinal cord injury; an unusual but devastating complication associated with this injury is the development of a spinal epidural hematoma. Hyperextension injuries frequently disrupt the anterior longitudinal ligament; if there is sufficient distraction during the course of such hyperextension (as from a massive blow to the chin), anterior displacement of the vertebral body above the injury may occur, resulting in a hyperextension fracture-dislocation that can be confused radiographically with a pure flexion injury.[2,11,14]

Hyperextension injuries may be divided into two subgroups, disruptive and compressive. The traumatic forces that underly the *disruptive hyperextension injury* are applied with the neck in extension, with or without rotation. Under such circumstances, there is disruption of the anterior longitudinal ligament; occasionally one observes a small avulsion fracture of the vertebral body at the site of the ligamentous disruption anteriorly. Clinically, one often observes the concomitant presence of a frontal cranial, facial, or mandibular injury, indicating the site of application of the injurious force. *Compressive hyperextension injuries* (including the above-described *hyperextension fracture-dislocation*) occur in the setting of anterior body separation in association with a compression fracture of the posterior bony elements, resulting in an associated horizontal facet fracture. These injuries may have associated fractures of the pedicle, lamina, or spinous process.

Application of *lateral* forces result in *spine injury* less frequently than the aforementioned mechanisms. However, such injuries may result in fractures of the articular processes, vertebral body, and transverse and uncinate processes as well as disruption of the oncovertebral joints. Such isolated injuries may cause damage to proximal nerve roots or blood vessels (particularly the vertebral artery); major damage to the spinal cord under such circumstances, however, is unusual. These injuries frequently have a normal appearance on plain roentgenograms and require sophisticated radiographic assessment to define the anatomical integrity of pedicles, facets, and laminae.

Syndromes of Spinal Cord Trauma

The extent of spinal cord injury relates, of course, most directly to the amount of force applied to the spinal cord at the time of impact, although vascular consequences, both hemorrhagic and ischemic, secondary to the injury may contribute significantly to the ultimate clinical picture.

The most severe consequence of spinal cord trauma is the complete transverse myelopathy in which all functional activity below the level of the lesion is lost. This entity is frequently, if not always, associated with the finding of spinal shock in which there is total absence of all sensory and motor modalities as well as absent monosynaptic reflexes below the level of the lesion at the initial evaluation. This injury may occur as a consequence of true anatomical disruption of the spinal cord, physiological disruption of neural function because of compression or ischemia, or a combination of both. One may rarely see an extensive injury to the spinal cord, including even the clinical picture of a complete transverse myelopathy, that spontaneously resolves within 24 to 72 h after the injury. Such an occurrence obviously relates to transient physiological dysfunction secondary to trauma and may be considered a concussion of the spinal cord.

A second clinical syndrome is the anterior spinal cord syndrome. In this clinical setting, one observes dysfunction of those substrates of spinal cord function subserved by the anterior two-thirds of the spinal cord embracing the corticospinal tracts and the anterolateral spinothalamic systems. Under such circumstances one observes a loss of all voluntary motor activity along with absence of sensation to pain and temperature below the level of the lesion. On the other hand, posterior column function, as evaluated by proprioceptive responses, is generally preserved. Reflex activity below the level of such lesions is generally absent acutely, although one may see extensor plantar responses. The degree of the motor deficit in both the upper and lower extremities below the level of the lesion is generally equal. The pathophysiological process underlying the genesis of this syndrome has not been defined precisely. It may relate to stretch applied by the attachment of the dentate ligaments at the equatorial plane of the cord or ischemic injury generated by compromise of the anterior spinal artery whose blood supply is known to subserve the anterior two-thirds of the cord. Most likely there is an interaction between these phenomena in the genesis of the anterior cord syndrome.

The third most common clinical syndrome following acute spinal cord trauma is the central cord syndrome. This syndrome involves a focus of trauma lying within the centrum of the cervical spinal cord, therein involving those structures traversing this area. Underlying pathological substrates may involve a hemorrhagic contusion to the centrum of the cord, mechanical disruption, ischemia, or a combination of all three. Clinically, one observes disproportionate weakness in the upper extremities below the level of the lesion when compared with the lower extremities. Sensory loss is usually minimal, although this is variable and frequently occurs in no specific pattern. The extent of the motor deficit may be variable, the key clinical observation being that the motor deficit in the upper extremities is greater than that in the lower extremities. Deep tendon reflexes in the lower extremities are generally preserved and may show signs of an upper motor neuron pattern; deep tendon reflexes in the upper extremities at the level of the lesion will generally be absent. The central cord syndrome is frequently associated with radiographic evidence of degenerative disease of the cervical spine (cervical spondylosis) or a congenitally narrow spinal canal.[24]

The well-known entity of the Brown-Séquard syndrome of hemisection of the spinal cord is not commonly observed after blunt spinal cord trauma; we most frequently observe this syndrome secondary to penetrating injury.

Radiology of Cervical Spine Injuries

Optimal treatment of patients with cervical spine injury is dependent upon an accurate radiographic assessment of the traumatic bony abnormality both with respect to existent pathology and the underlying mechanism of injury. Failure to recognize a cervical fracture or evidence of cervical instability may result in the subsequent genesis of severe neurological sequelae. A single lateral plain x-ray film encompassing the area of C1 to T1 is probably the single most important film for the initial evaluation of the patient with a suspected or demonstrated cervical spine injury. Inadequate visualization of the cervical spine to the level of the upper portion of T1 is the most common cause of a suboptimal x-ray evaluation. Downward pull on the arms is often necessary to adequately visualize the C7-T1 area; if this is technically inadequate, a swimmer's view may suffice. Occasionally, if both of these methods fail, lateral tomography or xeroradiography will be required for adequate visualization of the C7-T1 area.

When the lateral cervical spine film is being reviewed, a number of areas must be addressed. The anterior prevertebral soft tissue width should be measured at the inferior aspect of C3. The normal width of the soft tissue at this level is less than 5 mm; any increase in soft tissue size should lead one to suspect retrotracheal hemorrhage secondary to cervical spine injury. Loss of the normal lordotic curve of the cervical spine may be an indication of cervical injury, although the normal cervical lordotic curve is absent in 20 percent of normal patients. Careful inspection of the relationship of the posterior aspect of the vertebral bodies as their alignment is visualized on the lateral roentgenogram provides good evidence for anterior or posterior displacement; in addition, close inspection for angular deformity or changes in the bony configuration of the vertebral bodies is essential. Abnormal separation anteriorly at the level of the interspace that may or may not be associated with an avulsion fracture of the adjacent vertebral body or increased separation between the dorsal spines posteriorly provides evidence of injury to the ligamentous structures supporting the vertebral column secondary to hyperextension or flexion injuries, respectively.

Anteroposterior (AP) views of the mid- and lower cervical spine are helpful in defining the presence of a unilateral facet dislocation that may not be evident on the lateral projection. Under such circumstances one must carefully view the spinous processes as they appear on the AP view, looking for rotation of the spinous processes toward the side of the dislocation above the level of the injury. One may also detect a widening of the oncovertebral joints as well as fractures of articular processes, vertebral bodies, and transverse and uncinate processes on the AP view. In the event that the clinical picture is suggestive but roentgenograms are not definitive of facet dislocation, oblique views of the cervical spine taken with the physician in attendance may lend further support in establishing a diagnosis.

Between 15 and 20 percent of patients who have cervical spinal cord injuries will have no overt radiographic spine injury evident on plain films. Two-thirds of such patients will demonstrate radiographic abnormalities when thin-section computed tomography (CT) of the spine is subsequently added to the radiographic evaluation. In addition, in more than 50 percent of patients such tomography will demonstrate more extensive factors than are visualized on plain x-ray films.[15] In a study by Maravilla et al. in 1978, such tomographic evidence resulted in an alteration in the mode of treatment in 18 percent of cases studied.[19] Thin-section or computed cervical tomography therefore may be of help when used to (1) clarify suspicious findings noted on plain x-ray films, (2) identify additional factors that may not be evident on adequate plain films, and (3) visualize associated fractures in patients with known fractures and fracture-dislocations.

X-ray films demonstrate a static situation with respect to the pathology of the cervical spine. Even though major disruptions of ligamentous structures may strongly argue that a given fracture is unstable, demonstration or proof of instability may require manipulation of the cervical spine under fluoroscopic or x-ray visualization. Flexion-extension views are recommended only in conscious patients and preferably, when one has direct visualization of the cervical spine during flexion and extension movements. These maneuvers are only done under direct supervision of a physician in those situations in which there is no subluxation and in which ligamentous injury is suspected. It should be emphasized that, in patients with major spinal injury, any radiographic evaluation of the patient, especially any involving transportation to an x-ray table, should be under the direction of a physician; cervical immobilization with a head holder, cervical collar, or sandbag should be used to reduce neck motion prior to and during x-ray evaluation. In a patient with major muscular spasm, frequently observed after cervical spine injury, it may be impossible to adequately assess instability of the spine because of the paravertebral muscle spasm. Our practice has been to place such patients in traction or a restrictive cervical collar until such spasm abates in order to more adequately assess spinal stability, with the physician, once again, in attendance during this assessment.

The evolution of high-resolution computed tomography has added another positive dimension to our radiological armamentarium for the assessment of cervical spine injury. This study, which can be performed while the patient is in traction, can be rapidly performed with minimal manipulation of the cervical spine. Of particular importance is the capacity of the studies to demonstrate the projection of bone and/or disc material into the spinal canal and the presence of nondisplaced fractures of the laminae, pedicles, facets, and body. Combined with the intrathecal administration of the water-soluble contrast agent metrizamide, CT myelography has essentially replaced conventional cervical myelography in our institution for the assessment of intraspinal contents. The contrast agent may be administered atraumatically via a lateral C1-2 puncture with subsequent CT evaluation giving a precise assessment of the bony structures around the spinal canal as well as the contents of the spinal canal. This can be particularly helpful in assessing the potential posterior displacement of disc fragments into the spinal canal during the course of the evaluation of such patients. The CT scan is also helpful in defining the presence of spinal stenosis whatever the underlying cause.[9,12]

One can readily appreciate that radiographic evaluation can provide information concerning two areas in the evaluation of the patient with a cervical spine injury. Impingement upon the intraspinal contents may be defined by plain x-ray films; if any questions exist, CT scanning, with or without a water-soluble contrast agent, can provide meticulous definition of the spinal canal. Our present feeling is that CT scanning can be done more easily and rapidly than conventional polytomography, and it has consequently become our secondary mode of diagnostic evaluation. Total understanding of the extent of spine injury, however, requires an assessment of stability. Radiographic findings indicating disruption of ligamentous structures may provide sufficient indirect evidence of instability to warrant therapy on that basis alone; normal plain roentgenograms in the face of potential spinal instability demand dynamic evaluation by either flexion-extension films or cineradiography in an appropriate setting.

Management of Cervical Spine Injuries

Care of the patient who has sustained an injury to the cervical spine is designed to minimize the potential for further injury and to provide an environment that will maximize the opportunity for recovery of spinal cord dysfunction. Such a program demands that one be alert to the possibility of the existence of a cervical spine injury so as to take measures radiographically and clinically to evaluate this potential. The presence of a complete transverse myelopathy involving the cervical spinal cord poses a major medical challenge to the physician charged with the care of such patients; such challenges may also occur in the patient with a partial or incomplete cord lesion.

One of the major causes contributing to the worsening of a patient with a mechanical spinal cord injury is a superimposed ischemic injury to the spinal cord. Loss of sympathetic tone may result in peripheral vasodilatation with subsequent peripheral vascular pooling and hypotension. The frequent concomitant finding of a bradycardia may well compound the problem of spinal cord vascular perfusion. Attention to such problems with the judicious use of alpha stimulators, intravascular volume augmentation, intravenous atropine, and possible transvenous pacemaker utilization may avoid conversion of an incomplete or recoverable lesion to one that fails to respond to therapy. Interruption of the corticospinal system also impedes pulmonary function since the intercostal musculature is denervated, resulting in a decrease in pulmonary excursion. Frequent evaluation of arterial blood gases and pulmonary function at the bedside may alert the attending physician to the need for pulmonary support in advance of a potential castrophe from a hypoxic insult.

Sympathetic denervation will result in the loss of thermal regulation, allowing for the development of hypothermia with potential disastrous cardiovascular consequences. Loss of bladder control after such injuries requires meticulous attention to a bladder drainage system. A massively distended bladder may never recover sufficient tone to function adequately even in the face of spinal cord recovery. We have adopted a policy of intermittent catheterization on a 6-h basis even in the acute phase in order to minimize the potential for urinary tract infection. However, use of an indwelling catheter during the acute care of the spinal cord–injured patient, particularly in the absence of a "catheterization team," may prove most effective in preventing the complications of bladder overdistension. Finally, careful attention to skin care in the complete cervical spinal cord injury is of paramount import. A number of mechanical devices allow maintenance of cervical traction while varying skin pressure (kinetic therapy) in order to minimize skin compression and possible necrosis.

One additional potential catastrophic complication of immobilization in the spinal cord–injured patient is development of deep vein phlebothrombosis and subsequent pulmonary embolization. Various measures have been utilized in an attempt to reduce this potential. Some claims have been made that the use of "constant motion" beds markedly reduces the incidence of pulmonary embolism, but this has not been verified. We evaluated the use of inflatable compression stockings applied to the legs of patients with spinal cord injury. Unfortunately, we found that these devices did not reduce the incidence of deep vein phlebothrombosis as measured by radioactive fibrinogen labeling of venous thrombi. Our present mode of preventive treatment of deep vein phlebothrombosis rests on the use of minidoses of heparin (5000 units subcutaneously twice daily).

Once stabilization of systemic parameters has been

achieved, attention should be directed to the need for alignment and immobilization of the spine. The use of skeletal traction for restoration and/or maintenance of the normal alignment of the spinal column is a long-practiced and effective approach in the treatment of patients with cervical spine fractures. Throughout the years a number of different cervical traction devices have evolved; recently the spring-loaded Gardner-Wells, Heifetz, and Trippi tongs have become popular because of their ease of application and maintenance. The spring-loaded devices may be applied directly in the emergency room, do not require any surgical manipulation, and can even be used in the face of a suspicious injury to maintain stability of the spine while an evaluation is in progress. Application is simple and poses minimal risk to the patient, particularly when compared with the potential for excess motion of the unprotected cervical spine. Some authors have expressed a preference for immediate application of the halo ring for traction in those patients in whom halo immobilization is anticipated for maintaining reduction of the cervical injury. With a defined lesion of the cervical spine, our practice has been to apply weight to the traction device with a maximum of 5 lb for each level below the occiput (C7 = 35 lb) based on the guidelines promulgated by Crutchfield many years ago in his evaluation of vigorous young male patients. Reduction of highly unstable cervical fractures under these circumstances is generally readily accomplished. Because of the potential for distraction at the fracture site, however, our practice has been to begin with 10 lb (for lesions at C4 or below) and then, under x-ray or fluoroscopic control, to add weights up to the maximum weight if necessary.

Reduction of unilateral and bilateral facet dislocations, however, has been difficult; other authors have recommended greater amounts of weight in order to accomplish such reduction. Under such circumstances the patient is taken to the radiology department and sedated. The fluoroscopic table is tilted upward, and the body weight serves as a countertraction to the pull of the tongs. The patient remains supine and transverse fluoroscopy is utilized. Constant fluoroscopic monitoring is used to recognize and avoid dangerous distraction while attempted reduction is carried out. With unilateral and bilateral facet dislocations, some authors have even advocated manipulation of the neck under fluoroscopic control while weight is applied in order to accomplish reduction of locked facets. In the face of a horizontal fracture through a facet, closed reduction may be impossible.

The critical consideration in such vigorous manipulations is the significance of reduction relative to the outcome from spinal cord injury. Although a number of authors have demonstrated their capacity to effect closed reduction even in the face of locked facets utilizing as much as 80 lb of weight for cervical traction, there is absolutely no evidence that such reduction has altered the outcome with respect to spinal cord function. Certainly, in the absence of spinal cord injury, rapid reduction is neither advocated nor necessary. Our policy has been to take the patient to maximum weights as defined above and then to allow persistent traction to overcome paraspinal muscle spasm in order to aid eventual reduction.

The major risk of attempting reduction by cervical skeletal traction is overdistraction with associated worsening of the neurological status of the patient. In older patients with cervical spondylosis and associated fracture-dislocation, overdistraction has been reported with as little as 15 lb of weight, resulting in a worsened neurological status because of this overdistraction.[25] Therefore, in elderly patients with degenerative changes and in patients with fracture-dislocation associated with significant ligamentous injury, weights less than those recommended by Crutchfield should be used initially.

Our European and Australian colleagues have advocated the use of general anesthesia in association with cervical traction in an attempt at closed reduction of all fracture-dislocations. This course of action has not been popular in the United States, where an attempt at reduction by the application of cervical traction with manipulation while the patient is awake remains the primary approach to the reduction of a fracture-dislocation.[15,21,22,26]

Once reduction has been accomplished, the question arises as to the best mode of therapy to assure healing with permanent stability at the fracture site. Application of a halo or rigid brace to the cervical spine may be satisfactory. This technique may be effective when there is adequate reduction of the cervical spine without persistent angulation due to extensive ligamentous disruption. In practice, the use of the halo device or an effective rigid cervical brace is probably the ideal method of immobilization and treatment in patients who are neurologically intact with reduced yet unstable cervical spine fractures and fracture-dislocations.

Some neck movement, however, does occur despite halo immobilization.[17] For this reason Norrell and others do not believe that immediate halo fixation and ambulation should be practiced after the reduction of a cervical fracture-dislocation.[21] Norrell recommends that the patient remain immobilized for 3 to 4 weeks after the reduction of a fracture-dislocation before being allowed to be ambulatory in a halo device. In practice, a loss of reduction following halo immobilization occurs infrequently; when loss of reduction does occur, it usually occurs early in the course of immobilization and is easily correctable by adjustments of the halo apparatus. In general, we think that the halo is an ideal instrument for traction, reduction, and long-term stabilization.[7,15,18]

Contraindications to the use of the halo include pre-existing infection of the scalp, severe restrictive respiratory expansion of the chest, and severe chronic pulmonary disease. The patient with a complete transverse myelopathy who has an anesthetic shoulder and chest may develop the complication of pressure necrosis under a halo vest, which is, in our mind, a relative although not absolute contraindication for the use of the halo apparatus.[7,15]

The major indication for early or acute surgical intervention in acute spinal cord injury is preservation or restoration of neurological function if this is deemed possible. Numerous studies have evaluated the impact of "decompression" of the spinal cord acutely after cervical trauma on eventual outcome of spinal cord injury. Unfortunately, those studies that have attempted to look at similar patients who underwent surgical or nonsurgical therapy have failed to demonstrate any evidence of improved neurological function from acute operative decompression of the cervical spine in the face of spinal cord injury. Most acute cervical spine cord injuries do not call for emergency open surgical intervention.[16]

However, selected patients may benefit from decompressive surgery performed after a significant period of observation. Those patients considered candidates for surgical decompression have preservation of some distal neurological function but either fail to improve under observation or demonstrate evidence of a progressive neurological deficit. Progression of a neurological deficit demands emergent intervention if a compressive lesion is demonstrated. Observation for a minimum of 7 to 10 days in the patient with a partial lesion has been our practice before deciding upon evaluation for a mechanical cause of failure to improve. In the event that a patient with an incomplete lesion fails to improve after observation for 7 to 10 days, a metrizamide CT myelogram is performed to assess for persistent extrinsic compression of the spinal cord within the canal, particularly from a herniated cervical disc, a depressed fractured lamina, or an osteophytic bar. Under such circumstances, removal of the offending agent may aid in neurological recovery. This has been particularly effective in the syndrome of the "chronic central cord" in which recovery begins and then reaches a plateau as a result of persistent impingement upon the cord that may be relieved by operative intervention. It should be stressed that attempts at definitive stabilization of the cervical spine should be made at the same time that any indicated operative decompression is carried out. We no longer undertake "decompression" in the face of an unimproved complete transverse cervical myelopathy.

The vast majority of operative interventions relate to procedures designed to stabilize the unstable cervical spine. Such procedures are undertaken when indicated at approximately 2 weeks after injury in order to minimize postoperative pulmonary complications, which occur frequently when operative intervention is undertaken within 7 days of the spinal cord injury. I recognize the extensive debate that has been maintained with respect to the optimal form of operative intervention for spinal stabilization.[1,3,5,10,21,22,24,27,29] Our approach has been to assess by radiographic and clinical criteria the underlying mechanism responsible for the spinal injury and to direct our operative intervention at that particular site. In the presence of a hyperextension injury with disruption of the anterior and possibly posterior longitudinal ligaments but with preservation of the posterior ligamentous support system (facet joint capsule, interlaminar and interspinous ligaments), we have favored an anterior approach with insertion of a bony strut graft at the site of the injury. However, if there is evidence of posterior ligamentous instability either because of a flexion, flexion-rotation, or distraction type of injury, we have preferred a posterior fusion using wire and bone to provide immediate and prolonged stability. When there is evidence of extensive bone damage either anteriorly, posteriorly, or both, we have recently grown more enthusiastic about the use of external immobilization as long as good alignment of the spine can be established with such a system. However, if there is minimal bony involvement but major ligamentous disruption, we have preferred operative efforts at stabilization. Because of the poor prognosis for stability in the face of extensive posterior ligamentous disruption as found with facet dislocations, we have generally favored operative reduction and fusion of these lesions from behind in order to assure long-term stability.

In the situation in which we are unable to satisfactorily reduce locked facets by closed reduction, we have favored posterior reduction and fusion in order to effect stabilization of the spine. We have not used anterior decompression with attempted reduction of locked facets, although several authors have addressed this mode of surgical intervention. A particularly complicated case is one in which there is posterior protrusion of disc fragments (which may occur in as many as 20 percent of cervical fracture-dislocations) in association with extensive disruption of posterior ligamentous structures. Primary posterior fusion, in this situation, may further compromise the diameter of the spinal canal, particularly if the jumped facets are holding the canal open in an angulated position. Under such circumstances, defined by CT evaluation at the fracture site, we would approach the protruded disc anteriorly, clean out the intraspinal compartment, and then fuse to solid bone anteriorly. Because of the posterior ligamentous disruption, we would maintain the individual in a halo brace for 6 weeks after the anterior fusion, assuming that the spine is in good alignment. If there is persistence of facet dislocation, either unilateral or bilateral, which could not be corrected by the anterior procedure, we would perform a secondary procedure to reduce the posterior locked facets and fuse posteriorly after the ventral intraspinal comminuted disc material or fragments have been removed.

Various pharmacologic treatment methodologies have been recommended in patients with both complete and incomplete cervical myelopathy secondary to trauma. Glucocorticoids, diuretics, biogenic amine synthesis blockers, local hypothermia, barbiturates, and, most recently, endogenous opiate antagonists have been effective in various experimental laboratory models. To date, however, no controlled clinical study exists evaluating the usefulness of these pharmacologic agents in spinal cord injury. Despite there being no proven clinical effect, glucocorticoids are frequently recommended for treatment of the edema associated with spinal cord injuries. Osmotic diuretics (mannitol or urea) have been recommended for the same purpose. Selected spinal cord injury centers are presently evaluating these agents in an objective protocol to provide a rational basis for such pharmacologic intervention. Of particular interest is assessment of the use of "megadoses" of glucocorticoid in the management of severe spinal cord injury. Sufficient data for analysis have not yet been reported. Until such evidence is forthcoming, it is fair to say that glucocorticoids, in conventional doses or megadoses, are frequently used in the clinical setting; justification for their use is yet forthcoming.

Prognosis for Neurological Recovery; Factors Influencing Prognosis

The single most important factor determining the eventual outcome from spinal cord injury is the initial extent of the injury. There is little evidence to indicate that any manipulations (operative, closed reductive, or pharmacologic) contribute in a statistically significant fashion to the outcome.[13,25,31] Anecdotal case reports of clinical improvement following immediate decompression after spinal cord injury are promulgated as indices of the therapeutic efficacy of such surgical ventures; other reports, however, indicate that 8 percent of nonoperated patients who initially have complete transverse myelopathy secondary to cervical cord injury end up with recovery of useful lower extremity motor function.[14] There has been no controlled study that indicates that any surgical venture can improve upon this grim prognosis. The most recent study by Wagner and Chehrazi confirms the lack of positive impact of acute surgical decompression on the outcome of spinal cord injury.[29] Ducker and his group reported a 34 percent 1-year mortality in patients with a complete cervical cord injury.[8] Prolonged immobilization while awaiting spontaneous fusion may result in significant morbidity and mortality from pulmonary embolism, infection, or renal problems. Early fusion and stabilization allowing mobilization may improve upon this parameter even if neurological function does not show a similar parallel improvement. Significant data to support even this thesis, however, are not yet available.

The optimism expressed about the outcome from central spinal cord injury also appears to be under some question. In a recent study, it was found that 23 percent of patients who were ambulatory at the time of initial discharge after sustaining a central cervical cord syndrome subsequently developed progressive lower extremity weakness resulting in the loss of ambulation.[14] The clinician must be aware of the potential development of the post-traumatic syrinx or the persistence of spinal cord compression as causes of a delayed increase in neurological deficit. Such a delayed progressive deficit may occur years after the initial trauma; early intervention under such circumstances may effect dramatic resolution of the additional deficit. In addition, recovery of useful hand function after central cervical cord injury is much less likely to occur (50 percent) than is recovery of sufficient lower extremity function to permit free ambulation. This may also relate to the presence of persistent cord compression due to cervical spondylosis at the level of the lesion; operative intervention under these circumstances may result in functional improvement. The anterior cord syndrome, on the other hand, has a poor potential for eventual free ambulation in spite of the fact that this does not represent a complete transverse myelopathy. Almost 50 percent of these individuals will not regain sufficient motor function of the lower extremities to allow free ambulation.[14] In those patients with complete myelopathy, Ducker et al. found that 6.7 percent gained useful recovery of motor function after 1 year; this was unrelated to the modality of therapy utilized.[8]

Well-documented instances of recovery of useful function after immediate and complete spinal cord injury occur but are rare. Reduction, fixation, and fusion of the vertebral column are worthwhile in their own right; but their role in enhancing neurological recovery is questionable at best. Cases of progressive loss of function after an incomplete lesion are almost invariably related to events external to the spinal cord such as protruded discs, bony spicules, vascular compression, or progressive distortion of the spinal canal; such events are rare, however. Complete lesions tend to remain complete; partial lesions usually show some improvement. If partial lesions progress, the problem most probably relates to significant external compression or vascular compromise rather than central hemorrhagic necrosis; these lesions must be evaluated vigorously for the existence of a surgically remedial lesion.

Cooling, irrigation, and the administration of dimethylsulfoxide, noradrenalin antagonists, barbiturates, etc., used in laboratory settings have no convincing effect in the clinical setting. Glucocorticoids and endogenous opiate antagonists, as mentioned earlier, may be of some value; but even this is not clear. The prognosis for severe myelopathy secondary to spinal injury is truly grim at our present level of sophistication. We can only look to those centers engaged actively in spinal cord injury research to provide the basis for rational new concepts for the management of spinal cord injury deserving of controlled clinical trials.

References

1. Alexander E Jr: Posterior fusions of the cervical spine. Clin Neurosurg 28:273–296, 1981.
2. Allen BL Jr, Ferguson RL, Lehmann TR, O'Brien RP: A mechanistic classification of closed, indirect fractures and dislocations of the lower cervical spine. Spine 7:1–27, 1982.
3. Bohlman HH: Acute fractures and dislocations of the cervical spine: An analysis of three hundred hospitalized patients and review of the literature. J Bone Joint Surg [Am] 61A:1119–1142, 1979.
4. Calenoff L, Chessare JW, Rogers LF, Toerge J, Rosen JS: Multiple level spinal injuries: Importance of early recognition. AJR 130:665–669, 1978.
5. Cancelliere M, Montinaro A, Cantisani PL, Armenise B: Surgical treatment of acute cervical fracture-dislocation. J Neurosurg Sci 25:79–83, 1981.
6. Clarke KS, Powell JW: Football helmets and neurotrauma—an epidemiological overview of three seasons. Med Sci Sports Exerc 11:138–145, 1979.
7. Cooper PR, Maravilla KR, Sklar FH, Moody SF, Clark WK: Halo immobilization of cervical spine fractures: Indications and results. J Neurosurg 50:603–610, 1979.
8. Ducker TB, Russo GL, Bellegarrique R, Lucas JT: Complete sensorimotor paralysis after cord injury: Mortality, recovery, and therapeutic implications. J Trauma 19:837–840, 1979.
9. Farber EN, Wolpert SM, Scott RM, Belkin SC, Carter BL: Computed tomography of spinal fractures. J Comput Assist Tomogr 3:657–661, 1979.
10. Foley MJ, Lee C, Calenoff L, Hendrix RW, Cerullo LJ: Radiologic evaluation of cervical spine fusion. AJR 138:79–89, 1982.
11. Gehweiler JA Jr, Clark WM, Schaaf RE, Powers B, Miller MD: Cervical spine trauma: The common combined conditions. Radiology 130:77–86, 1979.
12. Gonsalves CG, Hudson AR, Horsey WJ, Tucker WS: Computed tomography of the spine and spinal cord. Comput Tomogr 2:279–293, 1978.
13. Harris P, Karmi MZ, McClemont E, Matlhoko D, Paul KS: The prognosis of patients sustaining severe cervical spine injury (C2–C7 inclusive). Paraplegia 18:324–330, 1980.
14. Heiden JS, Weiss MH: Cervical spine injuries with and without neurological deficit: Part I. Contemp Neurosurg 2(12):1–6, 1980.
15. Heiden JS, Weiss MH: Cervical spine injuries with and without neurological deficit: Part II. Contemp Neurosurg 2(13):1–8, 1980.
16. Heiden JS, Weiss MH, Rosenberg AW, Apuzzo MLJ, Kurze

T: Management of cervical spinal cord trauma in Southern California. J Neurosurg, 43:732–736, 1975.
17. Johnson RM, Hart DL, Simmons EF, Ramsby GR, Southwick WO: Cervical orthoses: A study comparing their effectiveness in restricting cervical motion in normal subjects. J Bone Joint Surg [Am] 59A:332–339, 1977.
18. Kostuik JP: Judications for the use of the halo immobilization. Clin Orthop 154:46–50, 1981.
19. Maravilla KR, Cooper PR, Sklar FH: The influence of thin-section tomography on the treatment of cervical spine injuries. Radiology 127:131–139, 1978.
20. Murray GC, Persellin RH: Cervical fracture complicating ankylosing spondylitis: A report of eight cases and review of the literature. Am J Med 70:1033–1041, 1981.
21. Norrell H: The treatment of unstable fractures and dislocations. Clin Neurosurg 25:193–208, 1978.
22. Norrell H: The early management of spinal injuries. Clin Neurosurg 27:385–400, 1980.
23. Riggins RS, Kraus JF: The risk of neurologic damage with fractures of the vertebrae. J Trauma 17:126–133, 1977.
24. Schneider RC, Crosby EC, Russo RH, Gosch HH: Traumatic spinal cord syndromes and their management. Clin Neurosurg 20:424–492, 1972.
25. Shrosbree RD: Neurological sequelae of reduction of fracture dislocations of the cervical spine. Paraplegia 17:212–221, 1979.
26. Sonntag VKH: Management of bilateral locked facets of the cervical spine. Neurosurgery 8:150–152, 1981.
27. Stauffer ES, Kelly EG: Fracture-dislocations of the cervical spine; instability and recurrent deformity following treatment by anterior interbody fusions. J Bone Joint Surg [Am] 59A:45–48, 1977.
28. Surin VV: Fractures of the cervical spine in patients with ankylosing spondylitis. Acta Orthop Scand 51:79–84, 1980.
29. Wagner FC Jr, Chehrazi B: Early decompression and neurological outcome in acute cervical spinal cord injuries. J Neurosurg 56:699–705, 1982.
30. Young JS, Chesire JE, Pierce JA, Vivian JM: Cervical ankylosis with acute spinal cord injury. Paraplegia 15:133–146, 1977.
31. Young JS, Dexter WR: Neurological recovery distal to the zone of injury in 172 cases of closed, traumatic spinal cord injury. Paraplegia 16:39–49, 1978.

213
Psychological Aspects of Whiplash Injury
Henry Berry

The term *whiplash injury* is widely applied to a variety of clinical syndromes that follow a musculoskeletal strain of the neck, the adjacent portion of the vertebral column, and the shoulder region as a result of a vehicular accident. As a mechanism of injury, the term is imprecise, and it can refer to hyperextension-flexion strains or jolts as well as angular or axial forces, with or without interposed blows from a headrest, window, or other structure. Although originally applied to rear end collisions, in practice the term comes to be applied to a wide spectrum of twists, strains, falls, and blows and to collisions from different angles. As a diagnosis, the term is even more general and imprecise and has about the same value as a diagnostic conclusion of neuralgia or madness. The differential diagnosis and precise meaning, when properly considered, should include conditions such as acute cervical musculoskeletal strain, post-traumatic neurosis with anxiety, prominent musculoskeletal symptoms and depression, compensation neurosis, exacerbation or precipitation of symptoms in pre-existing cervical degenerative changes, and frank malingering. To put it in another way, the term *whiplash injury* must be analyzed further in order to have any useful or precise meaning. Recently, the term *soft tissue injury* has come into increasing use by doctors and lawyers involved in accident work, and this term is equally imprecise and objectionable.

Epidemiology

Approximately 15 percent of automobile accidents are rear end collisions, and a clinical picture of acute, short-lived musculoskeletal strain occurs in the majority of patients. A minority of patients go on to a chronic picture that lasts for months to years. This chronic syndrome is poorly understood, is the subject of much misinterpretation, and requires further study from a physical, psychological, and situational point of view. At this stage in our knowledge, we know that the prevalence of the syndrome varies considerably from country to country. It is common in the United States and Canada and is rare in the United Kingdom. The syndrome does not occur in the context of a sport where physical conditioning is good and where motivation for recovery is understandably high. The chronic form of the syndrome is usually seen in patients involved in a personal injury claim against an insuring firm or workers' compensation board, and fashion in diagnosis and prevailing medicolegal practices appear to be important epidemiologic factors. The condition usually subsides when the medicolegal issue is resolved. There is a growing awareness that this chronic form of disability is in most instances, a type of accident neurosis, a medicolegal artifact of our time, arising in susceptible patients and further suggested, aggravated, and perpetuated by well-meaning but misguided lawyers, doctors, and other therapists.

Clinical Syndrome

The clinical picture of acute cervical strain is readily understood. Muscle stiffness and pain develop within hours and may be severe the next morning. There is tenderness and limitation of neck movement, and cervical x-ray films reveal straightening of the vertebral column due to muscle spasm. A number of other symptoms may also be encountered; tingling of the long, ring, and little fingers, apparently on the basis of spasm of the scalene muscles, headaches, nonvertiginous dizziness, blurring of vision, tinnitus, fatigue, and a profound sense of exhaustion occur in a minority of patients. Acute cervical strain is readily distinguished from cervical fracture or dislocation, acute cervical disc herniation, head injury with postconcussive symptoms, vertebrobasilar insufficiency, and benign postural vertigo. In the older age group, where there is pre-existent cervical spondylosis, the accident may have precipitated a recurrent bout of neck pain. Recovery occurs in several days to a few weeks.

Symptoms become chronic in some patients, and careful questioning will disclose a wide range of symptoms.[2] Nervousness, a sense of muscle tension, excitability, and tremulousness are found in about 80 percent of patients, with an equal incidence of neck pain and headache. In some, there is no neck pain as such but an altered sensation of the head being too heavy for the neck, and a sense of pulling, tightness, or clicking of the neck is present. Fatigue, loss of interest and libido, poor memory, numbness of the hands, dizziness, sudden episodes of weakness, faintness, nervousness, and palpitation, and symptoms of blurring of vision, hand weakness, and tinnitus are encountered in a minority of patients. In the anxious person who is prone to nervousness, depression, and muscle tension symptoms, these chronic symptoms develop and persist as part of a post-traumatic anxiety state. In the hypochondriacal or neurasthenic patient, headache, nervousness, forgetfulness, worry, fatigue, and pain and tension about the neck and shoulders will persist. The angry, embittered, or demanding patient becomes preoccupied with symptoms and discomforts in the region of the former strain, as well as with other bodily sensations and with a quest for justice and compensation. Interference with work and other activity and financial difficulties may also contribute to the development of the chronic syndrome. Overconcern and overtreatment by the attending physician, confusion in diagnosis, and unnecessary restriction of activities, coupled with the patient's knowledge of the liability of the other driver and insurance company, an awareness of the financial settlements that can be obtained (a motivation for financial gain and opportunity), and the promptings of an overzealous counsel, may all too readily foster a concern with trivial symptoms and lead to exaggeration and disability. The neurological examination in the chronic state is usually entirely normal; in my experience, a functional (nonorganic) type of weakness or sensory loss is seen in the upper limb in about 10 percent of patients and limited neck movement in about 10 percent.[2] Cervical x-ray films are also negative or reveal changes in keeping with the patient's age. Psychiatric assessment reveals features of chronic anxiety in the majority of patients, with superimposed acute episodic exacerbations and with obvious hysterical behavior in a few.[2] Malingering can be suspected when there is an obvious discrepancy in findings such as the presence of pain and limitation of movement on formal examination but its absence when the patient is distracted. Exaggeration and overreaction are common in such patients while litigation is pending.

Evidence for a Psychological Basis

As in other syndromes of altered or disturbed behavior, the argument on behalf of the role of psychological and social factors in the chronic whiplash disability syndrome is based upon a combination of positive and negative evidence. In my experience, careful assessment of the emotional state and life situation will usually reveal the findings of emotional symptoms and significant stresses within the marital, familial, financial, or vocational areas. Although depression and anxiety can be secondary to genuine pain from an undiagnosed physical cause or illness, repeated examinations do not reveal any significant physical abnormalities. Experimental studies in animals have been extrapolated to humans to indicate chronic changes, but these, as well as the diagnosis of soft tissue injuries with chronic changes, have not been confirmed histologically at the time of operation or postmortem examination.

Direct evidence of motivation in human behavior as a causative factor is difficult to demonstrate. It is recognizable, however, that acute neck strains commonly occur in the course of body contact and other sports activities and do not pass into a chronic phase of disablement. The chronic syndrome is also not seen in the context of a demolition derby, where hundreds of whiplash injuries may be witnessed in one evening of this car-crashing sport.[10] Although physical conditioning may play a role, these observations suggest that motivation is an important influence in the development of the chronic condition. Studies in medical sociology provide information on illness behavior,[9] and it is known that illness behavior is altered when there is an opportunity for blame, for financial gain, or for increased dependency or helplessness. It is also recognized that the natural history of conditions involving pain and disability is altered by the availability of insurance disability schemes and workmen's compensation acts.[1,7] Exaggeration and simulation are recognized by medical and legal authorities as a provable basis of symptoms and disability in a significant number of patients, although there is a natural reluctance to make such a diagnosis.[3,4,8,11]

Factors That Perpetuate Symptoms

A neurotic predisposition or a previous history of anxiety, depression, or other emotional difficulties may result in delayed recovery or chronic disability on the basis of a genuine emotional disturbance. Residual anger toward the offending driver, a sense of grievance or unfairness about the event, a tendency to blame one's life failures upon others, as well as character traits of laziness, irresponsibility, and opportunism, will all contribute to the development of an accident or compensation neurosis in which exaggeration is prominent. Iatrogenic influences such as excessive caution and undue restriction of activity by the physician, the suggestion that symptoms may be prolonged and that permanent injury has occurred, recourse to unnecessary and painful investigations, excessive physiotherapy and chiropractic treatment, and prolonged work absence will all contribute to the development and persistence of a chronic disablement syndrome. It must be recognized that illness behavior is influenced by others and by external events. Counsel can at times be seen to become actively involved in the assessment and management of their clients, and by focusing their client's attention upon relatively minor symptoms and arranging for additional specialist attention and investigation, counsel can prolong the condition. The prospect of returning to an unsatisfactory or boring job, stresses within a marriage or family, financial difficulty, and other illness and health problems unrelated to the accident may all affect the patient's sense of well-being and ability to tolerate minor residual discomforts, and these factors can impair motivation for recovery. Confusion and delay in diagnosis, conflicting opinions, and statements that suggest that there has been permanent injury to the nerves, vertebral bodies, or spinal cord, or that a certain type of work must be permanently avoided, may serve to perpetuate symptoms and limit recovery.

Management

In the usual acute form of injury, the patient should be reassured that a sprain has occurred and that this should subside completely. The patient should be warned that the neck may be stiff and painful on the day after the accident but that this is not serious and will gradually subside. Analgesics and mild sedation may be helpful, and the patient should be encouraged to continue at work and with his or her usual activities as much as possible. The value of physiotherapy and various forms of cervical immobilization is not clearly established. A therapeutic collar in some patients appears to perpetuate the problem and is best avoided.[6]

As in any other form of actual or suspected accident neurosis, management of the patient with chronic disablement is logically based upon a 10-point assessment of factors in causation and perpetuation, as noted in Table 213-1. The history of the accident must be taken in detail, as this helps to define the mechanical forces involved and the possibility of an undiscovered physical basis for the symptoms. Severe angular forces may result in fracture or significant disc injury, whereas the usual hyperextension-flexion strain does not lead to any permanent changes. A clear recognition of the physical diagnosis will place the degree and duration of symptoms and expected disability in better perspective and permit a more accurate assessment of the patient's difficulties. Psychological trauma may be understandably severe in some forms of injury but is transient and relatively mild in the ordinary rear end collision. Pain and suffering following

TABLE 213-1 Emotional Disturbances following Trauma; A Schema of the Evaluation of Factors in Causation and Perpetuation

1. Nature of trauma (physical, psychological)
2. Physical diagnosis
3. Extent of physical treatment, complications, suffering
4. Emotional symptoms and psychiatric illness
5. Underlying personality, attitudes, motivation
6. Situational stresses (familial, marital, financial, work)
7. Iatrogenic (diagnosis, investigations, treatments, restrictions)
8. Effects of litigation
9. Motivation for gain or blame
10. Degree of exaggeration and simulation

such a collision are usually short-lived and, except in the vulnerable patient, do not lead to a significant emotional disturbance. When a genuine emotional disturbance along with muscle tension symptoms does develop, management becomes that of the treatment of an anxiety state with muscle tension symptoms. Explanation as to the nature of the symptoms, reassurance, and medication to diminish anxiety and depression are required. Physiotherapy has usually been tried without effect in such patients, but relaxation therapy and training may prove helpful. Most patients with significant emotional symptoms do not require formal psychiatric treatment, although antidepressant medication along with a degree of support and explanation may be helpful. In my experience, the degree of emotional disturbance serves as a useful index of the genuineness of the disability, and significant emotional symptoms are absent in patients in whom exaggeration or simulation are prominent. Underlying personality characteristics, feelings of anger and vengefulness, poor work motivation, irresponsibility, poor social and work adjustment, and drug or alcohol dependency may all contribute to the development of chronic disability. Situational stresses before and after the accident, with family or marital difficulty, business failure, financial problems, and disagreeable or unsatisfactory work arrangements, will serve to perpetuate symptoms and ailing. Iatrogenic factors have already been commented upon and must be considered in evaluating the causative factors in the individual patient. It is appropriate to inquire as to the stress of repeated examinations by different specialists, the effects of dealing with lawyers and legal assessments, and apprehension over possible appearance at trial, as these may represent major and recurring sources of emotional distress to the patient. Some patients readily admit a strong sense of anger and blame toward the other driver, and this may be the dominant emotion that underlies the anxiety and muscle tension symptoms or the exaggeration of symptoms and disability. Motivation for gain is difficult to assess but can usually be deduced from the overall clinical picture and assessment of individual causative factors. Evidence of exaggeration and simulation can be considered as an indirect indicator of a striving for secondary gain. Exaggeration during history taking and findings and reactions of a functional or nonorganic type should be looked for; weakness, tenderness, and limited movement may be found on formal examination but may be absent when the patient is distracted, dressing, or performing other acts. The writings of earlier authors dealing with accident neurosis contain detailed descriptions of various examination procedures that would detect simulation and functional findings with respect to weakness, sensory loss, and alterations of movement.[3] When motivation for financial gain or invalidism is strong, the physician can do little except avoid iatrogenic contribution. The physician should assert satisfactory physical health and urge an early settlement of the accident claim. The prognosis is considerably influenced by the causative factors that have contributed to the development of the chronic syndrome. Those patients disabled by genuine emotional symptoms usually improve with the passage of time; in compensation neurosis, where motivation for gain or blame is strong, patients fail to improve or become worse up until the time that the medicolegal issue is resolved.[5]

References

1. Bailey P: Injuries and disorders of the nervous system following railway and allied accidents, in Petersen F, Haines WS, Webster RW (eds): *Legal Medicine and Toxicology*, 2d ed. Philadelphia, Saunders, 1923.
2. Berry H: Psychological aspects of chronic neck pain following hyperextension-flexion strains of the neck, in Morley TP (ed): *Current Controversies in Neurosurgery*. Philadelphia, Saunders, 1976, pp 51–61.
3. Collie J: *Malingering and Feigned Sickness*, 2d ed. London, Arnold, 1917.
4. Collie J: *Fraud in Medico-Legal Practice*. London, Arnold, 1932.
5. Culpan R, Taylor C: Psychiatric disorders following road traffic and industrial injuries. Aust NZ J Psychiatry 7:32–39, 1973.
6. Eastwood WJ, Jefferson G: Discussion on fractures and dislocation of cervical vertebrae. Proc R Soc Med 33:651–660, 1940.
7. Huddleson JH: *Accidents, Neuroses and Compensation*. Baltimore, Williams & Wilkins, 1932.
8. Lawton F: A judicial view of traumatic neurosis. Med Leg J 47:6–17, 1979.
9. Mechanic D: Response factors in illness: The study of illness behavior. Soc Psychiatry 1:11–20, 1966.
10. Melville PH: Research in car crashing. Can Med Assoc J 89:275, 1963.
11. Reed JL: Disorders of conscious awareness: Compensation neurosis and Munchausen syndrome. Br J Hosp Med 19:314–321, 1978.

214
Cervical Traction
Albert B. Butler

The primary aim of therapy in the treatment of the patient with acute spinal cord injury is that of decompression of the spinal cord by restoring the normal sagittal diameter of the spinal canal. This is particularly important in patients sustaining incomplete lesions of the cervical spinal cord where the neurological deficit is found to be increasing. Restoration of the spinal canal to a nearly normal anatomical position accomplishes relief of spinal cord compression by displaced bone and may also alleviate pain and motor dysfunction by reducing nerve root compression resulting from tension on the nerve root as it exits through the intervertebral foramen between the dislocated vertebrae. Even when there is complete cord transection, cervical traction may benefit the patient not only by reducing pain, but also by restoring motor function mediated by cervical roots immediately above the level of the fracture-dislocation and cord transection. Although early operative intervention has enjoyed some popularity in the treatment of acute cervical fractures, the use of skeletal traction in the acute and longer-term management of selected cervical spine injuries remains a very safe and easily used method of reducing the fracture and maintaining the spinal canal in the best possible anatomical position.

Historically, earlier methods utilized wires or hooks anchored to the skull. Neubeiser devised a means of cervical traction in which modified fish hooks were surgically placed under the zygomatic arches, a method still used occasionally in instances where infections of the scalp or skull injuries contraindicate the use of skull tongs. The inherent disadvantage of this method of traction is the necessary anatomical placement of the hook in a position such that the plane of traction is anterior to that of the cervical articulations. Hoen, and 4 years later, Zorn, introduced a method of inserting wires extradurally through burr holes in the skull in order to place traction on the cervical vertebrae. This technique, however, also caused a number of complications, particularly those associated with epidural placement of the wires where undetected perforation of the dura occasionally resulted in CSF leakage, hemorrhage, and meningitis. Although these earlier methods were effective in achieving satisfactory cervical traction, their use had the disadvantage of requiring the placement of wires and zygomatic hooks, which required an often extensive and time-consuming operative procedure.

At about the same period of time, the introduction of skeletal tongs by Crutchfield provided a safe, effective, and easily used method of achieving similar aims.[1] The original Crutchfield tongs, the basic design of which has been maintained through subsequent modifications, were conceived and designed with the basic principle of ice tongs in mind. The earlier Crutchfield tongs utilized a pointed conical pin for insertion into the drilled hole in the skull and were occasionally responsible for dural perforation, CSF leakage, meningitis, and penetration of the brain. These complications were generally the end result of a sequence of events that started with the presence of a pointed end of the conical pin and then loosening of the pins secondary to necrosis of the skull resulting from prolonged pressure. This problem required frequent tightening of the instrument to compensate for loosening of the pin, which often resulted in perforation of the pointed pin through the inner table of the skull and adjacent dura. Later models of the Crutchfield tong were modified to use blunted cylindrical pins rather than the older pins with sharper points. They also incorporated a "squeeze" and "hook" principle in their design.[2] The "squeeze" was accomplished by the same cross-armed mechanism employed in the older tongs, while the "hook" principle was achieved by adding auxiliary screws to the articulated cylindrical pins so that with turning of the screws counterclockwise, the points of the pins could be directed medially upward away from the inner table of the skull. Variations on the basic design of Crutchfield tongs were also introduced by Cone, Barton, and Vinke. These tongs were designed to avoid the complications of penetration through the inner table of the skull and of sudden tong dislocation from the skull with prolonged usage or while using heavy weights. The tongs designed by Vinke, in particular, addressed the problem of tong release by incorporating an interlocking device between the inner and outer tables of the skull, thus more effectively securing the tong and minimizing the incidence of premature release.[5] Their application, however, usually required moving the patient to the operating room in order to assure proper insertion. The tongs of Cone, Barton, and Vinke have the particular advantage of a lower incidence of complications when compared with the earlier Crutchfield tongs. On the other hand, these tongs have the disadvantage that their width, projecting beyond the lateral limits of the skull, limits the extent to which a patient can be turned in order to avoid pressure necrosis of the scalp. The narrow profile of the Crutchfield tongs and the resultant lack of projection beyond the lateral limits of the head avoid this problem.

Methods of Cervical Traction

Halter cervical traction, although most widely used in the conservative management of cervical radiculopathy secondary to herniated disc or spondylosis, may also be used quite effectively in the acute management of cervical spine fractures. The use of cervical halter traction in the conservative management of cervical radiculopathy requires attention to several factors that significantly influence the effectiveness of this form of therapy for both the comfort of the patient and the relief of nerve root compression. For example, the effective use of halter traction requires attention to the equal distribution of pull of the sling between the chin and occiput for patient comfort. Precise adjustment of the traction cord through the pulleys and positioning of the occipital and chin straps are pursued with the patient's comfort and implementation of the correct axis of pull relative to the axis of the spine as the desirable end points.

Once the sling has been comfortably positioned, the following routine has been found to be most satisfactory for inhospital cervical traction. In most adults, the amount of weight used should range between 8 and 12 lb depending on the patient's size and, in particular, the muscular development of the neck. Lesser weights may be required initially in younger patients or those with a particularly thin neck. As weight is added to the pulley, it is important to make sure that the traction cord is positioned such that the line of force will be that of a straight line corresponding to a line through the axis of the spine. Traction is usually applied without interruption for a period of 2 h and then released for another hour. Traction is again reapplied for an additional 2 h and thus, on and off, throughout the waking hours. The apparatus should be disconnected at night while the patient is sleeping. During the initial 48 h of traction, the weight used may cause additional neck pain due to muscle and ligament stretching. This may be alleviated by the use of diazepam and the application of a heating pad to the neck. Although in many instances dramatic pain relief may occur early in the course of traction, it is usually considered best to continue this regimen for at least 7 to 10 days. During this time, the patient frequently requests longer periods of time in traction, especially if pain relief is readily apparent. Because of the potential for considerable irritation of the skin and resultant noncompliance, traction for periods longer than 2 h should not be used. The patient's comfort in traction may be aided by the application of foam pads to the inner surfaces of the sling that contact the skin. A small pillow placed under the lower part of the neck may also enhance patient comfort, particularly in the earlier days of cervical traction when neck pain may be increased.

Halter cervical traction, although most effectively used in a controlled hospital environment, may also be used at home. Halter traction kits, which may be purchased for use at home, include those that may be attached to the bed or used with the patient in the sitting position by placing the pulley over a door. The weight, in each instance, is usually provided by adding water to a calibrated bag. Although these methods of cervical traction are of benefit, they do suffer from the problems of patient compliance and discomfort related to inappropriate use of the appliance. Greater benefit from the use of these appliances can be expected when the physician is thoroughly aware of the directions for setting up the apparatus and discusses these in detail with the patient prior to its use. Additionally, if the patient is able to maintain close contact with the physician, simple adjustments in the setting up of the appliance may be discussed over the telephone and thus enhance the comfort and effectiveness of the halter cervical traction device at home.

Use of halter cervical traction in the treatment of acute spinal cord injuries must be considered only as a temporary measure, the benefits of which are its ready availability and ease of application in an emergency situation. This method, however, does not permit the use of heavier weights without causing great discomfort to the patient. In a situation where a patient may be uncooperative, or frankly combative, the possibility of easy removal of the halter sling by the patient contraindicates its use. The use of a sling for prolonged periods of time predisposes the patient to pressure sores beneath the chin and the occiput. The wide availability of Gardner-Wells tongs[3] or the University of Virginia modification of these tongs[4] (see below) should, in most instances, eliminate the need for halter cervical traction in the emergency treatment of acute spinal cord injury.

The newest generation of skeletal tongs, and probably

those currently in widest use, were introduced by Gardner in 1973.[3] The Gardner-Wells tongs were designed for emergency application, and they can be applied safely under antiseptic rather than aseptic conditions. The spring-loaded pin design and tilting of the pins in the direction of pull ensures a firm, prolonged grasp of the skull, limited penetration of the outer table of the skull beyond that attained within the first 24 h, and capacity to readily tolerate at least 65 lb or more of traction. The significant advantages of the newer tongs over earlier skull tongs include eliminating the need for shaving or incising the scalp and drilling holes in the skull. The further advantages of immediate application in the emergency room and ease of prolonged use are tempered somewhat by the disadvantage of the width of the tongs and a fixed interpin distance. The considerable extension of the lateral mass of these tongs interferes with the necessary turning of the patient and nursing care, while the fixed distance between the innermost extension of the pins does not allow use of these tongs on younger patients in the pediatric age group. Modified skull tongs recently developed at the University of Virginia combine the advantages of the Gardner-Wells tongs—those of ease of application and increased weight-handling capacity—with newer features allowing greater patient mobility and use in younger patients.[4] The University of Virginia skull tongs are low-profile tongs that may be used for emergency and short-term traction as well as for longer periods of time, tolerating up to as high as 90 lb without tong dislocation. The narrow-profile design allows the ease of turning possible with Crutchfield tongs, and the capacity to adjust interpin distance permits application of these tongs to skulls of different biparietal diameters.

Technique of Tong Application

Using either the Gardner-Wells or University of Virginia tongs, the hair and scalp should be cleansed with an antiseptic solution; hair removal is optional. The pins are positioned just above the pinna of the ear on both sides along an imaginary line drawn between the tip of the mastoid process and the external auditory canal. The location for pin insertion, usually just anterior to the highest portion of the pinna, is infiltrated with generous quantities of local anesthetic. Care should be taken to obtain x-ray films of the skull, particularly in the area of pin placement, to assess the possibility of bony abnormality at that site. Once the pins have been advanced into position and secured in place using the spring-loaded point of the Gardner-Wells tong or the combination of the central locking device and the locking knob of the University of Virginia tongs, appropriate weight is attached to a rope passed through the pulley device. The line of pull should in most instances be directed along a line passing through the cervical articulations and continuing through the point of attachment of the skull tongs. Maintaining this line of pull through the rope to the pulley device ensures the appropriate application of forces through intact ligaments, which, in combination with appropriate amounts of weight, adequately reduces the fracture and, with longer-term use, maintains the fracture site in a nearly normal anatomical position.

The amount of weight necessary to accomplish adequate reduction varies considerably, but as a rule less weight is required for higher cervical injuries and fractures demonstrating minor dislocation and ligament disruption. Initially, 5 lb of weight should be applied for each cervical vertebra above the level of fracture dislocation. The amount of weight initially applied, however, may require some adjustment as indicated by the position and stability of the fracture shown on the initial roentgenograms. In instances of highly unstable fractures in the lower cervical area and especially in the upper three cervical levels, the application of excessive weight may rapidly induce excessive distraction and further neural injury. Accordingly, when there is question about instability of a fracture, the initial use of lesser amounts of weight is recommended; the addition of further weight is considered only after repeat lateral x-ray films. In these and other instances, the use of the C-arm fluoroscope can significantly reduce the time required to make these judgments and permit more frequent and accurate assessment of the response to progressive increases in weight. However, the application of tongs and weight should not be delayed if a fluoroscopy unit is not readily available. For adequate maintenance of alignment, from 10 to 20 lb is usually required, the precise amount of weight being dictated by the level and stability of the fracture and the ease or difficulty of initial fracture reduction.

The rapidity with which reduction should be carried out, as well as the amount of weight required for reduction, remains controversial. Crutchfield employed the method of applying lesser amounts of weights over a longer period of time, whereas more recently others have advocated the more rapid reduction of the fracture dislocation using relatively greater amounts of weight. Certainly, in conditions of rapidly deteriorating neurological function associated with an obvious fracture-dislocation, reduction should be achieved as soon as possible. The advantages of immediate application of Gardner-Wells or University of Virginia tongs and the capacity for better and more frequent radiographic examination of the spine, especially with C-arm fluoroscopy, now considerably enhance the safety of rapid reduction. In utilizing the rapid-reduction technique, however, extreme caution must be exercised in the reduction of highly unstable fractures, particularly in the upper cervical spine.

Traction in the Management of Acute Spinal Injuries

While the above-described principles of tong application, addition of weight, and reduction of cervical fractures apply in most instances, particular fractures may require placement of the skull tongs anterior or posterior to the usual position of pin application in order to effect appropriate hyperextension or hyperflexion and may require variations in the timing or amount of weight application.

The treatment of fractures involving the upper cervical vertebrae, including odontoid fractures, is usually accomplished with pin placement and line of traction directed toward maintaining the spine in the neutral position. Weights varying from 5 to 10 lb, and occasionally up to 20 lb, may be all that is required to maintain adequate stabilization of these fractures for longer-term care. More recently, the use of halo immobilization or early operative stabilization has been advocated and offers much in terms of more rapid mobilization of the patient. Fractures involving the C2 or C3 vertebra, or a hangman's fracture, usually result from hyperextension injuries. Although some fractures of this type are simple, many are associated with major ligamentous disruption and bony fracture. Here, x-ray examination during reduction minimizes the likelihood of distraction and potentially lethal injury of the spinal cord. As with C1 and odontoid fractures, C2-3 fractures, although adequately treated by external stabilization for 6 to 8 weeks in traction, are now being treated more frequently with halo stabilization or early surgical stabilization.

Hyperextension injuries associated with rupture of the anterior longitudinal ligament, and thus an increased likelihood of instability, may require skull traction in which the patient's neck is maintained in a degree of hyperflexion obtained by positioning the pins somewhat posterior to the usual placement just above the pinna of the ear. The newer generation of tongs facilitate repositioning of the tongs as required by changes seen at the fracture site on repeat x-ray examination after initial placement and application of weight.

Bilateral, and especially unilateral, facet dislocations present difficult problems in management when using skull tong traction. Here, the goal is to reduce the dislocation as rapidly and completely as possible. Following the intravenous administration of diazepam or another muscle relaxant, traction is applied along the longitudinal axis of the cervical spine, the neck being maintained in a neutral position. While gradually adding weight, the clinician must repeatedly assess the patient's neurological status and utilize frequent radiographic examinations either by repeating lateral x-ray films or C-arm fluoroscopy in order to assess the effect of traction. As the nature of the injury causing facet dislocation is usually that of hyperflexion, the plane of traction required to aid reduction of the dislocation may require placing the neck in slight flexion by positioning the tongs posterior to the usual point of placement. Although manipulation of the spine has been advocated by some to aid in reduction of a unilateral or bilateral facet dislocation, it is generally considered safer to gradually increase the amounts of weight, up to as high as 75 lb, and then undertake operative reduction if restoration of the spinal canal to a nearly normal anteroposterior diameter cannot be attained within a period of 2 to 3 h. The rapidity with which weight is added in attempting to reduce the dislocation is directly related to patient discomfort and reduction of the dislocation as determined by x-ray examination after each increase in weight.

Long-term treatment of cervical fracture dislocations using skull traction usually requires 6 to 8 weeks of immobilization. Longer periods of time, up to 12 weeks, may be required for adequate healing of upper cervical fractures. In summary, although general guidelines have been provided for the treatment of various types of cervical fractures using cervical traction, it must be stressed that each case must be individualized. The initial plan for application of tongs and use of weight is dictated by the patient's neurological status and the severity of the fracture-dislocation, and thus its stability, as visualized on x-ray examination. Subsequent changes in the traction measurement are likewise mandated by changes in these same parameters.

Cervical Traction in Foster or Striker Frame at Operation

The ability to maintain adequate cervical traction prior to and during operation on the patient who is in frames of this type requires considerable attention. The use of C-arm fluoroscopy while turning the patient to the position required for a particular operative approach may considerably increase the safety of repositioning during this critical period of time. Similarly, the use of intraoperative fluoroscopy permits the more judicious addition or reduction of weights. When the patient is anesthetized particular care must be taken that the addition of weight does not cause distraction of a highly unstable fracture, a condition which is readily apparent when continuous fluoroscopy is being utilized.

References

1. Crutchfield WG: Skeletal traction for dislocation of the cervical spine: Report of a case. South Surgeon 2:156–159, 1933.
2. Crutchfield WG: Redesigned Crutchfield skull tongs: Technical note describing the combined "squeeze" and "hook" principle. J Neurosurg 25:656–657, 1966.
3. Gardner WJ: The principle of spring-loaded points for cervical traction: Technical note. J Neurosurg 39:543–544, 1973.
4. Rimel RW, Butler AB, Winn HR, Park TS, Tyson GW, Jane JA: Modified skull tongs for cervical traction: Technical note. J Neurosurg 55:848–849, 1981.
5. Vinke TH: A skull-traction apparatus. J Bone Joint Surg [Am] 30A:522–524, 1948.

215

Halo Immobilization of Cervical Spine Injuries

William T. Hardaker, Jr.

The halo was first introduced as a traction apparatus in 1959 by Perry and Nickel in the management of severe cervical instability secondary to poliomyelitis.[9] Over the ensuing years, its advantages over previous traction systems have been well recognized. The early halo systems have undergone significant modifications to expand its role in the management of a variety of spinal disorders, including traumatic instability.[1,2,4-10,12,14] Cervical stability can be achieved by attaching the halo to a body jacket by means of metal uprights. The halo-jacket system offers distinct advantages over previous traction and stabilization systems.

Crutchfield, Vinke, Barton, and Gardner-Wells tongs are effective in applying traction in only one direction. This limits these devices primarily to longitudinal traction. Complex cervical fractures and fracture-dislocations often require multiplanar forces to achieve satisfactory realignment of the spine and decompression of the neural tube. Some of the tong systems require skin incisions as well as cranial drill holes to achieve fixation. Motion occurs at the tong-skull junction, thus increasing the possibility for infection. In addition, calipers alone do not provide rigid external fixation for the unstable spine, necessitating prolonged bed rest until stabilization is achieved. This form of treatment increases the likelihood of thrombophlebitis, muscle atrophy, and demineralization, as well as renal and pulmonary complications. Hospitalization and rehabilitation time can be lengthy.

The plaster of paris Minerva jacket has been the traditional method of obtaining external fixation of the unstable cervical spine. However, even the most expertly applied Minerva jacket allows movement of the cervical spine. The jacket is heavy, hot, and uncomfortable, and adjustment of head or neck position is impossible once the jacket is applied. Radiological evaluation of the spine is difficult through the plaster of paris jacket. If surgery were to be performed, a small window could be cut in the cast. These windows provide, at best, barely adequate exposure for the surgeon.

The halo-plastic jacket system has distinct advantages over tongs as a traction device and over the Minerva jacket as a fixation device. The halo pins are applied directly to the skull without the need of a skin incision or predrilling. No motion occurs at the pin penetration site, thus allowing the patient less discomfort and providing a decreased potential for infection. The device can be applied quickly and, once in place, allows precise three-dimensional positioning of the cervical spine.

To allow rigid external fixation of the cervical spine, the halo can be mounted on a plastic vest. The halo-jacket allows the patient to sit, stand, and walk, thus decreasing the time of recumbency and its potential complications. The time and cost of rehabilitation can be reduced significantly. Adjustable aluminum uprights allow radiological examination of the spine, and surgical access is very satisfactory. In case of cardiac arrest the anterior portion of the vest can be removed quickly.

Indications

Over the past 20 years, the indications for halo traction–fixation have expanded to include a variety of unstable cervical spinal lesions, including traumatic, congenital, neoplastic, and arthritic conditions.[1,2,4-10,12,14] The indications for the halo include:

A. Reduction of cervical
  1. Fractures
  2. Fracture-dislocations
  3. Subluxations
B. Realignment of thoracic kyphosis and scoliosis using
  1. Halo-femoral traction
  2. Halo-pelvic traction
C. External fixation of the unstable cervical spine in
  1. Severe muscle paralysis
  2. Fracture-dislocation
  3. Rheumatoid arthritis
  4. Primary or metastatic neoplastic disease
  5. Extensive laminectomy
  6. Following arthrodesis
  7. Osteomyelitis

Description

Stabilization of the cervical spine is achieved in the halo-jacket system by externally fixing the skull in reference to the chest. The system consists of three major components: the halo ring and pins, the plastic vest, and the adjustable metallic uprights that connect the halo ring to the jacket.

The stainless steel halo ring is available in various sizes and contains an occipital offset to allow clearance for high cervical fusions (Fig. 215-1). The halo is attached to the skull above the eyes and ears in four quadrants using pins that penetrate the skin and outer table (Fig. 215-2). The pins have sharp points and require no skin incision on introduction. The pins rapidly flare into broad shoulders, thus

1723

minimizing penetration and increasing the contact area (Fig. 215-3). The pins and the channels within the halo ring are threaded to firmly fix the halo-pin assembly to the skull. Additional pin channels are available in each of the four quadrants to allow for alternate pin placement if the pins should migrate or loosen or induce inflammation. The pins are firmly locked to the halo by hexagonal nuts on either side of the halo ring (Fig. 215-1).

The halo ring and the jacket are connected to one another by aluminum turnbuckles on each side. The turnbuckles are adjustable to provide variable traction, flexion, extension, or cervical translation (Fig. 215-1).

The polyethylene body jacket is available in multiple sizes to permit optimum fit for the dissipation of forces and thus minimize pressure on the soft tissues. To further reduce the pressure on the soft tissues, the jacket is lined with synthetic lamb's wool (Fig. 215-1). The jacket allows full use of the arms, and the anterior compartment can be rapidly removed to gain direct access to the chest in case of cardiac arrest. Once in place, the system firmly fixes the cervical spine, allowing less than 4 percent of normal motion in flexion-extension and lateral bending, and less than 1 percent of normal rotation.[3]

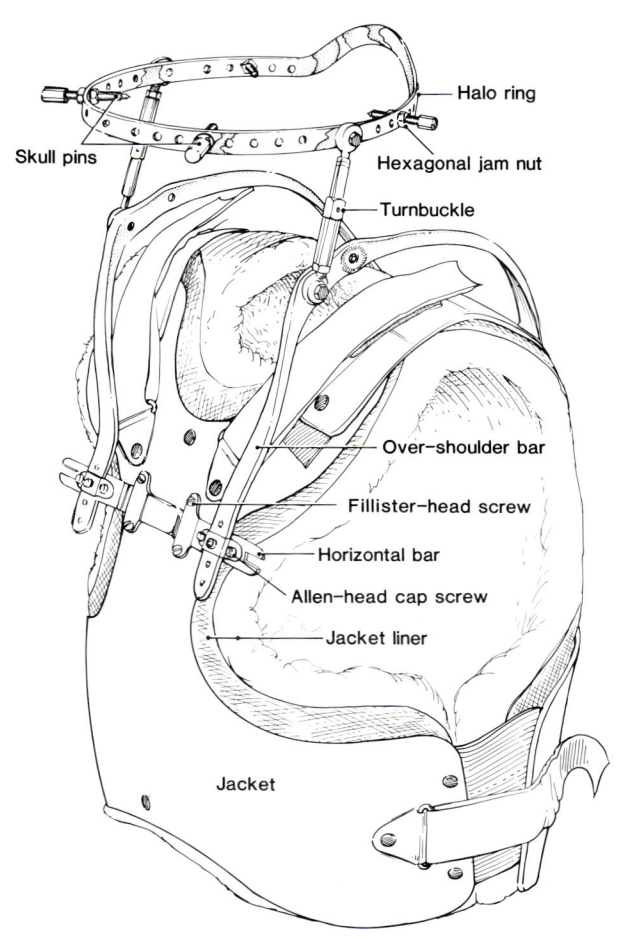

Figure 215-1 Components of the halo-jacket system.

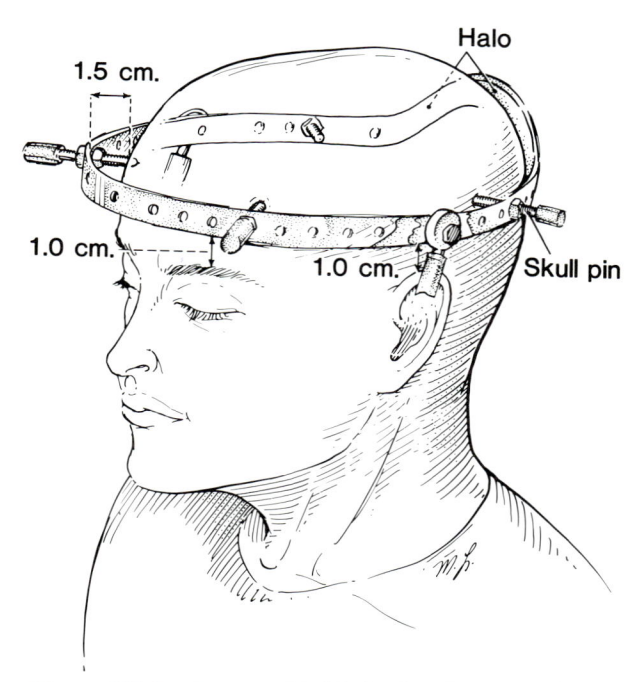

Figure 215-2 An assembled halo ring demonstrating correct pin placement.

Materials and Methods

The materials necessary for application of the halo-jacket system include:

1. Halo ring (stainless steel), available in multiple sizes.
2. Skull pins (stainless steel), available in two sizes.
3. Hexagonal nuts (stainless steel), to fix and lock the skull pins to the halo ring.
4. Turnbuckles (aluminum), to connect the halo ring to the jacket. They are radiolucent and adjustable to provide varying amounts of traction, and are available in various lengths.
5. Shoulder bars (aluminum), to allow the turnbuckle assembly to be fixed to the jacket. They are radiolucent and are available in multiple sizes to correspond with varying jacket sizes.
6. Jacket bars (stainless steel), to mount the shoulder bars to the jacket. Horizontal slots within the jacket bars allow for multiple adjustments.
7. Allen head screws, to hold the jacket bars to the shoulder bars.
8. Jacket (polyethylene), lined with synthetic lamb's wool.
9. Tools necessary for halo-jacket application (Fig. 215-4): two torque screwdrivers, two open-ended wrenches, and one Allen wrench.

Application

Patient Premedication and Positioning

On most occasions, a mild sedative and analgesic are helpful in relieving the anxiety and pain associated with halo application. In addition, the physician should thoroughly explain

Halo Immobilization of Cervical Spine Injuries

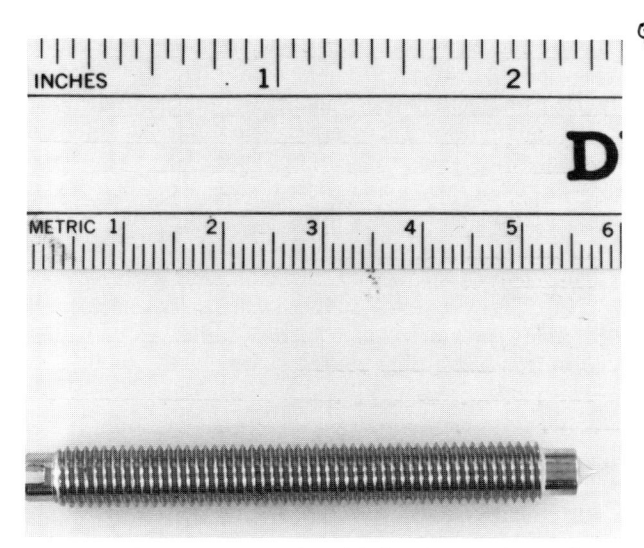

Figure 215-3 The halo pin with its sharp point and broad shoulder.

the procedure to the patient so that the patient will know what to expect.

The patient is positioned on a stretcher or bed with the head beyond the edge. The head is supported on a thin wooden board. Traditionally, the halo is held in position by the first assistant and the second assistant assists the surgeon with the materials. However, with a specially designed positioning fixture (Fig. 215-5), the entire procedure can be performed more effectively and with less assistance. The positioning fixture not only supports the head but also securely holds the halo in the correct position during application. Such a device obviates the need for positioning pins and the wooden board and allows the surgeon to apply the halo with only one assistant.

Halo and Jacket Selection

Halo rings are generally available in five sizes. Approximately 1 to 1½ cm of halo-to-skull circumferential clearance should be present, with the halo positioned just below the maximum diameter of the skull. When correctly placed, the halo is 1 cm above the eyebrows anteriorly and 1 cm above

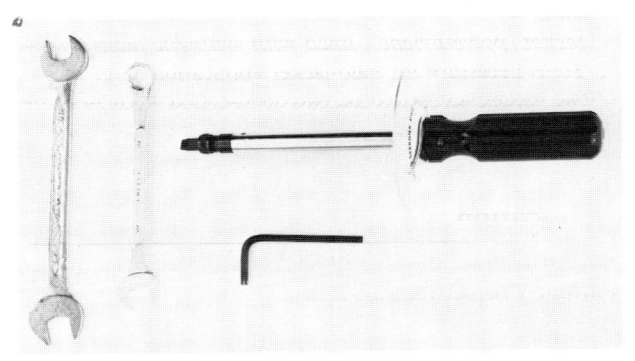

Figure 215-4 Tools required for the application of the halo-jacket system.

the pinnae of the ears laterally (Fig. 215-2). The polyethylene jacket is available in six sizes, based on chest circumference. Intermediate chest sizes are accommodated by adjustment of the Velcro straps connecting the anterior and posterior shells.

Skin Preparation and Local Anesthesia

The hair is clipped and shaved in a bandlike pattern just above and posterior to each ear in preparation for the posterior pins. Some surgeons have, in the past, placed the anterior pins within the hairline. This is not routinely recommended, however. These areas are characterized by relatively thinner and less supportive bone. In addition, the temporalis muscle must be penetrated, leading to patient discomfort while chewing and also a greater chance for skin and muscle necrosis and infection. Finally, if these sites are selected, there is a danger of directly injuring the superficial temporal artery.

The skin is thoroughly scrubbed, and the skin and underlying periosteum at the four pin sites are infiltrated with a 1% lidocaine solution. A trial positioning of the halo is recommended to ensure that the exact sites are well prepared and infiltrated.

Fixation of the Halo Ring

The autoclaved halo ring is held in correct position by the assistant, by positioning plates, or by the halo positioning fixture (Fig. 215-5). If the positioning fixture is employed, the positioning plates and screws and the second assistant will not be needed. With the halo properly centered on the head, the anterior pins are placed in channels overlying sites 1 cm above the lateral third of the eyebrows (Fig. 215-2). The posterior pins are diagonally opposite the anterior pins in channels approximately 1.5 cm posterior to the ears. Hexagonal lock nuts should be loosely placed on each pin between the ring and the skull prior to advancing the pin.

The skull pins are advanced by hand until just above the skin. The anterior and the diagonally opposite posterior pins are simultaneously tightened by hand. The surgeon and the assistant then simultaneously tighten each diametrically opposite pin using the torque screwdriver to a maximum torque of 6 kg. Alternate tightening of the halo pins is necessary to prevent displacement of the halo into an asymmetric position. The pins with their sharp points and broad shoulders are designed to penetrate the periosteum and impact into the outer table but not to penetrate into the inner surface. When the halo is in place, at or near the maximum diameter of the skull, the pins impact at 90 degrees to the skull surface, thus providing maximum fixation in order to prevent superior migration of the halo when traction is applied.

Once the pins have been placed, the inner hexagonal nuts are tightened using the open-ended wrench. An additional outer hexagonal nut is placed on each pin. These are tightened to further lock the halo firmly to the pins. Plastic caps are then placed on each pin to prevent impalement in sheets or bed clothing.

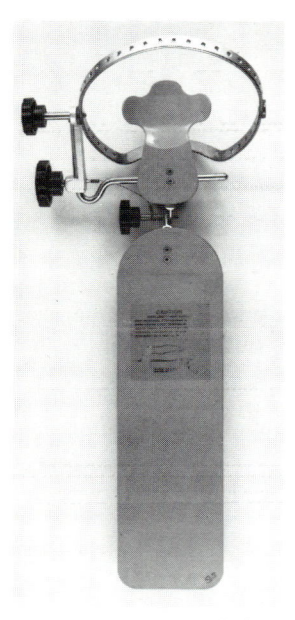

Figure 215-5 The halo positioning fixture.

Attachment of Traction or Jacket

The cervical spine may be placed in longitudinal traction using a traction hoop attached to a rope, weight, and pulley system. Alternatively, the surgeon may proceed immediately to fixation of the cervical spine by connecting the halo superstructure to a polyethylene jacket. When this is the case, the posterior half of the jacket is first gently placed under the patient. With the head supported, the anterior portion of the jacket is placed and secured to the posterior shell using Velcro straps. The turnbuckles are then adjusted to achieve the desired cervical translation and flexion or extension. The hexagonal open-ended screws are then placed to securely fix the turnbuckles to both the halo and the shoulder bars. The hexagonal open-end wrenches and the Allen wrenches should then be securely taped to the anterior aspect of the jacket. This assures their immediate availability should the anterior shell need to be removed in case of cardiac arrest.

X-Ray Views

Supine anteroposterior and lateral x-ray films of the cervical spine are then taken to assure that the desired cervical alignment has been achieved.

After Care

The hexagonal lock nuts should be loosened and the pins tightened using the torque screwdriver daily for 3 days. Continued tightening after 72 h is not recommended. The pin sites should be cleansed with peroxide several times daily to remove any coagulum at the pin-skin interface. Following pin irrigation, povidone-iodine solution should be applied with a cotton-tipped applicator to each pin site. The pins are left undisturbed otherwise. No surgical dressings or paste antiseptic solutions should be applied at the pin sites.

A pin may need to be replaced because of loosening or significant inflammation or actual infection of the pin site. Patients often detect a loose pin because of a "clicking" sensation at that site. Loosening can occur secondary to pressure osteonecrosis or from infection itself. Regardless, the involved pins should not be advanced further. To replace a loose pin, the new sterile pin is first placed in an adjacent channel in the halo and tightened before removal of the loose pin.

Complications

Complications associated with the halo apparatus relate primarily to the skull pins. In most cases, these potential complications can be prevented by strict adherence to the correct techniques of halo application and meticulous daily care of the pin sites.

Superior migration of the halo can occur if the halo is not placed below the maximum diameter of the skull. When properly placed, the pins impact the skull at right angles in thick cortical bone. Traction forces are then directed into a thickening bony mass rather than into a thinning, obliquely sloped cortical margin.

Skin necrosis can occur if the halo ring is allowed to contact the scalp or the ears. A circumferential clearance of 1 cm will allow room for edema following pin placement and will prevent contact with the scalp by the ring.

Infection of the pin sites is probably the most common problem associated with the halo device. Some pin drainage and mild inflammation is to be expected, but active infection requires early recognition and proper management or premature removal of the halo may be required.

Many pin problems can be avoided by correct application techniques. Great care should be taken to prevent tension on the skin and surrounding soft tissues at the time of pin insertion. Tension often leads to tissue ischemia and eventual necrosis. Tissue necrosis then provides the medium for bacterial infection. Loose pins similarly promote inflammation of surrounding tissues and should be replaced promptly. Properly placed pins still require meticulous daily care to prevent later infection. Peroxide debridement is routinely necessary to remove coagulum around the pins and to prevent the tracks from sealing and trapping bacteria within.

Soft tissue infection that does not respond to local care and antibiotics requires removal of the involved pin after first inserting a sterile fifth pin in a nearby channel. Local wound care will usually clear the infection from the involved pin track. Deep infection, involving bone, requires soft tissue debridement as well as removal of the underlying bony sequestrum. Following adequate debridement, these wounds can likewise be expected to heal. Brain abscesses, involving pins that have penetrated the inner table, have been described.[13] This is indeed a more serious complication and requires early diagnosis and aggressive management.

Other complications encountered with the halo apparatus relate to its use as a traction device. The halo is a powerful traction instrument capable of causing serious neurological damage.[6,11] Excessive traction can lead to cranial nerve, nerve root, and spinal cord injury. The sixth cranial nerve is quite sensitive to traction and is frequently affected early in the setting of improper traction.[4] Accordingly, lateral rectus function should be assessed periodically in all patients in halo traction.

References

1. Houtkin S, Levine DB: The halo yoke: A simplified device for attachment of the halo to a body cast. J Bone Joint Surg [Am] 54-A:881–883, 1972.
2. James JIP: Fracture dislocation of cervical spine. J R Coll Surg Edinb 5:232–233, 1960.
3. Johnson RM, Hart DL, Simmons EF, Ramsby GR, Southwick WO: Cervical orthoses: A study comparing their effectiveness in restricting cervical motion in normal subjects. J Bone Joint Surg [Am] 59-A:332–339, 1977.
4. Keim HA: Spinal stabilization following trauma. Clin Orthop 81:53, 1971.
5. Kopits SE, Steingass MH: Experience with the "halo-cast" in small children. Surg Clin North Am 50:935–943, 1970.
6. Nickel VL, Perry J, Garrett A, Heppenstall M: The halo: A spinal skeletal traction fixation device. J Bone Joint Surg [Am] 50-A:1400–1409, 1968.
7. O'Brien JP, Yau ACMC, Smith TK, Hodgson AR: Halo pelvic traction. J Bone Joint Surg [Br] 53-B:217–229, 1971.
8. Perry J: The halo in spinal abnormalities: Practical factors and avoidance of complications. Orthop Clin North Am 3:69–80, 1972.
9. Perry J, Nickel VL: Total cervical-spine fusion for neck paralysis. J Bone Joint Surg [Am] 41-A:37–60, 1959.
10. Prolo DJ, Runnels JB, Jameson RM: The injured cervical spine: Immediate and long-term immobilization with the halo. JAMA 224:591–594, 1973.
11. Ransford AO, Manning CWSF: Complications of halo-pelvic distraction for scoliosis. J Bone Joint Surg [Br] 57-B:131–137, 1975.
12. Thompson H: The "halo" traction apparatus: A method of external splinting of the cervical spine after injury. J Bone Joint Surg [Br] 44-B:655–661, 1962.
13. Victor DI, Bresnan MJ, Keller RB: Brain abscess complicating the use of halo traction. J Bone Joint Surg [Am] 55-A:635–639, 1973.
14. Zwerling MT, Riggins RS: Use of the halo apparatus in acute injuries of the cervical spine. Surg Gynecol Obstet 138:189–193, 1974.

216
Anterior Approach in Cervical Spine Injuries

Edward L. Seljeskog

As a general rule, the indications for surgery in cervical spine injury chiefly relate to two factors, decompression and spinal stabilization. Even these two general indicators have their relative merits, disadvantages, advocates, and antagonists, but a decision for surgical intervention must be weighed rather carefully. Beyond the specific considerations of the proposed surgery, including approaches and techniques, are those factors relating to coexisting conditions or injuries that must be taken into special account. In this regard, one should not risk aggravating a life-threatening situation by additional surgery, and under these circumstances cervical decompression or fusion should be postponed until the patient's condition permits its undertaking without major risk. Most importantly in this context are problems of respiratory insufficiency, especially those that are compounded by paralysis of the chest wall muscles of respiration. Nothing can be so disturbing to the surgeon who successfully completes a nonemergent cervical spine decompression or fusion, only to have it complicated in the postoperative period with respiratory failure. As a consequence, assessment of respiratory function is a necessary part of the preoperative evaluation of any cervical cord injury, and if respiratory function is significantly impaired, nonemergent surgery should be deferred. Many surgeons would consider a total vital capacity of less than 700 to 800 ml a contraindication to a nonemergent operation.

On the other hand, an ascending neurological level or progressive neurological dysfunction becomes a paramount factor, especially in the presence of an incomplete spinal cord injury. Under these circumstances decompressive surgery must often be considered under less than optimal circumstances. It must be emphasized, however, that except under unusual circumstances, treatment of life-threatening conditions is at the first level of priority in the patient's overall management.

In considering the specific arguments for surgical intervention in cervical spine injury, the need for decompression has traditionally been considered as a primary indicator. Experience has shown, however, that in most cases spinal canal compromise by bony elements is largely relieved during the course of traction and fracture reduction, obviating the need for decompression. Despite this usual radiographic improvement following fracture reduction, it is prudent in all cases of persisting neurological loss to further assess the need for decompression and to be absolutely assured that there is not continued spinal canal encroachment by retained bone fragments, disc material, or hematoma. In this regard, standard x-ray views and tomograms are useful, but of more value is a myelographic study of the area. This is best achieved with the patient in traction, in the prone position, and via a lateral C2 approach. Utilization of a mobile or portable C-arm fluoroscopy unit aids in the procedure and avoids the necessity of discontinuing traction and transferring the patient. Most importantly, however, the technique optimally visualizes the ventral aspect of the spinal canal, the usual site of retained bone or disc material (Figs. 216-1 and 216-2). Currently, CT scanning, usually with contrast CSF enhancement to precisely visualize the dural sac and spinal cord, is rapidly replacing traditional myelography in the assessment of these injuries. To be emphasized is the fact that these types of studies usually demonstrate relief of compromise of the spinal canal and spinal cord, with a free flow of the contrast material past the injury site (Fig. 216-3).

Anterior versus Posterior Approach

In the event that one demonstrates a persisting problem of disc or fracture-fragment herniation, either by tomograms, myelography, or CT scanning, decompression should then be considered. Depending on the location of the mass effect, an appropriate surgical approach can now be logically

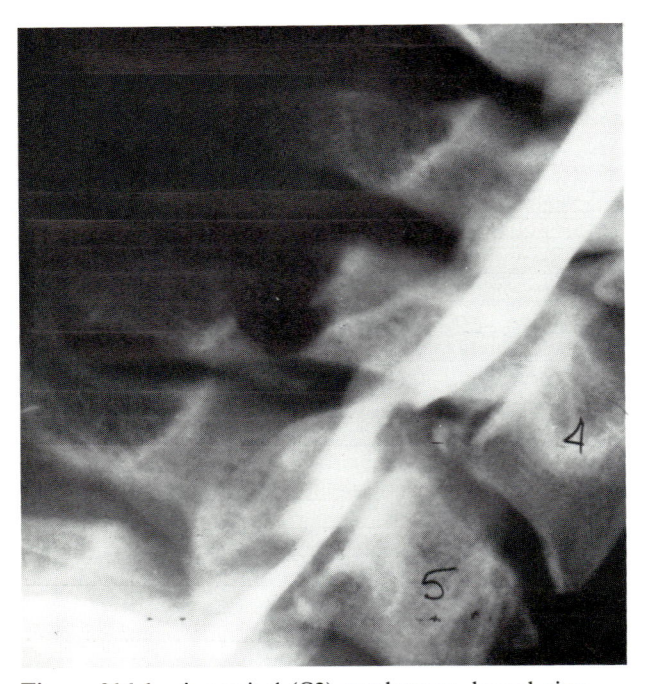

Figure 216-1 A cervical (C2) myelogram, lateral view, demonstrating a C4-5 traumatic central disc herniation.

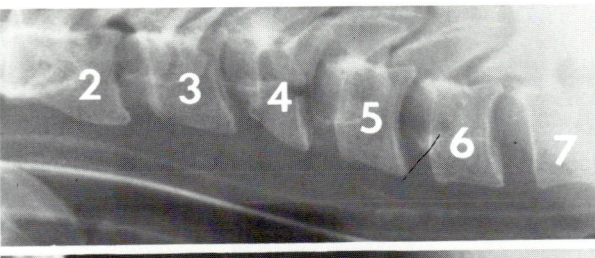

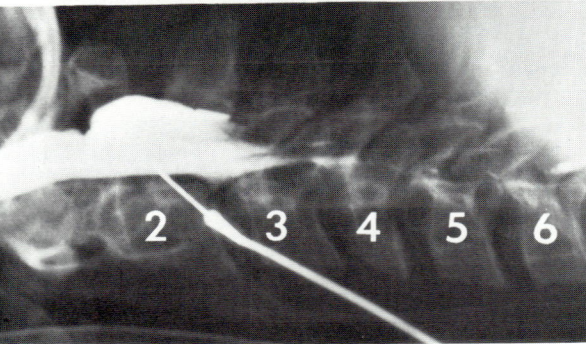

Figure 216-2 *Top:* An admission lateral cervical spine film demonstrating a comminuted fracture of C4. *Bottom:* Cervical myelogram, lateral view, revealing a complete block at the fracture level, secondary to ventral compression by hematoma, fractured bone, and disc material.

planned. Usually the problem is ventral to the spinal cord (Figs. 216-1 and 216-2). Under these circumstances, the preferred procedure is an anterior decompressive approach, either by excising the central portion of the fractured vertebral body or through the disc space if the vertebral bodies are intact. Demonstration of a ventrally located mass, then, creates a strong argument for an anterior approach. Attempted removal of any ventrally located fracture fragments from a posterior or posterolateral cervical approach is difficult and fraught with the potential risk of compounding the spinal cord injury. The need for decompression then becomes an indication for anterior surgery in most cases.

On rare occasion, one identifies cord compression from the posterior, by fractured laminar elements. Under these circumstances the more traditional laminectomy type of decompression becomes the preferred procedure. A second situation in which to consider the posterior approach is that of a significantly widened spinal cord, identified on myelography or CT scanning, reflecting a probable hematomyelia. Often these patients have a neurological level cephalad to their bony injury. Some of these patients will benefit from evacuation of a hematoma and necrotic material from within the spinal cord. However, one should not be erroneously led into a diagnosis of hematomyelia with spinal cord expansion, since it can be mimicked by a ventrally located mass in the spinal canal (Fig. 216-4). Careful scrutiny of both anteroposterior and lateral myelographic views is therefore mandatory. Further development of cervical CT scanning is proving to be of considerable help in the diagnosis and differentiation of this infrequent problem.

Finally, there is the question of whether the immediate and complete spinal cord injury should be considered for decompression when this is accompanied by radiographic evidence of persisting spinal cord compression (Fig. 216-2). The bleak outlook for recovery in virtually all immediate and complete spinal cord injuries is well documented. There is always, however, the anecdotal case of a miraculous change, which often relates to an incomplete initial neurological examination. Despite the irreversibility in the case of the immediate and complete neurological loss, a logical argument can still be made for decompression, in that one may at times be able to retrieve function of an additional adjacent nerve root level by decompression of the cord and removal of the offending intraspinal mass. This, then, seems to be reason enough to consider strongly the relief of persisting spinal cord compression, even in the case of immediate and complete injury, providing the patient's condition otherwise permits.

In summary, the initial, acute management of cervical spinal injury involves an early and complete radiographic assessment of the problem, followed by early and expeditious fracture reduction and realignment of disturbed spinal anatomy. This is followed in most cases, where there is persisting neurological loss, by a myelographic and CT evaluation of the area, to eliminate the possibility of continued spinal cord compression as well as to exclude an intramedullary mass at the injury site. In most cases, following traction and reduction, there is a free flow of contrast material, with only minimal alteration of the dimensions and contours of the spinal cord. As a result, in only a small number of cervical spinal cord injuries are there continuing indications for surgical decompression of the area; if identified this is usually best achieved by the anterior approach.

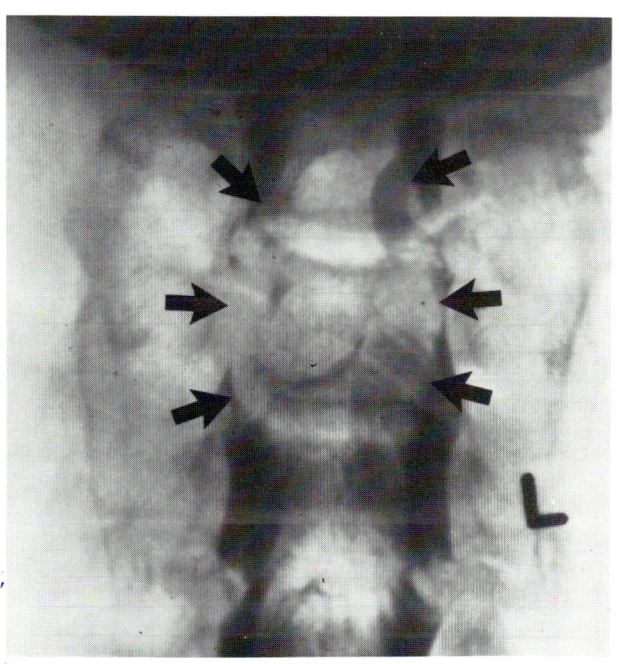

Figure 216-4 An anteroposterior myelographic view, revealing an apparent widening of the spinal cord (*arrows*) secondary to a ventrally located intraspinal mass.

Spinal Stabilization

One next considers the need for surgical stabilization of the area of injury, a decision that can be accomplished in a more leisurely fashion. The fundamental question is whether or not anything is to be gained by operative intervention and fusion. The disadvantages and complications of classical skeletal tong traction immobilization are well documented, including skin breakdown, respiratory problems, phlebitis, and pulmonary embolization, but in addition are the extraordinary costs of prolonged hospital care. With the development of the halo apparatus and halo vest, a very reasonable alternative was developed that avoids many of these problems.[5] Its major advantage relates to permitting much earlier patient mobilization; expedited patient transfer to a rehabilitation ward and earlier hospital discharge are additional benefits.

The halo apparatus has, however, its own disadvantages and complications. Fracture collapse and angulation with kyphosis are not infrequent, but they are potentially avoidable problems. In addition, poor tolerance of the device and local infection are common and bothersome. In the majority of cases, however, there is satisfactory fracture healing and alignment. The real question then becomes whether surgical fusion or stabilization has anything to offer over this now standard external type of immobilization.

In reviewing the experience of many surgeons, internal surgical stabilization and fusion appear to afford some advantage over the external halo technique in that fracture healing is more complete and more solid, with a smaller incidence of pseudarthrosis, fracture collapse, and late kyphosis.[1,2,3,6] It should be noted, however, that even with fusion,

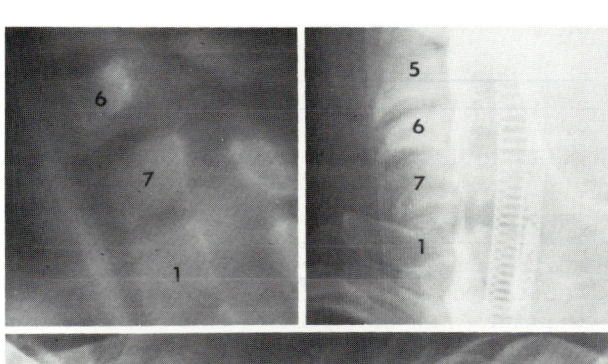

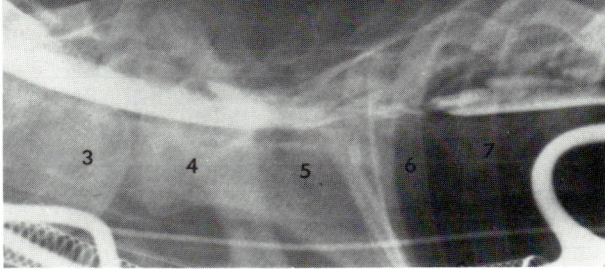

Figure 216-3 *Top left:* An admission lateral cervical spine film reveals a C6–7 fracture-dislocation prior to skeletal traction and fracture reduction. A cervical myelogram in the anteroposterior (*top right*) and lateral (*bottom*) views demonstrates a free flow of contrast material following fracture reduction. Fluoroscopy of the area revealed the small hematomas ventral to the spinal canal to be insignificant.

technical problems are not infrequent and, coupled with less than optimal postfusion immobilization, the potential for fracture collapse and angulation are still of significant concern.

In deciding which types of injuries might benefit most by surgery, the injury with major subluxation through the disc space and with intact adjacent vertebral bodies would seem to be a situation that would particularly be aided by surgical fusion (Fig. 216-5). Spontaneous healing in this type of injury is often fibrous in character, and bony fusion offers the possibility of greater long-term stability for the area. It certainly lessens the chance of pseudarthrosis or fibrous union with instability. In addition, following fusion there appears to be earlier stability, permitting external immobilization to be removed at an earlier date, compared with a group of patients treated only by external methods. One should bear in mind, however, that in major cervical spine injuries, with vertebral body comminution, collapse, and subluxation, one usually does not achieve immediate stability with the anterior technique. This is due to the significant ligamentous disruption and instability at the injury site. This is a major disadvantage of this anterior approach when dealing with this major type of injury. As a consequence, immobilization is often a very necessary part of the patient's postoperative management.

In conclusion, when there are solid and intact adjacent vertebral bodies and where the subluxation is purely through the disc space (Fig. 216-5), healing and stability seem to develop much earlier following anterior fusion, to the point where one can on occasion utilize only a cervical collar or brace postoperatively rather than the halo apparatus. Similarly, earlier discontinuance of external immobilization is common when compared with the group treated only by external methods. Late stability is definitely bettered by the operative intervention. As indicated, however, most major fractures are not immediately stabilized by anterior fusion, even though solid bony healing eventually occurs. In this situation one could consider the possibility that a posterior type of fusion would avoid this difficulty, but early stability, even utilizing rib grafts or other struts, is often difficult or impossible to achieve because of disruption and fracturing of posterior elements in these major injuries. In addition, posterior fusion can result in neurological deterioration as a result of inward displacement of fracture fragments or floating laminae beneath the fusion struts.

Another common injury for which to consider the anterior approach is that of the significantly comminuted cervical fracture, including the teardrop injury, especially when there is no major instability (Fig. 216-6). Here the argument for anterior stabilization and fusion relates to the significant propensity of these fractures for collapse and kyphosis, even with seemingly adequate external immobilization (Fig. 216-7). Certainly a posterior type of fusion would stabilize and prevent subluxation in the area, but with the vertebral body comminution, it would only minimally prevent late collapse and angulation. It is therefore reasonable to consider these patients for an anterior type of fusion, with central excision of the vertebral body fragments and their replacement with a solid block graft, keyed into the two intact adjacent vertebral bodies (Fig. 216-8). Some surgeons have advocated a fibular strut graft, but most prefer the block graft technique that includes the solid cortical bone of the iliac crest. This cortical portion offers significant support to the area and eventually forms a solid fusion (Fig. 216-6). Late fracture collapse should therefore be minimal.

In summary, the decision for operative stabilization in some cases of cervical spine injury is obvious, since the patient has evidence of spinal canal compromise and indications for decompression, usually via an anterior approach. Under these circumstances, placement of a dowel graft or bone block is a companion part of the decompressive procedure. In most cases of cervical cord injury, however, decompression is not required. This permits one to make a more measured decision regarding the merits of surgical stabilization, as opposed to the nonoperative external halo immobilization approach. Since the anterior technique is not technically difficult, it often is the preferred approach, even though in many of the more severely disrupted cases it does not give immediate stability. It has much in its favor when the vertebral bodies are relatively intact, with dislocation through the disc space, in which case a Smith-Robinson or Cloward technique is preferred. Similarly, in most cases where there is disruption and comminution of the vertebral body, typified by the teardrop fracture, a solid argument can be made for an anterior excision of the fracture fragments and a block type of fusion. With appropriate placement of the block graft and an appropriate period of postoperative immobilization, good healing should occur, and in most cases with a minimum of late spinal deformity.

Operative Technique

In the patient with evident spinal instability, the anterior decompression and fusion is carried out with the patient in skeletal traction, best accomplished in a circle bed or Stryker operative turning frame. In cases of significant instability, the patient is intubated under local anesthesia, while

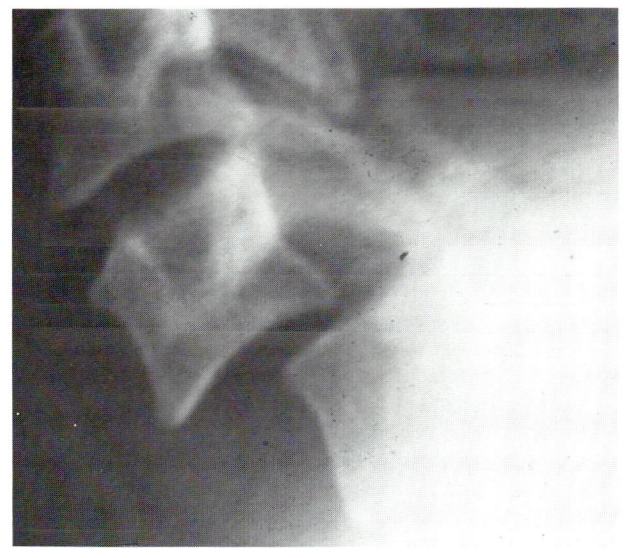

Figure 216-5 A lateral view of the cervical spine with major subluxation through the disc space and minimal involvement of the adjacent vertebral bodies.

Anterior Approach in Cervical Spine Injuries

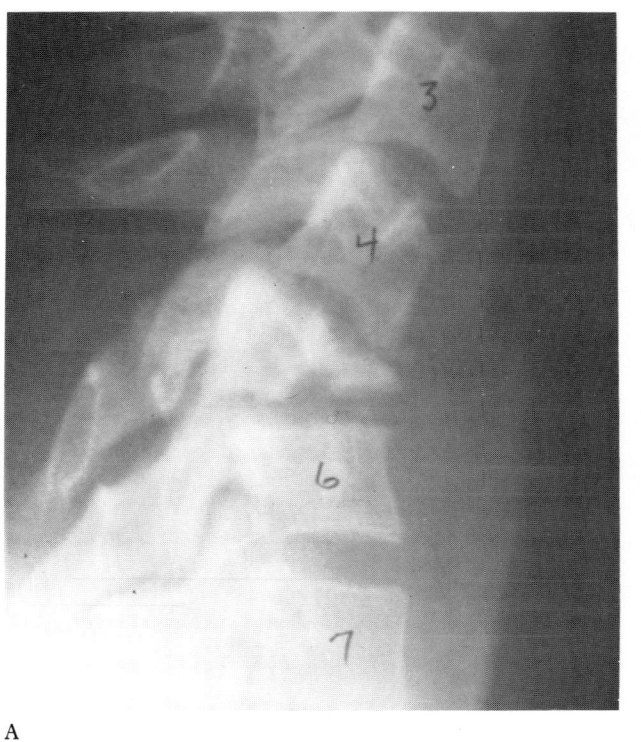

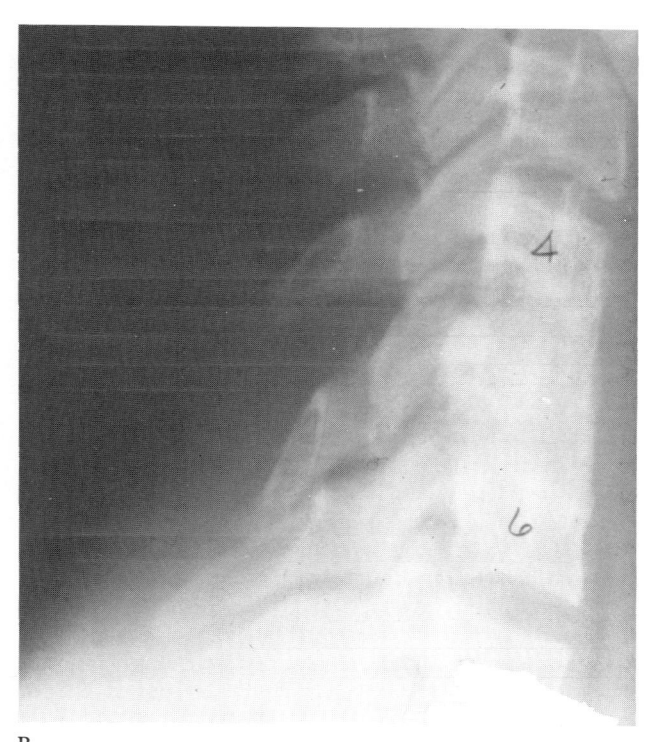

Figure 216-6 *A.* A lateral view of a teardrop fracture involving C5. *B.* A 6-month follow-up view after an anterior block type of fusion. Note the normal alignment and the lack of fracture collapse.

awake and in skeletal traction. This avoids unnecessary manipulation of the neck and cervical spine. In patients who are neurologically intact, or who have a partial spinal cord syndrome, monitoring of spinal cord function utilizing somatosensory evoked techniques is a reasonable adjunct to the procedure.

The patient is positioned with a small roll or pad behind the shoulders to optimize anterior exposure. The head and trunk are slightly elevated above the level of the heart to minimize cervical venous congestion. At the same time, the contralateral iliac crest is prepared and draped into a separate operative field. This permits harvesting of the graft during exposure of the cervical area.

The basic technique is well described by Cloward, Smith and Robinson, and other authors.[2,4,7] The level of the skin incision is varied according to the cervical fusion level, and skin towels are sutured in place to optimize x-ray viewing. In most fracture cases radiographs add little, since the level of injury is very readily identifiable and exposure is adequate. The skin and platysma are sharply incised, and with blunt and sharp dissection a plane is developed medial to the sternocleidomastoid muscle into the retropharyngeal area, avoiding trauma to the carotid arteries, larynx, esophagus, and laryngeal nerves. The longus colli muscle is split and the standard self-retaining retractors are placed, exposing the site of the injury. If the vertebral bodies are intact and in good alignment, a standard exposure through the disc space is accomplished. Direct visualization of the posterior longitudinal ligament is facilitated with vertebral spreading. Retropulsed posterior fracture fragments and disc material are then excised under direct vision. If the posterior longitudinal ligament is disrupted, it is opened further with a small punch for exploration and to remove any additional intraspinal fragments. If the ligament is intact and if one has found a

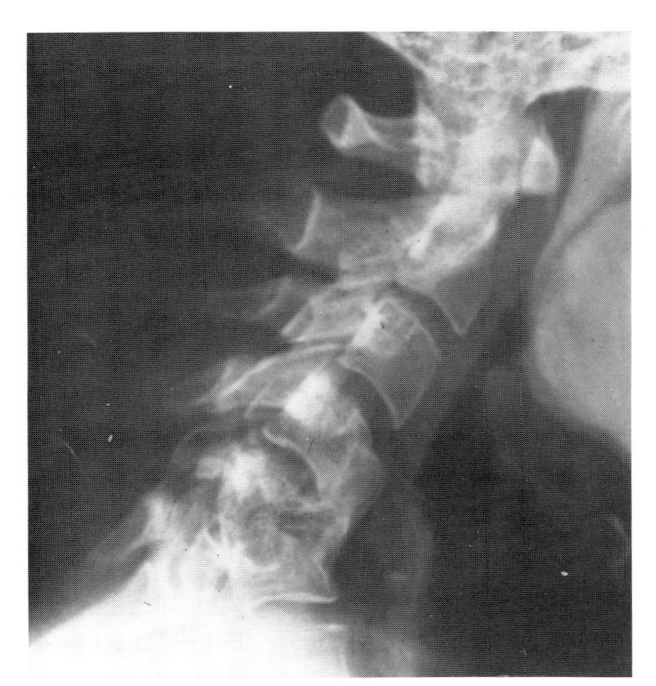

Figure 216-7 A lateral view of a teardrop fracture involving C5, 3 years following injury. Note the significant angulation and collapse.

sufficient explanation for any myelographic or CT abnormality, the ligament is left intact, since it serves as a barrier to inward displacement of the bone graft and its destruction significantly compounds spinal instability. A standard dowel or wedge fusion is then carried out in the manner described by several authors.[2,4,7]

In many operative cases, there is comminution of the vertebral body, necessitating its excision. In this situation, the intervertebral spaces are entered above and below the fractured vertebral body and the discs are carefully removed with curettes and forceps back to the posterior longitudinal ligament. The comminuted vertebral body is then excised in its central portion, leaving the lateral segments of the vertebral body undisturbed (Fig. 216-8). The lateral walls of the created cavity are tapered as one proceeds more deeply down to the posterior longitudinal ligament (Fig. 216-8). This lessens the chance of posterior displacement of the bone graft. Any additional disc material is then removed cephalad and caudad, and the cartilaginous end plates of the adjacent vertebral bodies are curetted away, undercutting the anterior cortical surface to allow a solid, keyed placement of the bone graft into the intact vertebral bodies. A wide exposure of this sort also affords one the opportunity to closely inspect the posterior ligament and to remove any retropulsed disc or bony fragments should decompression be necessary.

Once decompression has been assured, as now visualized directly, attention is directed toward placement of the graft. This has been harvested from the iliac crest, with the surgeon being certain to remove the graft subperiosteally, to allow for some degree of iliac regeneration. The graft is fashioned with tapered ends, and much of the thin cortical bone is removed laterally (Fig. 216-8). Exposure of cancellous bone will enhance healing and fusion; however, one must be certain to leave enough solid cortical crest to assure support. The graft should be fashioned so that it will only fit into the adjacent vertebral bodies with a bit of distraction. This is accomplished with the skeletal tongs and vertebral spreaders. The graft is then gently tapped into place, and ideally it should be snug at this point.

Following placement of the graft and inspection of the carotid artery, larynx, and esophagus, the incision is closed in a routine manner. Approximation of the longus colli muscles will further buttress the bone graft. Drainage is usually not necessary, since bothersome bone bleeding is quieted down with a bit of absorbable gelatin sponge or microfibrillar collagen and with seating of the graft. Depending on the degree of stability following fusion, as noted at the time of surgery, as well as from the preoperative x-ray assessment, the patient is immobilized in a cervical collar or brace (or in cases of significant instability, a halo device) until bony healing begins to occur. Mobilization is now possible immediately following the surgical procedure.

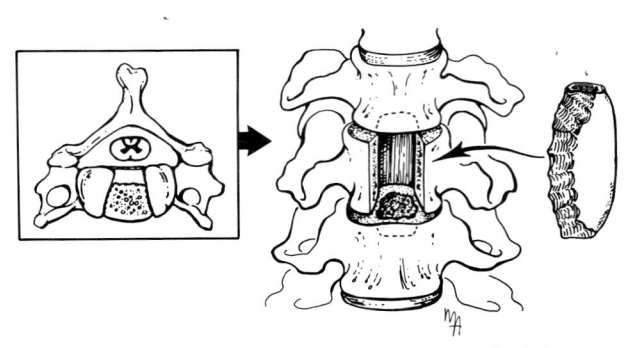

Figure 216-8 The technique of anterior cervical decompression and block graft fusion, particularly useful in the comminuted teardrop type of cervical fracture.

References

1. Braakman R, Penning L: *Injuries of the Cervical Spine.* Amsterdam, Excerpta Medica, 1971, pp 98–120.
2. Cloward RB: Treatment of acute fractures and fracture-dislocations of the cervical spine by vertebral body fusion: A report of 11 cases. J Neurosurg 18:201–209, 1961.
3. Horsey WJ, Hudson AR, Tucker WS: Indications, techniques, and results of anterior cervical fusion after cervical spine injury, in Tator CH (ed): *Early Management of Acute Spinal Cord Injury.* New York, Raven Press, 1982, pp 305–313.
4. Johnson RM, Southwick WO: Surgical approaches to the cervical spine, in Rothman RH, Simeone FA (eds): *The Spine.* Philadelphia, Saunders, 1975, pp 69–133.
5. Nickel VL, Perry J, Garrett A, Heppenstall M: The halo: A spinal skeletal traction fixation device. J Bone Joint Surg [Am] 50A:1400–1409, 1968.
6. Norrell HA: Fractures and dislocations of the spine, in Rothman RH, Simeone FA (eds): *The Spine.* Philadelphia, Saunders, 1975, pp 529–566.
7. Southwick WO, Robinson RA: Surgical approaches to the vertebral bodies in the cervical and lumbar regions. J Bone Joint Surg [Am] 39A:631–644, 1957.

217
Diaphragm Pacing
Ronald F. Young

The ability of electrical stimulation of the phrenic nerve to cause diaphragmatic contraction was described in 1937. Diaphragm pacing (DP) refers to the rhythmic electrical stimulation of the phrenic nerve to cause diaphragmatic contraction and thus respiratory exchange. Pacing is accomplished in humans by implantation of a radio frequency-coupled, battery-powered, phrenic nerve stimulator (see Fig. 217-1).

Indications

Two primary pathological processes produce physiological defects in respiration that may be treated by DP.[1,2] These are (1) malfunction of the respiratory pathways above the location of the phrenic motor neurons at C3-5 and (2) central alveolar hypoventilation. Recently it has been suggested that respiratory failure in certain selected cases of neuromuscular disease may also be treated by diaphragm pacing.[4]

Most patients seen by the neurosurgeon for DP will be in the first category.[5] Such processes as high cervical spinal cord injury, spinal cord tumors, medullary infarctions, bilateral high cervical cordotomy, and syringobulbia or syringomyelia may interfere with connections between the respiratory centers in the brain stem and the phrenic motor neurons, causing respiratory insufficiency. With complete high spinal cord injury due to trauma, the patient is apneic and requires permanent and continuous respiratory support. With partial injuries in the cervicomedullary region, patients may breath normally when awake but become apneic during sleep, the so-called Ondine's curse. If spinal injury or neuromuscular disease occurs at C3-5, damage to the phrenic motor neurons usually renders the phrenic nerve electrically inexcitable. In some cases, however, testing of phrenic nerve electrical function reveals residual electrical excitability, which may be enhanced by DP.[4]

Central alveolar hypoventilation is characterized by cyanosis, polycythemia, cor pulmonale, and often sleep-induced apnea. Ventilatory capacity is normal or near normal in such patients since the pathological process responsible for hypoventilation is a reduced central sensitivity to hypercarbia and hypoxia.[1]

Preoperative Evaluation

Preoperative testing of phrenic nerve and diaphragm function is strongly recommended prior to surgical implantation of a DP system.[3] In patients with some residual voluntary ventilation, fluoroscopic demonstration of a diaphragmatic descent of 5 cm or more confirms that successful diaphragm pacing can be effected. In patients with complete respiratory paralysis or with neuromuscular disease, electrical testing of phrenic nerve–diaphragm function is required.

The phrenic nerve is electrically stimulated in the neck, and conduction velocity to the diaphragm is recorded from surface or needle electrodes.[3,4] Normal conduction time is 8 to 10 ms. Moderate prolongation (12 to 14 ms) is not a contraindication, but marked prolongation or inability to record motor activity from the diaphragm contraindicates DP.

Technique

The DP system is composed of an implanted passive radiofrequency (RF) receiver with an attached cuff electrode and an external battery-powered RF transmitter with antenna (Avery Laboratories, Inc., Farmingdale, N.Y.). Adjustments to the transmitter permit control of respiratory rate, tidal volume, respiratory time, and stimulation threshold. The latter allows a gradually increasing electrical stimulus strength to activate the diaphragm in order to evoke a smooth diaphragmatic contraction and avoid sudden maximal diaphragmatic descent, which may be uncomfortable to the patient and produce poor gas exchange. Additionally the transmitter may be programmed to include respiratory "sighs," which are useful in preventing the atelectasis that may occur with a constant tidal volume.

Until recently the cuff electrode was applied by exposing the phrenic nerve through a small transverse incision in the neck about an inch above the midportion of the clavicle. At this level the phrenic nerve lies beneath the deep cervical fascia and on the anterior surface of the scalenus anticus muscle. Recently Glenn has recommended intrathoracic placement of the electrode for maximal phrenic nerve activation.[1] The cervical electrode placement does not allow stimulation of an accessory root of the phrenic nerve, which often joins the nerve trunk below the level of the clavicle.[2] Formerly, a bipolar stimulating electrode was employed, but a newer and smaller monopolar electrode is recommended to reduce dissection of the phrenic nerve and concomitant nerve injury, which may cause reduced electrical excitability and ineffective DP.[1,2] The RF receiver is implanted in a subcutaneous pocket over the lower chest wall.

Efficacy and Complications

DP is an excellent method of providing ventilatory support and should be almost universally successful in properly selected patients. Several precautions, however, are suggested for patients undergoing chronic DP. For patients with total

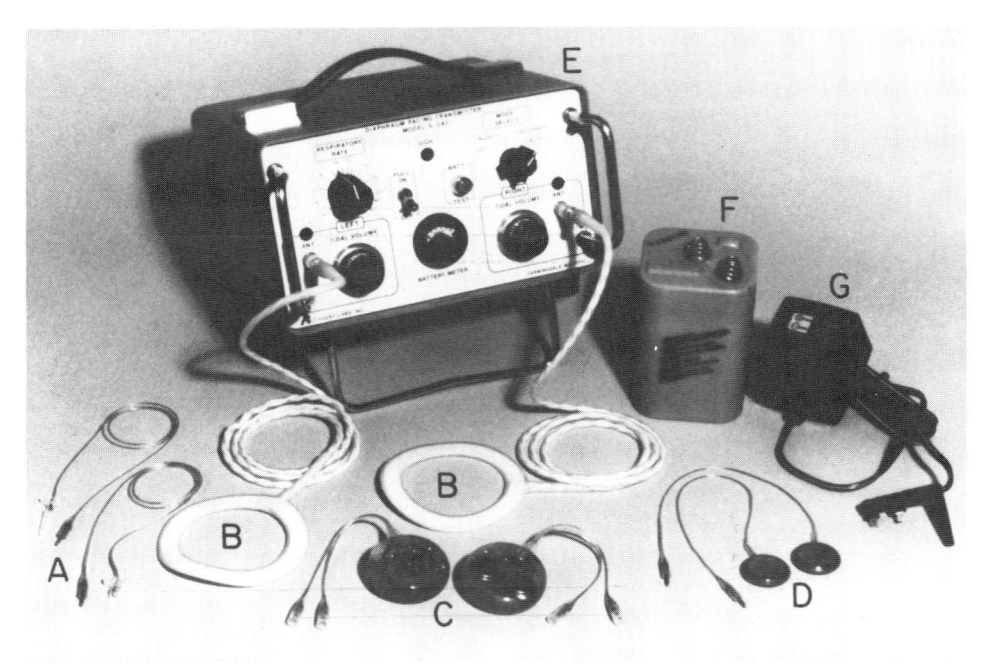

Figure 217-1 Complete apparatus for bilateral electrical stimulation of the phrenic nerves (diaphragm pacing): *A.* Monopolar stimulating electrodes (to be placed on phrenic nerves). *B.* Transmitter antennas. *C.* RF receivers. *D.* Indifferent stimulating electrodes. *E.* Dual-channel stimulator. *F.* Battery for stimulator power supply. *G.* Transformer used to power stimulator from line electricity.

respiratory paralysis a backup system of ventilation should be immediately available at all times, and an apnea monitor is extremely useful in detecting stimulator malfunction. The phrenic nerve and diaphragm can be electrically activated safely for a maximum of 12 h. Subsequently the diaphragm fatigues; thus bilateral implants and alternate side stimulation are required in patients with total ventilatory failure. Although injury to the phrenic nerve may occur at the time of electrode placement, prolonged electrical stimulation alone does not appear to cause nerve injury. Glenn has successfully employed DP for over 10 years in individual patients. Prolonged electrical activation of the diaphragm (over 12 h) will result in permanent irreversible injury to the diaphragmatic muscle with function reduced to less than 20 percent of normal.[2] Excessively high stimulus current strengths and frequencies may also produce diaphragm injury.[2]

Diaphragm pacing may provide gratifying freedom from an external ventilator for patients who are quadriplegic from high cervical spinal cord injuries. DP may obviate the need for permanent tracheostomy and allow the patient to communicate by speaking. It may also provide excellent respiratory assistance for patients with hypoventilation or sleep apnea from a variety of causes. The procedure is easily accomplished surgically and in properly selected patients is effective and reliable.

References

1. Glenn WNL: Diaphragm pacing: Present status. Pace 1:357–370, 1978.
2. Glenn WNL, Hogan JF, Phelps ML: Ventilatory support of the quadriplegic patient with respiratory paralysis by diaphragm pacing. Surg Clin North Am 60:1055–1078, 1980.
3. Lieberman JS, Corkill G, French BN: Phrenic nerve conduction studies in the evaluation of ventilatory problems in patients with cranio-cervical trauma. Surg Neurol 10:205–208, 1978.
4. Richardson RR, Roseman B, Singh N: Diaphragm pacing in spinal muscular atrophy: Case report. Neurosurgery 9:317–319, 1981.
5. Young RF: Diaphragm pacing as an adjunct in respiratory insufficiency. Neurosurgery 2:43–46, 1978.

218
Injuries to the Thoracic and Lumbar Spine

Wesley A. Cook, Jr.
William T. Hardaker, Jr.

Seventy percent of the injuries to the spinal cord result from trauma, whereas disease (neoplastic, neurological, or congenital) accounts for only 30 percent.[20,21] Trauma secondary to motor vehicle accidents is responsible for more than one-half of the total number of spinal cord injuries, which approaches 10,000 cases per year. The death toll from motor vehicle accidents in the United States is about 50,000 per year, and slightly more than one-half of these accidents are related to alcohol. In perspective the loss of life during a single year from motor vehicle accidents nearly equals the number of Americans lost during the entire Vietnam conflict.

The significance of these tragic figures is that the majority of deaths and major injuries from motor vehicle accidents are preventable. To diminish this highway tragedy, society must learn to dissociate drinking and driving. Furthermore, greater utilization must be made of existing restraint systems while driving. It has been demonstrated that serious and fatal injuries can be reduced 65 to 80 percent by employing restraint systems.[4,31] Despite such conclusive information, the insurance industry estimates that only 14 percent of the driving population regularly use lap-shoulder restraints.

Types of Thoracolumbar Injuries

The mobility of the thoracolumbar spine (T10-L5) is considerably greater than that of the thoracic spine (T1-9) because of the stability imparted to the latter by the rib cage and sternum. This mobility contributes to the more frequent occurrence of injury at the thoracolumbar junction.

Fractures of the thoracolumbar spine may be divided into three groups: wedge fractures, burst fractures, and fracture-dislocations.[14,17] The wedge fracture is the result of axial compression and flexion (Fig. 218-1). Mild wedge fractures are generally stable, whereas those with greater than 50 percent anterior wedging are potentially unstable. Instability in this case refers to the progressive flexion-angulation of the spine that may occur with the passage of time. Severe wedge fractures are often associated with fractures of the laminae, pedicles, or facets.

Burst fractures result from axial compression and are characterized by a decrease in the height of the entire circumference of the vertebral body (Fig. 218-2). Severe burst fractures are often associated with posterior element fractures, and the anteroposterior roentgenogram will demonstrate widening of the interpedicular distance (Fig. 218-3). Miller et al. have noted that dural lacerations are commonly associated with severe burst fractures.[26]

Posterior protrusion of the vertebral body into the spinal canal may occur with either severe burst or wedge fractures. In our series of patients, computed tomography has consistently demonstrated that the bone fragments compressing the dural contents arise from the upper portion of the vertebral body (Fig. 218-4). Similar findings have also been noted by Jelsma and associates.[17] This pattern should be recognized and considered when planning surgical decompression for these lesions.

When rotation is added to the force producing a fracture-dislocation, a so-called "slice fracture" often results. In this injury a "slice" of the lower vertebra remains attached to the upper displaced vertebra. The slice may be composed of a single bone fragment or multiple fragments attached to the annulus.[19]

A distinctive distraction injury of the thoracolumbar spine results from extreme flexion and is most often associated with lap belt injuries.[11,30,33] This type of injury is most likely to occur when the lap belt is worn above the iliac crests or when the belt slides up during the accident. The characteristics of this injury are listed in Table 218-1 and are shown in Fig. 218-5. A clinical analysis of this injury by Smith and Kaufer suggests that the axis for flexion is shifted

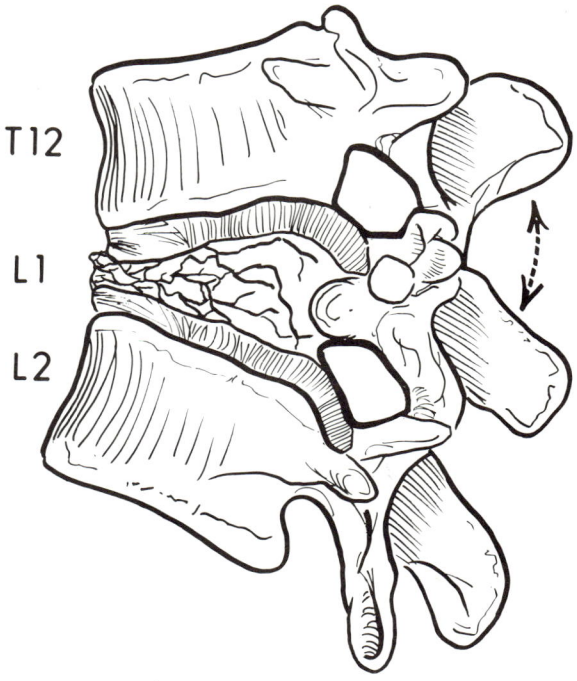

Figure 218-1 Wedge fracture of the first lumbar vertebra resulting from axial compression and flexion.

TABLE 218-1 Characteristics of Distraction Injuries

Disruption and separation of posterior elements, either ligamentous or osseous
Little, if any, anterior wedging of the vertebral body
Little, if any, anterior or lateral displacement
L1, L2, and L3 most commonly involved
Patient usually neurologically intact unless displacement occurs
Intra-abdominal injuries common

---

from the center of the nucleus pulposus in the normal situation to a point between the seat belt and the abdominal wall.[30] With the axis for flexion at the latter point, the spine is then subjected to a distractive force. It would also appear that an extreme degree of flexion is required to produce this type of injury, since only 1 in 24 cases involved the driver of the vehicle, the remaining cases being passengers. Presumably, the steering wheel prevented the required amount of flexion.

When only the posterior ligaments or posterior osseous elements are disrupted, the patient is usually neurologically intact (Fig. 218-5A). Less frequently, displacement of the vertebral bodies will occur, and then neurological damage can be expected. (Fig. 218-5B). Incomplete neurological deficits are unusual with this lesion. Patients are either intact or demonstrate a complete neurological deficit.

When fracture does occur, it is of the variety described by Chance, that is, a horizontal splitting of the spinous process and neural arch with extension of the fracture into the vertebral body (Fig. 218-5C).[1] Not all of these fractures are grossly unstable, and many will heal satisfactorily with a hyperextension brace. The more severe examples require posterior fusion augmented by compression instrumentation.

Abdominal wall ecchymoses will be noted in many patients with lap belt injuries, although their absence does not exclude this type of injury. Intra-abdominal injuries are common with lap belt injuries and should not be overlooked.

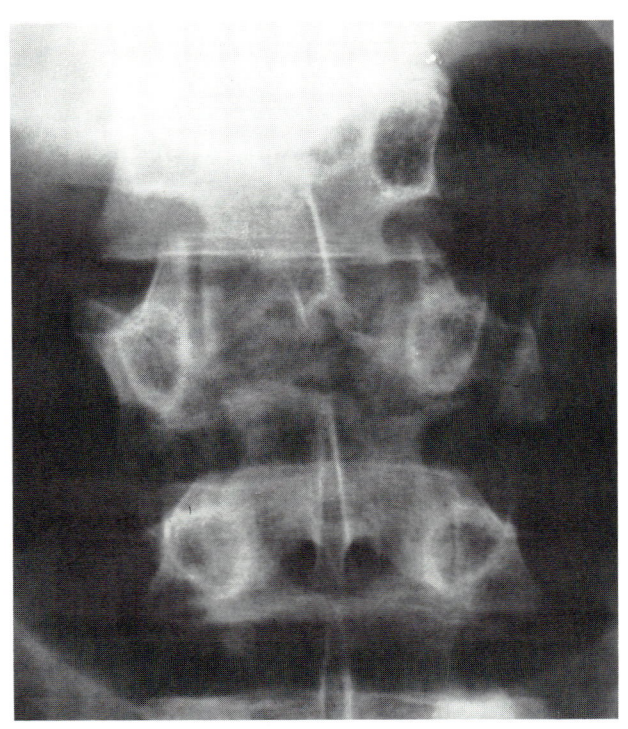

Figure 218-3 Anteroposterior roentgenogram of an L2 burst fracture showing widening of the interpedicular distance.

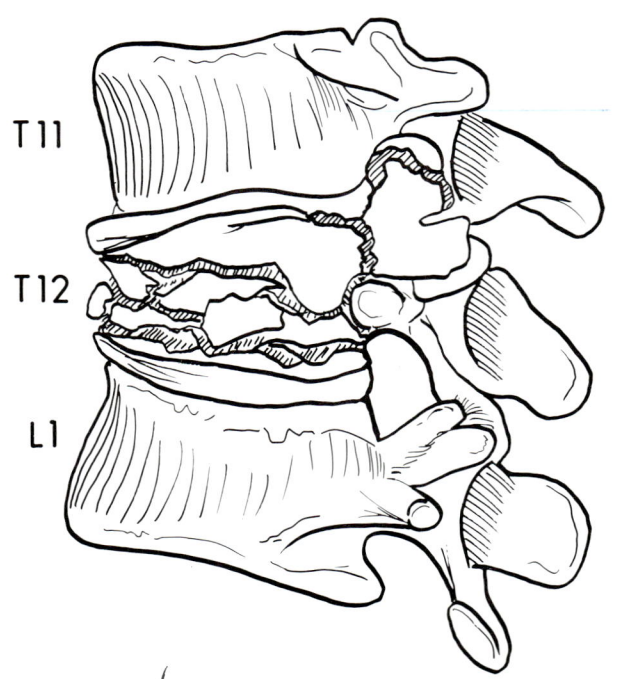

Figure 218-2 Burst fracture of the twelfth thoracic vertebra resulting from axial compression.

Radiology of Thoracolumbar Injuries

The roentgenographic evaluation of spine fractures has been revolutionized by the advent of computed tomography and water-soluble contrast agents. Following initial plain films, computed tomography of the injured spine will provide the necessary information in most clinical situations. The CT scan provides a more accurate picture of the degree of spinal canal compromise and is of less risk to the patient than conventional polytomography. The radiation dose is greater with polytomography, and with most tomographic units the patient must be shifted to a lateral position for the lateral tomography, which entails a certain risk if the spine fracture is unstable. A comparative study suggests that conventional polytomography is the procedure of choice only for suspected fractures of the pars interarticularis.[19]

Metrizamide myelography is indicated in those patients whose neural deficit is not consistent with the level or extent of vertebral involvement. Myelography is not necessary in cases of marked fracture-dislocation with an appropriate neurological level. On the other hand, a minimal burst fracture or dislocation with severe neurological damage is an indication for myelography, as is the situation in which the neurological level is not consistent with the radiological level of injury.

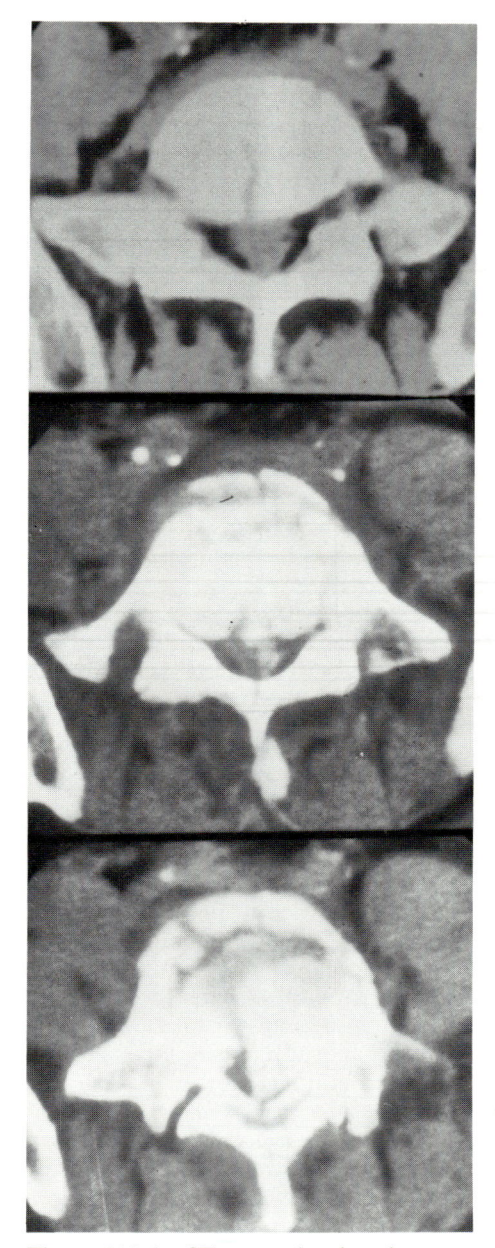

Figure 218-4 CT scans showing the amount of posterior protrusion of bone fragments at the caudal (*lower*), mid, and cephalad (*upper*) portion of the vertebral body of L5.

Therapy of Thoracolumbar Injuries

The question as to whether the final neurological outcome following spinal cord injury reflects the form of treatment or the extent of damage to the spinal cord at the time of injury remains controversial. While it would appear reasonable to assume that both factors are operative, the small number of complete spinal cord injuries that improve, irrespective of treatment modality, is considered to prove the importance of the initial injury by many investigators. However, interest and optimism have been stimulated by the observation that spinal cord blood flow decreases following injury, suggesting that evolving ischemia may, indeed, contribute to the irreversible nature of spinal cord injury. In the experimental animal, naloxone and thyrotropin-releasing hormone have been reported to improve the degree of neurological recovery following spinal cord injury.[6,7] These agents are opiate antagonists, and their beneficial effects are presumed to reflect increased spinal cord blood flow as well as other factors. Appropriate clinical trials with these agents are now in progress.

The utilization of high-dose steroid therapy is also controversial. Although the potential benefits and mechanisms of action have been well recorded,[13] the clinical utilization of high-dose, short-term steroid therapy is recommended by some groups but not by others.

The goals of therapy are listed in Table 218-2. Irrespective of the treatment modality employed, a team approach to the spinal patient is essential if these goals are to be achieved. Each patient should receive input from neurosurgical, orthopedic, urologic, nursing, physical therapy, rehabilitation, and social service specialists.

Essential to the initial management of the spinal cord–injured patient is an accurate recorded neurological examination against which future examinations can be compared. Improper movement of the patient, hypoxia, and hypotension must be avoided to prevent further damage to the spinal cord. Associated injuries must be recognized and treated. In thoracic fractures, injury to the lungs and cardiovascular structures is not uncommon. Thoracolumbar fractures may be associated with retroperitoneal or visceral injuries. It should be emphasized that the characteristic signs of peritoneal irritation may be abolished by spinal shock. Finally, the care of the bladder and anesthetic skin should begin immediately to avoid the debilitating complications of urinary tract infections and decubitus ulcers.

Nonsurgical Therapy

Postural reduction is a nonsurgical means of treating spinal fractures that was developed by Guttman in 1944.[12] Although this form of therapy has not gained widespread acceptance in this country, the contributions of Guttman and his colleagues to the care of the spine-injured patient have been considerable, and the degree of initial neurological improvement achieved by this means is similar to that reported in comparable surgical series. For example, in patients with thoracolumbar fractures and partial neurological involvement, Guttman in 1963[12] and Frankel in 1969[9] reported that 60 percent and 63 percent of the patients, re-

TABLE 218-2 Goals of Therapy

Preservation of remaining spinal cord function
Maximization of the degree of neurological recovery
Restoration of spinal alignment
Achievement of a stable and pain-free fracture site
Prevention of pulmonary, gastrointestinal, genitourinary, and cutaneous complications
Prevention of delayed neurological complications
Rapid mobilization and early rehabilitation
Cost containment

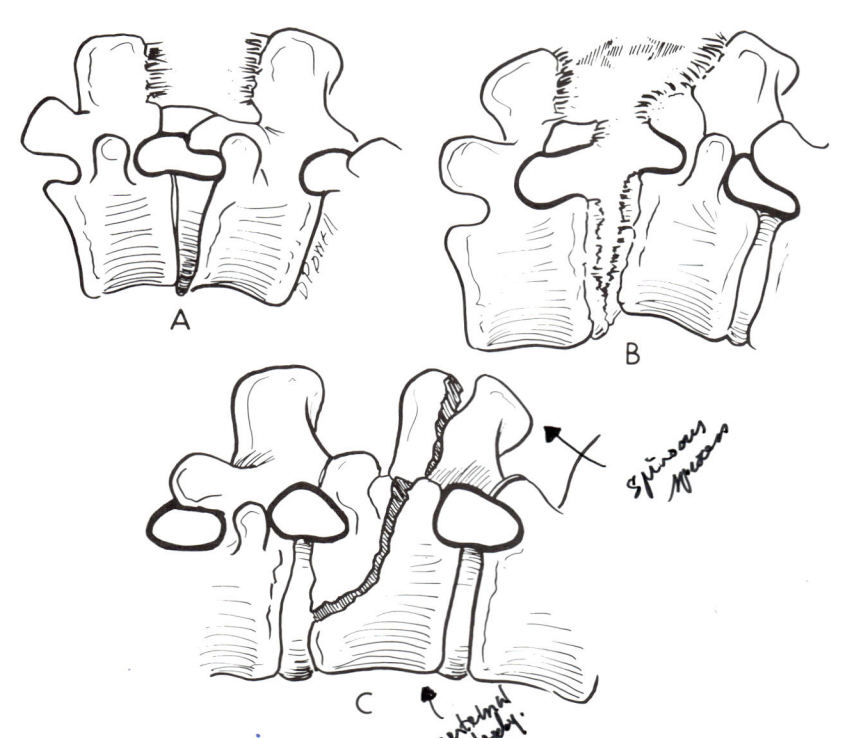

Figure 218-5 Distraction fracture-dislocations. *A, B.* Primarily ligamentous injury. *C.* Chance fracture.

spectively, improved one or more neurological grades (Frankel classification). Patients undergoing surgery (laminectomy with or without fusion) during the same period of time did not improve neurologically to any greater extent.[34] A more recent study reports improvement in 95 percent of patients treated by postural reduction.[3] In comparison, two recent surgical series (posterolateral decompression and Harrington instrumentation) report 90 percent or more improvement in a similar group of patients.[8,16]

For this form of therapy to be successful, a team approach is required, and the nursing staff must be both talented and dedicated. Disadvantages of postural reduction include a prolonged period of immobilization (9 to 13 weeks) and the complications associated with prolonged bed rest. Although the displacement of the fracture-dislocation can usually be corrected by postural reduction, the abnormal angulation of the spine will frequently recur. In the series of patients reported by Davies et al. the prereduction angulation of the spine measured 16 degrees.[3] This was reduced to 6 degrees by postural reduction but then increased to 18 degrees at follow-up.

Surgical Therapy

The primary indications for surgical intervention with thoracolumbar fractures are to relieve actual or anticipated neural compression and to stabilize the spine (Table 218-3). The universally accepted indication is progressive neurological deterioration due to a compressive lesion; however, this situation is not commonly encountered. The remaining indications continue to be controversial. It is our opinion that the spinal canal should be decompressed with removal of all bone and disc fragments to provide an optimum environment for spinal cord recovery. The compression of the spi-

nal cord or cauda equina may be actual or anticipated. In the latter case, the lumen of the spinal canal is reduced, and with healing of the fracture and further angulation of the spine, neural compression and deficit occur with time. Dural lacerations should be identified and repaired. Not infrequently, portions of the cauda equina will herniate through the laceration, and if the dura is not repaired, scarring and a chronic pain syndrome may result. Although many believe that the spinal canal should be decompressed and experimental evidence suggests that spinal cord recovery is related to both the force and duration of the compressing agent,[18] it must be recalled that, in terms of neural recovery, the results of operative and nonoperative therapy appear to be approximately the same.

Controversy also exists as to which fractures are stable and which are unstable (Table 218-3). This reflects, in part, the different definitions of the term *stability*. For example, some authors do not consider progressive angulation of the spine as a sign of instability, yet late progressive kyphosis may be accompanied by loss of neurological function.

When surgical intervention is indicated, timing is the next important consideration. Initially we attempted to operate within the first few hours following injury with the expectation that immediate decompression and stabilization

TABLE 218-3 Indications for Surgical Treatment

- Progressive neurological deficit
- Spinal cord compression
- Dural lacerations
- Unstable spine
  - Fracture-dislocation
  - Anteroposterior or lateral translocation
  - Severe wedge or burst fracture
  - Progressive angulation

would improve the degree of neurological recovery. This has not proved to be the case, either in our series or those of others.[8,16] We now believe a more orderly and complete diagnostic workup, stabilization of the patient, and therapy for associated injuries should be completed first. With this approach the majority of our spine fractures are operated upon within 3 to 4 days following injury. The result has been fewer complications and no detectable loss in the degree of neurological recovery.

A variety of intraoperative aids are available that improve the technical aspects of the surgery and diminish potential complications. These include improved lighting, magnification, high-speed drills of different configurations, and the monitoring of evoked potentials. The intraoperative monitoring of spinal somatosensory evoked potentials (SSEPs) is a useful, but not absolute, method of minimizing spinal cord injury during spine fracture surgery.[10] With stimulus intensities three times the motor threshold, the evoked potentials primarily reflect activity in the dorsal columns[10,24] and thus do not provide precise information regarding status of the more ventrally placed motor tracts. Varying degrees of motor paralysis have been reported to occur without significant change in SSEPs. We utilize SSEPs with this reservation in mind, and if there is any question, we awaken the patient intraoperatively to test motor function. Several recent reports of animal models suggest that this limitation of SSEPs may be overcome in the near future.[23,28]

Surgical procedures designed to decompress and stabilize thoracolumbar fractures are primarily anterior or posterior approaches. The anterior approach involves resection of the fractured vertebral body followed by fusion, and the posterior operative approaches include laminectomy, lateral extracavitary decompression (modified costotransversectomy), posterolateral decompression via the pedicle, and Harrington instrumentation.

Anterior Vertebral Body Resection

Anterior exposure of the vertebral body is gained by a transthoracic, a transabdominal, or a combined approach.[32] Since the portion of the vertebral body compromising the dural contents invariably involves the cephalad portion of the vertebral body, the resection should begin at the lower interspace where the anatomy is relatively normal. A high-speed drill and thin upbiting curettes are useful for this. Once the posterior longitudinal ligament and dura have been exposed, the resection is carried cephalad through the fractured vertebral body to the interspace above. The dura should be completely exposed from below to above and from one lateral gutter to the other. Iliac crest or fibular strut grafts are utilized for the fusion. Simple anterior fusion alone is often inadequate to prevent graft collapse and progressive angulation of the spine with weight bearing. Therefore, posterior Harrington instrumentation and fusion, as a staged or combined procedure, is recommended.

Laminectomy

Laminectomy as primary therapy for thoracolumbar fractures is being viewed with increasing disfavor in this country, and, although late in coming, this is a welcome trend. There are very few reasons to recommend laminectomy for this condition, and many reasons to condemn this practice. For example, the abnormality in the majority of thoracolumbar fractures is anterior to the spinal cord (Fig. 218-4), and laminectomy does little to relieve the traction of the spinal cord over an anterior lesion. Laminectomy may also add to the instability of a damaged spinal column. Removal of the interspinous and yellow ligaments increases the possibility of a progressive flexion deformity. There is also a risk of further damaging the spinal cord when a laminectomy is carried out for thoracic fractures. The diameter relationships of the thoracic spinal column and spinal cord are such that there may be insufficient space to safely insert the jaw of a rongeur between the lamina and the posteriorly displaced spinal cord. If there is any doubt regarding this point, the history of surgery for thoracic disc disease should be recalled. In our opinion, there is little justification for the routine use of laminectomy. The procedure should be reserved for those few specific situations where laminectomy will benefit the patient.

Posterior compression of the spinal cord resulting from bone fragments or epidural hematoma formation may be an indication for laminectomy. Preoperative utilization of the CT scan with water-soluble myelography will indicate whether the main lesion is anterior or posterior to the spinal cord. Another indication for laminectomy is the severe burst (impaction) fracture with associated dural lacerations.[26] This diagnosis is established by noting the widened interpedicular distance on the plain film. In this case laminectomy may be required to repair the dura, and if the fracture is caudal to the termination of the spinal cord, the fractured bone within the canal can be reduced by transdural impaction. This is accomplished by opening the dura and retracting the cauda equina to either side of the midline to permit transdural impaction of the fragments back into the vertebral body (Figs. 218-6 and 218-7). Following closure of the dura, Harrington rods are then inserted as described below.

The following technical points should be considered when laminectomy is utilized for fractures of the spine. The exposure for the laminectomy must be accomplished by sharp dissection and not by use of a periosteal elevator, which may drive bone fragments into the spinal canal. In some cases it is possible to remove the lamina with rongeurs, but in other cases, when the spinal cord has been displaced posteriorly, there is insufficient space to insert an instrument between the lamina and the dura. To prevent further damage to the spinal cord in this situation, removal of the lamina with a drill is advisable. In addition, lateral and central dural tack-up sutures should be employed to prevent postoperative epidural bleeding from compressing the spinal cord.

Lateral Extracavitary Approach

Another posterior approach to the spinal column is the lateral extrapleural or extraperitoneal approach.[22] This involves resection of the posterior portion of the ribs and the transverse processes to gain exposure to the lateral aspect of the spinal column. It will be recognized that this is a modification of the costotransversectomy originally developed to deal with tuberculous involvement of the spine. Once the

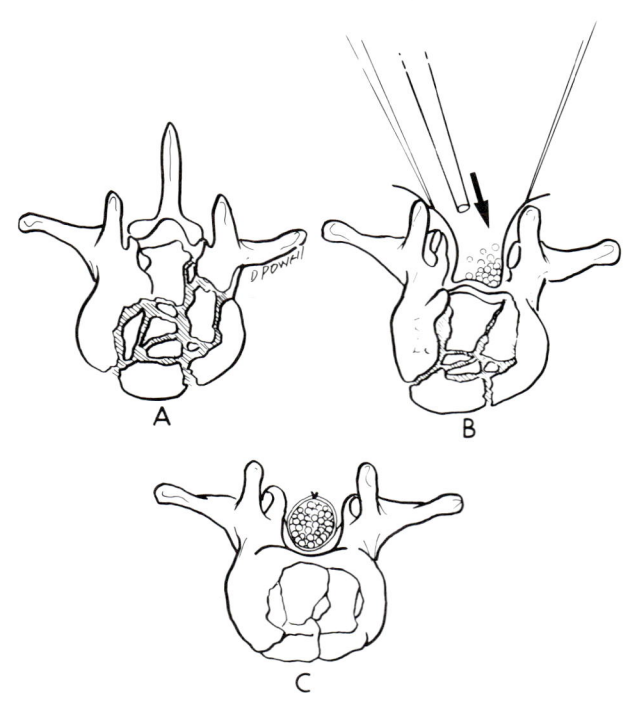

Figure 218-6 Transdural impaction for decompression of lumbar fractures. Following laminectomy the dura is opened, the cauda equina is retracted laterally, and the bone fragments are driven back into the vertebral body.

leaving a rim of bone. The remaining rim of bone is then fractured into the cavity with a thin downbiting curette and is removed with pituitary rongeurs. If complete decompression is not obtained, the procedure is repeated from the contralateral side. The decompression is confirmed by visual inspection and palpation, with intradural palpation being more accurate than extradural palpation, or by intraoperative myelography. Following placement of the Harrington instrumentation and fracture reduction, drains are placed and the wound is closed.

The following points regarding this operative procedure are worth emphasizing. During inspection of the fracture site, CSF leaks must be recognized, and if present, the dural

lateral aspect of the vertebral body is exposed, the posteriorly protruded fragments may be removed as described below.

Posterolateral Decompression

A posterolateral approach to the spinal canal through the pedicle provides direct access to the cephalad portion of the vertebral body while avoiding the disadvantages of laminectomy.[5,16,18,25,29] Furthermore, following decompression of the spinal canal, Harrington rods may be inserted, thus eliminating the need for a second procedure that is required when the fractured vertebral body is removed by an anterior approach. However, from the technical standpoint, the procedure is tedious, and meticulous attention to detail is required to achieve adequate decompression without further neural injury.

In this procedure, the patient is placed prone and is carefully positioned to avoid abdominal compression and brachial plexus stretch injuries. A midline incision of sufficient length to encompass the Harrington rods is utilized. Over the fracture site only sharp dissection should be employed to avoid driving bone fragments into the spinal canal with a periosteal elevator. The fracture is identified visually, and the level is confirmed by a lateral x-ray film. The pedicle is removed with a high-speed drill as shown in Figs. 218-8 and 218-9. Whether the right or left pedicle is removed is based on the configuration of the fracture as determined by the preoperative CT scan. The crucial step is leaving a thin rim of bone to protect the dural contents. The posterior portion of the vertebral body is then removed with the drill, again

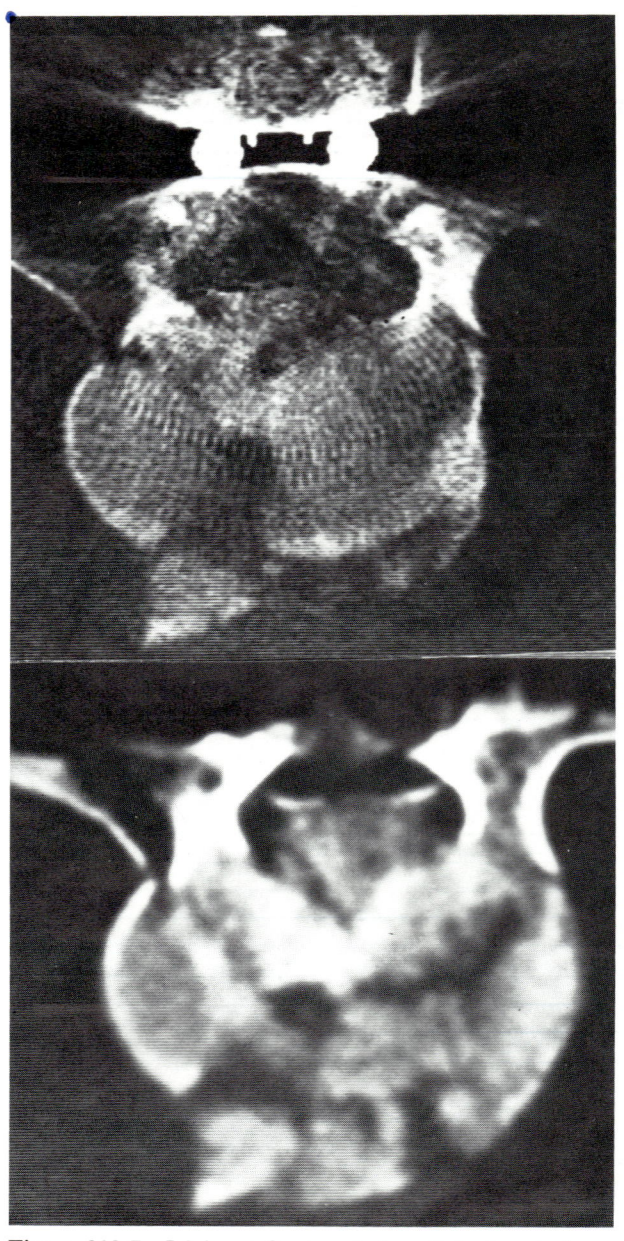

Figure 218-7 L2 burst fracture before (*below*) and after (*above*) transdural impaction and Harrington instrumentation.

Injuries to the Thoracic and Lumbar Spine

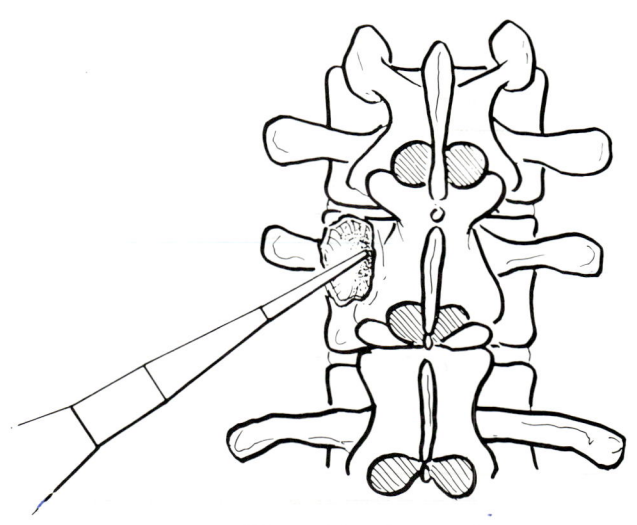

Figure 218-8 Posterolateral decompression via the pedicle. The pedicle and posterior portion of the vertebral body are drilled out lateral to the spinal cord.

lacerations must be repaired. With many of these fractures, the ligamentum flavum is torn, and if this is so, the ligamentum should be removed. If it is not resected, spinal realignment with the Harrington instrumentation may buckle the torn ligamentum inward and produce posterior spinal cord compression. A final point to recall is the relationship of the neurovascular bundle to the pedicle, so that the vessels and nerves are not damaged when the pedicle is drilled out.

Harrington Instrumentation

The Harrington instrumentation system has been a major contribution in the operative management of fractures and fracture-dislocations of the thoracolumbar spine. Initial reports suggested that realignment of the spinal column using the Harrington apparatus might effectively decompress the neural tube. Experience has demonstrated, however, that satisfactory decompression in most cases requires direct removal of bony and disc elements from the spinal canal and that Harrington instrumentation alone cannot be relied upon to achieve consistent and effective decompression. The primary role of Harrington instrumentation, therefore, is the realignment and stabilization of the spinal column.

Following decompression via an anterior or posterolateral approach, a single Harrington distraction rod is positioned and placed to distraction. The inferior hook is placed via a small laminotomy in a vertebral arch, in most cases two or three spaces below the fracture. The superior hook is inserted beneath the laminal arch of an intact vertebra three spaces above the injury site. The distraction system utilizing hooks placed just two spaces above and below the fracture will not effectively reduce some major kyphotic deformities or severely displaced fracture-dislocations.[15]

In injuries involving disruption of the interspinous and supraspinous ligamentous complex, we routinely fix the involved, displaced spinous processes using triple-braided 25-gauge stainless steel wire. During distraction and realignment, the spinous processes are approximated and fixed.

Restoration of height and alignment of the spinal column with the Harrington system utilizes both the principles of distraction and three-point bending.[15] These considerable mechanical forces, if not controlled, can be transmitted through the bony and soft tissue elements of the spinal column to the neural structures. Direct observation of the neural tube at the fracture site must be maintained to ensure that displacement of bone fragments into the spinal canal or overdistraction does not occur. In this manner, a safe, controlled realignment can be accomplished. Operative roentgenograms are employed to confirm satisfactory reduction. Somatosensory evoked potentials are closely monitored during the following realignment.

In some cases, the rods may require prebending prior to distraction in order to achieve satisfactory restoration of the normal kyphotic and lordotic contours of the thoracolumbar junction. When contoured rods are employed, the square-ended distraction rods and appropriate inferior hooks are recommended. During the following spinal alignment with the initial distraction rod, the injury site is inspected to ensure that complete decompression has been maintained. The second rod is then placed in conjunction with the standard posterior decortication and fusion using autogenous iliac bone grafts. The grafting is bilateral from the level of the superior hooks to the level of the inferior hooks of the distraction system. Graft material is placed medially between the rods and the borders of the spinous processes and laterally within the facet joints and spanning the transverse processes.

Suction drains are placed in the graft donor site and in the fusion site, and these are routinely removed within 36 to 48 h. Postoperatively, the patient is placed in a prefabricated plaster splint. At 5 days, the dressings are removed and the surgical wounds are inspected. The patient is then placed in a plaster body jacket awaiting fabrication of a polypropylene thoracolumbar spinal orthosis. Patients with insensitive skin are fitted with a bivalved polypropylene jacket held with Velcro straps. This facilitates periodic removal for

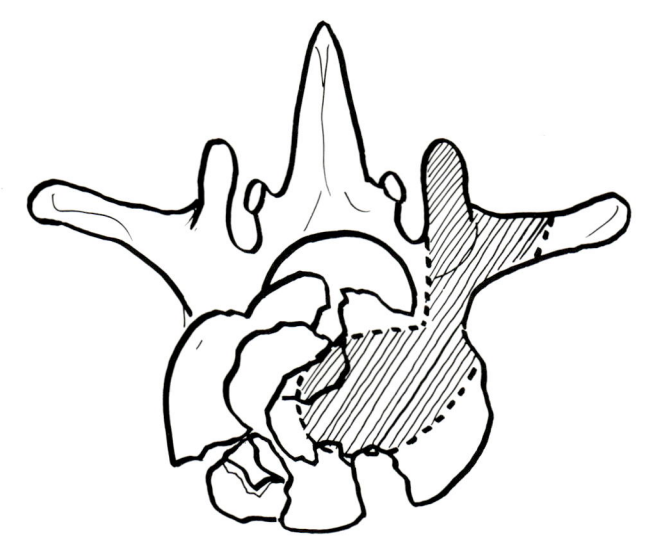

Figure 218-9 The shaded area indicates the extent of the drilling. The remaining fragments are fractured down into the cavity and removed.

skin inspection to prevent pressure skin necrosis. Neurologically intact patients are maintained in a riveted body jacket until satisfactory fusion can be demonstrated on x-ray films.

The results of posterolateral decompression and Harrington instrumentation for thoracolumbar injuries can be considered in light of the goals of therapy (Table 218-2). The immediate stabilization of the fracture by the Harrington instrumentation permits rapid weight bearing and early rehabilitation. This has reduced the acute hospital stay to approximately 10 days, with a corresponding reduction in cost and in the complications related to prolonged bed rest. The stabilization and fusion have eliminated the problem of progressive angulation of the spine and have diminished, but not abolished, pain at the fracture sites. Whether or not decompression of the spinal canal and repair of the dural lacerations will diminish the late complications of chronic pain, spinal stenosis, tethering, and intra- or extradural scarring[27] remains to be proved. The amount of neurological recovery that can be achieved by posterolateral decompression and Harrington instrumentation is greater that that obtained by postural reduction if the comparison is made with the earlier reports by Guttman[12] and Frankel et al.[9] A more recent report indicates an equal degree of improvement.[3]

Thoracic Injuries

The thoracic spine is stabilized by the rib cage, and a much greater force is required to produce fracture-dislocation here than for the more mobile cervical and thoracolumbar areas of the spine. Thus, thoracic fracture-dislocations are less common, but when they do occur, the spinal cord injury is usually complete. In addition to the stability imparted by the rib cage, two other factors contribute to the high percentage of complete thoracic spinal cord injuries. The first is that the diameters of the thoracic spinal column and thoracic spinal cord are nearly equal, so that minimal displacement results in cord compression. Secondly, the blood supply to the thoracic cord is such that watershed zones are present and thus ischemic as well as compressive damage may occur. Guttman has pointed out that complete thoracic spinal cord injuries have the least chance of any neurological return but that incomplete lesions have a greater degree of return than do incomplete cervical or lumbar spinal cord injuries.[12] The inherent stability of the thoracic spine may explain the better recovery rate for the incomplete injuries.

As for thoracolumbar injuries, the mechanisms of injury include flexion, extension, compression, and rotation. Most commonly, the major force is flexion, with the upper vertebra shearing forward on the lower vertebra. Because of the magnitude of the force, associated injuries are common and include damage to the lungs, great vessels, and myocardium.

Traumatic or nontraumatic compression fractures of thoracic vertebrae are frequently encountered in elderly patients. These fractures are generally not associated with neurological deficit and will respond to symptomatic therapy, which may vary from simple analgesics to a hyperextension brace.

In contrast to thoracolumbar fractures, thoracic (T1-9) fracture-dislocations are generally stable, and progressive angulation of the spine is an infrequent problem. Thus, many of these fractures can be managed by postural reduc-

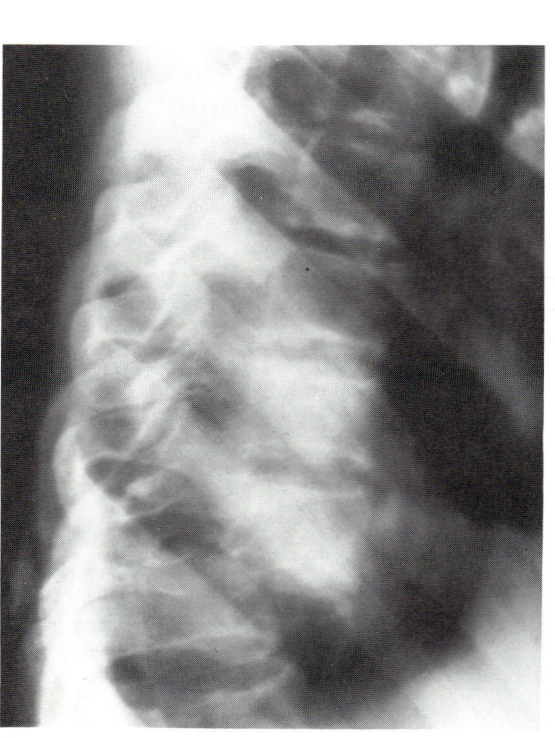

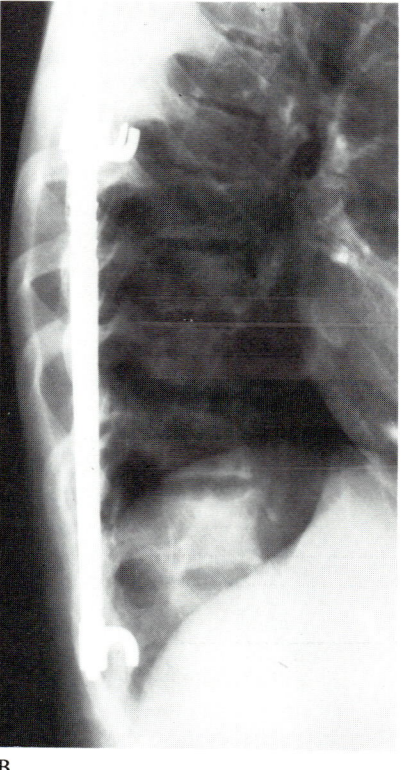

Figure 218-10 Thoracic fracture-dislocation before (A) and after (B) posterolateral decompression and Harrington instrumentation.

tion and external stabilization with an appropriate orthosis. When faced with a major unstable dislocation, operative reduction followed by Harrington instrumentation and fusion is the procedure of choice (Fig. 218-10). An alternative method of management is pin traction from the lower extremities. If this option is undertaken, particular attention must be paid to the patient's anesthetic skin due to the friction between the skin and bed created by the heavy traction.

Surgical decompression of the thoracic spinal cord in the face of complete neurological deficit is an unrewarding procedure. If the neurological deficit is incomplete, then posterolateral or anterior decompression may be indicated. As noted earlier, decompression by laminectomy is to be avoided.

Lumbar Injuries

Fractures of the lower lumbar spine and lumbosacral junction are encountered infrequently.[2] These fractures usually result from flexion and compression. A rotational component to the injury may also be present. With these injuries only the cauda equina is involved; thus the potential for neurological recovery is high. Our current practice includes decompression of the cauda equina, either by a posterolateral or transdural approach, and fusion. Usually a posterolateral bone fusion combined with wiring will suffice.

References

1. Chance GQ: Note on a type of flexion fracture of the spine. Br J Radiol 21:452–453, 1948.
2. Das De S, McCreath SW: Lumbosacral fracture-dislocations: A report of four cases. J Bone Joint Surg [Br] 63-B:58–60, 1981.
3. Davies WE, Morris JH, Hill V: An analysis of conservative (non-surgical) management of thoracolumbar fractures and fracture-dislocations with neural damage. J Bone Joint Surg [Am] 62-A:1324–1328, 1980.
4. Dooley BJ: The role of seat-belts in reducing the road toll. J Bone Joint Surg [Br] 64-B:518–519, 1982.
5. Erickson DL, Leider LL, Brown WE: One-stage decompression-stabilization for thoracolumbar fractures. Spine 2:53–56, 1977.
6. Faden AI, Jacobs TP, Holaday JW: Thyrotropin-releasing hormone improves neurologic recovery after spinal trauma in cats. N Engl J Med 305:1063–1067, 1981.
7. Flamm ES, Young W, Demopoulos HB, DeCrescito V, Tomasula JJ: Experimental spinal cord injury: Treatment with naloxone. Neurosurgery 10:227–231, 1982.
8. Flesch JR, Leider LL, Erickson DL, Chou SN, Bradford DS: Harrington instrumentation and spine fusion for unstable fractures and fracture-dislocations of the thoracic and lumbar spine. J Bone Joint Surg [Am] 59-A:143–153, 1977.
9. Frankel HL, Hancock DO, Hyslop G, Melzak J, Michaelis LS, Ungar GH, Vernon JDS, Walsh JJ: The value of postural reduction in the initial management of closed injuries of the spine with paraplegia and tetraplegia. Paraplegia 7:179–192, 1969.
10. Grundy BL: Monitoring of sensory evoked potentials during neurosurgical operations: Methods and applications. Neurosurgery 11:556–575, 1982.
11. Gumley G, Taylor TKF, Ryan MD: Distraction fractures of the lumbar spine. J Bone Joint Surg [Br] 64-B:520–525, 1982.
12. Guttman L: The conservative management of closed injuries of the vertebral column resulting in damage to the spinal cord and spinal roots, in Vinken PJ, Bruyn GW (eds): *Handbook of Clinical Neurology*, vol. 26. New York, American Elsevier, 1976, pp 285–306.
13. Hall ED, Braughler JM: Glucocorticoid mechanisms in acute spinal cord injury: A review and therapeutic rationale. Surg Neurol 18:320–327, 1982.
14. Holdsworth F: Fractures, dislocations, and fracture-dislocations of the spine. J Bone Joint Surg [Am] 52-A:1534–1551, 1970.
15. Jacobs RR, Asher MM, Snider RK: Thoracolumbar spinal injuries: A comparative study of recumbent and operative treatment in 100 patients. Spine 5:463–477, 1980.
16. Jelsma RK, Kirsch PT, Jelsma LF, Ramsey WC, Rice JF: Surgical treatment of thoracolumbar fractures. Surg Neurol 18:156–166, 1982.
17. Jelsma RK, Kirsch PT, Rice JF, Jelsma LF: The radiographic description of thoracolumbar fractures. Surg Neurol 18:230–236, 1982.
18. Jelsma RK, Rice JF, Jelsma LF, Kirsch PT: The demonstration and significance of neural compression after spinal injury. Surg Neurol 18:79–92, 1982.
19. Keene JS, Goletz TH, Lilleas F, Alter AJ, Sackett JF: Diagnosis of vertebral fractures: A comparison of conventional radiography, conventional tomography, and computed axial tomography. J Bone Joint Surg [Am] 64-A:586–595, 1982.
20. Kraus JF, Franti CE, Riggins RS, Richards D, Borhani NO: Incidence of traumatic spinal cord lesions. J Chronic Dis 28:471–492, 1975.
21. Kurtzke JF: Epidemiology of spinal cord injury. Exp Neurol 48 (Part 2):163–236, 1975.
22. Larson SJ, Holst RA, Hemmy DC, Sances A Jr: Lateral extracavitary approach to traumatic lesions of the thoracic and lumbar spine. J Neurosurg 45:628–637, 1976.
23. Levy WJ: Spinal evoked potentials from the motor tracts. J Neurosurg 58:38–44, 1983.
24. Macon JB, Poletti CE, Sweet WH, Ojemann RG, Zervas NT: Conducted somatosensory evoked potentials during spinal surgery: Part 2. Clinical applications. J Neurosurg 57:354–359, 1982.
25. McAfee PC, Yuan HA, Lasda NA: The unstable burst fracture. Spine 7:365–373, 1982.
26. Miller CA, Dewey RC, Hunt WE: Impaction fracture of the lumbar vertebrae with dural tear. J Neurosurg 53:765–771, 1980.
27. Osborne DRS, Vavoulis G, Nashold BS Jr, Dubois PJ, Drayer BP, Heinz ER: Late sequelae of spinal cord trauma: Myelographic and surgical correlation. J Neurosurg 57:18–23, 1982.
28. Powers SK, Bolger CA, Edwards MSB: Spinal cord pathways mediating somatosensory evoked potentials. J Neurosurg 57:472–482, 1982.
29. Schmidek HH, Gomes FB, Seligson D, McSherry JW: Management of acute unstable thoracolumbar (T-11–L-1) fractures with and without neurological deficit. Neurosurgery 7:30–35, 1980.
30. Smith WS, Kaufer H: Patterns and mechanisms of lumbar injuries associated with lap seat belts. J Bone Joint Surg [Am] 51-A:239–254, 1969.
31. Watson N: Road traffic accidents, spinal injuries and seat belts. Paraplegia 21:63–64, 1983.
32. Whitesides TE Jr, Shah SGA: On the management of unstable fractures of the thoracolumbar spine. Spine 1:99–107, 1976.
33. Williams JS, Kirkpatrick JR: The nature of seat belt injuries. J Trauma 11:207–218, 1971.
34. Young JS, Dexter WR: Neurological recovery distal to the zone of injury in 172 cases of closed, traumatic spinal cord injury. Paraplegia 16:39–49, 1978.

219
Injuries to the Sacrum and Pelvis

Barth A. Green
Ignacio Magana

A neurological deficit associated with injury to the sacrum or pelvis is rare. The reported incidence ranges from 0.75 to 11 percent, with the occurrence being more frequent in fractures of the pelvic ring that involve the sacrum in association with an anterior pelvic fracture or a fracture of the sacrum solely.[1,2,6]

Most fractures of the sacroiliac joint or sacrum are associated with an anterior fracture of the rami or symphysis pubis. Such patients often have multiple injuries of acute severity such that the initial evaluation does not reveal a neurological deficit. Reported instances of related system involvement are musculoskeletal, 85 percent; respiratory, 60 percent; central nervous system, 40 percent; and gastrointestinal, 30 percent. Respiratory failure and unrelenting hemorrhage are frequent complications that contribute to the overall mortality rate of 10 to 20 percent for closed pelvic injuries.[5] Pelvic visceral injuries are more accessible to diagnosis with the availability of high-resolution computed tomography combined with contrast injection (i.e., into the bladder, bowel, or vessels) and the use of high-resolution real-time ultrasound technology.

Open fractures of the combined type have a mortality rate of 50 percent.[5] Open sacral injuries may result in contamination of the subarachnoid space by genitourinary, gastrointestinal, or skin flora with a resultant meningitis.

Three types of forces have been described to produce sacroiliac dislocation or vertical fracture.[5] Less commonly, transverse fractures may result as well. Anteroposterior compression and a lateral compression usually arise from directly applied trauma. Vertical shear force may be transmitted through sudden deceleration forces applied to the lower extremities. The subsequent response of the posterior pelvic ring is a stress to the broad ligament of the sacroiliac joint or a vertical sacral fracture with sacroiliac joint instability. This may produce traction on the cauda equina and injury to the lumbar or sacral nerve roots.[3] Less commonly, bony compression, subluxation, or epidural compression from a hematoma can also result in damage to the sacral roots.[1,3]

The neurological sequelae to the combined injury may be varied. Most often, the patient presents with weakness of the posterior lower extremity muscle groups with an associated sensory deficit in the posterior lower extremity. Frequently ankle jerks and rectal tone are diminished. Neurogenic bladder (lower motor neuron), perineal hypesthesia, and sexual dysfunction are common and help to identify the process as involving the cauda equina.

Although many pelvic fractures are well defined on plain x-ray films, they can also present with only subtle changes. The pelvic ring should be studied by anteroposterior, inlet, and outlet pelvic films. The appearance of the upper sacral foramina and the posterior pelvic brim must be scrutinized. Plain x-ray techniques can be complemented by the use of conventional complex motion tomography in selected cases. In patients with neurological deficits, metrizamide myelography followed by a postmyelogram high-resolution computed tomography scan should be performed with sagittally reconstructed views added to the conventionally obtained axial images. If the dural sac does not extend to the body of S2, this study may be of limited value. Findings of meningeal diverticuli or rupture of the subarachnoid space suggest a nerve root avulsion injury. The sacral foramina may be compromised, with nerve root impingement. Finally, epidural compression from a hematoma can sometimes be appreciated.

Neurophysiological evaluation with nerve conduction studies and electromyography may aid in localizing the involved roots for clinical and radiographic correlation. Information regarding whether complete or partial nerve root avulsion is present may be useful in the therapeutic strategy as well as in the diagnosis. Serial evaluations can help assess the return of neurological function after injury. An associated neurogenic bladder can also be evaluated by electrophysiological techniques (i.e., urodynamics). Sphincter and bladder wall responses should be documented as a baseline and serially reassessed as another means of monitoring the status of the neurological injury.

Isolated sacral fractures with neurological injury are rarely reported in the literature. The mechanism of injury may be blunt trauma, penetrating injury, or indirect forces. Weaver et al. have classified closed isolated sacral fractures into two types according to location.[6] The pathological result is the product of the forces acting on the vertebral column and the maturity of the sacral ossification process.

Upper transverse sacral fractures usually occur in young patients under 25 years of age who have suffered a flexion injury of the lumbosacral spine while having the pelvis held fixed. These injuries have been reported following motor vehicle accidents in patients wearing a seat belt.[6] The injury is an anterior subluxation and fracture of S1 and S2, and occurs because the ossification of the sacrum begins caudad and moves cephalad, with completion upon reaching approximately 20 years of age.[6] Beyond this period, the upper sacrum becomes so rigid that isolated transverse fractures above the coccyx are rare.

The evaluation of the upper transverse fracture is similar to that of the combined anterior and posterior pelvic ring fracture. Neurological examination may reveal a similar distal cauda equina syndrome. These injuries may be associated with lumbar root deficits due to coincidental occurrence of lumbar pedicle or facet fractures from the same traumatic flexion injury. X-ray evaluation frequently reveals a distinct gibbus at the S1-2 junction. Again, as in combined anterior and posterior fractures, the use of metrizamide myelography, high-resolution computed tomography, and neurophysiological studies may be helpful in the evaluation of these injuries.

Direct forces of sufficient degree may result in a fracture of the coccyx, which is rarely associated with a neurological deficit. More severe cases may be complicated by tears in the rectal mucosa, saddle anesthesia, and rarely bladder or bowel symptoms.[1] Occasionally, this type of injury may be complicated by a pseudarthrosis resulting in chronic rectal pain or coccydynia. Evaluation of this type of fracture is limited to plain x-ray films and computed tomography scanning as myelography does not adequately define the distal sacral region.

Lourie has recently described the entity of spontaneous osteoporotic fracture of the sacrum.[4] Geriatric patients with severe osteoporosis may be at risk of developing stress fractures of the lower lumbar and sacral spine. The syndrome is reported to consist of marked sacral tenderness with pain in lumbar or sacral distribution. Neurological exam may not be contributory, and plain x-ray films may not be diagnostic. However, computed tomography, especially with sagittal reconstructed views, and radioisotope bone scanning may be helpful in establishing the diagnosis.

The anatomical characteristics of the pelvic-sacral region present many unique problems in cases of traumatic injury. The treatment of pelvic fractures is well documented in the literature dealing with orthopedic and surgical trauma. These injuries may require treatment ranging from prolonged bed rest to surgery with internal or external fixation. Associated compromise of the nerve roots of the distal cauda equina should be treated aggressively with regard to surgical decompression. This approach is based on the fact that the sacral roots are composed of peripheral nerve fibers capable of self-repair or regeneration under favorable circumstances. This translates into creating adequate decompression of the nerve roots and stabilization of the sacrum and pelvis to allow such recovery to progress. A direct blow to the sacrum resulting in displacement of its roof onto the underlying nerve roots can be simply treated by a posterior approach with decompressive laminectomy. In fractures associated with posterior displacement of sacral body elements into the canal with ventral compromise of the nerve roots, an anterior decompression via a posterolateral approach with partial sacral corpectomy is recommended. Both of these approaches are enhanced by the use of the illumination and magnification of the operating microscope and microsurgical technology. Although the primary purpose of such surgery is the decompression of the nerve roots, at the time of operation any rents in the dura should be repaired to prevent the postoperative occurrence of pseudomeningocele or cerebrospinal fluid fistula. Microanastomosis of severed sacral roots is technically feasible, but the effectiveness of this manuever has not been demonstrated. Because many of these injuries are associated with direct trauma to the sacral area with soft tissue and skin disruption and because of the frequent need for prolonged bed rest, we have found the use of the Roto Rest Treatment Table (Kinetic Concepts, San Antonio, Tex.) and kinetic therapy a valuable tool in the care of these individuals.

Two case histories will illustrate the management of these injuries:

Case 1 A 35-year-old male suffered multiple injuries after being struck by a truck. He was transferred from another hospital 6 days after the accident complaining of persistent pain in both hips and paralysis of the right leg. Examination revealed an areflexic, flaccid right lower extremity; rectal tone and perianal sensation were intact. Plain x-ray films revealed a combined anterior and posterior pelvic fracture with malalignment of the right sacroiliac joint.

He underwent metrizamide myelography and computed tomography, which showed an extensive epidural collection of metrizamide from L3 to L5 (Fig. 219-1). Nerve conduction studies were normal, but electromyography revealed increased insertional activity, sharp waves, and fibrillation in the iliopsoas, adductor longus, vastus medialis, and anterior tibial muscles of the right lower extremity. These studies suggested an incomplete avulsion of the lumbar plexus associated with the classic myelographic appearance of nerve root avulsions.

The patient received intense physical therapy without surgical intervention. Approximately 2 weeks after his initial evaluation he was able to move his leg proximally and distally against gravity. Follow-up EMG showed minimal denervation activity. He subsequently improved to an ambulatory status.

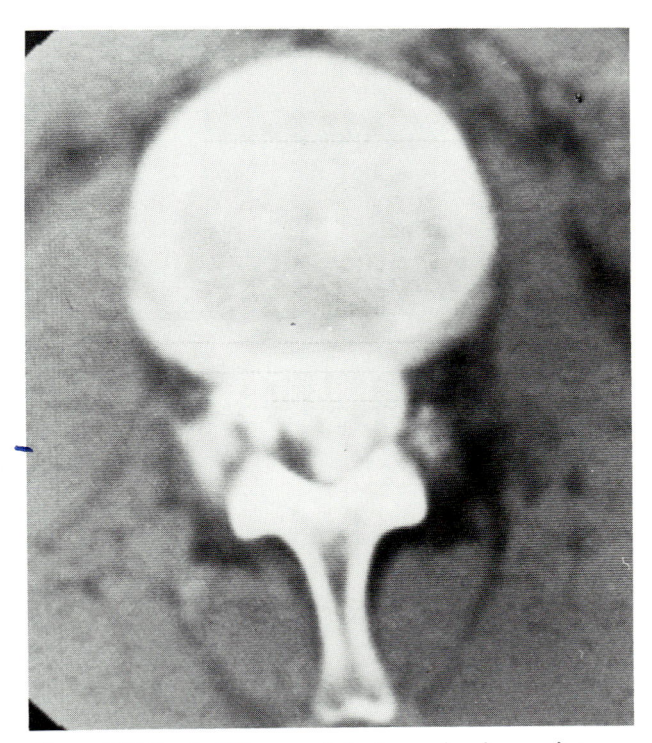

Figure 219-1 A CT scan of the lower lumbar region after metrizamide injection showing extravasation of the medium into the epidural and paraspinal areas. The subarachnoid space and cauda equina appear distorted.

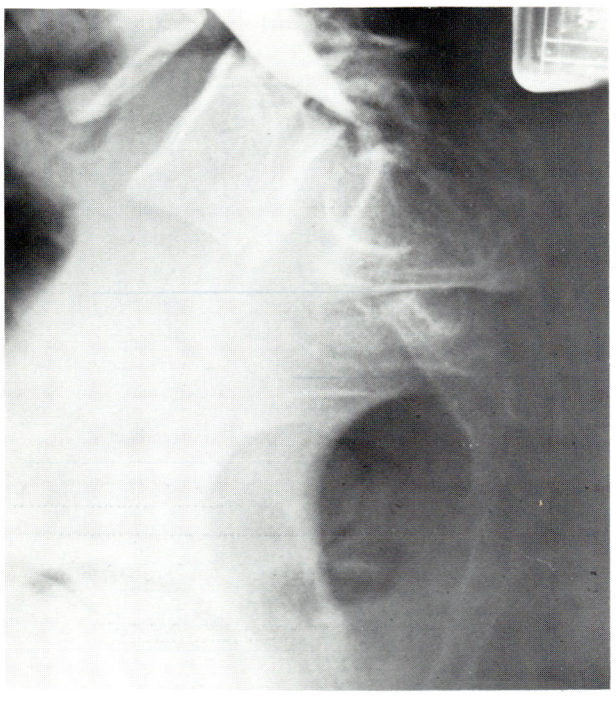

Figure 219-2 Lateral view of the lumbosacral spine from a metrizamide myelogram showing a transverse fracture at S2-3 with displacement of the distal segment and an epidural block of the metrizamide at the lumbosacral junction.

Case 2 A 27-year-old female suffered multiple injuries in a motorcycle accident, including a left hip fracture and a combined anterior and posterior pelvic fracture. She was taken for emergency laparotomy, and postoperatively she complained of vague paresthesias of the lower extremities and severe pelvic area pain. Her physical examination revealed a tender sacrum, saddle anesthesia, absent rectal tone, absent ankle jerk reflexes, and weakness of the gluteus, hamstring, and gastrocnemius muscles bilaterally. X-ray films revealed a fracture of S2-3 with anterior and proximal dislocation of the distal fragment (Fig. 219-2).

Three weeks after injury the patient underwent a sacral unroofing with a partial corpectomy via a posterolateral approach with decompression of the sacral nerve roots. A small sacral epidural hematoma was removed. Crushed but intact sacral nerve roots were noted, with the exception of total severance of the S2 root on the left. One year later the patient is ambulatory with a normal gait and has experienced partial recovery of sphincter function and saddle sensation.

References

1. Byrnes DP, Russo GL, Ducker TB, Cowley RA: Sacrum fractures and neurologic damage. J Neurosurg 47:459–462, 1977.
2. Goodell CL: Neurological deficits associated with pelvic fracture. J Neurosurg 24:837–842, 1966.
3. Huittinen VM: Lumbosacral nerve injury in fracture of the pelvis: A post-mortem radiographic and patho-anatomical study. Acta Clin Scand [Suppl] 429, 1972.
4. Lourie H: Spontaneous osteoporotic fracture of the sacrum. JAMA 248:715–717, 1982.
5. Rubash HE, Steed DL, Mears DC: Fractures of the pelvic ring. Surg Rounds, Aug: 16–30, 1982.
6. Weaver EN Jr, England GD, Richardson DE: Sacral fracture: Case presentation and review. Neurosurgery 9: 725–728, 1981.

220
Penetrating Wounds of the Spine
Carole A. Miller

In this chapter I will review penetrating injuries of the spinal column, with emphasis on gunshot wounds to the spine. Stab wounds have never been particularly prevalent (except in South Africa), but they are becoming more common in certain areas of the United States.

Perhaps the most famous missile wound of the spine was that to Admiral Nelson at the Battle of Trafalgar. After sustaining the injury, Nelson fell on his side and turned to the flag-captain and gasped "They have done for me at last, Hardy." "I hope not," said Hardy. "Yes," said Nelson, "my backbone is shot through."

This type of injury was nearly universally fatal until World War II and the advent of antibiotics. On the other hand, spinal stability is rarely a problem with penetrating injuries as compared with those from vehicular accidents, falls, etc.

Incidence

The incidence of traumatic spinal cord injury per se is unknown because it is not uniformly documented and reported by the hospitals that handle acute conditions. Several studies have been done, however, that indicate an overall incidence of 50 cases per 1 million population every year—

50 percent due to vehicular accidents, and 12 percent due to penetrating wounds. Gunshot wounds are the third most common cause of spinal cord injuries. They were previously ranked sixth but have increased in the past 5 years. In several metropolitan areas with large inner-city populations, gunshot wounds of the spinal cord exceed automobile injuries as a cause of spinal cord injury. In south Florida, 40 percent of spinal cord injuries are due to penetrating wounds, with 28 percent secondary to vehicular accident.

Sex and Age Distribution

There is a marked predominance of males over females in spinal cord injuries due to penetrating wounds. The vast majority of these injuries are also in victims who are less than 35 years of age. In a series of 59 civilian gunshot wounds to the spine, Six et al. reported 77 percent males, with 57 percent younger than 35.[4] In a review of 450 stab wounds of the spinal cord, Peacock et al. reported a male incidence of 84 percent, with 70 percent younger than 35 years of age.[3]

Weapons Causing Gunshot Wounds

The weapons most commonly used in civilian gunshot injuries are handguns. Cartridges used in automatic pistols are typically full metal-jacketed, are round-nosed, have lower velocity, and penetrate but do not shatter. Cartridges used in revolvers are half-jacketed, are hollow-point or flat-nosed, have higher velocity, and may expand and shed fragments during penetration. The .22, .25, .32, .38, and .357 calibers are most common. The .38 and .357 cartridges have identical diameter and are mainly used in police guns; the .357 has a longer casing, giving it a larger gunpowder capacity and higher velocity. The .22 caliber gun is often used for hunting small game and for practice shooting. The .44 is used mainly for hunting and silhouette shooting; it has a range greater than 200 m. The .45 is used mainly for military purposes. The .22, .32, and .45 caliber bullets are used in either automatics or revolvers. However, the .22 is most commonly a revolver cartridge, and the .32 or the .45 an automatic cartridge.

Wounds from .22 or .38 caliber handguns are relatively low velocity injuries. In general, the caliber of the bullet is not considered to be a significant factor in the degree of damage. The energy of the projectile expended upon the target is the major factor. Although the weight of bullets from side arms and rifles may be similar, energy imparted by rifles is higher because the velocity is greater. High-velocity missiles may destroy spinal cord function even if the missile, bone fragments, or resulting hematoma does not impinge upon the nervous tissue. In addition to the energy imparted, the degree of spin of the bullet and fragmentation are important.

The impact of the bullet is a product of the mass and the velocity squared (kinetic energy = $\frac{1}{2}mv^2$). Bullets from high-velocity military weapons may injure the cord by transmitted shock waves without actually penetrating the cord.

By contrast, most civilian casualties are from handguns of much lower muzzle velocity, and direct injury to the cord or closely adjacent vertebral structures is required to produce neurological deficit.

Neurological Deficits

The majority of penetrating injuries of the spinal column are to the thoracic region. Of civilians sustaining gunshot wounds, it is estimated that 50 percent have an immediate and complete neurological deficit.[1,4] In the series of 450 stab wounds of the spine, 21 percent were complete and 79 percent were incomplete injuries.[3]

Neurological symptoms and signs relate to the level and severity of the injury. These include motor and sensory dysfunction as well as loss of sphincter control. Among civilians with gunshot wounds, four syndromes are identified:

1. Immediate, clinically complete loss of spinal cord function above the conus medullaris
2. Incomplete nonprogressive spinal cord deficit
3. Progressive spinal cord deficit
4. Injuries of the conus medullaris or cauda equina with an initial neurological deficit, varying in severity

Groups 1 and 4 are by far the most common. To these may be added cases in whom significant partial improvement or complete recovery occurs, which are reported principally in the military literature.

In the acute phase, flaccid paralysis is the rule. Partial conus medullaris and cauda equina injuries with neurological signs are occasionally difficult to differentiate from wounds isolated to the lumbosacral plexus. Bloody cerebrospinal fluid on lumbar puncture is helpful with the differential diagnosis. Vertebral injury, bilateral neurological findings, and sphincter dysfunction also assist verification, or the lesion may be proved by surgical exploration.

With stab wounds of the spine, as many as 70 percent of the incomplete lesions are of the Brown-Séquard type of hemisection. Many of these are not of the classic pattern, showing occasionally bilateral weakness, with one leg more severely involved than the other, or with bilateral dorsal column loss, indicative of damage to more than half the cord. The reason for the high incidence of damage to only half the cord, considering it is a narrow structure, can be explained by the anatomy of the vertebral column.

Associated Injuries

The direct trajectory of the missile may cause associated injuries of the blood vessels in the neck, the trachea, or vital structures within the thorax or abdomen. Such associated injuries as a result of a single missile or stake usually take precedence in treatment over the spinal cord injury since immediate and complete cord lesions rarely improve after surgery. Abdominal and thoracic lesions take precedence in the acute phase. These complications occur in approximately 25 percent of civilian cases, but 67 percent of military cases have associated injuries. Chest injuries causing hemopneumothorax are the most common, followed by gastrointestinal and renal lesions. Traumatic spinal fluid fistulas resulting from bullet wounds have been described in thoracic injuries but are relatively rare. Such fistulas are generally self-limited but may require thoracentesis and/or later closure of the dural or pleural rent. A missile that has passed through the bowel may cause meningitis and/or osteomyelitis.[2]

Because stab wounds that damage the spinal cord are aimed haphazardly, other structures are sometimes involved. Stab wounds are often also multiple. Stab wounds of the lower cervical and dorsal region may penetrate the thoracic cage and injure the lung, producing a pneumothorax, hemothorax, or hemopneumothorax. Penetrating abdominal stabs may injure almost any abdominal organ. Occasionally the diagnosis of an intra-abdominal injury is difficult, e.g., if the patient is already quadriplegic.

Diagnosis

Routine roentgenograms of all suspected areas are obtained for the purpose of exact localization of the bullet; fragments may also indicate the trajectory. Tomograms and CT scanning may identify vertebral fractures that cannot be seen by routine films. In some patients the trajectory may indicate that the spinal canal has not been transgressed by the missile. In those cases, where there is actually no bony disruption, shock waves are presumed to cause loss of neurological function, although it is possible that deflection of the bullet may have occurred and the straight line between the radiological location of the metallic fragment and the area of entrance may not represent the true bullet path. Also, it is theoretically possible that a bullet may transgress the spinal cord without bony injury. Metrizimide myelography may be helpful if spinal fluid leakage is suspected.

Management

All patients receive large doses of one or more parenteral broad-spectrum antibiotics and tetanus prophylaxis. Steroids in large doses have been administered without any apparent increase in infection rate; whether this helps reduce cord edema is unknown.

The biggest argument in the management of penetrating spinal cord injury is whether to subject the patient to laminectomy. It is interesting that all war-related spinal cord injuries of the Vietnamese conflict were operated upon within hours of the injury. There was 0 percent operative mortality and an overall mortality of 2.3 percent. Most civilian reviews of this topic are very pessimistic about the advisability and neurological benefit of surgical intervention.[1,3-5] No review cites any significant improvement in neurological outcome in operated versus nonoperated cases.

There is no denying that an aura of pessimism justifiably shrouds this unfortunate condition. However, the following guidelines may help neurosurgeons in the decision as to whether or not surgery should be undertaken.

Obvious compression of neural elements (spinal cord, nerve root, or cauda equina) by bone fragments, bullet fragments, the bullet itself, or hematoma should be relieved as soon as possible. Appropriate radiological techniques should be employed early to determine the possible presence of such compression. Manipulation can be more vigorous than with other spinal cord injuries because the spine is stable. It must be remembered that postlaminectomy instability can occur, and if laminectomy is undertaken, it is important to preserve stability.

One may sometimes avoid chronic problems in patients with missile wounds of the spinal cord by identifying bony fragments within the spinal canal that may result in chronic scarring and pain. The occasional copper-jacketed bullets cause severe inflammation and scarring, and should be removed. Decompression of the swollen spinal cord, opening of the dura, placing of a patch graft, and myelotomy are not commonly accepted modes of decompressing the spinal cord.

Another reason for exploration is to prevent infection by debridement of devitalized tissue and to close spinal fluid leaks, although these are admittedly rare.

Psychological benefit to the patient and the family by allowing them to feel that everything possible has been done has also been cited as a reason for operative intervention. Such factors should be left to the judgment of the surgeon in the individual case.

In a review of stab wounds of the spine only 4.4 percent of these were explored, usually to remove retained fragments of the weapon. As noted above, the prognosis with stab wounds of the spine from the standpoint of neurological recovery is much better than the prognosis of injuries due to gunshot wounds. Cauda equina injuries are injuries to peripheral elements rather than to the cord itself, and they should be treated aggressively by decompression and dural repair since recovery of function is much more likely and root herniation with chronic pain can be prevented.

References

1. Heiden JS, Weiss MH, Rosenberg AW, Kurze T, Apuzzo MLJ: Penetrating gunshot wounds of the cervical spine in civilians: Review of 38 cases. Neurosurg 42:575–579, 1975.
2. Matson DD: *The Treatment of Acute Compound Injuries of the Spinal Cord Due to Missiles.* Springfield, Ill, Charles C Thomas, 1948.
3. Peacock WJ, Shrosbree RD, Key AG: A review of 450 stab-wounds of the spinal cord. S Afr Med J 51:961–964, 1977.
4. Six E, Alexander E Jr, Kelly DL Jr, Davis CH Jr, McWhorter JM: Gunshot wounds to the spinal cord. South Med J 72:699–702, 1979.
5. Suwanwela C, Alexander E Jr, Davis CH Jr: Prognosis in spinal cord injury, with special reference to patients with motor paralysis and sensory preservation. J Neurosurg 19:220–227, 1962.

221

Posterior Lumbar Spinal Fusion

J. Leonard Goldner

Spinal fusion procedures of various types have been performed for many years.[1-14] The reader may consult the references at the end of the chapter for the details of some of these operations, especially those relating to posterior lumbar spinal fusion.

Selection of Patients

Fusion of the lumbar and lumbosacral spine segments, when indicated, provides stability, diminishes painful incongruity, and lessens or eliminates back pain.[1-4,6-11] The best results occur when the lesion is identified and when definite indications for spine fusion are determined.[6] If an anatomical cause for pain is not determined, a spinal fusion procedure will not succeed.[4,7,10,12-14]

Data gathering includes a detailed history, a meticulous physical examination, and appropriate laboratory studies. These are essential in determining the location of a pathological condition. The emotional characteristics and personality profile are also essential items in the preoperative investigation.[6,7]

Helpful Adjuncts to the Patient's History

Certain adjuncts are very helpful in verifying and extending the history obtained from the patient. (1) The prior medical records are reviewed to obtain information about the past history, prior treatment, findings at operation, and the patient's progress. Details of the initial onset of the current complaints and comments about the patient's cooperation are helpful in determining the pathomechanics involved and the kind of lesion suspected. (2) Old operative notes are helpful in reconstructing the characteristics of the original lesion. (3) The initial x-ray films, myelogram, and other invasive and noninvasive studies aid in reconstructing the patient's original condition. (4) Information about the postoperative course, pain pattern, frequency and kind of medications, and rapidity of recovery are helpful in determining the patient's response to treatment. This information describes the original lesion as being well-defined or nondescript. (5) A current day-to-day pain diary is obtained. The pain pattern is separated into morning, afternoon and evening and correctly compared with the subjective pain during the past several months. The patient's pain threshold is assessed and the medication requirements are noted.

Historical and Physical Items that Require Special Precautions

If pain is constant, being described as never changing during a 24-h period, the examiner must be cautious. A malignant tumor is suspected but a psychosomatic problem may be the basis for this pain pattern.

If the physical examination is essentially negative, but the patient requires large doses of opiates, requests antidepressants or tranquilizers, and must have medications for sleep, a significant emotional component probably exists.

If the patient has had one or more operative procedures in the absence of strongly positive preoperative findings, and if the pain relief obtained was slight or none, or, conversely, in the absence of positive preoperative diagnostic data total relief of pain was obtained, either event must be viewed with suspicion and more attention given to the patient's emotional profile.

If the physical examination reveals bizarre hypersensitivity of a scar; or a stocking-type hypesthesia, the patient's problem should be viewed with both concern and suspicion.

A patient with a bizarre gait not consistent with a specific pathological lesion requires psychiatric and psychological assessment. The surgeon may suspect conversion or malingering, but if the clinical psychological studies are normal then the problem must be reassessed. However, occasionally a normal psychological study occurs in the presence of clinical findings consistent with conversion reaction or malingering. A special review of this requires further communication between the surgeon, the psychologist, and the psychiatrist.

Inconsistent sciatic or femoral nerve stretch tests which show, for example, positive complaints of pain at 30 degrees of straight leg raising when the patient is supine but none with 90-degree straight leg raising when the patient is sitting requires careful assessment of the patient's complaints and a repeat of the examination.[7]

Over-reaction to palpation, percussion, or manipulation during the examination is reason for careful assessment of the patient's complaints.

Diagnostic Studies that are Helpful in Determining a Pathological Lesion of the Spine

Plain x-ray films are taken to assess bone density, and also to document motion of the vertebral bodies and posterior elements. (Lateral flexion and extension films and anteroposterior right and left lateral bending projections are helpful in determining the degree of motion between the vertebral bodies and the presence of a pseudoarthrosis).

Lordotic projections of the sacroiliac joints may show

evidence of ankylosing spondylitis. The plain anteroposterior projection may not allow the subchondral sclerosis to be visualized.

A metrizamide myelogram followed by computed tomography in the horizontal and vertical planes will provide much information about the facet joints, the size of the canal, and the relationship of a nerve to the canal and the exit foramen.

Electromyography, if positive, gives helpful information that determines whether the lesion is recent or old and whether there is denervation or reinnervation of the muscles involved. Careful communication should occur between the surgeon and the electromyographer.[7]

Serological studies are helpful if an inflammatory condition is suspected. Rheumatoid factor and antinuclear antibody assessment, a special blood smear for lupus cells, a uric acid level (for gout), and the determination of the erythrocyte sedimentation rate (for nonspecific inflammatory conditions) are important. Assessment of the HLA-B27 locus 40 is helpful in determining the presence of ankylosing spondylitis.

A technetium-99 bone scan will provide information about degenerative arthritis, trauma, infection, and inflammation. The study must be interpreted in conjunction with the other radiographic and physical and laboratory findings.

Thermography has been helpful as a screening test in determining an inflammatory process of the spine. This test complements the bone scan and is particularly helpful if the sedimentation rate is elevated.

Clinical psychological and psychiatric assessment are valuable in providing information about the patient's emotional profile, secondary gain, and behavioral deviations. An operative procedure, if indicated, is performed, but the prognosis for time of recovery and the way the patient responds to the operation from a behavioral standpoint will be clarified.

Diagnostic nerve root blocks or facet injections with a local anesthetic, and a differential spinal anesthesia test may provide information that is helpful in assessing the patient's pain complaints and in determining the validity of these complaints.[7]

A discogram done with the aid of an image intensifier may show disorganization of the intervertebral disc bond, will provide information about reproduction of the patient's pain complaints, and will be helpful if an enzyme is to be used in treating the patient's radiculopathy.[7]

A pain test employing Pentothal (thiopental sodium, Abbott Laboratories, North Chicago, Ill.) gives the surgeon information about the validity of the patient's complaints with reference to straight leg raising, manipulation of the extremity, and movement of the spine. If the patient is partially asleep after Pentothal induction, and if the straight leg raising can be performed without pain whereas prior to the injection of the Pentothal the patient had severe pain, then the interpretation of the patient's pain demands reassessment.

Indications for Lumbar Spine Fusion

The major reasons for spine fusion are segmental instability and segmental incongruity.[1,4,6,9,14]

Pain

The rationale for stabilization of the spine is determined by the factors which cause pain. *The anatomical structures* that might be involved are the posterior longitudinal ligament, the ligamenta flava, the facet joints and their synovium,[5] the subchondral bone of the vertebral body or the facet joints, and the interspinous ligaments. Reactive fibrosis and osteophytes may occur as a result of a pathological process in the intervertebral disc space or the facet joints or due to avulsion of the ligaments.[4,6] Determination of whether or not these radiographic findings are significant depends on the many factors already mentioned. Also, the deep ligaments between the laminal arches and the transverse processes may be affected by tearing or fibrosis. This is meaningful only in the acute stage of an injury as these ligaments usually heal within several weeks after the original injury.

The individual motor and sensory nerve roots, the sensory ganglia, the combined common roots, and the sinuvertebral nerves, alone or together, may be responsible for pain. Combinations of lesions involving bone, ligaments, and neural tissue, as noted in adult scoliosis, spondylolisthesis, or intervertebral disc excision followed by interspace narrowing, may be responsible for the pain syndrome.[5,14]

Other structural changes that may cause pain are facet degeneration, facet sclerosis,[5] exit foramen narrowing, or radicular canal stenosis.[4] The nerve root may be affected by any of these alterations and require bone decompression.[4] If several roots are involved or if the entire cauda equina is compressed, then the laminal arches are removed. If decompression is extensive at one interspace or over several interspaces and if the disc bond is abnormal, then spinal fusion may be indicated.[3,4,6-8,12-14]

Although an exact correlation between the patient's complaints and the anatomical site of pain is not always possible, enough information is available to allow a reasonable speculation concerning the site of pain as it relates to the patient's complaints. There are many documented syndromes that demonstrate correlation between the cause of back or extremity pain and elimination of this pain after treatment. Examples of this will suggest clinical indications for or against spine fusion:[4,6,7]

The pain relief that follows removal of a large disc fragment causing root irritation is dramatic. Fusion is not indicated initially.

Pain due to nerve root fibrosis caused by prior trauma is temporarily eliminated by nerve root block which indicates that the sensory receptors in a particular location are affected and cause pain.

Diffusion of contrast during a discogram associated with disorganization of the nucleus and annulus may be associated with two kinds of pain: Fullness in the back, buttocks and thighs, a heavy feeling in the back, and a deep vague discomfort in the lumbosacral region are associated with a disorganized interspace. This occurs without leakage outside the interspace. If the contrast leaks posteriorly, it irritates the adjacent roots and causes pain. Either of these kinds of pain may reproduce the patient's original complaints. If the discogram needle touches a nerve root the radicular pain provides a sensory pattern recognized and described by the patient as different from or similar to the prediscogram pain.

Pain in spondylolisthesis due to manipulation of a loose laminar arch or movement of the isthmus defect are both relieved temporarily by flexion of the trunk and permanently by successful decompression of the nerve roots and spinal fusion.[9,11]

Pain caused by sclerotic intervertebral subchondral plates, affected by prolonged flexion, and usually relieved by extension or unloading, is frequently relieved by anterior interbody fusion.[10] Root decompression may not be necessary if the radicular canal is opened slightly by the interbody fusion.[7]

Pain associated with vertebral body translation, intervertebral disc disorganization, and nerve root irritation is relieved by both rest and spine fusion.[1,4,6,7,11-14]

Low back tightness, stiffness, and pain during sitting and after significant activity are usually relieved by rest. The early relief of pain by stretching the collagen and strengthening paravertebral musculature demonstrates relief of this kind of discomfort, which is different from facet pain, nerve root irritation, or vertebral interbody pain.

The surgeon should attempt to pinpoint one or several reasons why pain is present. Flexibility in decision making is an important aspect of managing the painful lower back. There are specific indications for the use of different spine fusion techniques.[1-4,8,9,12,13] The surgeon should be aware of the several techniques so that each problem can be managed by either anterior discectomy and bone grafting or posterior decompression and posterolateral fusion or a combination of both of these depending on the pathological lesion. The surgeon's familiarity with a particular procedure or enthusiasm for a particular approach should not interfere with the concept of selecting anterior or posterior or a combination of approaches in order to provide adequate nerve root decompression and stabilization of the vertebral bodies and the facet joints.

The Pathological Lesion

Opinions vary and experiences differ among surgeons. Pain tolerance varies from one patient to another. The decision to proceed with stabilization of the spine is made by performing the appropriate diagnostic studies and by determining one or more locations of pain. Our experience during the past 30 years with over 1,000 patients who have had spine fusion has shown that the prediction for lessening or eliminating pain by a spine fusion depends on the pathological lesion.

Fusion for *spondylolisthesis* will usually eliminate all or most of the pain. We recently reviewed 116 adolescents with spondylolisthesis who had had decompression and spine fusion within the past 30 years. After the first operation, 90 percent had excellent or good results; and after a second operation for pseudoarthrosis the other 10 percent were elevated to a good or excellent status. Although the degree of improvement varied from one patient to another, the overall trend was that of improvement.

Spine fusion for *failed intervertebral disc surgery* will result in improvement in about 80 percent of the patients. The degree of improvement varies but does justify this approach to solving the problem. Whether the fusion is anterior, posterior, or combined depends on the extent of the pathology and the surgeon's experience. Among our patients, those who have had extensive perineural fibrosis or arachnoiditis have done less well than those who have had segmental instability or incongruity. Furthermore, patients with personality deficiencies, emotional instability, and secondary gain factors have not responded as well as individuals who are emotionally stable and have good motivation.

The decision to perform a spine fusion is one that takes deliberation, careful diagnostic study and a cooperative, emotionally stable patient. Technical excellence will assure a maximum degree of bone healing. The following pathological abnormalities are likely to be improved by fusion of the spine:

1. Spinal instability—segmental, with secondary soft tissue or ligamentous changes and perhaps nerve compression. (*a*) Posterior element hypermobility associated with spondylolisthesis. The hypoplastic or loose fragment is excised partially or completely and a single space posterolateral fusion is performed.[13] (*b*) Anterior instability due to an isthmus defect associated with spondylolisthesis and a failed posterolateral fusion is stabilized by anterior interbody fusion.[7] (*c*) Instability associated with extensive central and lateral decompression causing iatrogenic spondylolisthesis is managed by anterior interbody fusion and a second stage supplementary posterolateral fusion. An alternative is posterior lumbar interbody fusion (PLIF) and supplementary posterolateral fusion.[4] The latter has the disadvantage of requiring nerve root and cauda equina manipulation during the procedure. (*d*) Destructive lesions of the posterior and anterior elements of the vertebra associated with metastatic tumor are stabilized by posterolateral decompression and Harrington metallic fixation and either autogenous or homologous bone or methyl methacrylate. (*e*) Instability associated with narrowing of the disc bond and with facet erosion and stretching of the interspinous ligaments requires stabilization by either facet and posterolateral fusion; or posterior interbody fusion; or anterior interbody stabilization and supplementary posterior fusion if necessary.

Spinal instability is detected by lateral flexion-extension films and anteroposterior right and left lateral bending films. A CT scan alone or even myelography without flexion and extension may not determine instability. Dynamic diagnostic studies are essential.

2. Incongruity of the spine without significant instability. (*a*) Facet joint degeneration and hypertrophy are the primary problem; or these lesions are combined with intervertebral disc bond narrowing.[5] (*b*) Foraminal encroachment occurs after discectomy and is combined with interbody narrowing and pain. (*c*) Interbody irritation may occur after intervertebral disc removal or with irregularity of the annulus and nucleus without localized extrusion. (*d*) Degenerative intervertebral disc disease causes secondary sclerosis of the vertebral bodies, subchondral cyst formation, and desiccation of the annulus and nucleus with resulting sequestration. (*e*) Inflammatory reaction associated with bacterial infection or granuloma not responding to antibiotics, rest, and anti-inflammatory medications causes incongruity. Occasionally, the bacterial discitis or interspace infection

postoperatively is aborted by antibiotics, but firm union of the vertebral bodies may not occur and the persistent limited motion causes pain with axial loading or spinal torque. (f) Spine fusion should be considered when interbody pain is a major persistent cause of the patient's complaints. Facet joint pain with or without nerve root irritation that does not respond to limited nonoperative treatment is successfully managed by nerve root decompression and localized arthrodesis. If the disc bond is stable, localized lateral resection may be performed without spinal fusion. Extensive posterior central and lateral compression associated with an insufficient intervertebral disc bond anteriorly will result in instability and incongruity, and spinal fusion is indicated.

3. Incongruity and instability. (a) *Trauma* combines the lesions described under incongruity and instability. Even minor translation of the vertebral body or the posterior elements results in pain because of incongruity. The anterior, middle, and posterior columns of the spine should be congruous and stable but if not, pain might occur. For example, in a severe compression fracture of the third lumbar vertebra with the posterior elements involved, the primary goal is stabilization by spontaneous or surgical arthrodesis to prevent further collapse of the vertebral body and the intervertebral disc spaces, and incongruity of the middle and posterior columns of the spine. Decompression of the exit foramina, the radicular canals, and the posterior central canal may be necessary as an associated step in providing stability and diminishing incongruity.[6] (b) *Pseudoarthrosis:* Fibrous union of an attempted fusion may cause persistent pain. The pain is not due to instability but rather localized incongruity. The same pathological lesion may occur after a fracture which affects the interspace but does not result in spontaneous fusion. The lesion may cause pain because of mechanical malalignment and incongruous joints posteriorly and anteriorly. Spinal fusion is indicated and may require mechanical realignment in addition to bone grafting.[6,7] Use of internal fixation is optional as this depends on the kind of problem occurring.[2,8,9] (c) *Perineural fibrosis* (adhesions of the epineurium and compressive lesions of the nerve root due to external and internal fibrosis): Stabilization of the interspace and the facets diminishes local contusion of the neural elements and decreases elongation of the nerve. An analogy is at the wrist, for example, where an immobile wrist joint diminishes the stretch and irritation of a compressed median nerve. (d) *Arachnoiditis* may result in tethering of several nerve roots on one or both sides or even the entire cauda equina. Elimination of motion at the lower three lumbar vertebrae may diminish the tethering by decreasing localized stretch of the nerve roots. The elimination of motion has in certain patients diminished radicular pain. This had occurred with anterior discectomy and fusion with or without additional posterior and posterolateral decompression. This indicates that diminution of motion is a prominent factor in diminishing pain of neural origin.

Surgical Techniques

In the following paragraphs I will describe the pertinent steps in performing a posterolateral fusion in a patient who has had posterior and lateral decompression for posterior and/or lateral stenosis, or a patient with a grade I, II, or III spondylolisthesis.

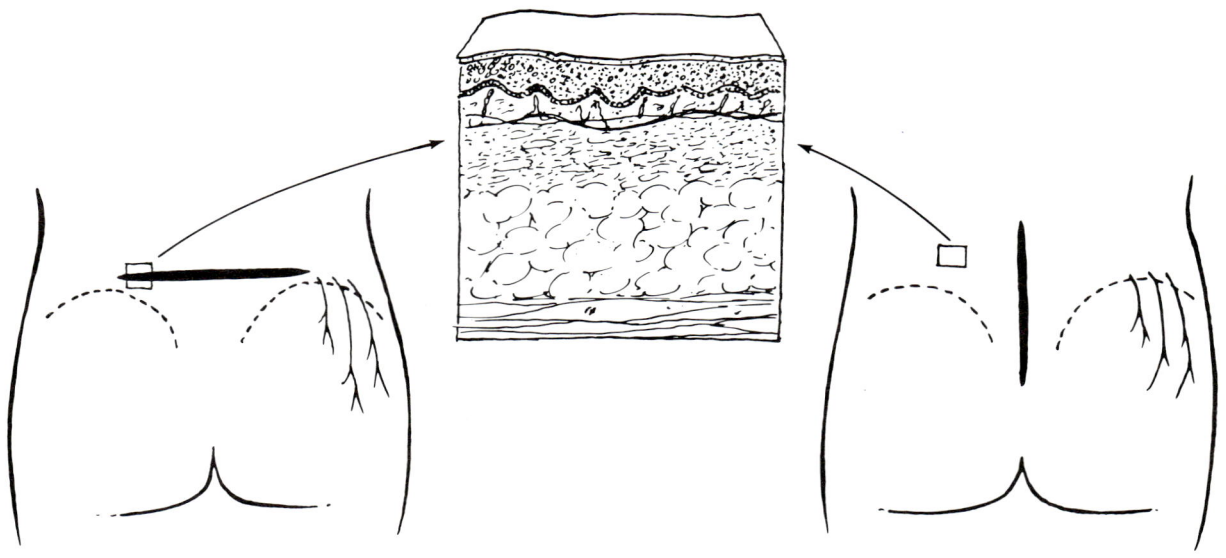

Figure 221-1 Skin incisions and donor site of fat graft. The horizontal skin incision provides exposure to the iliac crest and the transverse processes with minimal skin stretch. This skin incision is particularly useful in young individuals who are not obese. L4, L5, S1, and S2 are easily exposed through a vertical midline incision in the deep fascia. The lateral fascial cuts are made as noted in Fig. 221-2. The vertical incision avoids the cluneal nerves, as does the horizontal incision. For the same reason special attention is given to taking the bone graft from the midline horizontal or vertical incisions.

Skin Incision

The skin may be incised either horizontally, extending from one posterior iliac spine to the other, or vertically, in the midline over the spinous processes (Fig. 221-1). The cluneal nerves should be avoided in the horizontal incision. The advantages of this incision are: (1) Easier exposure of the transverse processes and lateral masses. (2) A direct approach to the posterior superior iliac bone graft. (3) The incision is in line with the skin creases.

The Posterior Spinous Ligaments and Paravertebral Fascia

A stable spinous process should be identified. If the spondylolisthesis is located at L5–S1, the initial dissection should be at the L4 spinous process. Electrocautery is used to isolate the tip of the spinous process. The fascia is separated subperiosteally and Hibbs sponges are inserted along the spinous process. A dissector is used to advance the sponges laterally, which cleans off the attached fascia and muscle. The incision is widened and the small sponges are replaced by larger Mikulicz pads which are forced laterally with a large Cobb elevator. The pad is compressed and forced laterally with a periosteal elevator and a mallet. The elevator forces the pad ahead and the mallet is used rather than manual dissection. The fascia over the paraspinal muscles is then incised horizontally opposite the L5 interspace and the L4 spinous process (Fig 221-2). This diminishes contracture of the long muscles and allows easier retraction of the muscles by self-retaining retractors.

The fascial attachment of the paraspinal muscles is then released from the sacrum, bleeding points are coagulated, the sacroiliac joint is avoided, and the bony surface of the sacrum is identified. Dissection is then continued from distal to proximal. An occult spina bifida may exist in conjunction with spondylolisthesis and midline dissection over S1 is performed carefully. The lateral bony elements are identified first and the midline dissection is completed last.

Removal of the Loose Posterior Element

The loose posterior element is grasped with a towel clip and stabilized while it is identified, isolated and either partially or completely excised. If the element is hypoplastic, it is removed completely. If it is large and moderately hypermobile then partial laminectomy and isthmus removal are performed beginning at the L4–5 space for an L5–S1 spondylolisthesis and following the L5 root through the radicular canal and out the exit foramen.

Preparation of the Site for Fusion

Lateral retraction is obtained on both sides by placement of Taylor retractors adjacent to the L5 transverse process which is located about 8 mm cephalad to the spinous process of L5 (Fig. 221-2). The length of this transverse process is determined preoperatively from an anteroposterior x-ray

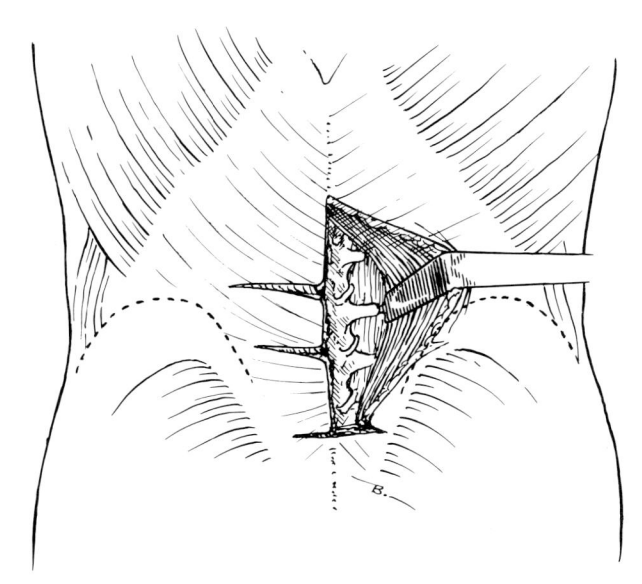

Figure 221-2 Detail of the midline incision. The paravertebral muscles have been dissected subperiosteally, exposing the facets and the transverse processes. The Taylor retractor is lateral to the L4 transverse process. The horizontal incisions are in the lumbodorsal fascia. This allows muscle retraction with less force. The fascial incisions also increase the postoperative range of motion and diminish the tightness and tension of the lumbar fascial attachments to the spine.

film. If the process is very short, then the L4 transverse process must be included in the fusion. Usually only L5 is included in the fusion to the sacrum for spondylolisthesis grades I–III. The transverse processes are cleaned with a periosteal elevator and a $\frac{1}{2}$ in. osteotome. Fracture occurs easily if too much pressure is applied. The concavity (lateral gutter) of the pedicle is identified, and a rough surface is formed with a double-action rongeur, a small curved osteotome, and a Cobb elevator. The L5 nerve root is caudad to the L5 transverse process and is avoided. The articular cartilage of the first sacral facet is removed and 1 mm thick, 10 mm long flaps are elevated from the sacrum and rotated cephalad to bridge the gap between the sacrum and the transverse process. The roughened bone surface includes the sacrum, the transverse process, and the lateral gutter on both the right and left sides.

The L4–5 facet joints are not included in the single space fusion. Bone is not placed over this facet joint. Stripping does not include the articular cartilage of this joint and bone in the lateral gutter is below the facet joints so that encroachment does not occur. Creeping or encroachment of the fusion on this joint may cause pain.

Grafting from the Posterior Superior Iliac Spine

The posterior superior iliac spine is identified lateral to the sacroiliac joint (Fig 221-3). Periosteal stripping is performed with electrocautery, and a Mikulicz pad is inserted along the concave surface of the ilium toward the sciatic notch. The inner aspect of the ilium is also freed of fascia and muscle

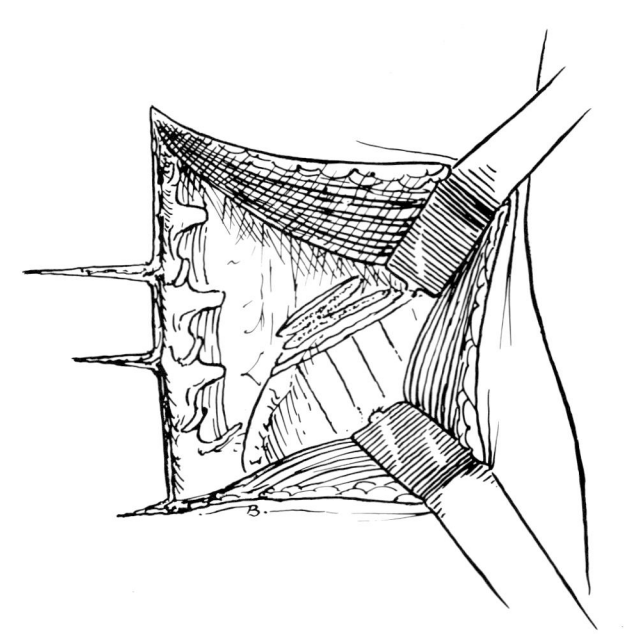

Figure 221-3 The posterior superior iliac spine is exposed through the midline incision. The paravertebral muscles are shown here retracted laterally for diagrammatic purposes. However, the iliac spine is exposed by subcutaneous dissection from the midline incision, during which bone is removed but the paravertebral muscles in the midline are left adjacent to the spine.

attachments and 3-mm-thick flat segments of bone are shaved from the wide surface of the ilium. Four flat grafts measuring 3 × 10 × 25 mm and including both cortices are taken from the widest portion of the posterior ilium. The cancellous bone and the outer cortex are then removed by making vertical cuts with a ½-in. osteotome 12 mm apart and extending downward about 3 cm (Fig. 221-3). A curved osteotome is used to remove the cortex, and then the cancellous bone in strips, until the medial cortical surface is encountered. Additional bone located between the cortices is removed with a curette.

The bone graft site is packed with a Mikulicz pad and the bone graft is shaped and placed on the recipient area (Fig. 221-4). The grafts are long enough to bridge from the L5 transverse process to the sacrum but are not small enough to drop into the exit foramen. The grafts must be bent about 20 degrees to fit the contour of the sacrum and the transverse process. The bone strips are laid adjacent to each other and gently compressed by the surgeon's thumb. Cortical and cancellous bone strips are placed in the lateral gutter. The width of the grafted surface should be about 3 cm on each side. If all soft tissue has been removed, the contact between each bone graft and the recipient site will include only bone touching bone without soft tissue interposition. The single layer contact is more important than a massive amount of bone that does not touch the recipient site.

The Bone Graft Donor Site

After the bone graft is placed on the recipient area, the donor site is inspected. Bleeding points are electrocoagulated and plugged with a thin layer of bone wax. Surgicel (oxidized regenerated cellulose; Johnson & Johnson Products Inc., New Brunswick, N.J.) is used to cover the cancellous bone. The muscles are inspected for bleeding and a suction tube is inserted into the bone graft site. The tube

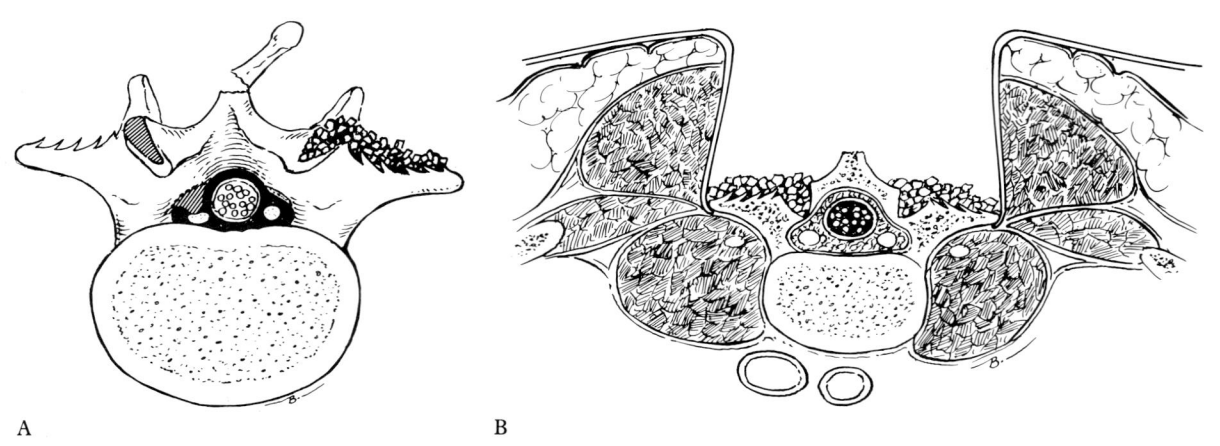

Figure 221-4 *A.* Axial view of posterior lateral fusion. Soft tissue has been removed from the laminae, the facet joints, and the transverse processes. The facet joint articular cartilage is removed meticulously. The outer cortex of the transverse process is roughened superficially. Combined cancellous-cortical grafts are impacted in the facet joints and compressed over the transverse processes. The spinous processes may be retained and stabilized with braided wire and interspinous bone grafts; or they may be removed if an extensive laminectomy is performed. *B.* Posterior lateral fusion after paravertebral muscles have been retracted, transverse processes have been cleaned and roughened, facet joints have been resected, and iliac cancellous chips have been inserted to cover the exposed lateral bone surfaces. The laminal arches are not included in the fusion in order to avoid bony ingrowth into the spinal canal.

Posterior Lumbar Spinal Fusion

exits just superior and lateral to the gluteus maximus muscle, away from the cluneal nerves. If bleeding is persistent, then a wide tube is used with one suction unit. The muscle is closed firmly with nonabsorbable sutures to obliterate the dead space.

The Fusion Site

The fusion site is then irrigated, and a free fat graft measuring 1 × 3 × 3 cm is placed over the exposed dura where the laminal arch has been removed. Bleeding points are coagulated, particularly in the lateral muscles, and the muscles are pulled together and closed with nonabsorbable sutures. The cuts in the paravertebral fascia are left open, allowing for expansion and improved postoperative flexion. The subcutaneous tissues are closed with absorbable sutures and skin clips are used for either the vertical or the transverse incision. A suction drain is placed in the lateral muscular recesses, one tube on either side, and is attached to a wide tube connected to a suction unit. A separate suction unit is used for the bone graft donor site. Abdominal pads are applied and paper tape is used to hold the compression dressing in place.

Postoperative Management

Position The patient is kept in the supine position with the hips flexed 45 degrees and knees flexed 70 degrees. A small pillow is placed under the head. A trapeze is attached to the bed to assist the patient is shifting his trunk. He is rolled as a unit to the right or left through 30 degrees and propped with pillows after 2 h. Foot motion, leg motion, and deep breathing are encouraged. After 24 h the patient may lie on one side or the other. He is mobilized gradually after 24 hours, and may sit on the edge of the bed with a corset on, and may stand with assistance, preferably with the aid of a walker and a person.

Dressings A compression dressing is used for 24 h. Then all dressings are removed and a light sterile pad is placed over the wound and one over the suction drainage site. Suction drains are removed when the drainage stops, but are kept in no longer than 24 h, if possible. The open dressing technique is followed after 48 h. A sterile pad covers the wound only to prevent moisture while the patient is lying on his back.

Urine If a Foley catheter is used during the operation, it is left in place for 24 h. If a catheter is not used, then intermittent catheterization is practiced until the patient can void. If the catheter is left in place, then an antimicrobial agent is given while the catheter is in place and for 72 h after it has been removed.

Anticoagulation A heparin-Coumadin regime is used in the adult patients and has been since 1970. Heparin is given subcutaneously, 5,000 units on call and 3,000 units every 6 h beginning 4 h postoperatively or when the wound drainage diminishes and depending on the activated thromboplastin time determination. The thromboplastin time is monitored and is held at 10–20 percent longer than normal for the patient. Coumadin (Warfarin sodium; Endo Laboratories, Inc., Wilmington, Del.) is given as 5 mg orally on the fifth postoperative day and then daily until the prothrombin time reaches a 1.4 to 1.6 ratio. When that ratio is reached, the heparin is discontinued. The patient is discharged on Coumadin under the care of his family physician and continues the Coumadin for a total of 4 weeks from the time of the operation. If the patient has diabetes, a bleeding tendency, an ulcer or some other problem, then this form of anticoagulation might not be used.

Other mechanical methods of preventing venous thrombosis include antithromboembolic hose, continuous lower extremity elevation while in bed, and active motion of the extremities.

Fluid and Food Intravenous fluid is given until the patient has bowel sounds and flatus. Paralytic ileus may occur after a spine fusion and can usually be resolved by withholding oral food and fluid. Intravenous fluid includes appropriate blood replacement, and postoperative transfusions are given as indicated, maintaining the hematocrit above 30 percent. Vitamins D and C are added to the intravenous fluids postoperatively.

Antibiotics A wide spectrum antibiotic is given preoperatively on call and postoperatively for 48 h. The antibiotic is given longer if an indwelling catheter is necessary.

Pain Control Morphine complemented with a phenothiazine is used for 24 h. Chloral hydrate is given for sleep. Anti-inflammatory, salicylate, or other medication is given as soon as the patient tolerates medications by mouth. A transcutaneous stimulator applied immediately postoperatively has been helpful in diminishing pain at the bone graft site and from the spinal operation. A double blind study is currently underway, but early results are in favor of the stimulator.

Mobility Straight leg raising is initiated at 24 h. The overhead trapeze is used to assist the patient in moving. If perineural fibrosis has been present, straight leg raising to the point of maximum tolerance is begun early and anti-inflammatory medicine supplements the exercises. The patient is up out of bed when this is tolerated and as many times a day as he is able to stand, walk, and move. Pelvic tilt exercises are initiated on the third day. Sitting is avoided. A commode extension is used in the hospital and at home for 8 weeks. The patient is kept from driving an automobile for 6 weeks. Sexual activity is limited for 6 weeks. A corset is worn when the patient is up as a reminder to avoid twisting or bending the spine. The patient is given instructions in knee bending and hip flexion, is allowed to shower at 1 week with assistance. Sutures are removed at 2 weeks.

Patients who have had Harrington rods or more extensive fixation for instability are managed differently according to the problem involved. Postoperative splinting, a polypropylene jacket, and variations of trunk support are used if necessary. In most instances, with internal fixation, mobilization and walking are possible within a week after the operation.

Pulmonary Care Deep breathing, blow bottles, and coughing are used to maintain lung function. This program is the same for adolescents or adults who have had posterior stabilization for spondylolisthesis or a localized fusion for instability or incongruity.

Modifications of Surgical Techniques for Special Situations

Spondylolisthesis Greater than 50 Percent

Spondylolisthesis with greater than 50 percent forward displacement of the vertebral body may require inclusion of the transverse process of L4 and the inferior facets between L4 and L5 in the fusion (Fig. 221-5). The surgical technique is the same as described above and additional steps include fusion of the articular facets between L4 and L5, but not inclusion of the superior facets between L4 and L3. The bone graft extends from the transverse process of L4 and L5 and from L5 to S1.

If the laminal arch of L5 is large and is not completely removed, then the laminal arch of L4 is wired to the laminal arch of L5 by twisted stainless steel wire placed through the base of the spinous process of L5 and tightened with a wire twister. A bone graft measuring about 1×1 cm (combined cortical and cancellous bone) is placed between the spinous processes prior to tightening the wire. This prevents excessive tilting of the laminal arch and avoids compression of the dura (Fig. 221-6).

Spinal Stenosis

Posterior and posterolateral decompression is performed for spinal stenosis and stenosis of the exit foramina. All of these areas are decompressed and the cauda equina and nerve roots are freed by extensive resection of bone. (Fig 221-7A). If this is done at two spaces, then posterolateral fusion is performed, as already described under the spondylolisthesis technique (Fig. 221-7B). If decompression of four spaces is required, then a Harrington rod is placed on either side of the spine from L1 to S1, placing the hook in the sacrum and prebending the rod to conform to the normal lumbar lordosis (Fig. 221-8A). An alternative to the Harrington rod is the prebent unit Luque rod (Fig. 221-8B), which extends above the fusion and is prebent along either side of the lumbar vertebrae, with the caudal extension directed into a hole in the ilium on either side. The rods are then anchored to the spine by passing wires through the foramina or around the transverse processes.

My preference for stabilization of the spine that has undergone extensive posterior and lateral bone removal for stenosis is anterior interbody fusion as a primary procedure followed, if necessary, by posterolateral reinforcement with rods or bone graft alone. Once the anterior fusion is stable, a posterolateral reinforcement without metallic fixation is usually sufficient. However, the Harrington rod or the supplementary single or double Luque rod will reinforce an unstable spine and allow the patient to be semisitting after a few weeks and walking with external support at about 6 weeks.

Autogenous Bone Grafts vs. Methyl Methacrylate for Fusion

Autogenous Bone

We favor autologous and supplementary homologous frozen bone for spinal fusions in patients who do not have a malignant bone tumor. The advantages of autogenous bone are:

1. It is nonreactive and is not rejected.
2. It is biological in its ability to establish trabeculae and react to stress.
3. If assimilation of the graft occurs with host bone, the stress on internal fixation is eliminated and the need for internal fixation is less essential, both initially and secondarily.
4. The bone graft, once assimilated with host bone, tends to hypertrophy and provides additional protection against stress and strain as time passes.

The disadvantages of autogenous bone can be summarized as follows:

1. The bone graft site is a source of pain.
2. There is a limited source of bone for multiple procedures.
3. The bone may be of insufficient density in an osteopenic patient to provide significant support.
4. Nonunion may develop between the bone graft and the host site.

Methyl Methacrylate

The advantages of this substance are the following:

1. Immediate fixation.
2. The material can be reinforced with wire or metal.
3. Methacrylate can serve as a method of stabilization while radiation is given to surrounding tissues.
4. Methacrylate is useful in reinforcing severe bone defects and osteopenic bone in patients with rheumatoid arthritis for posterior stabilization of C1–C2.
5. This substance will serve as a space filler when bone has been destroyed by a malignant tumor. Metallic reinforcement is necessary, in addition to the methacrylate, in order to provide adequate strength.

Disadvantages of methyl methacrylate are as follows:

1. It does not bond to bone.
2. A membrane develops between methacrylate and bone which may externally absorb bone. The methacrylate may then loosen.
3. Methacrylate must be reinforced by metal in order to tolerate significant stress.
4. This material may serve as an impervious membrane between the host and a bone graft and prevent union from occurring. A Gelfoam (absorbable gelatin sponge; The Upjohn Company, Kalamazoo, Mich.) insert over the bone graft may protect the bone graft and the host bone from being invaded by the methacrylate.

Posterior Lumbar Spinal Fusion

Figure 221-5 *A.* Grade I spondylolisthesis, L5–S1. The isthmus defect is shown. On each side, the posterior lateral fusion extends from the sacrum to the transverse process of L5. Bone is placed in the lateral gutter after the fibrocartilage from the isthmus is removed and after the laminal arch is partially or completely removed. If the L5 spinous process is spared, it is fixed with wire and an interspinous process bone graft (as demonstrated in Fig. 221-6) to S1. The ilium is not included in the bridging graft, and the facet joints at L4-5 are avoided. *B.* Grade II spondylolisthesis. The isthmus defect is visible. The vertebral body is forward about 25 percent of the width of the body. The fusion is performed between L5 and S1. The bone graft on each side is more horizontal than in a mild displacement. The interspinous ligament wire and bone graft between L5 and S1 is used if possible. After the roots are decompressed, the laminae and the interspinous ligaments are parts of a free fragment but are stabilized by the wire. *C.* Grade III spondylolisthesis requires a fusion from L4 to S1. When the transverse processes of L4 and the facets at L4–5 are included in the fusion, the vertebral body of L5 is stabilized in spite of the isthmus defect. On each side, the fact that the bone graft extends from S1 to the L5 transverse process as well as the L4 transverse process gives a greater chance of stability. However, when two spaces are included, the incidence of nonunion is greater. An anterior interbody fusion may be necessary if pseudoarthrosis develops. *D.* Grade IV spondylolisthesis requires bridging from L4 to S1. The angle of the cauda equina is sharp and the roots are angulated. The nerve roots should be decompressed completely. The laminal arch of L5 is removed, and the fusion includes L4 to S1. If anterior reinforcement is necessary, bone is placed between the inferior body of L5 and the anterior surface of the sacrum, and the L4–5 interspace is included in the fusion; or, the vertebral body of L5 is resected and the vertebral body of L4 is allowed to settle and posterior Harrington rods are used for stabilization and reduction. *E.* The complete outline of the L4 posterior elements articulating with L5. On the left, the isthmus defect at L5 has been removed, the transverse process of L5 has been roughened, and the L5 nerve root passing caudad to the facet joint has been unroofed. In this instance, the fusion will include the L4 transverse process, which has not yet been roughened, the L5 transverse process, the L4–5 facet joint, the laminal arch of L5, and the S1 segment, which is not included in the drawing. On the right, the bone graft extends from the inferior articular process of L4 to the superior articular process of L5, including the transverse process of L5 and laminal arch of L5, and bridging the L5 root. Additional bone will be added between the transverse processes of L4 and L5 superiorly and from the transverse process of L5 to S1 inferiorly. This diagram represents the inclusion of L4, L5, and S1 in the posterior lateral fusion.

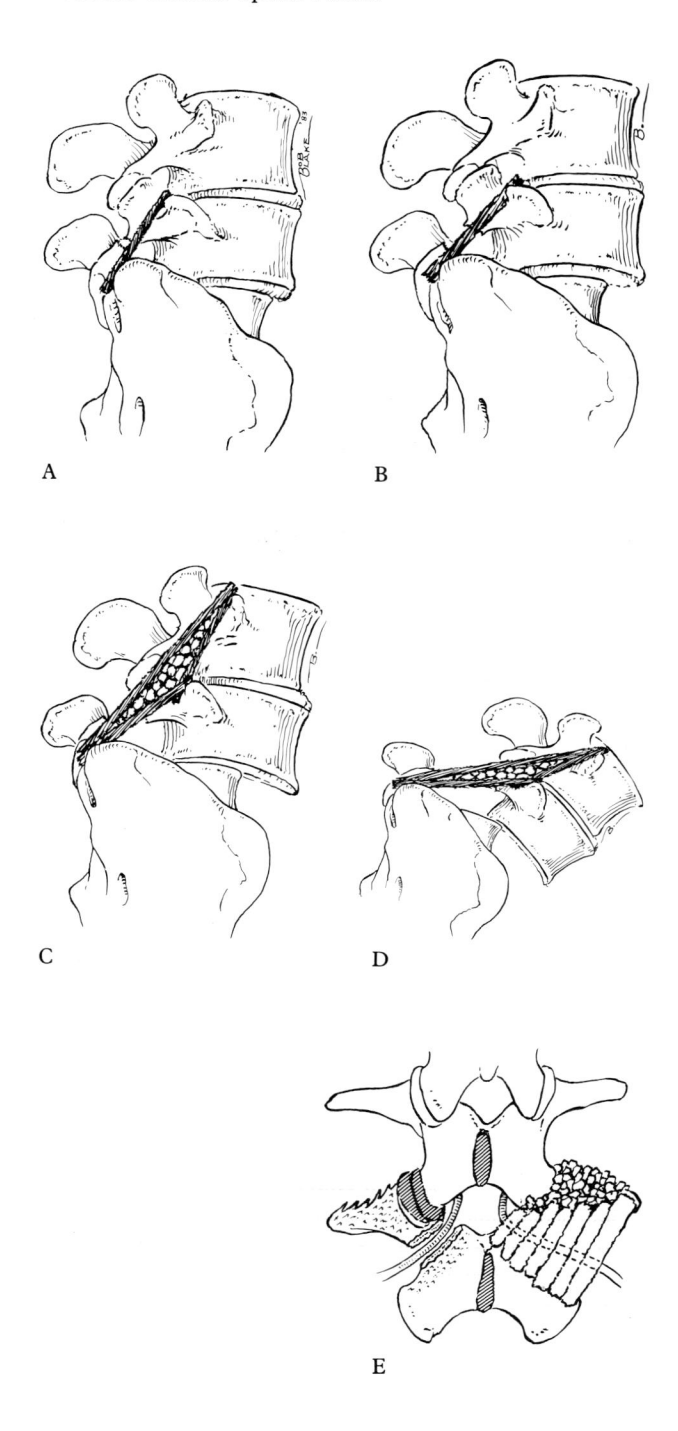

Currently, sintered metal is being used as an alternative to methacrylate for fixation of metal endoprostheses. Bony or fibrous growth occurs into the interstices of the irregular surface of the metal. Another technique is porous coating, which consists of covering a prosthesis with particles of metal by intense heat. The prosthesis with its irregular surface is press-fit into bone or adjacent to bone, and bony ingrowth occurs from the bone to the metal. This provides biological fixation without addition of material. Development of ways to use sintered metal and porous-coated metal for spine fixation is currently underway.

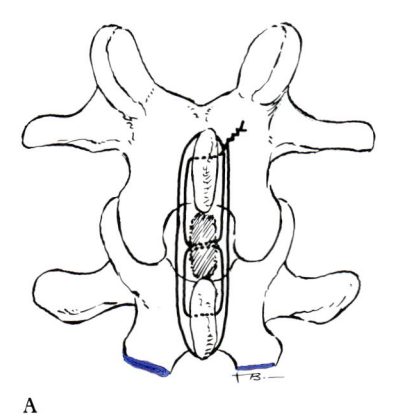

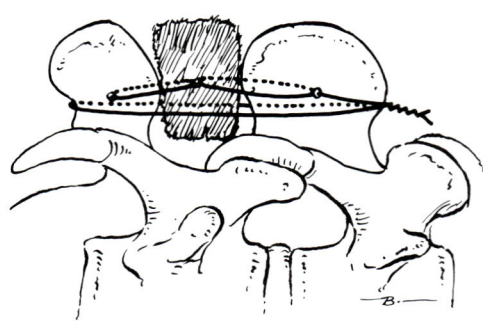

Figure 221-6 *A.* A method of stabilizing the spinous processes by insertion of an interspinous cancellous-cortical bone graft, which prevents hyperextension of the posterior elements. Fusion in hyperextension may cause the laminal arch to compress the dura, and it exaggerates lordosis. There are three strands of no. 25 stainless steel wire twisted in a drill chuck and passed through holes in the spinous processes and the bone graft. This diminishes torque and improves stability during the early postoperative period. This technique is used for posterior lateral fusion for degenerative arthrosis or for spondylolisthesis if the posterior element is not completely removed. *B.* Lateral view of a technique for providing spinous process–laminal arch stability and preventing hyperextension of the laminal arch. The holes in the spinous processes are made with an air drill or a punch. The bone graft is bicortical from the posterior ilium.

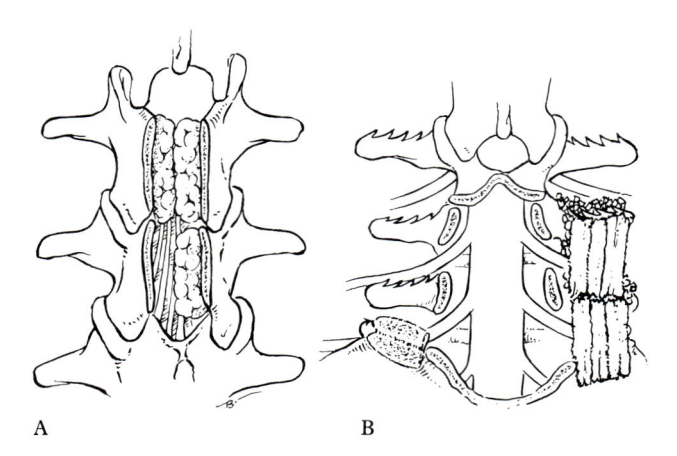

Complications Associated with Posterior Spine Fusion

Nonunion Any time a bone graft is performed, the possibility of nonunion exists. However, posterolateral fusions for spondylolisthesis are successful in about 85 percent of the patients in grades I to III. The spine can be stabilized for patients who have a nonunion after the first operation by anterior discectomy and fusion.

Pain Posterolateral fusion does not provide immediate spinal support against axial loading or torque. Postoperative pain may be significant and limited motion is essential for several weeks.

Nerve Compression or Injury; Dural Tear Bone grafts may compress the nerve roots or the dura at the time of the fusion or during the early postoperative period. Placement of the grafts must be done in order to avoid nerve compression. Nerve root or cauda equina contusion may occur during the initial exposure or subsequent decompression, and dural tears or cysts may develop during the course of decompression and/or fusion.

Infection The surgeon should attempt to avoid infection by operating in a room in which there is modern controlled air conditioning. Limitation of tissue trauma, appropriate wound closure, and suction drainage diminish the chances of infection. Prophylactic antibiotics protect temporarily against septicemia from the urinary catheter, endotracheal tube, or other sources of bacteria. Laminal air flow and ultraviolet lights may also be employed to enhance the air quality.

Figure 221-7 *A.* Laminectomy for spinal stenosis and for radicular canal stenosis may not affect stability if the facet joints are intact and if the anterior disc bond is strong and stable. After the necessary bone is removed, fat grafts, taken from locations designated in Fig. 221-1, are placed over the dura and nerve roots. *B.* If the facet joints are sacrificed, the disc bond is unstable, and the nerve root foramina are unroofed completely, then posterior lateral fusion is indicated at one or several interspace levels. The transverse processes of L3, L4, and L5 have been cleaned of soft tissue and cortical bone has been roughened. The articular cartilage has been excised from the remaining facet joints from L3 to S1. On the left, a flap of cortical-cancellous bone elevated from the sacrum acts as a bridge between L5 and S1. On the right, the space between L5 and S1 has been bridged by bone posterior to the nerve root, with special care taken to avoid bony compression of the root. Iliac bone struts have been extended from the sacrum to L5 and from L5 to L4. Facet joints have been packed, and bone will be added from L4 to L3. Laminae and spinous processes have been removed.

Posterior Lumbar Spinal Fusion

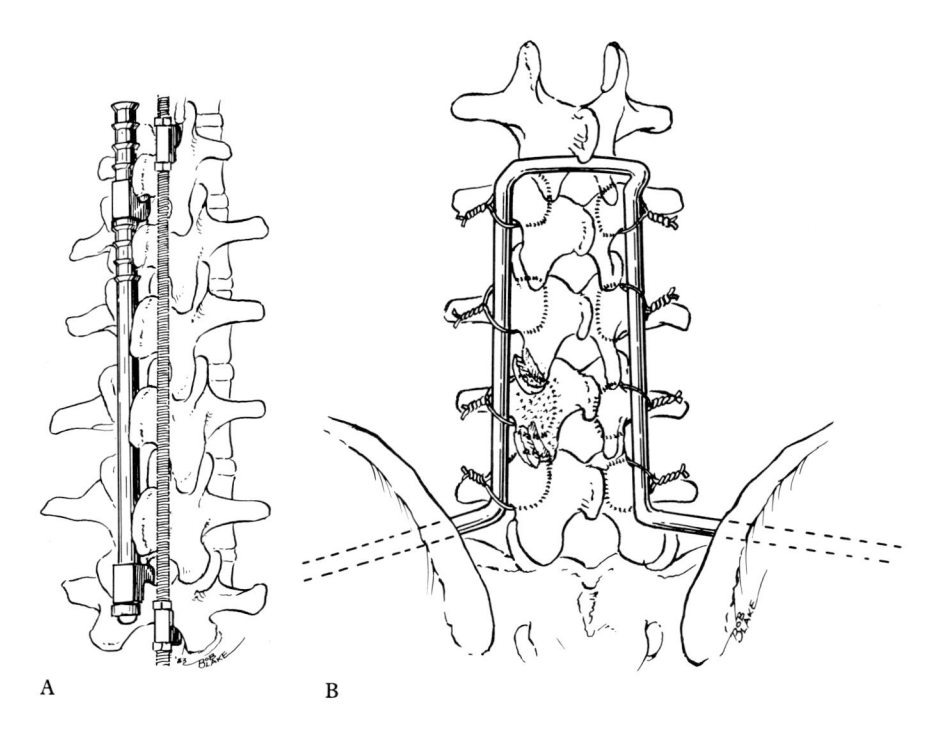

Figure 221-8 Spinal stabilization by rods. *A.* When several lumbar vertebrae are included in the stabilization, use is made of the Harrington technique, which is represented here by a distraction rod on the left and a compression rod on the right. The facet joints are excised and filled with cancellous bone. The spinous processes and the laminae are included in the fusion mass, and, if necessary, bone is placed on the transverse processes and in the lateral gutters. If a midline laminectomy is necessary, the emphasis is on lateral fusion. The rods maintain stability. They can be prebent to contour to the lumbar lordosis. *B.* The Luque rod system uses interlaminar wires and a prebent rod that is anchored into the ilium on either side. This provides strong lateral fixation and diminishes torque. Facet joint fusion and posterior lateral fusion are added to this internal fixation.

Postoperative Bleeding The patient's past history will usually give evidence of a bleeding tendency. Fibrinogen deficiency, platelet deficiency, or abnormal clotting factors, such as occur in von Willebrand's disease, may cause unexpected intraoperative and postoperative bleeding. Postoperative hemorrhage may cause cauda equina compression or nerve root irritation or adhesions.

Phlebothrombosis The incidence of thrombophlebitis and phlebothrombosis of the lower extremeties or the vena cava is 2–3 percent with clinical recognition and probably higher with nonclinical recognition. Prophylactic anticoagulation should be considered and the various options, in addition to elastic hose, elevation of the lower extremeties, hydration, and early walking are (1) aspirin alone, (2) aspirin and dipyridamole, (3) dextran and aspirin, (4) therapeutic adjusted low-dose subcutaneous heparin and Coumadin, and (5) Coumadin pre- and postoperatively.

Sequelae after Posterolateral Fusion

There is about a 7 percent nonunion rate following a single-space posterolateral fusion. The nonunion rate for a two-space posterolateral fusion is approximately 15 percent.

Early degeneration of the space above the fusion site does not always occur and depends on the characteristics of the patient's connective tissue. Patients have been observed who have had a single-space fusion at L5–S1 and who, 25 years later, show no greater narrowing of the interspace above the fusion than one would expect with their age. However, if the interspace tends to narrow as a part of the aging process, then the added stress of the fusion below hastens the development of changes at the movable space above the fusion site.

Creeping fusion to the facet joints proximal to the fusion may occur if bone reaction after placement of the bone graft is proliferative and rapid, or if the bone grafts are adjacent or over the facets even though the cartilage is not removed, or if cleaning the facet joints during the overall exposure causes bone reaction to occur at the site of subperiosteal dissection.

The sequelae after posterolateral fusion, when the central segment of the spine is not included in the fusion procedure, are much fewer than when the laminae and spinous processes are included in the fusion. This is particularly true for degenerative joint disease and postoperative intervertebral disc disease. The problems such as "napkin ring constriction" at the superior edge of the fusion, or overgrowth of the entire fusion resulting in compression of the cauda equina by central spinal stenosis, are less likely to occur when posterolateral fusion is performed rather than midline fusion. Also, metal rods with hooks under the laminal arches may infringe on the available space for the cauda equina, and the hooks may contribute to stenosis.

Long Term Results

Results are based on alteration of certain factors, including (1) relief of pain, (2) successful bony fusion, (3) maintenance of satisfactory daily activities, and (4) return to work or similar kind of activity.

Spondylolisthesis

Posterolateral decompression and fusion performed in 116 adolescent patients during the past 30 years resulted in an 88 percent primary fusion rate. The 12 percent who did not have a primary union were stabilized by anterior discectomy and fusion, so that all patients eventually reached a satisfactory union. Eighty percent of the total 116 patients were in the excellent and good group, which meant full unlimited activity. Twenty percent were limited in certain physical activities and had intermittent episodes of aching and discomfort. All were carrying out activities of daily living without difficulty. Those in the 20 percent group were less active in athletics and heavy work. None was worse. There were no infections (all patients were surgically treated in operating rooms with an ultraviolet light environment).

Failed Intervertebral Disc Surgery

Adults who had posterolateral fusion after failed intervertebral disc surgery showed a 78 percent primary union rate and 22 percent nonunion. The nonunion patients were treated by repeat posterior bone grafting or anterior discectomy and fusion, and a high percentage of these procedures resulted in union. Relief of back pain occurred in about 80 percent of the patients and relief of lower extremity pain occurred in about 85 percent of the patients. The remaining patients had varying degrees of persistent back and lower extremity aching, and many had a chronic pain pattern syndrome. Other procedures were used to attempt to diminish their pain.

Failed Posterior Decompression or Attempted Posterolateral Fusion

Patients referred from elsewhere with failed posterolateral fusions or extensive posterior decompression without fusion and with segmental instability were usually treated by anterior discectomy and fusion. This procedure was supplemented about 20 percent of the time by posterolateral decompression and fusion, and the ultimate fusion rate was over 90 percent.

Adult Scoliosis with Pain, with or without Root Compression

Spine fusion for adult scoliosis with internal fixation is successful in relieving extremity pain and diminishes back pain. About 80 percent of the patients were relatively free of pain for activities of daily living and 20 percent had moderate discomfort with increased physical activity. Those who developed pseudoarthrosis required repair of the pseudoarthrosis.

Anterior Discectomy and Fusion, Followed by Posterolateral Decompression and Fusion

My preference for management of the patient with persistent pain and segmental instability for incongruity associated with prior intervertebral disc surgery is to perform an anterior discectomy and fusion and then supplement that at 6 to 12 months by posterior decompression and reinforcement of the posterolateral fusion if diagnostic studies and the patient's symptoms indicate a need for additional treatment.

References

1. Albee FH: Transplantation of a portion of the tibia into the spine for Pott's disease: A preliminary report. JAMA 57:885–886, 1911.
2. Baker LD, Hoyt WA Jr: The use of interfacet vitallium screws in the Hibbs spine fusion. South Med J 41:419–426, 1948.
3. Bosworth DM: Clothespin graft of the spine for spondylolisthesis and laminal defects. Am J Surg 67:61–67, 1945.
4. Cloward RB: The treatment of ruptured lumbar intervertebral discs by vertebral body fusion: 1. Indications, operative technique, aftercare. J Neurosurg 10:154–168, 1953.
5. Ghormley, RK: Low back pain: With special reference to the articular facets, with presentation of an operative procedure. JAMA 101:1773–1777, 1933.
6. Goldner JL: The role of spine fusion. Spine 6:293–303, 1981.
7. Goldner JL, Wood KE, Urbaniak JR: Anterior lumbar discectomy and interbody fusion: Indications and technique, in Schmidek HH, Sweet WH (eds): *Operative Neurosurgical Techniques: Indications, Methods, and Results.* New York, Grune & Stratton, 1982, pp 1373–1397.
8. Harrington PR: Treatment of scoliosis: Correction and internal fixation by spine instrumentation. J Bone Joint Surg 44–A: 591–610, 1962.
9. King D: Internal fixation for lumbosacral fusion. Am J Surg 66:357–361, 1944.
10. Macnab I: The blood supply of the lumbar spine and its application to the technique of intertransverse lumbar fusion. J Bone Joint Surg 53–B: 628–638, 1971.
11. Rombold C: Treatment of spondylolisthesis by posterolateral fusion, resection of the pars interarticularis, and prompt mobilization of the patient: An end result study of seventy-three patients. J Bone Joint Surg 48–A: 1282–1300, 1966.
12. Watkins MB: Posterolateral fusion of the lumbosacral spine. J Bone Joint Surg 35–A: 1014–1018, 1953.
13. Wiltse LL, Hutchineson RH: Surgical treatment of spondylolisthesis. Clin Orthop 35:116–135, 1964.
14. Wiltse WW: The place of spinal fusion in lumbar intervertebral joint disease, in Cauthen JC: *Lumbar Spine Surgery.* Baltimore, Williams and Wilkins, 1983, pp 128–160.

222
Post-Traumatic Syringomyelia

Joseph H. Piatt, Jr.

In 1898 in one of his very earliest literary efforts, Cushing reported a nonprogressive syringomyelic syndrome in a young woman who had suffered a cervical gunshot wound.[5] He viewed hematomyelia as the pathological substrate of both acute and delayed post-traumatic syringomyelia. Reporting his observations of battlefield injuries in 1915, Holmes described "curious cavities" in the segments of the spinal cord adjoining traumatic lesions, and he speculated that such secondary changes might be responsible for late progression of neurological deficits.[7] Improved understanding of the clinical and pathological features of delayed post-traumatic syringomyelia did not occur until the antibiotic era and prolonged survival of large numbers of paraplegic and quadriplegic patients. In 1966 Barnett and colleagues drew on their experiences at a major center for the rehabilitation of patients with spinal cord injuries to report eight cases of late, progressive neurological deficit referable to the cervical cord,[2] and the subsequent monograph by Barnett, Foster, and Hudgson[3] led to wide recognition of and interest in this syndrome. Our current understanding of post-traumatic syringomyelia continues to evolve as heightened clinical awareness and sophisticated neuroradiological techniques augment our experience with this devastating but treatable complication of spinal cord injury.

Post-traumatic syringomyelia is a clinical syndrome characterized by delayed progression of neurological deficits corresponding to spinal cord segments distant from the level of a preceding injury. The prevalence of this syndrome among spinal cord–injured patients appears to be about 1.3 percent.[3,21] The mean latency from injury to the development of new symptoms has been reported to be between 4 and 9 years, and although a recent report has described a subgroup of patients who deteriorate slowly but continuously after the original injury, a prolonged static hiatus between the initial trauma and subsequent progression is the rule.[3,16,18,21,22]

The most common initial complaint is pain, appearing months to years after the original injury and usually localized to the chest wall or upper extremity. It may be acute in onset and is frequently related by the patient to coughing or straining. In the presence of spinal cord tethering by arachnoiditis at the site of injury, movements of the head and neck or spinal motion during transfer from a bed to a wheelchair may activate the pain. Other symptoms include paresthesias, numbness, weakness, and hyperhidrosis. Examination reveals hypesthesia, especially to pain and temperature, extending cephalad from the old spinal level, although clinically normal segments may be interposed. Depressed reflexes accompany the sensory changes cephalad and precede weakness and atrophy. Bulbar involvement may be heralded by facial hypesthesia and progress to dysphonia, dysphagia, and atrophy of the tongue. Less frequently noted are Horner's syndrome and neurogenic arthropathy of the joints of the upper extremity. If the original spinal injury was incomplete, progression of spasticity in the lower extremities and loss of retained bowel, bladder, and sexual function may occur. Like the pathological changes, the symptoms and signs of post-traumatic syringomyelia are usually unilateral in onset and remain asymmetric with the passage of time and the progression of the neurological deficits.

The natural history of this condition is not well documented in the literature. Progression is to be expected, but clinical features predicting the rate of progression have not been identified.[20] The early symptoms and signs tend to ascend, and pain may eventually be replaced by hypalgesia. Barnett et al. mention two patients whose symptoms remitted spontaneously. Of their 18 patients, 3 others were tolerating minor to moderate disability. The remainder either were submitted to surgery or had died.[3]

Well-studied autopsy cases of post-traumatic spinal cord cavitation remote from the site of injury are few. Holmes described cylindrical cavities adjoining the injured segment, extending as many as four or five segments cephalad or caudad, and situated posteriorly and laterally.[7] He believed these cavities to be under pressure. The age of these changes was not explicitly stated but was probably a matter of weeks. A more recent case studied 2 months after injury exhibited an angular cavity in the posterolateral quadrant extending cephalad and caudad from the level of the trauma.[9] The walls of the cavity were lined with macrophages and incipient glial proliferation; there was no iron pigment. Autopsy material further removed in time from the initial injury demonstrates long tubular cavities adjoining the injured segment and extending through the cervical enlargement, where they attain their greatest dimensions. These lesions can reach the caudal medulla, and in one report the syrinx opened into the fourth ventricle.[14] Communication with the subarachnoid space has not been observed in autopsy material. At levels where the anatomy of the cord is not totally obliterated, these syrinxes tend to be situated posterolaterally, separate from the central canal and without an ependymal lining. Gliosis with or without collagen constitutes the walls. The ends of the cavities are blunted and capped by thick fibroglial scar, and similar glial scar tissue forms internal septations. More than one channel may develop.[3,14]

The pathogenesis of post-traumatic syringomyelia remains fascinating and obscure, and only a cursory outline of current speculation can be presented here. It is expedient to consider three aspects of syrinx development separately: initiation, extension, and maintenance.

Holmes believed that the cavities that he observed probably not long after injury were created by transuded fluid and degeneration products tracking away from the site of injury under pressure along paths of least resistance.[7] He alluded to a possible role for vascular factors, and subsequent work has confirmed that the ventral posterior columns and posterior horns are an arterial watershed zone.[19] This anatomical arrangement may be responsible for the "en crayon" pattern of central cord infarction and may have a role in the initiation of syrinxes.[23] Venous infarction of the cord assumes a similar central pattern,[8] as does traumatic hematomyelia. On a subcellular level, autolysis of neural tissue by lysosomal enzymes transported to the site of injury along traumatized axons appears to have a role in cord cavitation.[10] The relative importance of these pathological processes in the initiation of post-traumatic syrinxes is unclear.

Mechanical considerations best explain the extension of syrinxes into segments remote from the original injury. Fluid injected into a cadaver spinal cord under pressure tracks preferentially through the gray matter of the posterior horns, which as a region of terminal capillary beds lacks the mechanical support provided by larger vessels.[11] Williams et al. have proposed that coughing and straining cause transmission of pressure from the abdomen to the thoracolumbar epidural venous plexus and thence to the cyst fluid, which is forced cephalad through the tissue planes that offer the least resistance.[22] Tethering of the cord at the level of injury by a meningeal cicatrix may also play a role.[12] Movement of the head and neck may stretch the tethered cord, narrowing it and, like Chinese handcuffs, transmitting pressure to its cystic contents.

The origin and maintenance of the syrinx fluid have been investigated as well. Ball and Dayan injected India ink at low pressure into a cervical syrinx at necropsy and observed percolation of the dye particles centrifugally along dilated perivascular Virchow-Robin spaces.[1] Perivascular centripetal passage of dye particles has been demonstrated in experimental animals.[4] Thus even in the absence of gross cyst-subarachnoid fistulas, cyst fluid may be in relatively free communication with the cerebrospinal fluid and would be expected to contain normal or only moderately elevated amounts of protein, as is true of samples obtained at surgery and during endomyelography.

Recent advances in neuroradiology have made the confident diagnosis of post-traumatic syringomyelia simple and safe. Conventional myelography with gas or iodinated contrast materials has been useful in demonstrating subarachnoid block, arachnoid adhesions, arachnoid cysts, and cord enlargement. Gas myelography has the further potential of demonstrating the collapsing cord sign, which, as it is thought to signify communication of the cyst with the fourth ventricle, is infrequently seen in post-traumatic syringomyelia. Percutaneous endomyelography provides exquisite pathoanatomical detail, but it is reluctantly performed in the absence of cord swelling or in the presence of preserved neurological function below the level of interest.

It is evident that the sensitivity of these conventional procedures depends on the prevalence of cord enlargement, and it is in this respect that computed tomographic (CT) techniques are proving most useful. Only 5 of 11 patients submitted to conventional myelographic examination exhibited an enlarged cervical cord in the series of Barnett et al.[3] Seibert and associates first reported uptake of metrizamide into traumatic spinal cord cysts, producing what has come to be called the *target sign*.[17] They used CT scanning delayed 2 to 5 h after the instillation of the contrast medium to demonstrate syrinxes in nine patients, only three of whom had an enlarged cord. Osborne and colleagues studied a series of post-traumatic paraplegic patients with intractable pain utilizing CT myelography with metrizamide.[15] They were able to visualize three thoracic syrinxes, at least two of which were in atrophic cord segments (Fig. 222-1). They also found this technique useful in demonstrating related spinal lesions, such as cord tethering, arachnoid adhesions, loculated subarachnoid cysts, and extradural fibrosis. Recently, Quencer et al. reported 16 patients collected from a regional spinal cord injury center over an 18-month period and studied to rule out post-traumatic spinal cord cysts.[16] Syrinxes were demonstrated in all patients, but the spinal cord at the segment of maximal cyst diameter was enlarged in only two. Their technique, which included sagittal reconstruction, provided fine pathoanatomical detail. They confirmed the previously noted predilection of post-traumatic cysts for the dorsal half of the cord; they documented two or more cysts in 25 percent of their patients; and they measured cyst length. In the 13 patients submitted to surgery, operative findings correlated well with these radiographic details. The speed with which this group collected 16 cases and the paucity among them of enlarged cords, formerly the radiographic hallmark of the condition, raise the issue of serious underdiagnosis of post-traumatic syringomyelia in the pre-CT era.

The possibility of effective intervention makes correct diagnosis imperative. The characteristic ascending asymmetric pattern of neurological deficit in a patient with an old

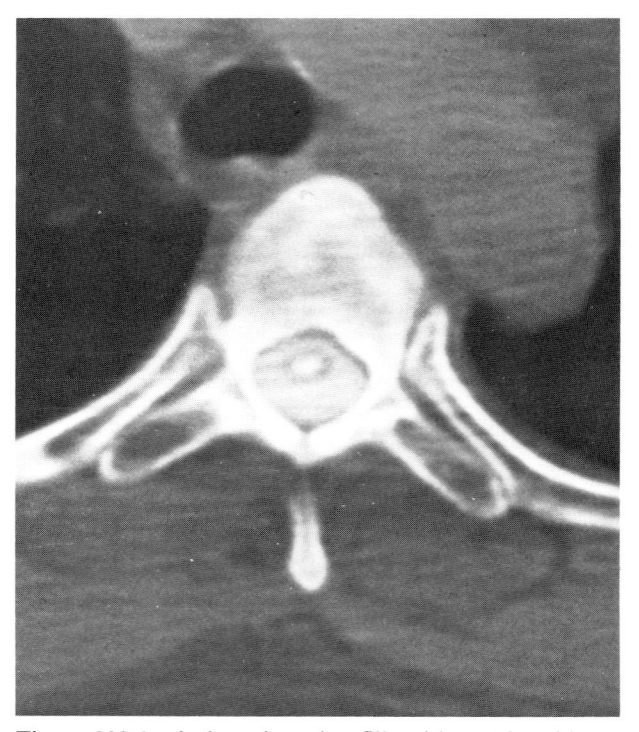

Figure 222-1 A thoracic syrinx fills with metrizamide to display the target sign about 4 h after the subarachnoid instillation of metrizamide. This middle-aged man was rendered paraplegic 30 years before by a midthoracic fracture.

cord injury is unmistakable, but the delayed onset of pain in such a patient has a nontrivial differential diagnosis.[6] Of particular interest in this regard is a central pain syndrome encountered in 5 to 10 percent of patients with spinal cord or cauda equina injuries, usually gradual in onset, continuous, diffuse, and severe. This syndrome can usually be distinguished from an ascending syrinx by the distribution of the pain below the level of cord injury. It is treated effectively by dorsal root entry zone (DREZ) lesions.[13]

Without a firm understanding of the natural history of post-traumatic syringomyelia, it is difficult to assess the value of surgical intervention. Nevertheless, because of the relatively low morbidity of the suggested procedures, two indications recommend themselves: development of pain and progression of neurological deficit. Whether to intervene before the neurological deficit results in major loss of function remains a matter of judgment.[3] Both syringostomy and, in cases of complete functional cord transection at the level of injury, cordectomy have proponents in the literature.[16,18] Published surgical results indicate almost invariable relief of pain and frequent improvement in motor and sensory function, but essentially no long-term follow-up is available. An alternate approach to the pain of syringomyelia is DREZ lesioning, either at the time of syringostomy or in the event of recurrence of pain.[13] Consensus on the optimal surgical intervention now awaits the wider experience that increased clinical suspicion and improved radiological techniques are beginning to provide.

References

1. Ball MJ, Dayan AD: Pathogenesis of syringomyelia. Lancet 2:799–801, 1972.
2. Barnett HJM, Botterell EH, Jousse AT, Wynne-Jones M: Progressive myelopathy as a sequel to traumatic paraplegia. Med Serv J Can 22:631–650, 1966.
3. Barnett HJM, Foster JB, Hudgson P: *Syringomyelia*. Toronto, WB Saunders Company Ltd, 1973.
4. Brierley JB: The penetration of particulate matter from the cerebrospinal fluid into the spinal ganglia, peripheral nerves, and perivascular spaces of the central nervous system. J Neurol Neurosurg Psychiatry 13:203–215, 1950.
5. Cushing HW: Haematomyelia from gunshot wounds of the spine. A report of two cases, with recovery following symptoms of hemilesion of the cord. Am J Med Sci 115:654–683, 1898.
6. Donovan WH, Dimitrijevic MR, Dahm L, Dimitrijevic M: Neurophysiological approaches to chronic pain following spinal cord injury. Paraplegia 20:135–146, 1982.
7. Holmes G: The Goulstonian Lectures on spinal injuries of warfare. Br Med J 2:769–774, 1915.
8. Hughes JT: Venous infarction of the spinal cord. Neurology (Minneap) 21:794–800, 1971.
9. Jensen F, Reske-Nielsen E: Post-traumatic syringomyelia: Review of the literature and two new autopsy cases. Scand J Rehabil Med 9:35–43, 1977.
10. Kao CC, Chang LW: The mechanism of spinal cord cavitation following spinal cord transection: Part 1. A correlated histochemical study. J Neurosurg 46:197–209, 1977.
11. Leyden-Goldscheider: Die Erkrankungen des Rückenmarkes und der Medulla Oblongata. Wien, 1895, cited in Cushing HW: Haematomyelia from gunshot wounds of the spine: A report of two cases, with recovery following symptoms of hemilesion of the cord. Am J Med Sci 115:654–683, 1898.
12. McLean DR, Miller JDR, Allen PBR, Ezzeddin SA: Posttraumatic syringomyelia. J Neurosurg 39:485–492, 1973.
13. Nashold BS Jr, Bullitt E: Dorsal root entry zone lesions to control central pain in paraplegics. J Neurosurg 55:414–419, 1981.
14. Oakley JC, Ojemann GA, Alvord EC Jr: Posttraumatic syringomyelia: Case report. J Neurosurg 55:276–281, 1981.
15. Osborne DRS, Vavoulis G, Nashold BS Jr, Dubois PJ, Drayer BP, Heinz ER: Late sequelae of spinal cord trauma: Myelographic and surgical correlation. J Neurosurg 57:18–23, 1982.
16. Quencer RM, Green BA, Eismont FJ: Posttraumatic spinal cord cysts: Clinical features and characterization with metrizamide computed tomography. Radiology 146:415–423, 1983.
17. Seibert CE, Dreisbach JN, Swanson WB, Edgar RE, Williams P, Hahn H: Progressive posttraumatic cystic myelopathy: Neuroradiologic evaluation. AJNR 2:115–119, 1981.
18. Shannon N, Symon L, Logue V, Cull D, Kang J, Kendall B: Clinical features, investigation and treatment of post-traumatic syringomyelia. J Neurol Neurosurg Psychiatry 44:35–42, 1981.
19. Turnbull IM, Breig A, Hassler O: Blood supply of the cervical spinal cord in man: A microangiographic cadaver study. J Neurosurg 24:951–965, 1966.
20. Vernon JD, Silver JR, Ohry A: Post-traumatic syringomyelia. Paraplegia 20:339–364, 1982.
21. Watson N: Ascending cystic degeneration of the cord after spinal cord injury. Paraplegia 19:89–95, 1981.
22. Williams B, Terry AF, Jones HWF, McSweeney T: Syringomyelia as a sequel to traumatic paraplegia. Paraplegia 19:67–80, 1981.
23. Zülch KJ: Réflexions sur la physiopathologie des troubles vasculaires médullaires. Rev Neurol (Paris) 106:632–645, 1962.

Part IX Disorders of Peripheral and Cranial Nerves and the Autonomic Nervous System

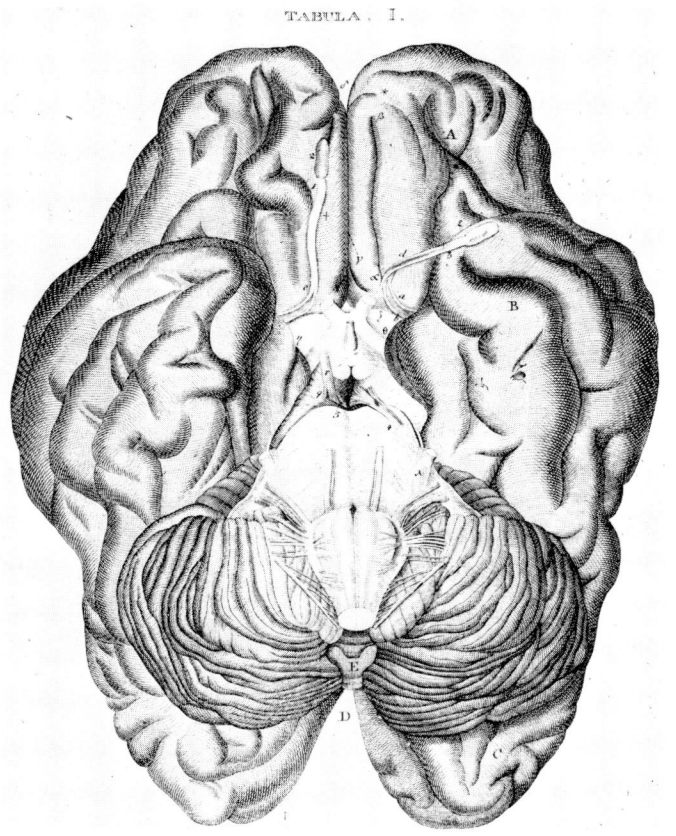

Soemmerring S. T. *De Basi Encephali*. Goettingen, A. Vandenhoeck, 1778. Our system of 12 cranial nerves was introduced by Soemmerring in this work, his dissertation.

SECTION A

Entrapment Neuropathies

223

Thoracic Outlet Syndromes

Russell W. Hardy, Jr.
Asa J. Wilbourn

One of the more elusive and controversial areas of surgical practice is the diagnosis and surgical treatment of the various forms of thoracic outlet syndrome. Throughout the past several decades some enthusiasts have performed a large number of operations for this condition, other surgeons have used narrowly defined operative indications, and still others have believed that surgical treatment is rarely indicated.

In order to understand the complexities of diagnosis, an understanding of the anatomy of the thoracic outlet is essential. The osseous elements of the outlet consist of the vertebral column (posteriorly), the first rib (laterally), and the sternum and clavicle (anteriorly). The anterior and middle scalene muscles arise from the cervical vertebral column and insert on the first rib, forming a triangle. Through this triangle pass the subclavian artery and the elements of the brachial plexus (Fig. 223-1). The subclavian vein crosses the first rib anterior to the scalenus anticus. While crossing the rib, the artery, vein, and neural elements pass between the clavicle and first rib; these then continue beneath the pectoralis minor into the arm.

Compression of the neurovascular bundle might theoretically occur at several sites. First, compression could occur within the triangle formed by the scalene muscles and first rib; second, between the first rib and clavicle; and third, beneath the pectoralis minor muscle.

In fact, several thoracic outlet–type syndromes have been described, each of which is said to be caused by compression at these various sites. These syndromes have been described as the hyperabduction syndrome, the costoclavicular syndrome, the thoracic outlet syndrome, and the cervical rib (compressive cervical band) syndrome.[8]

The simplest and perhaps least controversial are the hyperabduction and costoclavicular syndromes, which result from compression that occurs when the patient assumes an unusual posture.

In 1945 Wright described several patients with the hyperabduction syndrome.[12] The patients presented with diffuse paresthesia, pain, and (rarely) gangrene in the fingers, which appeared when the arms were habitually hyperabducted during activity or sleep. On physical examination the patients had a normal neurological examination; on hyperabduction of the arms, pallor appeared in the hands and fingers. Obliteration of pulses was also described, although it was noted this could also occur in normal individuals. The symptoms were said to be caused by compression of the brachial plexus and subclavian artery by the pectoralis minor when the arms were hyperabducted. Relief of symptoms occurred when the patients were forced to sleep with their arms at their sides or abandoned activities requiring chronic elevation of the arms.

A second positional syndrome (the costoclavicular syndrome), was described by Falconer and Weddell in 1943.[4] They reported a syndrome of numbness, paresthesias, and pain in the hands, coupled with cold intolerance. These symptoms were produced when the patients braced their shoulders or hyperextended their neck. Physical examination in these patients revealed decreased arterial pulsation in the hands, cyanosis, and a normal neurological examination.

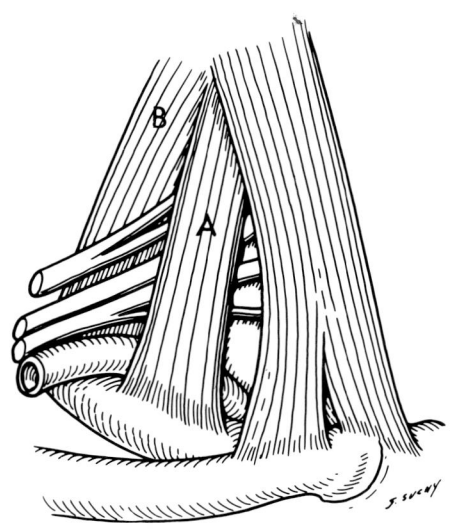

Figure 223-1 The brachial plexus and subclavian artery pass over the first rib between the anterior scalene (A) and middle scalene (B) muscles.

The presumed mechanism involved compression of the neurovascular structures between the clavicle and first rib; Falconer and Weddell reported that this occurred in soldiers forced to assume a military posture of hyperextension while wearing a backpack. In one instance the symptoms were relieved by resection of the first rib but in another the patient was relieved merely by cessation of activities that provoked symptoms.

It is noteworthy that in the same report Falconer and Weddell described patients with muscle wasting and a cervical compressive band similar to that observed in the cases to be discussed below.

Compression of the brachial plexus and subclavian artery or vein between the clavicle and first rib also has been described in patients who have had fractures and subsequent distortion of the clavicle.[7] Symptoms may be relieved in such patients by resection or realignment of the clavicle or by a first rib resection.

Patients with nonspecific symptoms attributed to neurovascular compression in the scalene triangle have for several decades been diagnosed as having a thoracic outlet syndrome. In 1927 Adson and Coffey described a series of patients with pain, atrophy, disturbances of sensation, and circulatory abnormalities in the upper extremity.[1] Many of the patients described had anomalies such as cervical ribs but a number of the patients were treated simply with anterior scalene section, which reportedly relieved the symptoms. Similar patients were later reported by Naffziger and Grant, who described some patients who did not have cervical rib abnormalities but reportedly had compression symptoms similar to those patients with a cervical rib.[9] These patients also were said to have been relieved by section of the anterior scalene muscle. Following these reports a large number of anterior scalenotomies were performed for various upper extremity symptoms, but in recent years operations on the anterior scalene muscle have fallen into disfavor, and few, if any, are done at the present time. On the other hand, resection of the first rib is now often advocated for indications similar to those previously employed for scalenotomy. The logic behind this operation rests on the assumption that first rib resection will correct neurovascular compression from several possible sources. Resection of the first rib would theoretically serve to relieve compression within the scalene triangle and also between clavicle and first rib. As described by Urschel and Razzuk, candidates for operation present with a variety of neurovascular complaints, the majority being attributable to neurological compression.[11] They report that pain and paresthesias occur in 75 percent of cases, and 90 percent occur in an ulnar nerve distribution. They further report that objective motor weakness is a relatively uncommon finding. Symptoms of vascular compression (coldness, weakness, easy fatigability, pain in the arm, and Raynaud's phenomenon) are relatively infrequent. It is noteworthy that a percentage of their patients have a cervical rib or evidence of other bony anomalies of the shoulder.

Urschel selects candidates for first rib resection by measuring ulnar motor conduction velocity across the thoracic outlet. Urschel and Razzuk report a normal velocity of approximately 72 m/s and recommend surgery in those patients in whom the velocity is reduced below 60 m/s. Subjective postoperative improvement is greatest in those in whom the postoperative conduction velocity shows the greatest improvement.[11]

It should be noted that the validity of this measurement as a useful indicator for surgery has been challenged by a number of electromyographers.[2,3] Roos evaluates patients solely on clinical grounds and believes that electromyography (EMG) and nerve conduction studies are of little benefit in patients being considered for first rib resection.[10]

We agree that there is a group of patients with arm pain who may benefit from first rib resection. The principal problem is patient selection; we believe that only a small number of patients qualify for operation. Such patients are selected largely on the basis of symptoms. Appropriate candidates for surgery demonstrate pain in the arm and shoulder, often in an ulnar distribution. They may complain of fatigue or numbness on use of the arm in normal anatomical positions. Patients who have symptoms only on elevation of the arm are not offered surgery unless their work requires chronic elevation of the arm. Rarely, patients may have symptoms of venous compression or Raynaud's phenomenon.

Physical examination usually is normal. Some patients may have reduced pulsation on Adson's maneuver (but this also occurs in normal individuals). Reduced arterial pulsations may be significant if they occur *pari passu* with the onset of symptoms. Reduced pulsations on extreme elevation of the arm is of minimal significance. A few patients may have signs of venous engorgement and a rare patient will have a supraclavicular bruit. In the absence of a demonstrable cervical rib or prominent C7 transverse process, we have not encountered a patient with an objective neurological deficit.

Arteriography is not performed unless symptoms of distal microembolization are present or a supraclavicular mass suggestive of an aneurysm is palpated. Recently, noninvasive vascular studies have been utilized, and these may demonstrate reduced distal blood flow in some individuals. We agree with Cherrington that the conduction slowing across the thoracic outlet is a doubtful criterion for patient selection and do not employ this measurement in selecting patients for operation. Similarly, in the absence of a cervical rib or prominent C7 transverse process, we have not seen an abnormal EMG examination in a single patient referred with this diagnosis in a laboratory performing over 2500 examinations per year.

Provided that a patient is significantly disabled by pain, that other correctable lesions have been excluded, and that the patient has not responded to conservative treatment, a first rib resection may be offered. This can be performed via a supraclavicular or transaxillary approach with good results in carefully chosen individuals.

Although we are cautious about performing surgery for thoracic outlet syndrome, we do believe that the cervical rib syndrome (compressive cervical band) is a rare but well-defined entity and is clearly responsive to surgical treatment. The association of neurological deficit, arm pain, and cervical ribs has been known since antiquity and extensively reported in the early part of this century by a number of writers. This syndrome was well recognized and described by these early authors although there were occasional instances of confusion between compression at the level of the cervical

Thoracic Outlet Syndromes

rib and lesions such as a carpal tunnel syndrome or ulnar compression at the elbow. More recently, with the advent of electromyography and nerve conduction studies, the syndrome has been well defined electrically and clinically by Gilliatt.[5] It is his belief, as well as ours,[6] that in the majority of patients the symptoms are not due to the cervical rib per se but rather to an anomalous compressive fibrous band, continuous with the medial edge of the scalenus medius, which causes symptoms. This band extends from the rib or elongated transverse process of C7 to the first rib and produces symptoms by compression of the lower portion of the brachial plexus (Fig. 223-2).

The syndrome consists of arm pain, motor weakness, and variable sensory loss, which is caused by compression of the lower trunk of the brachial plexus. The symptoms are caused by the sharp angulation and compression of the lower roots, particularly the T1 root, which must pass anteriorly over the sharp edge of the band.

The onset of symptoms typically occurs in young to middle-aged females, males being only occasionally affected. In most but not all patients there is a pain or aching sensation along the medial aspect of the arm and forearm. This is followed by atrophy in the hand, beginning in the thenar eminence and invariably in the abductor pollicis brevis. In some patients there are associated complaints of paresthesia or a cold sensation along the medial aspect of the arm. In a minority of patients, atrophy occurs with minimal, if any, antecedent arm pain.

The atrophy may be limited to the thenar eminence or include the hypothenar eminence and other intrinsic hand muscles and sometimes the medial forearm muscles. Patients tend to seek assistance because of arm pain and will often tolerate a surprising degree of atrophy before seeking medical attention.

Physical examination reveals atrophy at least in the thenar muscle groups. Weakness is particularly evident in the abductor pollicis brevis and the opponens pollicis. Sensory testing may reveal no deficit or at most slight diminution in the fourth and fifth digits and the medial portion of the forearm. There is no evidence of cyanosis, pallor, or other symptoms of arterial or venous insufficiency. In some patients supraclavicular palpation will reveal tenderness over the lower portion of the plexus.

X-ray films of the cervical spine will reveal either frank cervical ribs or prominent C7 transverse processes (Fig. 223-3). We have not observed this syndrome in the absence of C7 anomalies.

The diagnosis that has been suspected on clinical and radiographic evidence is confirmed by electromyography. The typical patient will show evidence of a chronic axonal loss lesion involving the fibers of the lower trunk of the brachial plexus. Nerve conduction studies reveal a very low-amplitude median motor response, normal or relatively low ulnar motor responses, low or at least relatively low ulnar sensory amplitudes, and normal median sensory responses. These changes are logical if one remembers that the motor fibers to the hand are derived from the C8 and T1 roots, as are the sensory fibers in the medial portion of the hand, whereas the sensory fibers to the lateral part of the hand are derived from the C6 root. Motor and sensory latencies and conduction velocities are normal. Specifically, no proximal

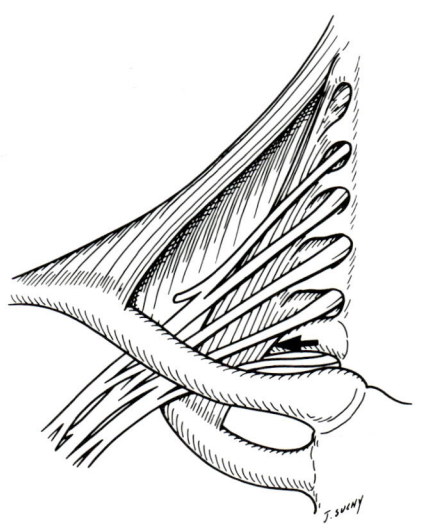

Figure 223-2 The anterior scalene muscle has been removed to show the brachial plexus crossing the scalenus medius. The compressive band is continuous with the medial edge of this muscle, as shown by the arrow.

slowing along the ulnar motor fibers between Erb's point and the axilla is seen. On needle examination there are chronic neurogenic motor unit potential changes and occasional fibrillations in the abductor pollicis brevis and to a lesser extent in the other muscles innervated by the lower trunk fibers, including the first dorsal interosseous, abductor digiti minimi, and, variably, the flexor pollicis longus, extensor indicis proprius, and extensor pollicis brevis.

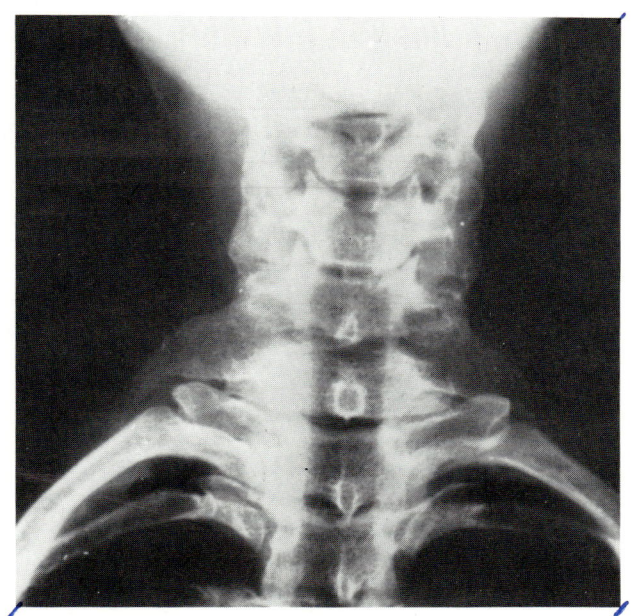

Figure 223-3 Prominent transverse processes of C7 in a patient with a compressive cervical band.

We believe that the diagnosis is made if a characteristic clinical picture is accompanied by typical x-ray and electromyographic findings. We do not believe that in the typical case a myelogram or subclavian arteriogram needs to be performed. The syndrome may be confused with intraspinal lesions such as syringomyelia or amyotrophic lateral sclerosis or with compressive mononeuropathies at the elbow or at the carpal tunnel. Indeed, in two of our patients inappropriate operations were performed before the correct diagnosis was made. In one case, a carpal tunnel release was performed and in the other the patient underwent an anterior cervical discectomy and fusion, an anterior scalene release, and an ulnar transposition before the compressive cervical band was diagnosed and resected.

Operation is recommended in these patients for relief of arm pain and sensory symptoms and to prevent further progression of intrinsic hand atrophy. Preoperatively we caution patients that they cannot expect return of muscle function once lost and to date we have not seen any return of motor function, although this has been described in a few cases in the early literature.

The cervical band is approached through a supraclavicular incision over the lower portion of the posterior triangle. Dissection is carried down to the plexus by retracting the omohyoid, care being taken to preserve the small sensory nerves to the anterior chest wall. In some cases the anterior scalene needs to be partially divided to gain exposure although in most it may simply be retracted (Fig. 223-4). In none of our cases has the anterior scalene been totally divided. When dividing this muscle care should be taken to preserve the phrenic nerve by traveling on the anterior aspect of the anterior scalene.

When the plexus has been identified, dissection is carried slightly inferiorly to expose, and if necessary isolate, the subclavian artery. At this point the compressive band may be easily felt beneath the artery and plexus. In some patients the band may be divided superior to the subclavian artery after care has been taken to identify and avoid the lower roots. In other patients it is easier to perform the section inferior to the subclavian after it has been retracted with umbilical tapes (Fig. 223-5). In either case we section approximately ½ to 1 in. of the band and this is usually sufficient to produce visible relaxation of the stretched and compressed neural structures. In no case to date have we found it necessary to remove the associated rib anomaly.

To date we have treated 12 patients with this anomaly. Ten of them have undergone operation, one declined operation, and for the other operation was not recommended because the case was so far advanced that pain had disappeared and the motor deficit appeared static. Good results were obtained in the 10 patients who underwent surgical treatment. In all patients who had preoperative pain or paresthesia, these symptoms cleared following operation. In most cases the improvement was immediate although in one the pain relief occurred over the several weeks following the operation. One patient had a slight increase in weakness postoperatively but this cleared within a few days. Otherwise, there has been no progression of preoperative weakness, although as noted we have not seen improvement in any patient. We saw immediate and lasting pain relief in the two patients who had undergone inappropriate operations prior to the section of the cervical band.

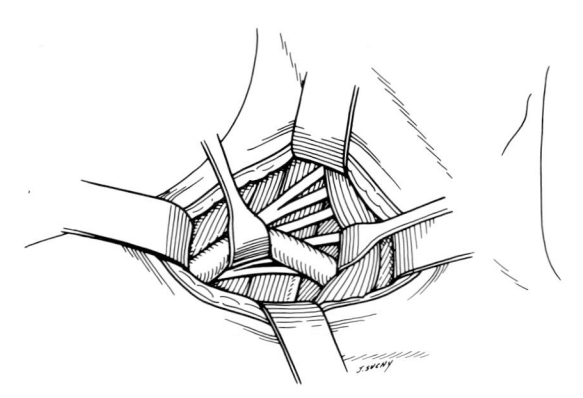

Figure 223-4 Exposure of the cervical band by elevation of the subclavian artery. The anterior scalene is retracted medially.

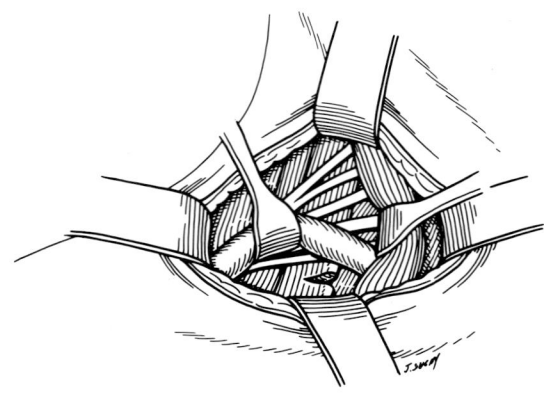

Figure 223-5 Section of the compressive band.

References

1. Adson AW, Coffey JR: Cervical rib: A method of anterior approach for relief of symptoms by division of the scalenus anticus. Ann Surg 85:839–857, 1927.
2. Cherrington M: Ulnar conduction velocity in thoracic-outlet syndrome. N Engl J Med 294:1185, 1976.
3. Daube JR: Nerve conduction studies in the thoracic outlet syndrome. Neurology (NY) 25:347, 1975 (abstr).
4. Falconer MA, Weddell G: Costoclavicular compression of the subclavian artery and vein: Relation to the scalenus anticus syndrome. Lancet 2:539–544, 1943.
5. Gilliatt RW: The classical neurological syndrome associated with a cervical rib and band, in Greep JM, Lemmons HAJ, Roos DB, Urschel HC (eds): *Pain in the Shoulder and Arm: An Integrated View*. The Hague, Martinus Wyhoff Publishers, 1979, pp 173–183.
6. Hardy RW Jr, Wilbourn A, Hanson M: Surgical treatment of compressive cervical band. Neurosurgery 7:10–13, 1980.
7. Howard FM, Shafer SJ: Injuries to the clavicle with neurovascular complications: A study of fourteen cases. J Bone Joint Surg [Am] 47A:1135–1346, 1965.
8. Hudson A, Berry H, Mayfield F: Chronic injuries of peripheral nerves by entrapment, in Youmans JR (ed): *Neurological Surgery*, 2d ed. Philadelphia, Saunders, 1982, pp 2430–2474.

9. Naffziger HC, Grant WT: Neuritis of the brachial plexus mechanical in origin. The scalenus syndrome. Surg Gynecol Obstet 67:722–730, 1938.
10. Roos DB: New concepts in the etiology, diagnosis and surgical treatment of thoracic outlet syndrome, in Greep JM, Lemmons HAJ, Roos DB, Urschel HC (eds): *Pain in the Shoulder and Arm: An Integrated View*. The Hague, Martinus Wyhoff Publishers, 1979, pp 173–183.
11. Urschel HC, Razzuk MA: Management of the thoracic outlet syndrome. N Engl J Med 286:1140–1143, 1972.
12. Wright IS: The neurovascular syndrome produced by hyperabduction of the arms. Am Heart J 29:1–19, 1945.

224
Entrapment Neuropathies
Setti S. Rengachary

Entrapment neuropathies, as the name implies, are a group of peripheral nerve disorders characterized by pain, paresthesias, or loss of function in the distribution of a nerve resulting from certain extrinsic anatomical constraints in the course of the nerve that allow sufficient, but marginal freedom to the nerve under healthy conditions but become pathologically restrictive when destined to be symptomatic. Two of the most common examples of such anatomical constraints are fibro-osseous tunnels such as the carpal or tarsal tunnel, and fibrotendinous arcades at the origin of certain muscles such as the supinator (arcade of Frohse), flexor carpi ulnaris (cubital tunnel), and flexor digitorum sublimis (sublimis bridge). In the former example (fibro-osseous tunnels), restriction in the available space may occur either from encroachment by the confining walls of the tunnel (e.g., thickening of transverse carpal ligament, callus from a healed carpal bone, etc.) or an increase in the size of the contents of the tunnel (e.g., tenosynovitis). Fibrotendinous arcades may impinge on the nerve under resting or static conditions but, more significantly, may cause a shutter-like constriction during active contraction of the muscle against resistance. Repetitive movements about the tunnel seems to be a significant predisposing factor in precipitation of symptoms; the fact that nearly all entrapment sites are located near major articulations in the limbs should not pass unnoticed. As a corollary, one would observe that spontaneous entrapments of nerves in the midarm, midforearm, midthigh, and midleg virtually do not occur.

Entrapment neuropathies constitute 10 to 25 percent of case material in contemporary neurosurgical practice. With appropriate diagnosis, careful case selection, and meticulous surgical technique, gratifying results are to be expected.

Continuing refinements in electrodiagnostic techniques have enabled more definitive and earlier diagnosis, long before objective sensory and motor findings become apparent. The reader is advised to review the chapter on electroneuromyography in this text before studying individual entrapment syndromes. Liquid crystal contact thermography is emerging as another valuable tool in the early diagnosis of entrapment neuropathies.

Pathophysiology

Over the past four decades, numerous elegant and ingenious experimental methods have been devised to elucidate the pathophysiology of peripheral nerve compression.[39] It is well recognized that both ischemia and direct pressure are the factors responsible for nerve fiber damage, although there is disagreement among various investigators as to the relative importance of each factor. Recent experimental results seem to point to direct pressure as a more significant factor in the pathogenesis.

When the cross section of a peripheral nerve that has undergone chronic compression is examined histologically, one notes that the fibers are not affected uniformly. The superficially located fibers tend to bear the brunt of compression, the central fibers being relatively spared. Large-diameter, heavily myelinated fibers are more sensitive to compression than poorly myelinated fibers. Thus, fibers subserving light touch and motor fibers are more likely to be involved in compression neuropathy than unmyelinated pain fibers.

The pathophysiological changes following nerve compression depend upon two critical factors—the degree of compression and its duration. The physiological and structural responses tend to be graded depending upon the severity of these two factors. Mild and brief compression produces a transient conduction block in the nerve, which normalizes soon after the pressure is relieved. There are no major structural changes in the nerve, but the axoplasmic flow is interrupted because of extrinsic pressure. There is impairment of centrifugal as well as centripetal axonal flow with blockade of metabolic products and enzymes at the margins of compression. Such impediment to axoplasmic flow is thought to lead to impaired membrane excitability and conduction block. With acute severe compression one observes a characteristic sequential invagination or telescoping of the myelin sheath, resembling intussusception in bowel.[28] The polarity of invagination is reversed at the edges

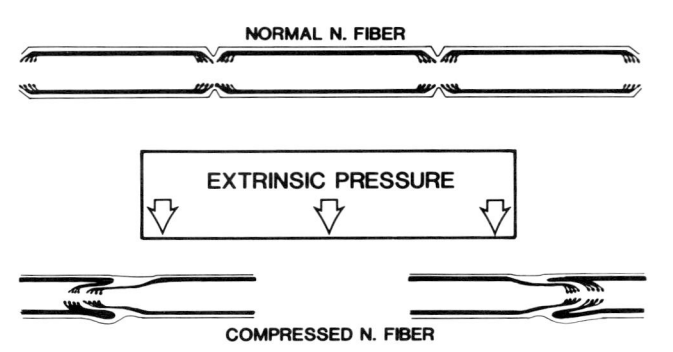

Figure 224-1 Invagination or telescoping of the myelin sheath as a result of extrinsic compression of a nerve fiber; the polarity of invagination is reversed at the edges of the compression.

of the compression (Fig. 224-1). With chronic compression, segmental demyelination occurs in the compressed segment. This accounts for the slowing of conduction velocity of the nerve observed clinically. In the early phases the nerve fibers distal to the compression show normal morphology but with sustained compression, axolysis occurs in the compressed segment, and wallerian degeneration occurs distally.

Median Nerve Entrapment at the Wrist: Carpal Tunnel Syndrome

Applied Anatomy

The carpal tunnel is a fibro-osseous tunnel located in the palmar aspect of the wrist. It extends from the wrist flexion crease to the distal border of the thenar eminence. The boundaries of the tunnel are formed of inelastic, unyielding structures. The dorsal and lateral walls are formed of the carpal bones, which by virtue of their contour offer a semilunar surface. This osseous trough is converted into a tunnel by the tough, fibrous flexor retinaculum (transverse carpal ligament). The retinaculum is attached to the pisiform and hook of the hamate medially and the tuberosity of the scaphoid and the crest of the trapezium laterally. The contents of the tunnel are the median nerve, the tendons of the flexor digitorum sublimis, flexor digitorum profundus, and flexor pollicis longus. The long slender tendon of the palmaris longus passes in front of the flexor retinaculum to become continuous with palmar aponeurosis. The thenar and hypothenar muscles arise in part from the flexor retinaculum, and in some muscular individuals, these almost meet in the midline. The ulnar nerve and artery do not pass through the tunnel but lie superficial to it in Guyon's canal (discussed elsewhere in this chapter). The palmar cutaneous branch of the median nerve, which innervates the skin over the base of the thenar eminence, arises a short distance proximal to the flexor retinaculum, pierces the deep fascia, and courses superficial to the flexor retinaculum to reach the skin; it is thus not involved in carpal tunnel compression. The palmar cutaneous branch of the ulnar nerve likewise courses superficial to the transverse carpal ligament. The motor branch of the median nerve in the hand arises under or just distal to the flexor retinaculum, and winds around the distal border of the retinaculum to reach hypothenar muscles and the lateral two lumbricals. Numerous variations in the branching of median nerve have been described (Fig. 224-2).[22] The sensory branches innervate the lateral three and one-half digits and the palm of the hand. The dorsal aspect of these digits beyond the distal interphalangeal joint is also supplied by the median nerve.

Historical Aspects

Paget in 1865 described a case of impairment of the median nerve resulting from an old fracture of the wrist. Hunt, in a series of reports from 1909 through 1914, described three cases of thenar atrophy and speculated that the motor branch of the median nerve was selectively compressed as it passed over the distal border of the flexor retinaculum. In 1913, Marie and Foix at the autopsy of an 80-year-old woman with stroke and bilateral wasting of thenar muscle demonstrated neuromata in both median nerves just proximal to the transverse carpal ligament and demyelination of the nerve under the ligament. They were the first to suggest decompression of the median nerve by sectioning the transverse carpal ligament to prevent paralysis of the thenar muscles. In 1946, Cannon and Love from the Mayo Clinic reported 38 patients with median nerve compression (tardy median palsy), nine of whom underwent section of transverse carpal ligament with good results. In the following year, Brain, Wright, and Wilkinson coined the term *carpal tunnel syndrome* and presented a series of patients with the typical clinical syndrome who improved with surgical therapy. Phalen has published one of the largest series of patients with this syndrome in recent times.[30]

Figure 224-2 Variations in the branching of the median nerve. *A.* Normal branching of the median nerve. *B.* Motor branch arising from the median nerve within the carpal tunnel. *C.* Motor branch piercing the transverse carpel ligament to reach the thenar eminence. *D.* Motor branch arising from the ulnar border of the median nerve. *E.* Motor branch running a recurrent course on the volar surface of the transverse carpal ligament before entering the thenar muscle mass. *F.* Two separate motor branches. *G.* High division of the median nerve with an intervening persistent median artery. *H.* High division of the median nerve with a very thick ulnar portion. *I.* High division of the median nerve with a thin ulnar portion. *J.* High division of the median nerve with an accessory lumbrical muscle between the two divisions. *K.* Accessory branch from the median nerve running proximal to the carpal tunnel. *L.* Accessory branch running proximal to the carpal tunnel after perforating the transverse carpal ligament. *M.* Accessory branch from the ulnar aspect of the median nerve proximal to the carpal tunnel. *N.* Two motor branches, a primary branch and an accessory branch, running directly into the thenar musculature. Despite these numerous variations, none is likely to be encountered at surgery if the incision depicted in Fig. 224-5 is used.

Entrapment Neuropathies 1773

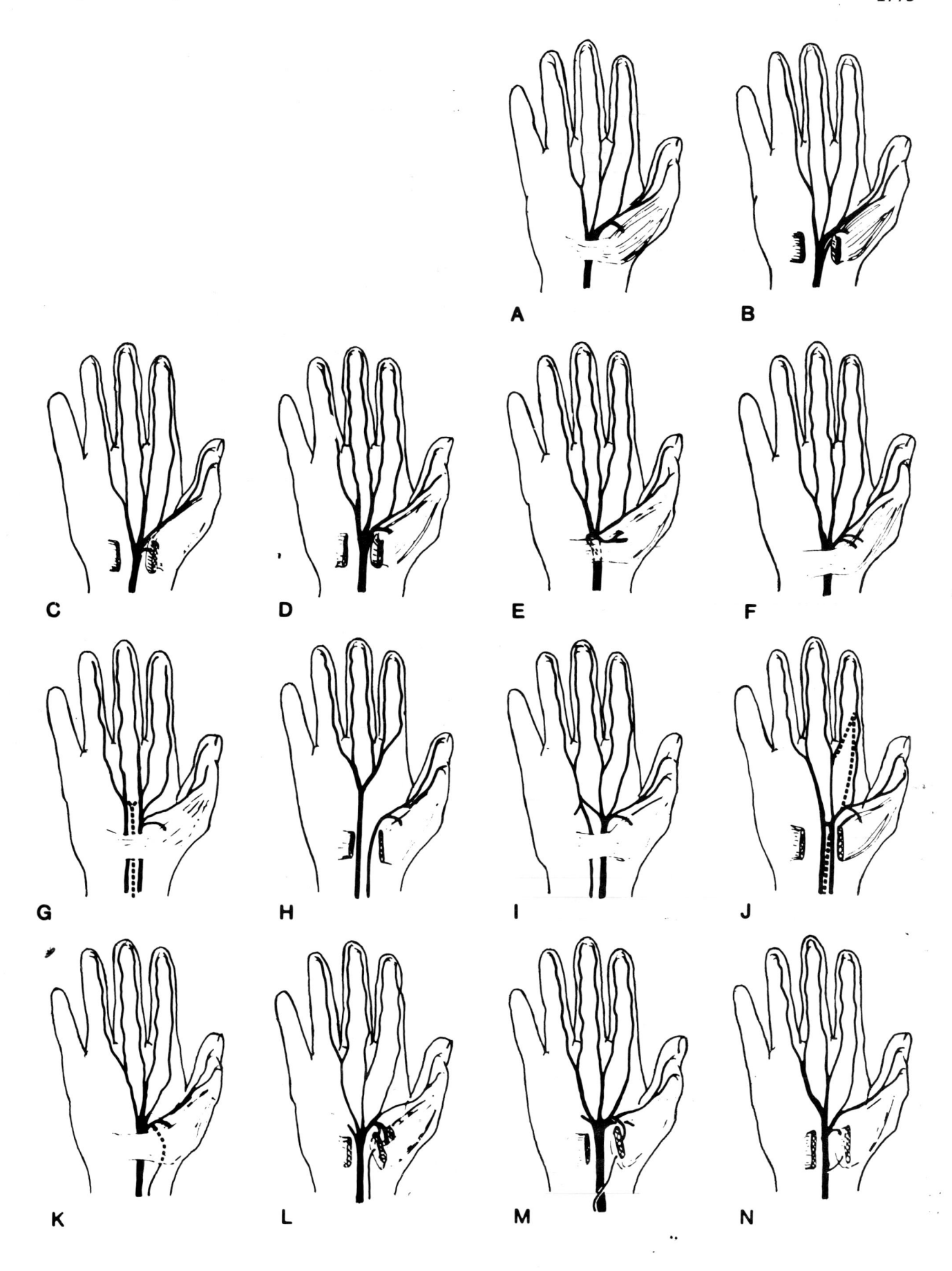

Clinical Features

The carpal tunnel syndrome (CTS) is more common in women than in men, with a ratio of 7:3. Most patients are between 40 to 60 years old at the time of onset of symptoms. The cardinal symptoms are aching, burning, tingling, and numbness in the hand, which is usually vaguely localized to the radial half of the hand and the lateral three digits. Not uncommonly these symptoms are present in the whole hand. Indeed in a few patients pain may be experienced in the forearm and shoulder. Typically the pain is worse at night. On awakening, the patient may have to shake the hand or massage the wrist to obtain some relief. Strenuous use of the hand nearly always aggravates the symptoms, although the symptoms may not be manifest until the patient has rested for several hours after activity. This syndrome is frequently bilateral but is usually worse in the dominant hand. Patients may complain of weakness or clumsiness in the hand, but this is seldom a prominent symptom, at least in the early stages. Paradoxically, the majority of patients with pain may not demonstrate any weakness, while a minority of patients may present with advanced weakness and atrophy with little or no pain.

A paucity of objective findings is the rule early in the course of the disorder. Tinel's sign may be elicited by lightly tapping over the median nerve at the wrist crease, but in itself this test is of dubious value in making the diagnosis because of a significantly high incidence of false-positive results.[4] Phalen's wrist flexion test is elicited by asking the patient to hold the forearms vertically and allow both hands to drop into complete flexion at the wrist for about 60 s. In this position the median nerve is compressed between the proximal edge of the flexor retinaculum and the flexor tendons and radius, and so aching pain in the hand is experienced. It is important that this test not be prolonged for more than a minute since healthy individuals may have pain in the hand with prolonged wrist flexion. Pain with wrist flexion may be absent in patients with profound sensory loss. Aggravation in pain has been shown to occur with the application of pressure in the arm exceeding patient's systolic pressure using a sphygmomanometer cuff. A sensory loss to light touch and pinprick may be detected in the median nerve distribution in the hand. Weakness of the abductor pollicis brevis and opponens pollicis muscle may be demonstrable. In advanced cases, atrophy may be noticeable in the thenar eminence, especially in the abductor pollicis brevis (Fig. 224-3). It is fair to say, however, that in contemporary neurosurgical practice the diagnosis of carpal tunnel syndrome is most frequently made based on suggestive history coupled with carefully conducted electrodiagnostic tests.

Pathogenesis, Etiologic Factors, and Associated Conditions (Table 224-1)

In the majority of patients with the carpal tunnel syndrome (CTS) a specific etiologic factor may not be identified. A common denominator in most patients appears to be repetitive wrist motion. Examples of manual activity that seem to predispose to or aggravate the symptoms are knitting, typing, scrubbing, dishwashing, driving, painting, and garden-

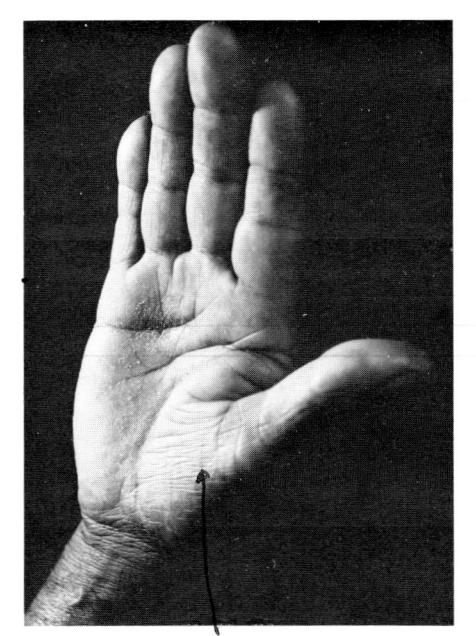

Figure 224-3 Thenar atrophy in a patient with the carpal tunnel syndrome.

TABLE 224-1 Conditions Associated with Carpal Tunnel Syndrome

Systemic Conditions
Pregnancy and lactation[27,42]
Menstrual cycles
Contraceptive pills
Menopause
Pyridoxine deficiency[10]
Toxic shock syndrome[34]
Maintenance hemodialysis[18]
Rheumatoid arthritis
Obesity
Amyloidosis
Mucolipidoses
Chondrocalcinosis[24]
Myxedema
Acromegaly
Athetoid-dystonic cerebral palsy[2]

Local Conditions
Increased volume of contents of the carpal canal
  Persistent median artery with or without thrombosis, aneurysm, or arteriovenous malformation[23]
  Anomalous muscles and tendons
  Tenosynovitis
  Acute palmar space infections
  Hemorrhage
  Masses: neurofibroma, hemangioma, lipoma, ganglion cyst, xanthoma, gouty tophus
Burns at the wrist[12]
Reduction in the capacity of the carpal canal
  Idiopathic or familial thickening of the transverse carpal ligament
  Malunion or callus following Colles' fracture or fracture of the carpal bones
  Unreduced dislocations of the wrist or intercarpal joints
  Improper immobilization of the wrist ("cotton loader position")
  Compression by cast

ing. Enthusiastic indulgence in a hobby that demands strenuous wrist motion or enforced manual activity in an unaccustomed new job are typical precipitating factors. Measurements of mean pressures within the carpal canal in patients with CTS compared with control subjects have shown that the resting values and values during extension and flexion of the wrist are significantly higher in patients than controls, and that these values normalize after section of the transverse carpal ligament.[15] Such abnormally high intracarpal canal pressures may interfere with capillary circulation within the median nerve and lead to conduction block and, if sustained, to demyelination and even axolysis.

Numerous clinical conditions are associated with CTS, and more are being recognized. They are listed in Table 224-1. A few factors deserve further comment.

The incidence of CTS in pregnancy has been reported to range from 1 to 25 percent. This wide range is due to the use of differing diagnostic criteria by various investigators.[27,42] When subjective hand symptoms alone are considered, 25 percent of pregnant women may be judged to have the syndrome. When strict electrodiagnostic criteria are used, only 7 percent of unselected pregnant women show positive results, implying that tingling and numbness in the hand in pregnant women may be nonspecific symptoms and may not always mean median nerve compression or that the electrodiagnostic tests may not be sensitive enough to pick up the very early syndrome. The occurrence of CTS in pregnancy is thought to result from fluid retention in connective tissue as a result of the effect of the putative hormone relaxin. The incidence of edema, pre-eclampsia, and hypertension are higher in the symptomatic women. In three-fourths of the patients the symptoms are bilateral. Patients with electroneuromyographic abnormalities tend to have a higher incidence of nocturnal pain; the presence of the latter symptom is a reliable clinical indicator of the presence of true CTS. Nerve conduction abnormalities may be detected in as early as the third month of pregnancy and as late as 20 months post partum, although typically symptoms tend to clear soon after delivery. In multigravidas, the symptoms may recur during each pregnancy. Because the symptoms are generally transient and improve soon after delivery, conservative measures are indicated; however, section of the transverse carpal ligament under local anesthesia may be a simpler solution in some selected women who have intractable pain, require large doses of analgesic drugs, and suffer from disturbed sleep at night.

Ellis and associates in a recent double-blind crossover study on seven patients with symptoms of CTS found that these patients suffered from pyridoxine (vitamin B_6) deficiency.[10] They based their conclusion on the low levels of specific activity of erythrocyte glutamic oxaloacetic transaminase (EGOT). With supplemental oral vitamin B_6, the symptoms improved in all patients concurrent with restoration of enzyme levels to the normal range. Several elements in their study design raise doubts about the validity of their conclusion. The number of patients entered into the study is extremely small compared with the frequency of this syndrome; electrodiagnostic studies were done in only five of the seven patients at the start of the study and were not done in any of the patients at completion. Four of the seven patients entered in the study showed poor compliance with vitamin intake.

There is a higher incidence of CTS in patients undergoing maintenance dialysis.[18] Early reports suggested that this was due to construction of arteriovenous access in the affected extremities. However, more recent studies find no correlation between the development of the syndrome and the site of vascular access. Instead, the thickening of the transverse carpal ligament and edema in the synovium demonstrated in these patients are thought to be responsible for the higher frequency of the syndrome.

A persistent median artery (Fig. 224-4) occurs in 10 percent of all upper extremities.[18] The artery may cause compression of the median nerve in the carpal canal if it is developmentally large, thrombosed, or the site of an aneurysm or arteriovenous malformation. Thrombosis of the persistent median artery usually presents as an acute CTS. If simply an enlarged artery is found at surgery, it should be left alone; a thrombosed artery or aneurysm may be excised. It is best to do a postoperative angiogram after the initial exploration to study the precise vascular anatomy of the hand before any vascular surgery is undertaken except for excising a thrombosed segment of the artery.

The median artery is the cardinal source of blood supply to the hand in early embryonic development. It represents the main branch of the primitive axial artery of the embryonic upper limb. Proximally the axial artery differentiates into the subclavian-axillary-brachial artery. Distally it becomes the anterior interosseous artery of the forearm leading to superficial capillary plexus in the hand. The median artery arises as the principal branch of the anterior interosseous artery and accompanies the median nerve distally. In the course of development, it briefly assumes the function of its parent artery, the anterior interosseous artery, and provides the main blood supply to the superficial capillary plexus of the hand. The ulnar and radial arteries start to develop and establish connection with the brachial artery. Gradually these arteries enlarge and assume the dominant role in sup-

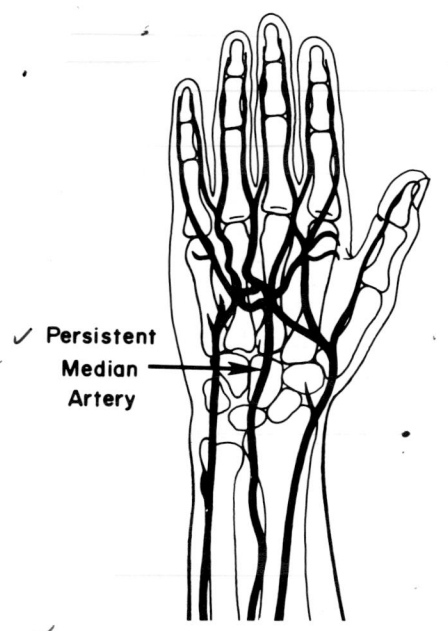

Figure 224-4 Persistent median artery.

plying blood to the hand, leaving the median artery as a slender vestigial remnant closely applied to the median nerve. Failure of such regressive changes to occur in the median artery results in the presence of an anomalously large median artery. Usually in such circumstances the ulnar artery may be reciprocally smaller. The relationship of the persistent median artery to the superficial palmar arch is quite variable.

Reports from certain burn centers suggest that burns at the wrist level are complicated by a high incidence of CTS and Guyon's canal syndrome.[12] This is not due to direct thermal injury to the median nerve but seems to be due to edema in the carpal tunnel with compression of the median nerve.

Electrodiagnosis

The most important, most sensitive, and earliest indicator of CTS is prolonged sensory latency; the sensory evoked response may show a diminished amplitude and is often absent. The distal motor latency is also prolonged, but this is not as sensitive an indicator as the sensory latency. Motor latency abnormalities tend to occur later in the course of the disease. Needle electromyographic examination may show loss of motor units and presence of denervation potentials in the thenar muscles. Although these abnormalities are present before clinically evident muscular atrophy sets in, they usually occur after distal motor latency is prolonged. The electrodiagnostic study is incomplete unless the ulnar nerve of the same arm is also evaluated to rule out the possibility of peripheral neuropathy.

Treatment

Although the majority of carpal tunnel entrapments are idiopathic in origin, every effort should be made not to overlook any systemic abnormalities listed in Table 224-1. Conservative treatment is justified under the following conditions: (1) short duration, (2) mild or intermittent symptoms, (3) when the symptoms are expected to be reversible—such as after termination of pregnancy, discontinuation of oral contraceptives, correction of endocrine abnormalities (myxedema or acromegaly), or avoidance of strenuous unaccustomed activities. Conservative treatment consists of the use of nonsteroidal anti-inflammatory drugs and the use of a wrist splint. Local injection of steroid medication is not recommended because of possible injury to the median nerve.

Indications for surgical therapy are (1) failure of sustained improvement with conservative therapy, (2) a typical clinical history to suggest CTS with confirmation by electrodiagnostic data, and (3) the presence of sensory loss, atrophy, or weakness.

Section of the transverse carpal ligament is a simple surgical procedure, but to avoid suboptimal results, a meticulous technique should be used based on sound knowledge of the anatomy of the region. The simplest anesthetic to use is local infiltration anesthesia. We prefer this over Bier block, axillary block, or general anesthesia. The use of a tourniquet is unnecessary. A curvilinear incision is made from the wrist crease to a point in line with the distal border of the fully extended thumb. The incision is generally placed 2 to 3 mm medial to the volar crease, in line with the long axis of the ring finger (Fig. 224-5). It is better to avoid an incision directly on the volar crease because it serves as a natural hinge in the skin during flexion of the thumb. An optional extension of the incision may be made into the wrist in an S-shaped curve, but this is seldom necessary. Subcutaneous fat generally protrudes out of the wound as the skin incision is completed. The first structure to be visualized is the palmar aponeurosis, which is incised sharply in line with the skin incision. All subcutaneous bleeding is controlled with bipolar coagulation, and self-retaining retractors are inserted. The transverse carpal ligament now is exposed, but this is generally obscured by the origin of the thenar and hypothenar muscles, which come into apposition in the midline. It is easier to start the section of the ligament distally, where it is thin. Division is started with a no. 15 blade knife. The median nerve covered by smooth epineurium pops into the wound. The remainder of ligament is divided by sharp heavy scissors. Section is extended proximally until the deep fascia of the forearm is reached. Firm retraction of the skin edge will facilitate this procedure. The most common cause of failure of surgery is the incomplete division of the proxi-

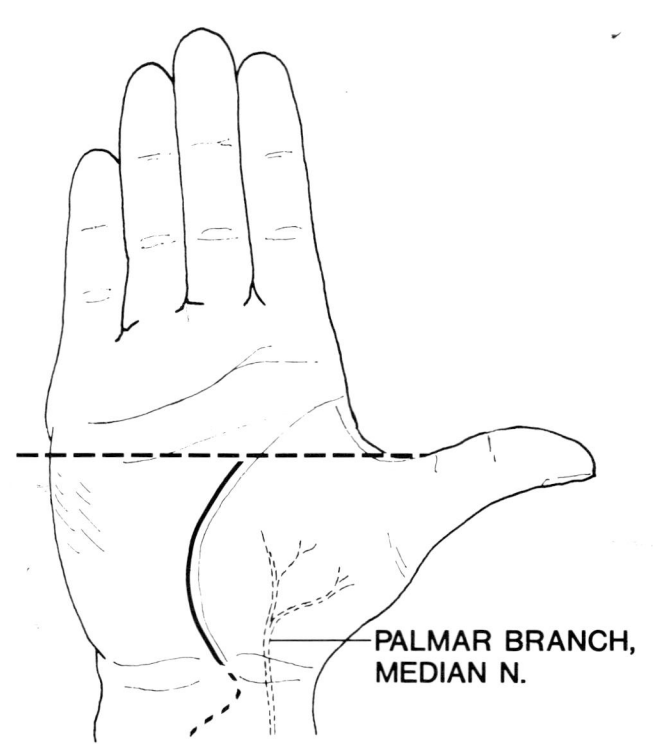

Figure 224-5 Skin incision used in the section of the transverse carpal ligament. The solid line indicates the incision commonly used and the curved interrupted line the optional extension. The horizontal interrupted line that is in line with the distal border of the outstretched thumb represents the distal limit of the incision. An incision directly in the volar crease should be avoided, and the palmar cutaneous branch of the median nerve should be preserved. Placement of the incision on the ulnar side of the volar crease tends to avoid the motor branch of the median nerve.

mal part of the ligament. It is unnecessary to perform a neurolysis of the median nerve. The wound is closed in two layers superficial to the divided transverse carpal ligament, and a bulky dressing is applied.

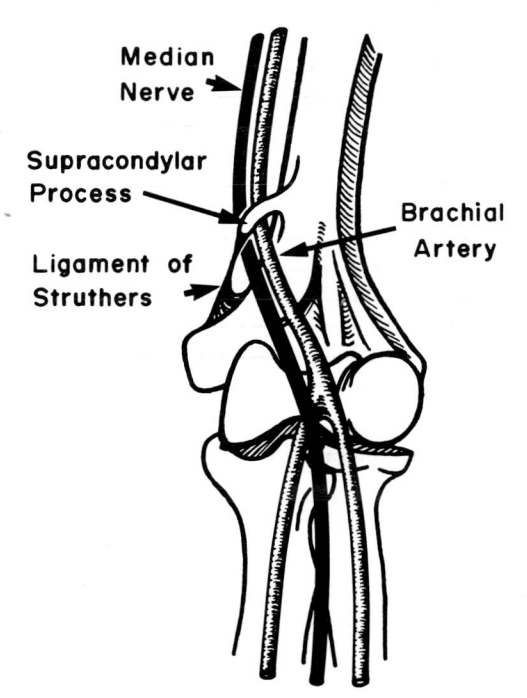

The Supracondylar Process of the Humerus and Struther's Ligament[3,21]

Applied and Comparative Anatomy

The supracondylar process is a rare, anomalous, beaklike bony process arising from the anteromedial surface of the humerus, 5 to 7 cm above the medial epicondyle (Fig. 224-6). The process generally projects downward, forward, and medially. The process has been variously referred to as supracondylar, supracondyloid, supraepitrochlear, or epicondylic. It is estimated to occur in 0.7 to 2.7 percent of the population, and is said to be more common in Caucasians than in blacks. A familial occurrence has been recorded. Not infrequently the process occurs bilaterally.

In most instances, a fibrous ligament (Struther's ligament) extends from the supracondyloid process to the medial epicondyle, enclosing a fibro-osseous foramen through which the median nerve and the brachial artery pass. Rarely, only the ligament may be present without the bony supracondylar process. The fibro-osseous bridge affords attachment to the lower part of the coracobrachialis; the pronator teres muscle has an anomalous origin from this ridge as well. It is said that Struthers' ligament represents the lower part of the tendon of a vestigial muscle (latissimocondyloideus), which is present in climbing mammals and extends from the tendon of insertion of the latissimus dorsi muscle to the medial epicondyle. The supracondyloid canal is thought to be a rudimentary homologue of a bony canal present in many lower animals.[17] It is present in many reptiles and mammals, especially marsupials and carnivores (the dog, and especially the domestic cat, are the best examples of the latter). Among primates, it is found in most lemurs, tarsiers, and many new-world monkeys, but not in old-world monkeys. Among anthropoid apes it is found in the orangutan and gorilla. In the lower forms, the supracondylar foramen serves to protect the neurovascular bundle passing through it and provides a large muscular attachment to the pronator teres muscle.

Clinical Features

Patients with a supracondylar process are generally asymptomatic. The lesion may be discovered accidentally by the patient or the examining physician as a palpable bony mass or during evaluation of x-ray films of the humerus for trauma to the elbow. Localized aching pain above the elbow may be present. Of neurosurgical interest, the median nerve may be compressed as it passes under the bony spur. The patient may complain of weakness in hand grip and in pronation, and tingling in the lateral three digits. There may be objective weakness in the pronator teres, flexor carpi radialis, flexor pollicis longus, flexor digitorum sublimis, the lateral half of the flexor digitorum profundus, and the thenar muscles. There may be sensory loss in the median nerve distribution. The presence of pronator weakness distinguishes this syndrome from the pronator and anterior interosseous nerve syndromes. Nerve conduction studies may show slowing in the conduction velocity in the median nerve in the arm; electromyography may show denervation potentials in the median innervated muscles in the forearm and hand. The clinical syndrome may be associated with symptoms and signs of ischemia in the distribution of the brachial artery.

The bony process may or may not be palpable. Tangential or oblique radiographic views of the humerus may show the supracondylar process to a greater advantage than routine anteroposterior and lateral views. A brachial angiogram may be necessary if vascular compromise is suspected.

Surgical therapy consists of excision of Struther's ligament and removal of the bony spur. Relief of symptoms invariably occurs.

Figure 224-6 Supracondylar process of the humerus and Struthers' ligament.

Entrapment of the Median Nerve at the Elbow and Forearm: Compression by Lacertus Fibrosus, Pronator Teres Syndrome, Compression by Sublimis "Bridge"

Applied Anatomy (Fig. 224-7)

The median nerve arises by two roots from the brachial plexus and crosses anterior to the brachial artery in the midarm from the lateral to the medial side of the artery. At the front of the elbow it lies behind the bicipital aponeurosis

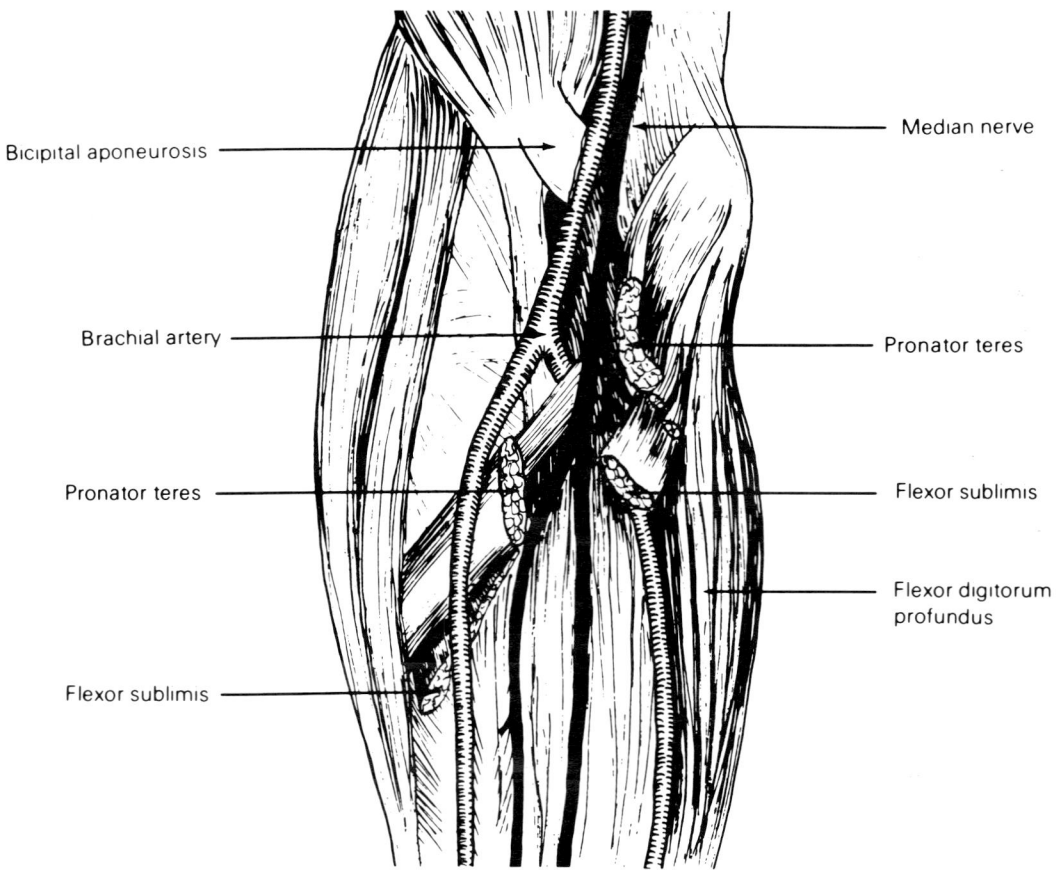

Figure 224-7 Anatomy of the median nerve in the cubital fossa. (From Laha RK, Lunsford LD, Dujovny M: Lacertus fibrosus compression of the median nerve. J Neurosurg 48:838–841, 1978.)

(lacertus fibrosus) and in front of the brachialis. The nerve enters the forearm between the two heads of the pronator teres. The anterior interosseous branch is given off from the posterior surface of the median nerve as it passes between the two heads of the pronator teres. The median nerve then passes under the fibrotendinous arcade that represents the origin of the flexor digitorum sublimis muscle. The median nerve descends in the forearm adherent to the undersurface of the flexor digitorum sublimis and lying superficial to the flexor digitorum profundus.

Clinical Features

The median nerve is vulnerable to compression by any one or a combination of three structures in the elbow and the proximal forearm: (1) the lacertus fibrosus, (2) the pronator teres, and (3) the sublimis "bridge."[17] Although subtle differences do exist, in most instances it is clinically impossible to differentiate which of these structures is responsible for median nerve compression. Indeed, exploration for entrapment of the median nerve in the arm may be considered incomplete unless all the three potential sites of entrapment are examined.

The symptoms are generally insidious in onset. The common precipitating factor is assumption of a new job that involves strenuous use of the forearm, especially in repetitive forceful pronation and supination, or overenthusiastic pursuit of a hobby on weekends by a sedentary worker. Commonly cited examples are hammering for a long time, using a manual screwdriver, scraping dishes, ladling food, practicing tennis serves, etc. The patient may complain of vague aching pain and easy fatigability of the forearm muscles. Weakness in the hand grip and poorly localized numbness and tingling in the index finger and thumb are the cardinal symptoms. Nocturnal exacerbation of pain is singularly absent unlike in the carpal tunnel syndrome. In fact, the complaints may be so vague and objective findings so minimal at the outset that even astute clinicians might suspect a functional disorder, unless they have a high index of suspicion for this entity. There may be tenderness on palpation of the pronator teres muscle; the latter may be brawny, firm, and indurated from work hypertrophy. Indeed some have considered the enlarged hypertrophic pronator teres muscle contained within the unyielding deep fascial sleeve to represent a dynamic compartment syndrome. Tinel's sign may be positive at the proximal edge of the pronator teres muscle. There may be mild to moderate weakness of median innervated muscles, especially the flexor pollicis longus, the radial half of the flexor digitorum

Entrapment Neuropathies

profundus, and the thenar muscles. In advanced cases, flexion of the radial three digits may be impossible, the hand assuming a benediction attitude (Fig. 224-8). Mild thenar atrophy may be present.

Nerve conduction velocity may be slowed in the forearm segment of the median nerve, but the distal sensory and motor latencies are normal unless there is an associated carpal tunnel syndrome. Needle examination may show denervation potentials in the median innervated muscles distal to the site of compression.

Treatment

It is most important to analyze in detail the patient's occupation or avocation to determine if it is causally related to his or her symptoms; should this prove to be the case, it is prudent to try to change the patient's work habits to the extent that is practical. Injection of a corticosteroid into the pronator muscle is said to offer temporary relief of symptoms. In intractable cases, the median nerve should be exposed and the three potential sites of compression mentioned earlier should be explored; if compression is present, the constricting bands should be generously divided.

The Anterior Interosseous Nerve Syndrome[36,38]

Applied Anatomy

The anterior interosseous nerve is principally a motor nerve. It arises from the median nerve at a variable point as it passes between the two heads of the pronator teres, descends vertically in front of the interosseous membrane between the flexor digitorum profundus and the flexor pollicis longus, supplying these two muscles, and finally terminates in the pronator quadratus near the wrist joint.

Clinical Features

The onset of symptoms may be acute or insidious. Vague aching pain in the elbow and forearm may be present. The patient's principal difficulty is moving the index and middle fingers. On objective testing there is weakness in the flexors of the interphalangeal joint of the thumb (flexor pollicis longus) and the distal interphalangeal joints of the index and the middle fingers (flexor digitorum profundus). This can be diagnosed by observing the pinch attitude of the hand. Normally, when an individual pinches something between the index finger and the thumb, the metacarpophalangeal and interphalangeal joints of the thumb and index finger are flexed (Fig. 224-9). With compression neuropathy of the anterior interosseous nerve, the terminal phalanges of the thumb and index finger are extended or hyperextended, and thus their pulps are brought into extensive apposition, but the metacarpophalangeal joint of the thumb and the interphalangeal joint of the index finger are flexed (Fig. 224-9).

The pronator quadratus muscle is difficult to test clini-

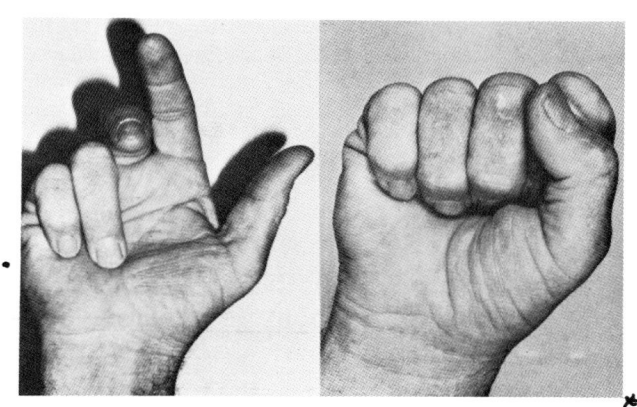

Figure 224-8 *Left:* When a patient with lacertus fibrosus compression of the median nerve attempts to make a fist, the hand assumes a "benediction attitude." *Right:* Postoperative photograph demonstrates return of function. (From Laha RK, Lunsford LD, Dujovny M: Lacertus fibrosus compression of the median nerve. J Neurosurg 48:838–841, 1978.)

cally because of the simultaneous contraction of the more powerful pronator teres muscle during the pronation motion; however, when the elbow is examined in flexion, the pronator teres is at a mechanical disadvantage, and any weakness of the pronator quadratus may become apparent.

Electromyography may show evidence of abnormal membrane irritability with loss of motor units in any or all of the muscles supplied by the anterior interosseous nerve. It should be stressed that needle examination of these muscles is difficult because of their deep location. Stimulation studies using needle recording electrodes have also been described.

Treatment

Except in circumstances where the etiologic factor is obvious (fracture of the forearm bones, penetrating wound to the forearm, paralysis following operative intervention such as plating, etc.), the syndrome should be treated conservatively

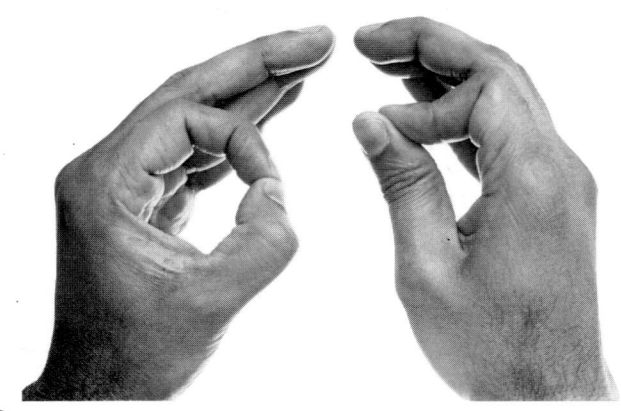

Figure 224-9 Pinch posture in the normal left hand contrasted with right hand with interosseous nerve palsy.

for 8 to 12 weeks because spontaneous recovery occurs frequently. In a refractory case the anterior interosseous nerve is explored and any constricting band (which is usually found near the origin of the nerve) is divided. On occasion no obvious constricting agent may be demonstrated at surgery.

Posterior Interosseous Nerve Entrapment: Entrapment at the Arcade of Frohse

Applied Anatomy

The radial nerve enters the anterior compartment of the arm lying deeply between the brachialis medially and brachioradialis and extensor carpi radialis laterally. In front of the lateral epicondyle it divides into its two terminal branches, the superficial radial nerve and the posterior interosseous nerve (Fig. 224-10).

The posterior interosseous nerve supplies the extensor carpi radialis brevis and the supinator muscles before entering the arcade of Frohse. This arcade is a tough fibrotendinous ringlike structure at the origin of the supinator muscle, and represents the usual site for entrapment of the nerve. This fibrous arcade is absent in full-term fetuses but is present in 30 percent of adult arms, suggesting "that the arcade is probably formed in the most proximal part of the superficial head of the supinator in response to repeated rotary movement of the forearm."[37] Anatomical studies by Spinner have shown that full pronation of the forearm produces pressure on the posterior interosseous nerve by the sharp tendinous edge of the origin of the extensor carpi radialis brevis muscle.[37]

The posterior interosseous nerve traverses the supinator muscle, and during the process winds around the lateral side of the radius and emerges on the dorsal aspect of the forearm in the interval between the superficial and deep extensor muscles. Soon after its emergence from the supinator muscle it arborizes into many muscular branches, which supply the extensor digiti minimi, extensor digitorum, extensor carpi ulnaris, abductor pollicis longus, extensor pollicis longus and brevis, and extensor indicis. It has no cutaneous sensory component.

Clinical Features

The pattern of paralysis, when it is typical and complete, is a reflection of the motor distribution of the nerve, and the examination offers a good exercise in neuroanatomy.[16] In contrast to radial nerve palsy, there is no wrist drop, because the extensor carpi radialis longus is supplied by the radial nerve proximal to its terminal branching. However, when the patient attempts to extend the wrist, the wrist deviates radialward because of the paralysis of the extensor carpi ulnaris supplied by the posterior interosseus nerve. The cardinal finding is the inability to extend the metacarpophalangeal joints of the fingers and thumb ("finger drop"). Extension at the interphalangeal joints of the fingers is possible because this is an ulnar and median innervated function. Extension of the thumb at the interphalangeal joint is not possible because of paralysis of the extensor pollicis longus. Sensory disturbances are entirely absent.

Needle electromyographic examination may show denervation potentials in the muscles innervated by the distal posterior interosseous nerve. The absence of such abnormal potentials in the brachioradialis, extensor carpi radialis longus, extensor carpi radialis brevis, and supinator muscles helps to pinpoint the lesion to the region of the arcade of Frohse. Nerve conduction velocity studies may show slowing across the site of entrapment.

Treatment

Surgical therapy, in refractory cases that do not improve after 4 to 8 weeks of conservative therapy, consists of exploring the posterior interosseous nerve and dividing the arcade of Frohse and any other constricting bands.

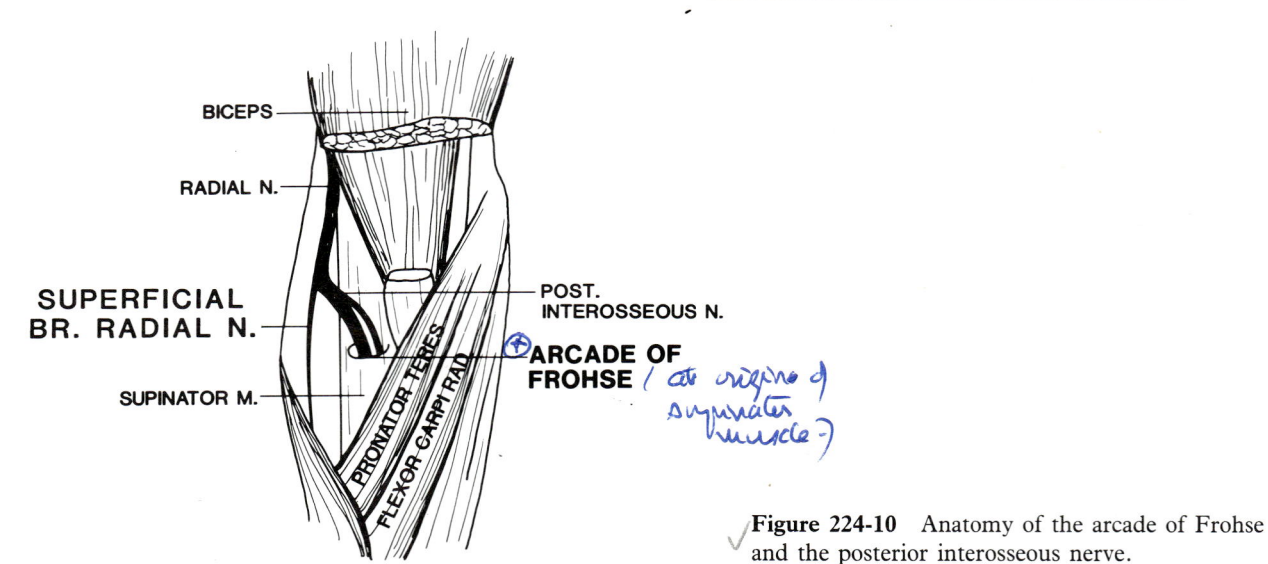

Figure 224-10 Anatomy of the arcade of Frohse and the posterior interosseous nerve.

Capener and others have championed the idea that the clinical syndrome of "tennis elbow" may represent a variant of the posterior interosseous nerve entrapment syndrome.[5,16] Exploration and neurolysis resulted in promising improvement in refractory cases.

Cubital Tunnel Syndrome: Tardy Ulnar Palsy, Feindel-Osborne Syndrome

Applied Anatomy

The ulnar nerve originates as a direct continuation of the medial cord of the brachial plexus, deriving its fibers from the eighth cervical and first thoracic nerve roots. It courses downward medial to the brachial artery. In the middle of the arm it pierces the medial intermuscular septum and descends in front of the medial head of the triceps. In about 70 percent of individuals, the nerve passes under the *arcade of Struthers*. This arcade is nothing but a flat, thin fibroaponeurotic band extending from the medial head of the triceps to the medial intermuscular septum. When present, it is situated about 3 in. above the medial epicondyle. (The *arcade* of Struthers is different from the *ligament* of Struthers, which is discussed above.) The arcade is not a site for entrapment under ordinary circumstances, but it may become a point of kinking if anterior transposition of the ulnar nerve is performed without adequately dividing this arcade and the adjacent medial intermuscular septum.

The ulnar nerve reaches a groove behind the medial epicondyle accompanied by the ulnar collateral artery. It then enters the forearm through a fibro-osseous tunnel, the cubital tunnel.[33] The roof of the tunnel is formed by the aponeurotic attachment of the two heads of the flexor carpi ulnaris, which spans in an arcade-like manner from the medial epicondyle of the humerus to the olecranon process of the ulna (Fig. 224-11). In the majority of instances the sharp proximal margin of this musculoaponeurotic arcade is the constricting agent in patients with the cubital tunnel syndrome.

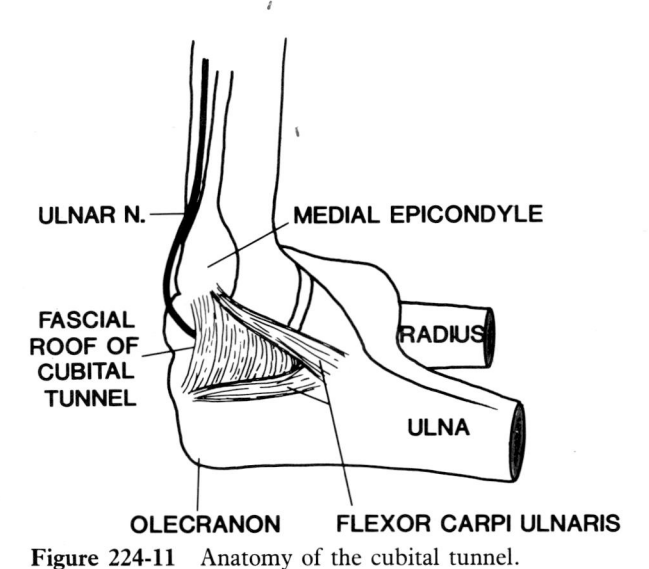

The floor is formed by the medial ligament of the elbow joint, which extends in a fanlike fashion from the medial border of the olecranon process to the base of the epicondyle. The ligament is attached distally to the coronoid process of the ulna, which delimits the distal end of the tunnel.

The volume of the cubital tunnel decreases, and extrinsic pressure over the nerve increases during *flexion* of the elbow; the reverse happens during *extension*. The mechanism is as follows: The aponeurotic roof of the cubital tunnel becomes maximally taut during flexion because the two points of its bony attachment (the medial epicondyle and the olecranon) are farthest apart during this position. The sharp free margin of the aponeurosis is thus stretched tightly over the nerve during flexion; this is aggravated if the flexion of the elbow is coupled with contraction of the flexor carpi ulnaris to initiate active wrist movement, as occurs during hammering or shoveling. During extension of the elbow, the bony points of attachment come very close together, relaxing the roof of the tunnel. An additional factor is the degree of tension in the medial ligament of the elbow joint, which forms the floor of the tunnel: during flexion, it becomes taut and compromises the capacity of the tunnel, and during extension it becomes lax and gives maximum room.

The ulnar nerve has no branches in the arm; at the level of the medial epicondyle before the nerve enters the cubital tunnel, it gives off the articular branches to the elbow joint. The branches to the flexor carpi ulnaris and the medial half of flexor digitorum profundus are given off distal to the entry of the nerve into the cubital tunnel, yet these two muscles are generally spared in the cubital tunnel syndrome. This paradox is probably accounted for by the fact that the fascicles that innervate these two muscles are situated quite deeply in the nerve compared with those innervating the intrinsic muscles or the skin. Chang and associates showed that the ulnar nerve had fusiform enlargement to varying degrees at the level of the medial epicondyle in about half of the 400 cadaveric ulnar nerves that they examined.[7] The ulnar nerve in such instances had the maximal diameter at the level of the elbow, more than at any other point. Histological examination of the fusiform area showed no pathological changes but showed an increase in the proportion of connective tissue in relation to neural tissue. It is probable that such fusiform enlargement may create the disparity between the size of the nerve and the size of the opening into the tunnel, contributing to the probability of the development of the cubital tunnel syndrome.

Clinical Features

The onset of symptoms is generally insidious. The average duration of symptoms before the patient seeks medical counsel is about 6 months to 1 year, although the range is anywhere from 1 month to 40 years. Men are affected three times as frequently as women. In about 12 percent of individuals the symptoms are bilateral, although the severity may not be of the same degree. The right arm is affected about as often as the left. The syndrome occurs most commonly between the ages of 30 and 60. It is exceptionally uncommon in children under 15, as is true with all other entrapment neuropathies. No particular occupation seems

Figure 224-11 Anatomy of the cubital tunnel.

to predispose to this condition; white collar workers are just as susceptible as blue collar workers.

In the early years when the disease was first recognized, deformity of the elbow from previous trauma appeared to constitute the major predisposing cause for this condition, although "idiopathic" cases were also reported. As late as 1947, in a series of 100 cases reported by Gay and Love, 57 percent of the cases were due to old fracture of the elbow and an additional 20 percent were caused by arthritis in this joint.[14] Symptoms generally appeared several years after the original trauma, and hence the term *tardy ulnar palsy*. The common lesions in the elbow were fracture of the medial epicondyle, malunited supracondylar fracture with cubitus valgus deformity, exuberant callus, or dislocation of the elbow. In contemporary neurosurgical practice, however, idiopathic cases are by far the most common. Less frequent causes include habitual leaning on the elbow(s), prolonged recumbency in bed from coma or major illnesses, improper positioning of the limb under general anesthesia, direct contusion to the elbow, rheumatoid arthritis of the elbow, ganglion cysts of the elbow joint, and the presence of a rare anomalous muscle, anconeus epitrochlearis.

Paresthesia consisting of tingling or burning along the inner border of the hand or in the fourth or fifth digits is the most common symptom. Unlike the carpal tunnel syndrome, pain is seldom a dominant feature, although infrequently there is some aching around the elbow or along the medial border of the arm or hand. Since the ulnar nerve at the elbow contains a greater proportion of motor than sensory fibers, motor symptoms and signs tend to be a significant part of the clinical picture. The weakness may be variously described as impairment of hand grip, clumsiness, difficulty in buttoning shirts, etc. Some degree of atrophy, especially of the interossei, is usually present by the time the patient seeks medical attention, which again contrasts with the carpal tunnel syndrome; the early onset of pain rather than motor weakness is the rule in the latter.

On objective testing, sensory loss to light touch and pinprick may be detected in the medial one and one-half fingers and the palm of the hand. There are varying degrees of weakness of the muscles of the hypothenar eminence, the interossei, the medial two lumbricals, and the adductor pollicis (testing of these muscles is described and illustrated in another chapter.* Weakness in the adductor pollicis may be demonstrated by asking the patient to grasp a piece of cardboard between the index finger and thumb against resistance. In patients with weakness of the adductor pollicis, there will be flexion of the interphalangeal joint of the thumb because of the substitution of the median innervated flexor pollicis longus for a weak adductor pollicis (Froment's sign) (Fig. 224-12). Weakness in the flexor carpi ulnaris and medial half of the flexor digitorum profundus is present infrequently, although these two muscles are innervated by the ulnar nerve distal to the site of entrapment.

Diagnosis

The electroneuromyographic features of the cubital tunnel syndrome are as follows:

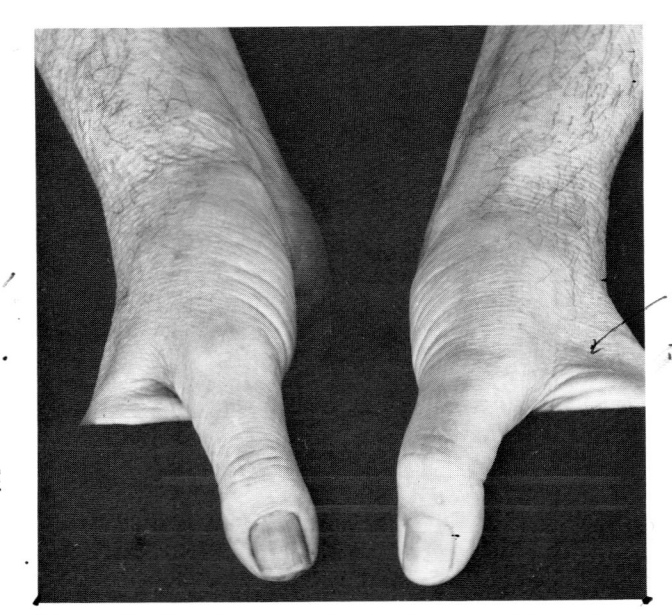

Figure 224-12 Froment's sign in a patient with a left cubital tunnel syndrome; observe also the atrophy of the left first dorsal interosseous muscle.

1. The conduction velocity in the ulnar nerve across the elbow is slowed compared with the velocity in the forearm segment. It is important to keep the elbow flexed 70 to 90 degrees during conduction measurements because in this position the nerve is optimally stretched, which allows accurate measurement of the across-the-elbow segment of the nerve; during extension the nerve buckles upon itself and is redundant, a factor that may lead to spuriously low computed values of conduction velocity. Demonstration of normal conduction velocity in the forearm segment is helpful in excluding intrinsic disease of peripheral nerves such as diabetic neuropathy.
2. The amplitude of motor response in the abductor digiti minimi is decreased and the duration of the response is prolonged with stimulation above the elbow compared with stimulation below the elbow. This finding is especially valuable in patients who may have normal conduction velocity across the elbow in spite of typical clinical symptoms.
3. The sensory latency (usually elicited antidromically) is prolonged.
4. Needle examination of the ulnar innervated muscles may show varying changes. An early finding is a reduction in the voluntary motor unit action potentials. When axonal degeneration sets in, positive waves and fibrillation potentials may be observed. With reinnervation, polyphasic action potentials or large-amplitude, long-duration motor potentials may be observed.

Several clinical conditions may mimic the ulnar nerve entrapment syndrome at the elbow. These include intrinsic spinal cord lesions affecting the C8 and T1 segments (syringomyelia, spinal cord tumor, ALS), extramedullary spinal lesions (cervical disc disease or spondylosis, neurofibroma, or meningioma), lesions of the brachial plexus involving the lower trunk or medial cord (Pancoast tumor), entrapment of the ulnar nerve distally at the wrist (in Guyon's canal), and polyneuropathy (most often secondary to diabetes or alcoholism). The problem becomes complex when some of these lesions coexist, such as the occurrence of the cubital tunnel syndrome in an elderly individual who also has evidence of advanced cervical spondylosis and diabetic polyneuropathy.

Intrinsic spinal cord lesions are generally painless, produce bilateral symptoms and signs, may be associated with Horner's syndrome, and produce sensory and motor loss in a segmental rather than peripheral nerve distribution. Thus, the wasting and motor weakness may be noticeable in the hypothenar and thenar muscles; the clawing posture involves the whole hand, not just the medial two fingers; and the sensory loss is not delineated by a boundary that splits the ring finger. Other evidences of involvement of the spinal cord, such as the "long tract signs," may be evident. Fasciculation in muscles may be prominent. The nerve conduction velocity across the elbow is in the normal range.

Extramedullary lesions produce characteristic root pains, may be associated with Horner's syndrome, and produce sensory and motor loss in a root distribution without alteration in nerve conduction velocity. Guyon's canal syndrome is diagnosed by careful assessment of the etiologic factors that led to the syndrome, such as the patient's occupation or hobbies, history of trauma to the wrist, etc., and by evaluation of distal motor and sensory latencies of the ulnar nerve. In polyneuropathy, symptoms and signs tend to be diffuse, affecting both arms and legs, with glove and stocking type of sensory loss. Paresthesias and burning pains are prominent symptoms. There is usually diffuse slowing of nerve conduction velocity.

Treatment

In the early cases, especially in those patients with minor symptoms and no evidence of motor atrophy, one is justified in pursuing a conservative approach. There is no specific nonoperative therapy, however, except to follow the patient carefully for lack of progression and with instructions to avoid any precipitating factors such as habitual leaning on the elbows. As a rule, once the symptoms set in, they tend to be progressive. Spontaneous improvement or fluctuation in symptoms occurs less often with the cubital tunnel syndrome than with the carpal tunnel syndrome. Surgical therapy should not be delayed once motor weakness or atrophy is apparent so as not to jeopardize the chances for complete recovery.

Historically there have been numerous methods of operative treatment for ulnar nerve compression at the elbow: supracondylar osteotomy, deepening of the bony ulnar groove, neurolysis, resection of a pseudoneuroma with end-to-end anastomosis of the ulnar nerve, medial epicondylectomy, anterior transposition of the ulnar nerve, and simple section of the roof of the cubital tunnel. In contemporary neurosurgical practice the choice is restricted to one of the two latter procedures, anterior transposition of the ulnar nerve or simple decompression of the cubital tunnel. The variety of operative approaches used for this condition over the years is in itself a testimony to the poor understanding of the pathogenesis of tardy ulnar palsy. Feindel and Stratford[11] and Osborne[29] deserve the credit for elucidating the pathogenesis of this syndrome and focusing our attention to the point of compression of the ulnar nerve, namely, at the entrance of the nerve into the cubital tunnel, by the sharp fibroaponeurotic edge of the flexor carpi ulnaris muscle. Over the years, numerous strong convictions have been and are being held pertaining to the pathogenesis and management of this entity. Some of these are stated sufficiently often by various authors that they are mistaken for established facts. Critical analysis of these convictions follows. Based on this analysis, I prefer a simple decompression operation over transposition of the nerve.

Conviction 1: Recurrent dislocation of the ulnar nerve out of its groove leads to ulnar neuropathy from repeated trauma; anterior transposition of the nerve in such instances protects the nerve from chronic damage by impingement against the epicondyle.

Childress in an analysis of 2000 apparently normal elbows found ulnar nerve dislocation in 162 individuals, almost always bilaterally (Fig. 224-13).[8] These were apparently normal individuals without symptoms of ulnar neuropathy. No apparent etiology was found for the dislocation. This anomaly occurs sufficiently commonly in normal individuals (16.2 percent) that it can be considered simply as a congenital variation due to laxity of the fascia binding the nerve. It has been suggested, but not proved, that this variation predisposes to ulnar neuropathy. To establish a causal relationship between recurrent dislocation of the ulnar nerve and ulnar neuropathy at the elbow one needs to demonstrate (1) a higher incidence of ulnar neuropathy in individuals with recurrent dislocation of the ulnar nerve than those who do not have this anomaly, and (2) a higher than 16.2 percent incidence of recurrent dislocation of the nerve in individuals with documented ulnar neuropathy at the elbow. This statistical information, however, is currently not available.

Conviction 2: Transposition of the ulnar nerve across the elbow offers a more direct course to the nerve.

Although this statement is true when the elbow is in flexion, it does not hold good with the elbow in extension (Fig. 224-14). Applying a simple mathematical axiom that the

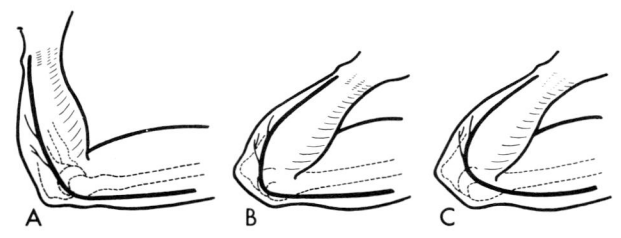

Figure 224-13 *A.* Ulnar nerve within the ulnar groove with moderate flexion. With further flexion there is partial (*B*) or complete (*C*) dislocation of the nerve. Partial or complete dislocation of the ulnar nerve occurs in 16.2 percent of the normal population. It is assumed but not proven that this anomaly predisposes to tardy ulnar palsy.

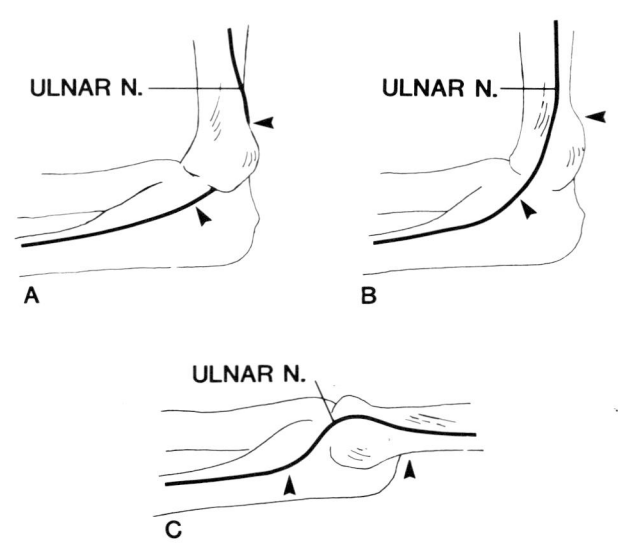

Figure 224-14 *A.* The normal course of the ulnar nerve. *B.* A transposed ulnar nerve with the elbow in flexion; the ulnar nerve seems to take a more direct course. *C.* A transposed ulnar nerve with the elbow in extension; the nerve does not take a direct course. The two arrowheads in each illustration define two points; the ulnar nerve depicted in (*B*) takes a straight course between these points, going through the shortest distance between them. This is not the case in (*C*).

shortest distance between any two points is a straight line connecting these two points, it becomes apparent that the course of the transposed nerve approximates a straight line during flexion but assumes a deviously curved course with the elbow in extension. Most neurosurgeons have recognized this fact during the transposition procedure when it is done with the elbow in extension. To do a proper transposition, one has to do fairly extensive mobilization of the nerve both proximally and distally, divide the medial intermuscular septum, dissect and mobilize the branches to the flexor carpi ulnaris, etc. Even with all these maneuvers, the nerve often appears taut, not redundant, after transposition. This is especially true in individuals with well-developed flexor muscles over which the nerve has to ride.

Conviction 3: The rationale for the transposition of the ulnar nerve from the ulnar groove to the anterior aspect of the elbow is to prevent frictional neuropathy. It moves the nerve from a vulnerable position to a more protected position in the arm.

The rationale for the transposition of the ulnar nerve is best appreciated when this operative procedure is reviewed with a historical perspective. In the early years of the original recognition of this syndrome, the most common etiologic factor that led to this syndrome was recognized to be a bony injury to the elbow with exuberant callus formation in the ulnar groove. This distorted the anatomical relationship of the nerve and allowed stretching of the nerve against the bony hump during flexion. The surgical cure for the lesion is to resect the callus or form a trough through the bony callus. Neither of these procedures was easy to perform. A simple alternative was to move the nerve away from the callus to the front of the elbow, that is, transpose the nerve. This reasoning is reflected in one of the pioneering papers on the subject written by 1918 by Adson: "Because of a tendency of overgrowth of callus which results in a condition similar to that for which the patient seeks relief, we have chosen as a surgical procedure the transference of the nerve to a position anterior to the internal condyle in preference to removing bony prominences or creating a new bony groove as has been done by several other surgeons."[1]

It became apparent in the later series that the bony injury to the elbow is an uncommon predisposing factor for ulnar neuropathy; indeed, most cases are "idiopathic." By now, however, the transposition operation had become an established procedure. The procedure was performed even in idiopathic cases with the unproven premise, almost an afterthought, that it prevents repeated trauma to the ulnar nerve against the normal medial epicondyle (not callus). Thus, the rationale for the transposition operation has changed insidiously and imperceptibly over the years; it has no proven basis for idiopathic cases of ulnar neuropathy.

Conviction 4: Preparing a trough in the flexor muscles and laying the nerve within the trough offers more protection to the nerve than leaving the nerve in the vulnerable subcutaneous position, especially in thin individuals.

Muscle tissue has very little regenerative potential in an adult. When muscle tissue is cut, it heals by fibrous tissue and not by new muscle fibers. Thus the trough created with the intention of offering more protection to the nerve forms a veritable tomb to the nerve. The nerve is encased and entrapped in dense fibrous tissue that severely restricts any longitudinal mobility of the nerve. Seddon likens the appearance of such a nerve observed on re-exploration to the "twisted ornamentation of a piece of Jacobean furniture."[35] With contraction of the muscles, the nerve is pulled and distorted, causing burning pain both locally and along the distribution of the ulnar nerve. Detaching the muscle from the common flexor origin, burying the nerve even deeper, with subsequent reattachment of the flexor muscle is a procedure that is even more traumatic but still has some advocates.

Conviction 5: The transposition operation is a superior procedure compared with simple decompression of the cubital tunnel; it should be performed in cases when the cubital tunnel decompression procedure has failed to relieve symptoms.

Although prospective randomized double-blind clinical trials comparing the efficacy of simple decompression versus anterior transposition have not been conducted, many large series comparing the short- and long-term results and morbidity of these two procedures are now available. They all show that the transposition procedure carries no advantage over simple decompression. Indeed, in some trials more complete neurological recovery occurred with simple decompression, and with less morbidity.[6,35] The evolving consensus is that the division of the roof of the cubital tunnel that is a prerequisite for the transposition operation is in itself salutary and the transposition itself adds no further benefit. This is suggested by the immediate improvement in symptoms after decompression alone.

In fact, one may cite numerous disadvantages of the transposition procedure that may lead to higher morbidity.

The transposition procedure requires a longer skin incision and wider exposure. The nerve has to be mobilized circumferentially through the length of the exposure with a risk of impairment of blood supply and ischemia of the nerve. Distal mobilization may require dissection of the motor branches to the flexor carpi ulnaris with a risk of injury to these branches. Although of little consequence, the articular branches of the ulnar nerve to the elbow usually have to be sacrificed to allow transposition of the nerve. The transposed nerve is at risk of being kinked at three points (1) the arcade of Struthers and the medial intermuscular septum, (2) in the front of the elbow where the nerve is anchored by some means to prevent relocation to its original site, and (3) at its entrance into the cubital tunnel, because of inadequate division of the roof of the tunnel.

Surgical Technique

The operative procedure may be done either with general anesthesia or with an axillary block. I have not considered a tourniquet to be necessary. A curvilinear incision, convex anteriorly, is made 5 cm above and below the elbow. With loupe magnification, the skin flap is reflected, protecting branches of the medial cutaneous nerves of the arm and forearm. Although this may appear unimportant, injury to the cutaneous nerve is one of the common causes of postoperative numbness and paresthesias. Injury to the basilic vein should also be avoided. The incision is carried to the deep fascia, and the skin flap is reflected. It is best to locate the ulnar nerve in the proximal part of the arm at the anterior border of the medial head of the triceps just behind the medial intermuscular septum. The nerve is traced distally until the point of entrance into the cubital tunnel is identified. The dense fascia forming the roof of the cubital tunnel is generously divided. Frequently the ulnar nerve will be seen to have a soft pseudoneuroma just proximal to the constriction (Fig. 224-15). With this technique it is not necessary to circumferentially isolate and mobilize the nerve.

If transposition of the nerve is decided upon, the nerve is traced further proximally to ensure division of arcade of Struthers and the medial intermuscular septum. The nerve is mobilized and moved anterior to the epicondyle. It may be necessary to dissect branches to the flexor carpi ulnaris and divide articular branches to facilitate mobilization. Transposition should be done without any tension in the nerve. The subcutaneous tissue in the medial flap is anchored to the fascia over the flexor muscles by one or two sutures to prevent relocation of the nerve.

Medial Epicondylectomy

Originally suggested by King and Morgan as an ideal procedure for tardy ulnar palsy, the procedure consisted of incising the periosteum over the epicondyle and excising the latter with a rongeur.[20] The periosteum was resutured. This allowed the previously mobilized ulnar nerve to easily slide forward without impediment during flexion. With a better understanding of the anatomy of the cubital tunnel and the pathogenesis of compression, medial epicondylectomy is seldom performed nowadays. This procedure is of historic interest only.

Results

Improvement occurs in 80 to 85 percent of patients either with decompression or transposition, although the neurological recovery tends to be complete with simple decompression. Factors that influence the outcome are (1) the age of the patient, (2) coexisting systemic peripheral nerve disorders such as alcoholic neuropathy or diabetic neuropathy, (3) the duration of symptoms and degree of muscle wasting before definitive therapy is undertaken, and (4) any precipitating event (patients with a history of acute trauma tend to do poorly).

Recurrent Ulnar Neuropathy

If symptoms of ulnar neuropathy fail to improve after a surgical procedure, the underlying factors that lead to failure should be analyzed carefully. Clinical examination and electrodiagnostic studies should be repeated and carefully interpreted to make certain of the original diagnosis and to ensure that proximal lesions such as cervical spondylosis or cord tumor or distal lesions such as the Guyon's canal syndrome are not overlooked. Patients with systemic peripheral nerve disorders such as alcoholic or diabetic neuropathy are unlikely to improve with further surgical therapy.

A painful syndrome is seen (fortunately infrequently) in individuals who have undergone transposition of the nerve. The transposed ulnar nerve is exquisitely tender to palpation, and the patient complains of distressing dysesthesias in the entire medial forearm and hand. The dysesthesias are constant and are resistant to most forms of therapy. The etiology of this syndrome is not clear; it may result from ischemia of the ulnar nerve from extensive mobilization, although this is only a conjecture. Another possibility is kinking of the nerve from inadequate immobilization. If the symptoms persist, as they often do, the nerve should be reexplored to exclude any kinking or tethering in the nerve

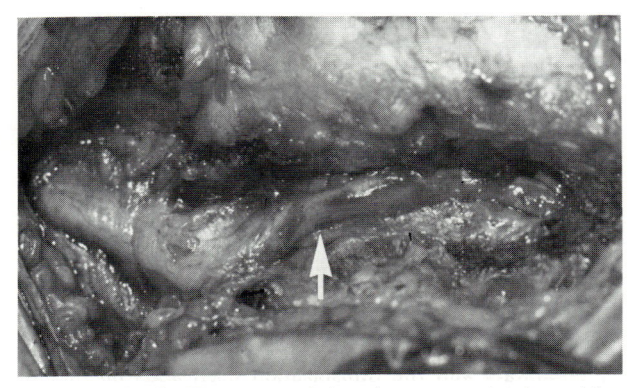

Figure 224-15 Exposure of the ulnar nerve in the cubital tunnel in a patient with tardy ulnar palsy. The arrow points to the focal area of constriction with a proximal pseudoneuroma.

and the nerve should be relocated in the groove, unless the groove is deformed by scar tissue or callus.

Ulnar Nerve Compression at the Wrist: Guyon's Canal Syndrome[31]

Applied Anatomy

The ulnar nerve descends in the distal forearm, lying just lateral to the flexor carpi ulnaris tendon but medial to the ulnar artery. About 5 to 8 cm above the wrist crease it gives off the dorsal cutaneous branch to the hand. At the wrist it enters Guyon's canal (loge de Guyon; ulnar carpal tunnel). This is an oblique fibro-osseous tunnel that lies within the proximal part of the hypothenar eminence (Fig. 224-16). The roof of this tunnel is formed by the palmar fascia (volar carpal ligament) and the palmaris brevis muscle. The floor is formed by the flexor retinaculum and the pisohamate ligament. The terminal part of the tendon of the flexor carpi ulnaris and the pisiform bone form the medial wall. The distal part of the lateral wall is formed by the curved ulnar surface of the hook of the hamate. In the proximal part, a lateral wall does not exist because of the fusion of the palmar fascia (volar carpal ligament) with the transverse carpal ligament. The canal contains the ulnar nerve and the ulnar artery embedded in loose fibrofatty tissue. At about the middle of the canal, the ulnar nerve divides into superficial and deep branches. The superficial branch proceeds distally in line with the main trunk of the nerve, and on exit from the canal, it supplies a small branch to the palmaris brevis muscle. Its terminal branches provide sensation to the little finger and the ulnar half of the ring finger. The deep motor branch, along with the ulnar artery, takes an acute lateral turn about the hook of the hamate. At this point it passes under a tough and unyielding fibrotendinous arch (pisohamate hiatus), which in part gives origin to the muscles of the hypothenar eminence. This is the most vulnerable site for compression of the deep motor branch of the ulnar nerve. The muscular branches to the abductor digiti quinti may arise either from the main trunk of the ulnar nerve or from its superficial or deep branch.

Clinical Features

The various etiologic factors that lead to the compression of the ulnar nerve at the wrist are summarized in Fig. 224-17. Occupational trauma and extrinsic compression from a ganglion cyst are the most common causes.

Depending upon the anatomical site at the wrist at which the ulnar nerve is compromised, three types of clinical syndrome may be encountered (Fig. 224-18). In the type I syndrome, the ulnar nerve is involved just proximal to or within the canal of Guyon. There is motor weakness of all of the ulnar innervated muscles in the hand. Sensory loss in the hand is in a typical ulnar nerve distribution. The dorsal aspect of the hand may not show sensory loss because of the sparing of the dorsal cutaneous branch of the ulnar nerve. The flexor carpi ulnaris and the medial half of the flexor digitorum profundus are not impaired, but these two muscles are so infrequently involved in cubital tunnel lesions that distinction between proximal and distal ulnar nerve lesions may not be made based on this finding alone. Electrodiagnostic studies may reveal the following findings: (1) normal motor conduction velocity of the ulnar nerve in the across-the-elbow and elbow-to-wrist segments, (2) prolonged distal latency to the abductor digiti minimi and first dorsal interosseus muscles, (3) prolonged sensory latency and diminished evoked sensory responses.

In the type II syndrome, the sensation is preserved but there is weakness in the muscles innervated by the deep branch of the ulnar nerve. The site of compression of the ulnar nerve in this syndrome is usually at the pisohamate hiatus. The branch to the abductor digiti quinti minimi and other hypothenar muscles is frequently spared because it originates just proximal to the pisohamate hiatus. Thus the hypothenar muscle bulk and strength may be normal while the interossei and adductor pollicis show marked weakness and atrophy. A "palmaris brevis sign" has been described that helps to differentiate between ulnar nerve compression at the cubital tunnel and at the wrist. When the patient abducts the little finger on volition, there is simultaneous contraction of the palmaris brevis. This contraction is absent if the entrapment of the ulnar nerve is at the cubital tunnel but is usually preserved when the ulnar nerve is compressed at the pisohamate hiatus. Electrodiagnostic studies may reveal the following: (1) normal motor conduction velocity in the ulnar nerve in the across-the-elbow and elbow-to-wrist segments, (2) normal sensory latency and sensory evoked responses, (3) normal distal motor latency to the abductor digiti quinti minimi (providing the branch to the hypothenar muscles is given off proximal to the pisohamate hiatus) and prolonged latency to the first dorsal interosseous, (4) denervation potentials in the first dorsal interosseous but not in the abductor digiti quinti.

In the type III syndrome, the rarest of the three syndromes, the compression is at the distal end of Guyon's canal. The sensory branch alone is affected.

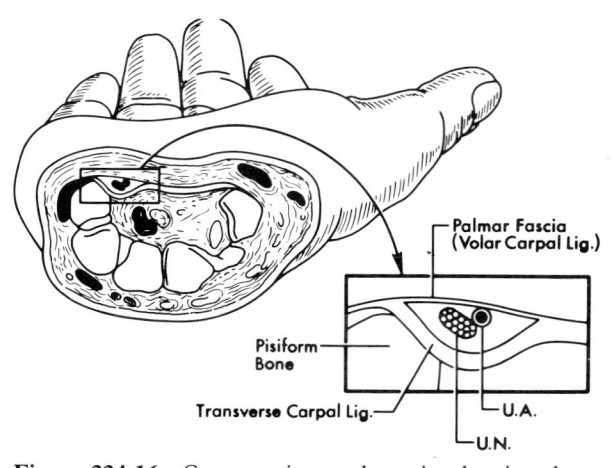

Figure 224-16 Cross section at the wrist showing the anatomical boundaries of Guyon's canal. U.A., ulnar artery; U.N., ulnar nerve. (From Rengachary and Arjunan.[31])

Entrapment Neuropathies

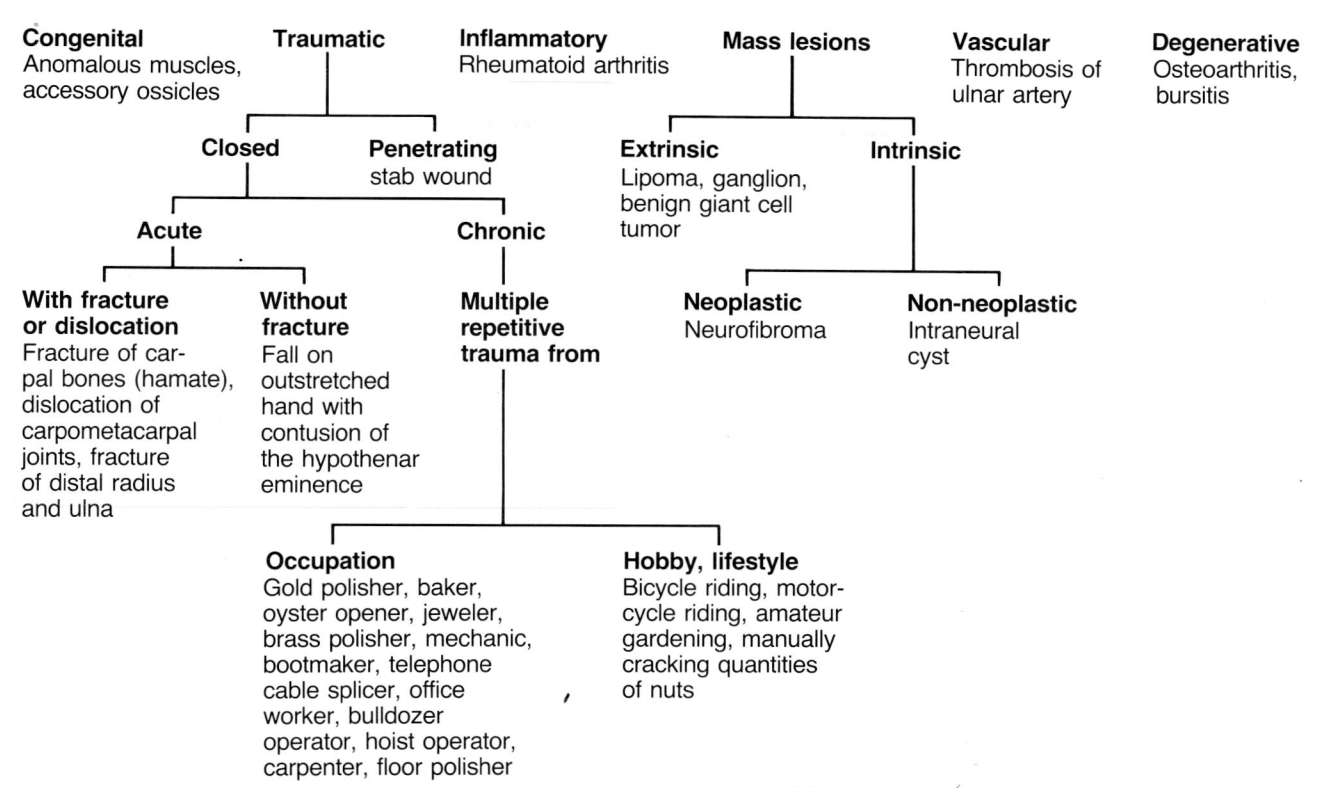

Congenital
Anomalous muscles, accessory ossicles

Traumatic
- Closed
  - Acute
    - With fracture or dislocation: Fracture of carpal bones (hamate), dislocation of carpometacarpal joints, fracture of distal radius and ulna
    - Without fracture: Fall on outstretched hand with contusion of the hypothenar eminence
  - Chronic
    - Multiple repetitive trauma from
      - Occupation: Gold polisher, baker, oyster opener, jeweler, brass polisher, mechanic, bootmaker, telephone cable splicer, office worker, bulldozer operator, hoist operator, carpenter, floor polisher
      - Hobby, lifestyle: Bicycle riding, motorcycle riding, amateur gardening, manually cracking quantities of nuts
- Penetrating: stab wound

Inflammatory
Rheumatoid arthritis

Mass lesions
- Extrinsic: Lipoma, ganglion, benign giant cell tumor
- Intrinsic
  - Neoplastic: Neurofibroma
  - Non-neoplastic: Intraneural cyst

Vascular
Thrombosis of ulnar artery

Degenerative
Osteoarthritis, bursitis

Figure 224-17 Causes of involvement of the ulnar nerve in the vicinity of Guyon's canal. (Modified from Rengachary and Arjunan.[31])

Treatment

Treatment of a patient with the Guyon's canal syndrome requires careful evaluation of the etiologic factor. If the syndrome results from occupational causes or from mechanical repetitive trauma for other reasons, the logical approach is to try to avoid pressure on the hypothenar eminence and watch for improvement. If mass lesions cause compression, the choice of therapy is clearly surgical (Fig.224-19). Mass lesions such as small ganglion cysts may not always be palpa-

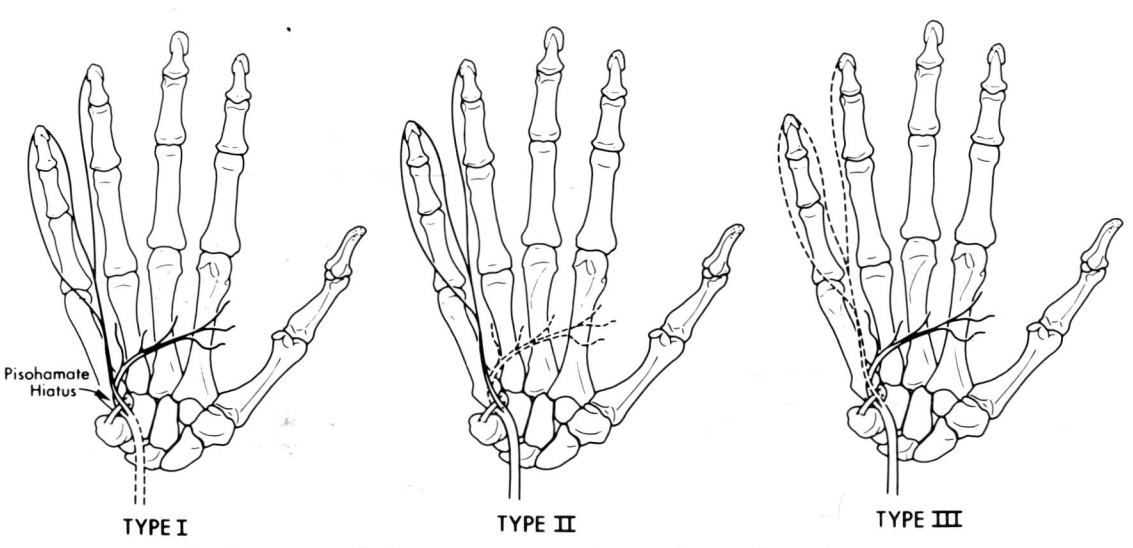

TYPE I TYPE II TYPE III

Figure 224-18 The three types of ulnar nerve compression syndromes about the wrist. In the type I syndrome the trunk of the ulnar nerve is involved just proximal to or within the canal of Guyon; in the type II syndrome the deep motor branch alone is affected as it passes beneath the pisohamate hiatus; in the type III syndrome, the sensory branch alone is involved. (Interrupted lines denote the segment of the ulnar nerve involved.) (From Rengachary and Arjunan.[31])

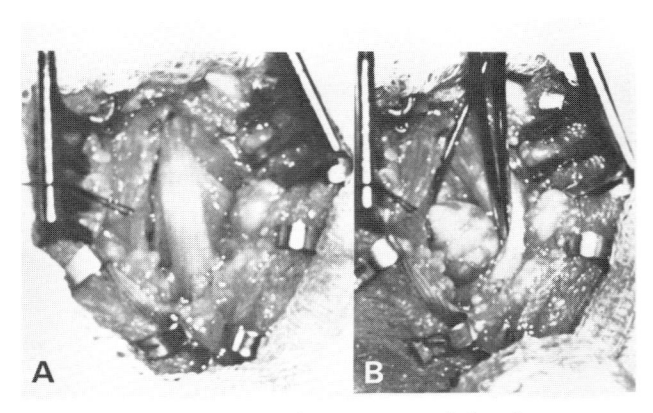

Figure 224-19 *A.* Operative exposure of the ulnar nerve in Guyon's canal. The nerve is humped tightly over the mass. *B.* On retracting the ulnar nerve, the mass (a soft tissue giant cell tumor) is well delineated. (From Rengachary and Arjunan.[31])

ble through the skin. Persistent signs of impairment of the deep branch of the ulnar nerve warrant surgical exploration.

Exploration of the Guyon's canal region is best performed through a Z-shaped incision starting vertically lateral to the flexor carpi ulnaris tendon, then horizontally along the wrist crease and extending vertically into the palm medial to the midpalmar crease. The ulnar artery and nerve are identified proximal to the wrist crease and traced distally. Guyon's canal is exposed by dividing the palmar fascia (volar carpal ligament). The sensory branch of the ulnar nerve forms the direct continuation of the nerve, whereas the deep motor branch dips dorsally through the pisohamate hiatus. If an obvious mass lesion is found, it is excised; otherwise, all constricting bands are divided and the pisohamate hiatus is unroofed.

Suprascapular Entrapment Neuropathy[32]

Applied Anatomy

The suprascapular nerve is a mixed peripheral nerve. Its motor component supplies the supra- and infraspinatus muscles. The sensory component has no cutaneous distribution, but supplies the posterior capsule of the shoulder joint (Fig. 224-20). Compressive lesions of the nerve therefore produce weakness and atrophy of the supra- and infraspinatus muscles and a poorly defined aching pain along the posterior aspect of the shoulder joint and the adjacent scapula (Fig. 224-21).

The suprascapular nerve arises as a large branch from the superior trunk (C5-6) of the brachial plexus. It crosses the posterior triangle of the neck deep and parallel to the inferior belly of the omohyoid, runs under the trapezius and through the suprascapular notch, below the suprascapular ligament, and into the supraspinous fossa. The suprascapular artery passes above the suprascapular ligament and joins the nerve in the supraspinous fossa. After supplying the supraspinatus muscle, the nerve curves around the lateral border of the spine of the scapula into the infraspinous fossa to enter the deep surface of the infraspinatus. The suprascapular nerve supplies articular twigs to the shoulder and acromioclavicular joints.

Clinical Features and Differential Diagnosis

The onset of symptoms may be insidious or be precipitated by an acute traumatic event. Shoulder pain is the most common presenting symptom. It results presumably from the compression of the articular branches to the glenohumeral and acromioclavicular joints. Thus the pain is deep and aching in character diffusely localized to the posterior aspect of the shoulder joint and adjacent scapula (Fig. 224-21). A striking objective finding is the presence of atrophy and weakness confined to the supra- and infraspinatus muscles (Fig. 224-22). Although both muscles are atrophic to the same degree, the atrophy in the infraspinatus muscle is more noticeable because the infraspinatus is essentially subcutaneous whereas the supraspinatus muscle is covered by the flat trapezius muscle. The diagnosis may be readily apparent on mere inspection of the scapular region.

Atrophy suggests a lower motor neuron lesion, and the distribution is clearly of the peripheral nerve type. Disease of the anterior horn cell, cervical root, or upper brachial plexus involving the fifth cervical segment will result in motor weakness of the rhomboids and deltoid. The absence of demonstrable sensory loss confirms the anatomical fact that the suprascapular nerve has no cutaneous distribution.

The demonstration of denervation potentials confined to the supraspinatus and infraspinatus muscles is the most helpful objective diagnostic test. Delayed conduction from Erb's point to the supraspinatus muscle, if demonstrable, is an additional corroborative finding, but a normal nerve conduction velocity does not necessarily negate the diagnosis; the latter simply implies that a few axons have escaped compression. The normal range of latency from Erb's point to the supraspinatus is 1.7 to 3.7 ms.

Clinical differentiation of suprascapular neuropathy from rotator cuff injuries may be difficult. In both instances patients have problems abducting the shoulder in the presence

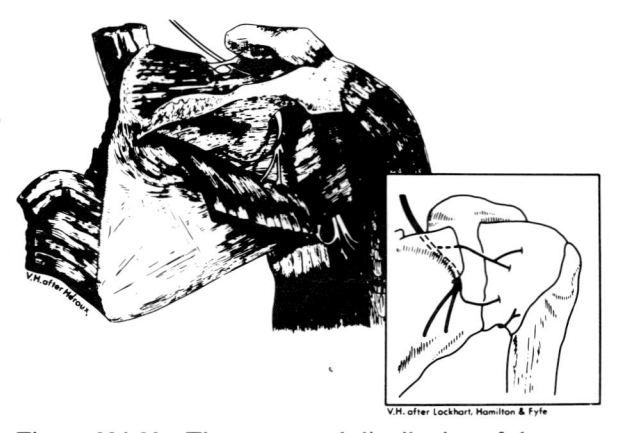

Figure 224-20 The course and distribution of the suprascapular nerve. The inset shows the articular branches to the shoulder joint. (From Rengachary et al.[32])

Entrapment Neuropathies 1789

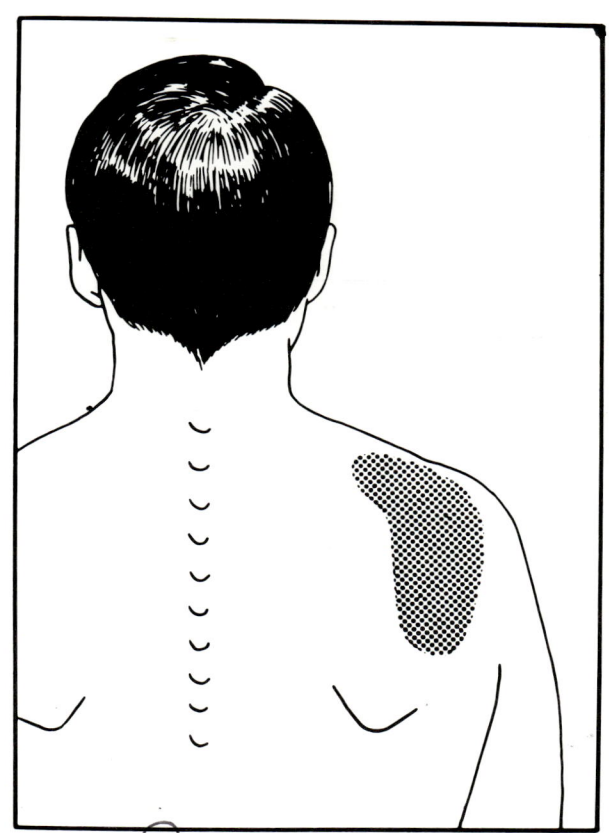

Figure 224-21 Location of pain in patients with suprascapular entrapment neuropathy. (From Rengachary et al.[32])

of normal deltoid contractions, and both conditions may show considerable atrophy of the supraspinatus and infraspinatus muscles. The ancillary diagnostic tests that are extremely helpful are electromyography, arthrography, and cinefluoroscopy. In patients with rotator cuff tears, electromyography shows no denervation potentials in the spinatus muscles because the atrophy represents disuse atrophy. Arthrography demonstrates the communication between the glenohumeral joint and the subacromial bursa through the tear in the cuff. On cinefluoroscopy, the humeral head is pulled into the glenoid upon attempts at active abduction.

Nontraumatic brachial plexopathy (discussed elsewhere in this text) may sometimes have to be differentiated from suprascapular nerve entrapment. In the former, muscle wasting and weakness is usually of the upper plexus type and cutaneous sensory loss may be demonstrable. In cervical spondylosis, muscle weakness tends to follow a root distribution; sensory and reflex changes are also present.

Treatment

Section of the suprascapular ligament is the treatment of choice if the symptoms do not improve with conservative therapy (Fig. 224-23). Under general endotracheal anesthesia, the patient is kept prone on chest rolls with the head turned away from the side of the lesion. The head of the table is elevated 30 degrees from the horizontal. A horizontal incision is made 1 in. above the spine of the scapula and parallel to it. The trapezius is split along its horizontal fibers by blunt dissection, and a self-retaining retractor is inserted. Care should be taken to avoid injury to the spinal accessory nerve, which runs at the medial end of the incision along the ventral surface of the trapezius. A constant fat pad covered by fascia overlies the supraspinatus. A horizontal incision is made in this fascia. Further dissection is guided by palpation of the sharp superior border of the scapula, which has essentially no muscle attachment except for the thin flat inferior belly of the omohyoid. Palpation is done from the medial to the lateral direction until the suprascapular notch and the ligament are identified. The notch lies at a deeper plane than the medial aspect of the scapula. It is neither necessary nor desirable to divide the supraspinatus. Dissection with a sharp periosteal elevator is done to clear the suprascapular ligament and the adjacent superior border of the scapula from the overlying fibrocollagenous adipose tissue. The ligament is unmistakably pearly white with horizontal fibers. The suprascapular artery and vein are usually embedded in adipose tissue. A dull nerve hook is passed under the ligament, which is excised in its entirety. No attempt is made to dissect the suprascapular nerve free from the surrounding fat. In the majority of instances, it is not necessary to resect the suprascapular notch to give added room to the nerve.

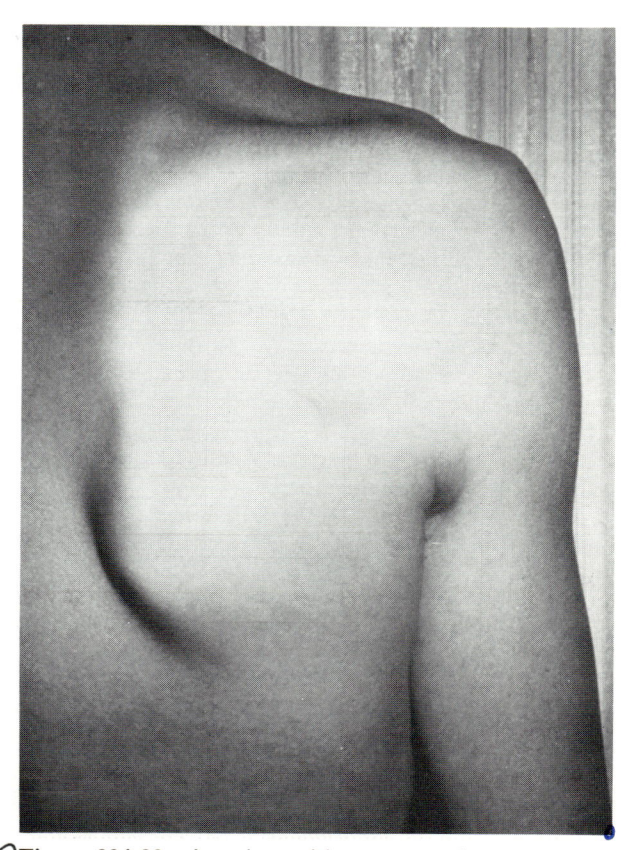

Figure 224-22 A patient with suprascapular entrapment neuropathy showing striking atrophy of the supra- and infraspinatus muscles. (From Rengachary et al.[32])

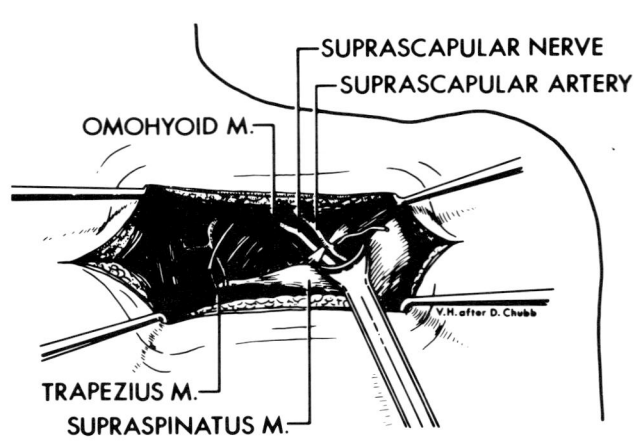

Figure 224-23 Operative exposure of the suprascapular nerve. (From Rengachary et al.[32])

The sequence of improvement in symptoms after operation consists of improvement of pain followed by gain in motor strength. Muscular atrophy is the last to reverse, if it improves at all.

Meralgia Paresthetica: Syndrome of the Lateral Femoral Cutaneous Nerve of the Thigh

Meralgia paresthetica is a clinical syndrome resulting from entrapment of the lateral femoral cutaneous nerve of the thigh in the inguinal region. The syndrome was first described by Bernhardt in 1895 and named meralgia paresthetica (meros, "thigh"; algos, "pain") by Roth in the same year. The famed psychoanalyst Sigmund Freud suffered from this disease; he published his own case report in 1895 as an example of Bernhardt's syndrome.[40] Understandably, he believed emotional factors to be responsible for the syndrome. His symptoms subsided over the years without treatment. It is of interest that one of his sons also presented with the same symptoms. Freud related this occurrence in a personal communication to Mendel, the Austrian geneticist, raising the question of heredity playing a role in its causation.

Early observers since Bernhardt and Roth were at a loss in explaining the causation of the disease, mistakenly attributing this condition to toxins and infections until Stookey presented the idea of a mechanical etiology for this syndrome in a landmark paper published in 1928.[41] He was struck by the marked angulation of the nerve as it emerged from the pelvis medial to the spine (Fig. 224-24). He compared this situation to the angular course of the ulnar nerve behind the elbow, with repeated movement of the nerve at the point of angulation, and a resultant "traumatic neuritis." Ecker and Woltman in 1938 presented their findings in 150 cases treated at the Mayo Clinic.[9] In 1962, Keegan and Holyoke presented detailed anatomy of this region based on dissection of 50 cadavers; they were the first to suggest section of the inguinal ligament and medial transposition of the nerve for treatment of meralgia paresthetica.[19]

Historical review of this entity is incomplete without a mention of Cushing's embarrasing failure after a surgical procedure for this condition in one of his famous patients, Simon Newcomb, a world-renowned astrophysicist and a colleague of Cushing at Johns Hopkins. The story is told in Cushing's own words:

> I had known little enough of Simon Newcomb and nothing of meralgia paresthetica—only that the old man was one of the peculiar geniuses of the early days of the University, large in brains but peculiar in habits. . . . Simon Newcomb had worn crutches for years or at least had possessed them for they were not always worn; for when he had to catch a crosstown horsecar he did so in lively fashion with the crutches under one arm. His story he tells in his own words in his MS. of May 10, 1900, evidently written for Barker and me to use, but we must have been thoroughly scared by the newspaper notoriety to which we had been subjected. I believe Barker saw him first about March 20th, and immediately recognized the condition as Bernhardt's "meralgia" of the external cutaneous nerve. As I recall it now, Bernhardt had reported the condition as having occurred to himself. I judge that the letter of March 26th was written before our conjoint examination when the operation was proposed. I was much interested at the time in local anesthesia and he highly approved of trying it, but it is evident that he procrastinated considerably. . . . What really happened was this. His operation went well enough and there was no difficulty in finding the nerve though the old gentleman was somewhat abdominous. He insisted on propping himself upon his elbows every now and then to see what we were doing, but unfortunately his centre of gravity intervened; despite this disappointment, however, he was much elated and kept up a running conversation during the procedure. He did well enough subsequently . . . was bursting with gratitude and wanted to give us a fee which of course we refused though both needed it badly

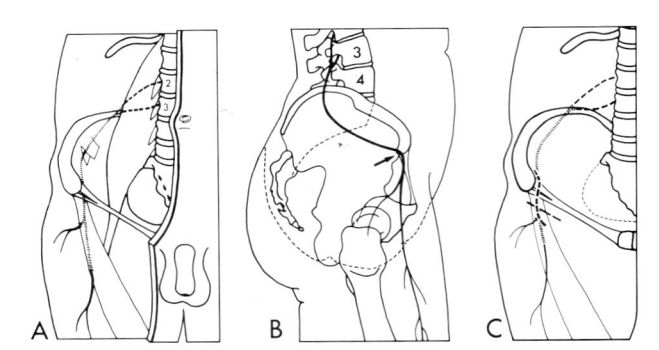

Figure 224-24 A. Course and distribution of the lateral femoral cutaneous nerve of the thigh. B. Side view of the pelvis showing angulation of the nerve as it exits from the pelvis into the thigh (arrow). C. Two types of incisions used to expose the nerve at the inguinal ligament (interrupted lines).

enough, Lord knows. I am sure it was out of the goodness of his heart that he retaliated as he did, for when he reached home he summoned the Washington representative of the N.Y. "American," most vile of all news-sheets, and gave him the whole story. I once had a copy—indeed many of them were forwarded to us to add to our shame—and remember there was a full page description with a large picture of the leonine S.N. directing an operation on his leg which two whiskered "Professors" of the J.H.H. were performing accordingly. It was long before we lived it down. . . . In spite of his great expectations—and possibly ours—he did not remain permanently well, though possibly as well as the neurasthenia of an intensive worker would permit; during my absence Finney operated again. . . ."[13]

Applied Anatomy (Fig. 224-24)

The lateral femoral cutaneous nerve is a pure sensory nerve. It arises from the second and third lumbar nerves of the lumbar plexus. It emerges from the lateral border of the psoas major muscle and runs obliquely forward and inferiorly across the iliacus muscle beneath the iliac fascia. The nerve then passes from the iliac fossa to the thigh, beneath the inguinal ligament, just medial to the anterior superior iliac spine. The nerve frequently passes between the two roots of attachment of the inguinal ligament to the iliac bone, in effect piercing through the ligament. On its entry into the thigh, it is in close relation to the anterior border of the sartorius muscle. This muscle often has a medial aponeurotic expansion from its tendinous attachment to the anterior superior iliac spine which attaches to the inferior border of the inguinal ligament. In such a situation contraction of sartorius muscle results in the depression of the lateral part of the inguinal ligament. The lateral femoral cutaneous nerve pierces this aponeurotic expansion of the sartorius muscle and descends down for a distance of 4 to 6 cm before it pierces the fascia lata and becomes subcutaneous.

Thus the lateral femoral cutaneous nerve is at risk of being compressed in the inguinal region by any one or a combination of the following fascial bands: (1) the anterior or (2) the posterior roots of the attachment of the inguinal ligament to the anterior superior spine, (3) the aponeurotic expansion of the sartorius muscle and the tendinous attachment of the muscle into the spine, and (4) fascial interconnecting bands between the fascia lata and the iliac fascia. Any factor or factors that causes pressure or a downward pull on the inguinal ligament tends to aggravate the pressure on the nerve. An obese and pendulous anterior abdominal wall tends to apply traction and strain on the ligament. Prolonged standing or walking accentuates the downward pull of the inguinal ligament by the fascia lata, whereas lying down, especially with the hips flexed, releases the tension on the ligament. Since the inguinal ligament provides attachment to the anterior abdominal muscles, contraction of these muscles (e.g., during coughing or straining) produces a shutter-like movement of the sharp border of the inguinal ligament against the nerve. In many instances a pseudoneuroma (a segment of the nerve containing excessive extrafunicular connective tissue) is present within the nerve as it traverses the inguinal ligament, presumably as a result of chronic irritation of the nerve from mechanical factors. Stookey emphasized the sharp angulation of the nerve as it passes from the iliac fossa into the thigh (Fig. 224-24). This may be an additional reason for the symptoms to get worse with extension of the leg (which accentuates the kink) and to be relieved with flexion or recumbency.

Clinical Features

This syndrome is most commonly seen in middle-aged men who are overweight. Men are three times more commonly affected than women. For reasons cited earlier, obesity and obstructive pulmonary disease with a chronic cough are common predisposing factors. The symptoms may appear transiently during the third trimester of pregnancy because of increased tension in the anterior abdominal wall; they tend to disappear after parturition. Young army recruits, who are not necessarily obese, may manifest the syndrome during strenuous basic training. Trusses, belts, binders, and corsets have been incriminated. It is doubtful that these external supportive devices cause direct pressure on the nerve since it is in a well-protected position just medial to the anterior superior iliac spine. A more likely explanation is that the very individuals who require these devices are those that have a lax, obese, or pendulous abdominal wall with poor muscular tone. Individuals whose occupation demands that they be on their feet most of the time (e.g., patrolmen, traveling salespeople, or mail carriers) are particularly affected.

The cardinal symptom is paresthesias in the anterolateral aspect of the thigh. The patient seldom uses the term *pain* to describe his or her symptoms except in response to a leading question but rather characterizes it as being disagreeably numb or as burning, stinging, crawling, tingling, pricking, "pins and needles," "like a hot poker," etc. In the early stages, the symptoms are mild and intermittent and are aggravated by standing or walking and relieved on recumbency. In advanced stages, the paresthesias tend to be replaced by sharp shooting pains that may become intractable and be present in any position. The distribution of paresthesias is typically along an oval area in the anterolateral aspect of the thigh, which is a much smaller area than the anatomical distribution of the lateral femoral cutaneous nerve of the thigh as depicted in standard anatomy texts. Curiously, the symptoms tend to be present most frequently in the distribution of the anterior branch of the nerve, although the division into the anterior and posterior branches occurs well below the inguinal ligament. This may be because the anterior division fibers are located immediately beneath the inguinal ligament and thus are more prone to direct compression. Infrequently, however, the pain may radiate to the gluteal region in the posterior distribution of the nerve. A blunting of sensation to pinprick and light touch may be demonstrated, but there is no motor involvement or alteration in muscle stretch reflexes. Some have observed loss of hair in the anterolateral thigh, a reflection of trophic disturbance. Focal tenderness may be present just medial to the anterior superior iliac spine.

Diagnosis

The diagnosis is based upon the clinical history and the demonstration of sensory loss strictly within the distribution of the lateral femoral cutaneous nerve. If the sensory loss extends beyond the distribution of the nerve or if there is motor atrophy or weakness, reflex alteration, or back pain, a more proximal lesion involving the lumbosacral plexus or cauda equina should be considered and ruled out by appropriate studies, including electromyography, metrizamide myelography, and computed tomography of the abdomen. A technique for studying the nerve conduction velocity orthodromically in the lateral femoral cutaneous nerve has been described, but in our experience, this is a difficult study to perform in obese individuals. A simpler diagnostic test is to administer a local anesthetic block by infiltrating 5 ml of 1% lidocaine just medial to the anterior superior iliac spine and observe for relief of symptoms.

Treatment

In the early stages, conservative management is indicated with an attempt to eliminate obvious causative factors. Weight reduction in an obese patient is an important therapeutic measure. Although most patients may agree to a weight reduction program, they are seldom willing to wait to see if this measure will bring about relief, especially if the symptoms are severe and persistent. Removal of tight binders, corsets, etc., may appear to be a logical measure, but this move is seldom of any benefit because, as indicated earlier, these external factors are not the real culprits. Injection with local anesthetic agents along with steroid medication seldom provides lasting relief but may be of benefit as a diagnostic test.

Surgical therapy should be resorted to in patients with persistent or severe pain. The options are either section or decompression of the nerve. We reserve the option of dividing the nerve only for the rare instances where decompression has failed. It has the disadvantage of producing an area of numbness, although this decreases in size over a period of a few months and seldom poses a serious problem. Formation of a neuroma at the site of nerve section is a possibility, although the actual incidence of this is unknown. In most instances, decompression of the nerve suffices. The surgery is performed under general anesthesia. Although a horizontal incision parallel to and below the inguinal ligament is generally recommended, we find a curvilinear vertical incision just medial to the anterior superior iliac spine most suitable, especially in obese individuals (Fig. 224-24). This allows easier retraction of the abdominal panniculus when exposing the inguinal ligament. The best place to locate the nerve is at the anterior border of the sartorius, *deep to the deep fascia.* Use of magnifying loupes (×3.5) is of considerable benefit in distinguishing the nerve from the adjacent adipose tissue. The nerve is traced rostrally to the inguinal ligament, and all the fascial bands that may actually or potentially constrict the nerve, namely the anterior and posterior slips of the inguinal ligament, the aponeurotic expansion of the attachment of the sartorius, and the fascial band connecting the fascia lata with the iliac fascia, are all generously divided. Adequate decompression is further checked by digital palpation around the nerve; one should feel only soft muscle tissue all around, and not the sharp edge of any fascia. There should be sufficient room around the nerve to permit insertion of a finger into the iliac fossa. The nerve is traced until it disappears beneath the iliac fascia. We have feared the potential development of a hernia through this defect, but this is not substantiated in the follow-up of our cases. Some have advocated transposing the nerve medially to allow for a more direct course of the nerve. It seems more important, however, to generously divide all constricting fascial bands than to attempt to alter the course of the nerve. The nerve is held in the iliac fossa by the overlying tough iliac fascia. Altering the course of the nerve immediately under the inguinal ligament will not alter the course of the iliac segment of the nerve; rather it will produce a kink in the nerve in the vicinity of the inguinal ligament. If division of the nerve is decided upon, traction should be applied on the nerve so that the part of the nerve proximal to the inguinal ligament is sectioned.

Saphenous Nerve Entrapment Syndrome[25]

Applied Anatomy (Fig. 224-25)

The saphenous nerve is a pure sensory nerve. It is the longest and the largest of the cutaneous branches of the femoral nerve. It arises just below the inguinal ligament, enters the adductor canal (subsartorial canal, Hunter's canal), crosses the femoral artery from lateral to medial, and leaves the canal by piercing its roof together with the descending genicular artery. *The point of penetrance of the subsartorial fascia* (the roof of the subsartorial canal) *is the site of entrapment.* After leaving the subsartorial canal, the nerve descends vertically behind the sartorius, pierces the deep fascia between the tendons of the sartorius and gracilis muscles, and divides into its two terminal branches, the infrapatellar branch, which supplies the anteromedial aspect of the knee, and the descending branch, which supplies the anteromedial aspect of the leg and ankle.

Clinical Features

The saphenous nerve entrapment syndrome occurs in young or middle-aged individuals, and in women more often than men. The onset may be sudden or insidious. Typically, the patient has intense pain along the medial aspect of the knee, which is aggravated by walking or climbing stairs and improves with rest. It is not uncommon for the patient to have undergone extensive evaluation of the knee joint with roentgenograms and arthroscopy, with negative results. On physical examination there is exquisite point tenderness at about a handbreadth above the medial aspect of the knee, which is roughly the point of emergence of the saphenous nerve from the subsartorial canal (Fig. 224-25). There may be variable

Entrapment Neuropathies

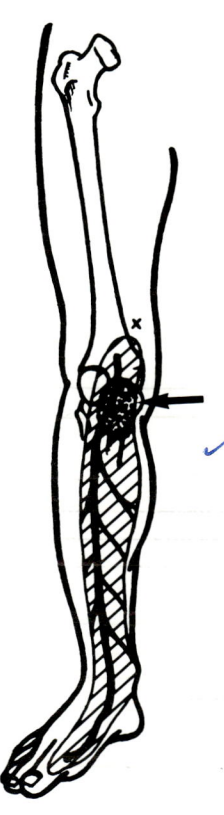

Figure 224-25 Saphenous entrapment neuropathy: X refers to the site of exquisite tenderness which overlies the point of emergence of the saphenous nerve from the subsartorial canal. The arrow pointing to a stippled area around the knee denotes the region where the patient has pain. The striped area conforming to the sensory distribution of saphenous nerve is the site of sensory alteration.

degrees of sensory loss over the medial aspect of the knee or shin. Muscle atrophy, weakness, and alteration in the muscle stretch reflex are absent.

A local anesthetic block at the site of maximal tenderness above the knee induces complete amelioration of symptoms. A technique to measure the conduction velocity along the saphenous nerve has been described but is seldom used. Electromyography and lumbar myelography may be indicated to rule out an L3 or L4 root lesion.

Treatment

In intractable cases, surgical decompression of the saphenous nerve by generous division of the subsartorial fascia is advised; recurrent cases may require division of the nerve. Under general anesthesia, a 5-cm curvilinear incision is made centered on the point of emergence of the saphenous nerve from the subsartorial canal. The deep fascia is divided at the anterior border of the sartorius muscle, which is retracted medially. The avascular plane between the vastus medialis and the sartorius is entered exposing the fascial roof of the subsartorial canal. The location of the femoral artery may be ascertained by palpation. The point of emergence of the saphenous nerve and the descending genicular artery is identified, and the fascia around it is opened generously. If nerve section is planned, it should be done quite proximal to its point of emergence through the subsartorial fascia.

Tarsal Tunnel Syndrome[26]

Applied Anatomy

The tarsal tunnel at the ankle is the counterpart of the carpal tunnel at the wrist. It is located posterior and inferior to the medial malleolus. The flexor retinanculum (the lancinate ligament), which is nothing but a condensation of the deep fascia spanning this area, constitutes the *roof* of the tunnel. It is not as thick as the transverse carpal ligament at the wrist. It extends from the medial malleolus above to the medial tubercle of the os calcis below. Its proximal and distal borders blend with the deep fascia of the leg and the plantar aponeurosis of the foot, respectively. The bony *floor* is formed by the medial aspect of the calcaneus and the posterior aspect of the medial malleolus. Unlike in the carpal tunnel, numerous fibrous septa extend from the roof to the floor of the tunnel, subdividing the tunnel into rather rigid fibro-osseous compartments that contain tendons with their synovial sheaths and neurovascular structures. The *contents* of the tunnel in the anterior to the posterior direction are the tendon of the tibialis posterior, the tendon of the flexor digitorum longus, the posterior tibial vessels, the tibial nerve, and the tendon of the flexor hallucis longus.

The posterior tibial nerve that is a terminal branch of the sciatic nerve descends vertically in the posterior aspect of the leg deep to the soleus muscle and enters the tarsal tunnel just behind the posterior tibial vessels. Either within the tunnel or at the distal border of the tunnel the nerve divides into its three terminal branches, the *calcaneal*, *medial plantar*, and *lateral plantar* nerves. The origin of the calcaneal branches is highly variable: they may arise proximal to the ligament, and may course superficial to the ligament to the skin of the heel; they may arise within the tunnel and perforate the ligament to become subcutaneous; or they may arise distal to the ligament. The calcaneal branches are purely sensory. The medial and lateral plantar branches pass through individual fibrous openings in the origin of the abductor hallucis muscles. Thus, these two terminal branches are at risk to be compressed individually at these fibrous hiati, distal to the flexor retinaculum. The medial and lateral plantar nerves supply the intrinsic muscles of the foot and provide sensory innervation to the sole of the foot. With regard to sensory distribution, the medial plantar nerve corresponds to the median nerve and the lateral plantar corresponds to the ulnar nerve (Fig. 224-26).

Clinical Features

A history of previous trauma to the ankle is elicited in about half of the patients. The injury might have been to the osseous or soft tissue structures. Tenosynovitis of any etiology (e.g., rheumatoid arthritis) may compromise the space within the tunnel and may induce pressure on the nerve. Venous stasis from prolonged standing may precipitate symptoms in some individuals. The original case report describing this entity was that of a young army recruit who had been undergoing rigorous basic training. Men and women

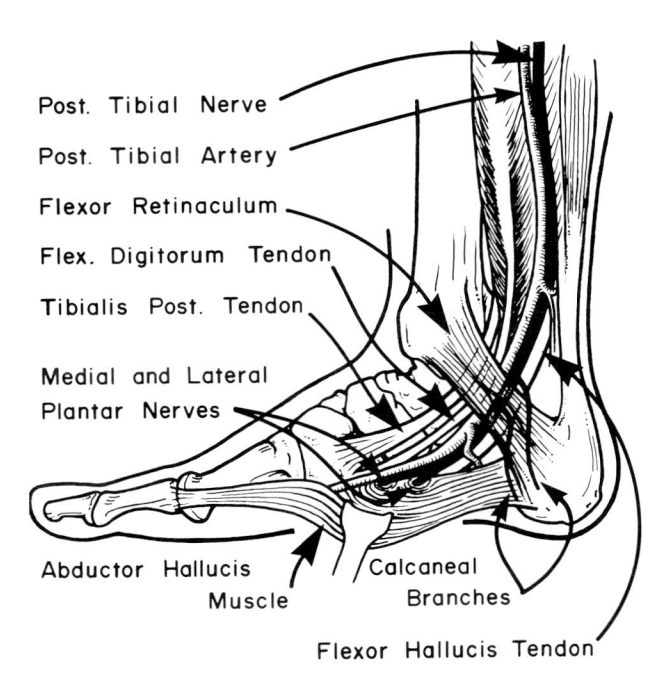

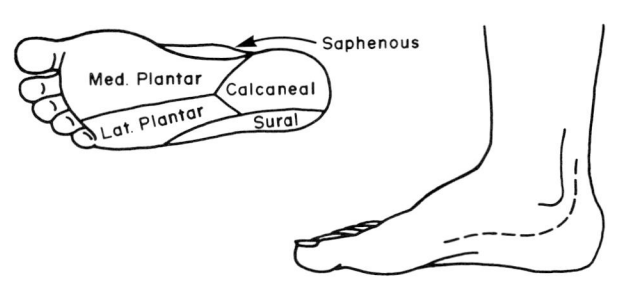

Figure 224-26 A composite illustration showing the anatomy of the tarsal tunnel, sensory innervation of the foot, and the incision used in exposing the tarsal tunnel.

are about equally affected. The symptoms usually consist of burning pain and paresthesias along the plantar aspect of the foot and toes. Frequently, the paresthesias may be confined to the medial or lateral aspect of the sole corresponding to the distribution of the medial or lateral plantar nerve. The heel is generally spared because the calcaneal branches often arise proximal to the flexor retinaculum and escape from compression (Fig. 224-26). The pain at times may radiate proximally to the calf. Exertion and activity aggravate the symptoms and rest relieves them. The pain is worse at night. Sensory impairment may be demonstrable in the sole in the distribution of the medial or lateral plantar nerve or both. There may be atrophy and weakness of the intrinsic muscles of the foot. Palpation along the proximal area of the tarsal tunnel may reveal an area of tenderness, and Tinel's sign may be elicited at this point.

In typical instances, the electrodiagnostic study will reveal the following:

1. Normal conduction velocity in the posterior tibial nerve in the leg.
2. Prolonged distal motor latency to the abductor hallucis, representing the medial plantar branch.
3. Prolonged distal motor latency to the abductor digiti quinti, representing the lateral plantar branch.
4. Decreased amplitude of evoked muscle potentials in the abductor hallucis or the abductor digiti quinti.
5. Absence of orthodromically induced sensory nerve potentials or decreased sensory nerve conduction velocity.

Treatment

Since foot pain is a very common symptom and arises from a host of heterogeneous causes, operative treatment should be undertaken only when the clinical features are typical and electrodiagnostic studies support the diagnosis. A block of the posterior tibial nerve with a local anesthetic agent just proximal to the flexor retinaculum may completely relieve the patient's symptoms, thus predicting a favorable operative result.

The operation may be done with general, spinal, or local infiltration anesthesia according to the surgeon's or patient's preference and the general condition of the patient. Use of a tourniquet is optional. A curvilineal incision is made 1.5 cm behind and below the medial malleolus (Fig. 224-26). The flexor retinaculum is divided, exposing the posterior tibial nerve. Deep fibrous septal prolongations from the retinaculum surrounding the nerve should be released as well. It is important to trace the medial and lateral plantar branches distally to the points where they disappear along the origin of the abductor hallucis. If there are any encircling fibrous bands at these points, they should be divided too.

References

1. Adson AW: The surgical treatment of progressive ulnar paralysis. Minn Med 1:455–460, 1918.
2. Alvarez N, Larkin C, Roxborough J: Carpal tunnel syndrome in athetoiddystonic cerebral palsy. Arch Neurol 39:311–312, 1982.
3. Barnard LB, McCoy SM: The supracondyloid process of the humerus. J Bone Joint Surg 28:845–850, 1946.
4. Bowles AP Jr, Asher SW, Pickett JB: Use of Tinel's sign in carpal tunnel syndrome. Ann Neurol 13:689–690, 1983.
5. Capener N: The vulnerability of the posterior interosseous nerve of the forearm. J Bone Joint Surg 48B:770–773, 1966.
6. Chan RC, Paine KWE, Varughese G: Ulnar neuropathy at the elbow: Comparison of simple decompression and anterior transposition. Neurosurgery 7:545–550, 1980.
7. Chang KSF, Low WD, Chan ST, Chuang A, Poon KT: Enlargement of the ulnar nerve behind the medial epicondyle. Anat Rec 145:149–155, 1963.
8. Childress HM: Recurrent ulnar nerve dislocation at the elbow. J Bone Joint Surg 38A:978–984, 1956.
9. Ecker AD, Woltman HW: Meralgia paraesthetica. JAMA 110:1650–1652, 1938.
10. Ellis JM, Folkers K, Levy M, Shizukuishi S, Lewandowski J, Nishli S, Schubert HA, Ulrich R: Response of vitamin B-6 deficiency and the carpal tunnel syndrome to pyridoxine. Proc Natl Acad Sci USA 79:7494–7498, 1982.
11. Feindel W, Stratford J: The role of the cubital tunnel in tardy ulnar palsy. Can J Surg 1:287–300, 1958.

12. Fissette J, Onkelinx A, Fandi N: Carpal and Guyon tunnel syndrome in burns at the wrist. J Hand Surg 6:13–15, 1981.
13. Fulton JF: *Harvey Cushing: A Biography*. Springfield, Ill, Charles C Thomas, 1946, pp 263–265.
14. Gay JR, Love JG: Diagnosis and treatment of tardy paralysis of the ulnar nerve. J Bone Joint Surg 29:1087–1097, 1947.
15. Gelberman RH, Hergenroeder PT, Hargens AR, Lundborg GN, Akeson WH: The carpal tunnel syndrome. J Bone Joint Surg. 63A:380–383, 1981.
16. Goldman S, Honet JC, Sobel R, Goldstein AS: Posterior interosseous nerve palsy in the absence of trauma. Arch Neurol 21:435–441, 1969.
17. Hartz CR, Linscheid RL, Gramse RR, Daube JR: The pronator teres syndrome: Compressive neuropathy of the median nerve. J Bone Joint Surg 63A:885–890, 1981.
18. Jain VK, Cestero RVM, Baum J: Carpal tunnel syndrome in patients undergoing maintenance hemodialysis. JAMA 242:2868–2869, 1979.
19. Keegan JJ, Holyoke EA: Meralgia paresthetica. J Neurosurg 19:341–345, 1962.
20. King T, Morgan FP: Treatment of traumatic ulnar neuritis: Mobilization of the ulnar nerve at the elbow by removal of the medial epicondyle and adjacent bone. Aust N Z J Surg 20:33–42, 1950.
21. Laha RK, Dujovny M, DeCastro SC: Entrapment of median nerve by supracondylar process of the humerus: Case report. J Neurosurg 46:252–255, 1977.
22. Lanz U: Anatomical variations of the median nerve in the carpal tunnel. J Hand Surg 2:44–53, 1977.
23. Lavey EB, Pearl RM: Patent median artery as a cause of carpal tunnel syndrome. Ann Plast Surg 7:236–238, 1981.
24. Lewis SL, Fiddian NJ: Acute carpal tunnel syndrome: A rare complication of chondrocalcinosis. Hand 14:164–167, 1982.
25. Luerssen TG, Campbell RL, Defalque RJ, Worth RM: Spontaneous saphenous neuralgia. Neurosurgery 13:238–241, 1983.
26. Mann RA: Tarsal tunnel syndrome. Orthop Clin North Am 5:109–115, 1974.
27. Melvin JL, Burnett CN, Johnson EW: Median nerve conduction in pregnancy. Arch Phys Med Rehabil 50:75–80, 1969.
28. Ochoa J: Nerve fiber pathology in acute and chronic compression, in Omer GE Jr, Spinner M (eds): *Management of Peripheral Nerve Problems*. Philadelphia, Saunders, 1980, pp 487–501.
29. Osborne G: Compression neuritis of the ulnar nerve at the elbow. Hand 2:10–13, 1970.
30. Phalen GS: Reflections on 21 years' experience with the carpal-tunnel syndrome. JAMA 212:1365–1367, 1970.
31. Rengachary SS, Arjunan K: Compression of the ulnar nerve in Guyon's canal by a soft tissue cell tumor. Neurosurgery 8:400–405, 1981.
32. Rengachary SS, Neff JP, Singer PA, Brackett CE: Suprascapular entrapment neuropathy: A clinical, anatomical, and comparative study: Part 1. Clinical study. Neurosurgery 5:441–446, 1979.
33. Roles NC, Maudsley RH: Radial tunnel syndrome. J Bone Joint Surg 54B:499–508, 1972.
34. Sahs AL, Helms CM, DuBois C: Carpal tunnel syndrome: Complication of toxic shock syndrome. Arch Neurol 40:414–415, 1983.
35. Seddon HJ: *Surgical Disorders of the Peripheral Nerves*. Edinburgh, Churchill-Livingstone, 1975, pp 112–129.
36. Smith BH, Herbst BA: Anterior interosseous nerve palsy. Arch Neurol 30:330–331, 1974.
37. Spinner M: The arcade of Frohse and its relationship to posterior interosseous nerve paralysis. J Bone Joint Surg 50B:809–812, 1968.
38. Spinner M: The anterior interosseous-nerve syndrome. J Bone Joint Surg 52A:84–94, 1970.
39. Spinner M, Spencer PS: Nerve compression lesions of the upper extremity. Clin Orthop 104:46–67, 1974.
40. Stevens H: Meralgia paresthetica. Arch Neurol Psychiatry 77:557–574, 1957.
41. Stookey B: Meralgia paresthetica. JAMA 90:1705–1707, 1928.
42. Voitk AJ, Mueller JC, Farlinger DE, Johnston RU: Carpal tunnel syndrome in pregnancy. Can Med Assoc J 128:277–281, 1983.

SECTION B
Acute Nerve Injuries

225
Anatomy and Physiology of Peripheral Nerves

Robert M. Worth

In many ways the neuron is unique among cells. One of the most important characteristics the remarkable cell possesses is the ability to generate and conduct action potentials, thus permitting rapid communication of commands over long distances. Furthermore, the neuronal soma is charged with the incredibly difficult mission of supplying the entire axon with metabolic products essential to the maintenance of the neurolemma and to intracellular communication and trophic control of other structures. In this chapter I will review certain aspects of the anatomy of the peripheral nerve and then discuss the electrophysiology of the neuron. The characteristics and mechanisms of axoplasmic transport will then be explored along with some recent information on the possible relationship between transport and axonal membrane function.

Anatomy

A peripheral nerve as visualized at the operating table is composed of many different axons of diverse diameters. This fact, well known to all students of elementary neuroanatomy, nevertheless causes much confusion in discussing the physiology of the neuron. The *axon* is a long projection from the perikaryon, which can extend for a distance of several feet. It is bounded by a semipermeable membrane called the *axolemma*. This is surrounded by a *basement membrane*, which, in turn, is encircled by the *myelin sheath* laid down by Schwann cells (Fig. 225-1). This latter structure has important effects on action potential conduction, which will be discussed below. The entire axon is then covered by *endoneurium*, the innermost layer of the peripheral nerve connective tissue structure. A number of axons are grouped together in a bundle called a *fascicle*, which is invested in another mesenchymal sheath called *perineurium*. The fascicle is the smallest segment of the nerve that is generally visible with the operating microscope. The perineurium itself is a semipermeable membrane and, as such, is the primary regulator of the intrafascicular environment.[4] The fascicles are grouped together to form a *peripheral nerve*, and this structure is covered by the outermost connective tissue layer, the *epineurium*, which is often used to hold sutures in peripheral nerve repairs.

The individual axons, as mentioned, are of different sizes, varying in diameter from 1 to about 20 μm. A number of different systems have been proposed to classify the fibers based on their diameter and the function that each subserves. Nerve conduction velocity (NCV) is proportional to the square root of fiber diameter. This allowed Erlanger and Gasser in 1937 to propose a classification of size based on Nobel prize–winning work in which they separated the components of the compound action potential.[5] This potential results from stimulation of a peripheral nerve (see below) and can be resolved into individual peaks conducted at different velocities related to the various diameters of the axons of which the stimulated nerve is composed. The largest myelinated axons produce the most rapidly conducted potential, which is designated by the letter A; these are thus known as *A fibers*. The A group can be further subdivided into alpha, beta, gamma, and delta fibers, again based on their size and respective conduction velocities. In actual practice only the A alpha and delta categories are readily distinguishable and have practical use. Erlanger and Gasser also noted slower conducted peaks that are carried by autonomic B fibers and unmyelinated C fibers.

In 1943, Lloyd introduced a classification using Roman numerals from I through IV in descending order of size.[7] Type I and type II fibers correspond to the large myelinated (A alpha) axons with diameters between 6 and 20 μm that consist of motor fibers and the larger sensory fibers. Group III, or A delta axons, have diameters of 1 to 6 μm and subserve pain conduction. Group IV contains the C fibers, which are small unmyelinated nerves that carry delayed-pain input, and the B fibers, which are preganglionic autonomic axons.

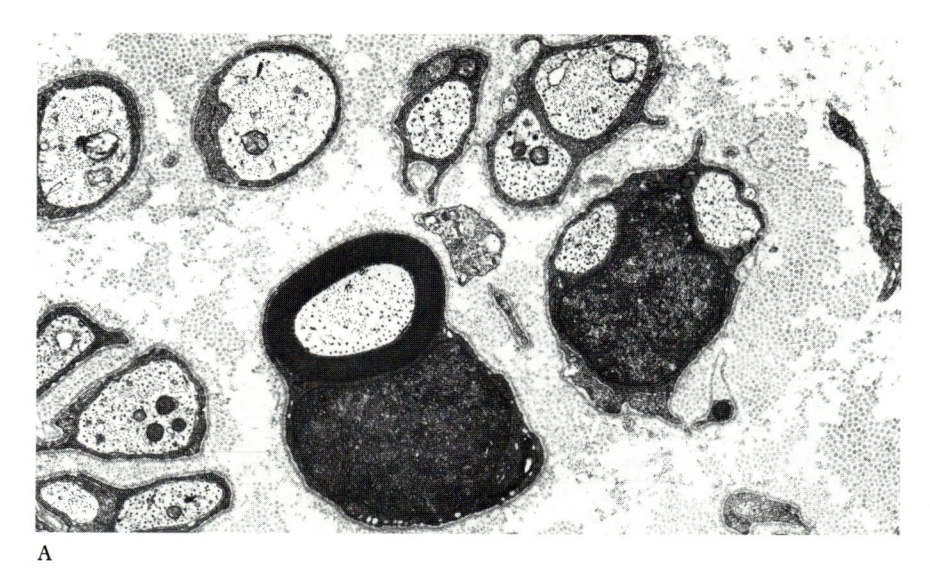

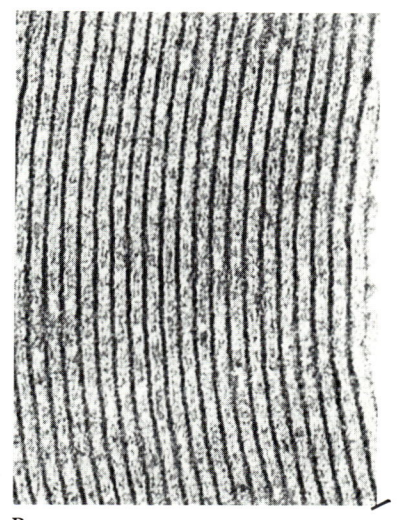

Figure 225-1 Electron micrographs of a peripheral nerve. *A.* Note two Schwann cells in the center of the field. The one at the left is encircling a typical large axon with a myelin sheath. The one at the right is investing two smaller nonmyelinated fibers. *B.* A magnified view of the myelin sheath, showing its lamellar arrangement.

A rough estimate of the conduction velocity of a given axon can be obtained by multiplying the fiber diameter by 6. Thus, a typical large group I motor nerve with a diameter of 15 μm will conduct at a velocity of about 90 m/s.

Physiology

Membrane Events

Action potential generation depends on an attribute that the axon shares with other excitable cells, the resting membrane potential. This is a steady potential difference across the neurolemma, with the inside of the fiber electronegative with respect to the outside environment. This potential is generated by the difference in concentration (technically the activity) of certain ions between the inside of the neurolemma and the outside. The most important ions involved are sodium (Na^+) and potassium (K^+). A concentration gradient develops in response to the differential permeability of the membrane to the ions, which allows the potassium that is present in high concentration within the cell to move down its concentration gradient to the outside. Negative charge within the cell is primarily mediated by large molecules such as proteins and amino acids that are not diffusible through the membrane. Thus, the potassium moves through the membrane until the outward force generated by its concentration gradient is precisely counterbalanced by the inward force produced by the developing negativity left inside the cell (Fig. 225-2). The electrical potential required to exert this restraint is called the *equilibrium potential* for potassium (E_{K^+}), and it can be calculated from the ionic concentrations on the two sides of the membrane by a formula known as the *Nernst equation*. This can be derived from the basic principles of thermodynamics and for practical purposes is expressed as $E = K \log [C_1]/[C_2]$, where E is the equilibrium potential in millivolts, $[C_1]$ and $[C_2]$ are the concentrations of the ion on the outside and inside of the membrane, respectively, and K is a constant resulting from the thermodynamic derivation of the equation. The equilibrium potential for potassium is about -88 mV, with the inside negative relative to the outside. Since sodium is present in higher concentration outside than inside the membrane, its equilibrium potential is about $+75$ mV; that is, the inside of the cell would have to be 75 mV positive relative to the outside to prevent inward diffusion of sodium along its concentration gradient. In the resting state, however, the membrane is much more permeable to potassium than to sodium; thus the resting membrane potential is about -80 mV, which is much closer to the potassium than to the sodium equilibrium potential. The fact that this value is slightly more positive than the potassium equilibrium potential reflects the fact that there is a small inward leakage of sodium that slightly discharges the potential difference.

In a series of landmark papers in 1952, Hodgkin and Huxley postulated that it is this differential permeability to sodium and potassium and the resultant resting membrane potential that provides for the axon's ability to generate and conduct the action potential.[6] When an electric current is applied to the axon, a small depolarization develops at the cathodal pole of the electrode; that is, the interior of the cell becomes slightly less negative relative to the outside. If the depolarization is great enough and occurs over a relatively short period of time, the axon reaches "threshold." When this occurs, there is a dramatic increase in the membrane permeability for sodium (Fig. 225-3). Since in the resting state both the electrical and the chemical gradient strongly favor sodium influx, there is a rapid, even "explosive," inflow of the ion down its electrochemical gradient. This moves the membrane away from the potassium equilibrium potential toward the sodium potential. The membrane po-

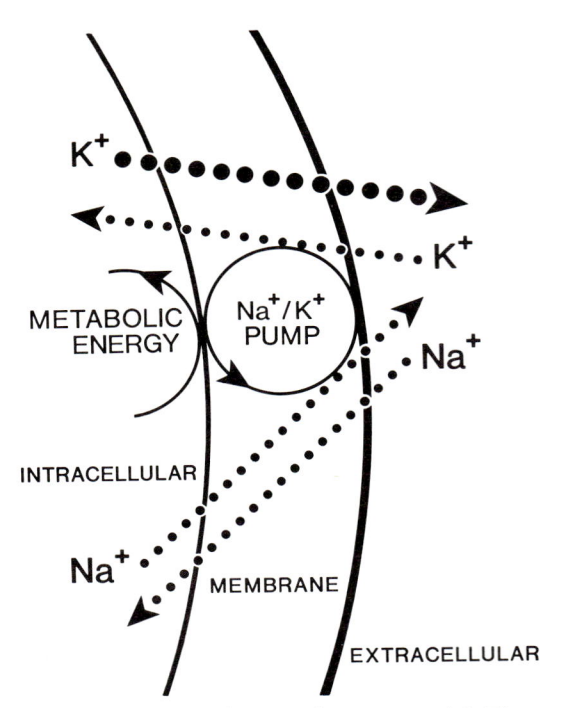

Figure 225-2 Resting membrane potential. The intracellular K^+ concentration is much greater than the extracellular K^+ concentration, and the ion moves down this concentration gradient until the efflux is counterbalanced by the attractive force of intracellular negativity that develops from anions that cannot penetrate the semipermeable membrane. In the resting state, the membrane is much more permeable to K^+ than to Na^+, but a high external Na^+ concentration produces a small influx that slightly raises the resting membrane potential to an average value of -80 mV. An active Na^+/K^+ pump operates to restore ionic balance after the passage of an action potential.

tential then moves from being strongly negative toward zero, and actually the inside of the cell becomes positive—that is, there is an "overshoot." This rapid influx of sodium soon ceases, the membrane permeability to sodium quickly turns off, and the potassium permeability increases and is again predominant. Since the interior of the cell is now much more positive than the potassium equilibrium potential, this ion is expelled in response to its electrical gradient, removing positive charges and consequently repolarizing the membrane. The end result of this entire process is to leave the cell interior with a slight increase in sodium ions and a corresponding decrease in potassium ions. Although the change in ionic balance produced by a single action potential is extremely small, it partially discharges the resting membrane potential, and if left unchecked would eventually depolarize the membrane, making the cell inexcitable. The proper internal-external sodium-potassium relationship is continuously restored through the action of the sodium pump. This is a membrane-bound enzyme that operates via an active process utilizing energy liberated by cleaving the high-energy phosphate bonds in adenosine triphosphate (ATP). The enzyme is a Na^+-K^+-ATPase that extrudes sodium from inside the fiber in exchange for potassium, which is pumped into the fiber, thereby restoring proper ionic balance. It is important to emphasize the fact that this is an active process requiring the use of metabolic energy as opposed to the purely passive events of the action potential that occur in response to the electrochemical gradients across the membrane. Furthermore, the activity of the sodium pump is a "housekeeping" function, and it does not participate in the rapid potential changes that constitute the passage of the action potential. In fact, for a large axon, many thousands of action potentials can still be elicited without a dramatic decrease in resting membrane potential after the sodium pump is poisoned with metabolic blocking agents.

Once the action potential is generated, it must be conducted along the axon. Upon development of an action potential, the interior of the membrane in the local area has an excess of positive charge relative both to the exterior of the membrane at that point and to the neighboring axoplasm inside the cell. This generates a local current flow that spreads down the axon in accordance with the "cable properties" of the nerve fiber.[1] This term refers to the passive electrical properties of the axon. The net effect of this local current is to depolarize the adjacent segment of the membrane so that it in turn reaches the threshold necessary to generate another action potential, beginning the process again and continuing the length of the fiber. Thus the action potential is conducted along the axon by a sort of "sequential depolarization and regeneration." The process has been termed an *all-or-none* phenomenon, referring to the fact that if the depolarization does not cross the requisite threshold, no potential is generated, but when this value is achieved, the potential develops with equal amplitude along the entire length of the axon and does not decrement during conduction.

From the above discussion, it will be realized that if each tiny membrane segment had to be sequentially depolarized for conduction to occur, this would be a very slow process indeed. According to the laws of cable theory, conduction velocity increases in proportion to the square root of fiber diameter, and thus faster conduction develops with an increase in the size of the axon. This is seen phylogenetically in lower animals, and the process reaches its zenith in the squid, where some of the axons in the mantle nerve are 0.5 mm or more in diameter.

Increasing conduction velocity by axon size is an inefficient process, and the conduction velocities necessary for functioning of more advanced species would not be possible unless a different method had evolved. Higher animals therefore have developed the myelin sheath that "insulates" the fiber. As noted above, this sheath is laid down by Schwann cells that are linearly adjacent to each other along the axon. At the junctions between the cells there is a small gap where the membrane is exposed to the surrounding extracellular fluid. It is at these gaps, the *nodes of Ranvier*, that the generation of the action potential occurs. In these myelinated fibers the local current that develops on excitation spreads along the axon to depolarize the membrane at the node instead of the next immediately adjacent membrane site. This allows the action potential to jump from one node of Ranvier to the next in the phenomenon known as *saltatory conduction*. This greatly increases the speed of transmission

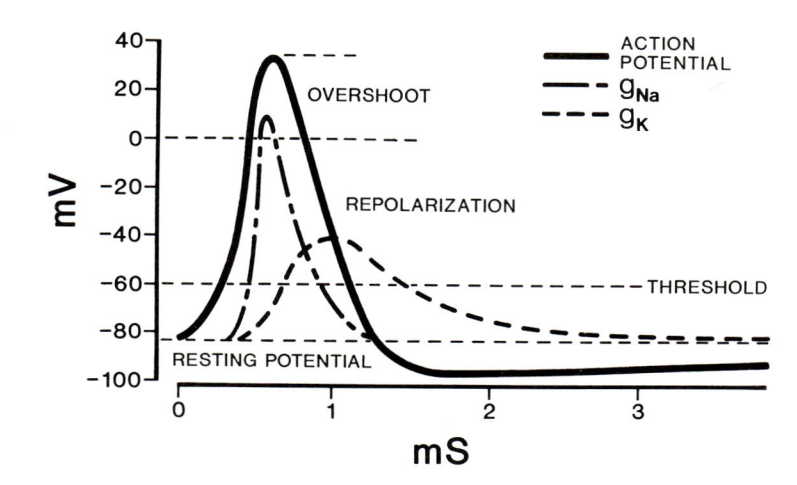

Figure 225-3 Curves of K⁺ conductance (g_K) and Na⁺ conductance (g_{Na}) superimposed on an action potential. Note that g_{Na} turns on at threshold and off just before the peak of the action potential and that g_K turns back on just as g_{Na} turns off, leading to repolarization.

and provides for the rapid conduction velocity necessary in the nervous systems of higher animals.

Axonal Transport

It has been demonstrated that the axon has very little synthetic capability, and thus the proteins and polypeptides necessary for maintenance of the neurolemma and internal organelles must be supplied from the cell soma. Furthermore, the substances expelled from the distal axonal terminals that are necessary for neurotransmission or for the trophic control of muscle fibers or other nerve cells must also be supplied by the perikaryon. The mechanism underlying this supply system has been largely elucidated in the past 10 years and is known as *axonal* or *axoplasmic transport*.[8] Theories of material flow in nerves date to the pre-Christian era,[10] but progressively more attention has been paid to this phenomenon since the work of Weiss and Hiscoe in 1948, which appeared to show accumulation of axoplasm proximal to a ligature placed about the nerve.[12] They concluded that the axoplasm (the cytoplasm of the axon) actually moved as bulk flow in a proximodistal direction. Subsequent work by many investigators has revealed that this concept is probably not correct but that, in fact, there is transport within the axon of a number of different specific substances synthesized in the cell body and necessary to the function of the axon and effector organs. This process appears to be remarkably uniform among fibers of different types and has been shown to move at the same rate in various-sized myelinated and unmyelinated fibers as well as in the autonomic nervous system. The synthesized materials consist largely of proteins and polypeptides and can be tagged by injecting radioactively labeled precursor amino acids such as [³H]leucine into the region of the neuronal cell bodies, e.g., into the spinal dorsal root ganglia or ventral horns of the cat. The precursor is then rapidly (within 15 or 20 min) synthesized into proteins and polypeptides and exported into the axon for transport distally. The rate at which these substances move can then be calculated from the time of appearance of the radioactivity in the axon and its movement distally (Fig. 225-4). This rate has been determined to be about 410 mm per day and is remarkably uniform among various species.[9] Much of this work has been done in cats, but when various animals including frogs, dogs, garfish, and primates have been studied and the data corrected to mammalian body temperature, very similar results have been obtained.

Fast axoplasmic transport can be studied in vitro by injecting the dorsal root ganglia of the seventh lumbar segment in the cat with [³H]leucine and then removing the entire sciatic nerve complex, including the dorsal roots and ganglia proximally and the peroneal and tibial branches distally. A period of about 2 h is allowed between the time of injection and removal of the nerve from the animal to permit incorporation of the amino acid precursor into proteins and polypeptides and their subsequent egress from the cell body into the axon. The nerve is placed in an environment in which transport will continue. In practice, two such systems are generally employed. The nerve may be placed in a flask of preoxygenated Ringer's solution to which can be added various agents whose effects on transport can then be assessed. Axoplasmic transport also continues if the nerve is placed in a sealed metal chamber in which the temperature and humidity are controlled. This device permits electrical stimulation of the nerve and the continuous monitoring of the resulting action potential. When the experiment is concluded with either system, the nerve is then removed and segmentally assayed for radioactivity to allow the computation of flow rates. In this way the effect of various experimental parameters on the characteristics of axoplasmic transport can be assessed. With these methods it has been demonstrated that if the oxygen in the atmosphere is replaced with nitrogen or if the nerve is exposed to metabolic poisons such as cyanide or dinitrophenol, transport fails within about 15 min. If one measures the concentration of high-energy phosphates in the nerve, it is noted to fall to approximately 50 percent of the control value at the time when axoplasmic transport stops. Coincidentally, action potential conduction ceases at about the same time. Agents that interfere with glycolysis or the citric acid cycle also interfere with transport, although the time delay is somewhat longer because of the ability of the nerve to utilize metabolites other than glucose. All of these data are consistent with the hypothesis that axoplasmic transport is an active process requiring the expenditure of metabolic energy. Furthermore, this energy must be available segmentally all along the axon because transport is blocked locally if a small segment of the nerve is covered with paraffin to prevent oxygenation. Thus, high-energy phosphates apparently are not capable of

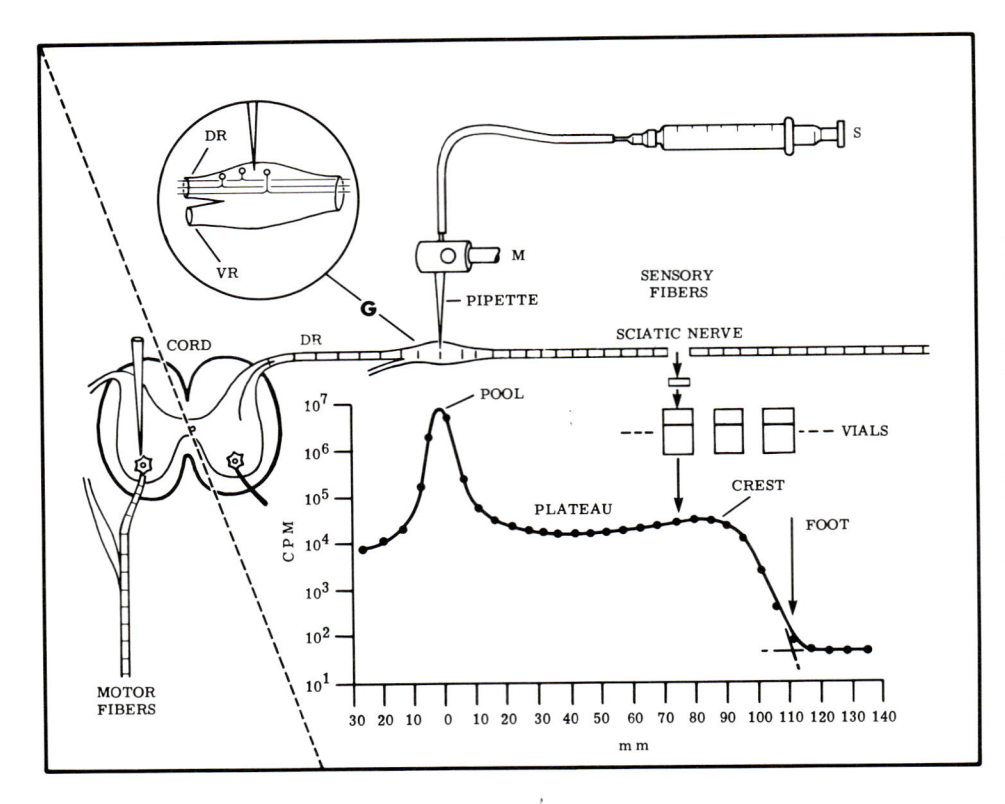

Figure 225-4 Study of axonal transport using a radioactively labeled amino acid precursor. [^{3}H]leucine is injected by micropipet into the region of neuron cell bodies. After time is allowed for the amino acid to be incorporated into the proteins and polypeptides, the sciatic nerve complex is removed, cut into 5-mm segments, and placed in a scintillation counter. The radioactivity per segment is then graphed on semilog paper as a function of the distance from the injection site. (From Ochs.[11])

diffusing from the oxygenated segments into adjacent hypoxic areas.

Although most experimental work has concentrated on proximodistal flow, it has also been demonstrated that there is a retrograde system capable of transferring substances from the periphery toward the neuronal soma. It has been postulated that interference with this mechanism is the signal for the chromatolysis that occurs in the cell soma when the nerve is injured.[11]

Much investigative effort has been expended in elucidating the mechanism by which a variety of substances might be transported in nerves of different diameters at the same fast rate. One important clue was the discovery that agents that impair the function of microtubules can alter axoplasmic transport. *Microtubules* are linearly arranged organelles with a diameter of approximately 25 nm that are present in many types of cells and underlie such vital functions as mitosis. They have been shown to extend throughout the entire length of the axon and are composed of individual protein dimer subunits called *tubulin*. It appears that there is a dynamic equilibrium between the soluble tubulin present in the cytoplasm and that which is assembled into microtubules. Certain chemical agents are capable of altering this equilibrium. Among these are colchicine, which precipitates the tubulin and has been useful in the experimental purification of the substance. Perhaps the most potent of these agents, however, are the vinca alkaloids, widely known in clinical medicine for their antimitotic effects in the chemotherapy of various malignancies. It has been shown that use of these drugs in concentrations as low as 1 μM can block axoplasmic transport.[3] Furthermore, this effect appears related to a loss of microtubular integrity. Interestingly, colchicine also interferes with axoplasmic transport.

Consideration of the experimental data discussed above allows one to construct a theoretical model of a mechanism by which different substances can be bidirectionally transported within the axon. This has been termed the *transport filament hypothesis* in analogy to Huxley's *sliding filament hypothesis* for muscle contraction and suggests that various components are bound to transport filaments, which in turn are moved along the stationary microtubules much like boxcars along a railroad track (Fig. 225-5). The transport filaments are moved by the action of cross-bridges, which utilize the energy stored in ATP. In apparent confirmation of this theory, a relatively high level of Ca^{2+}-Mg^{2+}-activated ATPase (an enzyme that hydrolyzes ATP) has been shown to be present in nerve fibers. Furthermore, nerve also contains high levels of the polypeptide calmodulin, which is capable of activating the enzyme in the presence of the micromolar levels of Ca^{2+} in the axon. This hypothesis then accounts for the dependence of axoplasmic transport on a local supply of metabolic energy and can also explain the sensitivity of the system to agents that "uncouple" microtubules.

From the above discussion it might be anticipated that satisfactory function of the axoplasmic transport system would require an optimum concentration of various ions in the extracellular fluid and consequently inside the cell. This is, in fact, true, although the mechanism for studying this point is complicated by the fact that the perineurium acts as a diffusion barrier to ions, as noted above. It was found that one could not alter the extra-axonal environment simply by changing ionic concentrations in the medium bathing the nerve. Therefore, a method was developed by which the perineurium could be stripped off the cat peroneal nerve under the operating microscope, allowing direct experimen-

Figure 225-5 A transport filament model. Glucose (G) via glycolysis and oxidative phosphorylation leads to ATP generation. ATP by means of high-energy phosphate bonds provides energy for both the sodium pump and the axonal transport filaments that move along microtubules (M) as a result of hydrolysis of ATP by Ca^{2+}-Mg^{2+}-ATPase. The latter enzyme is regulated by the intracellular Ca^{2+} level, which in turn is controlled by mitochondria (Mit), endoplasmic reticulum (ER), and calcium-binding proteins. A variety of substances are transported at the same rate, including organelles (a), small particles (b), and proteins (c). (From Ochs.[11])

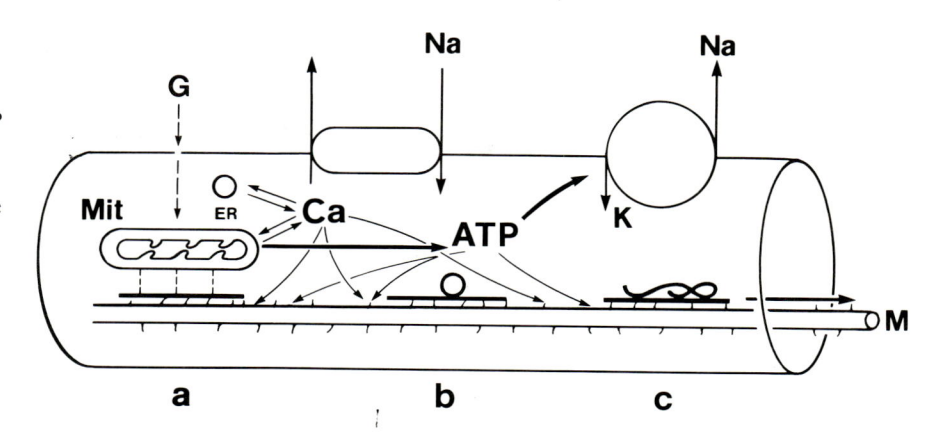

tal manipulation of both extra- and intracellular ionic environments. Using this technique, workers found that the concentration of calcium in the extracellular space must be maintained in the range normally found in vivo in order for axoplasmic transport to continue.[2] Magnesium is capable of lowering the calcium requirement somewhat but cannot substitute for it entirely. These data suggest that Ca^{2+} exerts a critical regulatory function and that its binding to calmodulin allows the latter to activate the Ca^{2+}-Mg^{2+}-ATPase present on the cross-bridges mentioned above.

Other ions may also be important, although their specific relation to the transport mechanism is more difficult to understand. The steroidal alkaloid batrachotoxin (BTX) has been shown to hold sodium channels open, thereby increasing intracellular sodium concentration. This produces depolarization of the cell membrane and also blocks axoplasmic transport in lower concentrations than any other pharmacologic agent yet tested, most likely by altering intra-axonal Ca^{2+} concentration.[14] This observation suggested that physiologically altering intra-axonal sodium by stimulating the nerve to conduct action potentials might also be capable of modifying axoplasmic transport. These experiments have been carried out in our laboratory and have demonstrated that, provided the rate of stimulation is high enough, the rate of transport decreases by as much as 15 percent.[13] Thus, the two basic axonal functions of electrical conduction and material transport are related through alterations in the intracellular ionic environment.

Clinical Implications

Certain aspects of peripheral neuropathology can better be understood in relation to the above discussion of axoplasmic transport. The phenomenon of wallerian degeneration has been discussed elsewhere, but it should be apparent that when the structural integrity of the axon is interrupted, the segment distal to the injury is deprived of the substances carried on the axoplasmic transport system that are essential for the maintenance of structural and functional membrane integrity. Hence, action potential conduction fails in this amputated distal portion of the fiber. Then the structure of the axon itself degenerates after a period of time. Furthermore, as noted above, the muscle fibers are dependent upon a continuous downflow of trophic substances from the cell body, and therefore both electrical and morphological alterations in muscle occur if it is deprived of its innervation.

Agents such as some of the pharmacologic compounds discussed earlier can also disrupt the axoplasmic transport system. This accounts for the widely recognized neuropathy that occurs with the administration of vincristine and significantly limits its use in antineoplastic chemotherapy. Some of the toxic industrial neuropathies also operate through the same mechanism.

Finally, in a more speculative vein, the finding that high rates of repetitive electrical stimulation can alter axoplasmic transport of neurotransmitters suggests that this might help to explain some of the beneficial effects of stimulation in the treatment of chronic pain.

Thus, although many of the characteristics of the electrical function of peripheral nerves have been known since the nineteenth century, the mechanism of axoplasmic transport has only been elucidated within the last decade or so, and much active research is still continuing. It is hoped that as data continue to accumulate, our understanding of this vital neuronal function will continue to increase and our patients will reap the benefit of this increased knowledge in the form of more effective treatment of peripheral neuropathies and more successful management of devastating peripheral nerve trauma.

References

1. Aidley DJ: *The Physiology of Excitable Cells.* London, Cambridge, 1971, pp 47–57.
2. Chan SY, Ochs S, Worth RM: The requirement for calcium ions and the effect of other ions on axoplasmic transport in mammalian nerve. J Physiol (London) 301:477–504, 1980.
3. Chan SY, Worth R, Ochs S: Block of axoplasmic transport *in vitro* by vinca alkaloids. J Neurobiol 11:251–264, 1980.
4. Crescitelli F: Nerve sheath as a barrier to the action of certain substances. Am J Physiol 166:229–240, 1951.
5. Erlanger J, Gasser HS: *Electrical Signs of Nervous Activity.* Philadelphia, University of Pennsylvania Press, 1937.
6. Hodgkin AL, Huxley AF: The components of membrane conductance in the giant axon of *Loligo.* J Physiol (London) 116:473–496, 1952.
7. Lloyd DPC: Neuron patterns controlling transmission of ipsilateral hind limb reflexes in cat. J Neurophysiol 6:293–315, 1943.
8. Ochs S: Fast transport of materials in mammalian nerve fibers. Science 176:252–260, 1972.
9. Ochs S: Rate of fast axoplasmic transport in mammalian nerve fibres. J Physiol (London) 227:627–645, 1972.
10. Ochs S: The early history of material transport in nerve. Physiologist 22:16–19, 1979.
11. Ochs S: Axoplasmic transport, in Siegel GJ, Albers RW, Agranoff BW, Katzman R (eds): *Basic Neurochemistry,* 3d ed. Boston, Little Brown, 1981, pp 425–442.
12. Weiss P, Hiscoe HB: Experiments on the mechanism of nerve growth. J Exp Zool 107:315–395, 1948.
13. Worth RM, Ochs S: The effect of repetitive electrical stimulation on axoplasmic transport. Soc Neurosci Abstr 2:50, 1976 (abstr).
14. Worth RM, Ochs S: Dependence of batrachotoxin block of axoplasmic transport on sodium. J Neurobiol 13:537–549, 1982.

226

Peripheral Nerve Injuries: Types, Causes, Grading

F. Gentili
Alan R. Hudson

Advances in instrumentation and microsurgical technique have improved our management of major peripheral nerve injuries. However the mechanism and extent of injury remain the chief influences on the degree of motor and sensory recovery.

To be useful, a classification of peripheral nerve injury should be simple, should correlate the degree of injury with symptomatology and underlying pathology, and should offer prognostic information to determine if and when operative intervention is needed or when spontaneous recovery is probable. There is no entirely satisfactory classification of the type and extent of nerve injury. Although classifications based on the degree of local nerve injury are of some use, they do not take into account the time between injury and operation nor the sequential changes that may occur in the nerve cell body, motor end plate, or target organ. Thus two injuries of identical local severity could have entirely different outcomes depending on the distance between the injury site and target organ and whether surgery is performed at, for example, 3 months or 2 years.

Codification of functional results after nerve injury adds to the difficulty in the design of a useful classification. No entirely satisfactory system of classifying motor or sensory function presently exists. The standard methods for grading motor power developed primarily for assessment of war injuries are only of limited usefulness (Table 226-1). Grading of sensory function is even more difficult because of its subjective nature and the need to score quality of sensation as well as the perception of the primary sensory stimuli (Table 226-1). Standard criteria and more precise objective methods for evaluation of functional motor and sensory recovery need to be developed.

Before World War II, a variety of ambiguous terms were used to describe nerve injuries. In 1943, Seddon introduced a classification of nerve injuries based on three fundamental types of nerve fiber injury.[11] While he admitted that his classification, in its simplicity, was only a rough approximation, his three original terms, *neurapraxia, axonotmesis,* and *neurotmesis,* have come to be widely accepted. Subsequently, Sunderland proposed a classification based on five degrees of injury of increasing severity (Table 226-2).[14] Both systems are based on the anatomy of the peripheral nerve and on the degree of injury to neural elements and connective tissue structures, the endoneurium, perineurium, and epineurium. Both attempt to correlate the degree of damage with clinical symptomatology (Table 226-3). However, neural injury is a continuum, and clear distinction between one grade and another is often not possible. Indeed, pure grades of injury may be seen only in the setting of the experimental laboratory.

Because it was not always possible to apply available grading systems at surgery, we and others[10] have proposed a classification based on intraoperative microsurgical assessment (Table 226-4).

TABLE 226-1 Assessment of Nerve Recovery—British Medical Research Council Classification

Classification	Description
	Motor Recovery
M0	No contraction
M1	Return of perceptible contraction in proximal muscles
M2	Return of perceptible contraction in both proximal and distal muscles
M3	Return of function in both proximal and distal muscles of a degree that all important muscles are sufficiently powerful to act against resistance
M4	Return of function as in stage 3 with the addition that all synergic and independent movements are possible
M5	Complete recovery
	Sensory Recovery
S0	Absence of sensibility in the autonomous area
S1	Recovery of deep cutaneous pain sensibility within the autonomous area of the nerve
S2	Return of some degree of superficial cutaneous pain and tactile sensibility within the autonomous area of the nerve
S3	Return of superficial cutaneous pain and tactile sensibility throughout the autonomous area with disappearance of any previous over-response
S3+	Return of sensibility as in S3 with the addition of some recovery of two-point discrimination within the autonomous area
S4	Complete recovery

Seddon Classification of Peripheral Nerve Injury

Neurapraxia

This term was proposed by Seddon to describe an often incomplete, transient loss of function in a peripheral nerve. The key feature is its reversibility within hours to several months of injury (average of 6 to 8 weeks). It represents a mild injury, and when it is incomplete, there is often greater involvement of motor than sensory function with sparing of autonomic innervation. When function is completely lost, neurapraxia can be distinguished from the more serious grades of injury only in retrospect and after recovery has taken place sooner than would be possible following wallerian degeneration. The usual cause of neurapraxic injury is mild compression or traction, blunt trauma, or the indirect effects of a high-velocity missile.

Experimental and clinical observations have suggested that more than one mechanism may underlie neurapraxia.[2,9,13] Biochemical ionic disturbance that produces a localized conduction block may be the substrate for the rapidly reversible clinical picture often seen with mild, transient compression. The finding of segmental demyelination and other perinodal myelin changes may explain the more lasting block (6 to 8 weeks) when it is accompanied by preservation of distal conduction. Although, by definition, denervation does not occur, a few fibrillation potentials are often seen on electromyography (EMG). Persistent neural deficit lasting more than 8 to 12 weeks indicates a more severe injury. Although any peripheral nerve can sustain a neurapraxic injury, the brachial plexus and radial, median, ulnar, and peroneal nerves are most commonly affected. Without doubt, a careful history and neurological examination are crucial in diagnosis. Although neurapraxia is not a surgical lesion, it may be associated with a more severe injury that requires surgical intervention.

Axonotmesis

Axonotmesis may be defined as a complete interruption of axon and myelin sheath with preservation of the connective tissue stroma of a peripheral nerve. The basement membrane of the axon, the perineurium, and the epineurium are preserved. Physiologically, the nerve is severed at the point of injury and complete distal wallerian degeneration follows. There is thus immediate and complete loss of all motor, sensory, and autonomic function distal to the lesion, with absent voluntary muscle potentials and EMG evidence of denervation after 2 to 3 weeks. Regeneration occurs spontaneously with axonal growth and myelin sheath formation along preserved endoneurial tubes. There is potential for return of function, which however will depend on the distance between the lesion and the end organ, the age of the patient, and the rate of regeneration, which on average occurs at a rate of 1 to 2 mm per day. While on initial clinical assessment this lesion is indistinguishable from more severe degrees of injury, the possibility of an axonotmetic injury must be considered since the result of natural repair is always better than that of surgical repair. This type of lesion in continuity is typically seen with skeletal fractures, moderate traction, compression, and injection injuries. A careful history and clinical and electrophysiological followup will help determine if axonotmesis is the cause of a complete nerve lesion.

TABLE 226-2 Sunderland Classification of Nerve Injury[14]

Classification	Description
Grade 1	Loss of axonal conduction
Grade 2	Loss of continuity of axons with intact endoneurium
Grade 3	Transection of nerve fiber (axon and sheath) with intact perineurium
Grade 4	Loss of perineurium and fascicular continuity
Grade 5	Loss of continuity of entire nerve trunk

TABLE 226-3 Classification of Peripheral Nerve Injury*

	Seddon		
	Neurapraxia	Axonotmesis	Neurotmesis
	Sunderland		
	First-degree	Second-degree, mild third-degree	Severe third-degree, fourth-degree, fifth-degree
Common mechanism	Mild blunt trauma Stretch Compression Missile Injection Ischemia	Compression Traction Missile Injection Ischemia	Laceration Crush Traction Missile Ischemia Injection
Clinical	• Often incomplete • Motor > sensory involvement • Sparing autonomic function	• Complete loss of motor, sensory, and autonomic function	• Complete loss of motor, sensory, and autonomic function
Electrophysiological findings	• Local conduction block • Preserved conduction distal to lesion • Rare fibrillation potentials	• Absent voluntary action potential • Absent distal conduction • Denervation with fibrillation at > 3 weeks	• Absent voluntary action potential • Absent distal conduction • Fibrillation > 3 weeks
Recovery	• Rapid (hours to weeks; average, 6 to 8 weeks) • Complete recovery	• Months to years Depends on level of nerve involved, age of patient (average, 1–2 mm/day)	• Prolonged • Never complete recovery • Surgical repair required

* Adapted from Seddon.[12]

Neurotmesis

Neurotmesis refers to complete anatomical severance of the nerve or to disruption of the neural and connective tissue elements to an extent incompatible with spontaneous recovery. A nerve may be left in continuity, but internal disruption could be so severe that it qualifies as a neurotmetic lesion. The clinical and EMG picture is identical with that of axonotmesis and includes complete loss of motor, sensory, and autonomic function and distal denervation. When the nerve is completely divided, axonal regeneration causes a neuroma to form in the proximal stump. While laceration and direct missile injury are common causes of this type of injury, severe crush, traction, chemical injection, and ischemic insults can result in neurotmesis. A neurotmetic lesion requires either direct repair or grafting if nerve function is to be restored. The prognosis depends on several factors, including the age of the patient, the duration of paralysis, the level of the lesion, the identity of the injured nerve, and the timing of surgery.

While it is useful in discussion to separate the different degrees of injury, in practice, mixed lesions are common. The high-velocity missile that penetrates the brachial plexus produces neurotmesis of the elements of the plexus that lie in its path and axonotmesis and neurapraxia of adjacent elements from its percussive effects. A compressive force applied for a short time may produce a neurapraxic injury, whereas neurotmesis will follow a more severe and longstanding compression.

Sunderland Classification of Nerve Injury

First-Degree Injury

The first-degree injury corresponds to Seddon's neurapraxia and involves a reversible, local conduction block at the site of injury without wallerian degeneration. Local demyelinization that has been shown experimentally to slow or block conduction may be the pathological substrate of a first-degree injury.

Clinically, a first-degree lesion may present as a mild paresis or complete motor and sensory paralysis. The key, however, is complete reversibility, usually beginning within hours or days with some sign of recovery by 4 to 6 weeks. When incomplete, motor involvement is often greater than sensory involvement. Of the sensory modalities, those subserved by large myelinated fibers, including touch and proprioception, are more involved than those related to small, nonmyelinated fibers (temperature and autonomic function). Electrophysiologically, the conduction block is confined to the injured area; distal conduction is normal.

TABLE 226-4 Intraoperative Grading of Peripheral Nerve Injuries

1. Divided peripheral nerve
   1a. Injury-to-examination interval less than 3 weeks
   1b. Injury-to-examination interval greater than 3 weeks
2. Lesion in continuity
   2a. Injury-to-examination interval less than 3 months
   2b. Injury-to-examination interval greater than 3 months
3. Mixed 1 and 2

Second-Degree Injury

In a second-degree injury (which corresponds to Seddon's axonotmesis), axon and myelin are interrupted but the endoneurial sheath and other supporting connective tissue stroma, including epineurium and perineurium, are preserved. Axonal interruption results in wallerian degeneration distal to the lesion and complete loss of motor, sensory, and autonomic innervation.

With preservation of endoneurial sheaths, a second-degree injury is compatible with good recovery, the rate of which will depend on the distance of the lesion from the structures innervated. Within a few days, there is complete loss of electrical excitability distal to the lesion. Recovery is often poor in high, proximal lesions when more than 18 months is required for the regenerative axons to reach their distal targets. The sequence of recovery is from proximal to distal. While the potential for complete recovery exists, residual deficits are often encountered and are due to reduced numbers of axons and failure of axons to regenerate. Recovery usually takes months or years.

Third-Degree Injury

A third-degree injury implies not only disruption of axon and myelin with distal wallerian degeneration but also damage to the internal structure of the fascicle with loss of endoneurial integrity. Preservation of perineurium and epineurium confers anatomical preservation of the nerve trunk. The fascicular pattern remains intact. A third-degree injury includes both axonotmesis and neurotmesis of Seddon's classification. A mild third-degree injury with minimal intrafascicular fibrosis, which permits significant regeneration, corresponds to Seddon's axonotmesis. On the other hand, damage to the intrafascicular structures causes fibrosis with obstruction to regenerating axons and puts the injury into the neurotmetic group. Thus, third-degree injuries are essentially intrafascicular lesions, most often produced by chemical injection, ischemia, or traction-compression mechanisms. It has been suggested that this may be the lesion of the chronic entrapment neuropathy. While wallerian degeneration occurs, as in second-degree injuries, the extent of intrafascicular fibrosis will determine the degree of regeneration and functional recovery. On gross inspection, the nerve may not appear heavily damaged, but, internally, there may be a significant third-degree injury.

Clinically, there is complete loss of motor, sensory, and autonomic function distal to the lesion with electrophysiological evidence of denervation. Recovery is usually delayed and incomplete depending on the severity of intrafascicular fibrosis; when severe, little if any recovery will result. A severe third-degree lesion should be suspected if there is no evidence of recovery or progressive regeneration when this would be expected to take place.

Fourth-Degree Injury

Fourth-degree lesions involve interruptions of all neural and supporting connective tissue stroma of a peripheral nerve except for the epineurium. The fascicular pattern is lost, and the nerve may appear as a thinned strand of connective tissue or as a neuroma in continuity. Regenerating axons enter grossly disrupted intrafascicular planes with few, if any, fibers reaching the distal trunk. There is complete motor, sensory, and autonomic loss. Surgical repair is mandatory and often requires nerve grafts.

Both fourth- and fifth-degree nerve injuries correspond to neurotmetic lesions in Seddon's classification.

Fifth-Degree Injury

A fifth-degree lesion implies loss of continuity of the nerve trunk involved, with complete motor, sensory, and autonomic dysfunction distal to the injury. Pathologically, outgrowth of regenerating axons in the proximal stump results in neuroma formation. A few axons may reach the distal stump, but this is usually not associated with any functional recovery. Although commonly seen with lacerations and incising injuries, fifth-degree lesions can occur from severe traction and compression forces that result in anatomical disruption of the nerve. Operative repair is required; however, even under the most favorable operative conditions, reduced numbers of regenerating axons and distortion of fiber pattern commonly result in some residual disability.

The Seddon and Sunderland classifications of nerve injury are based on a theoretical grading of nerve fiber pathology. The average human peripheral nerve is composed of thousands of nerve fibers contained in fascicles of varying caliber and number. While available grading systems imply pure grades, most injuries of a neural trunk are not of uniform severity either along or across the width of the nerve, with some fascicles and fibers being more severely involved than others. Moreover, a distinction between one degree and another is often unclear and is possible only in retrospect.

Intraoperative Grading of Peripheral Nerve Lesions

The application of existing classifications of peripheral nerve injury to the operating room setting has often been difficult.[10] A system based on the concept of fascicular integrity, taking into account the interval between injury and surgical intervention (injury-to-examination interval) is shown in Table 226-4. At operation, peripheral nerve injuries may be classified into one of three groups. Group 1 includes lesions associated with gross anatomical disruption of the nerve (Fig. 226-1). Group 2 includes lesions in continuity, and group 3 includes mixed lesions (Fig. 226-2).

Lesions in group 1 are associated with fascicular disruption that may be either complete or with the two ends connected by thin strands of connective tissue. This lesion corresponds to the grade 5 injury in Sunderland's classification. All group 1 lesions require resection and suture with or without grafting. With an injury-to-examination interval less than 3 weeks, the decision to repair a grade 1 lesion will depend to some extent on the mechanism of injury. An incised wound due to a knife, glass, scalpel, or other sharp object may be sutured primarily. When associated with extensive crushing, contusion, stretch, or contamination, re-

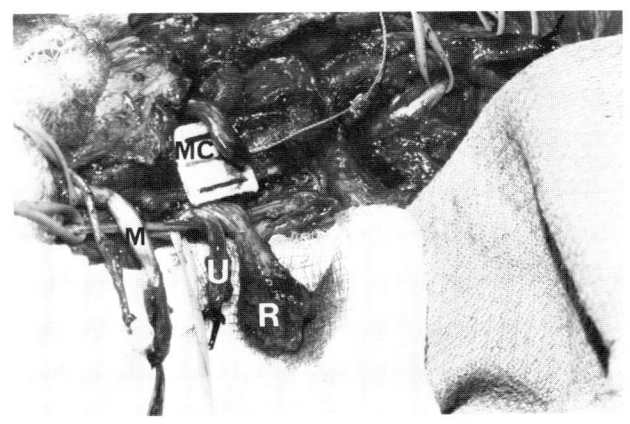

Figure 226-1 Divided peripheral nerves. Arm was thrust through a plate glass door, which severed all peripheral nerves in the lower right axilla. This was the appearance 2 weeks after injury. All elements repaired by epineurial suture, with the exception of the musculocutaneous nerve, which required grafting. R, radial nerve distal stump; U, ulnar nerve distal stump; M, median nerve distal stump; MC, musculocutaneous nerve distal stump.

pair of group 1 injuries should be delayed 3 to 4 weeks so that the full extent of the pathological lesion may be more readily defined (Fig. 226-3).

Group 2 lesions comprise the majority of civilian peripheral nerve injuries. On gross inspection, the nerve may look relatively normal, diminished in diameter, or swollen, as in neuroma in continuity (Fig. 224-4). Lesions in continuity can result from a variety of mechanisms, and include all degrees of nerve injury. In the majority of group 2 lesions, the severity of the pathological change, regardless of the mechanism of injury, is often unknown. In this circumstance, it is appropriate to wait for evidence of motor and sensory recovery. If no recovery has occurred by 3 months, it is reasonable to assume a serious injury to the nerve and to explore the lesion (Fig. 226-5).

At operation, external appearance alone may not be adequate to determine the function and regenerative capabilities of the nerve. Nerves that appear grossly abnormal in color, caliber, and consistency may contain fascicles whose continuity can be traced right through the lesion (Fig. 226-6). By contrast, a relatively innocent external appearance may disguise complete lack of fascicular and hence nerve fiber continuity within the structure of the nerve. While a hard consistency of the nerve on palpation suggests significant fibrosis and, by implication, fascicular disruption, this is not an absolute indicator of nerve fiber and fascicular integrity. With the use of magnification and careful microsurgical technique, epineurial and interfascicular dissection beginning from both proximal and distal normal nerve may help determine whether or not the fascicles are in continuity and the extent of epineurial and inter- and intrafascicular scarring. Intraoperative stimulation and recording techniques are useful in helping the surgeon decide the correct surgical treatment. If fascicular integrity is maintained and a measurable response is obtained across the lesion, or the first target muscle contracts to stimulation at the expected time, surgical resection and, indeed, extensive internal neurolysis

should be avoided. If no nerve action potential response is obtained across a group 2 lesion at 12 to 16 weeks, or fascicular integrity cannot be delineated by careful microsurgical dissection, neurotmesis must be suspected and appropriate resection and suture carried out. In group 3 lesions, careful internal neurolysis and intraoperative recording will help determine which fascicles are intact and which are irreparably damaged and will require repair.

Causes and Mechanisms of Peripheral Nerve Injury

Laceration and Contusion

Open wounds to an extremity commonly caused by knives, glass, and missiles are a frequent cause of nerve injury. The degree of damage may vary, but a high percentage suffer complete or partial division.[12,14] If the laceration is complete, the nerve injury falls into the classification of divided peripheral nerve. If the laceration does not involve the entire substance of the nerve, a lesion in continuity will result.

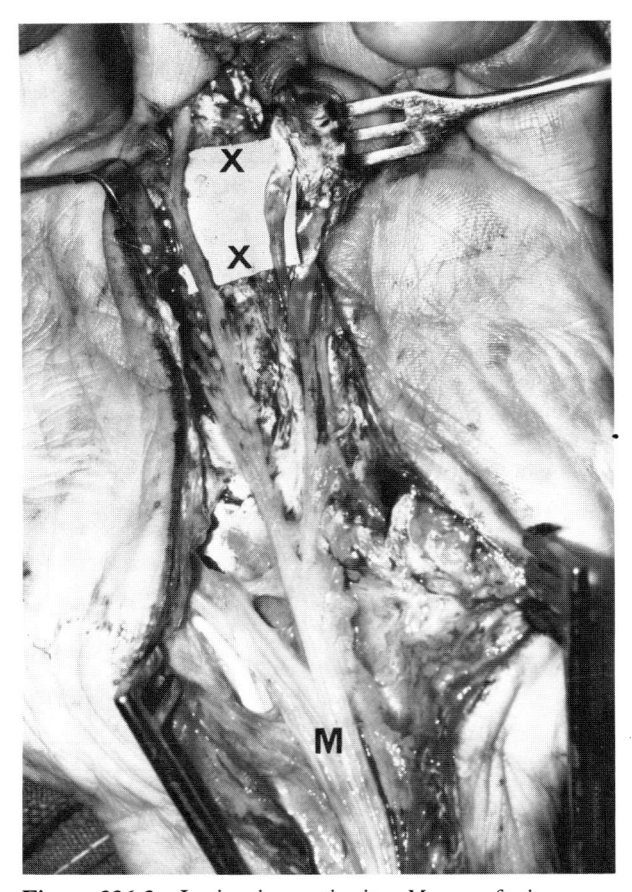

Figure 226-2 Lesion in continuity. Many soft tissues, including the median nerve, were injured in this paint spray-gun injury to the right palm. The branch X-X was irreparably damaged and had to be resected. It was repaired by grafting. M, median nerve at right wrist; X-X, paint in median nerve sensory branch.

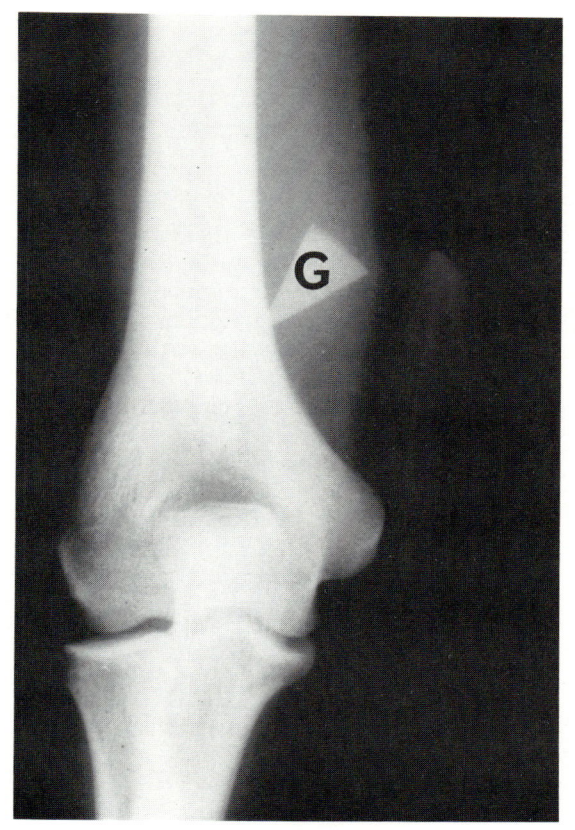

Figure 226-3 Divided peripheral nerve. Ulnar nerve was injured in automobile accident. Wound was grossly contaminated. Nerve repair was delayed for 3 weeks, at which time a fragment of glass, missed during the first debridement, was removed. All glass fragments are visible on x-ray, regardless of the lead content of the glass. G, glass fragment on course of ulnar nerve.

operative procedure is a more complex entity and requires careful analysis. In the latter circumstance, the nerve may have been divided by the surgeon's scalpel, may have been injured by prolonged retractor pressure or stretched during the manipulation of a fracture, or may have been subjected to thermal injury as a result of inappropriate coagulation near the nerve.

An exception to the general rule that immediate loss of function associated with a surface wound is in all probability related to division of the nerve is the situation attendant on missile injuries. Total immediate loss of nerve function following a gunshot wound may be associated with a lesion in continuity and not laceration of the nerve. Over 50 percent will regain some degree of useful function, so that an expectant attitude is usually advised. Laceration injuries caused by closed or open fracture or missile injury can be associated with extensive areas of contusion. A contusion injury can produce a wide range of neural damage, but when not severe or associated with laceration, there is a relatively good prognosis for return of useful function.

While a known mechanism of injury can have a prognostic implication, and neural contusion from blunt trauma, closed fracture, or the indirect effect of a missile wound would suggest that an initial nonoperative approach be taken, each patient must have a careful, initial clinical and electrophysiological assessment and regular follow-up. Conservative management must not be prolonged in those patients who do not exhibit the expected recovery at the appropriate period following injury (3 to 4 months).

Stretch and Traction

A common mechanism of injury, stretch or traction, can result in a wide range of neural damage. Although there is a certain elasticity of peripheral nerves that allows a degree of

When dealing with a lacerated nerve, it is important to consider the nature of the injuring agent. A specific issue is whether or not a laceration injury has resulted from a sharply incised wound or alternatively whether the laceration has been associated with extensive crushing, tearing, and contusion. With sharply incised wounds (knife, glass, scalpel, osteotome) the transverse and longitudinal extent of the lesion is usually obvious and the nerve may be sutured primarily. In injuries associated with extensive contusions or tearing of nerve fibers, as can occur with a chainsaw, wringer, or similar mechanism, repair must be delayed for 3 to 4 weeks so that the extent of the pathological change may be more readily defined under the operating microscope and only normal fascicles opposed during nerve repair. One should be reminded that if the injuring agent pursues an oblique course through the soft tissues, the surface wound may be at some distance from the lacerated nerve. The lacerating injury may also damage adjacent muscles and tendons, and the integrity of these structures should be routinely assessed at the time of injury. While complete loss of function of a peripheral nerve associated with a surface wound usually indicates that the nerve has suffered complete or partial division, lack of function in a peripheral nerve following an

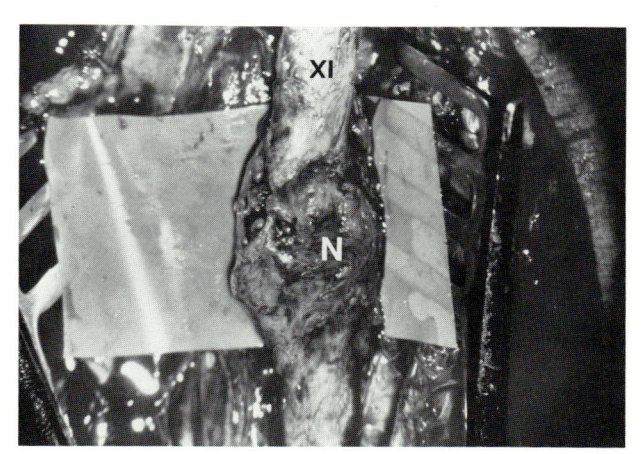

Figure 226-4 Lesion in continuity. Appearance of the accessory nerve in the posterior triangle following a lymph node biopsy. The neuroma in continuity probably resulted from a self-retaining retractor injury or partial incision by a scalpel. Intraoperative electrodiagnostic and/or microsurgical techniques are required to determine whether such a lesion should be resected. XI, accessory nerve; N, neuroma.

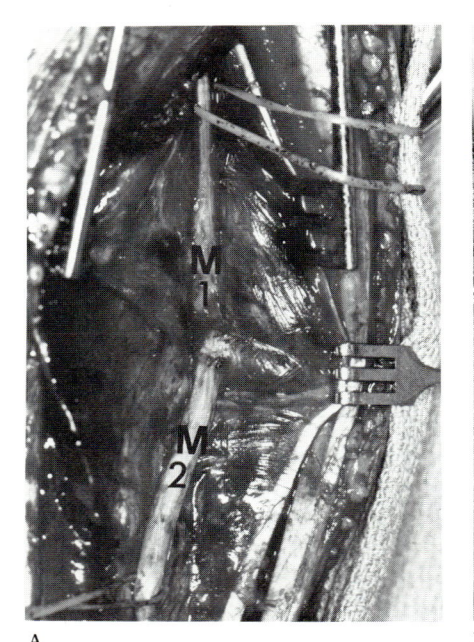

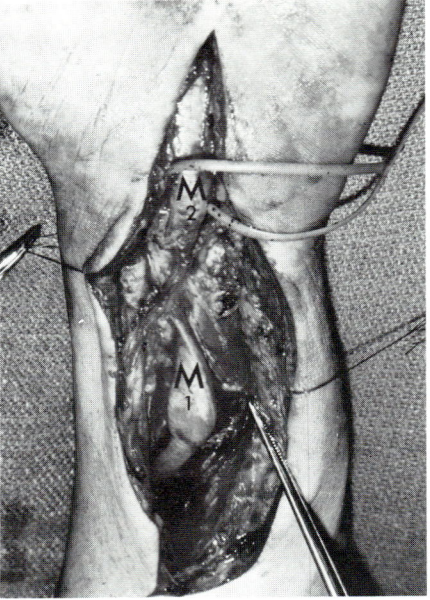

Figure 226-5 *A.* Lesion in continuity. There was no return of median nerve function following forearm fracture. Exposure at 3 months shows nerve trapped in fracture site. It was repaired by resection and epineurial suture. *B.* Divided nerve. There was no return of median nerve function following tendon graft. Exposure at 3 months shows median nerve harvested (erroneously thought to be palmaris longus). M1, median nerve proximal to lesion; M2, median nerve distal to lesion.

stretch, when the normal tolerance is exceeded, as can occur with fractures or joint dislocation, neural injury ranging from a mild neurapraxia to severe axonotmesis can occur. The severity will depend on the distribution of the stretch injury, which in turn is related to the degree and duration of the acting force. Mild focal traction injuries associated with fractures or surgical retraction have a good prognosis for useful recovery. More severe traction injuries are often associated with extensive intraneural fibrosis and will require operative intervention and extensive resection and grafting.

This mechanism of injury is commonly responsible for brachial plexus, radial, and peroneal nerve injuries. Femoral and sciatic nerves may sustain a traction injury during prolonged and difficult hip operations. Clinical examples commonly encountered are listed in Table 226-5.

The majority of stretch or traction injuries result in a lesion in continuity, but, on occasion, the force may be such that the nerve is torn apart. Stretch or traction is also a common mechanism in nerve injuries associated with skeletal fractures with and without dislocation. While one can never

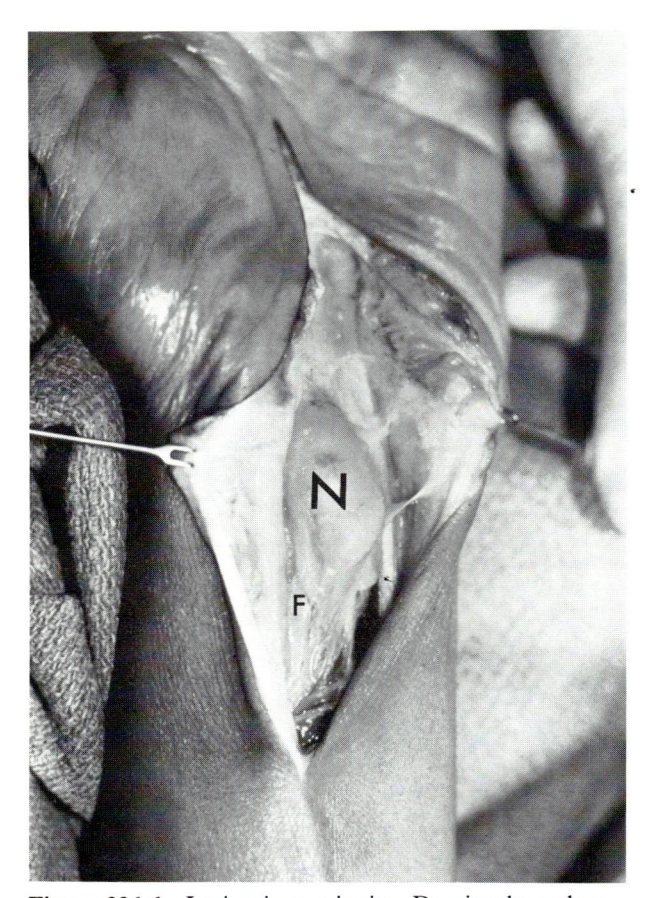

Figure 226-6 Lesion in continuity. Despite the rather dramatic appearance of this bulb in continuity, it was possible to trace three major groups of fascicles in continuity as they skirted the main neuroma. These fascicles were preserved. Continuity of the fascicles that participated in the neuroma formation was restored by grafting. N, neuroma; F, fascicles bypassing neuroma.

TABLE 226-5 Common Traction and Stretch Injuries of Peripheral Nerves

Nerve(s) Involved	Mechanism
Brachial plexus	
Infant	Birth injury (Erb, Klumpke)
Adult	Motorcycle accident
Axillary nerve	Fracture/dislocation (shoulder)
Radial nerve	Fracture (humerus)
Lumbosacral plexus	Fracture/dislocation (pelvis)
Femoral nerve	Hernia repair, hip surgery
Sciatic nerve	Hip surgery, fracture/dislocation (hip)
Peroneal nerve	Fracture/dislocation (knee), fibular fracture

be quite certain whether the lesion is due to the original injury or to manipulation during attempts at reduction, such injuries should initially be treated conservatively, as the majority will show spontaneous recovery within 3 to 4 months. Eighty percent of radial nerve injuries associated with midshaft fractures of the humerus improve spontaneously. Poor recovery is often related to trapping of nerve tissue at the fracture site or laceration of the nerve by sharp spicules of bone. Nerve injuries associated with fractures may also be due to excessive nerve retraction, misplacement of sutures, or blind coagulation during open fixation and plating. While nerve injuries resulting from stretch may be focal in nature, it is a characteristic feature of stretch injury that lesions can vary widely in their longitudinal extent, with relatively normal nerve intervening between two areas of irreparable damage.

As with a nerve injury from some other mechanism, management of a closed stretch or traction injury requires careful initial documentation of the neural deficit and close clinical and electrophysiological follow-up. If there is failure of adequate regeneration either on clinical or electrophysiological testing at a time when this would be expected, then surgical exploration is indicated and should not be delayed beyond 3 to 4 months.

Compression Ischemia

Peripheral nerve, like other neural tissues, is critically dependent on blood flow. Since it is rarely possible to compress a nerve segment without simultaneously affecting its blood supply, the relative role of ischemia and physical deformation in compression lesions remains unsettled. Recent evidence would suggest that while ischemia may be primarily responsible for the mildest type of rapidly reversible nerve lesion, direct mechanical distortion is the major factor underlying more severe, long-lasting forms of pressure palsy (Saturday night palsy, tourniquet paralysis.)[5] Nevertheless, it is likely that in most compressive lesions, including the chronic entrapment neuropathies, localized ischemia at the site of deformation plays some role. Ischemia can produce a wide range of nerve fiber lesions, and when severe and prolonged, will result in widespread axonal loss and wallerian degeneration. In less severe degrees of ischemia, reduction in nerve fiber density is characteristically the result of early dropout of large myelinated fibers. Although damage to a nutrient artery may lead to ischemic injury of a peripheral nerve, pure isolated ischemic neurogenic lesions, in humans, are uncommon. More commonly, nerve trunks are involved along with other soft tissue structures of the limbs, and the severity of the nerve injury will depend on the degree and duration of ischemia and compression. Studies on limb ischemia suggest that there is a critical period of approximately 8 h, after which irreversible nerve injury ensues.[6,7]

The vascular anatomy of peripheral nerves, with rich anastomoses between longitudinal vessels in the epineurium, perineurium, and endoneurium and regional segmental supply, allows the surgeon to mobilize long segments of nerve without producing ischemia. Nevertheless, extensive intraneural dissection by an inexperienced surgeon may jeopardize the microcirculation and result in ischemic damage. Evidence also suggests that a transected nerve or one under tension is more sensitive to ischemia and that one should minimize any interruption of regional segmental vascular supply or tension at the suture site.[8]

The sequential pathology of nerve fiber injury is rather stereotyped and occurs regardless of the injuring agent. An exception to this rule appears to be the nerve fiber pathology that results from more minor forms of compression. Compression of nerve fibers appears to produce myelinated nerve fiber changes that are peculiar to this mechanism. These include alterations in paranodal myelination, axonal thinning, and segmental demyelination.[2,5,9] Wallerian degeneration results from more severe degrees of compression.

The degree of recovery following compression ischemia injury may be accurately predicted in some clinical situations.

The characteristic "Saturday night palsy" results from compression ischemia of the radial nerve against the humerus. Total radial nerve palsy frequently results, but return of motor and sensory function occurs in the majority of cases without any need for surgical intervention. Most anesthetic palsies, or those related to improper application of plaster casts, are primary and second-degree injuries and carry a good prognosis for spontaneous recovery. The brachial plexus and the ulnar, sciatic, and peroneal nerves are most commonly affected. On the other hand, restoration of function following acute compression ischemia injury in other circumstances may be less certain. It may be difficult, for example, to predict the degree of recovery that follows evacuation of hematomas or relief of aneurysmal compression of such structures as the brachial plexus, femoral, or sciatic nerve. In these circumstances, multiple factors exist that affect the outcome of all peripheral nerve surgery. These include the identity and level of the nerve involved, the age of the patient, the degree of injury, and the timing of surgery.

Increased pressure within a fascial compartment as can occur with severe crushing injury, skeletal fracture with vascular compromise, and anticoagulant administration can lead to severe compression ischemic damage to peripheral nerves. A closed compartment syndrome with impending ischemic paralysis requires immediate decompression with properly placed full longitudinal fasciotomies. Delay in treatment will result in ischemic infarction of muscle, nerve, and other tissue, leading to contractures and other crippling deformities (Volkmann's ischemic contracture).

Thermal Injury

While not a common mechanism of peripheral nerve injury, thermal injury either by flame, fluid, steam, or hot elements can result in neural damage ranging from a transient neurapraxia to severe neurotmesis with extensive necrosis of neural and adjacent tissue. In patients with circumferential burns, neural damage may be related to delayed, constrictive fibrosis resulting in a tourniquet effect. Severe burn patients will present with complete motor and sensory loss. The clinical examination is often difficult because of associated soft tissue injuries and extensive skin loss. The degree of tissue necrosis, the degree of bacterial contamination, and the need for an adequate soft tissue bed makes immediate nerve reconstruction rarely feasible. Proper attention to the wound with repeated escharotomy, when indicated, will increase the success of secondary repairs. Unfortunately, in thermal injury, whether by direct effect or secondary to constrictive fibrosis, long lengths of nerves are often involved, necessitating nerve grafts. In such cases, particularly with extensive involvement of muscle and soft tissue, the prognosis for functional recovery is poor.

Electrical Injury

The relatively low tissue resistance to electricity of neurovascular structures predisposes peripheral nerves to electrical damage. Contact with a high tension wire usually results in severe and widespread neural and soft tissue injury (Fig. 226-7). Whether related to the direct action of the current or the associated thermal effects, severe electrical injuries are characteristically deeply penetrating in nature with extensive destruction of tissues that may include severe, irreversible damage to nerve trunks.[3]

Although there are no clear-cut guidelines for treatment, most authors advocate initial conservative management for the neural injury. While some injuries improve, others do not, and surgical intervention with extensive resection and grafting may be necessary. As with severe burn injuries, the often diffuse involvement of the nerve and the associated soft tissue damage reduce the chances of useful recovery.

Injection Injury

Injury to peripheral nerves complicating injections of therapeutic and other agents is common. The postulated mechanism of injury includes direct needle trauma, secondary constriction by scar, and direct nerve fiber damage by neurotoxic chemicals in the agent injected. Neurological sequelae can range from minor, transient, sensory disturbance to severe sensory disturbance and motor paralysis with poor recovery. The recommended treatment has ranged from a conservative approach of nonintervention to immediate operative exposure and irrigation, and has included early neurolysis and delayed exploration with neurolysis or resection. Recent experimental studies examining the effects of a wide variety of agents implicated in injection accidents have added to our understanding of the pathophysiology of this condition and have helped provide a basis for treatment.[4]

The sciatic and radial nerves are, by far, the most com-

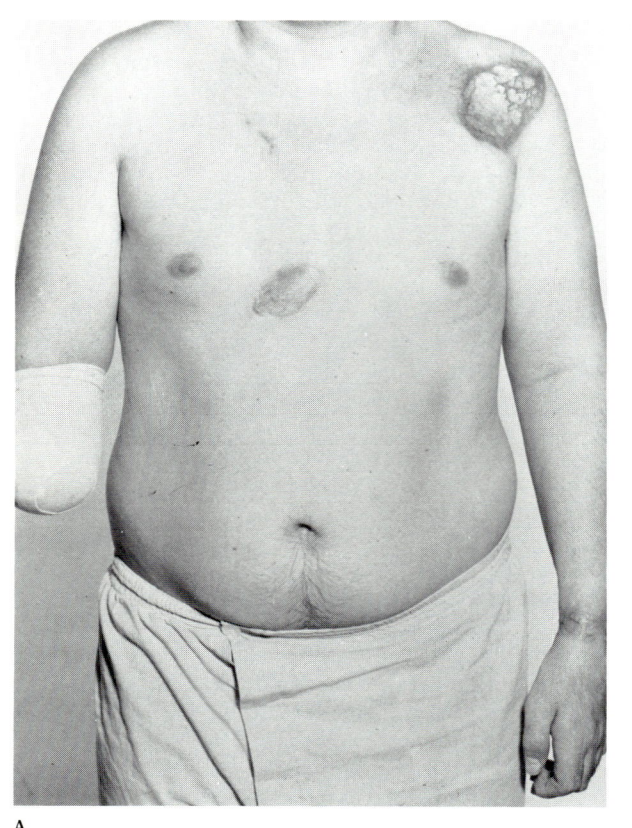

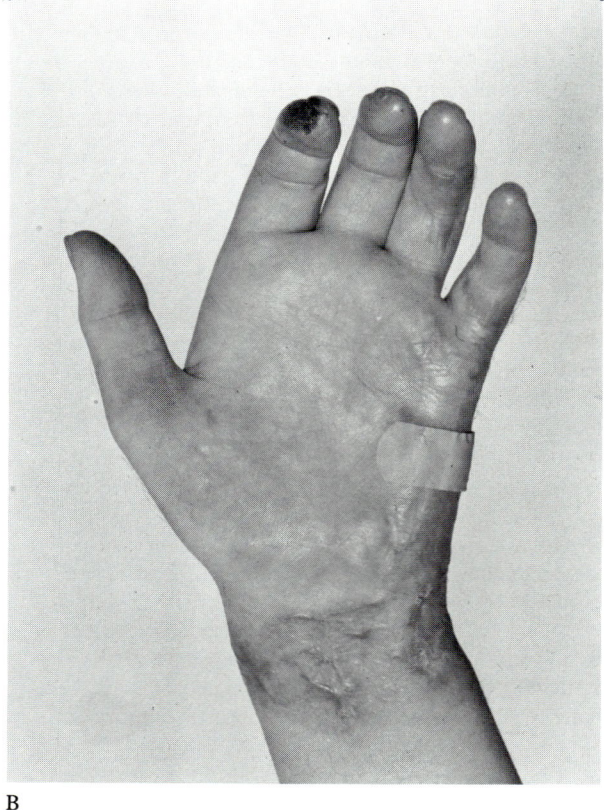

Figure 226-7 Electrical injury with lesion in continuity. *A.* Patient touched high-voltage line with right hand (amputated). *B.* Electrical current exited through the left hand. Total left median palsy resulted in a later superadded thermal burn to the left index finger and thumb. Median nerve was resected and grafted.

monly affected. Clinical features include the immediate onset of severe pain at the site of injection with, often, radiation along the course of the nerve affected. Motor and sensory disturbance, which may be partial or complete, follows rapidly.

The site of drug injection is the crucial factor in determining the degree of nerve fiber injury. Most moderate or severe injection injuries are the result of direct intrafascicular injection into the nerve trunk. The nature of the injected compound is also important, as certain drugs are much more damaging than others when injected into a peripheral nerve (Table 226-6). The toxic effect of the injected agent is related to direct injury of the nerve fiber unit, and more severe injuries are associated with wallerian degeneration.

Whereas experimentally regeneration is a constant finding in nerves damaged by injection injuries, clinically this is not always the case. The prognosis for recovery will, as with other injuries, depend to some extent on the specific nerve involved and the level of injection. Early return of function is important as a prognostic indicator for further subsequent recovery.

In view of the intraneural location of the pathological changes that begin quite soon following injury, any attempt

TABLE 226-6 Degree of Nerve Fiber Damage following Injection Injury (Rat Sciatic Nerve)

Agent	Degree of Nerve Fiber Injury	
	Extrafascicular Injection	Intrafascicular Injection
1. Gentamicin sulfate (Garamycin; Schering Co., Pointe Claire, Quebec, Canada)	+	++
2. Cephalothin sodium (Keflin; Eli Lilly Co., Scarborough, Ontario, Canada)	+	++
3. Benzylpenicillin (Penicillin G potassium; Ayerst Co., St. Laurent, Quebec, Canada)	+++	+++
4. Chloramphenicol succinate sodium (Chloromycetin; Parke, Davis & Co., Scarborough, Ontario, Canada)	+	++
5. Diazepam (Valium; Roche Laboratories, Chambly, Quebec, Canada)	++	+++
6. Chlorpromazine hydrochloride (Largactil; Poulenc Co., Montreal, Quebec, Canada)	++	+++
7. Meperidine hydrochloride (Demerol; Winthrop Laboratories, Aurora, Ontario, Canada)	+	+++
8. Dimenhydrinate (Gravol; Horner Co., Mount Royal, Quebec, Canada)	++	+++
9. Tetanus toxoid (Connaught Laboratories, Willowdale, Ontario, Canada)	++	+++
10. Iron-dextran (Imferon; Fisons Co., Scarborough, Ontario, Canada)	+	++
11. Potassium chloride (Glaxo Co., Toronto, Ontario, Canada)	+	+
12. Lidocaine hydrochloride (Xylocaine; Astra Chemicals Ltd., Mississauga, Ontario, Canada)	−	++
13. Bupivacaine (Marcaine; Winthrop Laboratories, Aurora, Ontario, Canada)	−	+
14. Mepivacaine (Carbocaine; Winthrop Laboratories, Aurora, Ontario, Canada)	−	+
15. Procaine (Novocain; Winthrop Laboratories, Aurora, Ontario, Canada)	−	+++
16. Dexamethasone (Decodrose; Merck Sharp & Dohme; Point Claire, Quebec, Canada)	−	+
17. Hydrocortisone sodium succinate (Solu-Cortef; Upjohn Canada, Don Mills, Ontario, Canada)	−	+++
18. Triamcinolone acetonide (Kenalog; Squibb Canada, Montreal, Quebec, Canada)	−	++
19. Methylprednisolone acetate (Depo-Medrol; Upjohn Canada, Don Mills, Ontario, Canada)	−	++
20. Physiological saline, 0.9%	−	−

Key: −, no nerve damage; +, minimal nerve fiber injury; ++ moderate nerve injury with focal axonal and myelin change; +++ severe nerve fiber injury with widespread axonal and myelin degeneration.

at early operative intervention would appear to be of little value. Both clinical and experimental data would suggest that initially the patient should be managed conservatively along the well-established lines for patients suffering from lesions in continuity. It is essential, however, that these lesions be followed closely and that conservative management not be prolonged in those patients who do not exhibit recovery at the expected time following injury. Follow-up studies of large series reveal that the majority of patients have some residual motor deficit.[1]

At operation, careful inspection of the nerve is important, although the external appearance may be misleading in view of the intraneural location of the pathology. Intraoperative electrophysiological studies are helpful in assessing the presence and rate of regeneration, and in deciding whether resection and suture is indicated. Care must be taken to appreciate the whole extent of the lesion, which often affects a much longer segment of nerve than might be expected. Rarely, severe causalgia-like pain will persist in the distribution of the injected nerve despite adequate motor recovery and require sympathetic block, sympathectomy, or surgical exploration. As with other iatrogenic nerve injuries, prevention must play a major role in the overall management of injection injuries.

References

1. Clark WK: Surgery for injection injuries of peripheral nerves. Surg Clin North Am 52:1325–1328, 1972.
2. Denny-Brown D, Brenner C: Paralysis of nerve induced by direct pressure and tourniquet. Arch Neurol Psychiatry 51:1–26, 1944.
3. DiVincenti FC, Moncrief JA, Pruitt BA Jr: Electrical injuries: A review of 65 cases. J Trauma 9:497–507, 1969.
4. Gentili F, Hudson AR, Hunter D: Clinical and experimental aspects of injection injuries of peripheral nerves. Can J Neurol Sci 7:143–151, 1980.
5. Gilliat RW: Physical injury to peripheral nerves: Physiologic and electrodiagnostic aspects. Mayo Clin Proc 56:361–370, 1981.
6. Lundborg G: Ischemic nerve injury: Experimental studies on intraneural microvascular pathophysiology and nerve function in a limb subjected to temporary circulatory arrest. Scand J Plast Reconstr Surg [Suppl] 6:1–113, 1970.
7. Lundborg G: Structure and function of the intraneural microvessels as related to trauma, edema formation, and nerve function. J Bone Joint Surg 57A:938–948, 1975.
8. Lundborg G: Intraneural microcirculation and peripheral nerve barriers. Techniques for evaluation—clinical implications, in Omer GE Jr, Spinner M (eds): *Management of Peripheral Nerve Problems.* Philadelphia, Saunders, 1980, pp 903–916.
9. Rudge P, Ochoa J, Gilliatt RW: Acute peripheral nerve compression in the baboon. J Neurol Sci 23:403–420, 1974.
10. Samii M: Fascicular peripheral nerve repair, in Ransohoff J (ed): *Modern Techniques in Surgery: Neurosurgery.* Mount Kisco, Futura Publishing, 1980, pp 1–17.
11. Seddon HJ: Three types of nerve injury. Brain 66:237–288, 1943.
12. Seddon HJ: *Surgical Disorders of the Peripheral Nerves.* Edinburgh, Churchill Livingstone, 1972.
13. Spinner M: *Injuries to the Major Branches of Peripheral Nerves of the Forearm,* 2d ed. Philadelphia, Saunders, 1978.
14. Sunderland S: *Nerves and Nerve Injuries,* 2d ed. Edinburgh, Churchill Livingstone, 1978, pp 133–141.

227
Pathophysiology of Peripheral Nerve Trauma

Thomas B. Ducker

The peripheral nervous system works with the central system as a single functioning unit. If the peripheral system is diseased, inadequate or incorrect information is passed to and from the periphery. Degenerative changes then occur in the distal peripheral nerves and muscles. In the pathophysiological events after peripheral nerve trauma, the normal metabolic and anatomical state is deranged within the central nervous system, at the cell body, along the axon, in the distal segment, and soon within the distal muscle and end organs. Many types of injuries occur to the peripheral nervous system, and different types of injuries will produce different symptoms and pathophysiological events. But to begin this chapter, I will discuss complete injuries of the nerve trunk.

Injury to a peripheral nerve axon that divides it in half involves removal of a large portion of nerve cell volume; however, the biochemical machinery for survival and repair remains intact within the central cell body in the spinal cord or dorsal ganglion. Nerve cells must synthesize large amounts of structural materials and transport these materials over relatively long distances. The mature nerve cell is among the most metabolically active cells in the body. In axonal injury, profound changes take place in the structure, biochemical properties, metabolic activity, and physiological properties of the central cell bodies.[5] Some of these processes are viewed as necessary for repair but others are not.[4,15] After axonal injury, chromatolysis, nuclear eccentricity, nucleolar enlargement, and cell swelling are the most obvious morphological changes seen during the retrograde response.[13] These changes have been associated with an enhanced formation of cytoplasmic ribonucleic acid (RNA) and a reorganization of these proteins to an active state directed toward the rebuilding of axoplasm and recovery of peripheral connections in the peripheral axon.[3]

Although injury to an axon may occur many centimeters from the central trophic cell, its effect is felt all the way back to the central cell body in the central nervous system. The transformation of DNA to RNA is the beginning of the rebuilding process. The RNA is translated into amino acids to yield appropriate polypeptides to make proteins in the axoplasm. Materials required for transmitter function are decreased, while materials required for regeneration of the axon are elevated during this time. For example, in adrenergic neurons there are decreases in monamine oxidase, dopa decarboxylase, and tyrosine hydroylase after axotomy.[4] Similarly, decreases in acetylcholinesterase and choline acetyltransferase have been reported in axotomized cholinergic neurons.[13] In contrast, the activity of glucose-6-phosphate dehydrogenase, a key enzyme for the biosynthesis of nucleic acids and lipids, is significantly elevated.[8,15] The proteins formed in the central cell migrate down the axon via axoplasmic transport or axoplasmic flow. The entire nerve depends on the central cells' ability to make these proteins.

A number of histochemical and biochemical studies have demonstrated that the activity of glucose-6-phosphate dehydrogenase is increased in the pentose phosphate pathway of spinal anterior horn cells, facial nucleus neurons, and sympathetic ganglion cells, all of which direct axons to peripheral structures.[15] Increases in this activity are not observed in neuronal perikarya, whose axons undergo wallerian degeneration without regeneration. The increases in glucose-6-phosphate dehydrogenase are associated with increased metabolism of glucose via the pentose phosphate pathway and occurs in the absence of any gross alteration in ATP utilization and oxygen consumption.[8]

The process of regeneration in nerve cell bodies is complicated by the simultaneous occurrence of extensive hydrolytic activity during increased biosynthetic activity. It appears that the increased hydrolytic activity is related to digestion of transmitter storage granules in the axotomized nerve cells. It is not known whether these particular changes are necessary for axonal sprouting and regeneration to occur.

The metabolism of nerve regeneration is influenced by many factors, for example, age. It is apparent that younger patients have better regenerative powers than older patients. Pertinent histological and temporal characteristics of the retrograde responses of various classes of neurons in young animals have recently been reviewed by Brodal.[4] Data concerning biochemical differences between young and mature axotomized nerve cells are minimal and do not clearly point out the mechanisms that account for the greater regenerative capacity in the neural tissue of immature animals. These differences reflect only one aspect of the major biological problem of the nature and control of cellular differentiation, which is itself not completely understood.

Glial cells, which form the supportive structure of the central nervous system, are thought to help to regulate the metabolic events external to the neuron. Glial cells in close association with axotomized neuronal perikarya undergo alterations that influence the metabolic changes accompanying neuronal regeneration. Shortly after axotomy, a proliferation of microglia close to axotomized perikarya can be found. Hypertrophy of astrocytes suggest activation of metabolism in the glia surrounding the injured neurons.[13]

After a peripheral nerve has been injured, the responses are at first degenerative and later regenerative. Strict classification of events as either degenerative or regenerative is not possible because of the interdependence of all parts of the nervous system. Regeneration of a damaged axon requires the restoration of large quantities of axonal lipids and proteins. Synthesis of these lipids and proteins occurs in the nerve cell body and they are delivered by one of many distinct transport systems to the growing axon. The materials are transported at different rates. The slower components of the system may be mediated by peristalsis in the nerve trunk plasma while the fast component involves active participation of microtubules. Results have been obtained from studies on the effect of axotomy on fast axonal transport.[10,11,14] Within 24 h material transported from the cell body accumulates at the injury site in the form of terminal bulbs. Subsequently, a growth cone is formed, which is a motile structure with a contractile mechanism involving actin and a myosin-like protein that leads the regenerating axonal tip.[10] It has been demonstrated in rats that rapidly transported proteins are carried past the level of axotomy into the regenerating nerve sprouts. Material moves down the sprouts at the normal rate of about 400 mm per day. Although rates of axoplasmic flow may not be altered in the regenerating axon, evidence has been obtained of an increase in the amount of protein transported. Material consolidates behind the tip and the physical characteristics of the growth cone are different from those of the rest of the axon. The tip is more fluid, more permeable to the movement of calcium ions, and higher in energy consumption and is pushed forward. There appears to be a reordering of proteins in the central cell body, as has been pointed out. The production of proteins associated with transmitter function is decreased, while that of proteins needed for the repair process is increased.[8]

When the nerve is disrupted, a gap between the separated ends fills either with hematoma or adjacent tissue. Within 1 h of cutting a peripheral nerve, the proximal end of the nerve swells and a retrograde response occurs to various degrees. The extent of the local retrograde changes depends on the kind of injury. The proximal swelling from the point of disruption is approximately 1 cm, an amount greater than previously realized. The cross-sectional area of the nerve increases threefold.[7] The swelling consists of both intracellular and extracellular edema with a gel-like amorphous substance, which contains large quantities of acid mucopolysaccharides. Subsiding slowly after a week, the swelling does not prevent the open end of the nerve from healing over, which occurs within the first 48 h after injury.

After a week, vigorous sprouting of axons can be seen. In traumatic blast wounds, the axonal sprouting may be 1 to 3 cm proximal to the point of the severed end.[6,8] In a clean operative sectioning, this occurs for only a few millimeters retrograde. After 1 to 3 weeks, axon buds begin to advance across the anastomosis of a primary neurorrhaphy.[12] The anabolic hypertrophic phase of the cell body in the spinal cord or dorsal ganglion occurs concomitantly with the onset of budding and regeneration. Most of the evidence to date indicates that there is a delay of a few days before the axon sprouts cross a repair site.[5,9,12] Thus, it would be ideal to repair an injured nerve when the regenerative efforts of the nerve are at their maximum.

Little information exists concerning the biological signal that initiates nerve sprouting. Considerable evidence exists that trophic interactions between nerves and target tissues regulate innervation.[10] One hypothesis of how this regulation works is that the target tissues continually manufacture a substance that serves to stimulate sprouting; the substance is neutralized in a negative feedback manner by the release of neural factors carried to the nerve endings by axoplasmic flow.[2] This hypothesis also serves to explain "denervation sprouting" and collateral sprouting.

Neurite elongation and transportation of chemical energy to sustain the process are central issues in nerve regeneration. Neurite elongation appears to originate at growth cones, situated at the tips of axons, which are characterized by a profuse elaboration of microspikes, which establish the direction for growth. The direction and amount of branching displayed by a growing axon are also influenced by adhesions between the cell surface and the substrate upon which it grows. Thus, initiation as well as maintenance of neurite elongation may involve changes in the cell surface. Factors in the immediate environment of the growth cone that influence the regeneration include not only the surround physical-chemical properties but also the presence of trophic and antitrophic compounds. These compounds in the immediate environment are apparently taken up by the axonal tip and alter the axonal metabolic state of the cell. Denervated muscle releases trophic factors, while dead cells, necrotic tissue, etc. release antitrophic or inhibitory factors.[10]

It is unlikely that sustained axonal growth could or would occur without increased metabolic activity during the retrograde reaction. This hypothesis is supported by the finding that the rate of axonal outgrowth is faster after the second of two successive axonal injuries.[10] Presumably, this occurs because the necessary metabolic adaptation for optimal axonal regeneration has taken place prior to the second injury.

Often, within hours and clearly within a few days after a nerve transection, the Schwann cells in the adjacent area begin to phagocytize their own myelin. Two or three days after injury, there is a cellular proliferation in both the proximal and distal stumps of nearly all elements; the Schwann cells, the perineural epithelial cells, and the epineurium increase in metabolic activity. The response of these cells is in part proportional to the severity of the injury.[9] Battle injuries of peripheral nerves are characterized by a marked inflammatory response and retrograde demarcation of the nerve anatomy several centimeters from the actual point of severance of the nerve. Conversely, the response of the Schwann cell is less in a clean operative injury or knife cut.

At the site of the injury, supportive cells from both stumps dominate the dynamic and metabolic action in the early post-traumatic period, when there are the earliest signs of axonal budding and regeneration. The orientation of the mesenchyme cells left behind after the debridement of Schwann cells is dependent on the state of the wound and on the local geometry rather than on processes such as chemotaxis.[12] There is good evidence that indicates that these cellular structures can be longitudinally aligned by mechanical devices such as wraps or tubes.[6,7]

Regardless of the timing, a nerve repair causes both proximal and distal stumps to swell, and the amount of the swelling may be up to three times the normal cross-sectional area of the nerve in humans.[7] Studies indicate that silicone rubber tubes possess physical properties that can force longitudinal alignment without constricting the nerve.[6,7] The larger tubes or cuffs allow for swelling in the immediate postrepair period and may provide the physical properties to force longitudinal alignment. Very carefully performed nerve anastomosis, with multiple small suture approximation of the epineurium, can accomplish the same goals. With careful repair of the epineurium, the biological properties of that layer in clean wounds surpasses any advantage gained by a mechanical cuff. As the edema decreases, the neuron bud advances and moves into the intercellular spaces. With the more direct axonal spanning there should be improvement in functional return.[9]

It must be stressed that the response to injury of the supportive structure is immediate, thick collagen being laid down 3 weeks after injury, and that the response of the neuron at the site of injury is often delayed until axonal budding and regeneration take place. Pathophysiologically speaking, a properly planned operative repair would place the injured neurons on a more equal footing with the supportive elements.

Wallerian degeneration of the nerve occurs from the death of all neuronal elements distal to the site of injury. Certain supportive peripheral nerve trunk substances survive. This term should not be applied to changes in the proximal stump or trunk. After nerve injury digestive enzymes are present in the axonal segments; the majority of neuronal elements break down within a week and the surrounding myelin undergoes fragmentation and is digested by the Schwann cells. By the end of 6 weeks, the cellular debris is phagocytized and debridement of the area is nearly complete. The fascicular anatomy persists in the distal nerve, although the endoneural sheaths either shrink or become nonexistent over a period of time. The entire nerve shrinks and in time the shrinkage may become irreversible and downgrade the prognosis of an unduly postponed nerve repair. The neuroectoderm and mesenchymal elements are in part dependent on the nerve fibers to maintain anatomical and metabolic existence.

With the penetration of new axons, the Schwann cell again increases in metabolic activity but not for phagocytic action. Fresh myelin is formed around the axon. As regeneration occurs, the original anatomy is reconstituted. If the axon regenerates successfully, the peripheral nerve never grows as large as it was originally. The smaller size accounts for the slower conduction times in the distal nerve trunk. Regeneration down most peripheral distal nerve trunks averages about 1 mm per day or 1 in. per month. Initially, however, there is a delay until the axon is clearly across the anastomosis; then, in some cases, regeneration may occur as fast as 3 mm per day. There is a slowing of the regenerative process with the formation of new connections with the muscle or sensory organs or both.

Practically all metabolites in the regenerating peripheral nerve trunk come from the central cell body by axoplasmic flow. The size of the central cell body and the metabolic activity may peak after the initial injury, but it peaks again at the end of the regeneration process when the myoneural junctions are being formed. In fact, the building of a new synaptic plate together with the return of a trophic perikaryal stimulus to and from the peripheral structures may cause metabolism to increase in the central cell body more than in the immediate post-traumatic period. Additional metabolites are required for maturation, formation of new myoneural junctions, attachments to sensory organs, and other processes.

Peripheral nerves influence biochemical and electrophysiological properties of skeletal muscles. After nerve injury, shrinkage of muscle cells occurs, endomysium and perimysium thicken, and atrophy of muscle spindles can be found. These changes may be ascribed in part to a loss of neurotrophic factors supplied to the muscles. The early alterations that occur after nerve section or injury include a decline in resting membrane potential, the appearance of extrajunctional acetylcholine sensitivity, and a decrease in muscle phosphocreatine.[1] The time course of these changes is dependent on the distance from the muscle at which the nerve is transected as well as on the type of muscle denervated. In general, these changes take place over the first 3 days after nerve section in small mammals. Muscle atrophy begins at 2 to 16 weeks in animals (somewhat later in humans). After 2 years or more, muscle fibers may fragment and disintegrate.[2] It must be noted that such changes take place despite good physical therapy or intermittent external electrical stimulation. Any denervation atrophy of the muscle is harmful because the thickening of the muscle sheath hinders end plate formation, and formation of fibrous tissue in and around the muscle interferes with nerve regrowth and muscle contraction. Thus, the sooner a nerve establishes connection with the muscle, the more likely it is that the metabolism and the anatomy of the muscle will be preserved. If reinnervation is delayed 1 year, function is poor. A delay of 2 years allows irreversible changes to occur in the muscle cells and negates any hope of motor return even with nerve repair.

As compared with muscles, the sensory end organs are less dependent on innervation for survival. In fact, a World War II study yielded no evidence that the time from injury to nerve repair has any influence on sensory recovery.

General factors influence the recovery from nerve injury. The age of the patient, the type of wound, and the type of nerve involved all affect regeneration. Of all these factors the age of the patient is the most important. There are no good statistical studies to verify that younger patients do better with regeneration following peripheral nerve injuries but all experienced surgeons have made this observation. Clinically, one suspects that growth hormone may be helpful. There is evidence that thyroid hormone promotes peripheral nerve regeneration; however, the clinical usefulness of thyroid hormone in patients with injured or transected peripheral nerves has not been fully evaluated.

The type of wound wherein the nerve was injured is important. Massive blast injuries result in thick scar formation and delayed healing. A regenerating nerve may become scarred in such injuries and motor recovery will fail. The blast injury can also result in distal ischemia of the limb with irreversible changes in all structures. Multiply injured patients may also suffer from a catabolic metabolic state, which will adversely influence nerve regeneration.

Another factor to consider is that the higher the animal on the phylogenetic scale, the more complex is the regeneration process and the less effective is the end result. Consequently, rat experiments cannot be readily applied to the human clinical situation. Within the human nervous system, certain neuronal pathways are phylogenetically older than others. Pain fiber regrowth may exceed proprioceptive fiber regrowth and leave the patient with pain and no useful function. Consequently, these systemic and general factors influence the final result, but the local injury and its extent are the most important.

Local injuries can be classified, like all nervous tissue injuries, into concussion, contusion, laceration, etc.

By definition, concussion of the brain means a transient neuronal dysfunction. The same term applies in the peripheral nervous system. Although concussions are rare, they usually occur as a result of an injury from a blunt object or a high-velocity missile in an area distant from the nerve. Not much information is available on the mechanism of this injury. The nerve may be grossly and microscopically normal. In some experimental studies, the large fiber myelin sheath close to the point of injury will become swollen and show a little disintegration while the nerve distal to the injury will remain normal and not have wallerian degeneration. In some cases the patient may be unable to use a nerve distal to the injury and yet the nerve will respond to an electrical stimulus. Motor and sensory functions return rapidly. When there is a prolonged delay in the return of function, the injury is probably not just a concussion. The metabolic processes just discussed are not called into play for the pathophysiology at most centers of a transient depression of conduction and segmental myelin repair.

The term contusion implies definite bruising of the peripheral nerve. Axonal disruption at the site of injury leads to complete disintegration of the distal axon. Regeneration must occur before function returns. During axonotmesis, in both the degeneration and the regeneration stages, much of the perineurium remains intact. At the site of injury, however, there is disruption of the axon, which then seals itself, buds, and regenerates back down the fascicle structure. While there is distal wallerian degeneration with nerve regrowth, remyelination takes place readily. The pathophysiological changes within the nervous tissue demand all the changes within the control cell, etc., but the adverse factors at the injury site are minimal. This type of contusion, in which regeneration takes place without an operation, can occur after blunt injuries, fractures, gunshot wounds, etc. It has also become apparent that this type of injury also occurs with injection injuries to the peripheral nerve that produce a chemical contusion.

A peripheral nerve can be contused sufficiently to disrupt all the fascicular anatomy but still have its external surface remain in continuity. There is complete severance of the axons and their myelin sheaths and gross derangement of the connective tissue. There is no successful regeneration. This injury is seen with high-velocity gunshot wounds, which can contuse the nerve's inner anatomy so badly as to destroy it. Direct chemical injury can also derange the fascicular anatomy. With this type of injury, the Schwann cell reacts and begins to digest all the myelin. Axonal segments degenerate, and connective tissue proliferates at the injury site, preventing anatomical anastomosis during axonal regeneration.

Once a human nerve has undergone complete physical division or *laceration*, there is no possible regeneration without operative repair. When the injury is by laceration, the associated tissue trauma is not great and the reaction is contained to the area, not extending proximally or distally. With gunshot wounds, derangement may extend in both directions. In both contusion without regeneration and laceration, operative repair is required for there to be any hope of regeneration into the distal nerve trunk.

When a nerve is pulled beyond the strength of the perineurium, a *traction injury* occurs. This injury is common in shoulder trauma. Nerve concussion, contusion, and disruption can all occur with brachial plexus injuries. At times the nerve roots may be pulled from the spinal cord. Often little can be done, and clearly no regeneration is possible when the central cell is literally pulled from its environment within the spinal cord.

Accidental contact with high-voltage electric wires can severely *burn* skin and deep tissues. The damage to the nerves in the area can be very extensive. The current can pass through the peripheral nerve even to the central cell bodies and cause central damage, which reduces any hope for regeneration.

Compression and ischemia injuries to a peripheral nerve can occur by many mechanisms, including hematoma formation and entrapment by bone. If compression is mild and of short duration, the nerve suffers only a concussion and/or mild contusion with regeneration. However, if compression is prolonged, the nerve may undergo a severe contusion without regeneration and may form a neuroma. In extreme cases, the nerve may undergo complete disruption. Generally if the fascicular anatomy is maintained and the local problem is corrected, the nerve will recover spontaneously by the mechanisms I have outlined.

In conclusion, in the care of peripheral nerve trauma one must consider both the central and the local pathophysiological responses, which are interdependent and together will influence the outcome of therapy.

References

1. Albuquerque EX, McIsaac RJ: Fast and slow mammalian muscles after denervation. Exp Neurol 26:183–202, 1970.
2. Aquilar CE, Bisby MA, Cooper E, Diamond J: Evidence that axoplasmic transport of trophic factors is involved in the regulation of peripheral nerve fields in salamanders. J Physiol (Lond) 234:449–464, 1973.
3. Brattgard SO, Edström JE, Hyden H: The productive capacity of the neuron in retrograde reaction. Exp Cell Res [Suppl] 5:185–200, 1958.
4. Brodal A: Anterograde and retrograde degeneration of nerve cells in the central nervous system, in Haymaker W, Adams RD (eds): *Histology and Histopathology of the Nervous System*. Springfield, Ill, Charles C Thomas, 1982, pp 276–362.
5. Ducker TB: Pathophysiology of peripheral nerve trauma, in Omer GE Jr, Spinner M (eds): *Management of Peripheral Nerve Problems*. Philadelphia, Saunders, 1980, pp 475–486.
6. Ducker TB, Hayes GJ: Peripheral nerve injuries: A comparative study of the anatomical and functional results following primary nerve repair in chimpanzees. Milit Med 133:298–302, 1968.
7. Ducker TB, Hayes GJ: Experimental improvements in the use of silastic cuff for peripheral nerve repair. J Neurosurg 28:582–587, 1968.
8. Ducker TB, Kauffman FC: Metabolic factors in surgery of peripheral nerves. Clin Neurosurg 24:406–424, 1977.
9. Ducker TB, Kempe LG, Hayes GJ: The metabolic background for peripheral nerve surgery. J Neurosurg 30:270–280, 1969.
10. Grafstein B, McQuarrie IG: Role of the nerve cell body in axonal regeneration, in Cotman CW (ed): *Neuronal Plasticity*. New York, Raven Press, 1978, pp 155–195.
11. Grafstein B, Murray M: Transport of protein in goldfish optic nerve during regeneration. Exp Neurol 25:494–508, 1969.
12. Kline DG, Hayes GJ, Morse AS: A comparative study of response of species to peripheral-nerve injuries. I: Severance. II: Crush and severance with primary suture. J Neurosurg 21:968–979, 980–988, 1964.
13. Lieberman AR: The axon reaction: A review of the principal features of perikaryal responses to axon injury. Int Rev Neurobiol 14:49–124, 1971.
14. Ochs S: Systems of material transport in nerve fibers (axoplasmic transport) related to nerve function and trophic control. Ann NY Acad Sci 228:202–223, 1974.
15. Robins E, Kissane JM, Lowe IP: Quantitative biochemical studies of chromatolysis, in Folch-Pi J (ed): *Chemical Pathology of the Nervous System*. Oxford, Pergamon Press, 1961, pp 244–247.

228
Brachial Plexus Injuries

Alan R. Hudson
B. Tranmer

The enthusiasm which greeted the application of modern electrophysiological and microsurgical techniques to patients suffering from brachial plexus injury has resulted in a false sense of optimism. The problem of major permanent motor and sensory disability remains. Although brachial plexus injury does not shorten life, it frequently results in permanent neurological crippling of a young, productive individual (Fig. 228-1).

Review of the extensive literature on brachial plexus injury reveals that there has been a tendency for practitioners to be polarized in their management strategies. On the one hand, an essentially nihilistic viewpoint is held, adherents of which claim that whatever improvement follows a traction brachial plexus injury is a result of the natural history of regeneration and healing of partially injured elements and that nerve grafting or other nerve operation cannot improve the outcome. The British World War II experience of open plexus injuries was reviewed by Brooks, who concluded that exploration of open wounds was rarely justified.[1] This conservative attitude is maintained to the present day, and Brooks emphasizes that congenital anatomical variation may account for many "successes" that follow surgery for either open or closed injury.

On the other hand, an aggressive viewpoint is espoused by those who claim that improvement following surgery is the direct result of this interference with the natural history following peri- and intraneural scarring and nerve fiber destruction. Narakas has reported extensive brachial plexus operations in a series of patients, including 615 with traction or crush lesions. Many of these cases would have been considered inoperable in the past. Critics of these extensive microsurgical procedures point to the lack of any randomized trial of the therapies.

A reasonable course for the surgeon in the next decade might well be a middle path on which the surgeon guides his patient to ensure that advantage is taken of every recent improvement in peripheral nerve surgical technique without adopting either an overly gloomy or an overly optimistic outlook. A proponent of this balanced approach is Kline who, with Judice, analyzed 171 cases and emphasized the necessity of an exact anatomical delineation of the injury.[11] Brachial plexus injury is an extremely broad term, which covers a wide variety of lesions affecting an infinite variety of plexus elements. Long a champion of intraoperative electrical measurement, Kline has used this technique, in conjunction with preoperative clinical and electrophysiological exclusion and inclusion criteria, to define more exactly which operative technique should be employed and what the extent of the operation should be.

Millesi has promoted the sequential microsurgical procedures of external neurolysis, internal neurolysis, and autologous grafting.[14] He has reported that these maneuvers and non-neural reconstructive procedures may give results superior to those of nonoperative approach if nerve injury is so severe as to prevent axonal transmission. This statement is particularly true of injuries to the C5 and C6 spinal nerves, upper trunk injuries, and posterior cord injuries. Unfortunately, severe injuries to the eighth cervical and first dorsal spinal nerves, the lower trunk, and the medial cord are still resistant to most forms of direct nerve surgery. A small

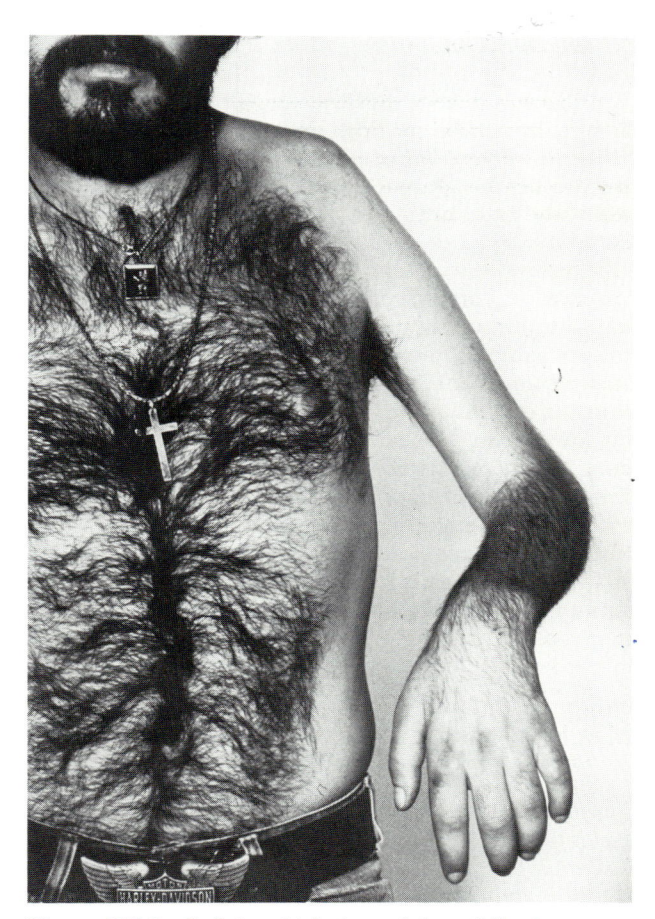

Figure 228-1 Left brachial plexus injury following a motorcycle accident. The swollen, shiny, anesthetic, paralyzed distal limb results from avulsion of the C7, C8, and T1 roots. Partial injury to the upper plexus elements is also present; weak elbow flexion is possible. Shoulder abduction, however, is accomplished by scapular rotation with minimal deltoid action. The abrupt alteration of this patient's masculine self-image had significant psychological consequences.

motor and sensory improvement can be of vital importance to the patient and may prevent subsequent arm amputation. However, the enthusiasm that greets these crucial improvements should not delude modern surgeons into thinking that the problem of brachial plexus injury is solved. A great deal of research is yet required in the basic neurobiology of nerve regeneration, and this is particularly apparent if one quantitates the loss, rather than the gain, which is apparent on review 2 years after a patient has suffered a serious brachial plexus injury.

Brachial plexus injuries are not uncommon. Our own experience involves 226 cases (174 males, with a mean age of 33 years, and 52 females, with a mean age of 34 years). These have been encountered among 1000 consecutive patients suffering from a significant nerve injury and examined by the senior author. Of the 226 brachial plexus cases, 145 had operative treatment and 49 received autologous nerve grafts.

Anatomy

The anatomy of the brachial plexus injury above the clavicle follows the standard text description in most cases. One of the major purposes of the clinical evaluation is that of defining whether the injury is to root, spinal nerve, trunk (situated in the posterior triangle), or cord (situated in the axilla). Surgeons should distinguish between the terms *nerve root* and *spinal nerve* with care, as this designation has particular significance in brachial plexus injuries.[18] Below the clavicle, the surgeon should not be surprised to find congenital variations in plexus anatomy. No surgeon should attempt brachial plexus surgery until he is totally "at home" in the posterior triangle and axilla of the cadaver. Once the vista of normal anatomy is clouded by scarring, considerable experience is required if the operator is not to cause further damage in the tedious dissection. The surgeon must be both a master of gross anatomy and microtechnique and must be prepared to devote many hours to the dissection of neural and vascular elements. It is stressed that current undergraduate anatomy courses do not provide the degree of facility required.

Mechanisms of Injury

The mechanism of injury resulting from a sharp plexus incision is the same as that encountered in any peripheral nerve. The effect of stretch on peripheral nerve is similar throughout the body, but specific anatomical relationships contribute to characteristic patterns of injury in the case of brachial plexus stretch.

The attachment of the rootlets to the spinal cord is best appreciated by the examination of an anatomical specimen. A neurosurgeon can observe the delicate rootlets during spinal operations and the radiologist can demonstrate these structures effectively by the use of water-soluble contrast material, provided sufficient concentration is maintained in the cervical area. Traction in the axis of the brachial plexus may quite literally tear these roots out of the spinal cord. Subsequent observation at open operation when performing a dorsal root entry zone procedure will reveal the absence of any dorsal proximal stumps and the presence of brownish staining of the pia in line with unaffected rootlets above and below the prime lesion. Clearly, avulsion of rootlets subtended by a single spinal nerve does not imply avulsion of all the rootlets subtending the brachial plexus, and a rootlet avulsion may coexist with brachial plexus injuries more peripherally placed in other elements of the plexus. Microscopic examination at the root entry zone reveals disruption of that site and gliosis, and it is thought that this might be a generator of a chronic pain syndrome.

Axial traction may cause tearing of the arachnoid and dura, which in turn gives rise to a characteristic pseudomeningocele formation seen at myelography. Nerve root avulsion and pseudomeningocele formation may occur independently of one another, giving rise to so-called false-positive and false-negative myelographic findings. With the advent of water-soluble contrast media, the physician is able to assess individually each root level and directly observe the rootlets, the presence or absence of subarachnoid adhesions, and the presence or absence of pseudomeningocele formation.

Axial injury may result in a proximally placed lesion, which is apparent in the presence of a normal myelogram. The spinal nerves run in the gutters on the upper surface of the transverse processes of the vertebra for which they are named and then angle inferiorly to appear between the scalenus anticus and scalenus medius muscles and thus gain the posterior triangle of the neck. The spinal nerves may be injured in a characteristic fashion just as they run off the lip of the gutter of the transverse process. The operator can palpate the tips of the transverse process during dissection and it is possible to graft onto the proximal stumps of the spinal nerves at this point. It is wise to confirm the structure of that spinal nerve before committing to a graft, as quick-frozen sections may reveal an abundance of scar or neuroma formation. On occasion the operator may be distressed to find that the quick section reveals dorsal root ganglion cells, which indicates that the posterior root has been stretched down the gutter and hence implies a lesion at a point more proximal than can be reached by conventional operation. Proximal axiotomy also induces a higher incidence of anterior horn cell death than a peripheral axiotomy, so operators should demand a normal fascicular pattern from their most proximally placed biopsy before contemplating grafting to that stump.

Stretch injury of the trunks in the posterior triangle usually results in neuromas-in-continuity and rarely in the actual tearing apart of these structures.

The clavicle, padded by the subclavius, has an important relationship to the plexus and it is extraordinary that the common clavicular fracture so rarely involves the brachial plexus. However, the entire plexus may be tethered at this point, and abduction and adduction of the arm at operation may show acute angulation of the nerve structures below the clavicle if they cannot move freely in the normal fashion. Callus from a healing clavicular fracture may on occasion impinge directly on the plexus, where it may cause a brachial plexus palsy in its own right or prolong or aggravate underlying nerve injury. Stretch injuries involving the divisions of the plexus may be extremely difficult to resolve because of the overlying clavicle, and it is in this unusual situation that we advise that the clavicle be divided to allow full exposure of all structures. Usually, by working alternatively above and below the clavicle and by pulling the clavicle forward on a sling, the operator is able to get a sufficient exposure, but this is not always the case.

In the axilla the most characteristic traction injury is that resulting from dislocation of the shoulder, which causes stretching, resulting in either avulsion or neuroma formation in the axillary nerve. The force may be transmitted directly to the posterior cord, injuring that structure, frequently subtotally. It is well to remember that the axillary nerve leaves the posterior cord at approximately the level of the coracoid process. The operator should search through the scar at that point, before dissecting down the quadrangular space. The overlying musculocutaneous nerve, issuing from the lateral cord, should be mobilized prior to this dissection on the back of the axilla or it will be compressed by the retraction used to gain exposure.

It is frequently possible to split the gross anatomical elements at the operating table. For example, the musculocutaneous nerve can be split up into the lateral cord for a considerable distance. It is possible to split the axillary nerve off the posterior cord for several centimeters. In the case of a low origin of the musculocutaneous nerve from the median nerve, it is usually possible to split that structure back via the median nerve, through the lateral head of the median nerve into the lateral cord. The suprascapular nerve may be split up the upper trunk for several centimeters. The purpose of such maneuvers is to isolate those nerve elements that are irreparably damaged and hence require excision and grafting from those elements that are composed of normal fascicles and hence require external neurolysis alone.

Characteristically, brachial plexus stretch injuries give rise to injury of more than one element. It is not unusual for injuries to roots, spinal nerves, trunks, divisions, and cords to coexist. Each case must be carefully assessed preoperatively by a combination of clinical, radiological, and electrical appraisal.

The lower spinal nerves and trunks of the plexus are intimately related to both the subclavian vein and the subclavian artery. Aneurysm formation may be related to both the subclavian vein and artery. Aneurysm formation may be the rare cause of progressive neurological disability following a peripheral nerve injury. On occasions, pseudoaneurysm formation may cause significant compression of the nerve elements in the face of a normal-appearing angiogram. Hemorrhage into the brachial plexus sheath following axillary angiography may cause a significant brachial plexus compression, and such a hematoma should be evacuated with dispatch if permanent neurological disability of the hand is to be avoided. Vascular surgeons do well to remember the intimate relationship of the cords to the axillary artery (indeed, they are so named with relationship to that artery as it passes beneath the pectoralis minor). Blind passage of vascular grafts deep to the pectoralis major or the attachment of grafts to vessels without adequate visualization and protection of the nerve structures is likely to result in permanent brachial plexus injury.

In the performance of either a supra- or infraclavicular plexus block with a local anesthetic, direct injection of the solution into a nerve element may result in temporary or permanent injury to the nerve fibers contained in that structure. We have treated patients suffering from permanent nerve damage as a result of nerve injection injury with a local anesthetic both above and below the clavicle.

Patients suffering from gunshot injuries to the brachial plexus frequently present with widespread neurological disability. These patients should be examined with the knowledge of the anatomical relationships of the pleura, vessels, and thoracic duct to the plexus, and injuries to those structures should be treated appropriately. Following injury with low-velocity civilian firearms, however, it may soon become apparent that much of the neurological disability is transient and presumably the result of the shock wave transmitted by the bullet. Persistence of neurological disability implies that the bullet or pellets have directly injured nerve structures, which then have to be managed appropriately.

The relationship of the first rib to the brachial plexus is an extremely close one, and semiblind, transaxillary resection of the first rib may lead to damage of the medial cord and permanent intrinsic hand muscle paralysis. We have very rarely seen significant nerve damage as a result of the normal anatomical relationship of the lower plexus elements to the first rib and have several examples of nerve damage caused by injudicious resection of that structure. The mechanism of injury in patients suffering from cervical rib compression of the plexus appears to be related to the drooping of shoulders that occurs in middle age. The relationship between the cervical rib and the plexus has of course been present since birth, and it appears likely that a combination of stretch and angulation and friction across the cervical rib or the band issuing from its tip is the mechanism of injury in those few cases that come to the surgeon's attention. It is essential that individual relationship of the particular rib to that particular plexus be established at operation, that the middle trunk and lower trunk and C8 and T1 spinal nerves be mobilized with care, and that the rib be adequately resected extraperiosteally so that the obvious anterior compression site is relieved as well as the less obvious posterior compression site.

The mechanism of injury following axillary operations varies. Thus, radical breast surgery may injure the plexus by incision, stretch, or cautery. It is essential that adequate incisions be made in biopsies of axillary masses. Such axillary masses are not inevitably lymph nodes. Schwannomas and neurofibromas have to be included in the differential diagnosis. The moment of production of the offending lump, with an 8-cm tail of nerve trailing behind, should not be the moment at which the diagnosis of nerve tumor is made.

In summary, the mechanism of injury of the brachial plexus is similar to mechanisms of injury to most peripheral nerves, with the additional feature of the influence of the peculiar anatomy of the brachial plexus. Each patient should be assessed and an attempt made to delineate which elements have been injured. Characteristic groupings of injury are readily recognized, such as the upper plexus injury which gives rise to Erb's palsy. Its purest form is seen in cases of obstetrical plexus stretch injury, with the limb being held in the characteristic "waiter's tip" position. If the lower plexus elements are injured (Klumpke), the disability is primarily experienced in the hand.

Pathology of Closed Injuries of the Brachial Plexus

Time and Diagnosis

A fundamental problem, for which as yet there is no solution, is that of prolonged denervation of end organs and muscle, leading to irreparable damage. Of necessity, distal limb structures suffer prolonged denervation in all but mild lower proximal brachial plexus injuries because of the time required for regenerating axons to travel from the plexus to the hand at the rate of 1 in. per month. Lack of sensibility in the hand is particularly important as a patient is usually reluctant to use the limb, regardless of proximal motor return, in the presence of an anesthetic hand. It is the exceptional case in which significant intrinsic hand muscle reinnervation occurs following a lower brachial plexus injury. This time-distance concept is of the utmost importance in the clinical management of brachial plexus injuries, as clearly any operative intervention must occur as soon as possible after injury if there is to be any hope of significant reinnervation of distal structures.

Site of Injury

The clinical distinction between intraforaminal root injury and extraforaminal spinal nerve or plexus injury is one of the first questions the surgeon must resolve on examining the patient, but it must be emphasized that a patient may harbor lesions at root, spinal nerve, and plexus levels coincidentally. Rootlet avulsion causes spinal cord injury, which is usually confined to the root entry zone. This injury may be the generator of a chronic pain syndrome.

The Lesion in Continuity

One of the major recent contributions has been an understanding of the pathology and management of lesions in continuity, which constitute the majority of the types of nerve injury seen by most civilian surgeons.[10] The nerve may be thickened, beaded, attenuated, or normal in appearance and is longitudinally in continuity. It is generally agreed that inspection and palpation of the nerve do not give a reliable indication of the pathology hidden by the surrounding epineurium. The nerve fiber injury contained within the lesion may be of the mildest proportions. For example, a fiber exhibiting segmental demyelination will contain an intact axon and a completely intact peripheral extension, synapse, and end organ and will merely require local remyelination for restoration of function. At the other extreme, a nerve, of identical outward appearance, may contain fascicles whose integrity has been completely disrupted, so that the pathway to regenerating axon sprouts is blocked by impenetrable scar. A characteristic feature of brachial plexus injuries is that sites of peripheral nerve injury are frequently multiple within the plexus structures, each composed of intrinsic injuries of varying severity. The key question is that of continuity of nerve fibers within the nerve rather than the external appearance of the structure.

In modern surgical practice it is unacceptable to ignore an injured element of the brachial plexus that has no hope of spontaneous recovery, and it is equally unacceptable to resect an injured component of the brachial plexus, which, if left alone, would be the route of superior, spontaneous regeneration. The two great contributors in this area have been Kline, who has emphasized the electrophysiological method of delineating the internal structure of the intact but injured nerve, and Millesi, who has emphasized microsurgical dissection technique for resolution of the mystery.[8-10,14] In contemporary practice, resolution of the clinical questions as to whether a patient will do better if essentially left alone or if submitted to operation and, of equal importance, the timing of these decisions, is now reasonably based on an understanding of the pathology and the microanatomy of brachial plexus injury.[9]

Diagnosis of Brachial Plexus Injury

History

The date of the onset of symptoms must be recorded prominently as it is from this point that all subsequent time measurements are made. In addition to the routine description of an injury, it is important to note the patient's report of the motor and sensory disturbance in the days immediately following the injury so that that situation can be compared with the findings obtained at the initial consultation by the neurosurgeon. The great majority of patients will report either improvement or no change. The rare occurrence of clinical deterioration of nerve function suggests the presence of a traumatic aneurysm compressing the plexus. Information regarding the patient's education, hand dominance, occupation, and avocations guides the overall management of the patient. The initial interview is of the utmost importance in establishing a good relationship with the patient, as this relationship is likely to be of at least 2 years' duration. A sense of realism must be injected at the initial consultation, as patients have frequently been recipients of either excessively pessimistic or optimistic advice. Many young patients are depressed as a result of the loss of function of a limb, so that a sympathetic appreciation of psychological factors is essential.

Physical Examination

The purpose of the physical examination, along with the history, is to delineate as accurately as possible the anatomical sites of injury in the brachial plexus. The examination itself is usually quite straightforward for those physicians who examine cases of plexus injury frequently. While there are usually no particular points of difficulty, surgeons may have some lack of fluency if they see this type of case only occasionally. As the clinical examination is critical to all planning, it is reasonable to emphasize certain key features that help the examiner to come to the correct conclusions as to which elements of the plexus are injured and whether the lesion is complete or partial. It is instructive to watch the patient undressing without aid. The practical effect of the disability can be judged and an estimation of the patient's ability to cope with motor loss can also be made provided the examiner makes allowance for the time the patient has had to practice various trick maneuvers. An estimation of the effect of pain on the patient's function may also be made at this stage.

Proximal Injury

Evidence of proximal injury should be sought at the outset, as this is a useful practical categorization of patients with brachial plexus injuries. While taking the history, the surgeon looks for evidence of a Horner's syndrome. As this is a most important physical sign, it is worth checking again at the beginning of the physical examination by dimming the lights in the consulting room. The unaffected eye will then show a dilated pupil and the affected eye will display the characteristic small pupil. If the examining room is brightly lit, this important feature may be overlooked. The presence of a Horner's syndrome implies a proximal C8-T1 injury, which is usually advertised by weak or paralyzed intrinsic hand muscles. The surgeon is virtually helpless in reversing this paralysis but may yet be able to help the patient if other elements of the plexus are reparable. Thus, a Horner's syndrome is not an absolute contraindication to surgery, but the surgeon must have a very strong indication for advising surgery in the presence of this syndrome.

The patient is then asked to face away from the examiner and attempts are made to assess the function of the rhomboid. This muscle is usually supplied from the C5 spinal nerve, so that paralysis of rhomboid function and a motor-sensory disturbance of the upper limb would indicate a proximally placed lesion. Contrariwise, display of rhomboid function in a patient with an upper plexus injury is immediately encouraging, as it suggests that the lesion is at least in a position available for surgical attack, should this subsequently be indicated. Unfortunately, the function of this muscle may be difficult to assess, even by an experienced examiner, if the overlying trapezius is excessively developed or the patient is obese. With the patient still facing away from the examiner, the serratus anterior is checked. This muscle is supplied by the long thoracic nerve derived from the C5, C6, and C7 spinal nerves, and paralysis of its function has the important connotation of a proximal lesion (Fig. 228-2). The surgeon should remember, however, that the serratus anterior may function on two of its three "motors" and possibly, weakly, on one of its motors.

By this stage, the examiner has already gathered a great deal of information concerning the proximal plexus. Although of grave prognostic importance, the finding of an abnormality in the proximal area of the plexus does not of itself exclude surgery. It is possible that reparable lesions exist in other parts of the brachial plexus subtended from normal proximal elements or that some form of neurotization may be available to the patient.

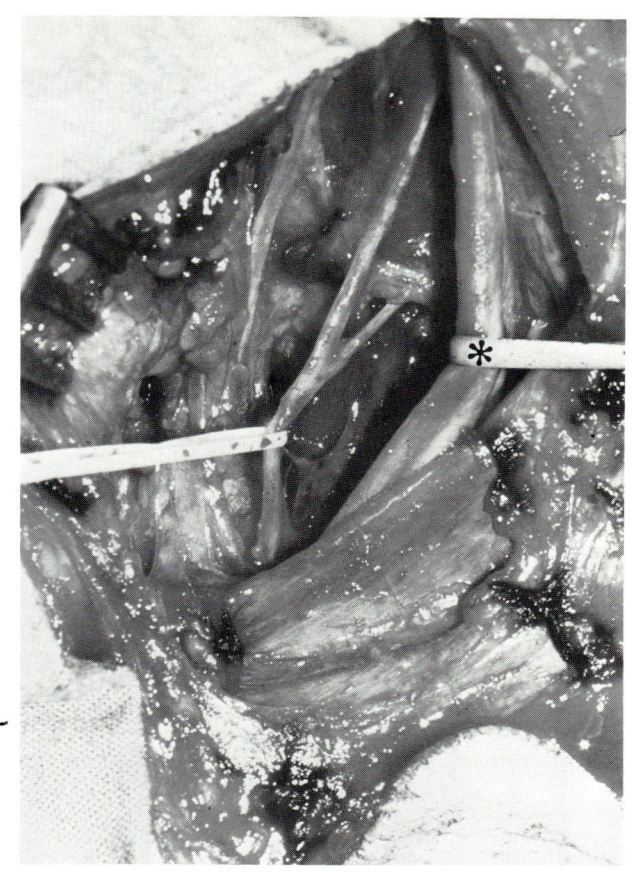

Figure 228-2 Right supraclavicular plexus exploration. The upper trunk has been pulled medially(★). The contributions from the C5 and C6 spinal nerves are seen arising from the substance of the scalenus medius and these fuse just above the sling. The contribution from the C7 spinal nerve joined the long thoracic nerve at a slightly lower level. The picture clearly illustrates that if serratus anterior palsy is present in a patient with a brachial plexus injury, the injury is at a proximal level.

Deltoid Function

With the patient still facing away from the examiner, the mass of the deltoid is next assessed. With severe paralysis, a characteristic groove is apparent between the tip of the acromion and the humerus, the result of the subluxing shoulder joint (Fig. 228-3). If this sign is present, the nerve lesion is usually at one of three sites, which is rapidly determined in the following manner. If the rhomboid is paralyzed, the lesion is proximally placed in the C5 root or spinal nerve. If the supra- and infraspinatus muscles are paralyzed (examined while the patient is still facing away from the surgeon), the lesion is in the upper trunk (the suprascapular nerve being the only branch of the trunks of the brachial plexus). In this setting, the patient will also have weakness or paralysis of elbow flexion, as the musculocutaneous nerve supplying the biceps and brachialis is a derivative of the upper trunk nerve fibers. (Very rarely, an upper trunk injury may exist distal to a proximal take-off of the suprascapular totally avulsed. Absence of an island of recovery in the presence of more general plexus recovery is one of the most important indications for surgical interference in brachial plexus injury, since this indicates that the patient clearly has irreparable injury to that particular element. The examiner must remember that some patients can abduct their glenohumeral joint by strong supraspinatus activity. In this circumstance, one of the best ways to test deltoid function is to passively abduct the humerus to 90 degrees, grasp the patient's deltoid, and then tell the patient to "take over." Any independent contraction of the deltoid can then be appreciated.

In our series of 226 brachial plexus injury patients (174 males and 52 females), we have 4 patients who exhibited evidence of combined suprascapular nerve and axillary nerve injury after shoulder dislocation. The clinical clue is that the patients have normal elbow flexion, ruling out an upper trunk injury, and normal rhomboid function, ruling out a proximal C5 injury.

We have seen two patients who exhibited solely combined deltoid and triceps palsy. There is only one place at which this injury can occur. The triceps branches leave the posterior cord in the axilla and at this point they are close in relation to the axillary nerve exiting via the quadrangular space.

Remainder of Limb Examination

Surgeons interested in brachial plexus will be sent many patients exhibiting mild to moderate periscapular wasting as a complication of shoulder joint pathology. Incorrect interpretation of minor electrophysiological changes may complicate the situation and it is not unusual to witness prolonged neurological investigation when correction of a simple orthopedic problem is all that is required. The correct diagnosis should be made at the outset and the appropriate orthopedic consultation obtained.

With the patient still facing away from the examiner, the latissimus dorsi function is assessed by having the patient cough while the surgeon grasps both latissimus dorsi muscles. The nerve supply of the latissimus dorsi is from the posterior cord in the axilla and, in the presence of a wasted deltoid, it is important to pinpoint the area of pathology as accurately as possible.

Finally, before the patient turns around, trapezius function is assessed. One of the options available to the patient might well be a shoulder fusion, so that it is important to assess at this stage the function of the great muscles acting upon the mobile pectoral girdle, as the trapezius, serratus anterior, latissimus dorsi, and pectoralis major may be called upon to be the main controllers of a fused shoulder joint.

The patient then turns around and the remainder of the motor examination is completed in routine fashion. The surgeon must be careful in assessing elbow flexion, as some patients with no musculocutaneous function (derived from the lateral cord) may have a fair degree of elbow flexion by way of the common flexor origin of the forearm muscles. Elbow flexion is assessed with care, as this movement is important to upper limb function. Elbow extension is not of nearly such clinical significance as the patient may merely release elbow flexion and obtain elbow extension by gravity.

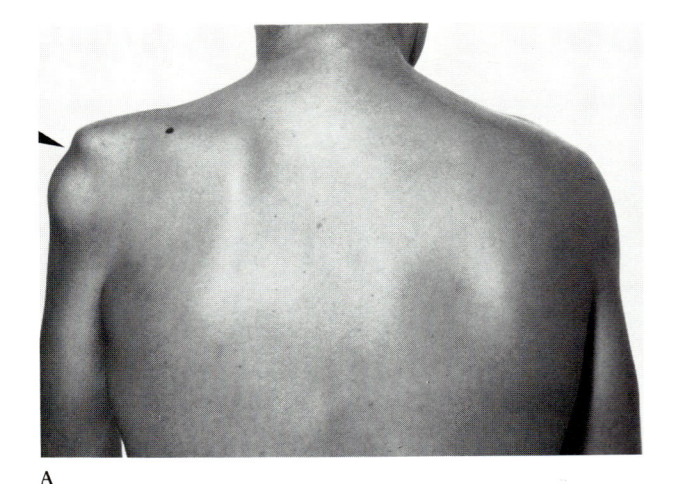

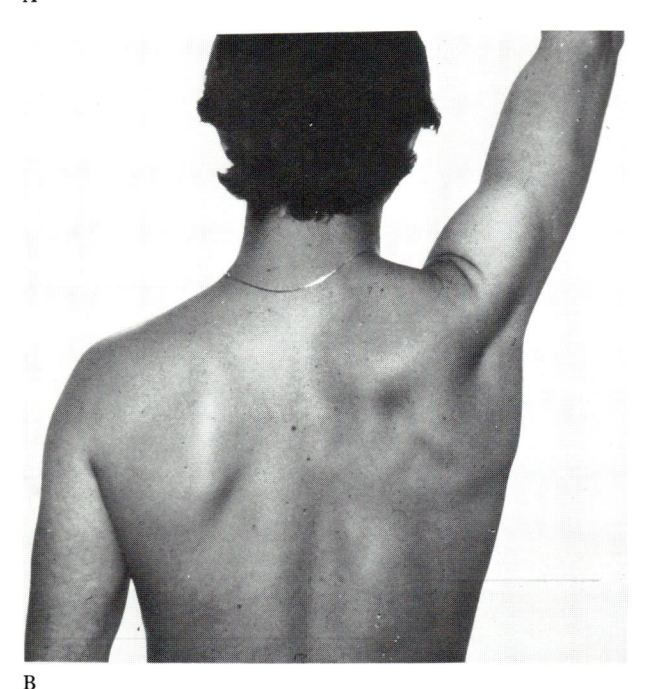

Figure 228-3 Deltoid palsy: *A.* The characteristic groove (*arrowhead*) occurs as a result of a subluxing humerus in a patient with total deltoid paralysis as the result of an upper trunk injury. *B.* Another patient 2 years after the grafting of an isolated axillary nerve injury on the right side.

nerve.) If the rhomboid is intact and elbow function is normal, an isolated deltoid paralysis is almost certainly the result of an axillary nerve injury. A not uncommon sequence of events in this latter situation is the patient's report of an initial wrist drop which rapidly clears, leaving the isolated deltoid palsy. The mechanism of injury is one of traction on the posterior cord by the axillary nerve, which takes the brunt of the onslaught from the subluxing or dislocating shoulder. It is of the utmost importance that the examiner not construe the sequence of events of improvement of wrist extension and elbow extension as evidence that all will be well, as in many instances the axillary nerve itself may be

Triceps weakness is usually seen in the context of a posterior cord injury and not a radial nerve injury. Wrist flexion and extension are assessed and the examiner should readily distinguish the wrist drop of a posterior cord lesion from the extension with radial drift observed in cases of posterior interosseous nerve palsy. Particular attention must be given to the long and the intrinsic muscles affecting the hand. It is well to remember that the medial cord gives rise to the ulnar nerve and hence controls the intrinsic hand muscles supplied by this nerve, as well as giving rise to the medial head of the median nerve, through which flows the motor median supply to the muscles at the base of the thumb. Thus, the simultaneous appearance of paralysis and wasting of the abductor pollicis brevis and abductor digiti minimi, in the absence of a Horner's syndrome, would suggest either a lower trunk or medial cord lesion. The lateral cord divides into the musculocutaneous nerve and the lateral head of the median nerve, so that injury to this structure will result in weakness of elbow flexion and anesthesia of the thumb.

The vascular supply to the limb is assessed in standard fashion. The sensory examination consists initially of assessing the patient's appreciation of pinprick and light touch. A careful appraisal is made of hand sensibility as this is one of the keys to the eventual outcome of limb function. Static and moving two-point discrimination should be recorded as baseline data. A medial cord injury may simulate an ulnar nerve injury, and an incorrect diagnosis of ulnar neuropathy at the elbow joint may be made. It is useful to remember that most, but not all patients with ulnar nerve pathology at the elbow joint will "split the ring finger" on sensory examination, whereas this is not a feature of medial cord injury. The presence of a wasted abductor pollicis brevis and weak opposition of the thumb immediately indicates to the examiner that a plexus injury and not an ulnar nerve injury at the elbow is involved. The presence of a sensory abnormality in the median distribution is of the utmost practical significance, whereas the sensory loss occasioned by posterior cord abnormality in the distribution of the radial nerve is of so little practical significance as hardly to be worth recording. It should be noted that the sensory loss of a C5 root injury is almost identical to that of an axillary nerve injury and is of no practical help in sorting out the two sites of pathology. Percussion in the posterior triangle over the plexus may yield useful information as intense dysesthesia within the distribution of the appropriate nerves indicates that the posterior root ganglion cells are attached to the spinal cord and hence a total root avulsion does not exist at that level.

As each joint is assessed while testing motor power, the opportunity is taken to assess the range of passive movement allowed. Particular attention must be given to the shoulder joint in upper plexus injuries and to the state of the small hand joints in lower plexus injuries. While making this assessment, it is advisable to impress upon the patient that he or she (and not the physiotherapist) is responsible for maintaining the full range of passive movement of all joints. Similarly, during the sensory examination, it is advisable to warn the patient repeatedly to guard anesthetic areas against burning. The neurological examination is then completed, particular attention being paid to the presence or absence of Brown-Séquard's syndrome, which may be present in mild degree with major nerve root avulsions in the cervical area.

At the completion of the physical examination the surgeon usually has an accurate idea as to the site of pathology and the extent of nerve injury at that particular point in time following the accident. Surgeons with a high incidence of brachial plexus cases in their workload retain the anatomical information, but for the average surgeon "spaghetti junction" is only vaguely remembered. Careful examination, followed by a refreshing return to a standard text of anatomy, will allow the diagnosis to be made in most cases on clinical data alone. The main decisions in management will be based on subsequent clinical appraisals, so it is important that these data be recorded in the initial report for future comparisons. It is essential that the recording be made by the surgeon personally and not only by paramedical colleagues.

At the initial consultation the surgeon should convey to the patient and the patient's family the seriousness of the situation and the likely duration of their relationship, which is at least 2 years. It is reasonable to tell the patient that the disability remaining 2 years after the event is likely to be the final disability. Plans for possible career reorientation and the importance of maximizing residual function rather than agonizing over lost function are discussed at this early stage and will form the basis for more detailed consideration at a later stage. Upgrading education should commence immediately if it is obvious that the patient's occupation will have to be modified, regardless of the final outcome. At this juncture, patients should receive a leaflet that describes nerve injury in lay terms and advises them of the tests they will undergo and the relationships they will develop with their surgeons, physiotherapists, occupational therapists, and electromyographers over a 2-year period.

Electrical Studies

If more than 8 weeks have elapsed from the time of injury, it is reasonable to obtain electrical studies. These studies rarely tell the surgeon anything new about the patient but the data may provide a useful base for future comparison. This electrical information is used to supplement the main guide to management, which is the repeated clinical examination. Under no circumstances does the electrophysiological estimation take the place of a careful clinical appraisal, and surgeons should only consult those who are truly expert in both the technical performances and interpretation of the electrophysiological studies. Confusion is added to an already difficult situation if anything less than an expert electrophysiological opinion is added to a poor clinical assessment. Electrical studies may show evidence of more widespread partial denervation than is apparent on clinical examination, and this pattern is compatible with the diffuse nature of plexus injuries. If the lesion is between the posterior root ganglion and the spinal cord, the peripheral axons of the posterior ganglion cells will be intact, and hence conduction along fibers will be possible. This occurrence may be important in cases with a proximal lesion as it implies root pathology, with its attendant poor prognosis.

Posterior cervical musculature electromyelographic (EMG) recordings cannot define segmental myotomes and are of limited clinical usefulness compared with a clinical appraisal. The clinical usefulness of somatosensory evoked potentials in the appraisal of brachial plexus pathology is not yet established. It is important that minor electrophysiological evidence of reinnervation not be greeted with unnecessary enthusiasm, as the reinnervation by a few nerve fibers of a few muscle fibers does not necessarily correlate with useful limb function in the future. Expert clinical appraisal, coupled with expert electrophysiological appraisal, is the best assessor of progress.

Other Tests

Standard x-ray films of the cervical spine, pectoral girdle, humerus, and diaphragm are obtained. Fractures of transverse processes, clavicle, scapula, or humerus may give a clue as to severity of the injuring force. These lesions may require appropriate management in their own right.

We have not found tests based on the axon reflex (histamine injection in anesthetic dermatomes) or sweating useful. Angiography is done after vascular injury or vascular surgery.

Management of Various Types of Injury

Closed Stretch Injury of the Plexus

Clinical Considerations

The principle underlying the timing of surgery is that irreparable lesions must be corrected as soon as possible so that the effect of chronic denervation on distal muscle and sensory receptors can be minimized. There is very little logic in waiting a matter of years to see what peripheral reinnervation will ensue and, on finding very poor reinnervation, contemplating brachial plexus nerve surgery. It is then far too late. In patients with closed injuries it is, however, appropriate to wait a reasonable period to allow the lesser forms of nerve fiber injury to give evidence of recovery. In the absence of recovery of an accessible element of the brachial plexus, it is then appropriate to explore the plexus, provided the operator has some method of assessing lesions in continuity on the operating table. Thus, we believe it appropriate that cases come to operation at approximately the sixteenth week following the injury (the mean interval in our series is 5.6 months). Unfortunately, this means that 16 weeks have been wasted if the lesion requires resection. The argument has been advanced, therefore, that the plexus should be explored as soon as possible after the injury, i.e., within a matter of days or weeks of the injury. In that so many of the elements of the plexus are in continuity in closed injury, it is difficult to understand how a surgeon would know whether or not to resect an intact plexus element, as at that stage there is no way in which axonal transmission through the lesion could have occurred. Admittedly, avulsed or grossly attenuated plexus elements could be repaired, but this is an unusual situation and the surgeon would therefore face the very real danger of resecting damaged elements that if left alone would make a reasonably good spontaneous recovery.

Suggested Plan of Management of Closed Plexus Injuries

The initial diagnostic interview and examination are made as soon as possible following the injury and the clinical diagnosis is supplemented by standard x-ray films. Diaphragmatic movement is assessed on an inspiration chest film. Appropriate splinting and physiotherapy are ordered. The patient is seen at monthly intervals and any motor or sensory improvement is noted. At about the eighth week it is appropriate to request electrophysiological testing.

At 12 weeks a careful appraisal of the situation should be made. At this stage it may be quite obvious that the patient is recovering in all areas, in which case surgical interference is unnecessary and the patient is followed at monthly intervals for the next 6 months towards good recovery, which may either be complete or, although incomplete, may be superior to that which could be achieved by any surgical interference. Contrariwise, the patient may show severe wasting, with no recovery whatsoever. A not uncommon pattern is to find recovery in certain muscle groups, with residual paralysis and anesthesia defined by irreparably damaged elements of the plexus in other areas. If there is no, or minimal, recovery of an element of the plexus, the patient should be admitted to the hospital for further investigation and treatment. The surgeon may be prompted to wait a few more weeks by minor motor or sensory change, but by the sixteenth week a definite decision must be made as to whether or not the patient is going to come to brachial plexus surgery. By this time the outcome of any concomitant cranial or thoracic injury can be determined.

The patient is then admitted to the hospital and careful clinical and electrophysiological reappraisals are made. Where appropriate, a myelogram is performed. The use of water-soluble contrast material may allow the rootlets to be delineated with accuracy, provided the contrast material is concentrated in the cervical area. The false-positive and false-negative results of cervical myelography are well known, so that the study must be interpreted with care. Root avulsion at one level does not imply root injury at all levels. Root avulsion, although of grave prognostic importance for limb function, does not of itself exclude a patient from consideration for surgery. To date, computed tomographic (CT) scanning has merely demonstrated traction diverticula, which were obvious with either conventional or water-soluble myelographic techniques.[17]

At this point it is appropriate to consider what might be achieved by brachial plexus surgery and what might be achieved by either bony or soft tissue reconstruction procedures. For example, if there is evidence of multiple nerve root avulsions in a patient considered unsuitable for neurotization, it might be preferable to proceed directly to reconstructive procedures without exploring the brachial plexus. Late referral may preclude any direct nerve surgery and in our hands is the commonest reason for exclusion of patients from the surgically managed series of cases. In marginal situations it might be appropriate to inspect the plexus at operation, perform the appropriate intraoperative recordings, and then, if faced with massive damage, retreat in favor of immediate reconstructive procedures, which are performed during the same hospital admission. As a general rule, however, the sequence of brachial plexus surgery, followed by reconstructive procedures approximately 18 months after the surgery, is preferred, as by that time reconstructive procedures may be totally unnecessary or alternatively may be of lesser magnitude so that they may be tailored more specifically to the partially recovered limb functions.

General anesthesia is used for the exploration but prolonged neuromuscular blockade is avoided, as the surgeon will want to stimulate the plexus elements directly and note muscle contraction. The patient is prepared and positioned as if a total plexus exploration with grafting will be the extent of the procedure. In fact, the procedure is frequently much more confined in scope and may involve solely a supraclavicular exploration or solely an intraclavicular exploration, and grafts may not be needed. Nevertheless, it is important that preparations for the full operation be made in every case, as it is extremely difficult to maintain aseptic technique should further fields of surgery be required during a plexus operation. Thus, the entire side of the neck, the side of the chest, and entire limb on the affected side are prepared and draped free so that incisions may be made both to gain exposure and to gain grafting material. The entire limb must be available for inspection of the results of direct intraoperative nerve stimulation. Both legs are prepared from the knee distally in case it is necessary to harvest sural nerves for grafting purposes. If the operator is certain that grafting will be required, it is easier to resect the sural nerve with the patient in the prone position with use of a minor surgery set-up and then to close the wounds, turn the patient over, and proceed with the plexus operation. This maneuver should be performed with caution, however, as the operator may find, unexpectedly, that grafting is not required or alternatively that appropriate grafts may be obtained locally (e.g., from the medial cutaneous nerve of the forearm).

Supraclavicular Exposure The supraclavicular exposure is made according to standard technique and in itself is a relatively simple operation. Indeed, the supraclavicular plexus can be inspected by doing little more than cutting the skin, so that the specific risk of surgery as a general rule should not be a major factor in deterring surgical exploration of these structures. The operator should not hesitate to resect the lateral inferior bony attachment of the sternocleidomastoid muscle, leaving a small cuff for subsequent reconstruction. It is advisable to be quite certain that the internal jugular vein is not adherent to the sternomastoid muscle before the muscle division is performed. The scalenus anticus muscle is characteristically palpable through the fat packing the posterior triangle, and this muscle should be approached with dispatch, as the phrenic nerve is plastered to its anterior surface by the prevertebral fascia and will not be injured while the adipose tissue is swept away. Arching branches of the transverse cervical artery are divided.

The point of junction of the fifth and sixth spinal nerves is a welcoming landmark and the touchstone to further dissection. The fifth and sixth spinal nerves should be dissected right up to the tip of the transverse processes, which are palpable at the end of the supporting gutters over which the spinal nerves flow. The proximal extent of the dissection is on the transverse processes. Unfortunately, patients may exhibit a normal myelogram and have proximal spinal nerve injuries at the level of the transverse process of the cervical vertebra. If nerve resection at this level is contemplated, quick sections of spinal nerves are essential, as the surgeon may be distressed to find either fibrous tissue, neuromatous formation, or posterior root ganglion cells, and there is no point in grafting to such material.

On occasion, excessive scarring may make this part of the operation difficult, in which case a useful maneuver is to pick up the phrenic nerve, usually clearly seen in front of the scalenus anticus, and dissect it up to its origin. This nerve will lead to the fifth spinal nerve and hence establish the plane between the scalenus anticus and scalenus medius, so that the operator can dissect from above down in that plane, displaying the spinal nerves that form the origin of the plexus.

The only branch of the trunks, the suprascapular nerve, characteristically arches posteriorly away from the upper trunk. The seventh spinal nerve and the middle trunk are usually displayed with ease, but the eighth cervical and first dorsal spinal nerves may provide a slightly greater challenge as they are frequently tucked down behind the arching subclavian artery. If there is any problem in exposure, it is a straightforward matter to define the phrenic nerve and protect this on a sling and then divide the scalenus anticus muscle, which reveals a clear view of the subclavian artery and the spinal nerves leading to the lowest trunk nestled in behind the artery. The surgeon should bear in mind that the thoracic duct will be bluish in color as there is seldom an intervening valve between it and the venous pathways into which the chyle flows. It is as well to remember the close relationship of the stellate ganglion to the first dorsal spinal nerve and also to remember to protect the vertebral artery. The pleural space is a normal occupant of the neck and is usually not a problem if Sibson's fascia is respected. Application of suturing or grafting techniques to these lower proximal plexus elements seldom gives significant clinical benefit, so that it is unlikely that the surgeon will be performing intricate microsurgical maneuvers on these elements of the plexus. The posterior approach to the brachial plexus may display these lower proximal elements to advantage in patients who have been subjected to previous surgery.[11]

In the relatively unaltered state, the supraclavicular dissection of the brachial plexus is straightforward, but if vascular grafts have been placed previously, if large neuromatous formations are present, or if previous surgery has been performed, the dissection may be both challenging and tedious (Fig. 228-4). The surgeon must have sufficient skill not to cause additional damage by either macroscopic or microscopic dissection. Absolute mastery of anatomy is mandatory. The surgeon embarking upon such a case must be prepared to handle significant vascular injuries, as large veins may be adherent to damaged neural elements. Particular care must be afforded if arterial grafts have been previously inserted, as they have a distressing tendency to fall apart if anything other than gentle technique is utilized. The distal extent of this dissection is usually close to the point of the

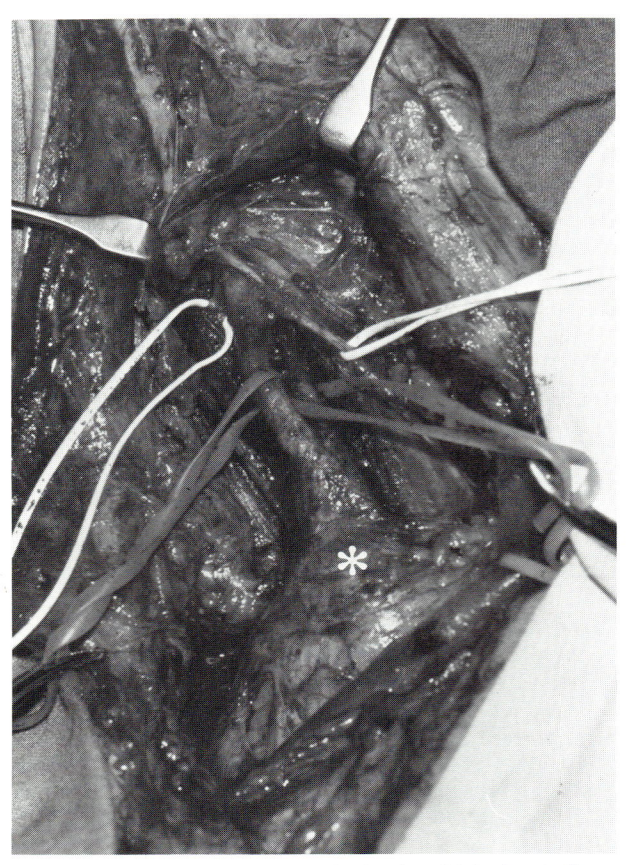

Figure 228-4 Right supraclavicular brachial plexus dissection. The white sling at the upper left surrounds the nerve to the rhomboids and the other white sling (*upper right*) surrounds the phrenic nerve. The two darker slings surround the fifth and sixth cervical spinal nerves. The upper trunk runs immediately after its formation into a massive neuroma(★). At this stage it was appreciated that the lesion could not be dealt with by this limited approach, so it was necessary to complete the infraclavicular dissection of the plexus before a safe resection was possible.

division of the various trunks of the plexus. If any difficulty is determined at the distal extent of the dissection, extra space can be gained by pulling down firmly on the limb. If there is any problem of adequate exposure, the surgeon should not hesitate to remove the lateral clavicular head of the pectoralis major from its attachment to the inferior border of the clavicle and dissect beneath the subclavius muscle. These extra centimeters may make all the difference to the ease and safety of dissection, and it is particularly useful to have peripheral control of the subclavian artery and vein at this juncture if the vessels are surrounded by scar tissue and stuck to the lower plexus elements. There may be a significant contribution to the plexus from the fourth cervical spinal nerve and the trunks may divide more proximally than anticipated, but beyond this congenital variations of the supraclavicular plexus are uncommon.

Infraclavicular Exposure The surgeon cuts boldly down to the cephalic vein, delineating the groove between the pectoralis major and deltoid muscles. The superficial fascia and the fascia immediately on the upper surface of the pectoralis major should not be mobilized, as this layer accepts sutures well in the subsequent reapproximation of the pectoralis major muscle. The incision is then swung on to the medial aspect of the arm for a short distance. Limited inspection of the axillary plexus can be had by placing a large sling around the pectoralis major and pulling it alternatively up or down. Any significant and detailed study, however, demands the release of the lateral attachment of the trifoil pectoralis major tendon. It is useful to place marker sutures for subsequent reapproximation, and the surgeon must be careful not to hook up the musculocutaneous nerve with the finger used to explore before dividing the tendon, leaving a centimeter cuff for future reconstruction. The coracoid process is readily palpable and is a useful landmark, as it is at approximately this level that the axillary nerve leaves the posterior cord, and it is to this structure that the pectoralis minor is attached.

The origin of the median nerve is immediately sought. The surgeon can then dissect up the lateral head and hence meet the musculocutaneous nerve. The medial head of the median nerve can then be displayed, which will lead the surgeon to both the ulnar nerve and the medial cutaneous nerve of the forearm, which is a useful donor nerve. The radial nerve and posterior cord are usually displayed without much difficulty by dissecting medial to and behind the great vessels. The surgeon should be careful not to cut the branches to the triceps, which come off in the axilla, while dissecting the posterior cord.

Dissection of the axillary nerve may pose greater difficulty, particularly if there is much scarring as a result of dislocation of the shoulder with concomitant hemorrhage and subsequent fibrosis. The following point may be of assistance. The first is that the shining tendon of the latissimus dorsi greets the surgeon on descending through the fat of the axilla, and the upper border of this silver tendon leads the operator to the quadrangular space. The second point is that if the great vessels are drawn medially, the circumflex humoral vessels will lead the surgeon down to the quadrangular space. It is important to remember that these vessels may be significant anastomotic channels if there is a proximal concomitant vascular injury. The third point is that the axillary nerve may leave the posterior cord at approximately the level of the coracoid and, once the pectoralis minor has been resected from the coracoid, the origin of the axillary nerve should be defined. In our series of patients exhibiting plexus injuries following shoulder dislocation, 10 of 16 with isolated axillary nerve injuries came to surgery and 5 of these 10 required nerve grafts. Six of seven patients with medial cord injury after joint dislocation were explored and none required grafting.

In dissecting through the scar in this area (Fig. 228-5), the surgeon must be particularly conscious of the nerve to the latissimus dorsi because an operative injury to this nerve would scarcely be in the patient's best interest. This nerve may flow from the posterior cord, may be part of a branch that gives rise to the nerve to the subscapularis muscle, or even on occasion may arise from the axillary nerve itself. Variations of structure are more common in the axilla than they are in the posterior triangle, so the surgeon should not

Brachial Plexus Injuries

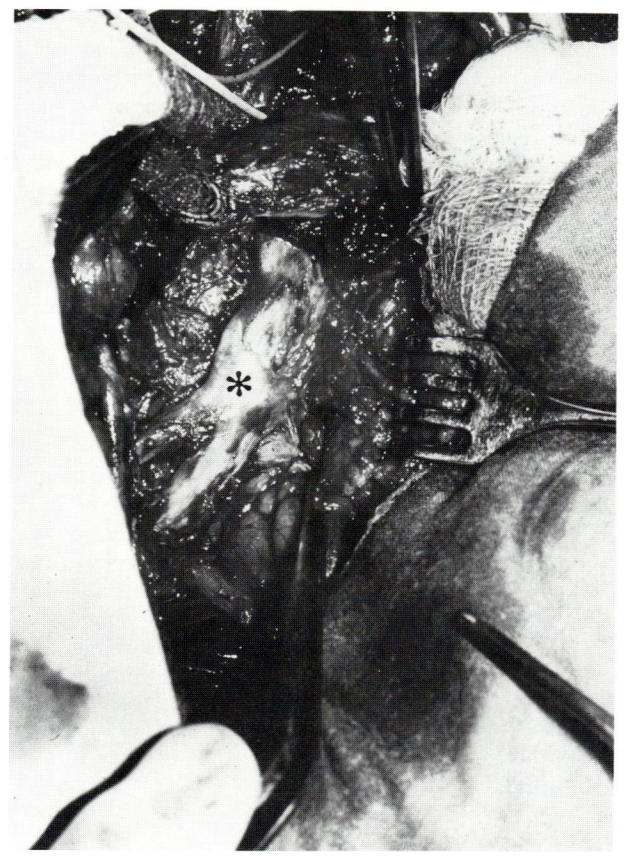

Figure 228-5 Right axillary dissection. This patient suffered from a carpal tunnel syndrome. The treatment offered for these symptoms was transaxillary first rib resection. Note the severe scarring of the medial cord(★), which resulted in permanent intrinsic muscular atrophy and paralysis in the hand.

be overly surprised to find the musculocutaneous nerve issuing from the median nerve or to find the absence of one or another of the heads of the median nerve.

Reconstruction of the pectoralis minor is not mandatory, but careful reapproximation of the pectoralis major is required. The musculocutaneous nerve must be respected, both in dividing the pectoralis major and particularly during dissection of the axillary nerve, as the assistant's retractor will be displacing both the biceps and brachialis and the musculocutaneous nerve. This nerve must also be respected during reapproximation of the pectoralis major.

Combined Approach Both supra- and infraclavicular exposures may be made initially or one component may be dissected and then extended as appropriate to the circumstances of the procedure. It is a rare situation in which the clavicle requires division. By the combined maneuver of abducting and adducting the undraped limb and elevating the clavicle by pulling upward on a sponge placed around that bone, most of the nerve structures can be dissected under the microscope. If the major pathology is directly in the line of the divisions, however, the clavicle should be divided in the usual way and considerable care given to its reapproximation at the end of the operation, as problems with delayed healing or nonunion may subsequently become a major nuisance.

Appraisal and Treatment of the Lesions Once the lesions have been dissected free of surrounding scar tissue, the decision must be made as to whether or not to resect the damaged portion of the plexus. Two fundamental tactics have been employed. The first is the intraoperative nerve action potential recording technique of Kline and the second is the sequential microsurgical technique of Millesi. In our opinion both techniques should be employed if the surgeon is operating on plexus cases at approximately the fourth month (i.e., long before it is possible for any regenerating axon to have made contact with an end organ at the periphery of the limb).

The initial procedure is to stimulate proximal to the lesion on each appropriate element of the plexus. If the appropriate muscle groups contract, the procedure is limited to a 360-degree external neurolysis of the scarred element. The prognosis for the return of useful clinical function is good. In the absence of contraction, the recording electrode is placed distal to the lesion and an attempt is made to evoke a nerve action potential across the lesion (Fig. 228-6). Where appropriate, the major elements are split, with the aid of the magnification provided by operating loupes. For example, it is possible to split off the origin of the axillary nerve at a considerable distance up the posterior cord. The medial and lateral head of the median nerve can be separated accurately and the musculocutaneous nerve can be split off the lateral cord. In certain circumstances it is thus possible to retain functioning elements and to isolate injured elements for appropriate repair.

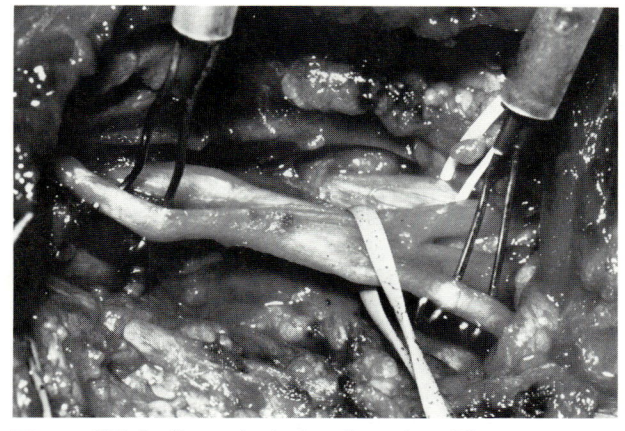

Figure 228-6 Supraclavicular dissection. The presence of axonal transmission through the upper trunk lesion (sling) is being tested by stimulating the C5 spinal nerve on one side of the lesion and recording off the suprascapular nerve on the other side. The resulting nerve action potential is displayed on an oscilloscope. Care is required to separate the appearance of the nerve action potential from the downsweep of the stimulus artifact because of the short distance between the stimulating and recording electrodes.

In the absence of a nerve action potential, the lesions are resected and grafted under the microscope using the sequential steps described by Millesi. It is seldom possible to mobilize the tissues sufficiently to obtain direct suture apposition. In the usual case, some of the elements will be subjected to external neurolysis alone, other elements to internal neurolysis, and still other elements to nerve resection and grafting.

Many factors influence the management of each particular element. Injuries to upper plexus elements and posterior cord elements are dealt with in an aggressive fashion. Lesions of the lower plexus elements and the medial cord are handled in a relatively conservative fashion. The younger the patient, the more aggressive and extensive the surgery, and the older the patient, the more conservative. The time interval between accident and surgery may be so prolonged as to negate the usefulness of nerve grafting. The appropriateness of the particular patient's remaining function for alternative, reconstructive procedures is assessed. The absence of suitable median or ulnar innervated muscles available for future tendon transfer might influence the surgeon to make an extremely aggressive attempt to repair elements leading to the posterior cord in a situation that might be considered inoperable in the presence of the potential for reconstructive procedures. The question of the extent of surgical intervention in brachial plexus surgery is a controversial issue and unfortunately is likely to remain controversial because of the difficulty of controlling multiple variables (for example, the length of the graft) in a study of a complex multifactorial situation.

Multiple Root Avulsion Cases In the past, patients with multiple root avulsions faced the prospect of amputation of the useless limb. It is not unreasonable to state that any procedure that stops short of amputation and provides a modicum of useful limb function should be construed as progressive. Each case requires particular individual assessment as to the particular roots avulsed, the degree of damage in the plexus elements subtended by the intact roots, and the alternative reconstructive procedures available. Motor drive can be led directly to peripheral nerve derivatives of the plexus via sural nerve grafts from intercostal nerves, and sensory input can be derived via sural nerve grafts from the cervical plexus to the median and ulnar nerve. Our present attitude is to offer these maneuvers to young patients within a few months of injury on the understanding that such procedures are not of proven value and that results have been unpredictable in our hands. Our most consistent success with these procedures has involved grafting into the musculocutaneous nerve in a young patient having good sensibility in the hand (Fig. 228-7). The exact place of these extensive procedures in the management of patients suffering from closed brachial plexus stretch injuries has yet to be determined but there undoubtedly are patients who benefit from them and hence avoid amputation.[3,19]

Open Brachial Plexus Injuries

In contrast to the policy that has evolved for the management of closed stretch injuries (i.e., waiting for 4 months prior to exploratory surgery), most surgeons agree that sharp lacerations of the plexus should be explored and repaired at the initial operation whenever possible. If major arterial or pulmonary injury precludes such surgery, the wound should be reopened within a few days as soon as the patient's general condition allows (Fig. 228-8). In this situation it is possible to suture sharply lacerated elements without the use of grafts. If the injury involves crushing as well as lacerating forces (e.g., a chain saw injury), it is advisable to wait 2 or 3 weeks to allow the transverse and longitudinal extent of nerve pathology to become plainly visible under the operating microscope before a repair is made, thus obviating the error of apposing damaged nerve elements.

Gunshot Injuries

Our experience with gunshot wounds of the plexus is limited to 2 of our 226 brachial plexus cases, a reflection of the social ambiance of the catchment area. Kline reported on 46 cases operated on in New Orleans; these patients were selected from a group of 77 gunshot plexus injuries because they displayed complete injury to plexus elements without evidence of recovery in the early months following wounding.[11] Other indications for surgery included aneurysm formation and intractable pain.

Radiation Injuries

The desperate plight of a patient suffering from carcinoma of the breast or a Pancoast tumor, presenting in the period after treatment by radiation therapy with excessive pain and progressive neurological disability of the limb, is a circumstance to which there is no easy answer. We have not found the particular brachial plexus element involved or the factor of the absence or presence of pain to be a sufficiently distinguishing feature to establish which patients are suffering from brachial plexus tumor invasion and which patients are suffering from postradiation fibrosis. In patients who show no evidence of metastatic spread and who are judged to have an acceptable life expectancy, consideration should be given to decompression of the plexus. The situation may be aggravated by radiation damage to the skin of the anterior chest wall and by perineural scarring of exceptional toughness and extent. Every effort should be made to leave the plexus against viable muscle tissue at the end of the procedure to promote vascularization of the neural elements. The value of pedicle or free vascularized flaps of omentum or muscle to the area following nerve decompression has yet to be determined.[2]

Iatrogenic Injuries

Iatrogenic injuries to the supra- and infraclavicular areas of the brachial plexus are encountered with distressing frequency (Fig. 228-9). The pathogenesis includes injection injury, retractor injury, cauterization injury, and direct laceration.[6] In addition to plexus injury occurring as a complication of operations in its general vicinity, the brachial plexus can readily be injured in injudicious biopsy of nerve

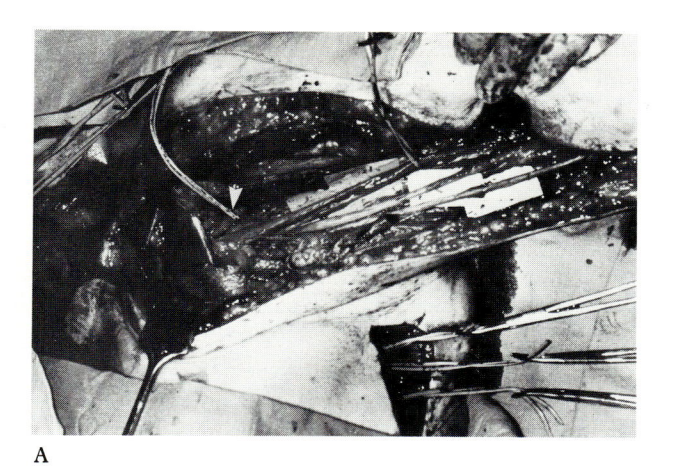

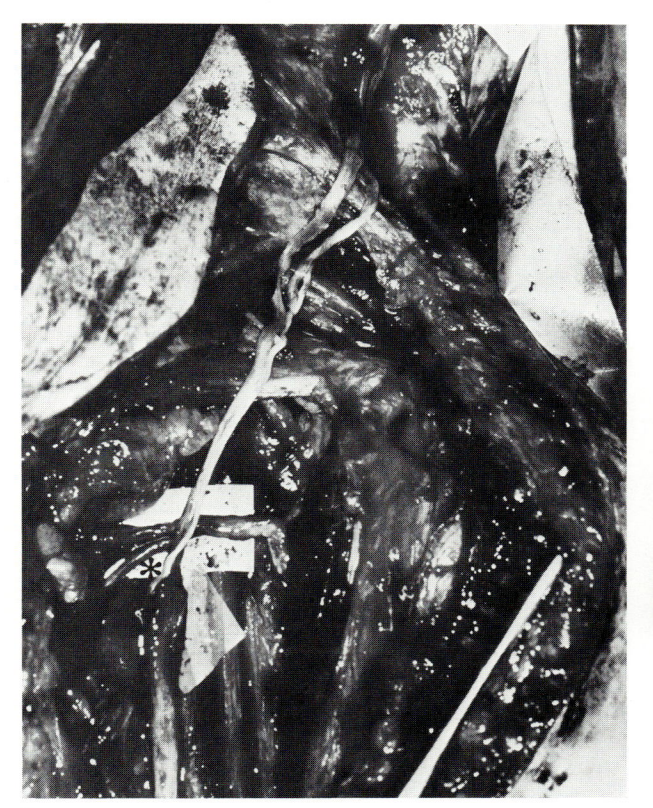

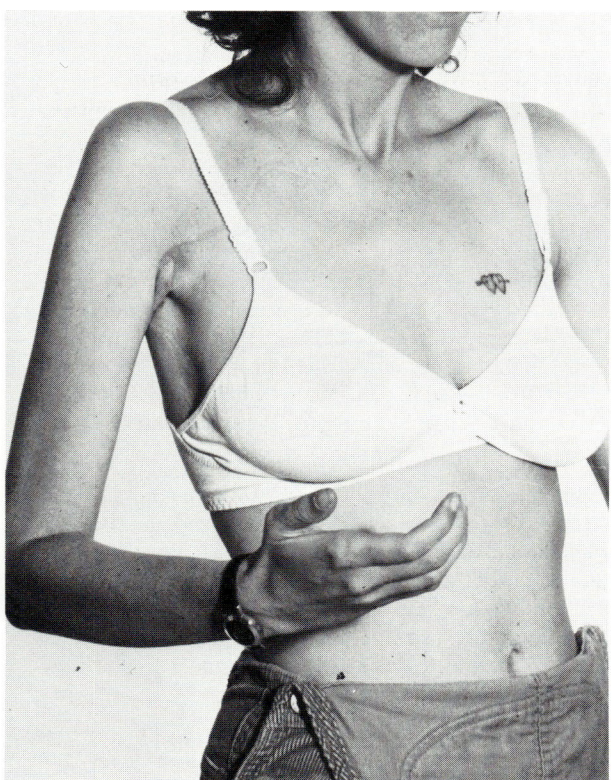

Figure 228-7 Neurotization: *A.* Infraclavicular dissection of the left brachial plexus. Three intercostal nerves have been dissected through a separate incision. They are surrounded by slings but cannot be seen in this illustration. Sural nerve grafts are subsequently placed from the intercostal nerves under the axillary skin to the musculocutaneous nerve (*arrowhead*). *B.* Cervical plexus branches have been turned down and anastomosed to sural nerve grafts, which at this stage are draped over the clavicle before they are routed to the lower anastomotic site (indicated by ★). *C.* Elbow flexion resulting from brachialis and biceps activity 2 years after an intercostal-musculocutaneous graft. The patient is taking a deep breath.

tumors whose true nature had not been appreciated by the operator. The plexus may be injured during transcutaneous angiography procedures, both in association with anticoagulants or in patients with normal blood coagulation (Fig. 228-10).

Birth Injuries

The incidence of congenital birth palsy of the brachial plexus has been reduced with improved obstetrical care. It is our feeling that the allowable interval between accident and

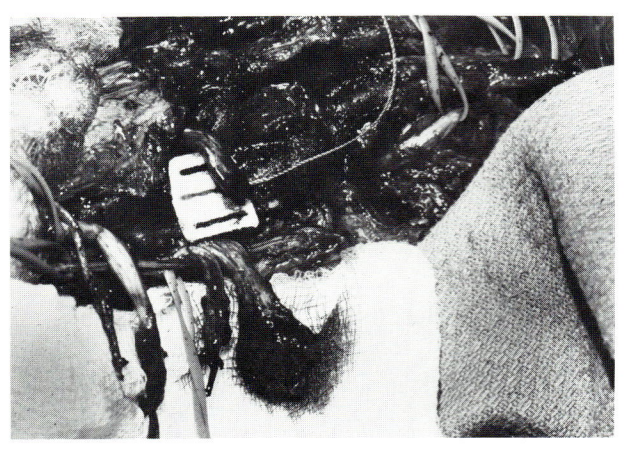

Figure 228-8 Right axillary plexus dissection after total division of the plexus-peripheral nerve junction by a plate glass window. The operation had been postponed for 2 weeks because of severe shock associated with the vascular injury. The operative exposure reveals the musculocutaneous nerve (on cottonoid) and the distal stumps of the median, ulnar, radial, and medial cutaneous nerves. The slings at the upper right are around proximal nerve elements. All nerves were repaired by direct suture, with the exception of the musculocutaneous nerve, which was grafted. Two years after operation, this 14-year-old boy was noted to have virtually normal elbow flexion and extension and grade 4 wrist flexion and extension, but weak intrinsic hand muscle action. He was able to write with a pencil. Protective sensation on the thumb and small finger was noted but fine discrimination was lacking.

regeneration is longer in children than it is in adults, so that a far more conservative attitude to this stretch injury is advised than in the adult situation. The place of a neurotization procedure in young children has yet to be determined, but the situation would appear to be an ideal circumstance for implementation of these strategies once it has been irrefutably determined that there is permanent loss of function in the limb of the infant.[15]

Rehabilitation

The rehabilitation of patients suffering from severe brachial plexus injury commences at the initial consultation. Well-qualified physiotherapists are invaluable colleagues in the management of these patients. They direct active and passive exercise, fashion active and passive splinting devices, and provide encouragement and direction. There is no proof that electrical stimulation of denervated muscle affects the outcome and the essential aim is to maintain a full range of active and passive movement of all joints and thus prevent contractions. The effectiveness of sensory re-education of hands with partial sensory return has not yet been determined and this concept requires randomized clinical study.[4]

A major requirement is for some form of therapy that would cause regenerating axons to grow faster as they course down the limb. Unfortunately, neither the physiotherapist nor the patient can alter the outcome in this regard, and there is as yet no evidence to prove that electrical or magnetic field application has any effect on clinical recovery.

The commonest error encountered in the rehabilitation phase of management is that of the patient in the situation where it is the physiotherapist who does the work and the patient has to attend the physiotherapy department to achieve benefit. Patients should be encouraged to do as much of the prescribed exercise program as possible at home and to maximize their residual function rather than bemoan their frequently substantial motor and sensory loss and assume a passive role in the first few years after injury.

Pain

Pain always accompanies a significant brachial plexus injury. This fact should be explained to the patient. The majority of patients with plexus injuries do not require an operation to deal solely with pain syndromes. It is our feeling that the amount of pain experienced, even in anesthetic limbs, is proportional to the freedom of movement of the joints. Whether this is a true physiological correlation or merely a reflection of an active patient displaying a positive attitude is not determined. Pain may be relieved by external neurolysis and this may be a welcome immediate result of surgery. The refinement of the dorsal root entry zone lesion operation by Nashold has been a major advance for patients who retain an intolerable chronic pain syndrome.

Reconstructive Surgery

The neurosurgeon must be intimately acquainted with the nature of the wide variety of soft tissue and bone operations available for the rehabilitation of the neurologically injured upper limb.[14] Until recently some surgeons thought that the results of reconstructive procedures (e.g., shoulder fusion) were far more predictable and rapidly achieved than those following nerve surgery, so they advocated these procedures as the initial procedures of choice. More recently, opinion has swung in favor of appropriate nerve surgery. This strategy has the disadvantage of requiring up to a year's hiatus before nerve repair evaluation can take place but has the decided advantage of avoiding reconstructive procedures in some instances and minimizing the extent of these procedures in others. Of the various procedures available to patients unsuitable for surgery (usually because of late referral) or in the circumstance of a poor neurosurgical result, we have found the combination of shoulder fusion (20 cases in our series) and common flexor plastic surgery (Steindler) particularly useful in patients whose hands have some sensory appreciation.

Long-Term Results

It is extraordinarily difficult to give a critical appraisal of the long-term results of surgical treatment of patients suffering from brachial plexus injuries.[11,14,15] The patient's age, the

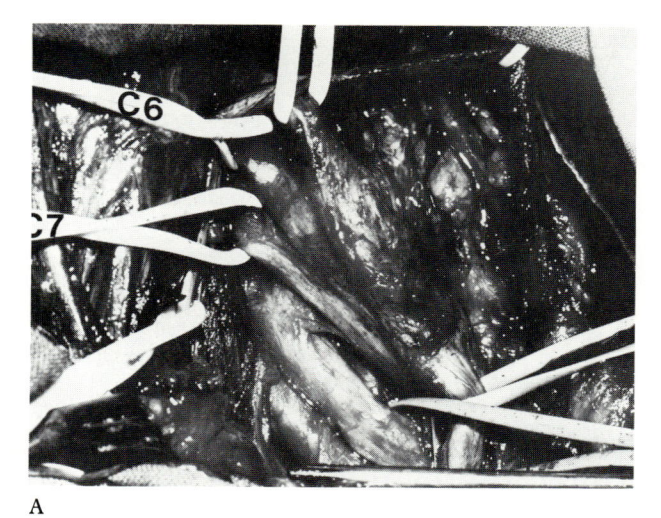

Figure 228-9 Supraclavicular exploration of the left brachial plexus. The patient had undergone a "scalenotomy" and awoke with paralysis of shoulder abduction and elbow flexion. *A.* Three slings (*left*) are around spinal nerves C5, C6, and C7. The sling at the lower left surrounds the phrenic nerve, which is nicely outlined in front of the intact scalenus anticus muscle. The slings at the lower right are around the upper and middle trunks. The lesion is at the junction of C5 and C6. *B.* A closer view of the lacerated upper trunk; proximal and distal end bulb neuromas have formed 2 months following the injury. *C.* After preparation of the proximal stump, the neuroma tissue has been resected and a healthy fascicular pattern is revealed through the operating microscope.

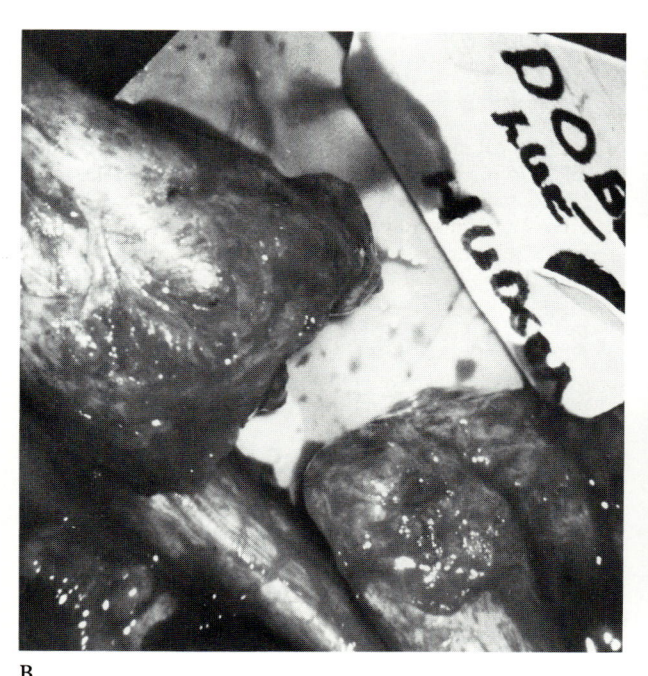

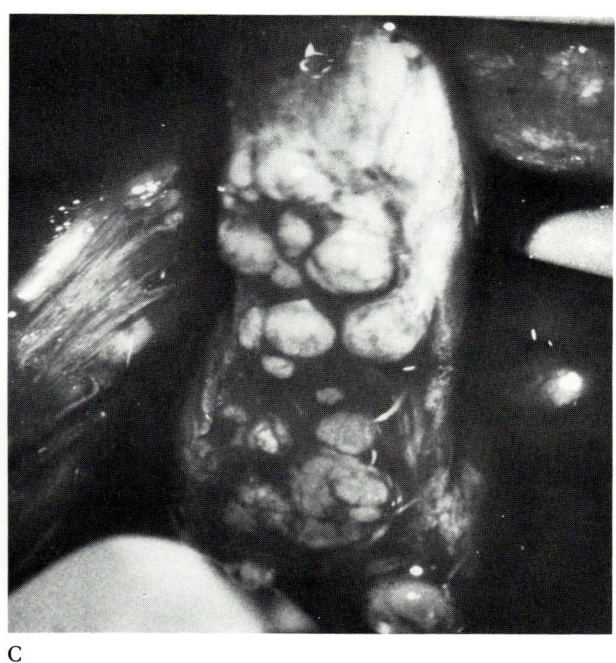

exact anatomical element of the plexus disturbed, and the accident-to-operation time interval are but a few of the variables which influence the final outcome. There is no common agreement on quantification of the end result according to the particular plexus element that was injured. Virtually none of the microsurgical techniques have been submitted to randomized clinical trial, although laboratory studies have given some guidance.[6] The examiner can never be certain that recovery following neurolysis occurred more rapidly or more completely than would have occurred in the absence of surgical interference.

Narakas reports 64 percent good or fair results following autologous nerve grafting of the supraclavicular plexus and 73 percent good or fair results following grafting of the infraclavicular plexus.[15] We have not been able to match the degree of success reported by this outstanding surgeon. Millesi reports useful recovery of elbow flexion in 9 of 18 cases following operation on a group of patients who suffered complete plexus palsy due to root injury. Reliable appraisers and reporters such as Kline, Millesi, and Narakas report current results that are superior to historical controls.[5,16]

It is hoped that progress will appear on three fronts. The first major requirement is a greater understanding of the neurobiology of regeneration following injury and the neurobiology of nerve immunology.[13] The second requirement is the establishment of an internationally recognized classification of brachial plexus injuries and an internationally recognized classification of methods of testing so that the re-

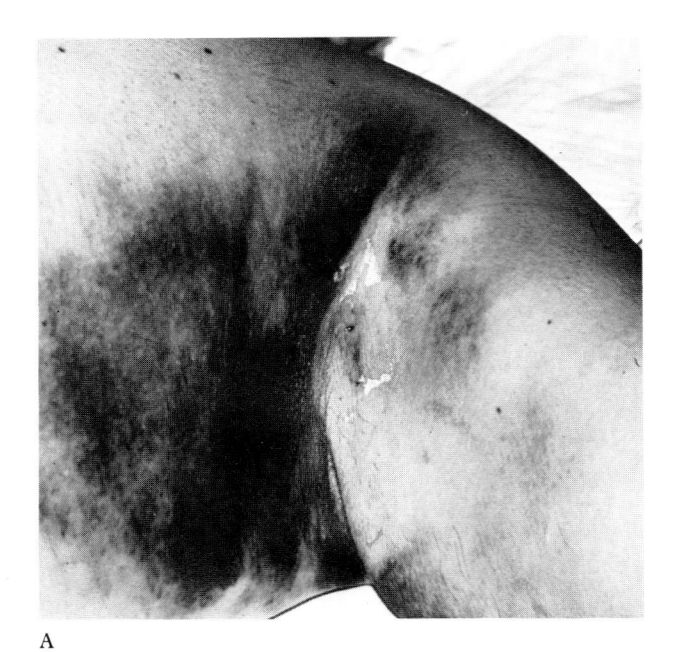

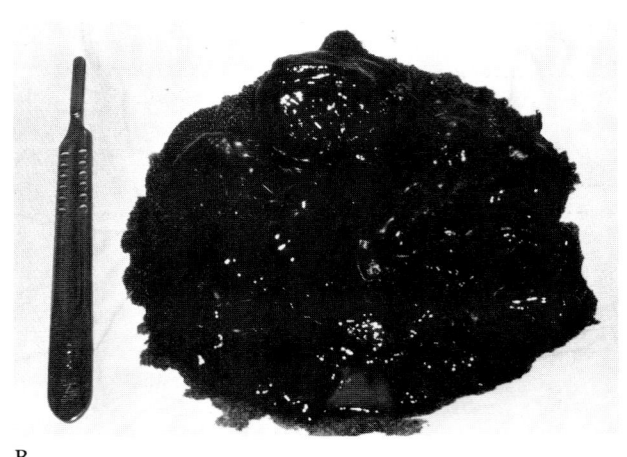

Figure 228-10 *A.* The axilla of a 65-year-old male patient subjected to a retrograde brachial angiogram 12 h earlier. The extensive swelling of the axilla was associated with a total axillary plexus palsy. *B.* A portion of the hematoma removed from the brachial sheath. Two years after operation, the patient had regained grade 4 elbow flexion and extension but had received no intrinsic hand muscle reinnervation. Protective sensation had returned to the hand but no sensory discrimination was found on clinical testing.

sults of various techniques can be compared and cooperative randomized studies performed. The third requirement is that of prevention of these injuries the majority of which are caused by traffic accidents.

References

1. Brooks DM: Open wounds of the brachial plexus, in Seddon HJ (ed): *Peripheral Nerve Injuries*, Medical Research Council Special Report Series, No 282. London, Her Majesty's Stationery Office, 1954, pp 418–428.
2. Brunelli G: Neurolysis and free microvascular omentum transfer in the treatment of postactinic palsies of the brachial plexus. Int Surg 65:515–519, 1980.
3. Brunelli G: Neurotisation of avulsed roots of the brachial plexus by means of anterior nerves of the cervical plexus (preliminary report). Int J Microsurg 2:55–58, 1980.
4. Dellon AL: *Evaluation of Sensibility and Re-education of Sensation in the Hand*. Baltimore, Williams and Wilkins, 1981.
5. Drake CG: Diagnosis and treatment of lesions of the brachial plexus and adjacent structures. Clin Neurosurg 11:110–127, 1963.
6. Hudson A, Kline D, Gentili F: Peripheral nerve injection injury, in Omer GE Jr, Spinner M (eds): *Management of Peripheral Nerve Problems*. Philadelphia, Saunders, 1980, pp 639–653.
7. Hudson AR, Hunter D, Kline D, Bratton B: Histological studies of experimental interfascicular nerve graft repairs. J Neurosurg 51:333–340, 1979.
8. Hudson AR, Kline DG: Progression of partial experimental injury to peripheral nerve. Part 2: Light and electron microscopic studies. J Neurosurg 42:15–22, 1975.
9. Kline DG, Hudson AR: Neuropathology and neurophysiology of the lesion in continuity, in Gorio A, Millesi H, Mingrino S (eds): *Posttraumatic Peripheral Nerve Regeneration: Experimental Basis and Clinical Implications*. New York, Raven Press, 1981, pp 175–181.
10. Kline DG, Hudson AR, Hackett ER, Bratton BR: Progression of partial experimental injury to peripheral nerve. Part 1: Periodic measurements of muscle contraction strength. J Neurosurg 42:1–14, 1975.
11. Kline DG, Judice DJ: Operative management of selected brachial plexus lesions. J Neurosurg 58:631–649, 1983.
12. Kline DG, Kott J, Barnes G, Bryant L: Exploration of selected brachial plexus lesions by the posterior subscapular approach. J Neurosurg 49:872–880, 1978.
13. Mackinnon S, Hudson A, Falk R, Bilbao J, Kline D, Hunter D: Nerve allograft response: A quantitative immunological study. Neurosurgery 10:61–69, 1982.
14. Millesi H: Trauma involving the brachial plexus, in Omer GE Jr, Spinner M (eds): *Management of Peripheral Nerve Problems*. Philadelphia, Saunders, 1980, pp 548–568.
15. Narakas AO: The surgical treatment of traumatic brachial plexus lesions. Int Surg 65:521–527, 1980.
16. Nulsen FE, Slade HW: Recovery following injury to the brachial plexus, in Woodhall B, Beebe GW (eds): *Peripheral Nerve Regeneration: A Follow-up Study of 3,656 World War II Injuries*. VA Medical Monograph. Washington, US Government Printing Office, 1956, pp 389–408.
17. Petterson H, Harwood-Nash DCF: *CT and Myelography of the Spine and Cord: Techniques, Anatomy and Pathology in Children*. New York, Springer, 1982, p 76.
18. Sunderland S: *Nerves and Nerve Injuries*. Edinburgh, Churchill Livingstone, 1978, pp 870–901.
19. Tsuyama N, Hara T, Maehiro S, Imoto T: Intercostal nerve transfer for traumatic brachial nerve palsy. Orthop Surg (Tokyo) 20:1527–1529, 1969.

229
Diagnostic Approach to Individual Nerve Injuries

David G. Kline

The diagnosis of nerve injuries and entrapments employs techniques common to other disease states such as an accurate history, a careful inspection, and then a thorough physical examination of the limb(s) involved, as well as selection of proper laboratory, radiological, and electrophysiological tests for confirmation. In addition, however, knowledge of the anatomy of the limb and thus the ability to localize as well as reconstruct the nature of the injury or disease affecting the nerve are of paramount importance. Once such limb anatomy is learned for peripheral nerve disease, it can be utilized to more accurately examine not only those patients with nerve injury but also those with spinal root, spinal cord, and even cerebral disorders. Such knowledge provides a breadth of clinical findings not available to the more casual diagnostician, who may record only reflex changes, drift of an extremity, decreased hand grip, or weakness in dorsiflexion of the foot as an index of a more central disorder affecting the limb.

A systematized approach helps in evaluating the limb with a neurological disorder, just as it does in reviewing a chest film or a cerebral CT scan. In this way the details are appreciated. Along the way one can not only document motor, sensory, and autonomic function of the limb but also develop a sense of joint mobility, vascular supply, soft tissue integrity and scar, and irritability of the nerves. The examiner dealing with peripheral nerve injury has a tremendous advantage, for he or she can usually compare function in the abnormal limb with that of the contralateral and usually normal limb.

Diagnostic considerations for brachial plexus lesions are presented elsewhere in this text, whereas those for the five major nerves of the upper limb, namely, the axillary, musculocutaneous, radial, median, and ulnar nerves and the lumbosacral plexus and its outflow, including the sciatic, femoral, and sural nerves, are included in this chapter.

Upper Extremity

Axillary Nerve

This nerve is usually the third major branch from the posterior cord, earlier branches being the subscapular to supply the subscapularis muscle and thoracodorsal to innervate the latissimus dorsi. It usually leaves the posterior cord at the clavicular level and along with the artery and vein penetrates the quadrilateral space to innervate the deltoid, a multipentate muscle capping the shoulder. Variations in origin and course do occur but are few. The sensory portion of the nerve supplies the cap of the shoulder. Sensory distribution is variable in extent, and injury usually results in a relative rather than an absolute loss in that area. The supraspinatus initiates abduction of the arm, for the first 15 to 20 degrees away from the side of the body, but the deltoid provides abduction to 180 degrees and then is aided by serratus anterior, rhomboids, and trapezius to provide both rotation and stabilization of the scapula for the next 90 degrees of abduction. Thus, in the presence of complete paralysis of the deltoid (which is the only muscle innervated by the axillary nerve), the patient with intact suprascapular nerve input to the supraspinatus can still initiate some abduction and even learn to "toss" or rapidly swing his limb upward beyond 180 degrees and to use scapular rotary muscles to provide some further abduction. The patient with axillary nerve palsy cannot maintain the limb at 180 degrees in true lateral abduction, particularly when downward pressure is applied (Fig. 229-1). Some degree of forward or anterior abduction of the limb can be achieved owing to contraction of the long head of the biceps, but this will not substitute for true lateral abduction. Within a few weeks of injury, inspection and palpation show atrophy as well as some droop of the shoulder, with lengthening of the deltoid muscle due to the unopposed gravitational pull of the limb. It should be obvious that other shoulder and limb muscles related to the origin and course of axillary nerve need to be examined, for this

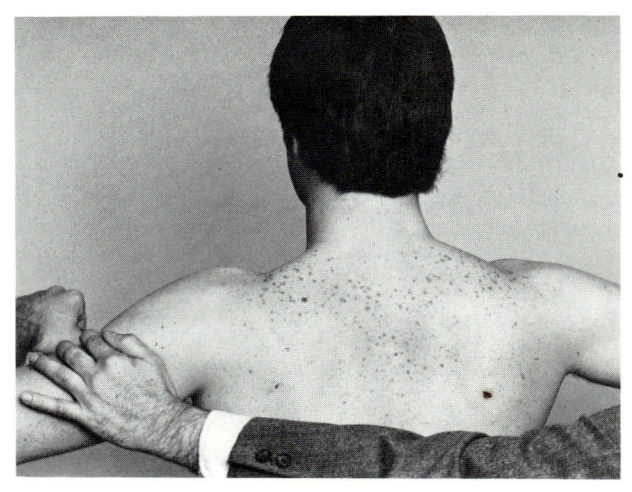

Figure 229-1 Testing deltoid function. The arms are roughly at 180 degrees of abduction.

1833

will localize the injury. It should be determined whether the supraspinatus and infraspinatus muscles contract, what the biceps brachialis function is, whether the latissimus dorsi (cough muscle) contracts, and what the function is of the radial nerve–innervated muscles.

Isolated axillary nerve paralysis is often due to milder degrees of stretch and distraction of the limb, particularly with hyperabduction of the arm with or without dislocation and/or fracture of the humeral head. Injections, particularly of serum or serum-related products, (whether given into the deltoid muscle or into the triceps) can lead to isolated deltoid paralysis, which does not always reverse with time. A recently identified syndrome, the *quadrilateral space syndrome*, can be associated with "spontaneous" axillary nerve palsy.[1] It is associated with stenosis or occlusion of the posterior humeral circumflex artery upon abduction of the arm.

Musculocutaneous Nerve

This nerve is one of the two major branches of the lateral cord in 88 percent of cases.[5] The other branch is the lateral branch to the median nerve, which supplies median-innervated forearm flexors and sensation in the median nerve distribution. In the remainder of cases, the musculocutaneous nerve originates from the proximal median nerve soon after the latter's formation by a lateral branch from the lateral cord and a medial branch from the medial cord. In the usual limb, the nerve angles laterally to penetrate the biceps-brachialis muscles, giving off fine coracobrachialis branches as it does so. Sensory fibers leave the nerve via the lateral cutaneous nerve of the forearm supplying the lateral border of the forearm to a variable extent. Injury can be direct, as in the case of penetrating wounds from a knife, glass, or bullet. Loss can also be seen as part of a distal stretch injury to the plexus at the level where cords change to nerves. A solitary injury to the musculocutaneous nerve is seldom produced by injection or fracture, presumably because of its medial locus and protection by the usually large and "fleshy" biceps muscle.

Testing for biceps-brachialis function should be done with the forearm and hand supinated or "palm up" so as to reduce input from the brachioradialis, which is innervated by the radial nerve. With intact musculocutaneous input, the biceps tendon can be readily palpated as it crosses the antecubital space, as can the muscle belly in the upper arm (Fig. 229-2). Most patients with musculocutaneous nerve loss but intact radial nerve input to the limb readily learn to substitute the brachioradialis and achieve very effective but, of course, not as strong flexion of the forearm on the upper arm, particularly when the hand is partially pronated.

Radial Nerve

The radial nerve originates in the distal axilla from the posterior cord after the latter gives off its subscapularis, thoracodorsal, and axillary nerves. It lies posterior and deep to the axillary artery and runs in a somewhat oblique direction toward the humeral groove. Its course is usually just medial to the profundus branch of the axillary-brachial artery, and

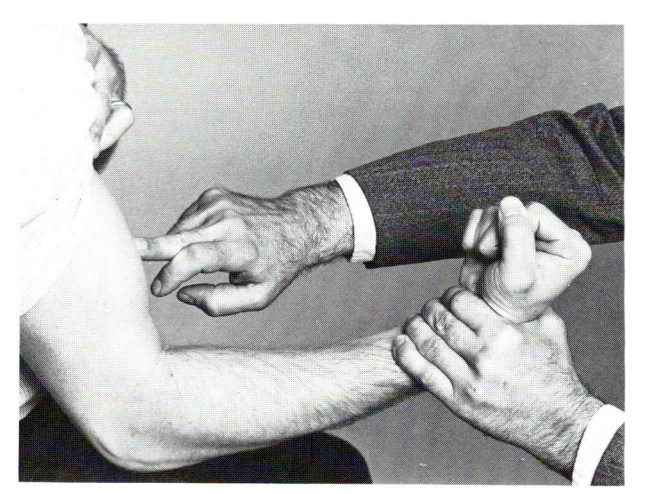

Figure 229-2 Biceps-brachialis testing. The hand and forearm are supinated and the elbow is resting on a firm surface.

usually just proximal to this point it gives rise to one or more triceps branches. The nerve passes superficial to the subscapularis muscle but may penetrate it. Arterial and venous branches of the axillary vessels are deep to the nerve and pass with it to the humeral groove. Injury at this level can be associated with a stretch to the distal brachial plexus outflow, can be caused by a gunshot wound, or can occur as part of a more complex sharp, penetrating injury; occasionally the radial nerve can be involved by an intrinsic tumor such as a neurofibroma or schwannoma. Compression of the axilla, such as occurs with crutch palsy or "Saturday night palsy" can also result in proximal damage. Key to the diagnosis of proximal radial nerve injury or disease is paralysis of the triceps together with loss in the distribution of more distal muscles innervated by the radial nerve. The triceps has three heads or parts and is the only effective extensor of the forearm on the upper arm other than gravity. The triceps is readily palpable in the posterior compartment of the upper arm and testing should always include palpation, since gravity can substitute for it.

The greatest incidence of radial nerve involvement is at the midhumeral level as the nerve winds around the humerus to take its position deep in the lateral, mid, and distal segments of the upper arm, between and somewhat beneath both the lateral triceps and the biceps-brachialis. At the midhumeral level, the usual mechanism of injury is humeral fracture. The hallmark of injury at this level is the sparing of triceps function in the presence of more distal radial distribution loss; including loss of brachioradialis function. Unlike the musculocutaneous nerve, the radial is relatively superficial from the mid-upper arm down and can be more readily injured by an inferiorly placed injection or by penetrating object. Radial palsy is an associated finding in up to 20 percent of humeral fractures.[14] The incidence increases with oblique fractures, compound or complex fractures, and fractures requiring open surgical manipulation for reduction. Branches to the brachioradialis leave the radial proximal to the elbow but in the adult limb at a point 3 in. or more distal to the midhumeral level, a consideration when

Diagnostic Approach to Individual Nerve Injuries

looking for signs of recovery in radial palsies associated with humeral fractures.[7]

Brachioradialis function is tested with the forearm and hand halfway between pronation and supination by asking the patient to flex the forearm on the upper arm. The biceps, if innervated, will, of course, also contract. The brachioradialis will rise up and be palpable along the radial aspect of the proximal forearm (Fig. 229-3).

Loss due to upper arm level involvement of the radial nerve will also include paralysis of the extensor carpi ulnaris, supinator, extensor carpi radialis, extensor communis including the extensor indicis proprius, and extensor pollicis longus muscles. Wrist drop and inability to extend the fingers and thumb are the more obvious findings (Fig. 229-4). If the extensor communis undergoes contracture owing to paralysis and poor splinting or care of the palsied extremity, some dorsiflexion of the wrist can be gained paradoxically by flexing the fingers while making a fist.[9] The radial nerve also innervates the anconeus at the level of the elbow. This is not a muscle of importance functionally but it occasionally is useful to an especially skillful electromyographer, who may be able to detect evidence of relatively early and proximal radial regeneration by needling this muscle.

At the elbow level, the radial nerve courses beneath brachioradialis, and usually a distal branch leaves the nerve to supply this muscle. In the proximal forearm the nerve divides into the superficial radial sensory and posterior interosseous nerves. A branch to the extensor carpi radialis provides the most proximal wrist extensor input from the radial complex and can either originate from the nerve before it branches or originate from the proximal superficial radial sensory branch.[5] The extensor carpi radialis provides radial extension of the wrist along with the extensor pollicis longus, and since it does not originate from the posterior interosseous nerve (PIN), its function is unimpaired in conditions involving this nerve (Fig. 229-5). Entrapment of the PIN can occur as it passes beneath the volar head of the supinator or by more proximal connective tissue or vascular bands. Contusion leading to swelling of the volar compartment of the forearm, with or without fracture of the radius and ulna, can also lead to compression of the nerve at this level, as can an occasional soft tissue tumor. Wrist extension is weak and the hand deviates in a radial direction since the extensor carpi ulnaris (ECU) and the extensor communis are paralyzed or weak. Just before the PIN runs beneath the volar head of the supinator, it gives off a branch to the ECU, which provides extension of the wrist in an ulnar direction. Extension of the thumb due to extensor pollicis longus function (Fig. 229-6) is lost with complete lesions at this level, while supination may or may not be weak. Since biceps contraction can provide some supinating movement to the forearm, true supinator function is best tested with the arm fully extended. The examiner grasps the patient's hand and asks the patient to try to turn the hand palm uppermost against some resistance.

The PIN courses somewhat obliquely and deep to the volar head of the supinator toward the dorsal compartment of the forearm, where it rapidly divides "pes-like" to supply

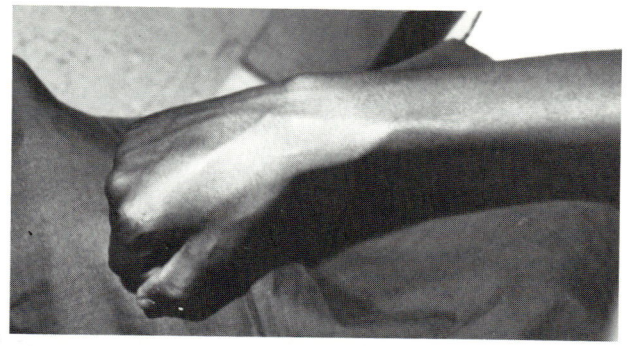

Figure 229-4 Wrist drop and inability to extend the thumb and fingers due to a proximal radial palsy secondary to a fracture of the humerus.

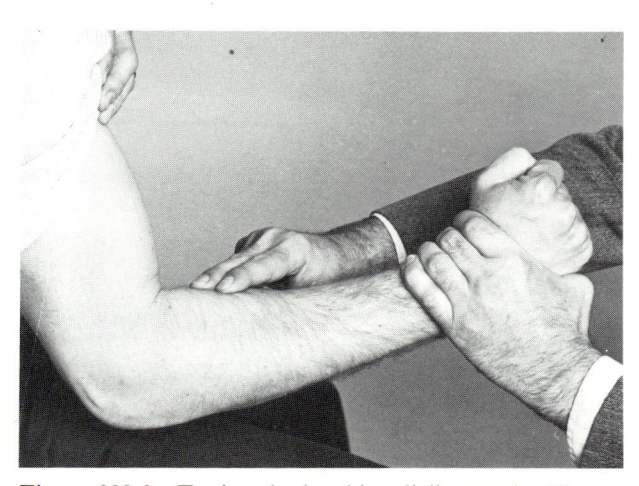

Figure 229-3 Testing the brachioradialis muscle. The forearm and hand are halfway between pronation and supination and the patient is asked to flex the forearm on the arm.

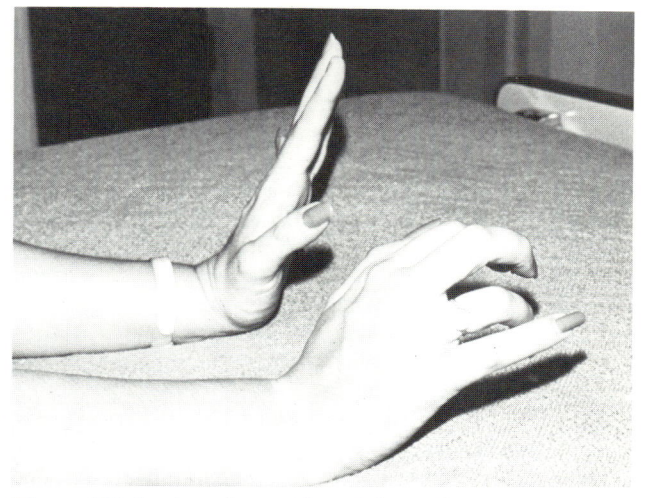

Figure 229-5 A patient with a right supinator entrapment of the posterior interosseous nerve. Normal left wrist and finger extension is seen. The right wrist extends only in a radial direction and extension of the fingers is partial.

the extensor communis and extensor pollicis longus.[6] These muscles are the terminals for the PIN branches. Involvement at this level is seen with penetrating wounds of the dorsal compartment of the forearm and an occasional fracture of the radius. Here, wrist extension is partially or completely preserved while extension of the fingers may be variable, with some of this function weaker in some fingers than in others and extension of the thumb usually absent. Useful function of the extensor communis is partially dependent on contraction and thus the ability of the median- and ulnar-innervated lumbricales to fix or set the metacarpal-phalangeal joints of the fingers so that extension of the distal phalanges can occur. As a result, if ulnar or median palsy is an associated finding, one must set the M-P joint by grasping it with finger and thumb or by placing the hand palm down on a flat firm surface and asking the patient to attempt to extend the fingers.

The radial sensory branch takes a more superficial course through the forearm than does the PIN and supplies a portion of the dorsum of the hand. Variability of the sensory distribution of this portion of the radial nerve is more the rule than the exception and it is possible to have complete radial nerve dysfunction with little or no discernible sensory loss. If loss is present it can usually be found in response to touch and/or pinprick over the region of the anatomic "snuffbox" bounded by the tendons of the extensor pollicis longus and the abductor pollicis (Fig. 229-6). Distal forearm injury, which is usually penetrating when it involves the radial sensory branch, may or may not cause discernible loss. However, since this is a sensory nerve, injury may lead to neuroma formation and often to a painful forearm and a very sensitive dorsum of the hand, with a mixture of hypesthesia and hyperesthesia on sensory testing.

Median Nerve

The median nerve originates at the lower axillary level from branches of the lateral cord (which supplies the median distribution sensation and sometimes the pronator teres and a portion of the flexor mechanism) and the medial cord (which usually supplies the flexors of the wrist and fingers and the median-innervated intrinsic muscles of the thumb). The nerve lies superficial to, but closely applied to, the brachial artery. Variations in lateral and median cord branches are not infrequent. For example, in 24 percent of cases, some of the lateral cord fibers intended for the median nerve travel in the musculocutaneous nerve for a distance before leaving it and returning to median.[5] Occasionally proximal Martin-Gruber anastomosis will occur in the upper arm. The lateral cord branch may also communicate with the medial cord branch before the median nerve is formed. The median nerve does not innervate any upper arm muscles but as it approaches the antecubital fossa, it does branch to innervate the pronator teres. Thus, upper arm lesions that are complete will paralyze all median-innervated muscles as well as produce a loss of sensation in the median distribution of the hand. Gunshot wounds, distal stretches (which usually involve other nerves as well), an occasional tumor, and penetrating wounds are the usual mechanisms of injury. Since the nerve is close to the brachial artery and vein, these struc-

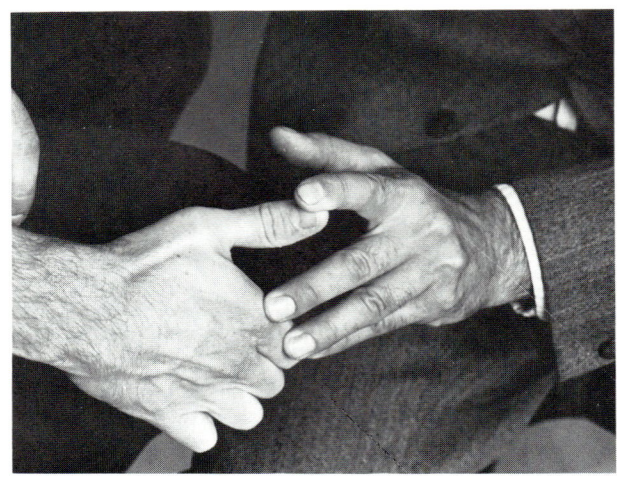

Figure 229-6 Testing the extensor pollicis longus muscle. Note that the tendons of this muscle and the abductor pollicis longus stand out in the region of the anatomist's snuffbox.

tures may be involved as well as the ulnar nerve, with which the median travels in the proximal portion of the upper arm.

Pronation is best tested with the upper arm extended; the patient should rotate the hand palm down while the examiner clasps it (Fig. 229-7). Supination can also be tested in a similar fashion.

The flexor carpi radialis, which supplies wrist flexion in a radial direction, is also paralyzed with a proximal median nerve injury. (However, in a few patients the musculocutaneous nerve can innervate this muscle as well as the pronator teres.) The palmaris longus, which is of little functional importance but which "corrugates" the palm of the hand, is paralyzed, as is the flexor digitorum sublimus, which flexes the middle phalanges of all four fingers. The distal phalan-

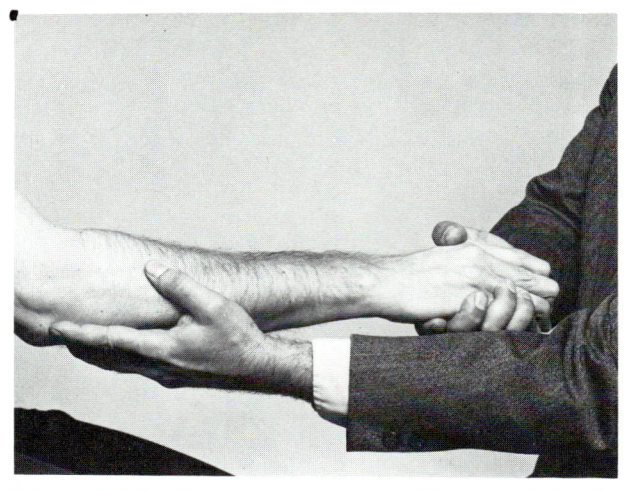

Figure 229-7 Testing for pronation. The patient's hand is clasped by the examiner's while the elbow is steadied with the other hand and the patient is asked to turn the hand palm down. Supination can also be tested with the limb in the same position.

Diagnostic Approach to Individual Nerve Injuries

ges must be kept as flaccid as possible when testing or otherwise the profundi will substitute for the sublimus. The nerve passes beneath the tendinous arch of the flexor superficialis and is usually somewhat adherent to it. The anterior interosseous branch usually, but not always, supplies the flexor profundus of the forefinger and long finger although the latter may also or alternatively be supplied by the ulnar nerve branch to the profundi or more distally may share a slip of tendon with that to the ring finger.[2] Profundus function to the long finger is seldom totally paralyzed with median nerve injuries or with anterior interosseous palsy. The profundi flex the distal phalanges and are best tested by placing the fingers palm up on a firm surface and holding the proximal and middle phalanges flat while asking the patient to flex the distal phalanx against resistance (Fig. 229-8). The anterior interosseous nerve also supplies the flexor pollicis longus, which provides flexion of the distal phalanx of the thumb. Injury or, less frequently, spontaneous entrapment of the anterior interosseous branch produces a very characteristic syndrome in which the usual pinch mechanism is lost and because of loss of distal flexion of the forefinger and thumb the patient is unable to form an "O." Although the median nerve is deep in the volar midforearm, it can be injured at this level in association with a fracture in the forearm (Monteggia fracture), a crushing injury or other lesion producing ischemia and edema of the forearm, and a penetrating injury due to a knife, glass, or bullet.[7]

Volkmann's ischemic contracture is the classic paradigm of secondary injury at the forearm level. With dislocation, with or without fracture, of the elbow, the brachial artery can be contused and/or go into spasm, producing ischemia. This results in some cases in infarction of the volar forearm musculature and in secondary compression, as well as in primary ischemia of the median nerve, producing a severe median palsy. On occasion, radial and even ulnar palsy can also result. Early signs of such a disorder include vascular symptoms in the fingers, severe and painful paresthesias in the hand, and then the onset of numbness. In time, contracture of the fingers with clawing occurs secondary to forearm flexor muscle shortening combined with paralysis of the intrinsic muscles of the hand.

In the lower third of the forearm, the median nerve innervates the pronator quadratus, which supplements the function of the pronator teres and is best tested with the forearm flexed on the upper arm.[11] As the median nerve approaches the wrist, it lies beneath the flexor carpi radialis and palmaris longus but superficial to the flexor superficialis. Injuries at this level are very common, particularly those due to glass or knife wounds and, of course, suicide attempts. Gunshot wound is an occasional etiology, as is the Colles fracture of the wrist. In these settings, the ulnar nerve can occasionally be affected as well as the median nerve. Median palsy due to lesions at this level will result in paralysis of the abductor pollicis brevis and opponens pollicis. Palmar abduction of the thumb utilizes not only the abductor pollicis brevis but also the flexor pollicis brevis (which has both median and ulnar input) and to a lesser extent the opponens pollicis (Fig. 229-9). The lumbricales of the forefinger and long finger are also paralyzed although these muscles may be entirely innervated by the ulnar nerve. In a few cases the long finger lumbricale may have dual input from

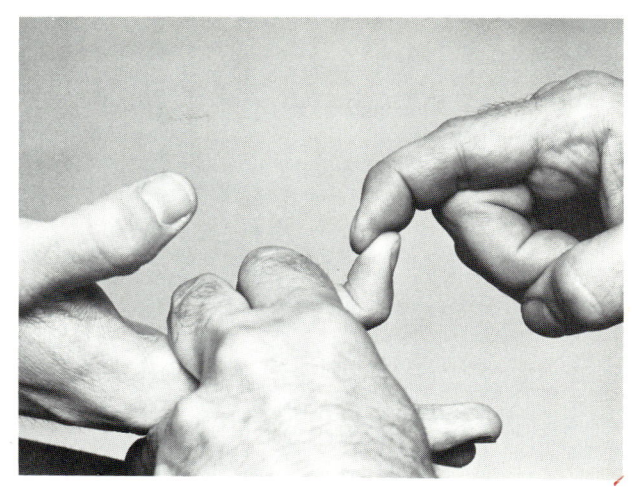

Figure 229-8 The flexor profundus of the forefinger is tested by fixing the metacarpal-phalangeal and proximal interphalangeal joints and matching the patient's distal phalangeal contraction against the examiner's. Note the concomitant flexion of the thumb.

both median and ulnar nerves. The lumbricale muscles are difficult to test by themselves since the extensor communis plays some role even when the metacarpal-phalangeal joint is held in hyperextension and the patient is asked to extend the middle or intermediate phalanx against resistance. With ulnar palsy, there is loss of the stabilizing influence of the little finger and to a lesser extent ring finger lumbricales on the M-P joints. Extensor communis function is ineffective and thus these fingers tend to claw. This is rarely the case with the forefinger or long finger even with a distal median nerve palsy.

The sensory distribution of the median nerve covers a portion but usually not all of the volar surface of the thumb,

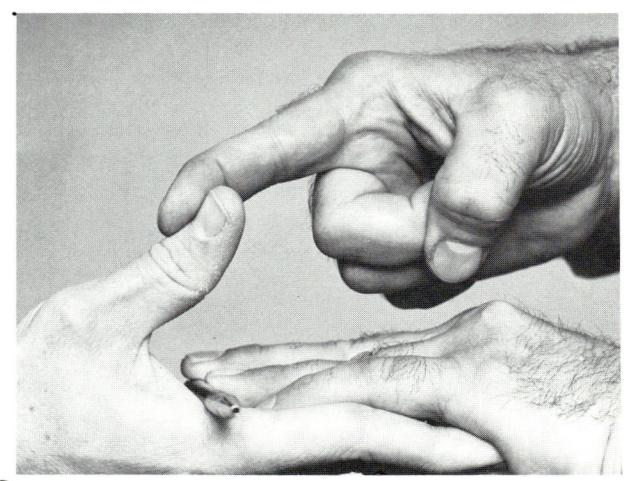

Figure 229-9 The abductor pollicis brevis is tested by asking the patient to lift the thumb away from the palm in a right-angled fashion. In this instance the examiner has placed a pen in the patient's palm. Sighting this helps the patient lift the thumb at a right angle.

the volar and dorsal surfaces of the distal two phalanges of the forefinger, and a variable portion of the volar and dorsal surfaces of the long finger, particularly its radial half (Figs. 229-10, 229-11). The sensory distribution extends to the palm, including a portion of the thenar eminence, and sometimes includes all of the long finger and the radial half of the ring finger. Inspection of autonomous zones with the ophthalmoscope while looking for the presence or absence of beads of sweat is also important.[4] The median nerve is frequently involved when true causalgia affecting the hand is present; this distinctive syndrome has been covered extensively elsewhere.[10,13,14]

Ulnar Nerve

Brachial plexus contribution to the ulnar nerve is entirely from the medial cord. As a result, the nerve lies medial to the course of the brachial artery and somewhat inferior to that vessel as well as the brachial vein. The ulnar nerve also lies close to the median nerve in the proximal upper arm but gradually courses somewhat obliquely to leave the company of that nerve and the major vessels and travel toward the olecranon notch. Along the way it travels beneath the intermuscular septum. Upper arm injury of the ulnar nerve is usually due to a knife or gunshot wound. Serious injury results in total ulnar palsy, which includes loss of flexor carpi ulnaris function, some flexor profundus loss (especially to the little finger), and loss of function in the abductor digiti quinti, opponens digiti quinti, lumbricales (partial), interosseous, and adductor pollicis muscles. The flexor pollicis brevis is paretic but seldom totally paralyzed since it also receives input from the median nerve.

An inch or so proximal to the elbow, one or more large branches leave the ulnar nerve to supply the flexor carpi ulnaris. The nerve at this level is often quite adherent to the

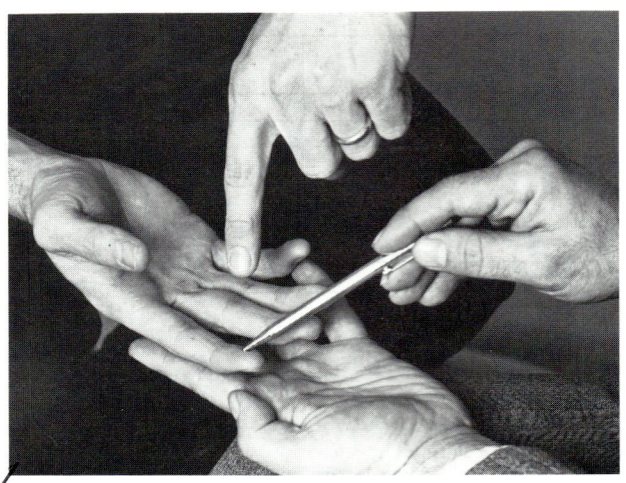

Figure 229-11 In this instance, the patient, whose eyes are closed, has been asked by the examiner to localize where touch applied in an autonomous area of the median nerve by the tip of a pen is occurring.

medial head of the triceps. Struther's ligament, if present, can entrap the proximal ulnar nerve just as it does the median nerve, although less frequently.

At the elbow, the ulnar nerve runs along the olecranon notch, with the vessels deep to the nerve. In some individuals the nerve may translocate out of the notch with flexion of the forearm on the upper arm. Since the nerve is often snug in the notch region to begin with, it can readily be entrapped secondary to repeated flexion and extension of the arm with or without a history of repetitive compression, to prior elbow fracture or dislocation, or to contusion with soft tissue swelling around the elbow. The onset of symptoms is usually insidious and the initial presentation is somewhat variable.[3] The most common presentation is with the onset of sensory symptoms in the ulnar distribution, consisting of paresthesias and, less frequently, complaints of numbness. Sensory testing shows a mixture of hypesthesia with hyperesthesia. The ulnar sensory distribution includes the little finger and usually all, but sometimes just the ulnar half, of the ring finger and even less frequently all of the ring finger and the ulnar half of the long finger. Autonomous zones include the volar and distal surfaces of the distal phalanx of the little finger and the volar surface of the middle or intermediate phalanx. Sensory change is most likely to be found in these areas. Most loss is variable. Since some but not all the branches supplying the flexor carpi ulnaris come off above the elbow, function of that muscle, which provides strong wrist flexion in an ulnar direction, is spared (Fig. 229-12). The ulnar nerve innervates a variable portion of the flexor profundi depending on median input. Thus, there may be connections between the anterior interosseous branch of the median nerve and the flexor profundus motor branch of the ulnar nerve which can affect loss seen in these muscles with either ulnar or median nerve injuries. The deep flexor to the little finger is, however, innervated by the ulnar nerve, and with complete injury this function will be lost. With entrapment it may or may not be weak. More certain with moderately severe and/or long-standing entrap-

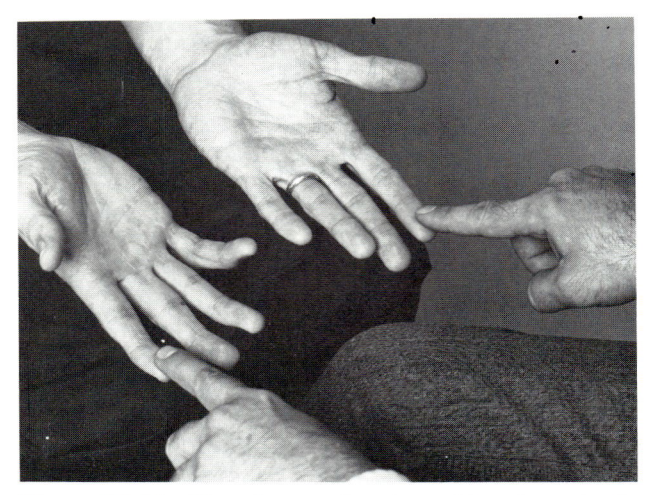

Figure 229-10 Here the examiner is stroking the patient's forefingers over a portion of the autonomous zones of both median nerves. The patient is asked to compare the touch on one side with that on the other. With this approach, the examiner can readily modulate the pressure applied and the area stroked.

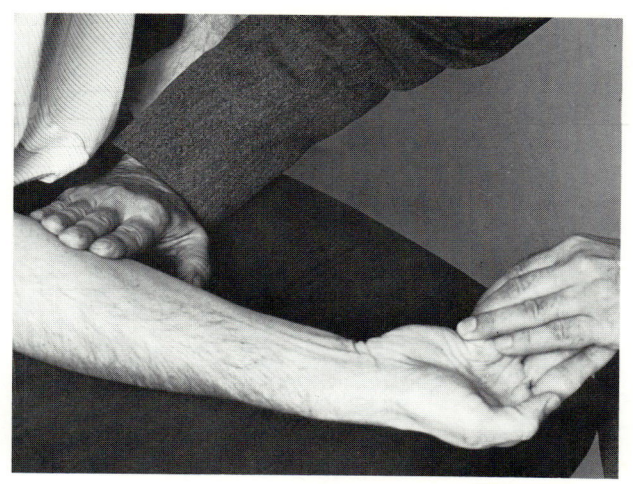

Diagnostic Approach to Individual Nerve Injuries

Figure 229-12 Testing for flexor carpi ulnaris function. The muscle belly is palpable in the proximal volar forearm as the hand is brought into flexion in an ulnar direction.

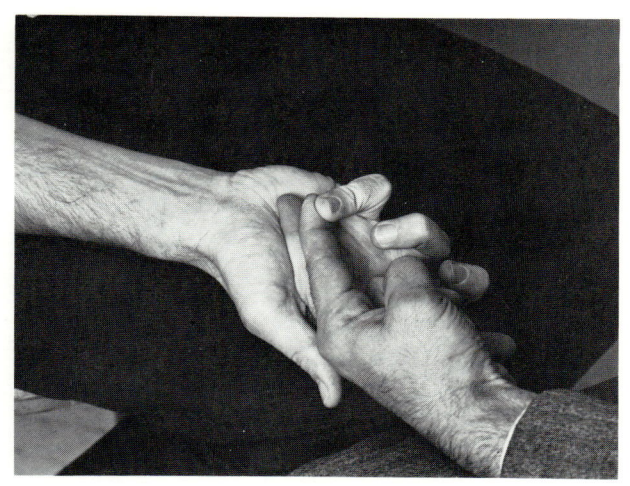

Figure 229-14 Opponens digiti quinti testing. The examiner's long finger and forefinger are placed one on top of the other in the midpalmar area and the patient is asked to flex his little finger down and press its distal phalanx into the examiner's fingers. In the adult with full opponens strength, the examiner should not be able to separate his forefinger and long finger. Using the same approach, the opponens pollicis of the thumb can be tested.

ment is weakness or loss of the intrinsic hand muscles innervated by the ulnar nerve. This loss includes the muscles of the hypothenar eminence, where atrophy will often be readily discernible. The abductor digiti quinti (Fig. 229-13) will be weak, as will also be the opponens digiti quinti (Fig. 229-14) and the lumbricale muscle to the little finger (Fig. 229-15). The lumbricale to the ring finger has a dual innervation from both ulnar and median nerves in 50 percent of cases and thus may not be weak.[14] The lumbricales provide important stabilization of the first M-P joint, permitting the extensor communis to extend the fingers. With their loss, the fingers are drawn down into a claw hand position because the flexor superficialis (and in more distal ulnar lesions the flexor profundi) are relatively unopposed (Fig. 229-16).

The interossei are usually the most severely affected and their loss can be appreciated by inspection of the dorsum of the hand, where atrophy, especially of the first dorsal interosseous muscle, may be evident, and by proper testing (Fig. 229-17). These muscles, along with the abductor digiti quinti minimi, provide abduction and adduction movements of small excursion necessary for fine manipulative movements of the hand, and thus their loss is quite disabling. In addition, the adductor pollicis will be weak or absent and

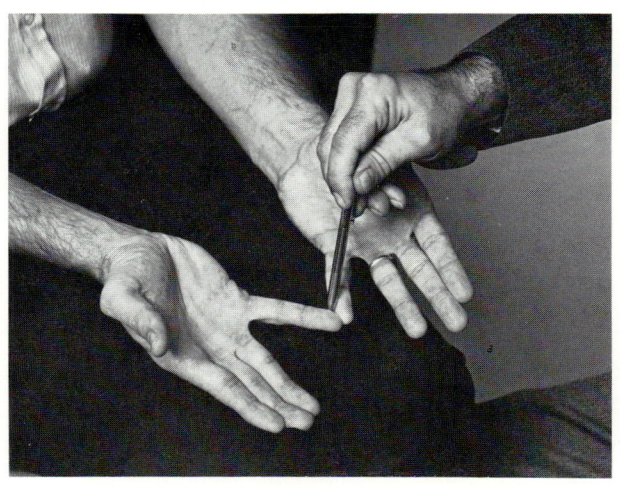

Figure 229-13 Abductor digit quinti function compared side to side. The patient is asked to bridge his little fingers together. An attempt is made to draw a pen through the "bridge." The weaker side will collapse and the pen will come through on that side.

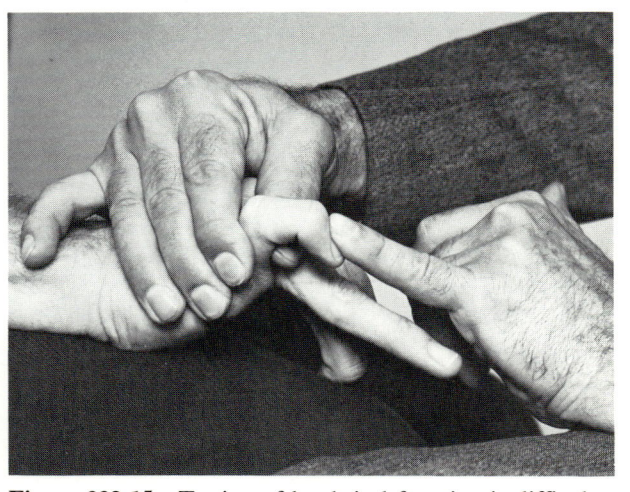

Figure 229-15 Testing of lumbrical function is difficult. In this case, the lumbrical to the little finger is evaluated by holding the metacarpal-phalangeal joint in extension and asking the patient to extend the intermediate and distal phalanges against the resistance of the examiner's little finger.

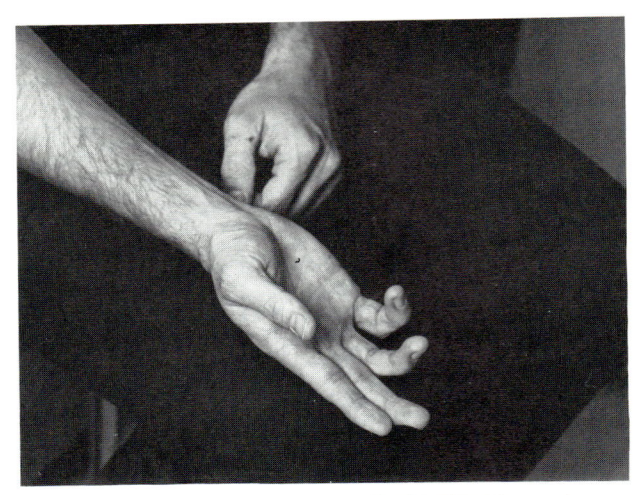

Figure 229-16 Typical posture of a hand with an ulnar palsy, with partial flexion or clawing of the little finger and the ring finger.

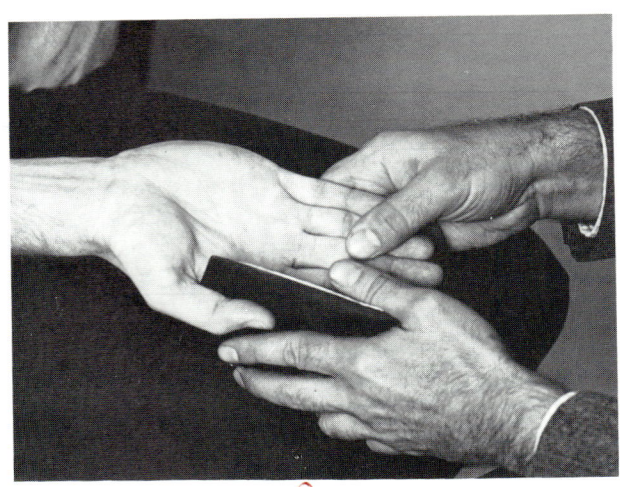

Figure 229-18 Testing for adductor pollicis function, which in this case is weak. As a result, the flexor pollicis has substituted, producing a classic Froment's sign.

adduction of the thumb parallel with the plane of the palm is difficult. As a result, the patient quickly substitutes the flexor pollicis longus, which is median-innervated, to provide a pinch against the side of the palm or forefinger (Froment's sign) (Fig. 229-18).

Branches to the profundi come off the ulnar nerve 1½ to 2½ in. distal to the olecranon notch in adults so that injury distal to this level will spare these muscles. Instead, sensory loss and dysfunction of the intrinsic muscles of the hand will be the principal findings. At a proximal or sometimes mid-forearm level, 15 percent of patients have a communication between either the whole median nerve or its anterior interosseous branch and the ulnar nerve, so that a portion of the median input to the hand travels in the ulnar nerve through a variable portion of the forearm. Input back to the median nerve may occur in the distal forearm or in the palm by a connection between the deep branch of the ulnar nerve and the recurrent thenar branch, the so-called Riche-Cannieu connection.[13] Similar connections in the palm between the median and ulnar sensory branches account for variations in ulnar sensory distribution.

The dorsal cutaneous sensory branch of the ulnar arises usually at the junction of the mid and distal thirds of the forearm. This branch supplies a relatively unimportant area, from a functional standpoint, on the back of the hand. However, injury often results in a painful neuroma as well as in paresthesias, which are especially bothersome when the dorsum of the hand is brushed against clothing or slid into a glove.[10]

Injury of the nerve at the wrist after the takeoff of the dorsal cutaneous branch results in hand intrinsic muscle loss and hypesthesia, at least in the autonomous zones of the nerve (Fig. 229-19). The mechanism of injury at this level is usually laceration due to glass or a knife and the ulnar artery is often involved as well, since it is anatomically close to the nerve. Less frequent are lesions due to gunshot wound or fracture.

The ulnar nerve enters the palm beneath an ulnar expansion of the transverse ligament and on the radial side of the pisiform bone through Guyon's canal. It divides into superficial and deep branches, the former supplying sensation and usually the hypothenar muscles and the latter supplying the other intrinsic muscles innervated by the ulnar nerve. Injury in this area can be due to entrapment (which is much less frequent than that at the elbow level) or to penetrating wounds of the proximal palm.

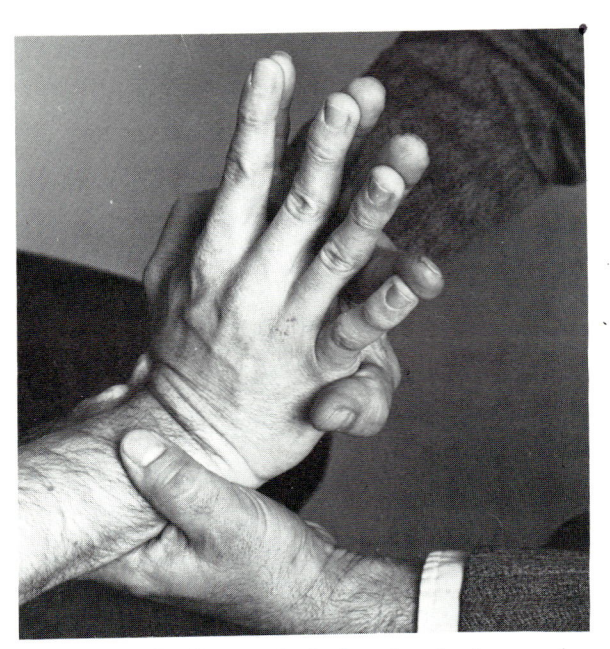

Figure 229-17 One method of testing the interossei where the wrist and fingers of the patient are placed in extension by bracing the examiner's fingers against the patient's. The patient is then asked to abduct and adduct his fingers against the resistance of the examiner's fingers.

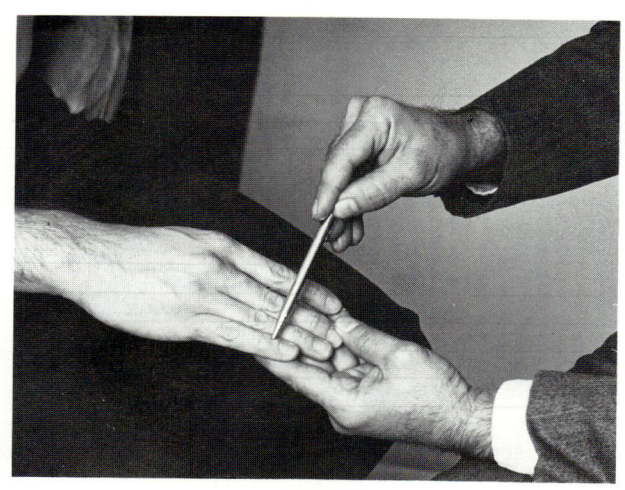

Diagnostic Approach to Individual Nerve Injuries

Figure 229-19 The examiner is stroking an autonomous zone in the ulnar distribution and asking the patient to localize sensation in that area with the eyes closed.

Lower Extremity

Lumbosacral Plexus

Fortunately, serious injury or tumor involving the lumbosacral plexus occurs much less frequently than similar conditions affecting the brachial plexus. Both are difficult to approach surgically and to repair but the lumbosacral plexus is especially so. Nonetheless, some understanding of the anatomical complexities of the plexus is necessary if one is to intelligently examine the peripheral nervous system of the lower extremity. The serious student should consult the drawings and the full text available in Haymaker and Woodhall's text.[2]

The lumbar portion of the plexus originates from the anterior primary rami, which are formed in turn by the roots of L1 through L4. L1 may receive a communication from T12, the subcostal nerve; the anterior primary ramus of L4 contributes to the sacral plexus by way of the lumbosacral trunk. Since the spinal cord usually terminates at the L1 level of the spine, both anterior and posterior divisions of the various roots have a variable length within the spinal canal. The latter are an extension of the central nervous system while the former are peripheral nerves even though they are in the spinal canal. The two divisions combine within the intervertebral portion of the root canal and exit the foramen as a single motor-sensory root just as brachial plexus roots do in the neck. Roots are located within the psoas muscle, which is innervated by branches from the anterior primary rami. The L1 root gives rise to the iliohypogastric, ilioinguinal, and genitofemoral nerves, the latter also receiving input in most cases from L2. L2 also contributes to the obturator nerve, as does L3, while the femoral nerve is formed by contributions from L2, L3, and L4. The lateral femoral cutaneous nerve is formed by L2 and L3. Lumbar plexus injuries result in a variable pattern of loss related to the sensory dermatomes and muscle myotomes corresponding to the above roots.

The iliohypogastric nerve passes through the psoas muscle and over the quadratus lumborum to reach the area superior to the iliac crest. There it lies between the transverse and internal oblique muscles, which it supplies in part. The nerve penetrates the internal and external obliques as it extends anteriorly. Its sensory distribution is via a lateral cutaneous branch to the skin of the superior gluteal region and via an anterior branch to the lower abdominal skin above the pubis. Injury to this nerve is usually iatrogenic, due to abdominal procedures, and results, unfortunately, in painful paresthesias or a sensory deficit in these distributions.

The ilioinguinal nerve circles the trunk just below the iliohypogastric and laterally is located between the transverse and internal oblique muscles. Part of its more medial course is along the inguinal ligament and then through the superficial inguinal ring and the external spermatic fascia. This nerve also supplies the internal oblique and transversalis muscles, but, more importantly, it supplies cutaneous sensation to the skin over the symphysis pubis, the dorsum of the penis, the upper scrotum, and the upper thigh medial to the femoral triangle.

The genitofemoral nerve, unlike the iliohypogastric and ilioinguinal nerves, takes a straight caudal course along with iliac vessels and forms two branches, the genital branch, which innervates the cremaster muscle and a portion of scrotal skin, and the femoral branch, which penetrates the fascia lata of the thigh to supply sensation to the skin in the region of the femoral triangle.

The femoral nerve is one of the major outflows of the lumbar plexus. After its formation by the L2, L3, and L4 roots, it courses several inches within the pelvis in a retroperitoneal position but superior and somewhat lateral to the psoas and iliopsoas muscles before passing beneath the inguinal ligament lateral to the femoral artery and vein. An inch or two distal to the ligament it divides pes-like into a number of branches supplying the quadriceps muscle, which is composed of the rectus femoris and the three vasti.[6] Sensory contributions from the femoral nerve go to the anteromedial thigh but also form the saphenous nerve, which courses obliquely along the medial thigh and knee and then branches to supply the medial surface of the lower leg and the medial aspect of the foot.

In the pelvis, branches of the femoral nerve supply the iliopsoas, which is a major flexor muscle of the thigh on the abdomen. This is best tested with the patient supine: the examiner holds the leg beneath the knee with the lower leg flexed on the upper and asks the patient to pull the thigh up or flex it against resistance. Less important are branches to the sartorius (tailor) muscle, which aides flexion at the hip and knee and assists lateral rotation of the hip. The function of the sartorius can be inferred from the fact that it arises from the anterior superior iliac spine above and inserts on the medial proximal tibia below.[2]

Injury to the femoral nerve within the pelvis may thus produce loss of hip flexion (iliopsoas) as well as an inability to extend the knee (Fig. 229-20). The latter loss interferes with a normal gait, the knee usually being hyperextended by the tensor fascia lata and gracilis muscles. Classically, going up stairs or climbing is very difficult or impossible under these circumstances. Pelvic level femoral nerve palsies due to penetrating lower abdominal injury caused by gunshot

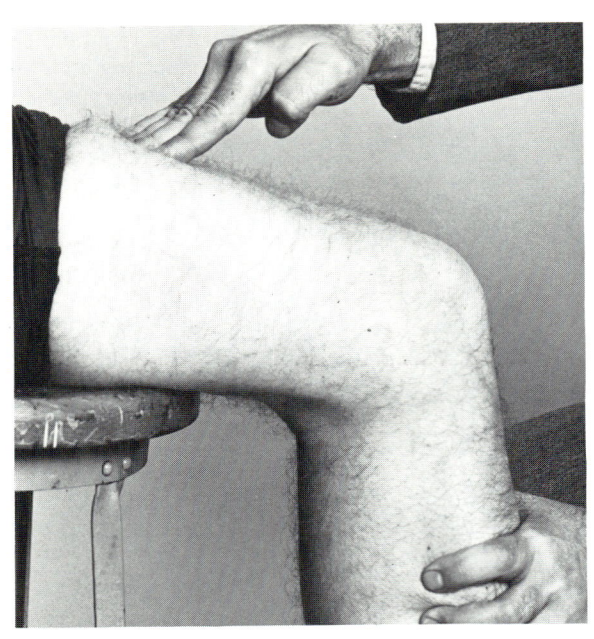

Figure 229-20 Palpation of the quadriceps femoris muscle as the patient attempts to extend the lower leg on the upper leg.

wounds, motorcycle handlebars, etc. have been seen in our clinic. Iatrogenic causes include packing of the pelvis or manipulation in association with bleeding during lower abdominal operations. A not infrequent cause is surgical section of a portion of the plexus for tumor removal, often either a benign neurofibroma or a schwannoma.[8] The femoral nerve can be mistaken for the lateral femoral cutaneous nerve and can be inadvertently resected in the treatment of meralgia paresthetica, or can be injured by investment with methyl methacrylate during hip repair. Sensory loss in the anteromedial thigh has been variable as has the degree of hip flexion weakness, but the absence of quadriceps function with loss of the knee jerk have been unmistakable. Thigh level injury in the region of the femoral triangle has been due to knife or glass wounds and less frequently to gunshot wounds (concomitant femoral artery and/or vein injury can be fatal). Iatrogenic causes include injury during femoral-popliteal bypass grafting or saphenous vein stripping. Sensory loss in the saphenous nerve distribution may or may not accompany the quadriceps loss, depending on the level and extent of injury.

The *lateral femoral cutaneous nerve* (lateral cutaneous nerve of the thigh) penetrates the psoas, crosses the iliacus, and at the level of the anterior superior spine of the ilium courses downward between the attachments of the inguinal ligament. It supplies sensation to the lateral thigh but when stretched or entrapped can give rise to the characteristic syndrome of meralgia paresthetica with a tingling burning pain in the lateral thigh and often severe hyperesthesia so that the lateral thigh is easily irritated by clothing or touch. Patients will often report pinprick sensibility but an increased and painful sensibility to touch testing.

The *obturator nerve* reaches the medial border of the psoas, travels below or deep to the iliac vessels, and takes a rather vertical course toward the obturator foramen. There, it divides into an anterior or superficial branch, which supplies primarily the adductor longus and gracilis muscles, and a posterior or deep branch, which supplies the obturator externus and adductor magnus muscles. Since the adductor magnus is also innervated by the sciatic nerve and the adductor longus sometimes by the femoral nerve, complete loss of adduction and complete atrophy are seldom seen with obturator nerve injury.[2] However, gait will be mildly disturbed since the leg will be externally rotated or will tend to swing outward. Damage to this nerve can occur as a portion of a lumbosacral plexus injury or, less commonly, as an isolated palsy associated with a pelvic fracture, and even less frequently secondary to surgical injury. Sensory loss is quite variable and unreliable in my experience as an index of involvement of this nerve; relative loss is sometimes present in a patchy distribution in the lower medial thigh but at other times there is no sensory loss at all.

Sacral Plexus

The L4 root of the lumbosacral plexus contributes to the sacral plexus via the lumbosacral trunk, as does all of L5 and the individual primary rami of S1, S2, S3 and a portion of S4, which also contributes to the coccygeal plexus. Each ramus receives postganglionic sympathetic fibers destined for blood vessels and sweat glands of the limb while S2, S3, and S4 includes parasympathetic fibers destined for the bladder and anal sphincter. As with the lumbar portion of the pelvic plexus, loss with sacral plexus injuries is variable but one can identify the contributions involved if one knows the sensory dermatomes and myotomes innervated by the various lumbar and sacral roots, especially in the lower extremity. The posterior divisions form the gluteal nerves and the peroneal division of the sciatic, while the anterior divisions form the tibial, hamstring pudendal, and posterior cutaneous nerves of the thigh. The sacral plexus lies deep and medial in the pelvis overlying the sacroiliac and sacrococcygeal junctions, its nerves for the most part exiting the pelvis by the greater sciatic foramen (sciatic, hamstring, gluteal, and posterior cutaneous nerves), while the pudendal reaches the perineum via the lesser sciatic foramen.

The *sciatic nerve* is the most frequently injured lower extremity nerve. High or buttock level sciatic nerve injury is associated with dislocation or fracture of the hip and occasionally results from attempts to repair these injuries. Other etiologies include injection injuries, occasional missile wounds, infrequent tumors, and, very rarely, subgluteal blood clots secondary to massive blunt trauma to the buttocks.[8] Despite the course of the hamstring nerve, which is medial and parallel to the sciatic nerve, function of the hamstring muscles is usually preserved except with severe penetrating injuries that have involved this branch as well as the sciatic nerve as a whole. Since the peroneal division is in a posterior position close to the ala of the sacrum as it leaves the notch, it is very prone to injury with fractures in that region. At this level and shortly after leaving the sciatic foramen, the sciatic nerve can lie anterior or posterior to the piriformis muscle, or its two divisions may split to go around or in a few cases through the belly of this muscle. It usually lies on top of the gemelli and the quadratus and of course is deep to the glutei between the greater trochanter and the ischial tuberosity. Severe injury at this level results in complete sciatic palsy so that plantar flexion and inversion of foot as well as toe flexion are absent, along with sensory loss on the sole of the foot in the tibial distribution. In the peroneal distribution, dorsiflexion and eversion of the foot are absent, along with extension of the toes, especially by the extensor hallucis longus. There is a variable amount of sensory loss on the dorsum of the foot. Since the sural nerve receives its primary contribution from the peroneal nerve in the lower popliteal space, as well as a variable amount of input from the tibial division, there will be sensory loss along the lateral foot and below the lateral malleolus as well as loss due to peroneal involvement over the dorsum of the foot. Hamstring muscle function will usually be spared even at this proximal level except for the short head of the biceps femoris (Fig. 229-21), and its loss signifies that this is a proximal lesion, at least to the peroneal division. Midthigh or more distal lesions of the sciatic nerve will spare this peroneal-innervated function.

Partial injury to the sciatic nerve at the buttock level is not at all uncommon, especially in association with fractures or dislocations or injection injury. Unfortunately, the peroneal division is the more sensitive to injury and the more likely to be involved. Recovery after injection of this division is difficult to obtain. Patients with injection injuries are often either constitutionally thin or chronically ill. Thus, poor gluteal covering predisposes to this type of injury, as does the use of a long needle, forceful placement of the needle, or selection of an area for injection other than the upper outer quadrant of the buttock. The pain pattern, extent of paresthesias, and amount of functional loss, as well as the subsequent course, will vary from patient to patient. In the usual situation the patient reports the immediate onset of painful paresthesias, radiating down the posterior thigh and lower leg and into the foot, with needle placement and then recrudescence of pain as the pharmaceutical agent is injected. The deficit is of rapid onset and may include the entire sciatic distribution or may involve the peroneal or tibial division alone. When the latter situation occurs, the injury is especially painful. The patient will complain of a burning hyperesthetic sole of the foot. Occasionally, a more delayed onset of symptoms may occur after injection injury so that paresthesias and then functional loss occur minutes to (in a rare case) hours later, presumably because the drug was not deposited intrafascicularly but rather into the epineurium or perhaps adjacent to the nerve.[8] There will be local tenderness and sometimes a Tinel's sign on percussion over the course of the nerve with either presentation.

Injury to the sciatic nerve at the thigh level is more common and the nerve was seen completely transected at this level in five instances in our experience.[9] It can also be injured by a gunshot wound or by a fracture of the femur with or without operative fixation. It can be partially injured by a less extensive laceration and sometimes because of ill-advised radical resection of a primary neural tumor such as neurofibroma or schwannoma. The loss will be in a portion or all of the tibial and peroneal distributions. Sural sensory loss may or may not be a concomitant of a midthigh sciatic injury. Of interest is the disposition of the two divisions at the level of the thigh. The point where they divide into two distinct nerves, tibial and peroneal, is variable.[8] (Even at the buttock level the nerve can present as two anatomically separate divisions.[12]) Thus, what appears to be a partial sciatic lesion at thigh level because one division's function is lost and the other's function is completely or incompletely spared may be a complete lesion to either the tibial or peroneal nerve with a partial injury or no injury to the other.

The *tibial nerve* takes a rather straight or vertical course through the popliteal space to reach the gastrocnemius musculature, which it penetrates and of course supplies. At the popliteal level, the nerve is closely associated with the popliteal artery and vein and thus concomitant injuries to these structures at that level are not uncommon. I have seen tibial nerve injury complicated by vascular involvement associated with femoral-popliteal bypass grafting and even secondary to arthroscopy in which the instrument penetrated the posterior knee joint and caught the nerve and vessels. An acute compressive hematoma or vascular injury leading to aneurysm or fistula formation are other uncommon mechanisms for injury to the tibial nerve in the popliteal region. A schwannoma or neurofibroma involving the tibial nerve at this level is also a possibility, and compression by the edge of a chair or recurrent blows to the area can cause paresthesias in the sole of the foot. Thus, one of our patients with a tibial nerve neurofibroma was asymptomatic except when hunting and then only when his dog, a retriever, grew excited and slapped the back of the patient's knee with his tail. The patient then noted a palpable mass and reproducible symptoms of paresthesias in the sole of the foot on percussion of the mass.

In the lower leg, the tibial nerve is deep to the triceps surae on top of the tibialis posterior, and posterior and slightly medial to the tibia itself. Because of its deep loca-

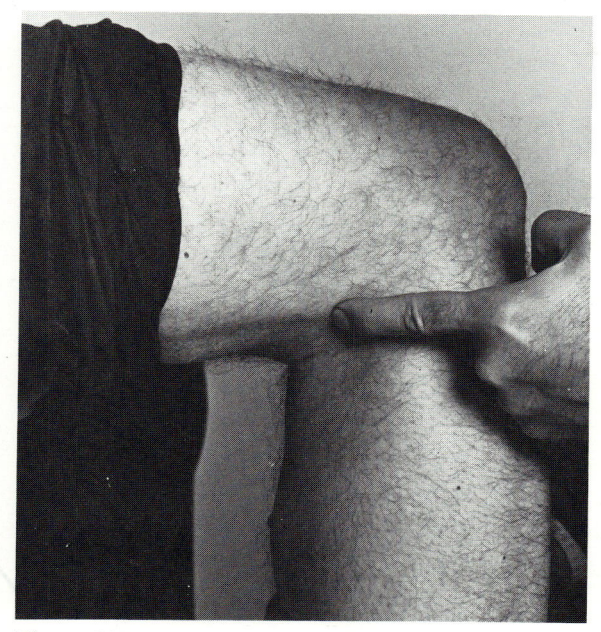

Figure 229-21 Palpation of the short head of the biceps femoris or hamstring while the patient flexes the lower leg on the thigh.

tion, significant injury at this level is uncommon but has been seen with penetrating wounds, especially gunshot wounds. The posterior tibial nerve then travels with the vessels beneath the medial malleolus and at the flexor retinaculum divides into medial and lateral and sometimes also posterior plantar branches. These branches supply the five intrinsic muscles of the foot, much as the ulnar and the thenar portion of the median nerves do for the corresponding hand muscles, (Fig. 229-22). They also supply sensation for much of the plantar surface of the foot, including the heel.

The tarsal tunnel syndrome secondary to entrapment of one or both of these branches as they run through the region of the instep is quite diagnostic. Patients present with paresthesias, usually burning in nature, on the sole of the foot. These symptoms are usually aggravated by weight bearing. There is a Tinel's sign below the medial malleolus or in the instep region and if compression is severe and persistent or actual injury has occurred to the nerves at this level, there will be paresis or loss of toe flexion, toe spreading, and other fine movements of the toes. Laceration or contusive injury to the nerves at this level, especially injuries associated with fracture of the ankle, occur not infrequently. Injury can also be secondary to attempts to repair the ankle or its ligaments.

The peroneal nerve, after leaving the sciatic, takes an oblique course toward the head of the fibula, which it crosses posteriorly. It then wraps around this structure laterally to enter the anterior compartment of the lower leg. The peroneal nerve in the lower leg is also known as the anterior tibial nerve. The nerve, distal to the fibula, has two divisions or branches. The superficial branch descends in the lower leg between the peronei and the extensor digitorum longus muscle and then in front of the fibula to eventually provide cutaneous sensation to the dorsum of the foot. Along the way, this branch innervates the peroneus longus and brevis muscles, the evertors of the foot (Fig. 229-23). The deep peroneal branch travels along the interosseous membrane and distal tibia. Superiorly it supplies the tibialis anterior, extensor digitorum longus, and extensor hallucis

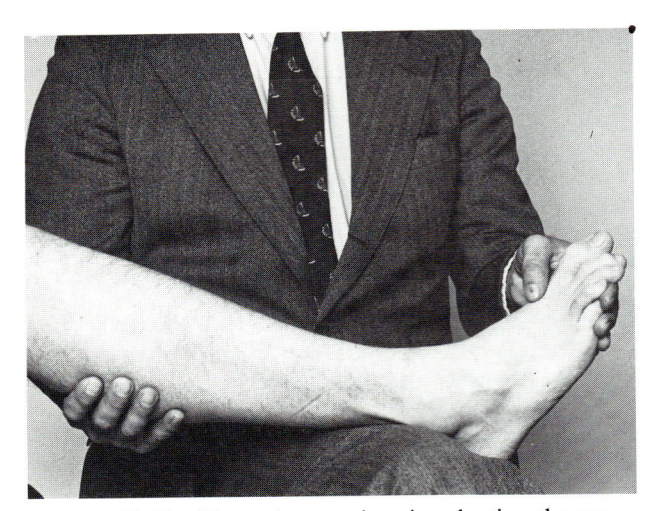

Figure 229-22 Here, the examiner is palpating the gastrocnemius muscle during plantarflexion of the foot and is also testing the ability of the patient to flex the toes.

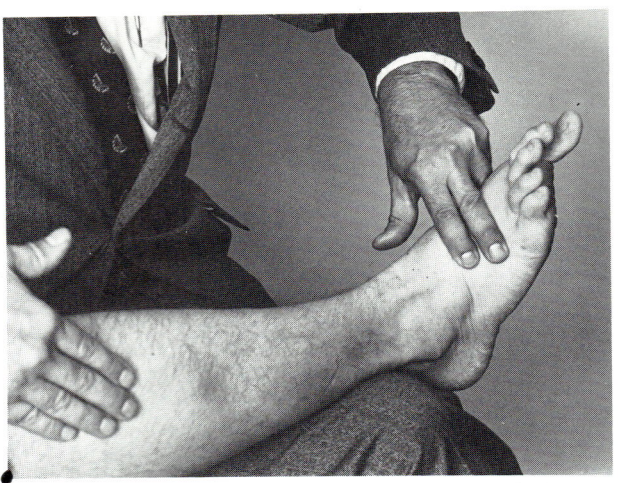

Figure 229-23 The peronei are palpated as the patient attempts to evert the foot.

longus muscles; after passing beneath the lateral malleolus, it gives off branches to the extensor digitorum brevis and first dorsal interosseous muscles and forms the dorsal digital cutaneous nerve supplying sensation to the lateral side of the great toe and the medial side of the second toe. Injury to the peroneal nerve either in the popliteal space or in the region of the head of the fibula is common and varies from the reversible neurapraxic lesions seen with a prolonged cross-legged position ("movie house drop foot") to severe stretch avulsive injuries seen in association with ligamentous tears or fractures or dislocations of the knee. The proximal peroneal nerve gives rise to much of the sural outflow, so the level of injury may be judged in some cases if there is sensory loss along the lateral foot. In addition, there will be a foot drop resulting in a "slapping" foot gait as well as inability to extend the toes, especially the great toe, and to evert the foot. This results in "steppage gait." Dorsiflexion of the foot and toes should be tested with the leg extended and with the patient supine so that the effect of gravity is minimized (Fig. 229-24). The same is certainly the case when testing tibial-innervated plantar flexion, for here if the lower leg is not extended to begin with, some of the extensor thrust of the quadriceps can be translated into apparent foot flexion.

The sural nerve runs beneath the fascia of the triceps surae and then in the proximal calf region penetrates this structure to run subcutaneously in a somewhat oblique fashion toward the lateral malleolus. It may sometimes branch proximally and travel distally as two or more branches. If its distal course is as a single branch, which is the most frequent case, then branching to supply the skin of the lateral lower leg begins as high as the midcalf region. The sural nerve is often closely applied to the vein and sometimes the artery and these structures can be all too easily mistaken for the nerve at the operating table. The major sensory supply of the nerve is to the lateral foot from beneath the lateral malleolus distally to the little toe. Loss on touch or pinprick testing will be found in this region, as well as sometimes along the lateral aspect of the lower leg. Injury is due to laceration or some other penetrating cause and when sufficient to pro-

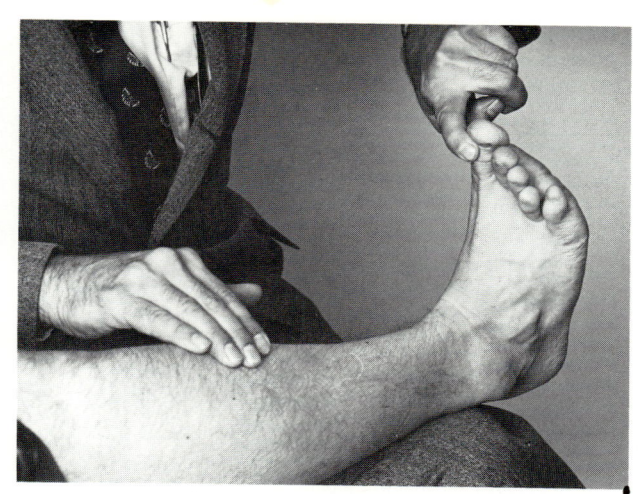

Figure 229-24 The extensor hallicus longus is palpable as the patient extends the large or first toe.

duce a neuroma, it is painful. We have seen several patients who have had the nerve lacerated as a result of exploding or dropped glass soda bottles, with a fragment of glass lacerating the posterior calf and the sural nerve. The patient reports paresthesias, often burning in nature, in the lower leg and lateral foot. Tapping or pressure on the injury site is usually quite painful but also quite diagnostic, for paresthesias will radiate to the lateral lower leg and the lateral surface of the foot. This nerve is most commonly removed for use as interfascicular grafts because of its accessibility and size and the small sensory deficit that results after removing it.

As the gluteal nerves leave the sciatic notch, the superior travels lateral to the sciatic nerve and upward to supply the gluteus medius and minimus. These muscles aid in abduction and medial rotation of the upper leg. Thus when the patient is recumbent, the leg tends to rest in an outwardly rotated position, while in walking the trunk is bent toward the side of the palsy. On standing, the contralateral pelvis drops down and thus there is a discrepancy in the height of the two anterior superior iliac spines. The inferior gluteal nerve exits the sciatic foramen somewhat medial to the sciatic nerve and supplies the gluteus maximus. An injury to this nerve results in weak extension of the hip and thus it is difficult for the patient to climb steps and to rise from a sitting position. Owing to sagging of the muscle belly the infragluteal fold is decreased or lost and with time atrophy of the buttock is obvious.

The pudendal or pubic nerve is seldom injured in an isolated fashion but loss can occur in its distribution when the sacral plexus is injured. It supplies sensation to the perineum and portions of the scrotum and penis, including the mucous membrane of the urethra and the perianal region. Motor fibers go to the external sphincter of the anus and the bulb and the corpus spongiosus of the penis. Owing to its input to the external sphincter of the bladder, it is concerned with voluntary control of urination.

References

1. Cahill BR: Quadrilateral space syndrome, in Omer GE Jr, Spinner M (eds): *Management of Peripheral Nerve Problems*. Philadelphia, Saunders, 1980, pp 602–606.
2. Haymaker W, Woodhall B: *Peripheral Nerve Injuries: Principles of Diagnosis*, 2d ed. Philadelphia, Saunders, 1953.
3. Hudson A, Berry H, Mayfield F: Chronic injuries of peripheral nerves by entrapment, in Youmans J (ed): *Neurological Surgery: A Comprehensive Reference Guide to the Diagnosis and Management of Neurosurgical Problems*, 2d ed. Philadelphia, Saunders, 1982, pp 2430–2474.
4. Kahn EA: Direct observation of sweating in peripheral nerve lesions. Surg Gynecol Obstet 92:22–26, 1951.
5. Kaplan EB, Spinner M: Normal and anomalous innervation patterns in the upper extremity, in Omer GE Jr, Spinner M (eds): *Management of Peripheral Nerve Problems*. Philadelphia, Saunders, 1980, pp 75–99.
6. Kempe L: *Operative Neurosurgery*, vol 2. New York, Springer, 1970.
7. Kline DG: Macroscopic and microscopic concomitants of nerve repair. Clin Neurosurg 26:582–606, 1979.
8. Kline DG: Operative experience with major lower extremity nerve lesions, including the lumbosacral plexus and the sciatic nerve, in Omer GE Jr, Spinner M (eds): *Management of Peripheral Nerve Problems*. Philadelphia, Saunders, 1980, pp 607–625.
9. Kline DG, Nulsen FE: Acute injuries of peripheral nerves, in Youmans J (ed): *Neurological Surgery: A Comprehensive Reference Guide to the Diagnosis and Management of Neurosurgical Problems*, 2d ed. Philadelphia, Saunders, 1982, pp 2363–2429.
10. Mayfield FH: *Causalgia*. Springfield, Ill, Charles C Thomas, 1951.
11. Medical Research Council, Nerve Injuries Committee: *Aids to Investigation of Peripheral Nerve Injuries*. MRC War Memorandum No 7, London, His Majesty's Stationery Office, 1943.
12. Prutkin L: Normal and anomalous innervation patterns in the lower extremity, in Omer GE Jr, Spinner M (eds): *Management of Peripheral Nerve Problems*. Philadelphia, Saunders, 1980, pp. 100–115.
13. Seddon HJ: *Surgical Disorders of the Peripheral Nerves*. Baltimore, Williams & Wilkins, 1972.
14. Sunderland S: *Nerves and Nerve Injuries*, 2d ed. Edinburgh, Churchill Livingstone, 1978.

230
Surgical Exposure of Peripheral Nerves

Charles L. Branch, Jr.
David L. Kelly, Jr.
George C. Lynch

Surgery of the peripheral nerves requires twofold expertise on the part of the surgeon. A knowledge of the anatomy and operative exposure of the nerve in question is necessary in addition to skill in the actual technique of nerve repair. The second skill is discussed elsewhere; in this chapter we attempt to provide fundamental knowledge about the anatomy and the surgical exposure of the major peripheral nerves. To this end we did thorough dissections of cadaver limbs, deriving from those dissections photographs and subsequently the illustrations that accompany the text.

When contemplating exposure of a peripheral nerve, the surgeon is well served by keeping in mind some of the following basic tenets:

1. First expose an anatomically normal segment of the nerve and then approach the pathological segment.
2. Dissect directly down to the nerve and then along it, avoiding the establishment of misleading or multiple fascial planes above the nerve.
3. Whenever possible, dissect between muscle groups and preserve vascular structures, especially those in close proximity to the nerve in question.
4. Provide for further exposure of the nerve or possible harvest of a cable graft when preparing and draping the limb or limbs at the start of the operation.
5. Consider the anatomy textbook an essential tool, both outside and within the surgical suite.[1-7]

Upper Extremity

Brachial Plexus

The brachial plexus is, as its name implies, a plexus or group of nerves arising from cervical and thoracic roots that consolidate to form the nerves responsible for motion and sensation in the upper extremity and the chest wall. Because of its relatively precarious position as it crosses from the cervical spine to the upper extremity, it is prone to various forms of injury. These include stretch or avulsive injuries secondary to athletic or motor vehicle accidents, blast injuries from gunshot wounds to the axilla or upper chest wall, incision injuries from stab wounds, and lacerations secondary to fracture dislocations near the plexus. Resultant paralysis and sensory loss are obviously related to the components of the plexus that are injured.

Anatomy

The brachial plexus is composed of components of roots C5 through T1. The plexus itself is subdivided into roots, trunks, divisions, cords, and individual nerves, the nerves being given off at various levels (Fig. 230-1). The cervical roots travel from the neural foramina of their respective vertebrae between the anterior and middle scalene muscles. At the root level, the long thoracic nerve arises from roots C5 through C7; it travels distally to supply the serratus anterior muscles. Also arising from root C5 at this level is the dorsal scapular nerve, which innervates the rhomboid muscles. The trunk level has three components: the upper trunk is formed from roots C5 and C6; the middle trunk from root C7, and the lower trunk from roots C8 and T1. Arising from the upper trunk while it is still supraclavicular are the supraclavicular nerve (to the subclavius) and the suprascapular nerve, the latter passing through the suprascapular notch to innervate the supraspinatus and the infraspinatus muscles. Deep to the clavicle, each trunk splits into an anterior and posterior division. No individual nerves arise from the division level. At this point the brachial plexus entwines itself around the axillary artery and lies just lateral to the axillary vein. It passes just deep to the pectoralis minor muscle and superficial to the subscapularis and teres major muscles.

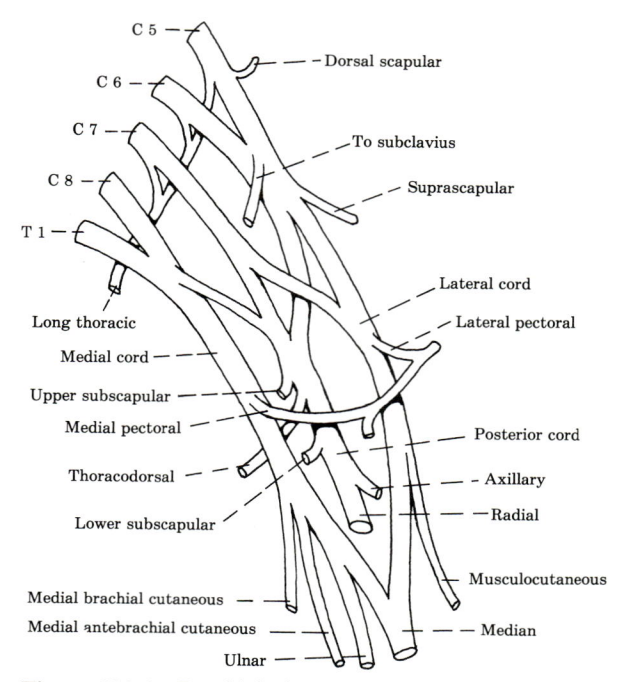

Figure 230-1 Brachial plexus.

The divisions unite infraclavicularly to form cords named for their relation to the axillary artery. The anterior divisions of the upper and middle trunks unite to form the lateral cord; the anterior division of the lower trunk continues as the medial cord; and the three posterior divisions unite to form the posterior cord. Aside from the portions of the medial and lateral cords that unite to form the median nerve, all branches of the plexus at the cord level are terminal nerves.

The lateral cord gives rise to the lateral pectoral nerve, which pierces the clavipectoral fascia and supplies the pectoralis major muscle, and the musculocutaneous nerve, which travels distally through the coracobrachialis muscle to supply this muscle and ultimately the brachialis and biceps muscles. A branch from the lateral cord is joined by a similar component from the medial cord to form the median nerve, the distribution of which is described under a separate heading.

The medial cord, in addition to its contribution to the median nerve, gives rise to the ulnar nerve, the distribution of which is also described under a separate heading. Other branches of the medial cord include the medial pectoral nerve, which supplies the pectoralis minor and major muscles, and the medial brachial and antebrachial cutaneous nerves, which provide sensory innervation to the arm and forearm.

The posterior cord gives rise to: the upper and lower subscapular nerves, which penetrate and innervate the subscapularis and teres major muscles; the thoracodorsal nerve, which runs distally on the subscapularis muscle to reach and innervate the latissimus dorsi muscle; and the axillary nerve, which rounds the subscapularis muscle laterally to pass posteriorly through the quadrilateral space and give off branches to the shoulder joint and the teres minor muscle and major branches to the deltoid muscle and the skin overlying the shoulder. The posterior cord then continues as the radial nerve, the distribution of which is described under a separate heading.

Surgical Exposure

The trunks and divisions of the plexus may be exposed through a supraclavicular approach, whereas the cord level is exposed through an infraclavicular approach. However, because injuries to the plexus are not always discrete and because the area of injury may have to be approached by identifying normal nerves proximal and distal to the injury, the surgeon should be prepared to perform, and the patient should be prepared and draped for, a transclavicular approach. The supraclavicular and infraclavicular approaches are limited versions of the illustrated transclavicular approach.

The patient is placed supine with the head and shoulders elevated to a position comfortable for the surgeon. The anterior chest wall, the neck, and the arm are prepared and draped; the arm may be at the patient's side or abducted and internally rotated as necessary. From a point approximately 7 cm above the clavicle, a lazy S incision is made along the posterior border of the sternocleidomastoid muscle to the clavicle, where it sweeps laterally to cross the clavicle at the junction between the middle and lateral thirds of that bone (Fig. 230-2A). It then extends distally and laterally along the deltopectoral groove toward the axilla. The skin and platysma are incised and separated supraclavicularly and the external jugular vein is identified, ligated, and divided. The supraclavicular nerve is identified and preserved if possible. Unless there is injury to the axillary artery, the transverse cervical artery may also be ligated and divided to provide exposure at the trunk level of the brachial plexus; in the absence of a patent axillary artery, however, the transverse cervical artery will be an important collateral vessel.

At this point, the fascia overlying the scalenus anterior muscle is divided and retracted medially, with care being taken not to injure the phrenic nerve. This retraction will expose the trunks of the brachial plexus, as well as the long thoracic nerve coursing along the scalenus medius muscle (Fig. 230-2B). The skin over the clavicle is then incised and divided, and the fascia and the subclavius muscle are stripped free of the clavicle subperiosteally. A 6-cm segment of clavicle is removed and the subclavius muscle and its accompanying artery and vein are ligated, divided, and retracted. The posterior belly of the omohyoid muscle will be found just superior to these structures and may be divided or retracted as necessary. At this point, the pectoral muscles may be retracted inferiorly, care being taken not to injure or avulse the lateral and medial pectoral (anterior thoracic) nerves as they arise from the medial and lateral cords and penetrate the superoposterior aspect of the pectoral muscles. This retraction will expose the trunk, division, and upper cord levels of the plexus (Fig. 230-2C).

If a more distal exposure is needed, the pectoralis major muscle may be divided superficial to the plexus and the pectoralis minor muscle divided approximately 1 cm from its insertion on the coracoid process. The brachial plexus will thus be completely exposed, along with all its terminal branches and the axillary artery and vein (Fig. 230-2D). Again, the nerves most susceptible to injury during exposure are the long thoracic and phrenic nerves during the upper exposure and the lateral and medial pectoral nerves in the infraclavicular or subclavicular aspect of the dissection. At the completion of the procedure, the clavicle may be replaced and fixed with stainless steel wire or a Steinman pin, although it also may be left out entirely. The pectoral muscles and the platysma are reapproximated epimysially before the skin is closed.

Median Nerve

The median nerve, perhaps the most important nerve to the hand, innervates the flexors of the thumb and the first two fingers, as well as the muscles of opposition of the thumb. It also provides the sensory innervation to the thumb and to the index and long fingers that is essential to any finely integrated function of the hand. Paralysis of this nerve leaves the victim with the so-called ape hand.

Anatomy

The median nerve arises as a consolidation of a medial branch of the lateral cord of the brachial plexus and an external branch of the medial cord of that plexus. It is composed of components from roots C6 through T1. It courses along the medial aspect of the upper arm in close association with the brachial artery. In the antecubital fossa, the nerve

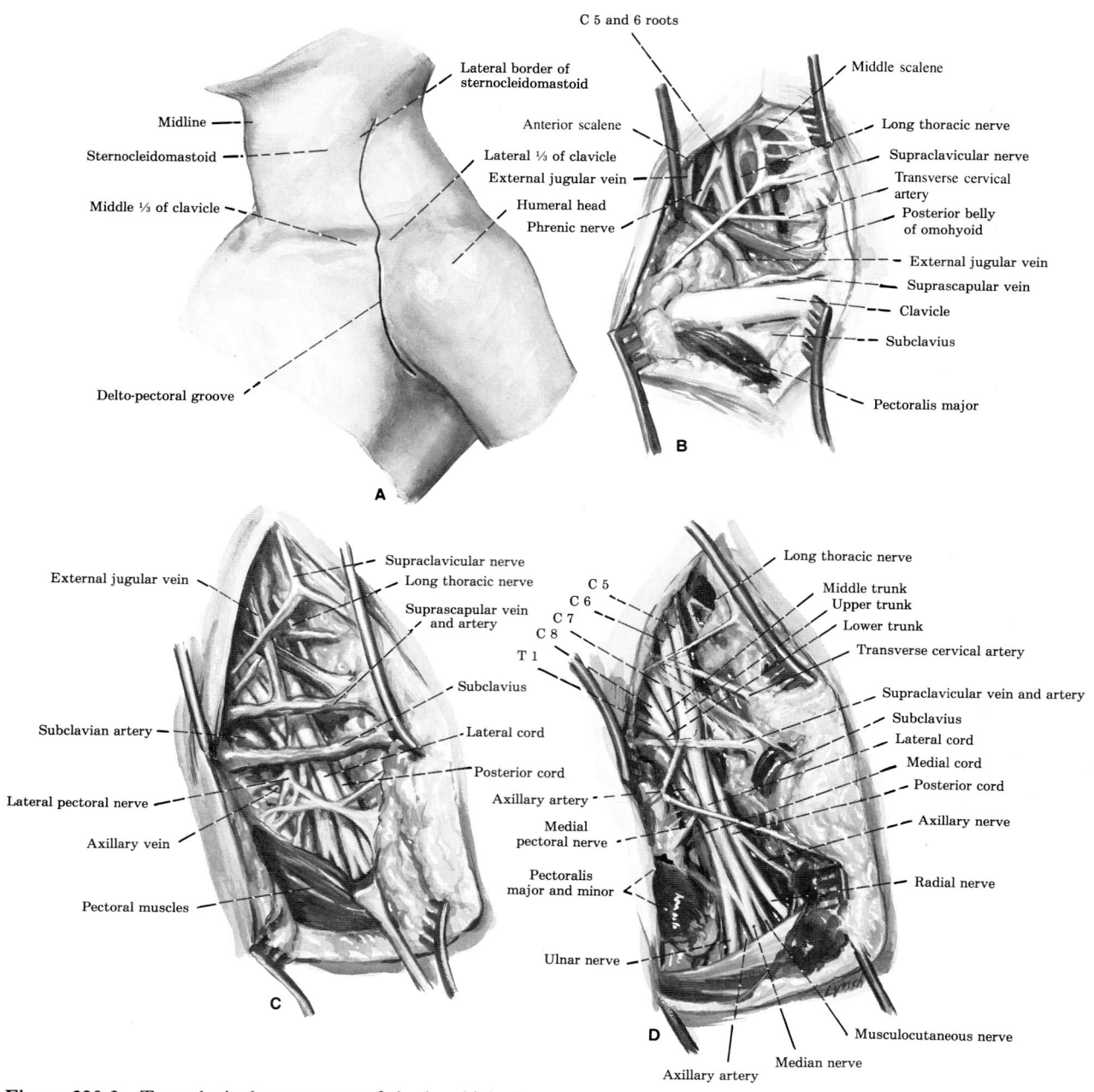

Figure 230-2 Transclavicular exposure of the brachial plexus.

courses laterally beneath the lacertus fibrosus and dives deep between the two heads of the pronator teres muscle, where it gives off branches to that muscle and to the flexor carpi radialis and palmaris longus muscles. The nerve then runs deep to the flexor digitorum superficialis, which it also innervates, and becomes relatively superficial again as it courses beneath the flexor retinaculum in the carpal tunnel at the wrist. In the forearm a major branch, the anterior interosseus branch, arises. This branch innervates the flexor digitorum profundus muscle to the index finger and the flexor pollicis longus muscle. At the carpal tunnel, a superficial palmar sensory branch arises to innervate the proximal aspect of the palm. In the tunnel or just distal to it the recurrent thenar branch arises; this motor branch innervates the opponens pollicis, the abductor pollicis brevis, and the flexor pollicis brevis muscles. In the palm the nerve divides into its distal branches, which provide motor innervation to the lumbrical muscles and sensory innervation to the first three digits.

Surgical Exposure

The patient is placed supine, with the arm abducted to 90 degrees and externally rotated so that the entire volar surface is exposed. For distal explorations Bier's block anesthesia is desirable since it provides a bloodless field. For more proximal explorations general anesthesia may be used.

Surgical Exposure of Peripheral Nerves 1849

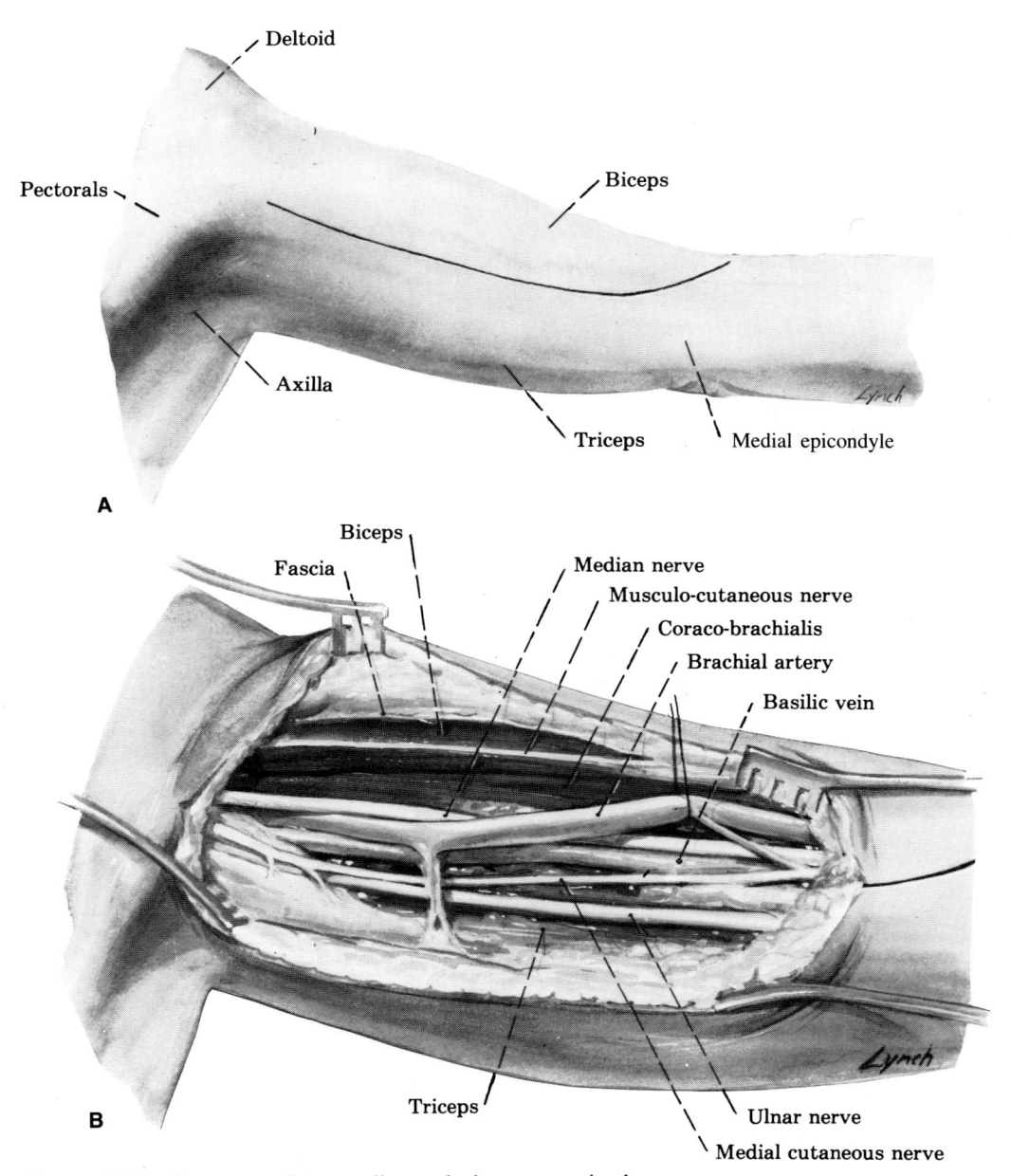

Figure 230-3 Exposure of the median and ulnar nerves in the arm.

In the arm, the neurovascular bundle is palpated between the biceps and triceps muscles on the medial aspect of the arm. A linear incision is made over the bundle from the axilla to a point 5 cm proximal to the medial epicondyle (Fig. 230-3A). The deep fascia is incised, and the coracobrachialis and biceps muscles are retracted laterally to expose the median nerve and the associated brachial artery (Fig. 230-3B).

At the elbow, the median nerve is exposed by an incision that extends distally from a point 5 cm proximal to the medial epicondyle and then laterally along a flexion crease in the antecubital fossa and finally curves downward along the medial border of the brachioradialis muscle (Fig. 230-4A). The skin is incised and undermined, care being taken to preserve the medial and lateral cutaneous nerves. The antebrachial fascia is incised longitudinally and the lacertus fibrosus is incised along the course of the skin incision (Fig. 230-4B). The nerve is exposed as it crosses the antecubital fossa superficial to the brachialis muscle. It dives between the two heads of the pronator teres muscle, and care must be taken at that point not to transect the branches to this muscle (Fig. 230-4C). Antecubital veins may be transected and retracted as necessary.

In the forearm, a linear incision is made along the medial aspect of the brachioradialis muscle, extending distally over the lateral border of the flexor carpi ulnaris muscle to a point 4 cm proximal to the flexor creases of the wrist. Through this incision, two approaches to the median nerve are possible. After crossing the antecubital fossa, the nerve passes deep to and between the two heads of the pronator teres

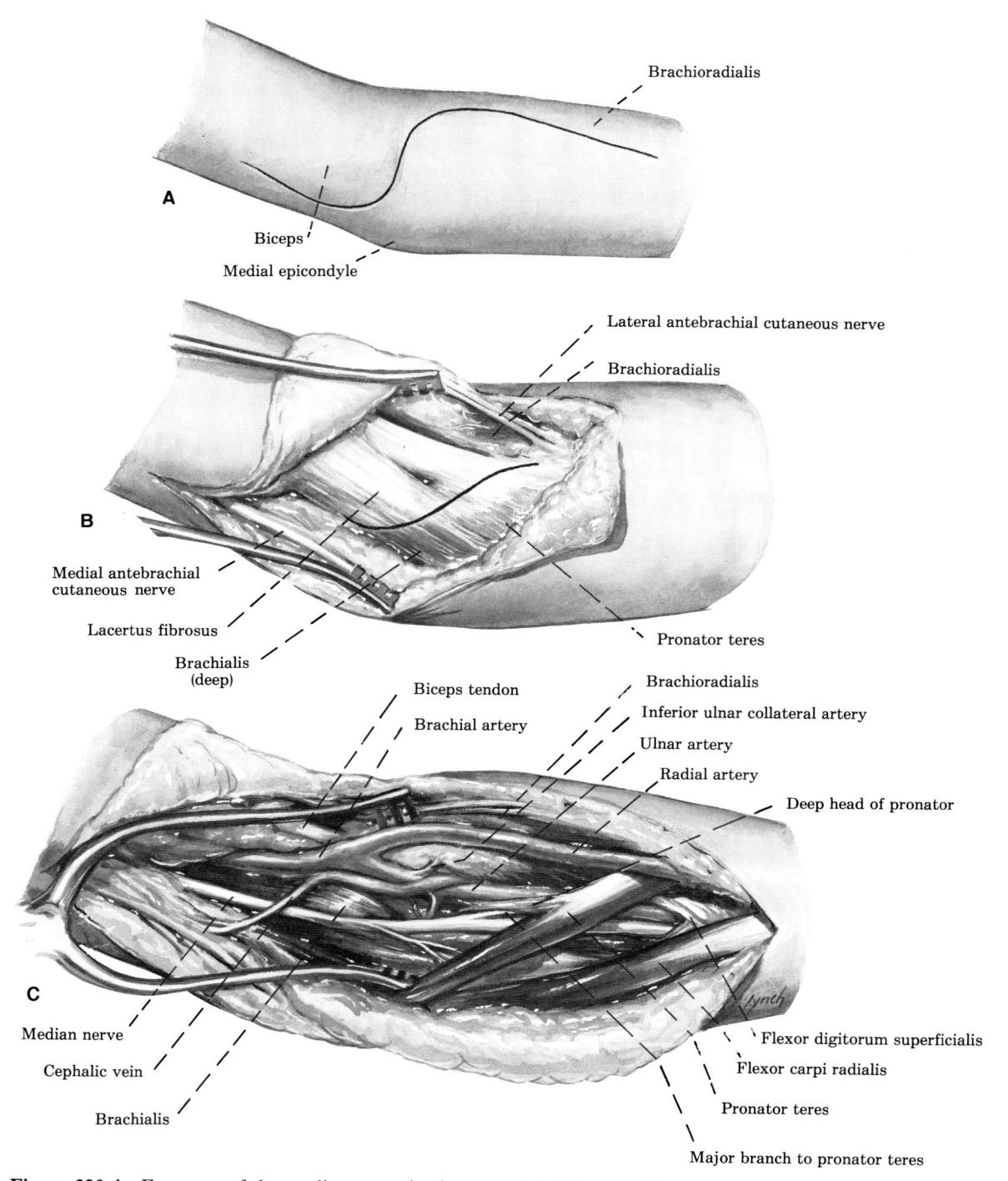

Figure 230-4 Exposure of the median nerve in the antecubital fossa and forearm.

muscle and then passes first deep to the flexor carpi radialis muscle and then deep to the flexor digitorum superficialis muscle (Fig. 230-4C). One approach to this nerve involves retracting the flexor carpi radialis and the flexor digitorum superficialis muscles medially and exposing the nerve along the undersurface of the flexor digitorum superficialis muscle. The second approach involves retracting the flexor digitorum superficialis muscle laterally and exposing the nerve in the same location but from the medial side. For lesions close to the antecubital fossa the first exposure is more advantageous, whereas for distal lesions the second approach is better. With either approach, care must be taken to preserve the anterior interosseous nerve, which branches from the median nerve and is accompanied by the median artery lying volar to the interosseous membrane.

At the wrist the median nerve is exposed through a Z-

Surgical Exposure of Peripheral Nerves 1851

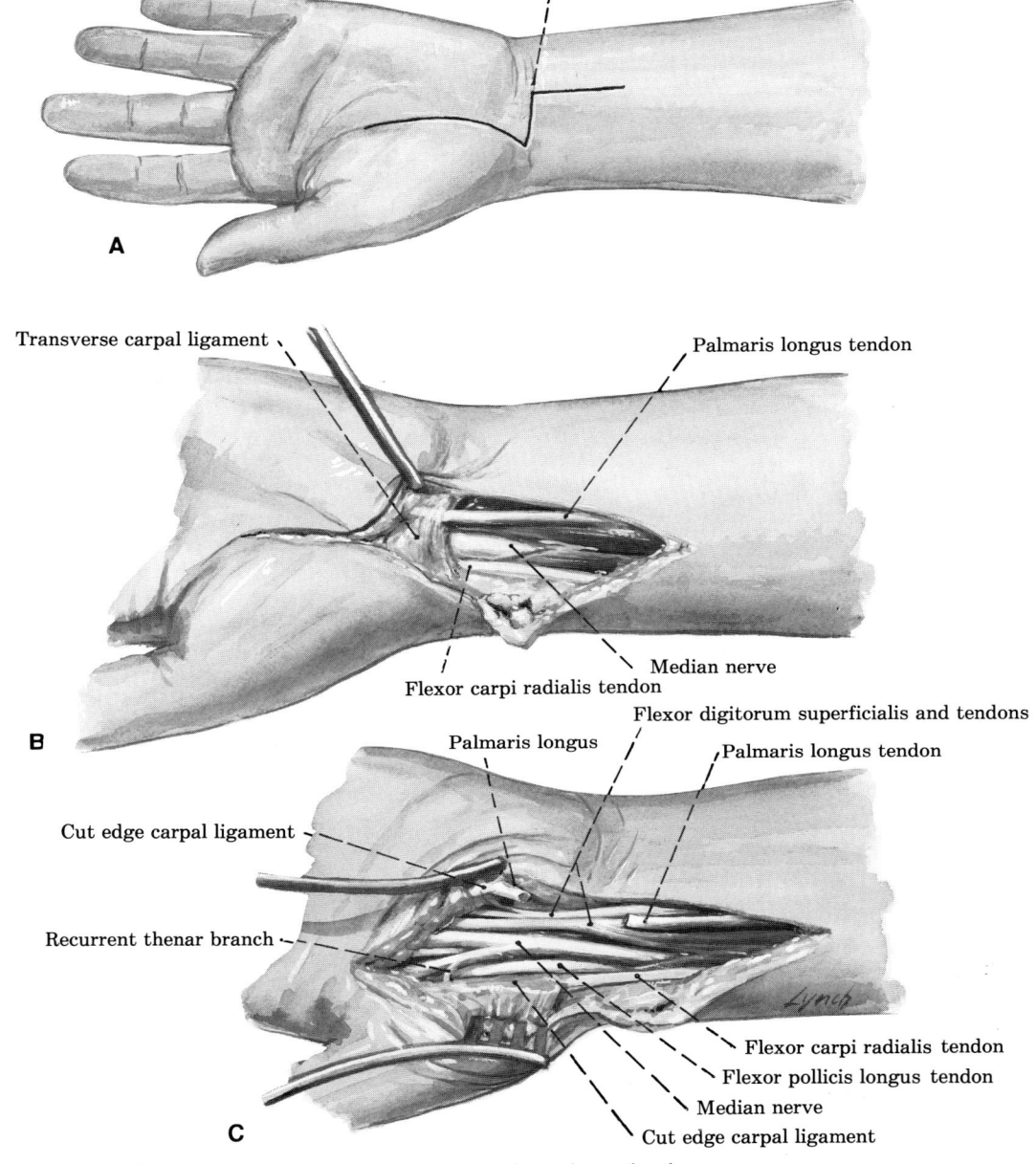

Figure 230-5 Exposure of the median nerve in the wrist and palm.

type incision, which is started on the ulnar aspect of the palmaris longus tendon approximately 4 cm proximal to the flexion crease, carried transversely across the crease, and then continued along the contour of the thenar eminence for several centimeters into the palm (Fig. 230-5A). The superficial fascia is then divided, which exposes the median nerve, the tendon of the palmaris longus muscle medial to the nerve, and the tendon of the flexor carpi radialis muscle lateral to the nerve (Fig. 230-5B). The thick transverse carpal ligament is then identified and incised along the ulnar aspect of the median nerve to avoid injury to the recurrent thenar branch, which leaves the median nerve on its radial side just distal to the carpal tunnel (Fig. 230-5C). The median nerve then divides into its three terminal palmar digital branches.

Ulnar Nerve

The ulnar nerve provides the major motor innervation of the interosseus muscles of the hand and the flexor muscles of the wrist and the fourth and fifth digits. Injury is most common at the wrist or at the elbow, secondary to trauma or entrapment. Lesions of the ulnar nerve may give the hand a claw-like appearance with chronic flexion of the fourth and fifth digits on attempted extension.

Anatomy

The nerve is composed of components of the C8 and T1 roots and arises from the medial portion of the medial cord in the brachial plexus. It traverses the medial side of the upper arm, lying dorsal to the median nerve, brachial artery, and intermuscular septum. At the elbow it lies in the ulnar notch on the medial epicondyle; it then dives between the two heads of the flexor carpi ulnaris muscle, which it innervates. Along the forearm it lies between the flexor carpi ulnaris and the flexor digitorum profundus muscles just medial to the ulnar artery. At the wrist it becomes superficial, lying just deep to the tendon of the flexor carpi ulnaris muscle. It passes into the palm superficial to the flexor retinaculum but deep to the palmar carpal ligament and the palmaris brevis muscle in Guyon's canal. Proximal to the wrist, the ulnar nerve gives off the superficial palmar branch to provide sensation for the medial aspect of the palm. In the palm, the nerve divides into a superficial branch, which primarily provides sensory innervation to the medial aspect of the palm and the dorsum of the hand, and a deep branch, which innervates the palmar and dorsal interossei, the third and fourth lumbricals, the adductor pollicis, and the abductor, flexor, and opponens digiti minimi muscles.

Surgical Exposure

The patient is placed supine with the arm extended and abducted to 90 degrees at the shoulder and the palm supinated.

In the upper arm the exposure is identical to that of the median nerve (Fig. 230-3A, B). The neurovascular bundle is palpated in the medial intermuscular groove, and an incision is made directly above it to a point about 10 cm proximal to the medial epicondyle. The ulnar nerve lies just inferior to the median nerve, passing deep to the intermuscular septum.

In the elbow an incision is made from the bicipital groove 7 to 10 cm proximal to the medial epicondyle and, following a gentle curve medial to the epicondyle, it is then continued 5 cm distally along the medial border of the flexor carpi ulnaris muscle (Fig. 230-6A). The nerve is exposed by incising the deep fascia overlying it (Fig. 230-6B, C). When the nerve is to be transposed, special attention should be paid to the dissection of the fibrous sheath surrounding the nerve as it dives between the heads of the flexor carpi ulnaris muscle and also as it arises from between the brachialis muscle and the intermuscular septum. If dissection is not adequate, the nerve will be kinked upon the fibrous sheath, which results in injury and poor relief of symptoms.

In the forearm the nerve lies between the flexor carpi ulnaris and the flexor digitorum superficialis muscles. It is approached by making an incision along the medial border of the flexor carpi ulnaris muscle. The fascia over the flexor carpi ulnaris is incised and after the nerve has been identified, the medial head of that muscle is incised and the muscle is separated from the flexor digitorum superficialis to further expose the nerve (Fig. 230-6D). The ulnar artery can be seen as it joins the nerve about halfway down the forearm; both become superficial in the wrist, passing to the radial side of the tendon of the flexor carpi ulnaris muscle. During this dissection attempts should be made to preserve the branches to the flexor carpi ulnaris muscle and the dorsal cutaneous branch to the hand.

In the wrist the nerve is found along the side of the ulnar artery. They pass by the radial aspect of the pisiform bone, superficial to the flexor retinaculum, and then deep to the palmaris brevis muscle. An incision is made around the hypothenar eminence, as shown in Fig. 230-7A, B, and the palmaris brevis muscle is incised and retracted to expose the nerve up to its bifurcation into a deep and a superficial branch (Fig. 230-7C).

Radial Nerve

The radial nerve, which is the major extensor nerve of the upper extremity, carries components of the C5 through T1 roots and innervates the extensor muscles of the forearm, hand, and digits. It is most commonly injured during a fracture of the humeral shaft in the upper arm or during repair of that fracture. Injury of the nerve at the humeral level produces the characteristic wrist drop with normal triceps strength.

Anatomy

The radial nerve is a direct continuation of the posterior cord of the brachial plexus. Before leaving the axilla, the radial nerve gives rise to the posterior brachial cutaneous nerves and to the motor branches to the long and medial heads of the triceps brachii muscle. With the profunda artery, it spirals around the humerus and courses distally in the radial groove beneath the triceps, innervating that muscle and giving off several cutaneous branches. Proximal to the elbow it pierces the lateral intermuscular septum and courses beneath the medial edge of the brachioradialis muscle, which it innervates. After crossing the elbow, the nerve sends branches to the extensor carpi radialis longus and brevis muscles and then divides into a superficial radial branch and a deep interosseous branch.

The superficial radial nerve continues beneath the brachioradialis muscle, becoming superficial in order to cross the wrist in the anatomist's snuffbox and provide sensory innervation to the dorsum of the hand.

The deep interosseous branch dives deep through the supinator muscle to pass around the radius. After emerging from the supinator muscle, which it innervates, the deep interosseous branch divides into motor branches that supply the extensor digitorum, the extensor digiti quinti proprius, the extensor carpi ulnaris, the abductor pollicis longus, the extensor pollicis longus, the extensor pollicis brevis, and the extensor indicis proprius muscles.

Surgical Exposure

The patient is placed supine. For upper arm exploration the limb is flexed at the elbow with the forearm resting on the chest or on a support. For elbow and forearm explorations the arm is abducted at the shoulder, extended, and pronated.

In the upper arm an incision is made from the posterior border of the deltoid to a point 5 cm proximal to the lateral

Surgical Exposure of Peripheral Nerves

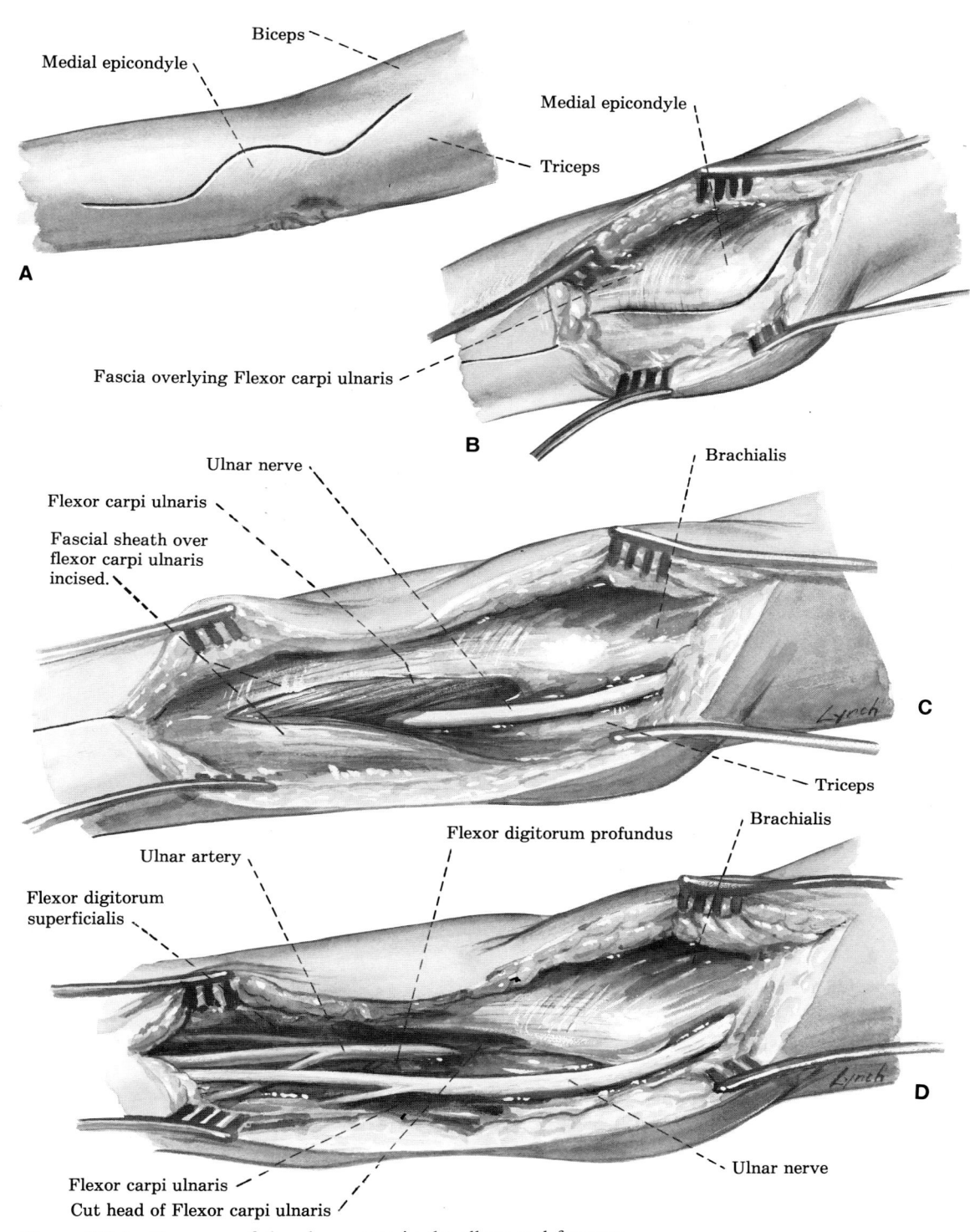

Figure 230-6 Exposure of the ulnar nerve in the elbow and forearm.

epicondyle (Fig. 230-8A). The fascia is incised, and the lateral and long heads of the triceps muscle are identified and separated bluntly to expose the radial nerve and the accompanying profunda artery (Fig. 230-8B,C). Distally the nerve pierces the lateral intermuscular septum above the medial head of the triceps muscle and can be found just beneath the medial edge of the brachioradialis muscle at the distal aspect of the incision. The posterior antebrachial cutaneous nerve will be found accompanying the radial nerve in this region.

At the elbow and forearm the incision begins 5 cm proximal to the epicondyle in the groove between the brachialis and brachioradialis muscles. It then extends along the medial border of the brachioradialis muscle to the extensor carpi radialis muscle (Fig. 230-9A). The skin and fascia are incised and the nerve is identified between the brachialis and the brachioradialis muscles (Fig. 230-9B). It is traced dis-

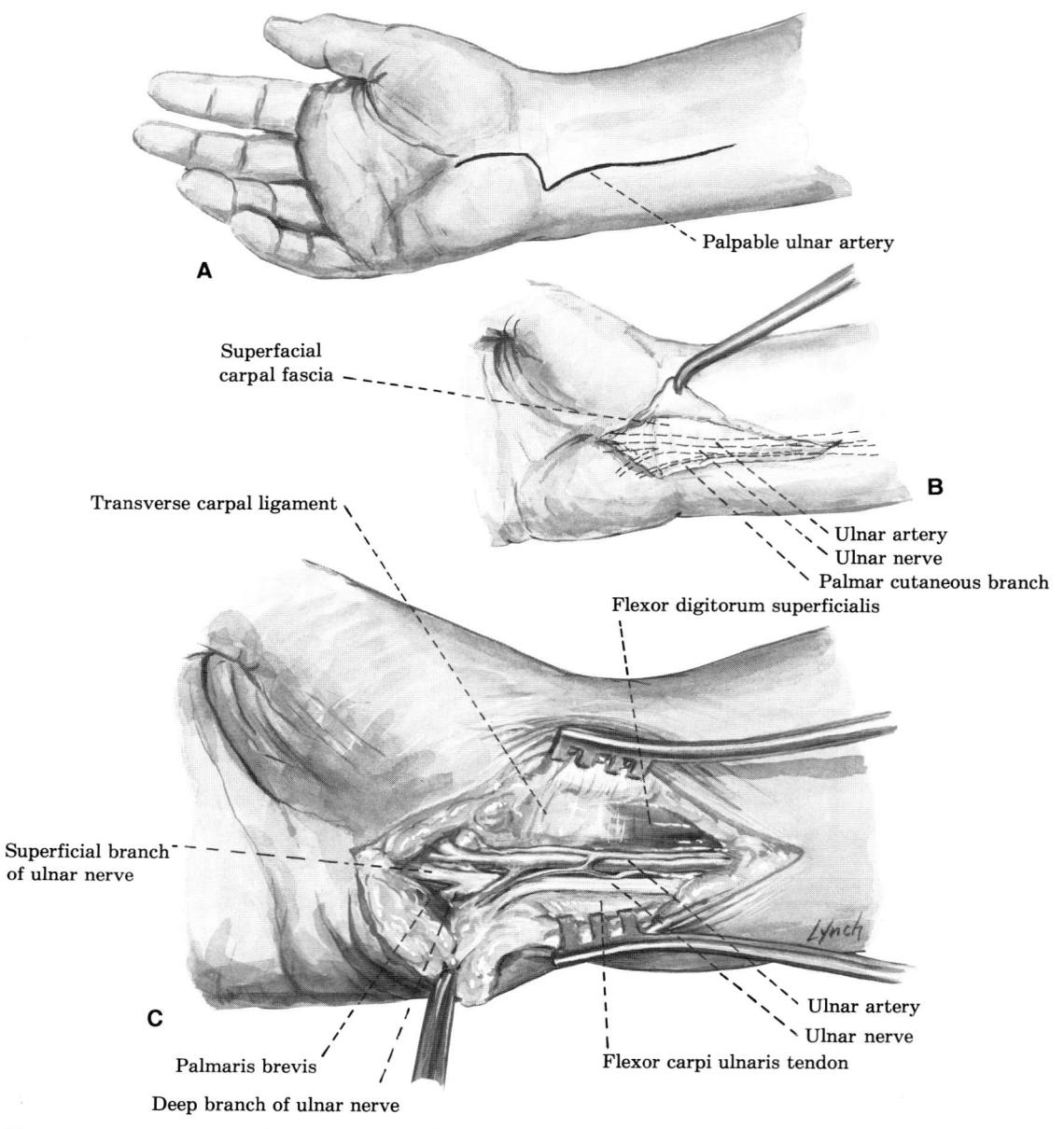

Figure 230-7 Exposure of the ulnar nerve in the wrist.

tally with blunt dissection while care is taken to prevent damage to its major branches to the brachioradialis muscle. If the brachioradialis is gently retracted laterally, the division of the nerve into its deep and superficial branches can be seen just distal to the antecubital fossa (Fig. 230-9C). Once the fascia over the supinator muscle is incised, the deep interosseous branch can be seen piercing the supinator muscle. Lateral retraction in the plane between the extensor carpi radialis longus and brevis and the extensor digitorum muscles exposes the distal aspect of the branch. The extensor carpi radialis muscles are retracted medially to expose the inferior surface of the supinator muscle and the major motor branches of the deep interosseous nerve, which pierce the extensor muscles. Henry describes a distal approach to the nerve.[1]

The superficial branch can be followed distally into the forearm on the inferomedial surface of the brachioradialis muscle. The nerve crosses the wrist superficial to the tendons of the brachioradialis and the extensor carpi radialis muscles (Fig. 230-9D) before entering the anatomist's snuffbox and dividing into its cutaneous branches.

Lower Extremity

Femoral Nerve

The femoral nerve innervates the quadriceps and sartorius muscles and is the major nerve for extension of the leg at the knee. Injury to this nerve may seriously affect the patient's ability to walk. The femoral nerve is most commonly injured

Surgical Exposure of Peripheral Nerves   1855

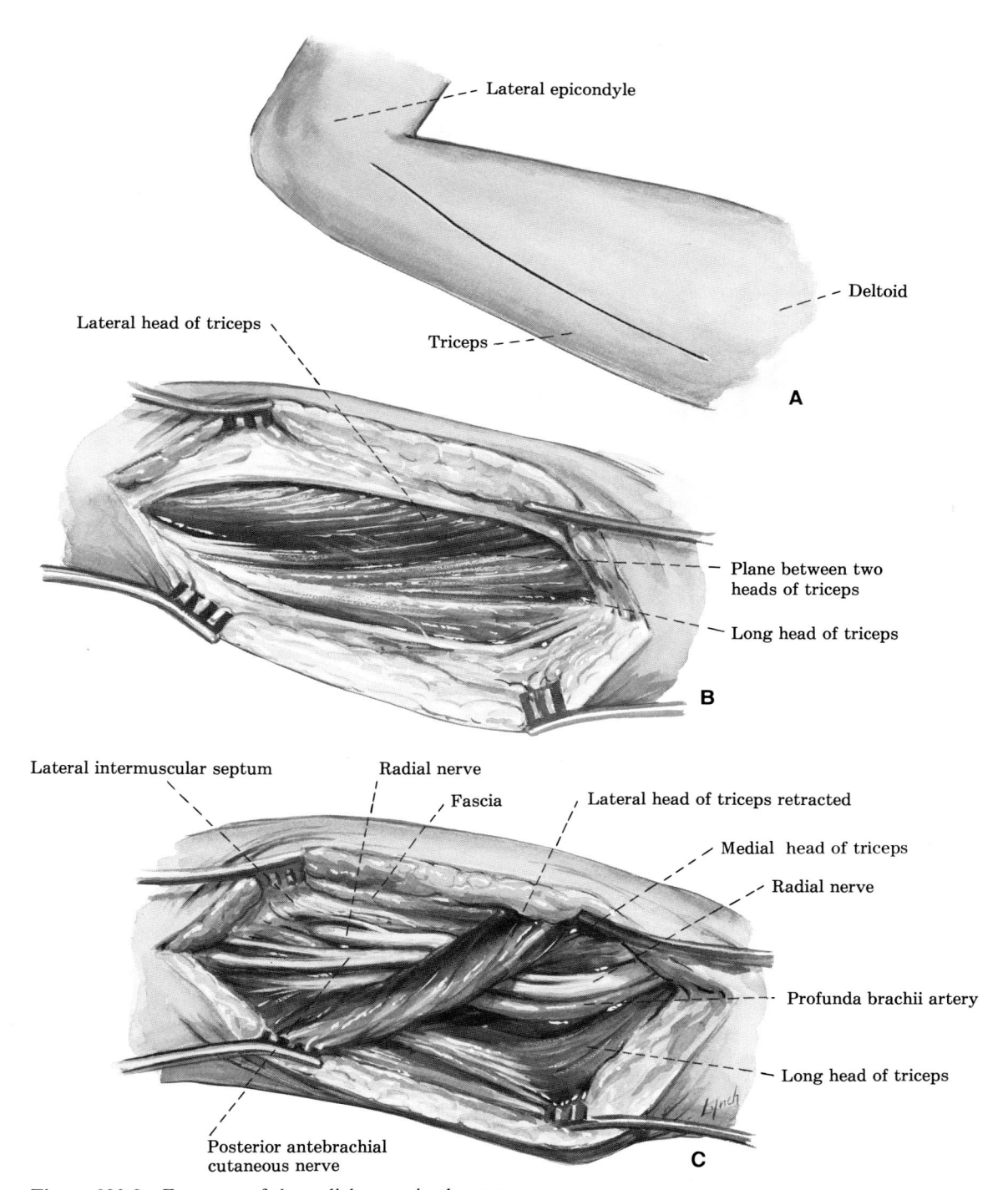

Figure 230-8 Exposure of the radial nerve in the arm.

by penetrating missile or stab wounds in the groin; concomitant major arterial injury is often seen.

Anatomy

The femoral nerve contains components of the L2 through L4 nerve roots. It courses retroperitoneally through the psoas major and then distally in the groove between the iliacus and psoas muscles, innervating the iliacus muscle. Thence it courses deep to the inguinal ligament just lateral and adjacent to the femoral artery but separated from it by the psoas and iliacus fasciae. Almost immediately after it passes under the inguinal ligament, it branches into its many motor and cutaneous branches. It provides motor function for the sartorius, the vastus lateralis, the vastus medius, and the vastus intermedius muscles and provides sensory innervation by giving rise to the saphenous nerve and to the intermediate and medial cutaneous nerves of the thigh.

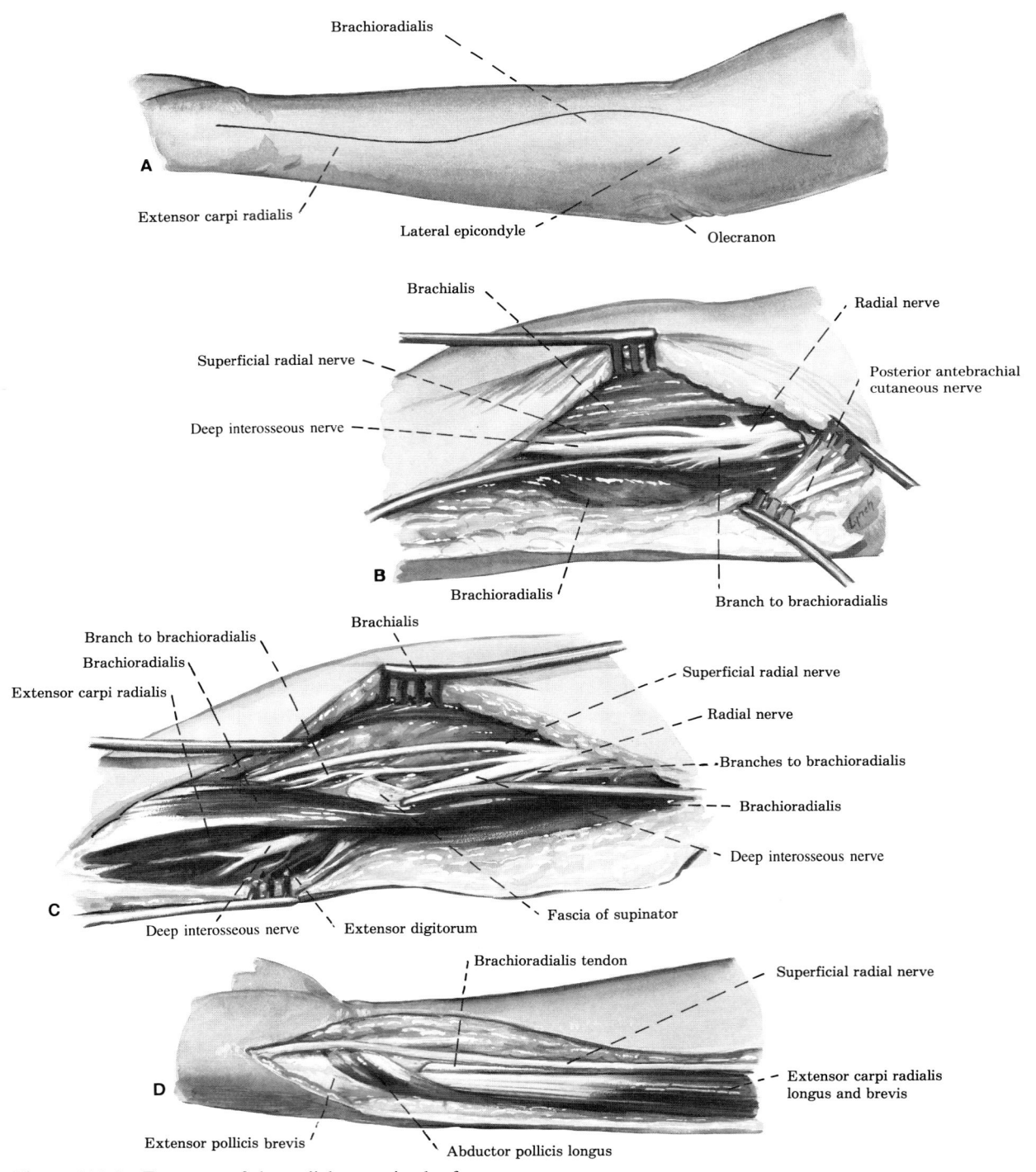

Figure 230-9 Exposure of the radial nerve in the forearm.

Surgical Exposure

The incision is made from a point over the inguinal ligament, midway between the anterior superior iliac spine and the pubic ramus, or 1 cm lateral to the palpable femoral pulse, and is extended inferiorly from the inguinal ligament for about 7 to 10 cm (Fig. 230-10A). The fascia lata is incised and the fascia iliaca is identified. The femoral vessels are dissected free of the femoral sheath to expose a crus of the fascia iliaca. The fascia iliaca is incised with a T or Y incision, as shown in Fig. 230-10B, from the lateral aspect of the crura around the femoral vessels. Retraction of the flap exposes the femoral nerve and its branches (Fig. 230-10C); further dissection is performed as necessary.

Surgical Exposure of Peripheral Nerves

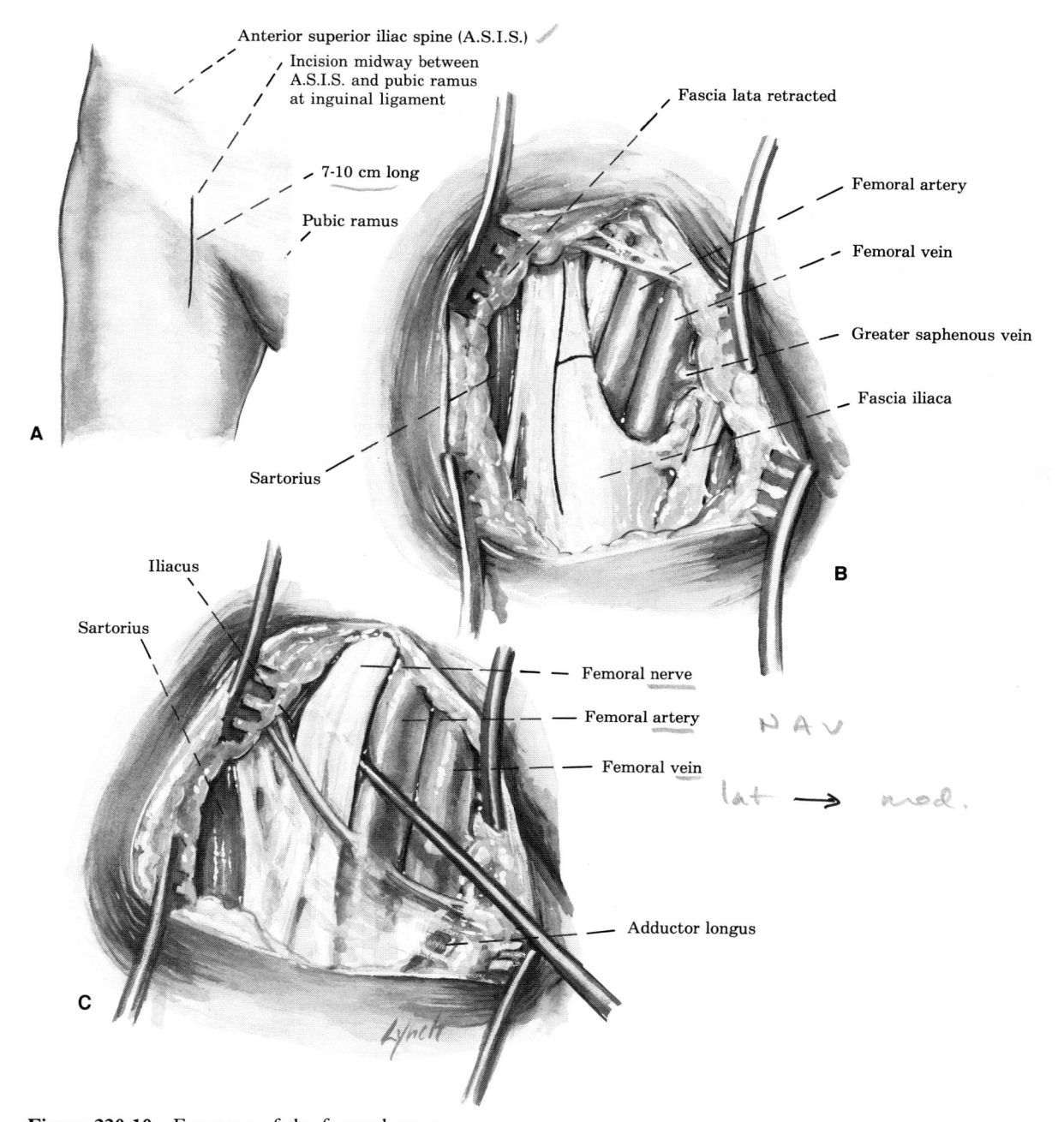

Figure 230-10 Exposure of the femoral nerve.

Sciatic Nerve

The sciatic nerve, the largest peripheral nerve in the human body, is responsible for the motor innervation of the entire lower extremity with the exception of the quadriceps muscles anteriorly, which are innervated by the femoral nerve. The sciatic nerve is most commonly injured in traumatic fracture dislocations of the pelvis or by deep penetrating wounds of the posterior aspect of the buttock or thigh.

Anatomy

The sciatic nerve is a consolidation of the major components of the lumbosacral plexus: the tibial component is composed of the anterior division of roots L4 through S3; the peroneal division is composed of the posterior divisions of roots L4 through S2. As these divisions consolidate in the sciatic nerve, the tibial group is usually medial and the peroneal lateral. Accompanied by the inferior gluteal artery and nerve and the posterior femoral cutaneous nerve, the sciatic nerve courses over the sacrum and leaves the pelvis through the sciatic notch inferior to the piriformis muscle. It then courses distally over the obturator internus, the gemelli, and the quadratus femoris muscles directly beneath the gluteus maximus muscle. Leaving the area of the buttock, it courses into the thigh just lateral to the biceps femoris and medial to the iliotibial tract, turning medially in just a few centimeters to cross distally deep to the biceps femoris and then to course between that muscle and the semitendinosus muscle.

In the mid to lower thigh, the division of the sciatic nerve into its tibial and peroneal components is anatomically complete, although even in the gluteal region those components often can be distinguished within the common nerve sheath. In addition to its two major branches the sciatic nerve gives off muscular branches to the long head of the biceps femoris, to the semitendinosus, and to the semimembranosus and ischial fibers of the adductor magnus muscle in the upper thigh.

Surgical Exposure

For exposure of the sciatic nerve in the gluteal region and upper thigh, the patient is prone, with the hips slightly flexed and the lower extremities extended. A question mark-shaped incision (Fig. 230-11A) as described by Henry,[1] is made, beginning about 2 to 3 cm lateral and inferior to the posterior superior iliac spine, curving laterally over the greater trochanter, returning to the midline, and finally extending along the posterior midline of the thigh. The adipose tissue and fascia are opened, and the fibers of the gluteus maximus muscle are split along a line running a few finger-breadths inferior to the posterior superior iliac spine toward the greater trochanter (Fig. 230-11B). The fibers inferior to this line are incised along the curved line over the greater trochanter, and the muscle is reflected medially to expose the sciatic nerve as it courses over the gemelli, the obturator internus, and the quadratus femoris muscles. The nerve may then be traced to its appearance from beneath the piriformis muscle, which may be retracted superiorly to provide additional exposure (Fig. 230-11C). When the gluteus maximus muscle is reflected, care must be taken not to injure the inferior gluteal artery and nerve as they course deep to and penetrate this muscle. The sciatic nerve may be followed into the upper thigh by retracting the fibers of the gluteus maximus muscle medially and tracing the nerve as it runs deep to the biceps femoris muscle. It must be remembered that the posterior femoral cutaneous nerve at this point lies superficial to the biceps femoris muscle, and its injury must be avoided as that muscle is retracted. After the sciatic nerve crosses deep to the biceps femoris muscle, it may be traced between that muscle and the semitendinosus muscle until it divides into its terminal branches 5 to 10 cm above the popliteal fossa.

Common Peroneal Nerve

The common peroneal nerve innervates the muscles of dorsiflexion, or extension, of the foot. It is most commonly injured by athletic or automobile accident–related trauma to the lateral aspect of the knee, where the nerve travels around the lateral aspect of the head of the fibula. Its injury results in a weakness characterized by a foot drop.

Anatomy

The common peroneal nerve is the lateral component of the sciatic nerve and arises from the L4 through S2 nerve roots. It is one of the terminal branches of the sciatic nerve, branching along with the tibial nerve at a variable distance above the popliteal fossa. The common peroneal nerve travels along the medial margin of the biceps femoris muscle (giving off a cutaneous branch and the sural nerve), wraps around the head of the fibula, and dives deep to the peroneus longus muscle. At this point, the common peroneal nerve divides into three branches: the recurrent articular branch, which provides sensory innervation to the knee joint and the tibiofibular joint; the superficial peroneal branch, which provides motor innervation to the peroneus longus and peroneus brevis muscles as well as sensory innervation to the lateral surface of the leg and the dorsum of the foot; and the deep peroneal (anterior tibial) branch, which extends toward the foot and provides motor innervation to the extensor muscles (the tibialis anterior, the extensor hallucis longus, and the extensor digitorum brevis). The deep peroneal (anterior tibial) nerve continues deep to the extensor digitorum longus to enter the anterior compartment of the leg. At this point, accompanied by but lateral to the anterior tibial artery, it travels distally between the tibialis anterior and the extensor hallucis longus muscles. It enters the foot by passing deep to the transverse crural ligament and then dividing into its terminal motor branches.

In the popliteal fossa, a lateral cutaneous branch of the peroneal nerve joins a medial branch of the tibial nerve to form the sural nerve, which innervates the skin over the lateral aspect of the leg and foot and the dorsal aspect of the leg.

Surgical Exposure

The peroneal nerve is best approached at the bifurcation of the sciatic nerve just proximal to the popliteal fossa. The patient is placed in the lateral decubitus position with the knee slightly flexed. A Z- or lazy S-shaped incision is made over the popliteal crease, with the superior limb of the incision extending up the midline of the thigh and the inferior limb extending toward the inferolateral aspect of the knee (Fig. 230-12A). The skin is incised and reflected from the underlying fascia in an attempt to preserve the posterior femoral cutaneous nerve, which travels beneath the fascia in the midline but penetrates the fascia with its superficial branches (Fig. 230-12B). The fascia is incised vertically over the plane between the biceps femoris and the semitendinosus muscles. These muscles are then separated and retracted to expose the sciatic nerve where it divides into the common peroneal and tibial nerves just above the popliteal fossa (Fig. 230-12C). With blunt dissection, the peroneal nerve is separated from the tibial nerve and followed laterally along the medial aspect of the biceps femoris muscle toward the head of the fibula (Fig. 230-12D). The lateral sural cutaneous branch may arise anywhere in the popliteal fossa and should be protected. The skin incision is continued around the lat-

Surgical Exposure of Peripheral Nerves　　　1859

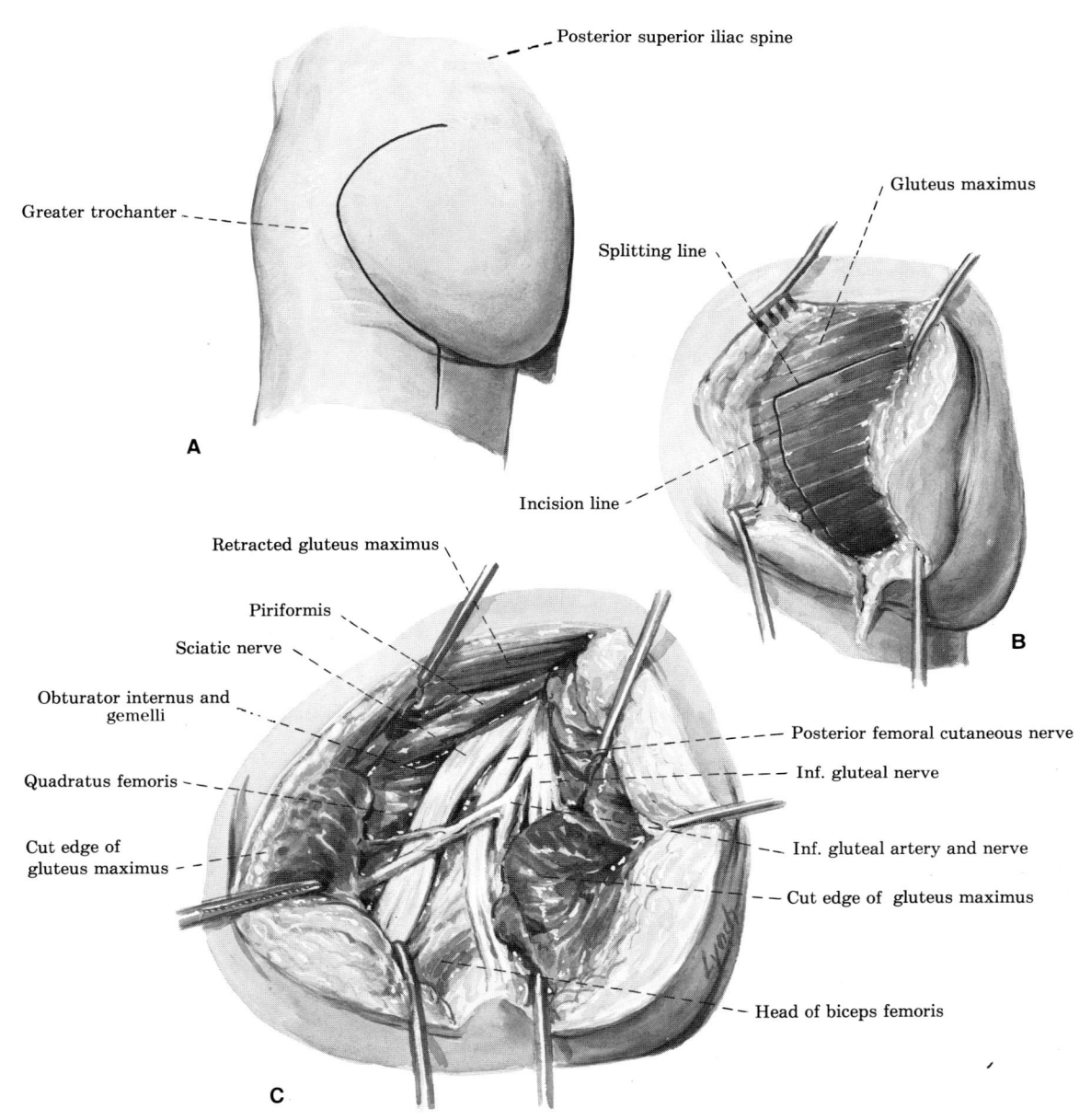

Figure 230-11 Exposure of the sciatic nerve.

eral aspect of the knee just inferior to the fibular head and then directed inferiorly in a line approximating the plane between the tibialis anterior and the extensor hallucis longus muscles (Fig. 230-13A). At the head of the fibula the fascia is exposed and the nerve identified as it penetrates the fascia (Fig. 230-13B). The fascia is incised to expose the nerve, and the nerve is followed to its entrance into the peroneus longus muscle between the superficial and deep heads of that muscle (Fig. 230-13C). The superficial aspect of the muscle is transected to expose the bifurcation of the common peroneal nerve into its recurrent articular, superficial, and deep peroneal branches. The superficial branch continues distally along the deep surface of the superficial head of the peroneus longus muscle while the deep peroneal (anterior tibial) branch dives deep into the anterior compartment of the leg to the extensor digitorum longus muscle (Fig. 230-13D). The incision is continued distally as far as necessary and the tibialis anterior and extensor hallucis longus muscles are separated to expose the deep peroneal nerve and the accompanying anterior tibial artery. This separation may be continued to the dorsum of the foot, if needed, but one must be careful to preserve all nutrient vessels to the nerve (Fig. 230-14A,B).

The sural nerve is particularly useful for nerve cable grafting. This nerve may be exposed and harvested through a linear incision or through multiple transverse incisions along the posterolateral aspect of the calf. The nerve is identified distally at the lateral aspect of the ankle, where it accompanies the lesser saphenous vein. It can then be traced proximally and the desired length obtained.

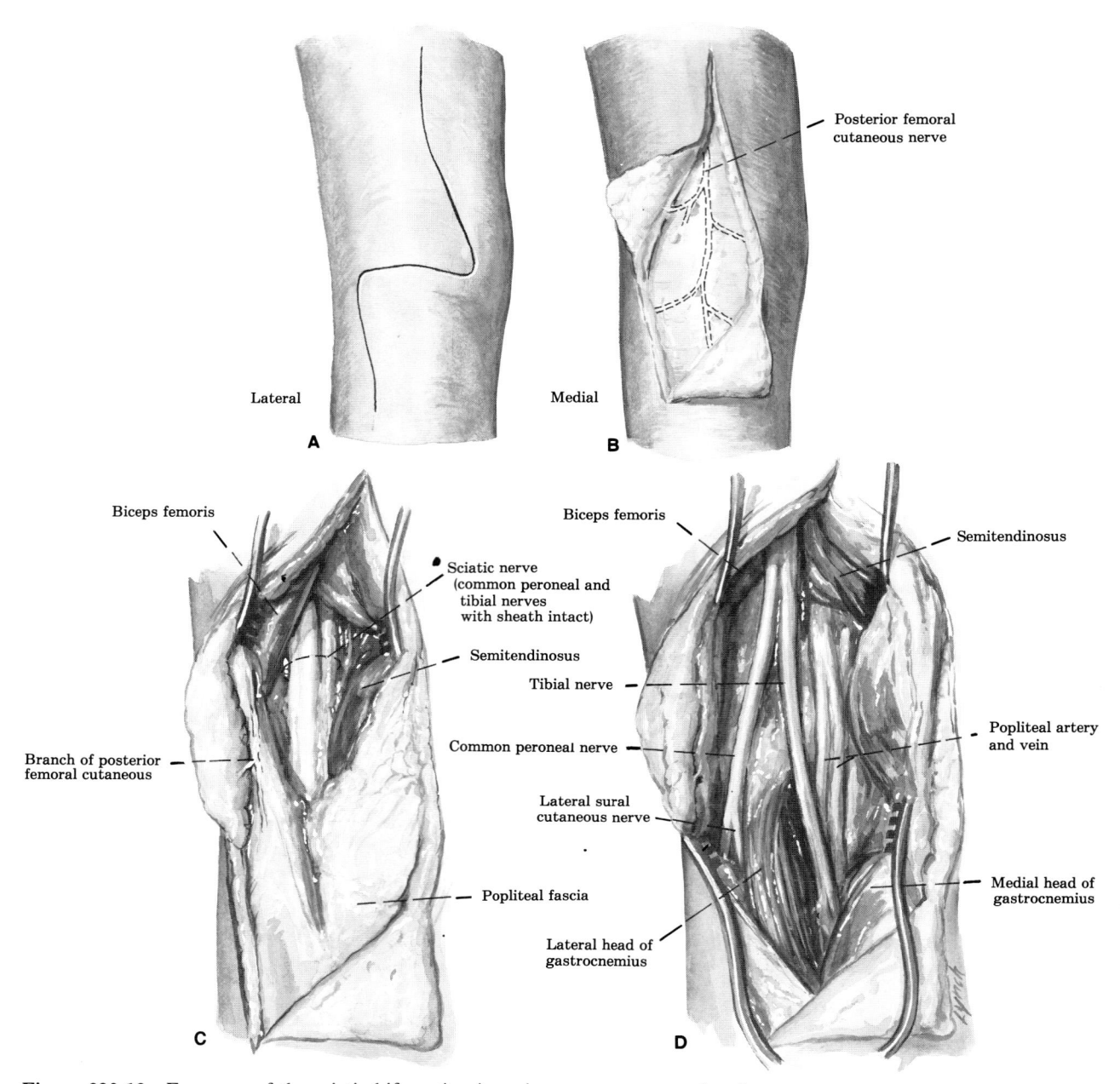

Figure 230-12 Exposure of the sciatic bifurcation into the common peroneal and posterior tibial nerves in the popliteal fossa.

Tibial Nerve

The tibial nerve is probably the most important nerve of the leg since it supplies motor innervation to the major muscles of the calf and the plantar flexor muscles of the foot. It also provides sensory innervation for the plantar surface of the foot. Injury to the nerve is uncommon, except by a penetrating wound of the popliteal fossa or by compression beneath the flexor retinaculum at the level of the medial malleolus, where it gives rise to the medial and lateral plantar nerves. This tarsal tunnel syndrome is characterized by burning pain on the ball of the foot.

Anatomy

The tibial nerve is the medial component of the sciatic nerve and is composed of the L4 through S3 roots. Like the common peroneal nerve, the tibial nerve (or posterior tibial nerve as it is sometimes called) is a terminal branch of the sciatic nerve and arises a variable distance above the popliteal fossa. The tibial nerve traverses the popliteal fossa in the midline between the plantaris and gastrocnemius muscles just lateral to the popliteal artery and vein. Within the popliteal fossa it gives rise to motor branches to the medial and lateral heads of the gastrocnemius, the soleus, the plantaris,

Surgical Exposure of Peripheral Nerves 1861

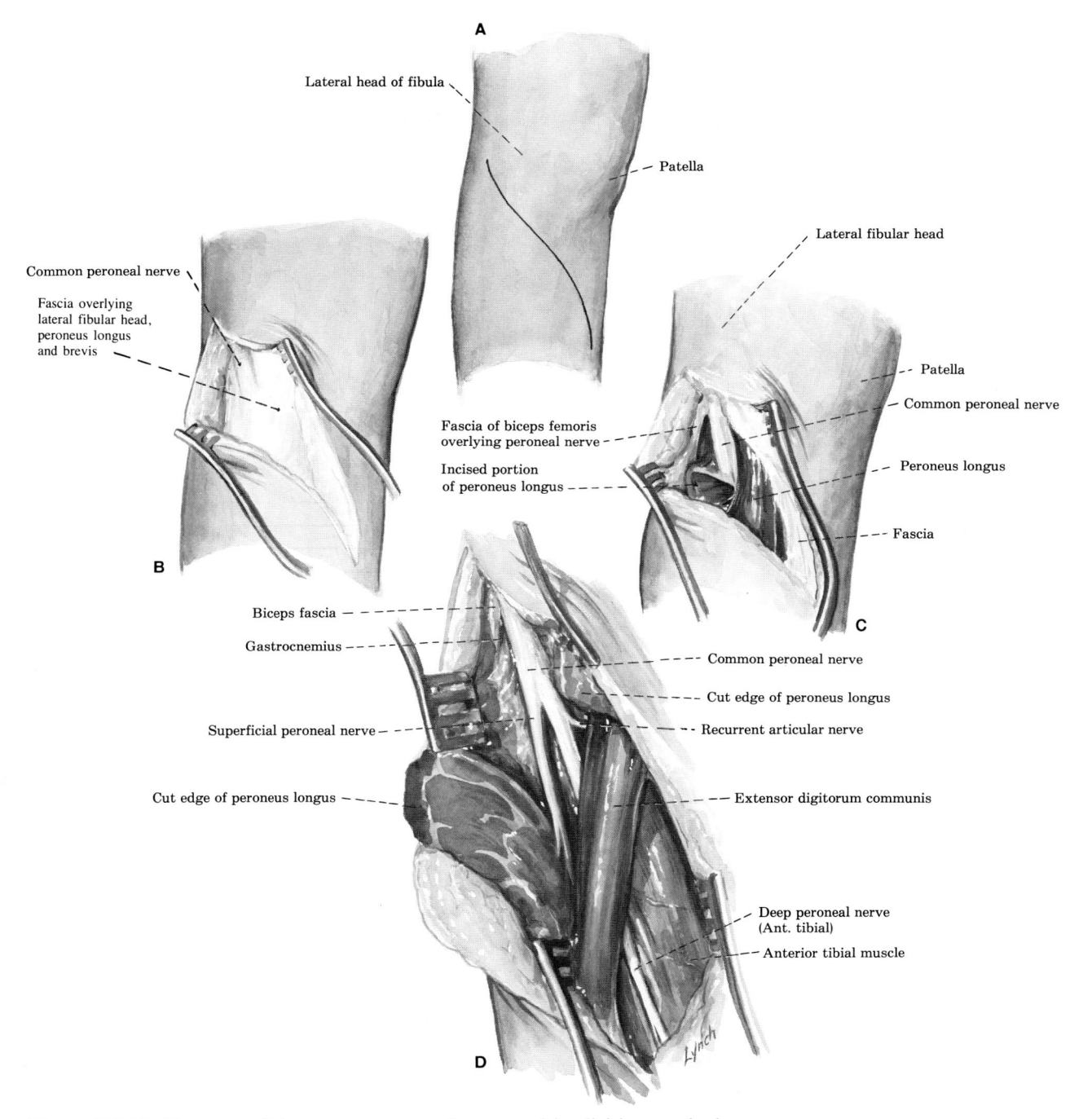

Figure 230-13 Exposure of the common peroneal nerve and its divisions at the lateral fibular head.

and the popliteus muscles and to sensory components of the medial sural cutaneous nerve, which joins with the branch from the common peroneal nerve to form the sural nerve. The tibial nerve leaves the popliteal fossa by diving deep to the soleus muscles but passes superficial to the popliteus and the tibialis posterior muscles. At varying intervals in the calf it gives off motor branches to the tibialis posterior, the flexor hallucis longus, and the flexor digitorum longus muscles. In the ankle the nerve travels deep to the flexor retinaculum and inferior to the medial malleous, where it divides into its terminal branches, the medial and lateral plantar nerves. The medial plantar nerve is responsible for motor innervation of the flexor digitorum brevis, the flexor hallucis brevis, and the adductor hallucis muscles, as well as the first of the lumbrical muscles. It provides sensory innervation to the medial aspect of the plantar surface of the foot. The lateral plantar nerve innervates the quadratus plantae, the abductor digiti minimi pedis, the flexor digiti minimi brevis pedis,

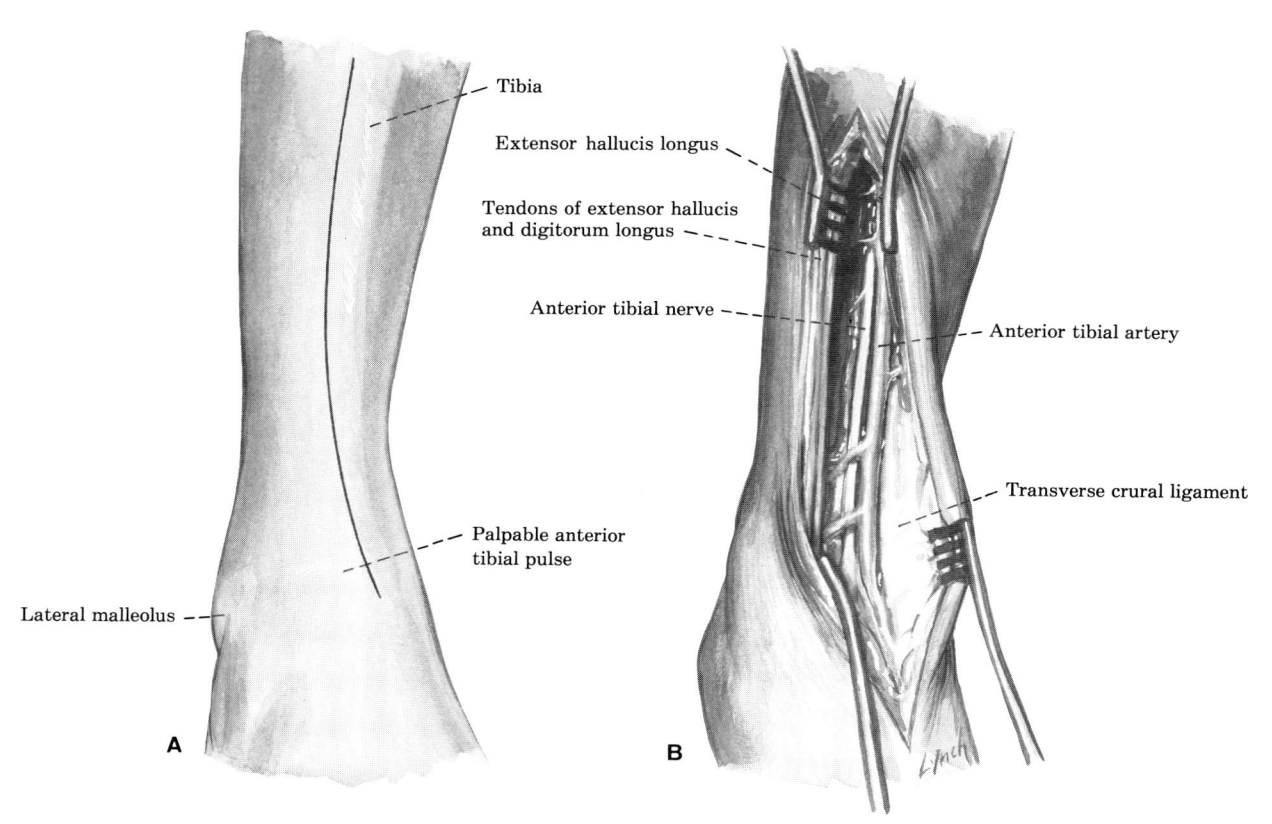

Figure 230-14 Exposure of the distal deep peroneal nerve.

and the adductor hallucis muscles, as well as the remaining lumbrical muscles and all the interosseous muscles. It provides sensory innervation to the lateral aspect of the plantar surface, with some extension onto the dorsum of the foot. The plantar distribution of the medial and lateral plantar nerves compares with the palmar distribution of the median and ulnar nerves.

Surgical Exposure

Surgical exposure of the tibial nerve, like exposure of the peroneal nerve, is through an S- or Z-shaped incision made over the popliteal fossa. The superior limb extends up the midline of the thigh and the inferior limb extends medially to continue over the medial border of the gastrocnemius and the soleus muscles as necessary (Fig. 230-12A). The nerve is identified in the distal thigh as it branches from the sciatic nerve and courses through the popliteal fossa. During retraction of the muscles care must be taken to preserve the vascular structures and the motor branches to the gastrocnemius, the plantaris, and the popliteus muscles. The medial head of the gastrocnemius muscle is retracted medially and the nerve is traced to the point where it dives deep to the soleus muscle but superficial to the popliteus muscle. In the popliteal fossa the nerve is lateral to the popliteal artery and vein, but as it progresses into the calf, it may be directly superficial to those two structures (Fig. 230-12C,D).

For exposure in the calf, the patient is prone, the involved leg is placed in full rotation, and the contralateral hip is elevated as necessary to provide adequate exposure of the medial aspect of the leg. The nerve is traced through the calf by extending the incision distally along the medial aspect of the leg along a line approximately 2 cm from the medial border of the tibia (Fig. 230-15A). The fascia is incised along the medial border of the gastrocnemius muscle, and the soleus muscle is retracted laterally to expose the transverse intermuscular septum. Longitudinal incision of this septum exposes the posterior tibial nerve and its accompanying artery, the posterior tibial artery, and the peroneal artery, all lying along the superficial aspect of the tibialis posterior muscle (Fig. 230-15B). Some of the fibers of the soleus muscle may need to be transected to obtain greater proximal exposure. The nerve is followed in this plane to the level of the ankle, where it becomes superficial to the flexor digitorum longus muscle and medial to the flexor hallucis longus muscle (Fig. 230-15C). It lies deep to the flexor retinaculum, passing around the medial malleolus to divide into terminal branches, the medial and lateral plantar nerves. A curvilinear incision tracing the approximate course of the nerve is made around the medial malleolus but must be kept well above the plantar surface of the foot. The flexor retinaculum is exposed and excised in the same curved incision and the tibial nerve and its medial and lateral plantar branches are identified. This step is facilitated by retracting the abductor hallucis muscle plantarward and the tendon of the flexor digitorum longus muscle dorsally.

If the exploration is confined to the ankle, the patient should be supine with the thigh externally rotated and the

Surgical Exposure of Peripheral Nerves

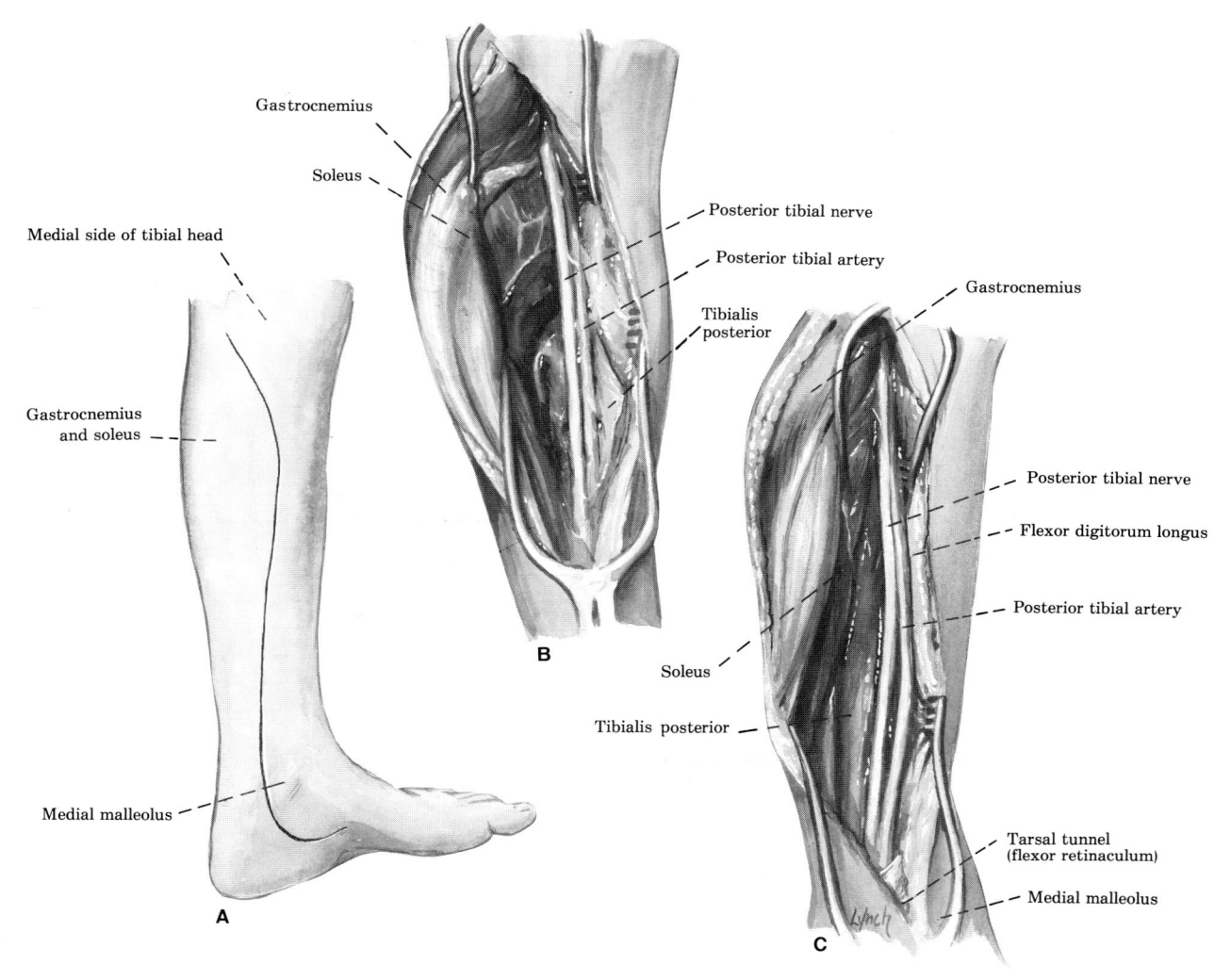

Figure 230-15 Exposure of the posterior tibial nerve.

knee flexed and elevated on a pillow. Because of the multiple vascular structures involved in this dissection, a tourniquet on the calf is invaluable.

References

1. Henry AK: *Extensile Exposure*, 2d ed. Baltimore, Williams & Wilkins, 1957.
2. Inglis AE: Surgical exposure of peripheral nerves, in Omer GE Jr, Spinner M (eds): *Management of Peripheral Nerve Problems*. Philadelphia, Saunders, 1980, pp 317–350.
3. Kempe LG: *Operative Neurosurgery*, vol II. New York, Springer, 1970.
4. Kline DG, Nulsen FE: Acute injuries of peripheral nerves, in Youmans JR (ed): *Neurological Surgery*, 2d ed. Philadelphia, Saunders, 1982, pp 2362–2429.
5. Pernkopf E: *Atlas of Topographical and Applied Human Anatomy*, vol 2. *Thorax, Abdomen and Extremities*. Philadelphia, Saunders, 1964.
6. Seddon HJ: *Surgical Disorders of the Peripheral Nerves*, 2d ed. Edinburgh, Churchill Livingstone, 1975, pp 250–286.
7. Seletz E: *Surgery of Peripheral Nerves*. Springfield, Ill, Charles C Thomas, 1951.

231
Management of the Neuroma in Continuity

David G. Kline
Earl R. Hackett

When a nerve is injured to the extent that major loss distal to the injury occurs, one of two conditions is found. The nerve is either transected or more bluntly pulled in half or it is left in some degree of gross continuity with a variable degree of internal derangement. The latter condition is by far the more common (60 to 70 percent of cases) and is the more difficult to manage.[10,25] When continuity is totally lost, function will not recover spontaneously except under very rare and extraordinary circumstances. As a result, management of such cases is straightforward; it is surgical and not conservative, and only the timing of and the technique used for such a repair involve any element of controversy or variability. This is not the case with lesions in continuity because some patients with such lesions may completely recover function in the distribution of the injured nerve with time alone. Other patients will recover partial function but less than might be gained by a good surgical repair. Still other patients will experience little or no improvement.[18] Thus, the decisions such as whether to intervene surgically, when to intervene, and what to do once the lesion is exposed are difficult, and management remains controversial (Fig. 231-1).

Neuropathology

When continuity is maintained despite serious injury, a spectrum of internal derangement can exist. For example, in up to 20 percent of cases with severe deficit distal to lacerating injuries, gross continuity to the nerve may be present. In many of these instances, there has been partial but of course incomplete division of the nerve, and dysfunction of the remaining segment may be due to contusion associated with the partial penetration of the nerve. Experimental evidence is available indicating that sharp and yet partial penetration of the nerve does not lead to static loss, for with time the original injury may progress to involve adjacent but originally noninjured areas, particularly if the perineurial barrier has been interrupted by the original injury.[13] Loss beyond the original injury may be due to an alteration in the blood-nerve barrier and edema formation, although other as yet unknown factors may play a role as well. Axons adjacent to but not included in the original injury undergo partial demyelination while others drop out entirely.[8] Over a period of weeks some restoration occurs in this zone, due to remyelination of some axons and regeneration of others. Recovery without surgical intervention is less certain in the original zone of laceration even in the nonhuman primate, let alone in the human. In a few cases, loss associated with a lacerating injury may be entirely due to contusion, the lacerating instrument bruising and/or stretching the nerve rather than lacerating it. Outcome then depends on the severity of the internal derangement of the nerve, just as with a lesion in continuity due to blunter forces.

The more common lesion in continuity produced by contusive and stretch injuries usually affects the entire cross section of the nerve. In its mildest form, the injury is neurapraxic and little or no structural damage is discernible on either light or electron microscopic examination, the temporary loss being secondary to a reversible block in conduction associated with milder and less prolonged degrees of compression than those that produce more serious injury. In some neurapraxic lesions (Sunderland grade 1), a portion of the axons that were compressed will show a localized thinning and some segmental demyelination but the neuropathological picture is a mild one in comparison with other grades of injury.[22] If the neurapraxic lesion is severe enough to come to clinical attention, a few of the fibers will sometimes be more severely injured and will undergo wallerian degeneration and eventually produce a few scattered denervational changes in more distal musculature. These fibers

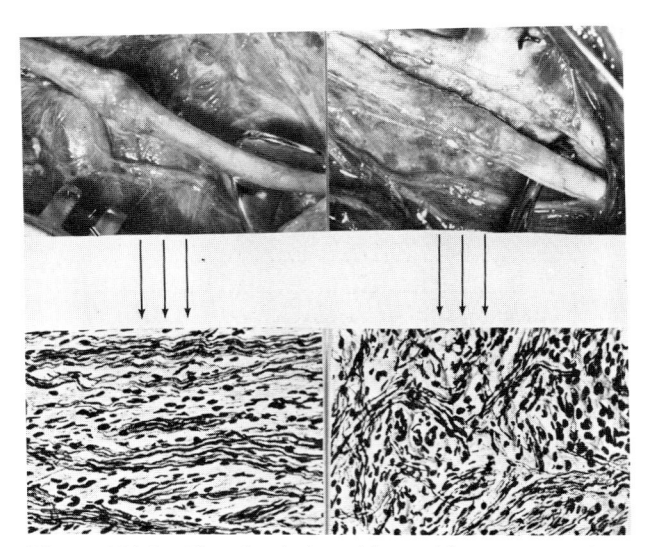

Figure 231-1 The classical problem with a neuroma in continuity is the extent of its internal derangement and its potential for significant regeneration. An irregular and firm lesion as shown at the upper left may be regenerating relatively well-organized axons (*lower left*) whereas that appearing smooth and modeled (*upper right*) may have a disorganized axonal structure with frequent branching (*lower right*) due to intrafascicular scar. (Taken in part from Kline and Nulsen.[15])

have invariably undergone axonotmetic change in which although axon continuity is lost, continuity of the endoneurial and other connective tissue framework is maintained and thus axons regenerate well over a period of several months. As a result, the few scattered distal denervational changes if detected initially in this setting, will gradually reverse.

In a small and unfortunately infrequent number of cases, injury, although affecting the entire cross section of the nerve, is mild enough that a significant number of axons are not lost and maintain their function while others are injured but usually in an axonotmetic fashion so that their recovery is assured. Still other fibers have only a neurapraxic block in conduction and may regain function in hours to days. Such patients have decreased function in the distribution of the nerve. No function is entirely lost but rather there is often a rather uniform reduction in motor power usually with minimal to no loss in the sensory sphere of the nerve. Recovery of full or near full function almost always occurs. Such lesions are usually due to more severe or prolonged degrees of compression than those producing a neurapraxic lesion or may be due to mild stretch, particularly that caused by a bullet that comes close to but does not strike the nerve.

A frequent lesion in continuity is one producing a predominantly axonotmetic lesion in which axon continuity is lost but most of the connective tissue framework of the nerve is preserved (Sunderland grade 2). There is a variable amount of endoneurial distortion although most of this fine tubular network of the nerve is preserved, as is the perineurial barrier and thus the overall integrity of the fascicles.[21] Since axonal continuity is lost, the wallerian process is very much in evidence with dissolution of axons and their myelin coverings and, over a period of weeks, phagocytosis of this debris. Schwann cells proliferate not only in the distal segment of the nerve but at the injury site itself. Regeneration is good, for the new regenerative units have a relatively well-structured framework to guide axons distally toward their original destinations. Moreover, the new axons are not forced to branch many times because there is relatively little in the way of connective tissue obstruction at the injury site. Recovery usually occurs without surgical intervention but the process may take many months depending on the nerve involved and on the locus of the injury.

Another frequent type of lesion in continuity is one in which the dominant pattern involves not only loss of axons but significant loss of connective tissue structure. Hemorrhage and edema, as well as frank necrosis of a portion of the cross section of the nerve, can also be seen. Such damage can be almost entirely intrafascicular, with little or no obvious disruption of the perineurium and thus of gross fascicular continuity, as is seen with some injection[3] and stretch[14] injuries (Sunderland grade 3). Unfortunately, the more common injury in this category distorts the extrafascicular as well as the intrafascicular structural characteristics of the nerve. The latter grade of injury (Sunderland grade 4) is the most severe lesion in continuity. In either case a degenerative picture ensues but regeneration of axons, although it does occur, is less successful than with other grades of injury. Owing to injury to the framework of the nerve, fibroblastic proliferation occurs and the connective tissue is laid down in a haphazard fashion, which obstructs successful axonal regeneration. Axons invariably penetrate these connective tissue barriers but do so slowly, are forced to branch many times, wind up in areas for which they were not originally intended, and seldom regain their original caliber or degree of myelination. Recovery of function thus seldom occurs and peripheral denervational changes persist in the absence of surgical resection and repair of the lesion.

Electrophysiology

For mild lesions in continuity that have a large element of neurapraxia, electrical studies are quite characteristic and diagnostic.[16] Stimulation of the nerve proximal to the area where compression occurred will produce little or no distal motor movement and one will not be able to evoke a nerve action potential (NAP) across the lesion. On the other hand, stimulation below the level of the lesion will produce full distal motor function and stimulating and recording below the level of the lesion will result in an NAP. As pointed out before, with time (e.g., 2 to 3 weeks from the onset of the neurapraxic injury) an occasional fibrillation or denervational potential will be recorded, but there will not be the widespread denervational pattern seen with more serious injuries and insertional activity will be maintained even though a muscle action potential cannot be elicited unless stimulation occurs below the level of the injury. In a relatively short time each of these electrical abnormalities will reverse although some of the more serious neurapraxic lesions can persist for a number of weeks, particularly those associated with gunshot wounds and some of the milder stretch injuries to the plexus.

Axonotmetic and neurotmetic lesions in continuity share most of the same electrophysiological characteristics. The principal difference is that one successfully regenerates and the other does not, so that the electrical concomitants of recovery are present in one and absent in the other. Both lesions lead to denervational changes distal to the level of the injury. Acutely, despite loss of axonal continuity at the level of the lesion, the nerve distal to the lesion can be stimulated and muscle contraction evoked. This response can persist for up to 72 h in some nerves because the wallerian process takes time to result in dissolution of the more distal axons and axon to motor end plate junctions.[15] When nerves are inadvertently injured at the operating table, one cannot therefore rely on the response of distal musculature as an index of integrity, particularly if one stimulates the nerve distal to the injury site. After 2 to 3 weeks, depending on how close the injury is to the muscle inputs to be tested, the electromyogram will show denervational changes with either type of injury. Insertional activity as the needle is placed into the muscle will either be reduced or absent. With the muscle at rest, there is spontaneous muscle fiber firing, presumably due to the release of acetylcholine. This spontaneous activity takes the form of fibrillations or denervational potentials and with the usual serious lesion in continuity has a widespread distribution in muscles normally innervated by the nerve distal to the level of the lesion. One also will not be able to evoke a muscle action potential by stimulating the nerve either proximal or distal to the level of the lesion, and of course when the patient attempts to voluntarily contract the muscle being tested, there is no electrical activity other than denervational change. In most cases dealt with by the neurosurgeon these changes persist for many months.[1,6,18]

In a nerve that is successfully regenerating (predominantly axonotmetic or Sunderland grade 2 and some grade 3 lesions), axons will penetrate the injury site in great number. Because of good organization and minimal branching, these axons readily reach the nerve distal to the lesion in continuity. Thus there can be thousands of axons greater than 5 μm in diameter, some of which have a degree of myelination present quite a distance down the distal stump. This occurs long before the muscle can contract in response to direct stimulation of the nerve and even before electromyographic studies show reversal of denervational changes.[12] At this point in time one can, however, record an NAP by stimulating proximal to the injury and tracing the recorded NAP through the injury and on into the distal stump of the nerve. This is usually 6 to 10 weeks after injury.[15] With more time, the evoked NAP can be tracked further distal to the injury in continuity. Absence of such a response by this time suggests poor regeneration and a more neurotmetic injury (some Sunderland grade 3 and most grade 4 injuries). The interval between the onset of recordable NAPs in the distal stump and reversal of denervational changes is greatest in proximal nerve injuries, where the first muscle innervated downstream is a relatively great distance away. Thus, the difference is greatest in brachial plexus lesions, especially those involving outflow to the median and ulnar nerves, upper arm injuries involving these nerves, and buttock and thigh level involvement of the sciatic nerve. With further time in the successfully regenerating nerve, axons will reach muscle, and after some degree of reconstruction of the axon-motor end plate-muscle fiber junction, needling of these muscles will show reversal of denervational changes and the onset of signs of reinnervation, such as nascent reinnervational units and early muscle action potential formation in response to attempts to voluntarily move the muscle.[1] It should be noted that muscle may be stimulated to contract by stimulating the nerve either above or below the level of the lesion sometime during this period. Thus, response to stimulation may antedate voluntary recovery of function by 2 to 6 weeks.[18,19]

In the nerve that is not successfully regenerating, these electrical signs of recovery will be absent. An NAP will not be recordable across the level of the lesion at 6 to 10 weeks, distal musculature will not respond to stimulation of the nerve even some months later, and electromyographic changes of denervation will persist. One must keep in mind that even in severe lesions in continuity some fibers do eventually succeed in reaching a distal locus so that occasionally some reversal of denervational change is seen depending on how thorough the electromyographic sampling is, but meaningful function seldom returns under these circumstances.[6,25]

Clinical Correlates

The question as to whether to operate on a lesion in continuity due to partial laceration can be difficult. If the function lost is not of great practical importance or if it is more extensive but can be readily and effectively replaced by other uninvolved motor and sensory modalities, then a conservative "wait and see" attitude is best. A good example is provided by the not infrequent occurrence of partial division of the median nerve at the wrist, where sensory function is spared but motor function is lost. To substitute for function of the thenar intrinsics, most patients can use ulnar- and radial-innervated thumb muscles. Such a course may be acceptable in the left and usually nondominant hand except for those patients who depend on both hands to do fine work. On the right or usually dominant side such an injury will require exploration and a split repair in which the intact portion is dissected away from the injured portion and the latter is trimmed back and repaired end to end or more frequently by the insertion of relatively short interfascicular grafts. By comparison partial division of the median nerve resulting in loss of sensory function should always be repaired and this can be done acutely or after a delay of several weeks.[20] Similar guidelines can be drawn up for the ulnar nerve but in a reverse sense, for here sensory function is much less important than motor function, which is of paramount importance. Here partial division leading to motor loss, especially that of the important intrinsic muscles of the hand "cries for repair," while that involving only the sensory portion may not unless painful paresthesias or hyperesthesia (implying incomplete sensory division or contusive injury) accompany the injury. Decisions concerning partial division of a nerve are not quite as straightforward for lesions involving the proximal median or ulnar or other nerves. At a more proximal level, the interfascicular mix of sensory and motor axons is greater than distally and thus division, even when partial, leads to a greater mix of sensory and motor loss.[22] When in doubt, the best thing to do is to explore the injury and do a repair.

Less divisive injuries that are partial affect the entire cross section of the nerve. Mild contusion with or without associated bony fracture and milder degrees of stretch can spare some degree of function in a widespread fashion. In this unusual setting there is partial loss of strength in each muscle or group of muscles innervated by the nerve distal to the injury site. Sensation may be partially lost or more commonly spared altogether. Such an injury usually is composed of a mixture of axonotmetic and neurapraxic damage, with little if any component of neurotmetic damage. Recovery is thus the rule and usually to a level superior to that afforded by resection and repair. The key to management of such injuries is frequent follow-up by both physical examination and appropriate electrical studies.[23] Function should improve in the early months after surgery. If it does not, then exploration may be in order, for the injury may be complicated by entrapment, particularly if it occurred at a site where the nerve is normally snug to begin with. Such a circumstance may apply with injury to the ulnar nerve close to the elbow or in Guyon's canal, the median nerve beneath the lacertus fibrosis or the edge of the pronator teres or close to the carpal tunnel, the radial nerve at the midhumeral level or its posterior interosseous branch near the supinator, or the peroneal nerve near the head of the fibula.

The majority of lesions in continuity are more serious than those mentioned above and are due to severe contusion or stretch.[9,10] Not only are axons disrupted but there is a variable amount of structural connective tissue damage both within and outside the fascicular environment. Such lesions can remain static, improve partially but to a level less than can be achieved by surgical repair, or improve considerably to a level superior to that achieved by suture or the use of grafts. All these lesions have an initially complete or nearly complete deficit distal to the level of the injury. Management includes a thorough baseline physical examination, early institution of physical therapy, and splinting where appropriate. After the lapse of several weeks, baseline electromyographic studies should be performed, including thorough sampling of the electrical activity of as many muscles distal to the lesion as possible. If no substantial clinical or electrical recovery occurs over a 2- to 3-month period, exploration is in order. Such a period gives time for reversal of any neurapraxic change and, more importantly, places the surgeon in a position to accurately test for the presence or absence of significant regeneration across the lesion in continuity once it is exposed at the operating table. A longer wait can jeopardize the result should resection and suture or graft repair be necessary.[2,7]

Exceptions are provided by severe stretch injuries, especially to the brachial or less frequently the pelvic plexus, where if continuity is present, which it is in the great majority of cases, spontaneous recovery takes longer. Thus, for such recovery to be documented at the operating table, the interval from injury to operation must usually be 3 to 4 months.[14] In an occasional instance, exploration of a lesion in continuity may be delayed because of wound infection or the need to obtain good soft tissue coverage of the area of injury.[25] Generally, the need for stabilization of the extremity or planned operative fixation of fracture(s) should not delay the neural operation. The fracture site can be protected during the operation and, if need be, can often be stabilized by the orthopedist at some point during the same procedure.

Operation

At exploration, the nerve should be exposed both above and below the injury site. It is best to work in both directions toward the injury, saving dissection of this for last. Dissection is most expeditiously done sharply. The bipolar coagulator is used to control bleeding points. Although collateral vessels can be sacrificed, every attempt should be made to preserve the longitudinal blood supply, which is subepineurial and deeper within the nerve.[11,17] For adequate inspection as well as intraoperative electrophysiological testing, the nerve should be exposed completely, which means dissecting entirely around it. The injury site is dissected loose from the surrounding scar, usually with a no.15 blade on a long-handled, narrow scalpel. The injury site is then inspected and gently palpated. Swelling greater than twice the normal diameter of the nerve suggests a neurotmetic or Sunderland grade 4 lesion, whereas less swelling can be compatible with either a neurotmetic or axonotmetic lesion. On palpation, a firm or hard lesion favors heavy internal scar and thus a neurotmetic rather than an axonotmetic lesion.[26] Unfortunately, many exceptions to these simple guidelines exist. Thus, enlargement or firmness may be minimal with injection injuries and some contusive, stretch injuries and yet internal derangement will be severe. In other cases, the neuroma may appear large and even feel firm because of a proliferation of connective tissue at an epineurial and interfascicular epineurial level and yet the intrafascicular architecture will be fairly well preserved and will be found to be regenerating in a relative longitudinal and mature fashion (Fig. 231-1). It is well to keep in mind that the derangement of the internal architecture is almost always worse than it appears on inspection and palpation. Lateral neuromas suggest partial division or laceration of the nerve, particularly if function in the distribution of the nerve is known to be partially spared by preoperative clinical or electrical testing.

A number of surgically oriented maneuvers have been suggested in the past for evaluation of the usual lesion in continuity that involves the entire cross section of the nerve.[20] Injection of saline or other physiological solutions to see if the fluid will dissect beyond the confines of the lesion does not make sense, for much of the scar interfering with regeneration and secondary axonal disorganization is within the fascicles themselves and this test does not delineate such changes. In addition, at least in the laboratory, the injection of saline can at least temporarily decrease or even obliterate electrical activity and thus this is not advisable even though the changes are usually reversible. For similar reasons, microscopic dissection of fascicles proximal and distal to the lesion followed by attempts to trace them through a severe lesion is seldom advisable. Fascicular continuity does not prove intrafascicular axonal continuity or regeneration of healthy and functionally useful axons. Even when done most meticulously, such dissection can on occasion be damaging to a proportion of the axons, especially in seriously swollen and scarred lesions in continuity. Trial section of the neuroma has been suggested. Here, the surgeon sections through the epicenter of the neuroma, stopping only if fascicles are encountered. Again, the presumption is that if fascicles are present in the center of the lesion, recovery will occur without resection and repair, and conversely if there are none, resection can be completed and repair done. Unfortunately both these tenets can be incorrect under a number of circumstances. Again, fascicular continuity can be maintained under some circumstances despite severe intrafascicular derangement requiring resection. On the other hand, fascicular continuity can be totally lost through a portion of the injury site and yet successful regeneration can be occurring, for example, through the center of a successfully sutured nerve.

Thus, after inspection and gentle palpation of the injury site, we prefer to test the usual lesion in continuity by electrophysiological means.[9] Bipolar electrodes are used to stimulate the nerve first above and then below the level of the lesion. Such stimulation can have a retrograde as well as an anterograde effect, particularly when applied to the proximal nerve. Thus, muscles with innervation proximal to the lesion can contract, possibly misleading the surgeon. However, if special attention is given to positioning and draping the limb, the site of muscle contraction can be seen as well as palpated and its origin noted. One looks, of course, for contraction of muscle both innervated by the nerve in question and distal to the lesion itself. If too much voltage is used or its duration is too long, impulses can spread to adjacent and possibly intact nerves, especially at the level of the brachial plexus or proximal upper arm, where other relatively intact

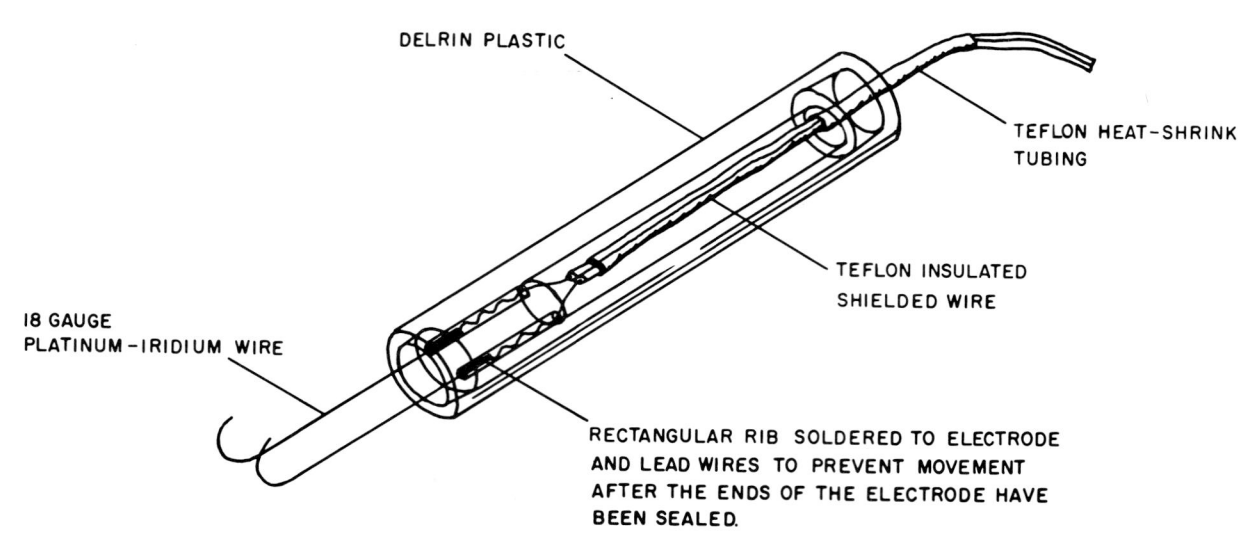

Figure 231-2 Construction of a bipolar electrode used for stimulating and recording from peripheral nerve lesions in continuity. The drilled-out center of the Delrin rod is sealed with acrylic cement after pulling electrodes soldered to shielded wire into the lower portion of the rod. The unit may be heat- or gas-sterilized. (From Kline.[9])

nerves may be located. The electrodes that we use for stimulation are bipolar and are usually made of no.18 stainless steel wire or platinum alloy, with the end of each electrode bent like a shepherd's crook in which the nerve nestles (Fig. 231-2). The other ends of the electrodes are soldered to shielded bipolar wire and the soldered junction and the wire are passed through a Delrin rod, the center of which has been drilled out. The ends of the rod are sealed with acrylic cement. The rod provides a good handle with which the electrodes can be held. The electrode unit can be either heat- or gas-sterilized. Stimulation is provided by a Grass S55 stimulator with an SIU 6 stimulus isolation unit (Grass Instrument Co., Quincy, Mass.). This set-up provides a square wave impulse of which the voltage, duration, and frequency can be easily varied by the clinical investigator. Stimulus duration and especially voltage applied to the nerve are gradually increased until a distal muscular response is obtained. The same instrumentation can be used to trigger an oscilloscopic trace should one want to record nerve action potentials beyond the stimulation site. While stimulating, it is best to elevate a short segment of nerve onto the crooks of the electrodes and to keep the site moist with saline and free of blood. Once the response of the nerve to stimulation is tested and particularly if there is no muscle contraction, the surgeon is ready to proceed with NAP recording.

In the early weeks after injury, axons can regenerate through the lesion and be present in great numbers in the distal stump. For the usual human nerve injury in continuity, many more weeks to months will be required for axons to reach distal targets in enough numbers and with enough maturity so that regeneration can be appreciated by simple stimulation of the nerve or by electromyographic studies. For this reason, it is necessary to stimulate and record across the lesion in continuity if relatively early evidence for or against adequate regeneration is desired (Fig. 231-3). At the present time this can be done most reliably at 8 or more weeks after injury. Intraoperative NAP recording requires bipolar electrodes, a good stimulator, and an oscilloscope with differential amplifiers. Two sets of electrodes are constructed as described above. The Grass stimulator and stimulus isolation unit are used to provide a brief duration shock and the stimulator triggers a sweep on an oscilloscope. We have used for a number of years a Tektronix (Tektronix, Inc, Beaverton, Ore.) 565 dual-beam oscilloscope with 3A9 differential amplifiers so that both an evoked NAP and any evoked and more distal muscle action potential (MAP) could be recorded on the two traces of the oscilloscope. Newer models are available and we now have in use a Tektronix 7704 oscilloscope with two differential amplifiers, 7B70 and 7B71 time bases, a 7M13 readout for displaying information

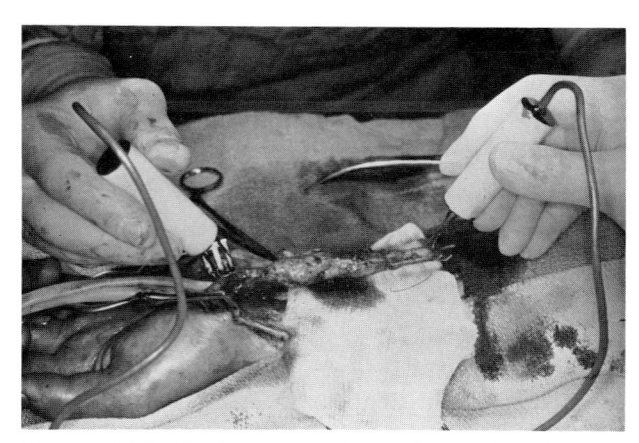

Figure 231-3 Bipolar stimulating and recording electrodes placed proximal and distal to a severe median nerve lesion in continuity. The stimulating electrodes lead out from a stimulus isolation unit and a stimulator while recording electrodes lead to an oscilloscope with a differential amplifier.

Management of the Neuroma in Continuity

about the patient on the screen, and a C53 Polaroid camera to make a record of the traces. Output from the stimulator must be interfaced with the oscilloscope so that with each stimulus a trace is triggered across the face of the oscilloscope. Other set-ups can certainly be used and many have used (with the addition of electrodes that can be sterilized) one of the more recent model electromyographic machines, which are commercially available and which provide suitable stimulation and recording parameters. Frequency filters on the differential amplifiers are usually set at or below 3 Hz for the upper filter and 1 Hz for the lower filter. Amplification necessary to record NAPs will vary between 20 μV and 0.5 mV per division and the time frame for the trace is usually set somewhere between 0.5 and 2.0 ms per division. The duration of the stimuli used should be relatively brief (0.01 to 0.06 ms) since the distance between the stimulating and recording electrodes is relatively short. This produces a shock artifact that is high in amplitude because increased voltage is necessary to evoke a recordable response. Voltage necessary with such brief stimuli will range from 1 to 125 V. By using a brief shock, the stimulus artifact runoff is decreased so that the fast following NAP, if present, can be viewed with minimal interference. Ground is usually provided by a lead from the Bovie plate beneath the patient, which is plugged into one of the ground sites on the oscilloscope after turning off the Bovie machine.

The initial step in NAP recording is to attempt to record a potential proximal to the lesion. If the system is working properly, such a potential should be recordable from the proximal and thus more healthy portion of the nerve. Occasionally, stretch or lengthy contusion to the nerve may extend proximal to the more obvious lesion site and this will make it difficult to record a healthy proximal NAP. When exposing stretch injuries involving the roots of the brachial or pelvic plexus, it is also difficult to stimulate and record proximal to the lesion.[14] Usually, however, a good proximal potential can be recorded and then the recording electrodes are moved distally across the injury site and onto the distal stump to see if the NAP can be evoked through the injury (Fig. 231-4). Both the voltage and the amplification used may have to be increased to evoke and to record a small response across the lesion. The rate of stimulation is enough to produce consecutive but slow traces that can be viewed comfortably, usually 1 to 2 per second. A Polaroid camera is then used to make a more permanent record of a single trace.

If a potential is recorded immediately distal to the neuroma in continuity, the recording electrodes are moved farther down the distal stump to see how far the potential, and thus also regenerating axons of adequate size and structure, extend. It should be emphasized that with very high-fidelity instrumentation, summation of many responses, and espe-

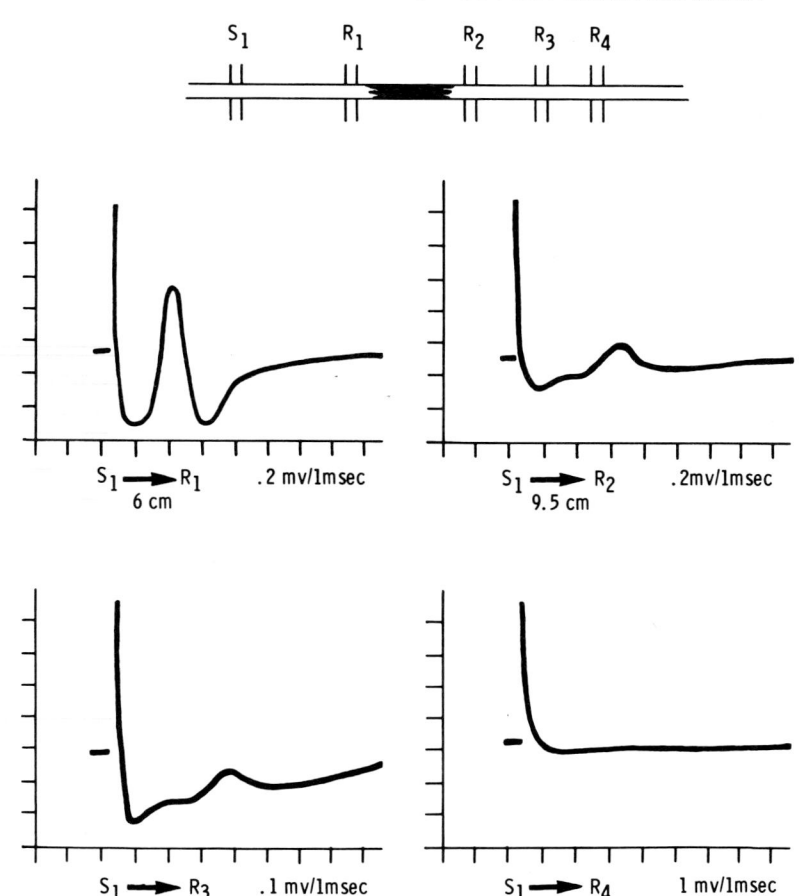

Figure 231-4 Nerve action potential (NAP) recordings from the ulnar nerve 3 months after an accidental injection injury. Early significant regeneration is documented since an NAP could be traced several centimeters distal to the injury site. As a result only an external neurolysis was done and the patient has subsequently made an acceptable recovery.

cially the integration provided by some computerized systems, intraoperative NAPs can be recorded from fine fibers within days to weeks after injury in a regenerating nerve. Such fibers may or may not eventually take on enough caliber and myelin to produce a functional result. Thus, if one is looking for evidence of functional regeneration it is better at this point in time to use a less sophisticated set-up. Studies available using the simpler set-up indicate that a recorded potential beyond the lesion correlates with a minimum of 2000 to 3000 axons at least 5 μm in diameter and with some early myelination.[12] This type of fiber population, particularly when documented at 6 to 10 weeks after injury, indicates a lesion in continuity that is undergoing satisfactory spontaneous regeneration. If an NAP cannot be recorded, this indicates a lesion that is not undergoing satisfactory regeneration and justifies resection and repair.[9] To date, in over 300 lesions in continuity in which resection has been done without the presence of NAPs across the injury and at 8 or more weeks after injury, histological study has proved a neurotmetic or Sunderland grade 4 picture and thus no possibility for useful recovery. On the other hand, 350 lesions in continuity have been found to have NAPs 8 or more weeks after injury, and more than 90 percent of the patients have had recovery in the distribution of that nerve to a functional grade of 3 or better.

When stimulation produces contraction of muscle either proximal or distal to the lesion in continuity, this can sometimes be recorded by the distal NAP electrodes. It should not be mistaken for an NAP, since such an NAP will have a longer latency, require less amplification, and generally have a more rounded peak than an NAP. If an NAP cannot be recorded distal to the injury, voltage and amplification are gradually increased until the portion of the trace after the stimulus artifact is difficult to visualize. Attention should be paid to electrode contact, and blood should be irrigated away from the region of the electrodes. Generally, the nerve should be elevated away from surrounding soft tissues by means of the hand-held electrodes, but if necessary the nerve can be stimulated and recordings made by isolating short segments on either side of the lesion in continuity, leaving the latter surrounded by soft tissue.

There are many instances in which fractional evaluation by NAP recording is helpful. Thus, if an NAP is recorded from a sciatic lesion in continuity, the latter should be split into its two divisions, tibial and peroneal, for one and not the other may be responsible for the NAP. If sciatic injury is close to but above its natural division into the tibial and peroneal nerves, then it can be evaluated by stimulating the whole sciatic nerve proximal to the lesion and recording from each of its outflows below. A similar approach can be used with most brachial plexus lesions. For example, lateral cord lesions can be evaluated by recording from the more distal musculocutaneous and median nerves and medial cord lesions can be evaluated by using recordings from the branch to the median as well as its larger input to the ulnar nerve. At a more proximal level of the plexus, roots are stimulated and recordings are made from divisions to cords or from the cords themselves (Fig. 231-5). A forearm level injury to the radial nerve can be evaluated by recording from both the superficial sensory and posterior interosseous branches. Such studies can lead to split repair of the lesion

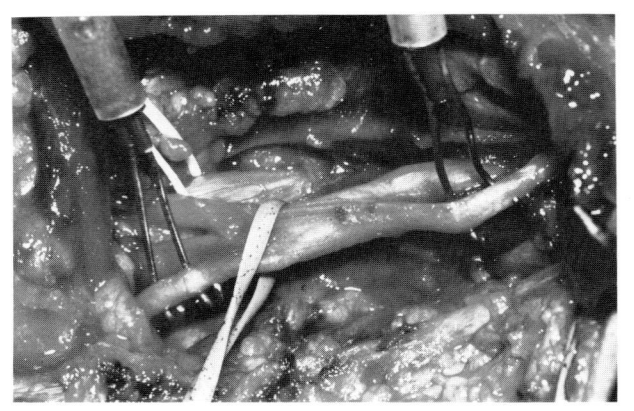

Figure 231-5 NAP recording from a brachial plexus lesion in continuity. (Photograph courtesy of Dr. Alan R. Hudson, Toronto.)

in continuity where a portion of the cross section of the lesion is maintained and a portion is split away and repaired. Williams and Terzis have described a variation on this theme in which the nerve is split into fascicles and fascicular recording is done; there are a few indications for this, particularly with wrist level lesions involving the median or ulnar nerve.[24]

If recording is done 6 or more months after injury and a potential through the lesion is found, its significance in terms of a reliable index of useful regeneration is less. This is particularly so if it cannot be traced well down the distal stump, if the amplification necessary to record it is high, and if it conducts at less than 20 m per second. Under these circumstances and depending on the clinical setting, the lesion may still need resection despite the presence of an NAP. Decision making once NAP recording has been done intraoperatively at an earlier time is more straightforward, for if no NAP is present across the lesion, resection is necessary. With the usual injury it should be present by 8 weeks if adequate regeneration is occurring. Stretch injuries are exceptions for such successful spontaneous regeneration may take up to 4 months. Thus, we currently delay exploration of such lesions in continuity for that period of time. In addition, nerves with partial injury will by definition have an NAP, and its presence does not mean that the injured portion is regenerating or will necessarily do so. In this case the injured portion can be split away from the noninjured or less injured portion and evaluated electrically in a separate fashion.

In summary, there are techniques available today to prove or disprove the presence of significant and potentially useful regeneration through a neuroma or lesion in continuity in the early weeks after injury. Use of such techniques at the operating table requires some experience and undoubtedly better and more readily achieved techniques will be developed in the future to evaluate lesions in continuity. Noninvasive or skin level stimulation and recording of NAPs has been developed and discussed elsewhere.[4,5,9] To date, there is an incidence of false-positive and -negative results (8 percent) not seen with intraoperative recording, and because of the disposition of many nerve injuries at proximal sites and very deep to the skin level, the noninvasive approach is not as applicable.[9]

References

1. Bowden REM: Electromyography, in Seddon HJ (ed): *Peripheral Nerve Injuries*. Medical Research Council Special Report Series No 282, London, Her Majesty's Stationery Office, 1954, pp 263–297.
2. Brown PW: Factors influencing the success of the surgical repair of peripheral nerves. Surg Clin North Am 52:1137–1155, 1972.
3. Clark K, Williams PE Jr, Willis W, McGavran WL III: Injection injury of the sciatic nerve. Clin Neurosurg 17:111–125, 1970.
4. Dawson GD: The relative excitability and conduction velocity of sensory and motor nerve fibers in man. J Physiol (Lond) 131:436–451, 1956.
5. Gilliatt RW, Sears TA: Sensory nerve action potentials in patients with periphral nerve lesions. J Neurol Neurosurg Psychiatry 21:109–118, 1958.
6. Grundfest H, Oester YT, Beebe GW: Electrical evidence of regeneration, in Woodhall B, Beebe GW (eds): *Peripheral Nerve Regeneration*. Washington, US Government Printing Office, 1956, pp 203–240.
7. Gutmann E, Young JZ: The re-innervation of muscle after various periods of atrophy. J Anat 78:15–43, 1944.
8. Hudson AR, Kline DG: Progression of partial injury to peripheral nerve. Part 2: Light and electron microscopic studies. J Neurosurg 42:15–22, 1975.
9. Kline DG: Evaluation of the neuroma in continuity, in Omer GE Jr, Spinner M (eds): *Management of Peripheral Nerve Problems*. Philadelphia, Saunders, 1980, pp 450–461.
10. Kline DG, Hackett ER: Reappraisal of timing for exploration of civilian peripheral nerve injuries. Surgery 78:54–65, 1975.
11. Kline DG, Hackett ER, Davis GD, Myers MB: Effect of mobilization on the blood supply and regeneration of injured nerves. J Surg Res 12:254–266, 1972.
12. Kline DG, Hackett ER, May PR: Evaluation of nerve injuries by evoked potentials and electromyography. J Neurosurg 31:128–136, 1969.
13. Kline DG, Hudson AR, Hackett ER, Bratton BR: Progression of partial injury to peripheral nerve. Part 1: Periodic measures of muscle contraction strength. J Neurosurg 42:1–14, 1975.
14. Kline DG, Judice DJ: Operative management of selected brachial plexus lesions. J Neurosurg 58:631–649, 1983.
15. Kline DG, Nulsen FE: The neuroma in continuity: Its preoperative and operative management. Surg Clin North Am 52:1189–1209, 1972.
16. Licht S (ed): *Electrodiagnosis and Electromyography*. New Haven, E Licht, Publisher, 1961.
17. Lundborg G: Structure and function of the intraneural microvessels as related to trauma, edema formation, and nerve function. J Bone Joint Surg [Am] 57A:938–948, 1975.
18. Nulsen FE, Kline DG: Acute injuries of peripheral nerves, in Youmans JR (ed): *Neurological Surgery*, 1st ed. Philadelphia, Saunders, 1973, pp 1089–1140.
19. Nulsen FE, Lewey FH: Intraneural bipolar stimulation: A new aid in the assessment of nerve injuries. Science 106:301–302, 1947.
20. Omer GE Jr, Spinner M: Peripheral nerve testing and suture techniques. Instr Course Lect 24:122–143, 1975.
21. Seddon HJ: *Surgical Disorders of the Peripheral Nerves*. Baltimore, Williams & Wilkins, 1972.
22. Sunderland S: *Nerves and Nerve Injuries*, 2d ed. Edinburgh, Churchill Livingstone, 1978.
23. White JC: Timing of nerve suture after a gunshot wound. Surgery 48:946–951, 1960.
24. Williams HB, Terzis JK: Single fascicular recordings: An intraoperative diagnostic tool for the management of peripheral nerve lesions. Plast Reconstr Surg 57:562–569, 1976.
25. Woodhall B, Nulsen FE, White JC, Davis L: Neurosurgical implications, in Woodhall B, Beebe GW (eds): *Peripheral Nerve Regeneration*. Washington, US Government Printing Office, 1956, pp 567–638.
26. Zachary RB, Roaf R: Lesions in continuity, in Seddon HJ (ed): *Peripheral Nerve Injuries*. Medical Research Council Special Report Series 282, London, Her Majesty's Stationery Office, 1954, pp 57–81.

232
Techniques of Nerve Repair
John E. McGillicuddy

Few subjects have produced as much debate and produced as few clear-cut conclusions as the proper method of repairing divided peripheral nerves. A wide variety of repair techniques and schemes for the timing of repair have been proposed, none of them universally accepted. The principal reason for this controversy is the number of factors that bear upon the successful outcome of peripheral nerve suture.

Those variables that significantly affect the end result of nerve repair have been enumerated by Sunderland.[24] They include the specific nerve injured, the level of the injury, the severity and extent of the injury, the severity of associated local tissue injury, the age of the patient, and the response of the cellular elements of the nerve to injury. These factors are already determined at the time of injury and cannot be changed by intervention. Two aspects of outcome are under the control of the surgeon: the timing of repair and the technique of repair. While manipulation of these two aspects has some effect on the end result, any assessment of their importance must be considered in the light of all the factors involved. To isolate one variable such as the technique of repair and causally relate it to the quality of recovery is to greatly oversimplify the situation.

Three fundamental concepts should be remembered in

any consideration of nerve repair; these include the intricate internal anatomy of nerve trunks, the unique nature of axon regrowth and reinnervation, and the reaction of neural connective tissue to injury. These have been discussed in detail in other chapters and only a brief review of pertinent points will be considered here.

The internal anatomy of the nerve is not homogeneous but is made up of varying combinations of axons and connective tissue. The latter may account for 20 to 60 percent of the cross-sectional area of a nerve trunk.[25] The axons are gathered and enclosed within sheaths of perineurium, forming fascicles (Fig. 232-1). Each fascicle, containing up to 10,000 axons, pursues an irregular course along the nerve trunk, changing its position within the nerve and engaging in plexus formation with other fascicles by interconnecting branches[24] (Fig. 232-2). Because of this plexiform arrangement the cross-sectional appearance of a nerve may be quite different at levels only a few millimeters apart. Motor and sensory axons are scattered diffusely within the fascicles in the proximal nerve, becoming segregated into functionally related motor and sensory fascicles as they progress distally (Fig. 232-3). This internal heterogeneity makes a perfect matching of identical fascicles theoretically possible but practically unattainable in nerve repair.

The very nature of peripheral nerves demands a complex reparative process after nerve division. Regenerating axons from the proximal stump must cross the anastomosis and find their way down the endoneurial tubes of the distal nerve to reach their appropriate end organs—sensory receptors or motor end plates. Clinical recovery will result only if axons grow down the proper endoneurial tube; a motor axon must grow down an endoneurial tube that terminates in a muscle. Axons advancing down inappropriate endoneurial tubes or advancing into the connective tissue of the distal nerve end will be wasted. Only a perfect pairing of every axon with its original endoneurial tube in the distal nerve end could result in total restoration of function—a theoretical ideal that will never be achieved.

The responses of the connective tissue of an injured nerve will also have a major effect on the results of nerve suture. The proliferation of intraneural connective tissue is as important a determinant of successful nerve repair as the better known processes of axon regeneration and wallerian degeneration. The amount of connective tissue formed is roughly proportional to the severity of the initial injury. Scars form at both the proximal and distal nerve ends. Connective tissue will also increase in response to rough handling at surgery or to excessive tension at the suture line.[14] In all cases this overgrowth of connective tissue can effectively block or distort the path of regenerating axons.

The basic goal of nerve repair is to provide, within the limits of those variables mentioned above, the optimum conditions for the passage of regenerating axons from the proximal nerve end to their appropriate destinations in the distal nerve with the least wasting of axons and with minimal scar formation. The technique that most closely approaches this ideal will be the most effective. The favored technique may very well be different in different clinical situations.

History

The repair of peripheral nerves has had a long and erratic history. Arabic physicians in the ninth and tenth centuries were likely the first to attempt union of divided nerves by suture. In the subsequent development of western medicine during the Middle Ages, the technique was largely ignored and attempts at nerve repair were extremely rare. Until the middle of the nineteenth century it was widely believed that nerves would regenerate spontaneously and that manipulation and suture would cause "convulsions" or at least impede the return of function.

The work of Waller and others in the middle years of the last century demonstrated the breakdown of axons and myelin sheaths in the distal segment of a divided nerve (wallerian degeneration) and the outgrowth of axons from the proximal end. Surgeons were thereby stimulated to attempt the repair of divided nerves. Hueter in 1873 described repair of nerves by sutures placed in the epineurial sheath. This technique, with some refinements, was the standard method of nerve repair until very recently. The results of nerve suture in those early years were discouraging. Infection was a frequent cause of suture line disruption, damaged tissue was inadequately resected, and nerve ends were often sutured under excessive tension.

The importance of resection of damaged nerves and the necessity of end-to-end contact without tension became rec-

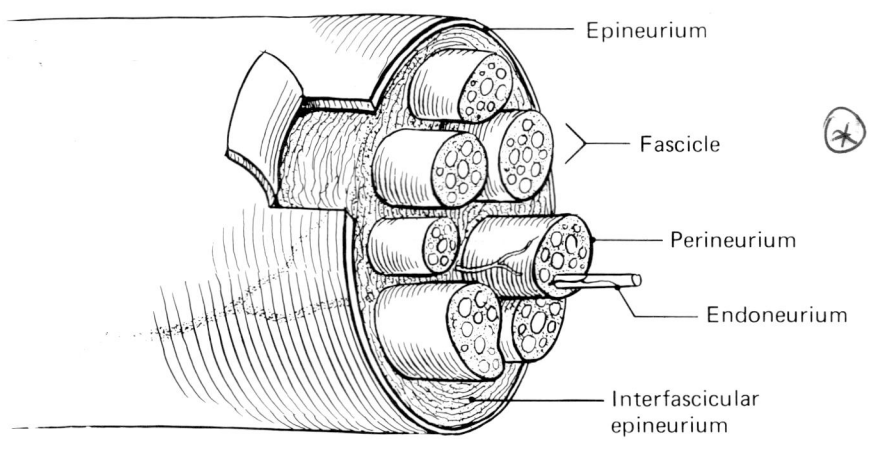

Figure 232-1 The surgical anatomy of a peripheral nerve. The axons are surrounded by sheaths of endoneurium and are gathered into fascicles each surrounded by a sleeve of perineurium. The space between the fascicles is filled with connective tissue, the interfascicular epineurium. The sheath of epineurium surrounding the nerve trunk is readily separated, as shown, from the fascicles and intrafascicular epineurium.

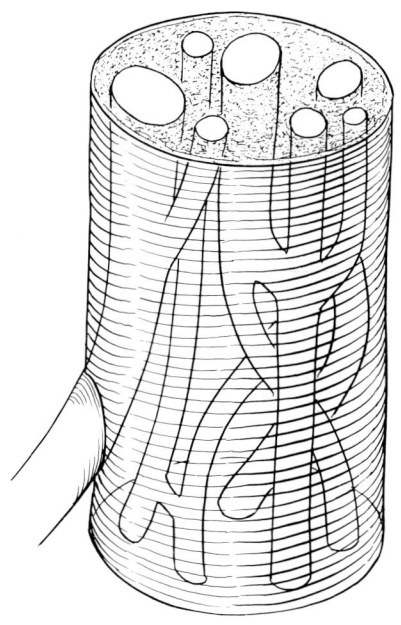

Figure 232-2 Schematic view of funicular topography. The funiculi are interconnected by small branches, forming a funicular plexus. The funiculi alter their position within the nerve, occupying different quadrants of the nerve at different levels. A funiculus is seen on the left leaving the nerve as a branch.

ognized during World War I.[21] Adherence to these principles led to vigorous attempts to close nerve gaps caused by destruction or resection. Lengthy nerve mobilization, transposition, and bone shortening were widely used but the most common technique involved flexion of adjacent joints to shorten the course of the nerve. After an interval to allow for healing of the nerve suture, the joints were slowly extended to "stretch" the nerve to its original length. Gaps of up to 18 cm could be closed in this manner. Nerve grafts, first used by Foerster in 1916, were rarely used and rarely successful. The use of grafts was considered only when all other methods of closing a nerve gap had failed.[18]

During World War II it quickly became apparent that end-to-end repair with marked joint flexion did not result in acceptable recovery. Highet and Sanders showed that postoperative stretching of a healed sutured nerve caused massive intraneural fibrosis and axonal disruption.[8] They also demonstrated that permanent elongation of the nerve did not take place; each extension of the joint caused a new, probably cumulative, neural traction injury.

In response to these findings, Seddon and his group at Oxford began to use interposed nerve grafts to fill large nerve gaps.[21] Both cutaneous nerves and major nerve trunks such as the ulnar were used. Good results were obtained both in war wounds and in civilian nerve injuries.[20] Nonetheless, nerve grafting was still considered to be a last resort.[24]

In 1964 Edshage found that the neat external appearance of the common epineurial repair often concealed very poor apposition of the fascicles.[6] Fascicles were buckled or failed to make contact and the gap filled with connective tissue. Careful perpendicular transection of the nerve ends was only a partially successful remedy.

The possibility that nerve fascicles could be aligned and sutured individually by sutures placed in the perineurium had been suggested as early as 1917[12] and was again put forward by Sunderland in 1953 as a development of his studies on the internal fascicular topography of nerves.[23] Such a repair was nearly impossible with the techniques available at the time. In 1964 Smith introduced the operating microscope into peripheral nerve surgery.[22] Fascicles could now be identified and isolated and sutures could be placed in the perineurium. Bora in 1967 performed fascicle-to-fascicle anastomosis in the cat and claimed an improved clinical recovery resulted.[1] The theoretical advantage of fascicular repair—a more anatomical alignment of fascicles—was quickly realized. However, the delicate perineurial repair could not be accomplished if there was tension at the anastomosis.

In the late 1960s Millesi demonstrated that connective tissue proliferation at a nerve anastomosis was derived from the epineurium and that the degree of proliferation was directly related to the amount of tension on the nerve repair.[14] To circumvent this problem he advocated the use of nerve grafts. Cutaneous nerves were used to fill the nerve gaps, each nerve graft being apposed to corresponding fascicles or fascicle groups at the nerve ends and sutured to them without tension. The results of this interfascicular nerve grafting technique were claimed to be better than those of epineurial or fascicular repairs done under tension.[14,15]

The development of techniques for nerve repair has thus resulted in three basic types of neurorrhaphy: epineurial

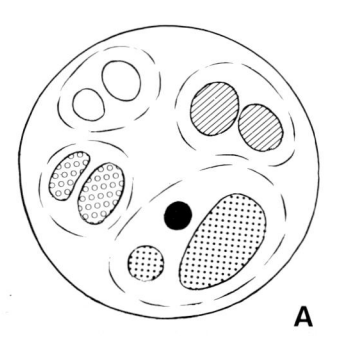

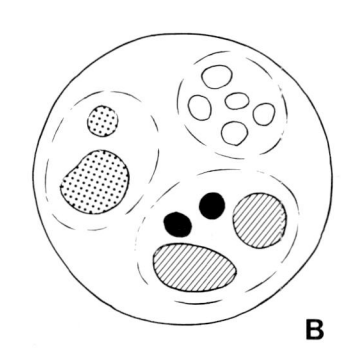

Figure 232-3 Schematic cross sections, about 1 cm apart, through a hypothetical nerve. *A* is the proximal cross section, *B* is the distal. The fascicles are separated into groups by condensation of the interfascicular epineurium (interrupted lines). One fascicle group has left the nerve as a branch between these two levels. The migration of related fascicle groups from one quadrant to another is exaggerated for emphasis, as is the change in number and location of the fascicles within a fascicle group.

anastomosis, perineurial or fascicular anastomosis, and interfascicular nerve grafting. Each repair has its advocates and its advantages but no one type appears superior in all situations. The common denominator in this diversity has been the increasing use of magnification in nerve repair. This modality has provided a better view of the internal structure of nerve trunks, led to a more accurate apposition of fascicles, and resulted in improved outcomes for all types of nerve repair.

Timing of Nerve Repair

The proper time at which to repair a severed peripheral nerve has been the subject of considerable debate. Some authors have advocated immediate repair; others prefer to delay repair for up to 3 weeks after injury.[5,7,9,11,13,20,24] The previous strong tendency to favor secondary repair was derived in large part from experiences with wartime injuries. These injuries were often associated with major soft tissue destruction, contamination, and ragged, contused nerve lacerations. Under such circumstances a delay to allow proper wound healing and to deal with infection was understandable. The vast majority of civilian nerve lacerations are clean cuts due to glass or sharp knife injuries and involve relatively little soft tissue damage.[4,20,24] The difference in injury pattern considerably alters the rationale for timing of nerve repair. In sharp, clean lacerations, good results may follow either immediate or early secondary repair. The choice of time of repair will depend upon the severity of the nerve transection, as indicated by contusion, shredding or hematoma at the nerve ends, the longitudinal extent of injured nerve beyond the ends, and the degree of local tissue damage and contamination. When one or more of these conditions is present, delayed repair is indicated.[9]

A major advantage of delayed or secondary repair is that it allows the injured nerve segment to demarcate. Exact location of reactive intraneural fibrosis can thus be established and the nerve resected back to healthy, pouting fascicles. Delay also allows an emergency procedure to become an elective one performed under optimum conditions. There are also some theoretical conditions favoring delayed repair. The metabolic activity of the central neuronal cell body is at its peak 2 to 3 weeks after injury and axonal regeneration across the nerve repair should then be most rapid.[5] These apparent advantages are offset by a progressive decrease in the diameter of the endoneurial tubules and fascicles of the distal stump, which will limit penetration and maturation of the regenerating axons. The disadvantages of delayed repair include the necessity for a second operation and the permanent fibrous shortening of the retracted nerve ends. If end-to-end repair is desired, nerve mobilization or transposition will then be required. Although mobilization has not been shown to have major ill effects on a nerve, it is best to limit dissection and possible interruption of the vascular supply.[10] Those surgeons favoring nerve grafting have less reservations about delayed repair.

If the nerve injury is sharp, clean, and less than 24 h old, primary repair should be considered. Primary repair has the advantage of an operation performed in normal anatomy without scar tissue. The ends of a sharp division will have retracted only minimally and can be brought together without mobilization and with only slight tension. Primary repair has two apparent biological advantages as well: it brings about the earliest axon crossing of the anastomosis and the axons can enter normal-sized endoneurial tubes. Grabb has demonstrated experimentally that primary repair gives better results than delayed repair of identical injuries.[7] The principal disadvantage of immediate repair is the difficulty in evaluating the degree to which the two nerve stumps have been damaged. A primary repair of contused stumps will result in major scar formation at the anastomosis.

If the conditions for primary repair are met, it should be strongly considered in lesions of the brachial plexus and proximal sciatic nerve.[11] In these areas retracted nerve ends cannot later be brought together readily by either mobilization or positioning of adjacent joints. In addition, the great distance from the lesion to the peripheral end organs demands the earliest possible repair if any degree of effective reinnervation is to occur. Primary repair is also strongly advised in very distal lesions. Here the segregation into motor and sensory fascicles allows identification of fascicle type by electrical stimulation of the proximal and distal fascicles.[4] Distal muscle contraction on stimulation identifies the motor fascicles in the distal stump. With the patient awake, a sensory response to stimulation of proximal stump fascicles can localize the sensory fascicles. This technique, which effects a more accurate pairing of corresponding fascicles, can only be utilized in the first 72 h after injury, before wallerian degeneration begins.

In many instances, especially in combined neural and vascular injury, it may be advisable to explore the nerve acutely. If the clinical conditions appropriate for primary repair are present, there is no reason to avoid it. If the nerve is ragged or contused, the ends should be tacked to local tissue under slight tension to minimize retraction of the stumps and repair should be made after the wound has healed. This discussion has considered only the treatment of a nerve that is known to have been severed. The waiting period necessary to rule out spontaneous recovery and the intraoperative assessment of a lesion in continuity is discussed in another chapter.

Repair Techniques

Epineurial Repair

Epineurial repair, the standard method of nerve repair for many years, still has a prominent place in nerve injuries today. The technique of epineurial repair is the least complicated of present methods but magnification and careful attention to detail are nonetheless required. The standard epineurial repair is performed in the following manner. The nerve stumps are identified in an atraumatic fashion by dissecting tissue away from the nerve. In a secondary repair, the nerve is identified in an uninvolved area and uncovered toward the injured nerve end. Preparation of the nerve ends is the most important step in epineurial repair. The nerve must be transected perpendicular to its axis so that a uni-

Techniques of Nerve Repair

form flush surface is produced. This is best accomplished by snugly wrapping the nerve end in a thin film of polyethylene or paper secured along one side of the nerve with a hemostat. The soft, deformable nerve is thereby given a firmer substance. Before trimming the nerve ends, two marking sutures may be placed 180 degrees apart and 1 to 2 cm back from the nerve ends to help align the ends during repair.[4] The pattern of the epineurial vessels may also be used to align the nerve. The two nerve ends are then brought together with a minimum of tension. Some limited mobilization may be required. The epineurial edge is grasped with jeweler's forceps and slightly everted. The surgeon places two sutures of 8-0 nylon 180 degrees apart, taking a full thickness of epineurium but avoiding the underlying fascicles (Fig. 232-4). The sutures are tied carefully so that the flush faces barely touch; they may be left long to aid in rotating the nerve. Two or three sutures of 9-0 or 10-0 nylon are then placed through the epineurium of both the anterior and the posterior surface of the repair. The ends are brought together gently, as excess tightness will distort and buckle the fascicles.

Upon completion of the repair, the marking sutures are removed. After wound closure, the limb is splinted for 3 to 4 weeks. If any joint flexion was required, the joint is slowly extended at 10 to 15 degrees per week after the splint is removed. The repair is best done with magnification to inspect and align the fascicular pattern of the cut faces and to monitor suture placement. The operating microscope is ideal although magnifying loupes are quite adequate. We have not found a tourniquet necessary and bleeding is controlled by bipolar coagulation and gentle pressure.

Fascicular Repair

The microsurgical repair of the internal components of a nerve has been given a confusing variety of names—perineurial repair, funicular repair, fascicular repair, group fascicular repair, and bundle repair. There are in reality but two types of end-to-end microrepair. In *fascicular* repair individual fascicles are connected with sutures in the perineurium. In the more common *group fascicular* or *bundle* repair, groups of contiguous fascicles are matched. In this type of repair the sutures are placed in the interfascicular epineurium, a condensation of intraneural connective tissue that separates groups of fascicles from one another (Figs. 232-1, 232-3). Both techniques are designed to provide optimal anatomical alignment of the fascicles at the nerve ends.

Fascicular suture, most useful in nerves with a few large fascicles, requires high magnification and microinstruments. After the nerve ends have been isolated, they are prepared by incising the superficial epineurial sheath and excising it circumferentially for a few millimeters back from the nerve end with a sharp microscissors and jeweler's forceps (Fig. 232-5). Each fascicle is carefully dissected free of its surrounding connective tissue. This dissection can only be performed in normal nerve; fibrotic nerve ends must be excised back to pouting fascicles. It may at times be preferable to begin epineurial resection and internal dissection in normal nerve and advance toward the nerve end. Only a few millimeters of fascicle length need be exposed; excessive dis-

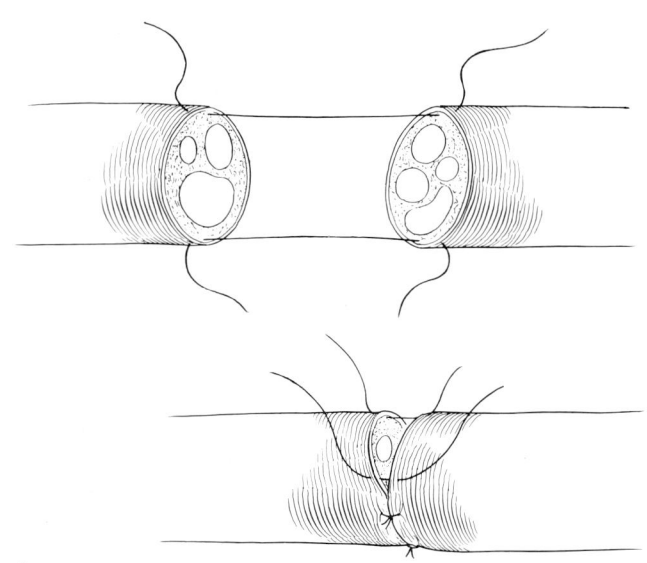

Figure 232-4 Epineurial repair. Two guide sutures 180 degrees apart have been placed in the upper drawing. These serve to maintain the original axial alignment between the two nerve ends. Two or three epineurial sutures are placed in each half of the circumference to complete the repair.

section results in increased intraneural scar and may also divide interfascicular crossing fibers. Proximal and distal fascicles are then matched according to size and location. A sketch of the components of each stump may be helpful here.[13] Each fascicle pair is then joined lightly end to end

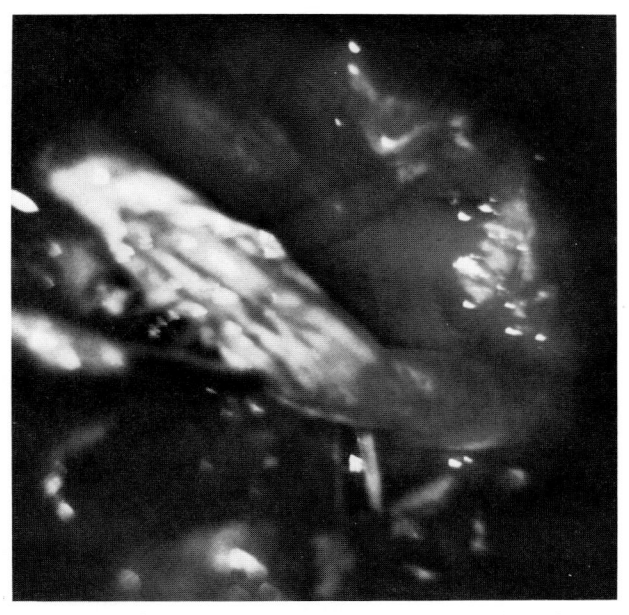

Figure 232-5 In this view through the operating microscope, the fasciculi of the radial nerve are seen after removal of the epineurial sheath. A few interconnecting fascicle branches can be seen.

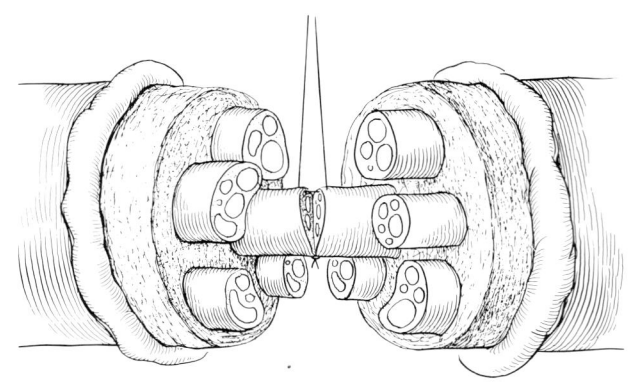

Figure 232-6 Group fascicular repair. The epineurial sheath has been resected back from the nerve ends and short lengths of the fascicular groups are isolated from the intraneural connective tissue. Sutures are placed through the condensed intrafascicular epineurium surrounding the groups. A similar technique is used to join individual fascicles by sutures placed through the perineurium.

with one or two sutures of 10-0 or 11-0 nylon (Fig. 232-6). If heavier suture is required, there is too much tension and grafting should be considered. A 50-μm needle (Ethicon BV50-3, Ethicon, Inc., Somerville, N.J.; Davis and Geck TE50, American Cyanamid Co., Wayne, N.J.) is best for this repair; a full thickness bite of perineurium with minimal penetration into fascicular contents is desired. The soft fascicular contents often protrude from the perineurial cuff and should be trimmed flush with the perineurium prior to suturing.

The technique of group fascicular repair is very similar. The epineurial sheath is incised and resected as described. Again, this dissection can only be carried out in normal nerve. Intraneural dissection separates groups of fascicles surrounded by interfascicular epineurium. The arrangement in groups may be more clearly seen if dissection is begun at the nerve face. After the groups and any large single fascicles are dissected out, they are paired by size and location. The corresponding bundles are joined by two sutures of 10-0 nylon through the interfascicular epineurium (Fig. 232-6). A 75-μm needle (Ethicon BV75-3 or Davis and Geck TE70) is preferable for this repair, done in firmer connective tissue. The groups should just lightly touch one another when the knot is tied. Tension at the anastomosis indicates the need for nerve grafting.

Both repairs require fine-tip (no. 5) jeweler's forceps for grasping the perineurium or interfascicular epineurium and everting it during needle penetration. A spring-loaded needle holder may be used; we prefer a wide-tip (no. 2) jeweler's forceps. A chip of razor blade in a blade holder and a sharp-pointed dissector are best for the intraneural separation of fascicles and groups. Any bleeding is handled by bipolar coagulation with fine-tip forceps or by light pressure on a cotton patty. Repairs are done under 10X to 16X magnification. A tourniquet is not required. After both types of repair the limb is placed in a splint for 2 weeks. Active and passive limb movement is begun after splint removal.

Closure of Nerve Gaps

When a nerve is transected by any means, a nerve gap is created. Even a clean, sharp division of a nerve produces an immediate gap of about 1 to 2 cm as the nerve stumps retract because of their inherent elasticity.[4] Although these stumps can initially be apposed with minimum tension, reactive intraneural fibrosis will eventually decrease their elasticity and the stumps will become permanently shortened. A fixed nerve gap is thus created and additional maneuvers will be required to bring the ends together. In more severe trauma, nerve segments may be avulsed and the longitudinal extent of intraneural scarring increased. Excision of the scarred nerve ends at operation will further lengthen the nerve gap. A tension-free anastomosis can only be created by increasing the relative lengths of the proximal and distal nerves or by decreasing the distance they must travel.[19]

Relative length of a nerve can be increased by stretching the nerve or by mobilizing or transposing it. Stretching the nerve is the simplest but least useful of these maneuvers. It is chiefly employed to bring together fresh, clean transections in primary repair, overcoming the natural elasticity that has caused the gap. A force of only 6 to 10 g is required to accomplish this, providing a nerve repair under only slight tension.[13] The elasticity of a nerve trunk allows an increase of about 6 percent of its free length by stretching.[20] Beyond this limit, internal disruption of the nerve occurs. Even before a nerve has been stretched to this degree, significant force is required to maintain its increased length, leading to considerable tension at the repair site.

Mobilizing a nerve by dissecting it free from its filmy connections to surrounding tissue can increase its length by taking up the slack naturally occurring along its course.[24] Mobilization is limited by the motor branches of a nerve, which tether it to the muscles along its course. Thus the technique is best used in those areas where there are relatively few motor branches, as in the median and ulnar nerves in the upper arm. Mobilizing a nerve separates it from its collateral vascular supply and may cause some degree of ischemia. Although the longitudinal epineurial vessels are usually able to provide adequate blood supply, mobilization should be limited to about 6 to 8 cm of dissection along the nerve.[10] If a nerve is mobilized in an area of motor branching, the segment of nerve distal to the branches should be mobilized. Dissection of the branches back into the nerve trunk by an intraneural separation will provide extra length to the branches, allowing the main trunk to be advanced distally.[19] An increase of 2 to 4 cm in nerve length can be provided by mobilization. This technique can be used to varying degrees on any nerve in any location.

In contrast, transposition or rerouting has more limited applications. With this method the nerve is effectively lengthened by moving it to a new location so as to give it a straighter course. The ulnar nerve, for example, may be transposed anterior to the medial epicondyle to facilitate the closure of a nerve gap at or distal to the elbow. Ulnar transposition has the additional advantage of placing the nerve on the flexor rather than the extensor surface of the elbow joint so that elbow flexion may further narrow the nerve gap. Ulnar transposition alone can add 3 to 5 cm to the effective length of the nerve. The median nerve can be transposed anterior to the pronator teres, adding up to 2 cm to its length.[19] This may be helpful in median nerve repairs in the antecubital fossa. The radial nerve may also be replaced anterior to the humerus between the biceps and the brachialis when the nerve is lacerated by a humeral fracture in the spiral groove. This transposition allows repair to be performed in a clean bed away from callus formation and increases the nerve length by about 3 cm. The relatively straight course of the other peripheral nerves precludes their transposition.

Nerve gaps may also be closed by positioning adjacent joints in such a way as to shorten the course of the nerve along the limb. In nearly all cases this implies placing the joints in flexion. Joint flexion will bring the nerve ends together and provide a tension-free repair only as long as the flexion is maintained.[8,18] When the joint is extended, traction will be placed on the repair and on the nerve itself. The amount of tension that will occur can be decreased by limiting the amount of flexion and by extending the joint gradually. Flexion of the knee and elbow should be limited to 90 degrees and flexion of the wrist to 40 degrees.[20] Following healing of the suture line, a flexed joint should be extended at no more than 10 degrees per week. Nevertheless, the use of joint flexion to close a nerve gap ensures that some degree of tension will eventually be placed on the repair. This degree of tension may be sufficient to cause a neural stretch injury, with resultant intraneural fibrosis and a poor outcome.[8] If more than minimal flexion is required to close a nerve gap, it is advisable to abandon attempts to secure end-to-end repair; a nerve graft should be used instead.

Bone resection and shortening to secure closure of a nerve gap is only rarely indicated. Its use is best limited to those occasions when extensive compound fracture or nonunion of the humerus requires open repair and some degree of bone loss is inevitable.[24] Under these circumstances, resection of 5 or 6 cm of humerus may be acceptable to close gaps in the nerves of the arm if mobilization and anterior transposition cannot do so. Resection of normal intact bone to close a nerve gap can no longer be considered allowable. Bone resection in the forearm and in the lower extremities should not be contemplated. It is difficult to conceive that bone shortening can be preferred over nerve grafting, and its use should probably be abandoned.

Before undertaking any major procedure to effect closure of a nerve gap, the likelihood of bringing about end-to-end union must be assessed. Seddon has stated that nerve gaps of greater than 5 to 7 cm cannot be closed by end-to-end union without seriously prejudicing the chances for recovery.[21] This critical gap length is approximately equal to the degree of nerve lengthening that can be brought about by vigorous mobilization and nerve transposition. If the nerve gap seen at secondary repair exceeds 7 cm, it is best to abandon attempts at end-to-end closure and resort to nerve grafting.

Nerve Grafts

Nerve grafting to fill nerve gaps has become increasingly common in the last decade and the poor reputation that nerve grafts have held in the past has largely been erased. This reputation was in fact undeserved; the early failures of nerve grafts were generally due to their employment in marginal situations when all other methods to close large nerve defects had failed. The circumstances of their use, not the grafts themselves, were responsible for the high failure rate.

The experimental studies and favorable clinical series of Millesi and Samii, among others, have been largely responsible for the current change in attitude toward nerve grafts.[13-15,18] Recent success with this modality is based on an understanding of the biological prerequisites of successful nerve grafting outlined in their studies. The ideal nerve graft must cover the cross-sectional area of the nerve trunk and must survive intact. Thin cutaneous nerves survive well but cannot alone match the area of a major nerve end. Grafts using segments of major nerves cover the cross-sectional area but often undergo central necrosis and fibrosis. A nerve graft is a devitalized tissue; in order to survive and undergo wallerian degeneration, an active metabolic process, it must be revascularized. Initially its nourishment is provided by diffusion from the tissues of its bed. After 1 week the ingrowth of vessels from the nerve ends, and especially from the bed, will supply its needs.[4] The thicker the graft, the less likely that its central axis will be adequately supplied before avascular necrosis and fibrosis occur there. The critical diameter for success appears to be less than 2 to 5 mm.[18] While the metabolic and area requirements can be partially met by assembling a bundle or cable of individual thin nerves, anastomosis of this group to the nerve ends is technically quite difficult and the fascicular matching is poor.[21]

Reluctance to use nerve grafts has also been based on the difficulties posed by the need for regenerating axons to cross two suture lines to reach the distal stump. Recent studies have shown, however, that axons cross two tension-free anastomoses better than one anastomosis performed under moderate to marked tension.[13-15,18,26] This favorable result is due to the elimination of tension at the graft anastomoses; tension results in increased connective tissue proliferation at the suture line, with consequent impairment or obstruction of axonal regrowth. This advantage of tension-free repair appears sufficient to overcome the disadvantage of two suture lines.

The increased acceptance of nerve grafting has also been spurred by major refinements in technique. Interfascicular nerve grafting, introduced by Millesi, apposes small-diameter cutaneous nerve grafts to individual fascicles and fascicle groups at the nerve ends.[4,13] The problems of difference in cross-sectional area, of fascicular apposition, and of adequate graft revascularization are thus largely eliminated. This technique requires the use of the operating microscope. The nerve ends are readied for grafting by initially resecting the epineurial sheath circumferentially back along the stumps for about 5 to 10 mm. Resection can only be performed in normal nerve. It may be started at the fresh normal nerve end after resection of the fibrous end bulb or it can be started in the normal nerve beyond the scar and advanced toward the nerve end. Resection of the epineurium removes the presumed major source of connective tissue proliferation from the area of the suture line and also allows intraneural dissection among the fascicles and fascicle groups.

After epineurial resection, the ends of the fascicles and the fascicle groups are separated from one another as previously described. Fascicle groups are generally clearly distinguishable and are contained in a recognizable sheath of condensed interfascicular epineurium (Fig. 232-3). The isolated fascicle groups at each nerve end are then paired by size. A sketch of the configuration of fascicle groups at each end is a great aid in this process. Once the fascicle groups have been paired, cutaneous nerve grafts are inserted between each pair and are sutured in place (Fig. 232-7). The grafts should be cut about 15 percent longer than the nerve gap to allow for shrinkage of the grafts. Millesi advocates transecting the fascicle groups at different lengths so that the suture lines are not all at the same level. This results in interdigitation of the grafts; the suture lines are bounded laterally by protruding fascicle groups or by graft segments. This technique gives a measure of lateral stability to the repair and disperses the mass of suture material. The grafts are sutured with one or two stitches of 10-0 nylon at each end of the graft. A 75-μm needle is preferred. The interfascicular epineurium surrounding a fascicle group is grasped with fine-tip forceps, and a full thickness bite of tissue, avoiding the fascicles, is taken. The suture is then passed through the epineurium of the graft. When the suture is tied, the graft should just touch the fascicular group without any tension. The full cross-sectional area of the fascicle group should be covered by the graft. Millesi and Samii believe that one suture at each end of the graft is sufficient. The grafts are largely stuck to the nerve ends by natural fibrin clotting. In our experience, two sutures at each end give better apposition.

The number of grafts required will vary with the nerve involved but generally four to six grafts are required for the ulnar, radial, and median nerves. In some cases, clearly defined fascicular groups are absent or the nerve may be composed of only a few large fascicles. The graft anastomoses will have to be modified accordingly.[13] In nerves with a few large fascicles, more than one graft may be apposed to each fascicle (Fig. 232-8A). In nerves with many fascicles but without group arrangement, the nerve face is arbitrarily divided into approximately equal sectors and one graft is sutured to the face of each sector (Fig. 232-8C). No attempt is made to dissect out the fascicles in this latter repair. After the grafts have been placed and the wound closed, the limb is splinted in place and the splint is left on for 10 days. Following removal of the splint, active and passive motion of the limb may be begun at 2 weeks.

The sural nerve is the most common donor nerve. It furnishes a long graft (20 to 30 cm) with little resultant neurological deficit. The nerve may be exposed in the subcutaneous tissue posterior to the lateral malleolus at the ankle by a horizontal incision. The nerve is posterior to the lesser saphenous vein, with which it may be easily confused. After dividing the nerve, gentle traction on its proximal end will allow its subcutaneous course along the posterior calf to be palpated. The nerve is easily removed through a series of horizontal incisions along its course, pulling the distal nerve out through each incision. After removal of loose connective tissue and fat, the sural nerve is ready for grafting. Other acceptable graft donors are the superficial radial nerve, the medial or lateral cutaneous nerve of the forearm, the lateral cutaneous nerve of the femur, and the medial cutaneous nerve of the arm.

The principal indication for nerve grafting is the presence of a nerve gap. The length of the gap requiring a nerve graft is a subject of debate. While most peripheral nerve surgeons would agree that a gap of 4 to 6 cm or more requires a nerve graft for repair, Millesi states that any gap of greater than 2 cm requires unacceptable tension for end-to-end closure and should be grafted.[13]

Interfascicular nerve grafting is nearly always performed as a delayed procedure. It is neither necessary nor helpful in the repair of acute clean transections. The wound must be clean, the soft tissues healthy and well vascularized, and fibrotic nerve ends cleanly resected before this technique can be used successfully.

Comparison of Results

Attempts to compare the various techniques of nerve repair in terms of their end results are complicated by the effects of other factors that, regardless of the method of repair, have a major influence on the outcome. The most important of these factors are the nerve injured, the level of injury, the age of the patient, and the interval between injury and repair. Results will generally be better in relatively pure motor or sensory nerves (radial nerve, median nerve at the wrist) than in mixed nerves (ulnar nerve in the forearm) and better in distal lesions than in proximal ones. Nerve repairs in children yield much better results than those in adults. Nerve repairs done within 6 months of injury have a better outcome than those done later.[20,24] The numerous clinical series reported have included consideration of these factors to varying degrees. Some series that have categorized injuries by nerve, location, and age of patient have relatively few cases of each type; those series considering only overall success rates may not adequately reflect the effects of the non-surgical variables. The absence of a uniform method of grading the degree of motor and sensory recovery makes comparisons among the reports quite difficult. Finally, no

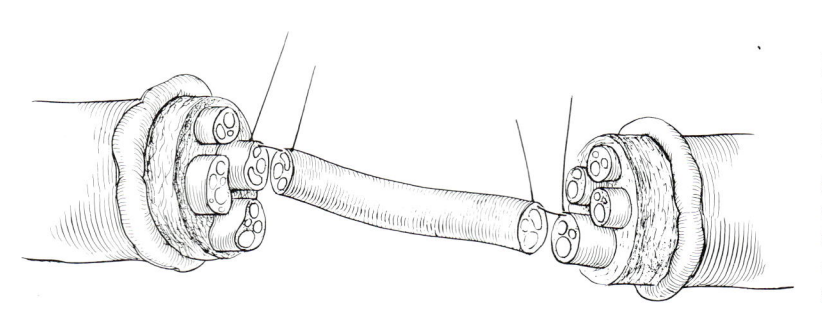

Figure 232-7 Interfascicular nerve graft. A segment of sural nerve is sutured to a fascicle group at each nerve end. Every attempt must be made to match corresponding fascicle groups from each nerve end. Grafts are then sutured serially to each pair of groups. Grafting between matched pairs provides the closest possible approximation to the original anatomical continuity.

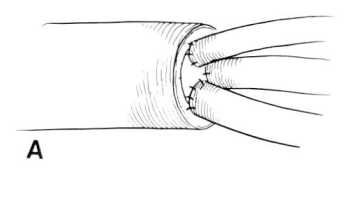

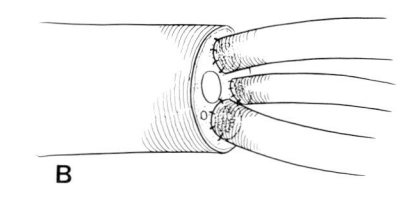

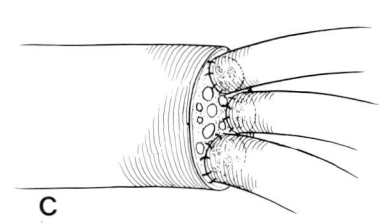

Figure 232-8 Interfascicular nerve graft techniques in relation to the fascicular anatomy of the nerve end. *A.* Fascicles are large and few in number. Two or three sural nerve grafts may be needed to cover one large fascicle. *B.* Many fascicles are arranged in groups. One sural nerve is sutured to each fascicle group. *C.* Many fascicles are present, without a group arrangement. The nerve end is arbitrarily divided into sectors and a single graft is used to cover each sector. (After Millesi.[13])

true comparative prospective study has been done as each author has presented results obtained by a favored technique rather than comparing results obtained by different methods.

Seddon has shown return of useful function in 67 percent of his series of epineurial repairs of the median and ulnar nerves.[20] Useful function returned in more than 80 percent of repairs when the injury was at the level of the wrist. Kline and Hackett had similar success with epineurial repair; more than 70 percent of their repairs resulted in useful improvement.[9] Millesi et al. have reported equally good results with interfascicular nerve grafts.[14,15] They claim substantial improvement in 85 percent of their patients with grafts. Samii, also using interfascicular nerve grafts, has had substantial improvement in 90 percent of his repairs.[18] In all these reports the percentage of good results was different depending on the nerve involved. There were also significant differences between the degree of motor and sensory return in each type of nerve injury. In view of the substantial difficulties involved in comparing these results, only one conclusion

can be drawn. In experienced hands a good outcome can be obtained both with epineurial repair and with interfascicular grafting. There is no report available that compares the clinical results of epineurial and fascicular end-to-end nerve repairs.

Many of the problems inherent in trying to analyze clinical results are eliminated in the experimental studies comparing repair techniques. Here the repairs can be performed on identical nerve injuries. Outcome may be evaluated in terms of objective findings, such as the number of regenerating axons in the distal segment, the strength of muscle contraction, and the measured nerve conduction velocities and nerve action potential amplitudes. Epineurial and fascicular repair have been compared in cat ulnar nerves, both after clean division and after excision of a short segment of nerve.[3,17] In both circumstances comparison of muscle strength and weight and of the number of regenerating myelinating axons distal to the anastomosis showed no significant difference between the types of repair. A similar study of the same techniques by Orgel and Terzis showed no differences in nerve conduction velocity or in the amplitude of the nerve action potential in the two types of repair.[16] When these same measurements were applied to a study of epineurial repairs under varying degrees of tension and to fascicular grafts, the best results were found with epineural repair performed under no tension.[26] Epineurial repairs with slight tension had results about equal to those of fascicular grafts. Repairs done under greater tension had markedly decreased conduction velocities and nerve action potentials. Bratton et al. compared end-to-end repairs, both epineurial and perineurial, and fascicular grafts in terms of nerve action potentials and muscle strength.[2] At 12 months after nerve suture there were no differences among the repairs although the nongraft repairs were superior at 6 months.

At present there thus appears to be no major difference in the effectiveness of the three common types of nerve repairs and no reason to favor one over the others on either a clinical or an experimental basis. Nonetheless, differences in the internal anatomy of the nerve trunks provide some theoretical basis for favoring certain techniques of repair in particular situations.

A sharp proximal nerve transection is best repaired by mobilization of the nerve and epineurial repair. Here the diffuse distribution of functionally related axons throughout the fascicles allows no advantage to fascicular nerve repair. The nerve can ordinarily be easily mobilized for end-to-end closure without tension and nerve grafts are not necessary. Fascicular end-to-end repair is favored in sharp, fresh distal injuries when the nerve can be easily apposed without tension and the segregation of axons into functionally related fascicles or fascicle groups makes anastomosis of corresponding fascicles worthwhile. Fascicular repair is also quite useful when a nerve has been partially divided with sparing of some fascicles or groups (Fig. 232-9). The delayed repair of a ragged, scarred proximal nerve laceration is best performed by mobilization of the stumps, resection of the fibrotic ends, and epineurial repair. If this repair can only be obtained with considerable tension or marked flexion of adjacent joints, interfascicular nerve grafts are more appropriate. In the delayed repair of a distal untidy nerve transec-

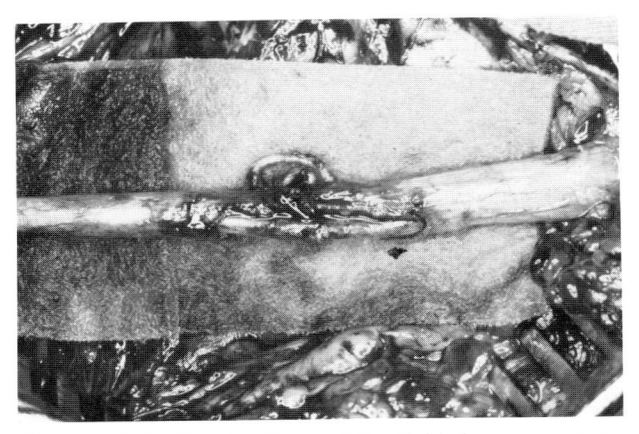

Figure 232-9 Repair of a partially divided common peroneal nerve. A single fascicle, at top, was spared. The remaining fascicles and fascicle groups were dissected free after excision of the epineurium. Matched groups were sutured with 10-0 nylon. Sixteen months after repair the patient had nearly normal strength in the tibialis anterior and the peronei.

tion, resection of scarred nerve ends and interfascicular nerve grafts seem most appropriate. A small nerve gap is created. Localization of related axons in fascicles or groups at this level is exploited and preserved by connecting corresponding fascicles or groups through the nerve grafts and thus overcoming the gap without tension on the repair. It should be stressed that these are only theoretical considerations and that a carefully performed repair of any type with attention to proper axial alignment and close approximation of the nerve ends or grafts is likely to give acceptable results.

Alternate Techniques

This chapter has been specifically concerned with the three major forms of nerve repair. A variety of other techniques have been proposed and used. These include guide sutures, nerve homografts, and sutureless nerve union.

Guide sutures are used to align central fascicles in combination with epineurial suture repair. The guide sutures are placed through the epineurium a few millimeters from the nerve end, penetrate into the interfascicular epineurium, and exit the nerve face beside a fascicle or group. The suture is then passed into the intraneural connective tissue beside the corresponding fascicle or group of the other nerve end and brought out through the epineurial sheath. Three or four sutures of this type serve to guide fascicular apposition and prevent axial rotation. The sutures are not tied and are brought out through the skin. They may be withdrawn a few days after repair.

Cadaver nerve homografts have been investigated actively in the hope of producing a source of full-thickness nerve trunk grafts. Unfortunately these grafts are not immunologically compatible and are quickly rejected by the host. Despite attempts to decrease the antigenicity of homografts by radiation, freeze drying, and lyophilization, the results of homograft use in humans have been disappointing and they are not currently recommended.

Sutureless nerve union has been attempted by a variety of methods in an attempt to minimize the fibrous tissue reaction initiated by sutures. The use of a fibrinogen-rich plasma to tack nerve ends together began during World War II. This "plasma clot" method was often used in the past and was the principal method used to perform the cable or bundle graft repair. The principal disadvantages of this method were its complexity and the fragility of the anastomosis. Plasma clot union could not be performed if there was any tension on the nerve repair. The current use of very fine suture material has reduced fibrous tissue reactions considerably and plasma clot union has subsequently declined. There has been some recent interest in the use of synthetic cyanoacrylate adhesives to hold a nerve union. The use of these materials has been hampered by their apparent histotoxicity. At present no form of sutureless nerve union compares favorably with microsurgical suture repair.

Complications

There are relatively few complications of peripheral nerve surgery aside from wound infection. The most common undesirable result is failure of the repair to result in reinnervation. This may be due to a poorly performed nerve suture, excessive tension on the repair, or an inordinate delay between injury and repair. As a general rule if there are no signs of reinnervation by 6 to 8 months after repair, the suture line should be explored and evaluated by either nerve stimulation or nerve action potential recording. A neurolysis or resection and resuture is then performed if indicated.

References

1. Bora FW Jr: Peripheral nerve repair in cats: The fascicular stitch. J Bone Joint Surg [Am] 49A:659–666, 1967.
2. Bratton BR, Kline DG, Coleman W, Hudson AR: Experimental interfascicular nerve grafting. J Neurosurg 51:323–332, 1979.
3. Cabaud HE, Rodkey WG, McCarroll HR Jr, Mutz SB, Niebauer JJ: Epineural and perineural fascicular nerve repairs: A critical comparison. J Hand Surg 1:131–137, 1976.
4. Daniel RK, Terzis JK: *Reconstructive Microsurgery*. Boston, Little, Brown, 1977.
5. Ducker TB, Kauffman FC: Metabolic factors in the surgery of peripheral nerves. Clin Neurosurg 24:406–424, 1977.
6. Edshage S: Peripheral nerve suture: A technique for improved intraneural topography. Evaluation of some suture materials. Acta Chir Scand [Suppl] 331:1–104, 1964.
7. Grabb WC: Median and ulnar nerve suture: An experimental study comparing primary and secondary repair in monkeys. J Bone Joint Surg [Am] 50A:964–972, 1968.
8. Highet WB, Sanders FK: The effects of stretching nerves after suture. Br J Surg 30:355–369, 1943.
9. Kline DG, Hackett ER: Reappraisal of timing for exploration of civilian peripheral nerve injuries. Surgery 78:54–65, 1975.
10. Kline DG, Hackett ER, Davis GD, Myers MB: Effect of mobilization on the blood supply and regeneration of injured nerves. J Surg Res 12:254–266, 1972.
11. Kline DG, Hudson AR: Surgical repair of acute peripheral nerve injuries: Timing and technique, in Morley TP (ed): *Cur-*

12. Langley JN, Hashimoto M: On the suture of separate nerve bundles in a nerve trunk and on internal nerve plexuses. J Physiol (Lond) 51:318–346, 1917.
13. Millesi H: Reappraisal of nerve repair. Surg Clin North Am 61:321–340, 1981.
14. Millesi H, Meissl G, Berger A: The interfascicular nerve-grafting of the median and ulnar nerves. J Bone Joint Surg [Am] 54A:727–750, 1972.
15. Millesi H, Meissl G, Berger A: Further experience with interfascicular grafting of the median, ulnar, and radial nerves. J Bone Joint Surg [Am] 58A:209–218, 1976.
16. Orgel MG, Terzis JK: Epineurial vs. perineurial repair: An ultrastructural and electrophysiological study of nerve regeneration. Plast Reconstr Surg 60:80–91, 1977.
17. Rodkey WG, Cabaud HE, McCarroll HR Jr: Neurorrhaphy after loss of a nerve segment: Comparison of epineurial suture under tension vs. multiple nerve grafts. J Hand Surg 5:366–371, 1980.
18. Samii M: Modern aspects of peripheral and cranial nerve surgery. Adv Tech Stds Neurosurg 2:33–85, 1975.
19. Schultz RJ: Management of nerve gaps, in Omer GE Jr, Spinner M (eds): *Management of Peripheral Nerve Problems.* Philadelphia, Saunders, 1980, pp 388–409.
20. Seddon H: *Surgical Disorders of the Peripheral Nerves,* 2d ed. London, Churchill Livingstone, 1975.
21. Seddon HJ: The use of autogenous grafts for the repair of large gaps in peripheral nerves. Br J Surg 35:151–167, 1947.
22. Smith JW: Microsurgery of peripheral nerves. Plast Reconstr Surg 33:317–329, 1964.
23. Sunderland S: Funicular suture and funicular exclusion in the repair of severed nerves. Br J Surg 40:580–587, 1953.
24. Sunderland S: *Nerves and Nerve Injuries,* 2d ed. Edinburgh, Churchill Livingstone, 1978.
25. Sunderland S: The pros and cons of funicular nerve repair. J Hand Surg 4:201–211, 1979.
26. Terzis JK, Faibisoff B, Williams HB: The nerve gap: Suture under tension vs. graft. Plast Reconstr Surg 56:166–170, 1975.

233
Clinical Signs of Peripheral Nerve Regeneration
Irvine G. McQuarrie

Nerve regeneration occurs as a stepwise process, with axonal outgrowth being followed by end organ reconnection and recovery. Most of the signs of functional recovery appear late in the process and reflect the maturation of a majority of the original axon–end organ units.[9] If spontaneous regeneration is expected but these signs fail to develop, a nerve repair is indicated. By then, however, it may be too late to expect a good result.[9]

There are two main strategies for resolving this dilemma. The first is the subject of this chapter: to acquire a thorough knowledge of the stages of axonal regeneration and end organ recovery so that tests of nerve regeneration can be applied in a timely manner and interpreted accurately. The second is to know when the nerve is likely to be interrupted so that early repair can be carried out. For example, a policy can be adopted of exploring the nerve within a month of injury whenever a skin wound is present and the status of the nerve is unknown, unless neurapraxia has been diagnosed in the meantime. To aid in the application of the first strategy, electroneurography has recently been developed to the extent that it permits the early detection of axonal outgrowth[3]; in most cases the test can be carried out noninvasively. To understand the rationale behind electroneurography and other tests of nerve regeneration, it is appropriate to begin with a brief overview of axonal regeneration.

Rate of Regeneration of Axons

When a peripheral nerve injury disrupts connective tissue elements as well as axons (neurotmesis), axonal regeneration occurs in the following stages[9]:

1. The *initial delay*, the time required for axons to sprout and advance as far as the lesion site.
2. The *scar delay*, the time required for axons to cross the lesion site or anastomosis.
3. The *intermediate delay*, the time during which axons traverse the distal nerve stump by following the persistent endoneurial tubes (Schwann cell basement membranes).
4. The *terminal delay*, the time during which axon–end organ connections mature sufficiently to subserve function.

When there has not been any disruption of the connective tissue elements at the injury site (axonotmesis), there is no scar delay and the uninterrupted endoneurial tubes direct each daughter axon sprout to the end organ that had originally been contacted by the parent axon.[9] Following these crush-type lesions, nerve regeneration is spontaneous; this is commonly seen after nerve injuries due to bone fractures.

Of necessity the stages of axonal regeneration have only been analyzed carefully in experimental animals. In the rat sciatic nerve, for example, the leading or fastest-growing sensory axons can be located accurately by using the nerve pinch test[2,6,9] which is a laboratory variant of the Hoffmann-Tinel test described below. Outgrowth distances are found to increase as a linear function of time after allowing for the initial and scar delays (Fig. 233-1). The duration of these delays can be determined by simple extrapolation of the calculated linear regression (of distance or time) to zero outgrowth distance (Fig. 233-1). The outgrowth rate is the slope of the linear function, 4.3/0.1 mm per day. Following a crush lesion of the sciatic nerve of a rat, the initial delay is approximately 2 days (Fig. 233-1). Following nerve suture, the combined initial and scar delays total 4 days, indicating that the scar delay is 2 days.[2] Since the outgrowth rate is linear, the length of the intermediate delay is simply the length of the distal nerve stump multiplied by the outgrowth rate. These values for outgrowth rate and scar delay are consistent with those obtained for motor and sensory axons in a variety of nonprimate mammals by using the pinch test, axonal transport methods, histology, and electromyography,[2,9] but the initial delay may be several days shorter in the rat.[2] In nonhuman primates, the initial delay is 2 to 3 weeks and the scar delay is 1 to 2 weeks as judged from the time required for silver-stained axons to appear in histological sections taken immediately distal to the nerve lesion.[4,5]

Certain factors other than species differences influence the time course of axonal regeneration. If the wounding agent acts to stretch the nerve (as may occur with displaced fractures) or transmits pressure waves through adjacent tissues (as may occur with high-velocity missile wounds), then retrograde axonal degeneration will extend for several centimeters up the proximal nerve stump,[9] thereby prolonging the initial delay. At the lesion site itself scarring not only delays the arrival of axons at the distal nerve stump but acts to continuously retard their growth.[1,2,9] Thus, in the rat sciatic nerve the outgrowth rate for leading sensory axons is 4.3 mm per day after nerve crush but only 3.2 mm per day after nerve suture.[2] Sunderland has concluded that this is primarily due to a chronic constriction of the axons by scar tissue at the lesion site and is secondarily due to a higher incidence of neuronal atrophy and death following neurotmesis compared with axonotmesis.[9] Proximal lesions also cause a higher incidence of neuronal atrophy and death than do distal lesions.[9] On the other hand, neurons that recover from the metabolic effects of axonal loss and enter a growth mode can sustain a second axotomy more readily and produce the second crop of daughter axons more rapidly.[6,9] This *"conditioning lesion effect"*[6] is usually associated with accelerated axonal outgrowth. Finally, aging has been shown to have a retarding effect on axonal outgrowth.[8,9]

Clinical Signs of Nerve Regeneration

The only sign that is available for detecting ongoing axonal outgrowth in the distal nerve stump is the Hoffmann-Tinel sign.[9] It is based on the 100-fold greater sensitivity of outgrowing axon tips to mechanical pressure compared with the more proximal axon shafts.[2,6] To elicit this sign, the degenerated nerve is subjected to light tapping at a distal point that regenerating axons could not yet have reached. Stimuli are continued proximally in 5 to 10 mm steps until the patient suddenly notes a strong tingling sensation that radiates to the cutaneous areas normally served by the injured nerve. This is a positive Hoffmann-Tinel sign; it locates the farthest advance of a few sensory axon tips. The progress of outgrowth can be charted by examining the patient at fortnightly intervals and plotting the distance from the lesion site to the various positive response sites as a function of time.[9] The outgrowth distances in humans do not increase as a linear function of time as they do in experimental animals, but rather as a function of the logarithm of time.[1] This is attributable to the gradual decrease in nerve temperature at progressively more distal sites in the extremity, since outgrowth rates are fairly uniform at a given distance from the body core regardless of the duration of outgrowth.[9] The rates of advance of the Hoffmann-Tinel sign that can be expected following axonotmesis are 3 mm per day above the elbow, 1.5 mm per day between the elbow and wrist (or the knee and ankle), and 0.5 to 1.0 mm per day below the wrist. The rates following nerve suture are 20 to 30 percent slower.[9] Since only a few sensory axons need enter the distal nerve stump to produce an advancing Hoffmann-Tinel sign,[9] eventual recovery is not assured.

Once axons reconnect with appropriate end organs, there

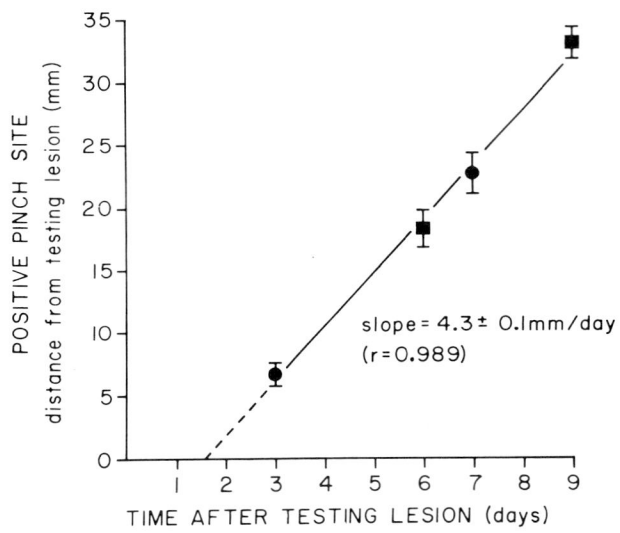

Figure 233-1 Normal sensory axon outgrowth after sciatic nerve crush as determined by using the nerve pinch test. The distance between the crush site and the positive pinch site is displayed on the ordinate. The outgrowth rate for leading sensory axons (4.3 mm per day) is readily calculated because the regression function of distance on time is linear (coefficient of correlation = 0.989). Extrapolation of this function to the abscissa yields the initial delay, which is the time required for injured axons to sprout and elongate as far as the lesion site. Filled circles and filled squares denote mean outgrowth distances for two different experimental series. Vertical lines denote the standard deviation of the mean. (From McQuarrie et al.[6])

is a terminal delay that precedes the onset of functional recovery. Events that are known to occur during this maturation stage of regeneration are: (1) reversal of end organ atrophy, (2) radial growth of axons, and (3) myelination of axons.[9] Often, a critical number of axon–end organ units must also have matured sufficiently to act "in concert" before signs of functional recovery can be elicited. Thus, those functions that require the action of only a few axon–end organ units and those that are normally subserved by small, unmyelinated axons involve the shortest terminal delays. Autonomic functions and certain sensory functions (perception of pain and temperature) are examples. To use the recovery of these functions as evidence of recovery due to nerve regeneration, testing must be confined to the autonomous sensory zones for the injured nerve in question. Autonomic function is best evaluated by examining the skin for sweat formation with an ophthalmoscope set at +20 diopters. The first sign of sensory recovery is the presence of muscle tenderness in response to deep pressure, since muscles are located more proximally than the autonomous skin areas. In these areas, the earliest sign of reinnervation is a high-threshold *protopathic* or *hyperpathic* response to pin stimulation: pain that is not sharp but is rather unpleasant, diffuse, and poorly localized.[9] Temperature appreciation is next to recover, followed by the recovery of light touch (at which point hyperpathia usually disappears). The sensory functions that are subserved by larger, myelinated axons (such as two-point discrimination and joint position sense) are associated with longer terminal delays. This level of recovery is heralded when two-point discrimination falls below 10 mm in the autonomous areas. While values of 10 to 20 mm reflect a degree of reinnervation, values of less than 10 to 12 mm are required before the patient will cease to employ visual control over most hand functions.[7]

A return of motor function requires the concerted action of a significant number of large myelinated axons, implying a long terminal delay. On that basis, the return of voluntary contractions would be expected to be a late sign of functional recovery. It is actually the earliest objective sign of functional recovery, since motor axons need regenerate only a short distance to reach the end plates of the nearest denervated muscle. By detecting the onset of voluntary contractions in that muscle, the examiner can be assured that satisfactory nerve regeneration is occurring. Conversely, the failure of voluntary contractions to develop in that muscle after an appropriate *latent period* is a clear indication for nerve exploration.[9] Estimation of the latent period, or interval between injury and the onset of voluntary contractions, requires a thorough knowledge of the variation in motor branch patterns for the nerve in question. This permits the clinician to accurately estimate the maximum probable distance from the lesion site to the motor end plates of any denervated muscle. Sunderland has compiled a comprehensive reference work that provides the necessary information for all noncranial motor nerves, which is based in each instance on the careful dissection of at least 20 cadavers.[9] Once the maximum probable distance has been estimated, it is divided by the appropriate axonal outgrowth rate (see above) to yield the intermediate delay. To this is added the number of days consumed by the *combined delay*, meaning all delays other than the intermediate delay.[9] Mean values for the combined delay have been calculated by Bowden and Sholl, who recorded the latent period for each reinnervated muscle in 14 patients with axonotmesis and 17 with nerve repair.[1] For each patient, the outgrowth distance was plotted as a function of the latent period; extrapolation to zero distance yielded the combined delay. After axonotmesis the mean delay was 64±6 days; after nerve repair it was 96±11 days.

An example will serve to illustrate how the latent period is estimated. With an injury to the radial nerve due to a fracture of the humerus at a level 10 cm above the lateral epicondyle, the brachioradialis is the nearest denervated muscle, and Sunderland's tables indicate that the shortest mean distance from the lesion site to the muscle is 82 mm, with a standard deviation (SD) of 15 mm.[9] Thus the maximum probable distance is 82 mm + 1SD, or 97 mm. Since spontaneous recovery is anticipated, this distance is divided by the outgrowth rate for axonotmesis lesions above the elbow, 3 mm per day,[9] to yield an intermediate delay of 32 days. This is added to the estimated combined delay for axonotmesis (64 days) to give an estimate of 96 days for the latent period. "One millimeter per day" is a convenient rule of thumb. That is, the latent period in days should not exceed the maximum probable distance in millimeters following axonotmesis.

Electrical Evidence of Regeneration

Two types of electrodiagnostic tests are used for detecting ongoing nerve regeneration prior to the return of voluntary movements. Electromyography (EMG) can detect the arrival of axons at the muscle end plates, an event that precedes the onset of recovery by 4 to 10 weeks because of the terminal delay.[9] Electroneurography can locate axons in the distal nerve stump before they have reached any end organs.[3] Variants of both tests can be applied intraoperatively.[3,4] EMG studies require the insertion of concentric needle electrodes into the muscle being tested; the motor-unit action potentials (MUAPs) are amplified electronically and monitored audiovisually by using a cathode-ray oscilloscope in series with a loudspeaker. MUAPs are recorded under four conditions: (1) during needle insertion, (2) at rest, (3) during mild voluntary effort, and (4) during maximal effort. Denervation is diagnosed by the absence of MUAPs during voluntary effort and the presence of two types of electrical activity at rest (when there is normally an absence of electrical activity): fibrillation potentials, which are nonvoluntary discharges of single muscle fibers, and positive sharp waves. The first evidence of axonal reconnection is a decrease in the frequency of fibrillations. This is followed in about 2 weeks by the appearance of low-amplitude polyphasic MUAPs, termed *nascent potentials*, on maximal effort. Within 2 to 4 weeks (axonotmesis) or 6 to 8 weeks (nerve repair), normal-appearing di- and triphasic MUAPs begin to be seen with mild voluntary effort, and visible muscle contractions are noted on maximal effort.[9] Soon after nascent potentials are first noted, it is often possible to elicit visible muscle contractions by stimulating either the regenerating motor nerve with needle electrodes or the proximal nerve stump with surface electrodes.[3]

With electroneurography, evoked nerve action potentials (NAPs) are used to determine the axonal outgrowth distance in the distal nerve stump; serial examinations make it possible to measure the axonal outgrowth rate. The distal nerve stump is stimulated with surface electrodes at sites that are increasingly removed from the lesion site; NAPs are recorded from the proximal nerve stump with needle electrodes and displayed on an oscilloscope.[3] The most distal stimulus that elicits a proximal NAP marks the farthest point reached by outgrowing axons. By adding a preamplifier and a signal-averaging computer to the test system, individual oscilloscope sweeps can be summated and averaged. The increase in the signal-to-noise ratio permits the use of surface recording electrodes instead of needle electrodes. Further increases in accuracy can be obtained by intraoperative electroneurography, since both the stimulating and recording electrodes can be applied directly to the nerve. This permits bypassing skin resistance as well as avoiding the MUAP artifacts that occur with the high-stimulus intensities necessary to stimulate the high-resistance outgrowing axons. Thus, stimulation can be carried out on the proximal nerve stump (where axons have a low resistance because of their large diameter) without producing muscle artifacts; recording is then done distally.[3] While intraoperative electroneurography cannot be done serially to obtain an outgrowth rate, it is the most efficient procedure for evaluating a suspected neuroma in continuity.[3] For this purpose it is done 8 to 10 weeks after injury, to allow sufficient time for the initial and scar delays to pass and to permit axons to grow a short distance into the distal nerve stump.

References

1. Bowden REM, Sholl DA: The advance of functional recovery after radial nerve lesions in man. Brain 73:251–266, 1950.
2. Forman DS, Wood, DK, DeSilva S: Rate of regeneration of sensory axons in transected rat sciatic nerve repaired with epineurial sutures. J Neurol Sci 44:55–59, 1979.
3. Kline DG: Evaluation of the neuroma in continuity, in Omer GE Jr, Spinner M (eds): *Management of Peripheral Nerve Problems*. Philadelphia, Saunders, 1980, pp 450–461.
4. Kline DG, Hackett ER, May PR: Evaluation of nerve injuries by evoked potentials and electromyography. J Neurosurg 31:128–136, 1969.
5. Kline DG, Hayes GJ, Morse AS: A comparative study of response of species to peripheral-nerve injury. II. Crush and severance with primary suture. J Neurosurg 21:980–988, 1964.
6. McQuarrie IG, Grafstein B, Gershon MD: Axonal regeneration in the rat sciatic nerve: Effect of a conditioning lesion and of dbcAMP. Brain Res 132:443–453, 1977.
7. Moberg E: Surgical treatment for absent single-hand grip and elbow extension in quadriplegia: Principles and preliminary experience. J Bone Joint Surg [Am] 57A:196–206, 1975.
8. Pestronk A, Drachman DB, Griffin JW: Effects of aging on nerve sprouting and regeneration. Exp Neurol 70:65–82, 1980.
9. Sunderland S: *Nerves and Nerve Injuries*, 2d ed. Edinburgh, Churchill Livingstone, 1978, chaps. 7, 8, 26, 41, 45, 54, 60.

234
Painful Neuromas
Suzie C. Tindall

Painful neuromas that have formed at the proximal ends of divided cutaneous nerves or within an amputation stump can be very disabling to a patient, rendering an otherwise functional extremity useless. Satisfactory treatment of such a lesion is frequently a challenge for even the most astute peripheral nerve surgeon. In this chapter, the histopathological events leading to the formation of a neuroma, the postulated mechanisms for pain in painful neuromas, and the clinical syndromes of painful neuromas and their treatment will be reviewed. Although neuromas in continuity are reviewed elsewhere, distal neuromas in the hand and the Morton's neuroma will be discussed here.

Histopathology and Pathophysiology

Formation of a bulbous neuroma at the proximal end of a severed peripheral nerve is a physiological attempt at spontaneous axon repair. Following section, the severed nerve fibers undergo wallerian degeneration back to the next proximal node of Ranvier as the nerve cell body undergoes chromatolysis and begins to manufacture new RNA to support the reparative process of axonal regeneration. As repair proceeds, fine axonal sprouts grow out from the cut end of the nerve, where they are greeted by a tangled mass of fibroblasts and regenerating Schwann cells. If these sprouts fail to enter the endoneurial tubules of the distal part of the cut nerve they form a neuroma. The neuroma contains poorly vascularized connective tissue infiltrated with large numbers of the sprouts of the parent axons. The neuroma may be well encapsulated in a fibrous sheath or it may be firmly attached to surrounding structures by fibrous adhesions.

Factors regulating the extent to which a neuroma will form are not well understood but it is thought that local tissue factors, anoxia, foreign material, or infected or necrotic tissue at each specific site play an important role in formation and symptomatology.[2] Obviously, a neuroma that is superficially located and vulnerable to repeated trauma or one that is attached to an adjacent tendon or surrounding scar and is constantly undergoing tension with wrist or finger motion is especially likely to be painfully symptomatic.

Only the minority of terminal neuromas become painful. Wall and Gutnick have studied the properties of afferent nerve impulses originating from a neuroma.[9] They point out that the membranes of the terminal axonal sprouts become spontaneously active and act as generators of abnormal electrical activity, which is transmitted to the central nervous system. They believe that this activity may be the source of pain in a neuroma and point out that such activity may be arrested or suppressed by electrical stimulation of the nerve proximal to the neuroma or by administration of alpha blocking agents.

Measures to Prevent Neuroma Formation

Over the years numerous measures have been tried to prevent neuroma formation either primarily at the time of amputation or secondarily when attempting to treat a painful neuroma. They include simple ligation; intraneural injection of hot water; heat and electrocoagulation; freezing; application of chemical agents such as alcohol, phenol, acids, or radioactive substances; burying the nerve endings within bone; and placement of epineural sleeves or caps of rubber or Silastic. Sunderland has long maintained that the perineurium presents an impenetrable barrier to the regenerating axonal sprouts,[8] and Battista and Cravioto have recently advocated microsurgical fascicular ligation as a method of perineurial closure for prevention of neuroma formation.[1] Unfortunately, no method can yet be relied upon to prevent neuroma formation.

It is well recognized, however, that neuromas forming in the primary wound cicatrix are much more likely to become symptomatic than those forming in minimally scarred, well-vascularized tissue well away from sources of superficial trauma or pressure. Consequently, optimum primary care of an amputation stump or of an irreparable nerve laceration is provision of the best possible tissue bed for the sectioned nerve to rest in as the neuroma forms.[2] This is accomplished by sharply severing all nerves, superficial and deep, as proximally as possible and permitting them to retract well away from the surface.

Clinical Syndromes

Painful neuromas may arise at almost any location but are particularly problematic when they develop within the oral cavity, where they are traumatized by chewing or dentures; on the digits or the superficial sensory branches of the median, ulnar, or radial nerve; or in amputation stumps, where they may interfere with the ability to wear a prosthetic appliance. It should be emphasized that the pain is not spontaneous or related to causalgia or the phantom phenomenon. Rather, the pain is provoked by pressure or traction on the neuroma and is characterized by radiation into the region originally innervated by the severed nerve. The neuroma is not always palpable.

Treatment

Pain from a neuroma may be temporarily blocked by flooding the neuroma and surrounding tissues with a local anesthetic solution. This maneuver is sometimes helpful in diagnosis, and because an occasional patient may obtain permanent relief from this treatment, it is usually worth a try.[1] Robbins has reported excellent results (successful treatment of 12 of 14 painful neuromas) with direct injection of triamcinolone into the neuroma, but the duration of follow-up in his cases is not reported.[6]

By and large the treatment for the painful neuroma remains surgical, and the form of surgical therapy will depend somewhat upon the location of the neuroma and the personal bias of the treating surgeon. For the oral cavity resection of the neuroma and sharp section of the nerve under traction constitute the treatment of choice.[7] For the hand Herndon and colleagues have had excellent results in 82 percent of patients by keeping the neuroma intact with its encapsulating scar and transposing it *en bloc* to an adjacent area that is free of scar and not subjected to repeated trauma.[3] For amputation stump neuromas some surgeons advocate neuroma resection. Because there is no consistently reliable method for controlling neuroma formation, the case for resection of the bulb rests on the expectation that the neuroma that develops the second time will be less troublesome than the first.[8] Whether the neuroma is resected or left intact, best results are obtained if the painful nerve end is embedded deeply into adjacent soft tissues so that it will no longer be subjected to local trauma or traction.

Morton's Neuroma

Morton's toe, Morton's neuroma, Morton's metatarsalgia, or Morton's neuritis are the eponyms usually applied to the clinical syndrome of pain between a pair of metatarsal heads with radiation into the corresponding toes. The affected individual is usually an adult female who complains that walking or standing precipitates the pain, while rest and removal of the shoe give relief. The left third intermetatarsal space is usually involved, although the second or fourth space may be the location and the condition is sometimes bilateral. Numbness and tingling of the toes are common complaints. Digital palpation in the affected cleft will elicit pain and a swelling may be palpable between the metatarsal heads. Sensory changes are occasionally detectable in the affected toes.

The cause of Morton's neuroma is trauma to the digital nerve where it traverses the intermetatarsal space beneath the deep transverse metatarsal ligaments. Walking in ill-fitting shoes is most often the precipitating traumatic factor. Histologically, the changes in the digital nerve are not those typical of the neuroma but rather consist of degenerative neural bands of various sizes surrounded by a greatly thickened perineurium, together with collagen bundles and thick-walled arterioles.[5]

Conservative treatment for this malady may provide temporary relief; such treatment usually consists of insoles, metatarsal bars, adhesive pads designed to spread the metatarsal heads, or injections of hydrocortisone or local anesthetics.[4,5] Most authorities recommend surgical excision of the neuroma through a vertical plantar incision as the most effective therapeutic option. Although exposure is a little more difficult, I prefer a Y type dorsal incision, which avoids a potentially painful scar on the sole of the foot. A symptomatic cure can be expected in approximately 85 percent of patients undergoing such a procedure.[5] Although the "neuroma" may recur after surgery, the incidence of recurrence is generally only 3 to 7 percent.[4]

References

1. Battista A, Cravioto H: Neuroma formation and prevention by fascicle ligation in the rat. Neurosurgery 8:191–204, 1981.
2. Eaton RG: Painful neuromas, in Omer GE Jr, Spinner M (eds): *Management of Peripheral Nerve Problems*. Philadelphia, Saunders, 1980, pp 195–202.
3. Herndon JH, Eaton RG, Littler JW: Management of painful neuromas in the hand. J Bone Joint Surg [Am] 58A:369–373, 1976.
4. Milgram JE: Morton's neuritis and management of post-neurectomy pain, in Omer GE Jr, Spinner M (eds): *Management of Peripheral Nerve Problems*. Philadelphia, Saunders, 1980, pp 203–215.
5. Morris MA: Morton's metatarsalgia. Clin Orthop 127:203–207, 1977.
6. Robbins TH: The response of tender neuromas and scars to triamcinolone injections. Br J Plast Surg 30:68–69, 1977.
7. Shira RB: Painful traumatic neuromas in the oral cavity. Oral Surg 49:191–195, 1980.
8. Sunderland S: *Nerves and Nerve Injuries*, 2d ed. Edinburgh, Churchill Livingstone, 1978.
9. Wall PD, Gutnick M: Properties of afferent nerve impulses originating from a neuroma. Nature 248:740–743, 1974.

235

Causalgia; Sympathetic Dystrophy (Sudeck's Atrophy)

William H. Sweet

Causalgia

Although the word *causalgia* [from the Greek *kausos* ("heat") and *algos* ("pain")] may be translated as "burning pain," this term was introduced by Weir Mitchell to describe only the circumscribed but at times dramatic syndrome seen after a minority of injuries to peripheral nerves.[23] His patients were soldiers wounded in the Civil War of 1861 to 1865. Gunshot or other injuries by foreign bodies to major peripheral nerves in the limbs are largely responsible for subsequent publications on the disorder. Thus its severe form, *major causalgia*, is most likely to occur in wartime, notably in wounds with high-velocity missiles.

Clinical Features

The pain is usually, but by no means invariably, burning in quality. In a critical analysis of their 52 patients, Kirklin et al. found that although 89 percent included the word "burning" to indicate the type of pain, the descriptions "throbbing," "aching," "pressure," "knifelike, stabbing," and "twisting, crushing" were also used by 10 to 48 percent of the patients.[15] The pain appears in the great majority of cases within 24 h of the injury. The worst pain is usually in the hand or foot, even though the causative wound is commonly much more proximal. Spontaneous and persistent, the pain may reach remarkable severity and give rise to extraordinary behavior, which the uninformed physician is likely to regard as exaggerated beyond reason. Thus, patients may insist on maintaining the entire affected limb immobile, not allowing the part to be examined. Often they seek relief by applying cold or, less often, warm wet cloths to the most painful area, usually the hand or foot. Apparently it is the moisture rather than the temperature that is needed for relief. In a few patients moderate temperature changes have no effect; in a few others either warmth or cold worsens the pain. Almost any sensory stimulus exacerbates the pain and the patient becomes a recluse in the attempt to avoid any light touch, vibration, loud sound, abrupt light, or even approaching footsteps. Not only minimal physical stimuli but emotional or other psychic stimuli become intolerable. In addition to worry and frustration, even normally pleasurable excitement from a movie or a book may intensify the pain. This may spread to the forearm or leg and beyond the territory of the injured nerve or nerves. Mitchell et al. described *causalgia* pain as varying "from the most trivial burning" to the "most terrible of all tortures which a nerve wound may inflict."[24] When the syndrome presents with less devastating intensity, the term *minor causalgia* has been used.

In some patients in whom the whole limb feels numb after the wounding, the pain may not appear until the numbness subsides hours or days later. Of Barnes's 48 patients, the onset of the pain occurred in 83 percent in the first 3 days.[3] Of Mayfield's 105, the onset was "instantaneous" in about 50 percent.[21] In the 70 patients of Omer and Thomas, over two-thirds had the pain by the end of the first week; in 16 percent it set in only after surgery.[26] Barnes described a steady, slow, spontaneous improvement of the pain in some patients. Sunderland states that the pain usually "subsides and vanishes" within 6 months, rarely persisting for more than 1 year.[31] On the other hand, Barnes, Leriche, Livingston, and many others point out that the pain may continue indefinitely for many years.[3,17,19] In any event, the severity of the pain and the worsening of the disability as long as it continues lead nearly all authors to recommend early aggressive treatment.

Vascular changes in the limb may be either vasodilator or vasoconstrictor in character, with a warm pink or a cold, mottled blue skin, respectively. A vasodilated state for days or weeks may be succeeded by a vasoconstricted state. Trophic changes, at least partly related to the immobility, include dry and scaly skin, stiffening of joints, thin, tapering fingers, ridged uncut nails, and either long, coarse hairs or loss of hair over involved parts. At times the skin is smooth and glossy with variable sweating ranging from anhidrosis to extreme hyperhidrosis. There is no correlation among skin temperature, a sense of burning, and degree of sweating. The extent of vasomotor and trophic changes tends to parallel the severity of the pain.

Detailed sensory and motor examination is often difficult because of the hyperesthesia and hyperpathia. However, appraisal after effective sympathectomy or surgical exploration of the injured nerves has revealed that the syndrome develops in the great majority only after partial nerve injuries. In fact, Barnes reports no total lesion of the nerve in any of his 48 cases.[3] Carayon and Bourrel record 17 percent total nerve sections in their 150 cases,[8] and Nathan notes 18 percent complete lesions in his 22 patients.[25] The extensive muscle wasting that may occur can be due both to voluntary protective immobility and to motor paralysis.

Multiple nerve injuries are often seen in war-wounded patients with causalgia (e.g., 24 of Barnes' 27 patients afflicted in an upper limb and 18 of 21 with the disorder in a lower limb had more than one major nerve trunk affected).[3] The pain is often associated with more than one of the involved nerves, as demonstrated by relief at times of only the relevant part of the pain when one of the nerves is blocked by an anesthetic agent. Perhaps related to the fact that injury of more than one nerve appears to be a predisposing factor, the causative wounds are likely to be in the proximal half of the limb, affecting the neurovascular bundle in the arm or the combined tibial and common peroneal components of the sciatic nerve in the thigh.

To the foregoing features of the pain, namely, spontaneity, severity, and remarkable aggravation by physical and psychic stimuli, must be added the crucial diagnostic criterion of relief by effective blockade of the appropriate sympathetic trunk. The physician is well advised to repeat the block several times and to do at least one placebo block in the series. Especially if relief is incomplete, tests for anhidrosis or the psychogalvanic reflex throughout the limb must be used to make sure that the block was complete. Before the first block the patient may have been tearfully pleading to be left alone. The abrupt alteration in a patient's whole demeanor and personality when the hot dry limb, signaling sympathetic blockade, appears, can be as gratifying and startling to the physician as to the patient and his ward mates. If a sympathetic block does not stop or greatly lessen the pain, it is, by definition of the term for many of us, not causalgia (i.e., it has some other pathogenesis such as direct irritation of somatic afferent fibers related to the lesion).

It seems reasonable to classify the pain on the basis of the principal sympathetic physiological pathogenesis, not only because this determines the treatment but also because the occasional patient with the characteristic clinical picture will have something other than a primary sympathetic neural abnormality and will require some other form of treatment.

Incidence

Most reports describe causalgia in 2 to 5 percent of peripheral nerve injuries in wartime. (For a summary of the incidence in 4435 cases, see White and Sweet,[36] Table XIX.)

Psychological Factors

A somewhat surprising finding in the few percent of patients suffering psychological effects is that analysis of their preinjury personalities tends not to reveal any predisposition to autonomic disturbances or an unstable personality.[21] Indeed, a relatively prompt return to normal activities is the rule once the unendurable painful state has been alleviated. Psychological studies made after successful treatment have rarely demonstrated predisposing factors. A number of investigators cite causalgia-afflicted soldiers with previous wounds that had healed uneventfully who had returned to a combat zone or soldiers with multiple nerve wounds but with causalgia related to only one of them. However a temperamental predisposition to this syndrome is apparently more likely after civilian injuries and illness (see below).

Treatment

On rare occasions, the clinical picture can be simulated by largely psychogenic mechanisms. Lidz and Payne cite a striking case of a young soldier who accidentally shot himself through the palm of the right hand: "He was experiencing uneventful wound healing when 49 days later he learned that a review board had concluded that the injury was deliberate to avoid combat. Greatly distressed that his comrades in arms, wife, and parents would also all think him a coward, he withdrew from all ward activities and began to have severe pain in the right hand, which he stopped moving. In 10 days it became deeply flushed, cold, edematous, and soaked with perspiration. The delay in appearance of the syndrome led to consultation by a psychiatrist, who concluded that the patient's anxiety that he had unintentionally disgraced himself was the main problem. Psychological support enhanced by physiotherapy resulted in prompt subsidence of the pain and objective signs. The man returned to his fighting unit in 6 weeks."[18]

Local Treatment at the Wound

Relatively soon after injury further surgery of the wounded area may cure the pain, particularly if the wound is more distal than usual. Thus Gordon describes a soldier who had the prompt experience of major causalgia after most of his second, third, and fourth fingers were shot off.[10] His burning pain and hyperpathia were confined to the distal portion of the hand. The edematous hyperpathic skin was excised and replaced by a direct pedicle flap from the abdomen after resection of the digital nerves to the involved fingers. The pain disappeared and recovery remained complete at follow-up 17 years later.

Omer and Thomas have instituted "periodic perineural infusions."[26] If they find one or more trigger areas of irritation at the site of the injury, they place an inlying catheter to the point that provokes the pain. A small dose of lidocaine, 0.5 ml of a 0.5% solution with epinephrine, is injected. If the causalgic pain is relieved, the injections are continued every 3 h for several weeks if necessary. Of the 17 of their 70 patients thus treated, 14 had "satisfying results."

Sympathetic Blocks

These "diagnostic" blocks at the stellate ganglion or of the lumbar sympathetic trunk become effective therapy in many of the patients in less severe pain. Bonica's search of the literature revealed that in 10 of 17 publications satisfactory lasting relief of pain from a succession of sympathetic blocks was reported in about 18 to 25 percent of cases.[5] In the other seven articles permanent relief from such blocks is reported as rarely occurring. The key to the discrepancy is probably given by the report of Rasmussen and Freedman.[27] Of their 48 patients in only moderate pain, 5 were fully and permanently relieved by a single injection, in 7 more the same result was achieved within 4 weeks after several injections, and in 26 of the remaining 36 the degree of relief afforded by blocks sufficed so that further treatment was not necessary. In their 43 patients with severe, almost immobilizing pain, only 2 had sustained relief long outlasting that at the height of the block.

A longer, somewhat more localized type of sympathetic block was introduced by Hannington-Kiff in 1974, and its clinical utility was documented in a series of articles that followed.[13,14] The agent used, guanethidine, displaces norepinephrine (NE), the neurotransmitter at the sympathetic nerve endings. It occupies the storage sites, thereby precluding the normal storage of NE and binding so strongly that its complete elimination from the body requires many days. For example, elevated skin temperature in a treated limb may persist for days or for a few weeks. Hannington-Kiff has introduced a general technique for a regional sympathetic block to a limb.[13,14] This consists of placing a cannula into a distal vein of that limb and then inflating a blood pressure cuff on the limb to 50 to 100 mmHg above the systolic pressure in that limb. Then 10 to 30 mg of guanethidine sulfate is injected into the venous cannula. During the 5 to 10 min in which the tourniquet is kept inflated, most of the guanethidine is fixed in the tissues, evoking and maintaining a greater rise in skin temperature of the treated than of the control opposite limb. Further details of management and the necessary precautions are given in the references cited by Hannington-Kiff.[13,14] Of the first 10 patients in whom he had diagnosed causalgia, each received two guanethidine blocks at 3-week intervals. In five of the patients, the causalgic pain had been present about 5 weeks and an average of about 80 percent relief was maintained 15 weeks after the first treatment. In the other five patients the pain had persisted an average of 15 weeks before the treatment. In them, there was less than 50 percent relief after another 15 weeks from the start of treatment. The principal confirmation is presented in a detailed account by Loh and Nathan.[20] Of their 45 patients studied with a single regional guanethidine block, they classified 5 as having a partial peripheral nerve lesion, 6 as having reflex sympathetic dystrophy, and 1 as having Sudeck's atrophy. The pain was relieved in all but two of these—one in each of the first two groups.

Sympathectomy

We owe to Leriche the concept that the disorder has its origin in the sympathetic nervous system. (Ref. 17, pp. 170–201). Because he regarded the vasomotor abnormalities as the main cause of the pain, he advocated through the years a high periarterial sympathectomy. Although he and at least 18 other surgeons (Ref. 17, p. 198) were able to report many cures of causalgia by that operation in soldiers wounded in World War I, sympathectomy of the relevant portion of the sympathetic chain has become the definitive therapeutic procedure because of its even more gratifying success rate, related no doubt to its providing more complete sympathetic denervation. The first three case reports in 1930 came from Flothow, Pieri, and Spurling working independently of each other.[29] Massive numbers of well-studied cases in World War II and since then permit the following comments:

Sympathetic denervation stops the pain in over 90 percent of the patients, although in a small percentage of these some tenderness, hyperalgesia, or hyperpathia persists. Some of the failures may have been due to inadequate denervation since many of the unrelieved patients were not studied further. However, the same patient may have other pain caused by mechanisms other than those related to the sympathetic nerves.

The results of local operations such as neurolysis, resection and suture of the damaged nerve segment, resection of obliterated arteries, or radiotherapy are grossly inferior to those of sympathectomy. An especially convincing report is that of Barnes.[3] An exception to this rule is the experience of Mayfield (i.e., complete relief in each of the five cases in which an injured segment of nerve was excised).[21]

The results of preganglionic and postganglionic operations have been compared. In two series, preganglionic sympathectomy of the upper limb by cutting of the rami communicantes to the second and third thoracic sympathetic ganglia and dividing the trunk below the third ganglion has been compared with the postganglionic operation, which includes the stellate ganglion. Barnes reported eight preganglionic operations and nine postganglionic procedures.[3] After his six operations of the preganglionic type in which denervation was complete, five patients had total relief of pain and one was much better. In the eight of the postganglionic group with complete denervation, five patients had complete relief and three were much better. In the preganglionic and postganglionic groups there were three patients with complete denervation who had persistent hyperalgesia. Rasmussen and Freedman had 14 in the preganglionic group in all of whom there was complete relief of pain within 1 month or less.[27] Of the 21 in their postganglionic group, only 10 achieved complete relief in 1 month. The results, especially those of the last-cited authors, suggest that the preganglionic procedure is preferable—the more so since the postganglionic operation includes the minor disadvantage of a Horner's syndrome. The standard operation for the lower limb of removing no ganglia below L3 is a preganglionic operation. A more extensive, probably preganglionic, operation via the transthoracic approach has been recommended by Buker et al.; this involves removal from the lower half of the stellate ganglion through the fourth or fifth thoracic ganglia.[7] This yielded success in all their nine patients, none of whom had a Horner's syndrome.

The importance of achieving complete sympathetic denervation is repeatedly emphasized. Failure to achieve this caused the only three failures among Barnes' 30 cases[3] and three among Whitcomb's cases.[21] A second operation completed the denervation in four of these five patients, with resultant relief in all four. Mayfield had nine patients with incomplete sympathectomies, all of whom were relieved by completion of the denervation. Of these, seven were in the lower limb and his standard L2, L3 or L2, L3, L4 ganglionectomy still permitted sweating in the foot. In three of these patients, removal of the L1 ganglion completed the denervation, but in the other four, D11 and D12 ganglia were removed before the limb was denervated. Complete relief was then attained in all seven cases. Other examples are cited by Bonica.[5] However, completing the denervation did not invariably bring success. Carayon and Bourrel had two continuing failures, one after a T2, T3 ganglionectomy was supplemented by stellate ganglionectomy and another after the reverse sequence of operations.[8]

Under pathogenesis, I describe a patient whose sympathetics regenerated so persistently that relief was finally secured only by a posterior rhizotomy.

Energetic physical therapy, possible once the pain has been significantly relieved, is essential to restore the mobility and power of the limb, the normal appearance of the skin, and the subsidence of edema. In some patients this regime alone may be the only therapy required.

A long duration of symptoms prior to operation does not necessarily preclude a useful result of sympathectomy, as attested by Barnes, who cites repatriated prisoners of war so treated after 6 years.[3] Some untreated patients of both Mitchell and Leriche (Ref. 17, pp. 182–183) were still suffering many years later.

Late follow-ups after sympathectomy show persisting relief. Mayfield reports continued freedom from burning pain in 15 of 24 patients 3 to 5 years after operation; pain was slight in the remainder.[21] White and Selverstone report results 2 to 8 years after sympathectomy in 45 causalgic veterans of World War II (Ref. 36, p. 96). The burning dysesthesia remained absent in all; however 15 had "various forms of residual discomfort such as one may find after any nerve injury."

Sympathetic Dystrophy (Sudeck's Atrophy)

A list of 26 German, 20 English, and 9 French terms under which disorders often termed *sympathetic dystrophy* or *Sudeck's atrophy* have been classified was assembled recently by Ascherl and Blümel.[2] Minor causalgia is one of the synonymous terms, so that what was said previously is applicable here. The disorders include the same variety of clinical features already described under *causalgia* with additional manifestations. A predominance of muscular or joint symptoms has led to such designations as *pseudorheumatism* and *pseudoarthritis*. Often there is osteoporosis of the affected part, a development that may appear surprisingly early, leading to the term *acute bone atrophy*. The osteoporosis, among other aspects of the picture, was emphasized by Sudeck in a comprehensive series of papers beginning in 1900 and extending over 42 years.[30] Hence his name designates the illness in many publications. The common denominator in all these clinical pictures is, as in classical causalgia, relief by effective sympathetic blockade. By 1943 Livingston had already concluded that "the post-traumatic pain syndromes seem to be identical in type with the minor causalgias."[19] Bonica has taken the logical view that effective treatment by sympathetic denervation justifies classifying the entire group under one rubric.[5]

The extremely varied clinical presentation of the patients, often with features not typical for sympathetic hyperactivity, may lead to protracted futile therapy, eventuating in a final stage of nearly irreversible trophic changes. In the early stages of the disorder a burning or dull pain, which is worse on motion or other modest kinds of stimulation, appears in some portion of a limb, often distal. The skin is likely to be red, warm, sweaty, and edematous, with increased growth of nails and hair and decreased muscle tone. Even as soon as 4 to 8 weeks later, x-ray films may show some rarefaction in the subchondral spongiosa as compared with the normal side. By roughly the third month the picture may change, with subsidence of the spontaneous pain, although pain on motion or weight bearing results in continuation of the relative immobilization of the limb. The skin may change to a reddish gray or pale color and become shiny, dry, and cool; this is accompanied by brittle nails and loss of hair. The edema becomes sclerotic; the atonic muscles atrophy. The x-ray films now show many bony rarefactions, with coarse residual lines of bone both in the shafts and the epiphyses (Figs. 235-1, 235-2).

Predisposing factors to such a picture are extraordinarily wide-ranging. Any kind of trauma to joints, bones, nerves, or any soft tissue may seem to set off the astonishing train of events described. Phlebothromboses or phlebitis, angina pectoris, myocardial infarction (shoulder-hand syndrome), pulmonary embolism, skin disorders such as scleroderma, and even drug toxicity have all been implicated as predisposing factors. There seems to be almost an inverse relationship between the severity of the injury and the magnitude of the abnormality. White and Sweet describe a patient who developed the syndrome successively in three limbs after trivial injuries to each.[36] She did have a long history of cool, cyanotic, sweaty hands and feet. Such a patient confirms

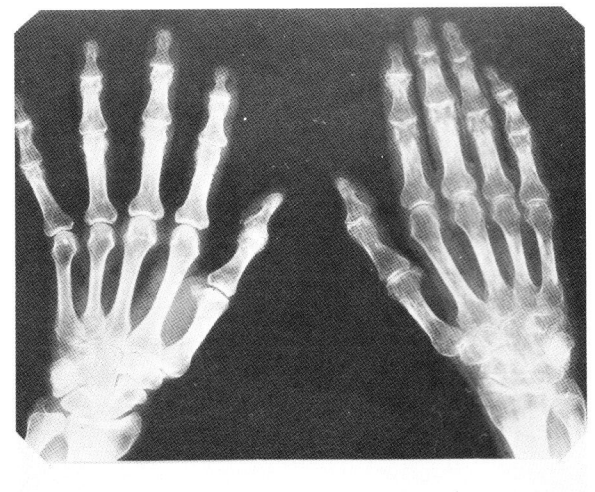

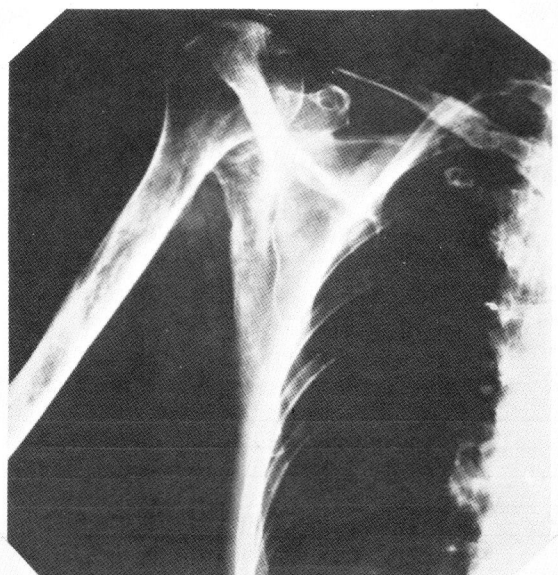

Figure 235-1 X-ray films of a 74-year-old male. He exhibits decalcification of the right hand, upper humerus, and scapula 2 years after the onset of crippling pain from a fall with dislocation of the right shoulder. He had pain throughout the limb distal to the elbow. His hand and forearm were kept constantly covered with a towel and supported on a pillow. He experienced intense pain on exposure of his hand and forearm to cool air or touch. (From White and Sweet.[36])

analysis of each case. Psychogenic factors are much more likely to confound the picture. Arieff et al. reported seven patients in whom determination to secure financial compensation appeared to be the dominant factor maintaining the trophic disturbances and disability.[1] Shaw presented a sobering account of "pathologic malingering" simulating a painfully disabled extremity.[28] Mounting jury or workmen's compensation awards after injury are magnifying the problem. Anxiety over potential disability leads to actual disability in some patients.

I enjoy the collaboration of a psychiatrist especially skilled and interested in problems of chronic pain, a general policy in many pain relief centers. Brihaye and Violon describe a dramatic success of psychotherapy sustained at 6 years following 2½ years of fruitless focal treatment for painful disability from a wound of an index finger.[6] How-

Leriche's conclusion that "causalgia is a disease which must be regarded as a function of the temperament of the individual."[17] Unlike causalgia, the exciting event often does not set off the adverse train of events until days or weeks later, with a more gradual buildup of symptoms and signs. A number of cases develop as complications of therapy such as injections into or near nerves, tight-fitting casts, or minor operations. It is clear that the number of patients in these categories whose clinical presentation suggests a sympathetic etiology vastly exceeds the number with major causalgia.

The definitive diagnosis, however, requires a careful

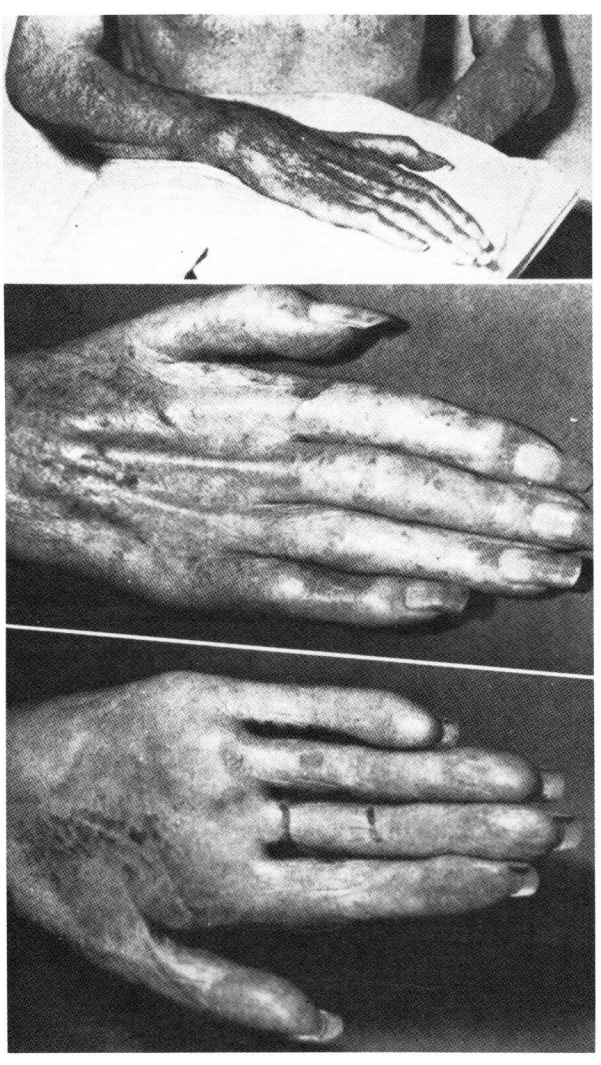

Figure 235-2 The patient whose x-ray films are shown in Fig. 235-1. The right hand shows atrophic skin and muscles. The fingernails are uncut because of pain. He had poor return of mobility to his rigid fingers despite lasting relief of pain from one block of the stellate ganglion. (From White and Sweet.[36])

ever, as in patients with major causalgia, many of these patients considered to have a psychalgia prove after consistent relief by sympathetic blocks to have a sympathalgia. Many more temporary sympathetic blocking procedures are advisable than are fruitful in major causalgia.

Thus at my fifth performance of a stellate block in one patient disabled by pain referred to an injured hand, I was called to the phone after barely putting the needle through the skin. I returned to find the patient pounding with his injured hand on the x-ray table and pronouncing this the best block yet. A more intensive exploration revealed major psychiatric problems in a man whom we had all assessed as a stable, stolid Swede.[36]

The sympathetic dystrophies are more susceptible to cure by single or oft-repeated blocks than the major causalgias. Bonica even estimates from seven publications an 80 percent cure rate by this approach, supplemented of course by vigorous physical therapy.[5] Of 17 patients treated by the regional intravenous guanethidine method of Hannington-Kiff, 7 "maintained great improvement" after one session and 5 more did so after the second session.[13]

The relief following block should be complete if sympathectomy is to be advised. But even full relief of pain after two or three technically successful sympathetic blocks is probably not an adequate basis to recommend the operation. We have made the mistake ourselves of moving too soon to surgery[36] and have seen many other patients in whom surgical sympathetic denervation has failed despite temporary relief after a block. The trivial character of an injury followed by severe pain widespread in a limb should not lead automatically to the assumption that sympathectomy is in order. We have seen one patient in whom pain following digital puncture with a rose thorn was unrelieved by T2–8 sympathectomy although the injury produced a hot, dry hand.[32] This caveat must, however, be followed by the same warm recommendation for sympathectomy that applies to major causalgia once the consistent benefit of temporary blocks is unequivocal and repetitions thereof are giving inadequate sustained relief. Wirth and Rutherford summarize the results of five reports in this type of patient; 95 of 108 patients were either totally relieved or significantly improved.[37]

A variety of other forms of surgical treatment have been advocated for causalgia and the various syndromes in the general category of sympathetic or Sudeck's atrophy or dystrophy. The failure to assess relief from sympathetic denervation as part of the diagnostic appraisal makes it impossible to compare these modes of therapy with those described here, the more so since some authors use the terms in a loose fashion to include many categories of burning or other pain.

Pathogenesis of Causalgia and Sympathetic Dystrophy

Since causalgic pain usually sets in soon after injury, it cannot be attributable to a slowly evolving process such as fibrosis or neuroma formation.

Damage to Non-Neural Tissues

The associated artery was damaged in 23 percent of Barnes' 48 cases of causalgia,[3] in 31 percent of the 70 cases of Omer and Thomas,[26] and in 25 percent of Carayon and Bourrel's 150 cases.[8] However 67 percent of the combined vasculoneural lesions of the latter authors occurred in those who developed causalgia. The mechanism whereby the arterial injury affects the nerve has yet to be demonstrated. Ischemic lesions in the tissues, hypothesized by many from Leriche onward, have not been shown to be etiologic.

Wound Infection

Although Mitchell believed that infection in the wound predisposed to causalgia, subsequent studies have not borne this out. However, infection is one of the factors predisposing to sympathetic dystrophy.

The "Artificial Synapse" of Injury

Granit et al. found in experimental animals that injury to a mixed motor-sensory nerve permitted efferent impulses descending the nerve to set off at the site of injury an afferent discharge, which was recordable from the sensory root when the motor root was stimulated.[11] Doupe et al. hypothesized that tonic efferent sympathetic impulses to such structures as blood vessels jump at the "artificial synapse" of injury to the adjoining small sensory fibers, including those mediating pain.[9] The known increase in tonic efferent sympathetic discharge accompanying physical or emotional stress would explain the characteristic increase in pain at such times. That afferent fibers from the limbs traveling via the sympathetic nerves are involved seems unlikely, since neither Walker and Nulsen[34] nor White and Sweet[36] have, except in rare instances, elicited pain in the upper limb in patients without causalgia by stimulating the upper thoracic sympathetic trunk or ganglia. However, the former authors demonstrated in three patients with causalgia that stimulation of the decentralized upper thoracic sympathetic ganglia caused a tingling burning pain, which developed slowly over 4 to 20 s and paralleled the pilomotor response. The great reduction during sleep of activity in the autonomic centers in the hypothalamus likewise explains why these patients tend to sleep well. Barnes has added the concept that antidromic as well as orthodromic conduction in the sensory fibers occurs at the artificial synapse.[3] The antidromic impulses cause release of a vasodilator substance at the periphery, which Barnes suggests may reduce the threshold of sensory stimulation or even itself set up centripetal impulses, accounting for the extreme sensitivity of the skin. This theory of the artificial or "ephaptic" synapse has enjoyed tentative widespread acceptance despite some facts that it does not explain. These are: (1) excision of the entire zone of nerve injury carried out in a few of the patients with a complete lesion has not always relieved the pain. For example, in the series of Kirklin et al. such an operation gave complete relief in two patients, some relief in one, and no sustained relief at all in two others.[15] (2) The pain may spread far beyond the domain of the impaired nerve or nerves. Loh and Nathan and Leriche cite examples of the spread of pain from a lesion of a single nerve to finally include the whole forequarter of the body.[17,20] (3) One standard type of successful sympathectomy for the lower limb does not include the first lumbar ganglion and tends to produce anhidrosis only from the knee down. Yet the wound in the great majority of patients is above the knee, so that at least some efferent sympathetic fibers probably remain intact at the site of the lesion.

A crucial observation is that the Hannington-Kiff regional guanethidine block procedure has relieved the pain even when the sphygmomanometer cuff has been applied distal to the lesion on the peripheral nerve.[20] Since artificial synapses at the site of injury would be unaffected by the distally injected drug, the pain should continue if these were the responsible mechanism. An abnormal action of norepinephrine (NE) at peripheral sympathetic terminals, producing hyperpathia and hyperesthesia, may prove the more likely explanation. Wall and Gutnick demonstrated that regenerating fibers after transection of a rat's sciatic nerve are constantly firing and that this response is increased by NE.[35] That a spreading hypersensitivity to the peripherally secreted NE occurs is indicated by the fact that guanethidine, replacing NE at all such terminals distal to the constricting cuff, stops all abnormal sensitivity below the cuff and not just that in the domain of the injured nerves. Moreover the 4- to 20-s delay in the slow buildup of pain in the three causalgia patients of Walker and Nulsen whose upper thoracic sympathetic ganglia were stimulated is better explained by a slow buildup of NE at the nerve terminals than by an instantaneous electrical excitation at the artificial synapse and prompt conduction back into the cord. As Hannington-Kiff points out, both patients with causalgia and those with the less circumscribed injuries of Sudeck's atrophy and sympathetic dystrophy may be successfully treated by regional blocks with guanethidine.[13,14] This makes it likely that the abnormal mechanism at the nerve terminals is operative in both types of patient. Hence a new mechanism need not be hypothesized to account for the sympathetic dystrophies. The unusual case of Gordon in which the successful surgical treatment was all distal also suggests abnormal response to the NE.[10]

Loh and Nathan have presented evidence that in 21 of 31 cases involving a variety of other hyperpathic states accompanied by constant pain, in which peripheral nerves, posterior root ganglia, nerve roots, or the spinal cord were involved, the pain and hyperpathia were relieved by sympathetic block.[20] This was true in only 2 of 15 such patients in whom the pain was not accompanied by hyperpathia. These observations point to a more general tendency to abnormal responses to NE as a cause of some of these painful states.

Torebjörk and Hallin have addressed the next logical question, namely identification of the structures responding abnormally to NE.[33]

> They studied a patient with causalgia of a hand recurrent after relief from a sympathectomy and recurrent despite removal of regenerating sympathetic fibers. Her temperature thresholds for pain with heat and with cold were greatly reduced in the painful hand as compared with the normal hand. An intracutaneous injection of only 1 μg of NE lowered these thresholds still further, triggering a severe attack of pain in the entire limb lasting hours despite large doses of intramuscular morphine. No such reaction was provoked from the healthy hand and does not occur in normal people. When local anesthesia of superficial cutaneous nerve endings was induced in her by topical application of Ketocaine, the intracutaneous injection of NE no longer produced an attack of pain or a substantial reduction in the thresholds of temperatures causing pain. This establishes that one major site of action of the NE is the cutaneous nerve endings. In further direct records from peripheral nerves on this patient they showed that populations of both A and C fibers were abnormally reactive to NE at nerve endings.

In four more causalgia patients studied after relief from their pain by sympathectomy, intracutaneous injections of NE into previously painful areas of skin still dramatically reduced the pain thresholds to both mechanical and cold cutaneous stimuli from normal levels.[12] When the limb nerves were compressed by inflating a blood pressure cuff, the hyperalgesia was abolished only after perceptions of touch and cold had disappeared. Warmth and delayed pain were still perceived. These results indicate that myelinated (A) fibers were signaling pain from the NE-sensitized skin rather than suppressing pain as described by Meyer and Fields.[22] Of their eight patients with causalgia, six obtained significant relief by electrical stimulation selective for the large fibers in the injured peripheral nerve proximal to the lesion.[16] In two patients this was so effective that neither required sympathectomy or surgery directly on the injured nerve. The mechanism responsible for the pain and hyperpathia in some afferent fibers related to the peripherally secreted NE remains to be elucidated.[16]

That impulses over afferent fibers in the posterior roots may be related to the pain in some areas is demonstrated by our patient Lillian T., whose pain was in the ulnar distribution.[36] She secured complete relief but for only several months after each of a series of five upper thoracic sympathectomies and a cervicothoracic ganglionectomy. With the fifth recurrence there was also return of sudomotor and vasoconstrictor reflexes. Our posterior rhizotomy at the C8-T1 level has kept her pain-free.

That abnormal central excitatory states in the spinal cord aggravate and sustain the problem has been urged on us by Livingston,[19] Sunderland,[31] and Loh and Nathan,[20] among many others.[32] However, critically designed and executed objective studies to support any of their hypotheses remain to be made.

That the neural impulses for pain in this disorder may traverse customary pathways for somatic pain is indicated by the patient of Birkenfeld and Fisher.[4] An incomplete sympathectomy did not relieve pain in the upper limb. These surgeons then carried out a bulbar spinothalamic tractotomy, producing contralateral analgesia up to the C1 level with relief of pain. The astounding ease with which a huge variety of physical and psychic stimuli trigger worsening of the pain in major causalgia certainly points also to a role for the cerebrum in these patients. Yet the abrupt success that so often attends peripheral sympathetic denervation makes it clear that this widespread hyperexcitability may happily be subject to a decisive, simply evoked peripheral control.

References

1. Arieff AJ, Bell JL, Tigay EL: Reflex physiopathic disturbances. Surg Gynecol Obstet 118:1029–1034, 1964.
2. Ascherl R, Blümel G: Zum Krankheitsbild der Sudeck'schen Dystrophie. Fortschr Med 99:712–720, 1981.
3. Barnes R: Causalgia: A review of 48 cases, in Seddon HJ (ed): *Peripheral Nerve Injuries*. Medical Research Council Special Report Series No 282, London, Her Majesty's Stationery Office, 1954, pp 156–185.
4. Birkenfeld R, Fisher RG: Successful treatment of causalgia of upper extremity with medullary spinothalamic tractotomy. J Neurosurg 20:303–311, 1963.
5. Bonica JJ: Causalgia and other reflex sympathetic dystrophies, in Bonica JJ, Liebeskind JC, Albe-Fessard DG (eds): *Advances in Pain Research and Therapy, vol 3*. New York, Raven Press, 1979, pp 141–166.
6. Brihaye J, Violon A: La douleur causalgique: À propos d'un cas. Acta Chir Belg 77:195–200, 1978.
7. Buker RH, Cox WA, Scully TJ, Seitter G, Pauling FW: Causalgia and transthoracic sympathectomy. Am J Surg 124:724–727, 1972.
8. Carayon A, Bourrel P: Indications et résultats du traitement chirurgical précoce de 150 causalgies. Ann Chir 17:554–560, 1963.
9. Doupe J, Cullen CH, Chance GQ: Post-traumatic pain and the causalgic syndrome. J Neurol Neurosurg Psychiatry 7:33–48, 1944.
10. Gordon S: Causalgia: A case report. Plast Reconstr Surg 28:417–419, 1961.
11. Granit R, Leksell L, Skoglund CR: Fibre interaction in injured or compressed region of nerve. Brain 67:125–140, 1944.
12. Hallin RG, Torebjörk HE: Observations on hyperalgesia in the causalgia pain syndrome. Presented at the 2d World Congress on Pain, Seattle, 1978.
13. Hannington-Kiff JG: Relief of Sudeck's atrophy by regional intravenous guanethidine. Lancet 1:1132–1133, 1977.
14. Hannington-Kiff JG: Relief of causalgia in limbs by regional intravenous guanethidine. Br Med J 2:367–368, 1979.
15. Kirklin JW, Chenoweth AI, Murphey F: Causalgia: A review of its characteristics, diagnosis, and treatment. Surgery 21:321–342, 1947.
16. Krainick JU, Biehl G, Fischer D, Loew F: Die Behandlung des Sudeck-Syndroms durch Neurostimulation. Dtsch Med Wochenschr 105:1637–1638, 1980.
17. Leriche R: *The Surgery of Pain*. London, Baillière, Tindall and Cox, 1939.
18. Lidz T, Payne RL Jr: Causalgia: Report of recovery following relief of emotional stress. Arch Neurol Psychiatry 53:222–225, 1945.
19. Livingston WK: *Pain Mechanisms: A Physiologic Interpretation of Causalgia and its Related States*. New York, MacMillan, 1943, pp 83–99.
20. Loh L, Nathan PW: Painful peripheral states and sympathetic blocks. J Neurol Neurosurg Psychiatry 41:664–671, 1978.
21. Mayfield FH: *Causalgia*. Springfield, Ill, Charles C Thomas, 1951.
22. Meyer GA, Fields HL: Causalgia treated by selective large fibre stimulation of peripheral nerve. Brain 95:163–168, 1972.
23. Mitchell SW: *Injuries of Nerves and Their Consequences*. Philadelphia, Lippincott, 1872.
24. Mitchell SW, Morehouse GR, Keen WW: *Gunshot Wounds and Other Injuries of Nerves*. Philadelphia, Lippincott, 1864.
25. Nathan PW: On the pathogenesis of causalgia in peripheral nerve injuries. Brain 70:145–170, 1947.
26. Omer G, Thomas S: Treatment of causalgia: Review of cases at Brooke General Hospital. Tex Med 67:93–96, 1971.
27. Rasmussen TB, Freedman H: Treatment of causalgia: An analysis of 100 cases. J Neurosurg 3:165–173, 1946.
28. Shaw RS: Pathologic malingering: The painful disabled extremity. N Engl J Med 271:22–26, 1964.
29. Spurling RG: Causalgia of the upper extremity: Treatment by dorsal sympathetic ganglionectomy. Arch Neurol Psychiatry 23:784–788, 1930.
30. Sudeck P: Über die akute entzündliche Knochenatrophie. Arch Klin Chir 62:147–156, 1900.
31. Sunderland S: Pain mechanisms in causalgia. J Neurol Neurosurg Psychiatry 39:471–480, 1976.
32. Sweet WH: Otfrid Foerster Lecture: Stimulation of the posterior columns of the spinal cord for the suppression of chronic pain. Adv Neurosurg 7:219–242, 1979.
33. Torebjörk HE, Hallin RG: Microneurographic studies of peripheral pain mechanisms in man, in Bonica JJ, Liebeskind JC, Albe-Fessard DG (eds): *Advances in Pain Research and Therapy, vol 3*. New York, Raven Press, 1979, pp 121–131.
34. Walker AE, Nulsen F: Electrical stimulation of the upper thoracic portion of the sympathetic chain in man. Arch Neurol Psychiatry 59:559–560, 1948.
35. Wall PD, Gutnick M: Ongoing activity in peripheral nerves: The physiology and pharmacology of impulses originating from a neuroma. Exp Neurol 43:580–593, 1974.
36. White JC, Sweet WH: *Pain and the Neurosurgeon: A Forty-Year Experience*. Springfield, Ill, Charles C Thomas, 1969.
37. Wirth FP Jr, Rutherford RB: A civilian experience with causalgia. Arch Surg 100:633–638, 1970.

SECTION C
Nerve Tumors

236
Neoplasms of Peripheral Nerves
Humberto Cravioto

Peripheral nerve tumors are growths that appear in cranial or other peripheral nerves, including the sympathetic chain and adrenal gland nerves. Most tumors of peripheral nerves, excluding those of the sympathetic nervous system, are the result of neoplastic transformation, usually benign, of Schwann cells. In those cases of Schwann cell tumors that involve a genetic abnormality (von Recklinghausen's disease) there are degenerative, hamartomatous, or neoplastic changes in other organs. In this disease single or multiple meningiomas and gliomas of the nervous system occur, in addition to nerve sheath tumors.[6,9,16]

Peripheral nerve sheath tumors (schwannomas) have been called *perineurial fibroblastomas* on the basis of the idea that these tumors arise from perineurial fibroblasts.[16] They have also been designated *neurinomas* or *neurilemmomas* because they arise in a nerve or nerve sheath. The terms *acoustic neurinoma* and *acoustic neuroma* have been used extensively to describe the schwannoma arising in the eighth cranial nerve. Peripheral nerve tumors in von Recklinghausen's disease have been considered mostly a disorderly arrangement of nerve fibers in a mass of connective tissue. Neurofibromas and plexiform neurofibromas have been thought to be variants of peripheral nerve sheath cells.[6] It has been suggested that the term *neurofibroma*, which has been applied to different neoplastic or even non-neoplastic conditions, be discarded.[6]

At our institution we prefer to call most of these peripheral nerve tumors *nerve sheath tumors*. In this chapter *schwannoma* has been used interchangeably with *nerve sheath tumor*.

On histological as well as ultrastructural and tissue culture grounds the cell of origin of most peripheral nerve sheath tumors is the Schwann cell.[2,3,16] This includes the solitary schwannoma as well as the so-called neurofibroma, usually seen in von Recklinghausen's disease. To every benign form of peripheral nerve tumor (and most of these tumors are benign) there corresponds a rare but distinct malignant form in which the cells of origin become anaplastic and, on rare occasions, may even invade neighboring structures or metastasize. Invasion and metastases are more common in tumors of the sympathetic nervous system.

Peripheral Nerve Tumors

Schwannoma

Peripheral nerve sheath tumors (Figs. 236-1 through 236-6) arise most frequently in sensory nerves and in females more often than in males (at a ratio of about 3:1). They frequently affect the acoustic nerve (vestibular branch), occasionally the trigeminal nerve, and rarely the oculomotor and other cranial nerves. The most frequent location of an intracranial schwannoma is the cerebellopontine angle. Intracranial schwannomas form about 10 percent of all primary intracranial tumors. Other frequent sites include the spinal sensory (very rarely motor) nerve roots and other peripheral nerves. Nerve sheath tumors occur in the distal portions of the cranial or spinal nerves and rarely penetrate the pia mater. Oc-

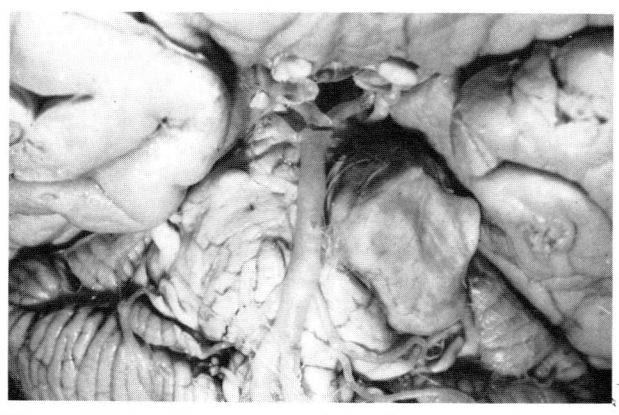

Figure 236-1 Schwannoma of the eighth cranial nerve (acoustic neuroma). Note the well-circumscribed, smooth, coarsely lobulated cerebellopontine angle tumor. (×0.5).

Neoplasms of Peripheral Nerves

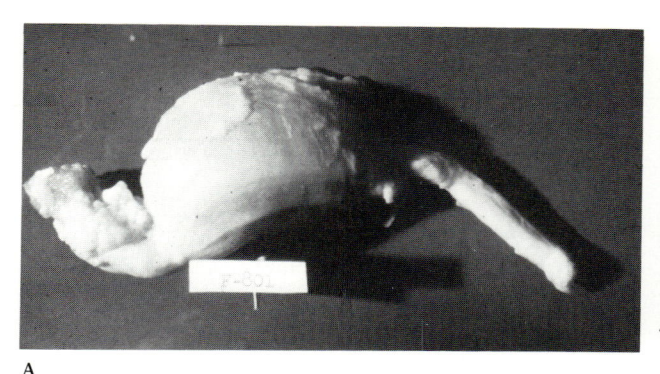

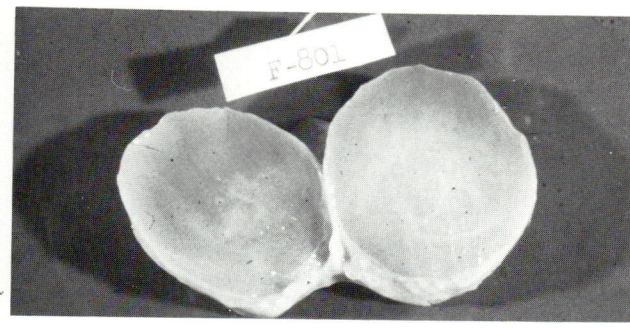

Figure 236-2 Schwannoma arising in the sciatic nerve. *A.* Note the marked enlargement of the middle of the nerve and the smooth outer surface of the tumor. *B.* On cross-section, note the diffuse growth of the nerve and the glassy appearance. (*A* and *B* ×2.7).

casionally there may be bilateral schwannomas of the acoustic nerve, in which case a forme fruste of von Recklinghausen's disease may be suspected. Solitary schwannomas may be part of full-blown von Recklinghausen's disease.

Gross Appearance

Schwann cell tumors are firm, well circumscribed, and apparently (although not actually) encapsulated. Cystic degeneration may occur when the tumor is large. The tumor may be lobulated. The cut surface is granular, with broad or punctate yellowish areas and at times areas of fresh hemorrhage. A rubbery texture, occasionally with a whorling pattern reminiscent of a meningioma, may also be seen. Clear distinction between a meningioma and a nerve sheath tumor arising in the cerebellopontine angle may be difficult on gross inspection only.

Microscopic Appearance

Schwannomas are usually composed of dense (Antony type A) and loose-meshed (Antony type B) tissues, which may be sharply distinct although they often merge imperceptibly into one another (Fig. 236-4). The dense areas appear as interwoven bundles of long bipolar cells with an ovoid, uniform, somewhat elongated nucleus and indistinct nucleoli. The cytoplasm forms long, thin, and usually pale processes. The cell bundles are frequently arranged in whorls of varying size, at times in an onionlike fashion. True palisading of tumor cells (Verocay body) formation, which may be characteristic of nerve sheath tumors, is noted more frequently in spinal than in acoustic tumors. Collagen and reticulin fibers are present throughout, usually alongside the tumor cells. The Antony type B tissue consists of polymorphic but usually stellate-shaped cells containing ovoid nuclei and widely separated from each other by a finely honeycombed eosinophilic matrix. Collagen and reticulin fibers are much less abundant than in the dense areas. Typical foam cells with a round eccentric nucleus and a distinct, irregularly round cell membrane (phagocytes) are present in both dense and loose-meshed areas but more frequently in the latter. The phagocytic cells contain abundant sudano-

philic birefringent lipid material, which stains bright red with Oil Red O in frozen sections of formalin-fixed material. Myelinated or unmyelinated axons are rarely seen. Cystic degeneration probably occurs more frequently in the loose-meshed than in the dense areas. It has been suggested that the loose-meshed areas as well as the phagocytes may represent areas of degeneration of the dense areas. A true connective tissue capsule forming a lamina distinct from the tumor is not seen in schwannomas, although these tumors are well circumscribed and sharply delineated from the nerve of origin. Blood vessels, often thrombosed (at times leading to small areas of necrosis), are also seen. In the stroma a few fibroblasts are noted, as well as old hemorrhage in the form of macrophages containing hemosiderin pigment. Mitoses are not seen. An occasional cell with a large, irregularly shaped, dense nucleus may be seen, but this is not a sign of malignancy.

Under the electron microscope both the dense and loose-meshed areas of schwannomas show cells in which the cytoplasm forms bundles of very thin, long processes in intimate contact with each other or with similar processes of neigh-

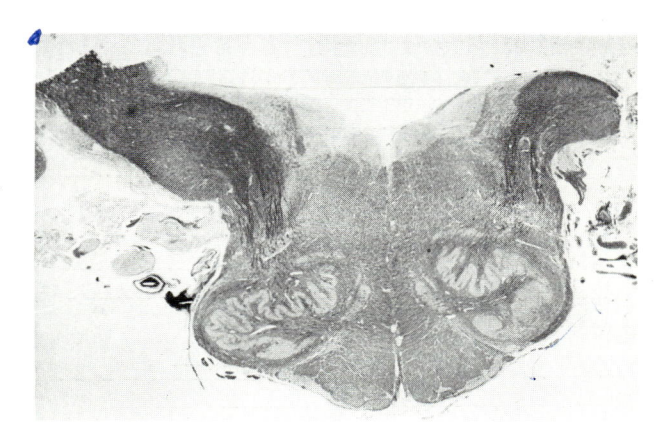

Figure 236-3 Bilateral schwannomas (neurofibromas, nerve sheath tumors) of the acoustic nerves in a 24-year-old female with multiple central and peripheral nerve sheath tumors and an early glioma of the cerebrum (von Recklinghausen's disease). Note the marked focal enlargement of the acoustic nerves (×3.7).

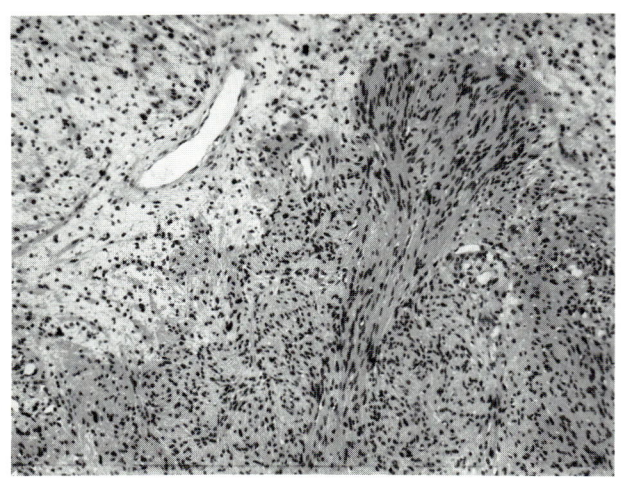

Figure 236-4 Light microscopic picture of a schwannoma. In the lower part of the picture is the dense cellular portion of the tumor with a tendency to form whorls; on the left is the loose-meshed area. There are no axons. (Hematoxylin and eosin, ×83.)

boring cells (Fig. 236-6).[3,4] The abundant smooth endoplasmic reticulum is responsible for the formation of these processes. The tumor cells appear surrounded by a basement membrane, native collagen, and a few fibroblasts. The intervening space in the loose-meshed areas either appears empty or contains fine granular material or bundles of fine filaments. The dense areas, and only rarely the loose-meshed areas, contain banded fusiform fibers of 1400-Å repeating macroperiods (long-spacing fibrous collagen). Some tumors, usually the very small ones, show a few myelinated as well as unmyelinated axis cylinders covered with hyperplastic Schwann cell cytoplasm. Schwann cells, not fibroblasts, appear to form the bulk of both dense and loose-meshed areas of nerve sheath tumors. This appears to be true of both solitary schwannomas, schwannomas in von Recklinghausen's disease, and so-called neurofibromas in the presence or absence of other pathological changes seen in von Recklinghausen's disease. The results of tissue culture studies of nerve sheath tumors also accord with the notion that nerve sheath tumors are derived from Schwann cells.[5]

By means of complement fixation tests and immunocytochemistry schwannomas have been shown to contain a high level of S-100 protein. This fact serves to indicate that Schwann cell tumors are of neuroectodermal origin.[11]

Malignant Schwannoma

Malignancy is a rare phenomenon in a solitary schwannoma, especially an intracranial schwannoma. It appears more frequently in the multiple peripheral nerve sheath tumors seen in von Recklinghausen's disease and in single nerve sheath tumors of the spinal roots and other peripheral nerves. The malignant schwannomas may be compared with fibrosarcomas involving peripheral nerves but are limited to the nerves themselves. These malignant tumors usually remain localized although at times they may infiltrate adjacent structures and even metastasize, usually to the lungs.

Malignant schwannomas have a tendency to recur. Anaplastic changes are noted microscopically. The Schwann cells are moderately to markedly increased in number, mitoses are frequent, and areas of necrosis are prominent. In areas the tumor cells are no longer bipolar and elongated but have become distinctly pleomorphic. Cartilage and osteoid tissue may appear. On occasion, a so-called triton tumor appears, in which case there seems to be transformation of a malignant schwannoma into a rhabdomyosarcoma.[17] This again is usually associated with von Recklinghausen's disease. Benign "triton" tumors in the absence of von Recklinghausen's disease have also been reported.[12]

Neurofibroma

A neurofibroma is a tumor of peripheral nerves composed of Schwann cells (Figs. 236-3, 236-5). It may, and frequently does, occur in a peripheral nerve of a patient with von Recklinghausen's disease (neurofibromatosis). The term *neurofibroma* has been applied to peripheral nerve neoplasms arising in the presence of von Recklinghausen's neurofibromatosis, to peripheral nerve alterations frequently seen in this disease, which may be degenerative or hamartomatous, and even to neoplasms not originating in but involving peripheral nerves.[6] Therefore, use of the term *neurofibroma* or *neurofibrosarcoma* to refer to a benign or malignant nerve sheath tumor in von Recklinghausen's disease probably should be discouraged.[6] The proper designation of such a tumor would be *schwannoma* or *peripheral nerve sheath tumor*.

So-called neurofibromas appear grossly as enlargements of a nerve. These are usually multiple and may affect intracranial, spinal, peripheral (neck, trunk, limbs), and sympa-

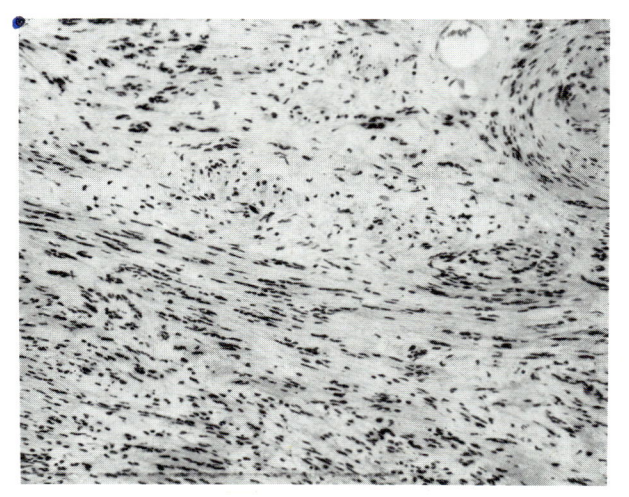

Figure 236-5 Light microscopic picture of a spinal (cervical) dumbbell-shaped schwannoma (neurofibroma) in a 52-year-old female with von Recklinghausen's disease. The patient had quadriparesis and a neurogenic bladder. A whorl is noted in the right upper corner. Note a "nerve" running through the middle of the field. There were many axons throughout this tumor. (Hematoxylin and eosin, ×83.)

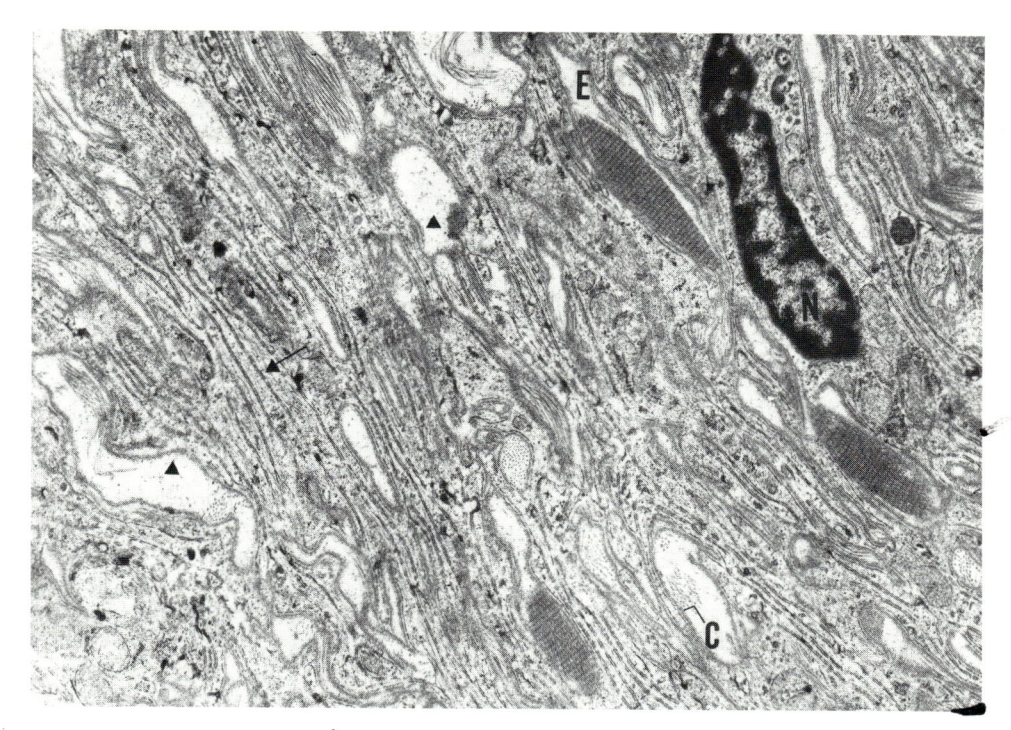

Figure 236-6 Electron microscopic picture of a dense area of a schwannoma of the eighth nerve (acoustic neuroma). Note the three banded structures (fibrous long-spacing collagen) in the extracellular space (E). The arrowheads point to the basement membrane. The arrow points to closely opposed cell membranes. N, nucleus of Schwann cell; C, collagen. (×11,620.)

thetic nerves. These enlargements may be cylindrical (plexiform neurofibroma) or fusiform. Occasionally they may be of great size, arising in the neck, mediastinum, or retroperitoneal spaces.

On cross section the granular or whorling pattern as well as the cystic degeneration characteristic of pure schwannomas may not be seen. The differences between pure schwannomas and neurofibromas consist in the scantier number of Schwann cells, the increase of collagen and reticulin fibers, and the constant presence of myelinated and unmyelinated axis cylinders in neurofibromas. In neurofibromas there is a wide separation of individual fibers by a relatively poorly cellular tissue lacking an orderly architectural arrangement. At times, an otherwise typical schwannoma is seen within a disorderly growth containing abundant collagen and axis cylinders (schwannoma within a neurofibroma). Melanin may on occasion be present in neurofibromas as well as in schwannomas.[16]

Malignant changes in neurofibromas are as frequent as or more frequent than those in schwannomas. Such changes usually occur in the presence of other manifestations of von Recklinghausen's neurofibromatosis. As with the schwannoma, malignant changes in a neurofibroma consist of an increased number of pleomorphic cells, multinucleated giant cells, mitoses, and necrosis. Also, blood vessels may become anaplastic. There may be metastatic lesions (usually in the lungs), which may take the form of angiosarcomas.

Granular Cell Myoblastoma

The granular cell myoblastoma has been described in peripheral nerves as a growth of Schwann cells.[1] It is not clear whether a granular cell myoblastoma is a true neoplasm or represents a lipid metabolic disturbance of Schwann cells giving a granular appearance to the cytoplasm of proliferated cells.[1,13] These tumors frequently appear as incidental autopsy findings in the neurohypophysis.[15] In this location they have been called *choristomas* or *pituicytomas*. Some authors have suggested that granular cell myoblastomas of the neurohypophysis probably represent granular cell tumors derived from Schwann cells.[15] Granular cell tumors, histologically and ultrastructurally similar to tumors arising in peripheral nerves, have also been described in the central nervous system.[13] It has been suggested that in central as well as in peripheral granular cell tumors more than one cell type may be involved.[13]

Hemangioma and Hemangioblastoma

These lesions have been described in peripheral nerves, at times in association with von Recklinghausen's disease. They are extremely rare.

Peripheral Neuron Tumors

Ganglioneuroma

This is a benign tumor composed of mature neurons, neuronal processes, Schwann cells, and collagen. It occurs in children and young adults. Care must be taken not to confuse these true neuron tumors with schwannomas or neurofibromas that in the course of their growth have incorporated a few neurons. Ganglioneuromas occur most frequently in the posterior mediastinum but also occur in the retroperitoneal area, the adrenals, and the dorsolumbar spinal ganglia. They are usually large, hard, well circumscribed, and relatively uniform. The spinal forms are usually dumbbell-shaped and may simulate a larger than normal spinal ganglion.

Microscopically, single neurons or groups of neurons, at times in rows, are noted. The neurons may show capsule cells and at times appear degenerated, with cyst formation, fatty change, and calcification. There is little or no Nissl substance in the neurons, which are often bi- or multinucleated. The tumors show a profusion of mostly unmyelinated axis cylinders, connective tissue in varying amounts, and foci of lymphocytes. These tumors contain abundant Schwann cells, but it is not clear whether they are reactive or neoplastic.[7] The ganglioneuroma is considered by some authors to be a form of maturation of a pre-existing neuroblastoma.[7] In this view, ganglioneuromas are embryonic tumors composed of cells that may continue to mature even after becoming neoplastic. Electron microscopy makes it possible to identify abundant endoplasmic reticulum and many dense-core vesicles, neurofilaments, microtubules, and synapses.[8] An association between ganglioneuromas and von Recklinghausen's disease has also been emphasized, especially in cases in which neurofibromas are seen in addition to single or multiple ganglioneuromas.

Neuroblastoma

The neuroblastoma is an embryonic neuronal tumor, usually found in children under the age of 4; it may even be congenital.[7,16] It is a malignant tumor which infiltrates adjacent structures and metastasizes. The adrenal gland and the abdominal sympathetic ganglia are the most frequent sites of origin of the neuroblastoma.

Such tumors appear grossly as gray, encapsulated, large, soft, frequently lobulated masses with well-defined borders; they may appear cystic, hemorrhagic, and even calcified. Microscopically, neuroblastomas appear composed of immature primitive neurons (neuroblasts). They show highly cellular areas of small dark cells with very little ill-defined cytoplasm. Homer-Wright rosettes (pseudorosettes), characterized by a group of dark tumor cells with their processes extending toward the center of a circle to form a tangle of fibrils there, are found not infrequently. Mitotic figures are seen. At times foci of necrosis and hemorrhage are extensive. Invasion of veins and perivascular lymphatics may be evident. Infiltration of adjacent tissues such as the inferior vena cava, aorta, kidney, pancreas, liver, para-aortic lymph nodes, and lumbar vertebrae may be seen. Metastatic lesions are frequently seen involving the liver, long bones, skull, and lungs. Metastases to the brain substance are extremely rare.

It is possible that a neuroblastoma may differentiate (maturing of neurons) into a ganglioneuroma; a malignant tumor then becomes a benign tumor.[7,16] This process would indicate that there is a transition (intermediate stages) between neuroblastoma and ganglioneuroma (ganglioneuroblastoma). Regression or spontaneous arrest of a neuroblastoma, even after metastases have become apparent, may occasionally occur.

Increased urinary excretion of catecholamines has been observed in patients with neuroblastomas and occasionally found in their relatives as well.[8,10] The amines excreted in the urine are dopa, dopamine, vanillylmandelic acid, homovanillic acid, and 5-hydroxyindoleacetic acid.

Neuroblastoma may develop in the nasal cavity near the ethmoid sinus, usually in young adults. It may spread and invade the brain. Although it is a slow growth, nasal neuroblastoma recurs after excision and may metastasize. This tumor has also been called *esthesioneuroepithelioma* or *esthesioneurocytoma*. Electron microscopy demonstrates cytoplasmic filaments, neurotubules, dense-core vesicles, dystrophic axons, and synapses. This tumor is allegedly sensitive to radiation therapy.

Ganglioneuroblastoma

This tumor shows characteristics of both ganglioneuroma and neuroblastoma. In addition, it may show tissues that superficially resemble the glial tissues of the central nervous system.[7] A continuum of changes from neuroblasts to fully mature neurons is noted in ganglioneuroblastomas. The amount of primitive or well-developed (mature) neurons varies in different tumors and even within the same tumor. Schwann cells appear frequently in ganglioneuroblastomas but have not been demonstrated in neuroblastomas. It is questionable whether the Schwann cells are neoplastic or reactive in ganglioneuroblastomas. Since there are opposing tendencies of the tumor tissue, one toward maturation (ganglioneuroma) and the other toward anaplasia (neuroblastoma), the prognosis in terms of survival is very difficult to evaluate.[7,16]

Chemodectoma

This is a tumor with a typical "Zellballen" microscopic pattern occurring in the carotid body, glomus jugulare, glomus aorticum, or glomus intravagale.[14] It has also been called *nonchromaffin paraganglioma*. Since a comprehensive discussion appears in another chapter of this book, chemodectomas will not be discussed here.

Pheochromocytoma

This tumor, also designated *chromaffinoma, functionally active paraganglioma* (*chromaffin paraganglioma*), or *medullary adenoma* of the adrenal gland, is a tumor that secretes epinephrine and norepinephrine. Characteristically, these two amines produce crises of paroxysmal or persistent hypertension. Pheochromocytomas affect the adrenal gland in a great majority of cases and occur with next greatest frequency in sites where aberrant adrenal tissue may be present, such as the kidney, ileum, or inferior mesenteric vessels (probably arising in the organ of Zuckerkandl). Occasionally pheochromocytomas may affect both adrenals. Most cases of pheochromocytoma occur in individuals between 30 and 60 years of age but children and the elderly may also be affected.

The great majority of pheochromocytomas are histologically benign. Grossly these tumors are usually small (about 5 cm or less in maximum diameter), but very small (less than 1 cm in diameter) as well as very large (20 cm in diameter) examples have been recorded. They are smooth, well encapsulated, and frequently show hemorrhages. The cut surface usually becomes darker with exposure to light. Microscopically, these tumors show cell masses forming alveoli and are separated from each other by strands of connective tissue and numerous thin-walled vessels. The tumor cells resemble the large cells of the adrenal medulla, with a finely granular cytoplasm. Multinucleated cells as well as large bizarre cells with large amounts of chromatin may be seen. The tumor is usually highly vascularized. Foci of lymphocytes may also be seen. On electron microscopy the tumor cells show 40 to 200 μm diameter dense-core granules.[8,10] No neuronal processes or synapses are noted. It is usually very difficult to determine on morphological grounds alone whether or not a pheochromocytoma will metastasize even in those cases that appear microscopically malignant.

References

1. Budzilovich GN: Granular cell "myoblastoma" of vagus nerve. Acta Neuropathol (Berl) 10:162–165, 1968.
2. Cravioto H: Studies on the normal ultrastructure of peripheral nerve: Axis cylinders, Schwann cells and myelin. Bull Los Angeles Neurol Soc 30:169–190, 1965.
3. Cravioto H: The ultrastructure of acoustic nerve tumors. Acta Neuropathol (Berl) 12:116–140, 1969.
4. Cravioto H, Lockwood R: Long-spacing fibrous collagen in human acoustic nerve tumors: In vivo and in vitro observations. J Ultrastruct Res 24:70–85, 1968.
5. Cravioto H, Lockwood R: The behavior of acoustic neuroma in tissue culture. Acta Neuropathol (Berl) 12:141–157, 1969.
6. Feigin I: The nerve sheath tumor, solitary and in von Recklinghausen's disease: A unitary mesenchymal concept. Acta Neuropathol (Berl) 17:188–200, 1971.
7. Feigin I, Cohen M: Maturation and anaplasia in neuronal tumors of the peripheral nervous system; With observations on the glia-like tissues in the ganglioneuroblastoma. J Neuropathol Exp Neurol 36:748–763, 1977.
8. Greenberg R, Rosenthal I, Falk GS: Electronmicroscopy of human tumors secreting catecholamines: Correlation with biochemical data. J Neuropathol Exp Neurol 28:475–500, 1969.
9. Harkin JC, Reed RJ: *Tumors of the Peripheral Nervous System*. Washington, Armed Forces Institute of Pathology, 1969.
10. Hermann H, Mornex R: *Human Tumours Secreting Catecholamines: Clinical and Physiopathological Study of the Pheochromocytomas*. Oxford, Pergamon Press, 1964.
11. Jacque CM, Kujas M, Poreau A, Raoul M, Collier P, Racadot J, Baumann N: GFA and S-100 protein levels as an index for malignancy in human gliomas and neurinomas. J Natl Cancer Inst 62:479–483, 1979.
12. Markel SF, Enginger FM: Neuromuscular hamartoma—A benign "triton tumor" composed of mature neural and striated muscle elements. Cancer 49:140–144, 1982.
13. Markesbery WR, Duffy PE, Cowen D: Granular cell tumors of the central nervous system. J Neuropathol Exp Neurol 32:92–109, 1973.
14. Murphy TE, Huvos AG, Frazell EL: Chemodectomas of the glomus intravagale: Vagal body tumors, nonchromaffin paragangliomas of the nodose ganglion of the vagus nerve. Ann Surg 172:246–255, 1970.
15. Popovitch ER, Sutton CH, Becker NH, Zimmerman HM: Fine structure and histochemical studies of choristomas of the neurohypophysis. J Neuropathol Exp Neurol 29:155–156, 1970 (abstr).
16. Russell DS, Rubinstein LJ: *Pathology of Tumours of the Nervous System*, 4th ed. Baltimore, Williams & Wilkins, 1977, pp 372–436.
17. Woodruff JM, Chernik NL, Smith MC, Millett WB, Foote FW: Peripheral nerve tumors with rhabdomyosarcomatous differentiation (malignant "triton" tumors). Cancer 32:426–439, 1973.

237
Ganglion Cysts of Peripheral Nerves

Suzie C. Tindall

Ganglion cysts are cystic masses that commonly occur near joint spaces and tendon sheaths. Characterized histologically by unilocular or multilocular cystic spaces lined by mesothelial-like cells with a myxoid matrix,[5] they may rarely communicate with or be attached to the synovium of a tendon sheath or a joint. Although its exact pathogenesis is not clear, this benign lesion probably forms from extra-articular synovial remnants unobliterated at the time of embryonic joint formation.[3] Ganglion cysts constitute the most common tumor of the hand, where they characteristically arise in the intertendinous spaces and protrude into the subcutaneous soft tissues. They may, however, be found near almost any joint space and have been reported to arise totally within tendons, muscles, semilunar cartilages, and nerves.

Ganglion cysts may cause neurological symptoms by one of two methods: extraneural compression from an adjacent mass or intraneural compression from expansion of the cyst within the nerve substance itself. Among benign extraneural soft-tissue tumors of the extremities that cause compression of nerves, lipomas are the most common and ganglion cysts are next in frequency.[1] External nerve compression by ganglia has been reported involving the ulnar nerve at the levels of the elbow and wrist, the median nerve at the wrist and palm, the common peroneal nerve at the knee, and the posterior tibial nerve at the ankle.[1,3] In these instances the clinical syndromes mimic those of the peripheral entrapment neuropathies.

Although spread of nerve fascicles by a slowly growing extraneural ganglion may sometimes simulate the effect of an intraneural ganglion, there are well-documented cases of the actual intraneural origin of ganglion cysts.[2-7] Intraneural ganglia have been reported in the posterior tibial nerve at the knee, the tibial nerve at the ankle, and the radial and ulnar nerves,[6] but by far the most common site is the common peroneal nerve at the knee. In the latter instance the most prominent symptom is always pain, usually around the knee and over the anterior tibial compartment. Tinel's sign may be present and a mass may or may not be palpable within the nerve. By the time the diagnosis is made, the patient has usually developed progressive weakness in the peroneally innervated musculature and perhaps altered sensation over the dorsum of the foot. Although nerve conduction velocity studies may be normal, electromyography of the tibialis anterior and extensor hallucis longus muscles usually shows denervation potentials.[4] It is important not to mistake this entity for the more common "crossleg palsy" or peroneal compression neuropathy. One should consider surgical exploration in instances of foot drop that are associated with a positive Tinel's sign, palpable mass, or pain at the head of the fibula.[4]

Treatment of simple ganglia causing nerve compression consists of excising the cyst and obliterating any fistulous communication with an adjacent joint space or tendon. If compression is at the elbow, the ulnar nerve may be transposed simultaneously. Intraneural ganglia will appear grossly as a fusiform neural dilatation. With longitudinal neurotomy, the cyst can be entered and its contents evacuated by gentle irrigation. If total resection of the cyst wall is possible by using microtechniques, this should be accomplished. However, most authors agree that destruction of nerve tissue to allow excision of the cyst wall is not advisable[4-6] and even if cyst wall is left behind, recurrence is rare. Surgical results are generally good, with at least partial improvement in the neurological deficit.[2,4-7]

References

1. Barber KW Jr, Bianco AJ Jr, Soule EH, MacCarty CS: Benign extraneural soft-tissue tumors of the extremities causing compression of nerves. J Bone Joint Surg [AM] 44A:98–104, 1962.
2. Barrett R, Cramer F: Tumors of the peripheral nerves and so-called "ganglia" of the peroneal nerve. Clin Orthop 27:135–146, 1963.
3. Brooks DM: Nerve compression by simple ganglia: A review of thirteen collected cases. J Bone Joint Surg [Br] 34B:391–400, 1952.
4. Cobb CA, Moiel RH: Ganglion of the peroneal nerve: Report of two cases. J Neurosurg 41:255–259, 1974.
5. Katz MR, Lenobel MI: Intraneural ganglionic cyst of the peroneal nerve: Case report. J Neurosurg 32:692–694, 1970.
6. Mahaley MS Jr: Ganglion of the posterior tibial nerve: Case report. J Neurosurg 40:120–124, 1974.
7. Stack RE, Bianco AJ Jr, MacCarty CS: Compression of the common peroneal nerve by ganglion cysts. J Bone Joint Surg [Am] 47A:773–778, 1965.

SECTION D
Neurovascular Compression Syndromes

238
Posterior Fossa Neurovascular Compression Syndromes Other than Neuralgias

Peter J. Jannetta

All the cranial nerves of the cerebellopontine angle are subject to vascular compression. The somatic sensory nerves and those with major autonomic distribution (nerves V, IX, and X) are considered elsewhere and will not be considered here. Of the remaining nerves in the cerebellopontine angle, nerves III and VI have been shown, starting with the observations of Cushing in abducens palsy, to be subject to loss of function as a result of compression and stretching by normal blood vessels with increased intracranial pressure (nerve VI),[3] posterior communicating and distal basilar artery aneurysms (nerve III), or normal or ectatic vessels (nerve III).[1] The somatic motor nerves are physically tougher and more resistant to gradually increasing compression than the sensory nerves. The abducens and hypoglossal nerves are frequently noted to be greatly stretched by hindbrain arteries, such distortion having caused no symptoms or measurable loss of function. All of the above leaves two nerves, VII and VIII, where vascular compression causes disabling symptoms, some of which are the subject of the present chapter.

In reviewing the older literature regarding those syndromes of nerves VII and VIII now thought to be caused by vascular compression, one is struck by the fact that ideas that were brought forth before technology was advanced to the state where they could be proved or disproved lay fallow. Such is the case with Gardner's observations on hemifacial spasm (Bell H: Personal communication).[4-6] Although the first observation on hemifacial spasm (HFS), made at postmortem examination by Schultze and reported in 1875,[25] implicated aneurysmal compression of the facial nerve as etiologic, and although Gardner and Sava[6] and Campbell and Keedy[2] demonstrated that ectatic and apparently normal arteries were distorting the facial nerve in some cases, the then current state of technology was not sufficient to prove or disprove the point. Indeed, Gardner observed the cerebellopontine angle using the binocular surgical microscope in one case; this is the only case in which he used the microscope, and he had no photographic equipment. In evaluating Gardner's series of facial nerve manipulations for hemifacial spasm where he found vascular compression of nerve VII in 8 of 19 operations,[4-6] it seems to me that of the 8 arteries implicated as causing contact with nerve VII, 7 were the lateral branch of AICA, which causes contact with nerves VII and VIII more peripheral than the brain stem region, usually in the middle or lateral third of these nerves in two-thirds of the older population. In any case, Gardner did not inspect the root entry zone of the facial nerve and treated the hemifacial spasm by neurolysis (deliberate controlled trauma). Scoville's observation that hemifacial spasm was relieved by separating a distal arterial loop from nerve VII in the cerebellopontine angle is intriguing.[26] One can postulate that the same vessel was causing root entry zone (REZ) compression and was mobilized away from the nerve as the more lateral portion was moved.

Thus, the clues regarding hemifacial spasm, as in most unsolved problems where new paradigms are developing, are in the older literature. It required the application of the binocular dissecting microscope to the treatment of hemifacial spasm for REZ vascular compression and the clinicopathological correlation to be clarified and treated systematically and effectively.[9-11,13-15,17,23,24]

The story of the auditory nerve is a bit different in several respects. Most of the thrust of our understanding of the mechanisms of tinnitus and especially of vertigo has come from the otolaryngologists, neuro-otologists, and auditory physiologists. Much excellent basic work has been done by these investigators who have studied normal and abnormal function of nerve VIII. A number of morphological studies of the portion of the nerve in the temporal bone have been performed in cadavers, the patients having had dysfunction of nerve VIII during life. Surgical treatment of vertigo, dysequilibrium, and tinnitus has been either ineffective (endolymphatic shunting procedures), destructive (labyrinthectomy, peripheral nerve section), or both. Even the peripheral destructive procedures (i.e., labyrinthectomy) have had a high recurrence rate of vertigo (50 percent) and have not been particularly effective for dysequilibrium or tinnitus. Again, with the application of the binocular microscope to the nerves in the cerebellopontine angle in patients with eighth nerve dysfunction, it has been shown that vascular compression of nerve VIII in the cerebellopontine angle is a common cause of these symptoms and that the symptoms can be relieved without injury to neural tissue and with preservation or improvement in function.[12,13]

Intraoperative brain stem auditory evoked potential (BSEP) monitoring[7,8,18,20,22] and direct monitoring of nerve VIII function[19] are necessary adjuncts to nerve VIII vascular decompression procedures. These monitoring techniques are also helpful in preventing hearing loss in operations on nerve VII.

Clinicopathological Correlations

Hemifacial Spasm

1. Classic HFS (i.e., onset in the orbicularis oculi muscles, with subsequent downward progression over the face): the offending vessel is at the brain stem on the anterocaudal aspect of the REZ.
2. Atypical HFS (i.e., onset in the buccal muscles, with subsequent upward progression over the face): the offending vessel is rostral to nerve VII or posterior to nerve VII (between nerves VII and VIII) at the REZ.
3. Peripheral blood vessels in the cerebellopontine angle do not cause HFS, although the more proximal part of the same arterial loop that is in contact with nerve VII close to the internal auditory meatus may be causing REZ compression.
4. The REZ of nerve VII extends caudally to the pontomedullary junction. Vessels compressing the brain stem in this region can be causal of classic HFS.
5. Small arterioles and venules (rare) can be the sole cause of HFS. Also, at reoperation in four patients who did not improve after microsurgical decompression of a larger vessel from the REZ, the implant was found to be pushing an arteriole across and into the REZ. The HFS was relieved by microvascular decompression (MVD) of the facial nerve from the arterioles in each case.
6. Even though a "scissors" configuration of vascular compression of the REZ, so common in trigeminal neuralgia, is rare in HFS, the entire circumference of the nerve VII REZ should be inspected in every case.
7. The offending vessel may lie away from the REZ by a millimeter or more at operation with the patient in the lateral decubitus position. The brain stem and blood vessels appear to move differentially with changes in head position. This may explain the frequent positional history noted in HFS patients.
8. The abnormalities are subtle.

Vertigo, Tinnitus, Dysequilibrium

1. If vertigo is present, the offending vessel is compressing the vestibular portion of nerve VIII at the brain stem.
2. If tinnitus is present, the offending vessel is compressing the cochlear portion of nerve VIII anywhere from the brain stem to the internal auditory meatus.
3. If dysequilibrium is present without frank vertigo, the offending vessel is compressing the vestibular portion of nerve VIII adjacent to but not at the brain stem.
4. If both vertigo and tinnitus are present, the offending blood vessel is compressing both portions of the nerve and is at the brain stem (unless there is more than one vessel, in which case all vessels should be decompressed).
5. The principles in parts 4, 5, 6, 7, and 8 above, which apply to hemifacial spasm, also apply to nerve VIII dysfunction.
6. Microvascular decompression of nerve VIII is the most difficult of the MVD procedures.

Technique of Microvascular Decompression

The patient, prepared with adrenal cortical steroids beginning 12 h preoperatively, is anesthetized and intubated with the head at the foot of the operating room table (to allow knee room for the surgeon). A central venous pressure line, arterial line, and Doppler ultrasound monitor are used. BSEP monitoring of auditory nerve function is instituted and used throughout. Direct nerve VIII monitoring is most helpful. A three-point headholder is attached to the head; then the patient is turned into the lateral decubitus position, and the headholder is attached to the fixation system with the connecting joints left loose. An axillary roll is put into place to protect the brachial plexus. The neck is slightly stretched, the chin is slightly flexed, the head is rotated slightly to the ipsilateral side, and the connectors of the headholder are tightened. It is important that the head not be brought forward and that there is no ipsilateral neck flexion if the occipital boss is to be easily accessible for exposure of the cerebellopontine angle (Fig. 238-1).

The shoulder is taped caudally and a bit forward. The back of the head on the ipsilateral side is shaved and prepped. The skin incision is marked out before draping. The incision is placed one finger breadth behind the mastoid eminence; it parallels the hairline and runs from the level of the rostral part of the ear caudally for 6 or 7 cm (up to 8 cm in heavily muscled, short-necked, or obese patients) (Fig. 238-2). The drapes are applied.

The incision is made and hemostasis is secured with Dandy clamps and electrocautery. A self-retaining Weitlaner retractor with posts (V. Mueller Co., Chicago, Ill.) is

Figure 238-1 Lateral decubitus position. The head of the patient is at the foot of the table. The neck is on some stretch, the chin is slightly flexed, and the head is slightly rotated to the up side.

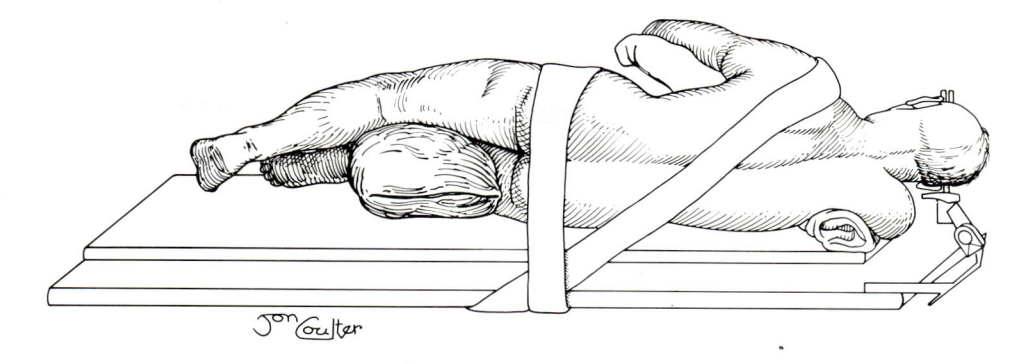

put into place. Emissary veins are waxed for hemostasis. The posteromedial aspect of the mastoid eminence must be cleared of soft tissue.

The craniectomy is performed (Fig. 238-3). It must extend to the sigmoid sinus, even if mastoid air cells are entered, and to the floor of the posterior fossa. It is especially important that the lower lateral corner of the occipital plate adjacent to the mastoid eminence be opened. The bone edges are heavily waxed, and any exposed mastoid air cells are sealed in this way.

The dura mater is opened obliquely and incised into the lower lateral corner. The dural flaps are sewn back out of the way (Fig. 238-4). The Weitlaner retractor with posts is secured to the drapes using a clamp and sponge strung through the handles for stability.

The narrow-bladed microsurgical retractor (V. Mueller Co.), attached with one connecting rod to the lower caudal post of the Weitlaner retractor, is placed inferolaterally over the cerebellum, which is protected by a piece of rubber dam under a cotton strip. A set of microsurgical angulated dissection instruments devised by the author has been found to be useful for these procedures. The microscope is utilized for the entire intradural portion of the procedure.

The cerebellum is elevated gently from the floor of the posterior fossa. The subarachnoid cistern over nerves IX and X is opened with a sharp hook. If a bridging vein from the cerebellum to the dura is found, it is coagulated and divided. The auditory nerve is identified. The technique of exposure of the REZ of nerve VII is to *elevate* the cerebellum from nerves IX and X rather than to retract it medially, putting the pia-arachnoidal trabeculi between the cerebellum and nerves IX and X on the stretch and dividing them with scissors, gradually placing the retractor tip more medially until it rests on the choroid plexus of the lateral recess of the fourth ventricle. The flocculus is not separated from nerve VIII but instead is elevated so that the brain stem and adjacent nerve VII can be visualized under nerve VIII.

The offending vessel or vessels (Figs. 238-5 and 238-6) will often be obstructing the view of nerve VII, which arises anterior to nerve VIII. The blood vessels may be a leash of several arterial loops, a single loop, a small artery that lies relatively free in the operative position, or a vein, usually a branch of the lateral pontomesencephalic vein crossing the nerve on the brain stem (Table 238-1).

The entire circumference of nerve VII must be inspected. This can usually be seen from the caudal exposure. Occasionally, one must inspect it from the rostral side as in the exposure for trigeminal neuralgia. The pontomedullary junction in front of nerve IX must be inspected.

The vessels are gently levered away (not grasped with forceps) and are held away with an implant. We currently use one or several pieces of shredded Teflon R felt (Dow Co., Midland, Mich.) These can be made of any size and shape and should be rolled loosely. Enough implant material

Figure 238-2 The retromastoid incision.

TABLE 238-1 Operative Findings in 229 Patients with Hemifacial Spasm (December 1979)

Abnormality	Number of Patients
Arterial	210
Mixed	10
Venous	4
Tumor	3
Aneurysm	1
AVM	1

AICA — most frequent.

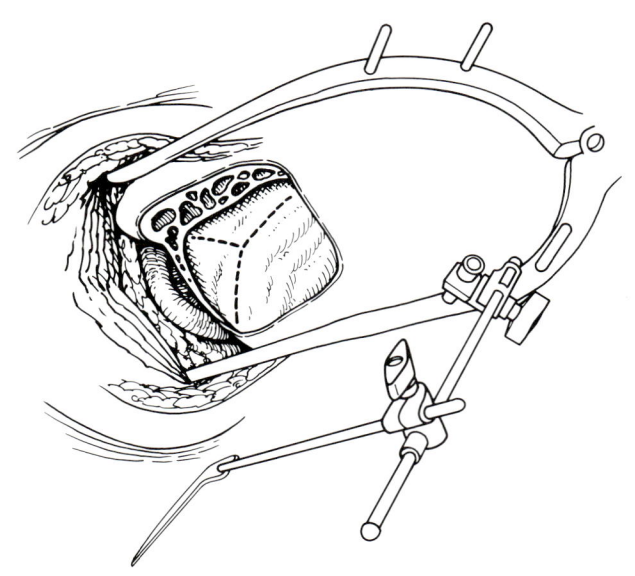

Figure 238-3 The retromastoid craniectomy, the lines of dural opening, and the retractor setup.

must be placed so that it will not float away in the cerebrospinal fluid. A piece of Gelfoam (The Upjohn Company, Kalamazoo, Mich.) may be placed around the area as a further guarantee of stability of the implant.

The nerves and vessels are inspected both before and during retractor removal to ensure that there is no kinking of vessels or excessive compression of the nerves. The Valsalva maneuver is performed several times, the retractor is removed, and the dura mater is closed in watertight fashion. The lower muscle layers are closed, and the bone chips are laid in over a piece of Gelfoam, which is first placed on the dura. The wound is closed in layers and a small wound dressing is applied. The head of the recovery room bed is elevated about 15 to 20 degrees.

The patient is kept in the intensive care unit overnight and then, if he or she feels well, is returned to a regular room. The patient may go to the bathroom with assistance the night of the operation. The steroids are discontinued after 48 h. Small doses of codeine sulfate are given as needed for incisional pain.

The spasm may be present postoperatively but should not be as severe as it was preoperatively. Alternatively, it may be absent, return slowly, plateau, and gradually disappear. If present postoperatively, it usually begins to decrease within 48 to 72 h. It should be considerably improved by the time of discharge. If the spasm is as severe postoperatively on awakening as it was preoperatively and does not begin to improve in 48 to 72 h, the presumption is that the vascular compression is still present and reoperation should be performed. Results and complications of operation in 229 patients are tabulated in Tables 238-2 and 238-3. We have now operated upon over 400 patients with no mortality.

The operative exposure and technique of MVD for auditory nerve dysfunction are similar to those for hemifacial spasm. Veins on the brain stem, usually the lateral pontomesencephalic vein and/or its branches, commonly cause tinnitus and/or vertigo. Such a vein may lie between nerves VII and VIII or posterior to nerve VIII (on the anteromedial side of the flocculus), and branches of the system may underlie the choroid plexus of the lateral recess of the fourth ventricle, cross in an anteroposterior direction between nerves IX and VIII, or lie on the rostral side of nerve VIII. The exposure of this area of nerve VIII and the adjacent brain stem both rostrally and caudally is especially difficult

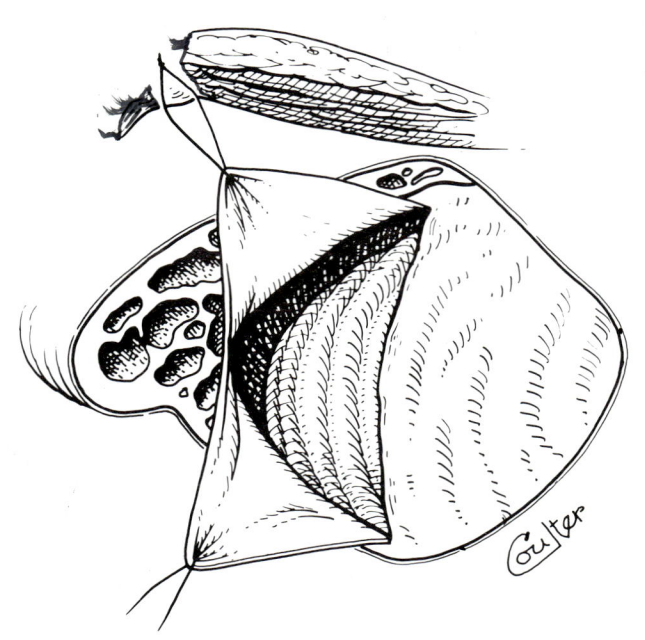

Figure 238-4 Dural retraction sutures hold back the inferior dural leaves.

TABLE 238-2 Operative Results in 229 Patients with Hemifacial Spasm (December 1979)

Operative Results	Number	Percent
No spasm after one operation	201	87.8
No spasm, second procedure necessary	12	5.2
Partially symptomatic (25% of preoperative level)	11	4.8
Failure of therapy	5	2.2

TABLE 238-3 Morbidity in 229 Patients with Hemifacial Spasm (December 1979)

Cranial Nerve	Deficit	Number of Patients
Trigeminal	Hypalgesia	1
Facial	Postoperative weakness	9 (6 persist)
	Postoperative late-onset weakness	7 (1 persists)
Acoustic	Hearing loss	18
	Deaf 8	
	Profound 8	
	Mild 2	
	Other Morbidity	
Wound infection		1
Persistent ataxia (mild)		2
Temporary ataxia		Not collated

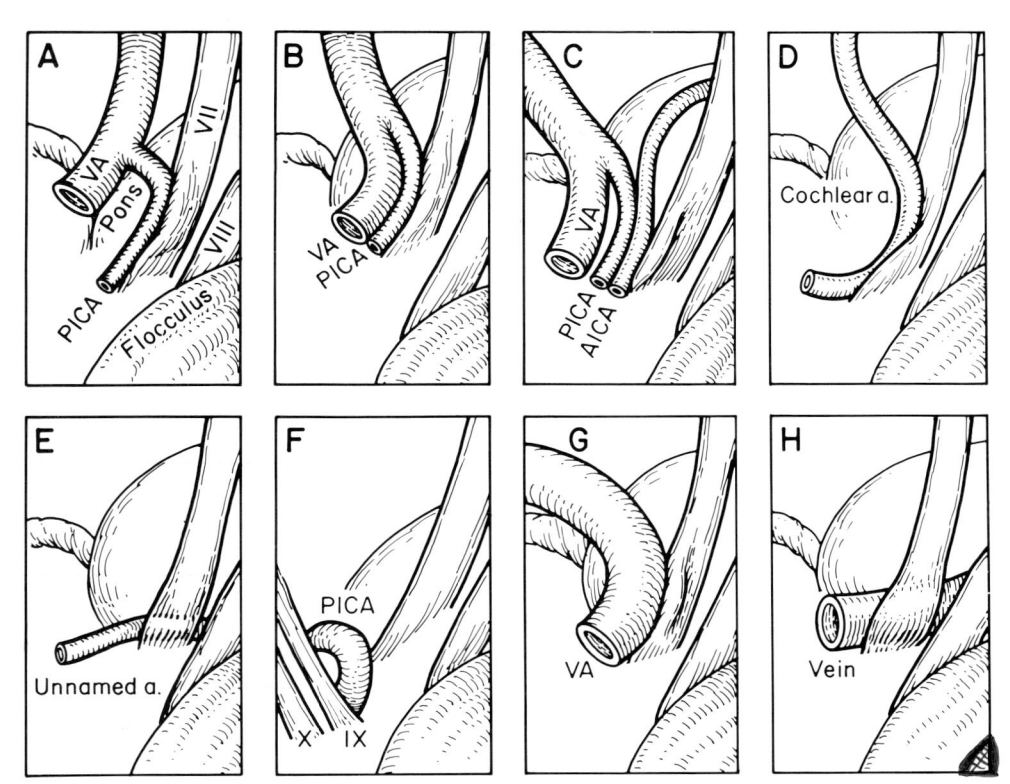

Figure 238-5 Depiction of various vascular configurations found in patients with typical (classical) hemifacial spasm.

if one is to see the abnormality clearly and treat it effectively without injuring neural tissue.

Operative findings, results, and complications of MVD for tinnitus and vertigo in the first 38 patients who have been followed for 3 years or more are collated in Tables 238-4, 238-5, and 238-6. We have now operated upon over 70 patients with no mortality and minimal morbidity.

About 40 percent of the patients develop a delayed headache, usually on the fourth to sixth postoperative day. A lumbar puncture should be performed. The cerebrospinal

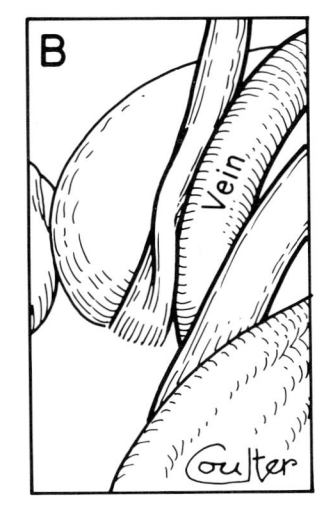

Figure 238-6 Depiction of two vascular configurations found in patients with atypical hemifacial spasm.

TABLE 238-4 Eighth Cranial Nerve Dysfunction

Operative Findings		Number of Patients
Offending vessel		
Artery		26
Cochlear	6	
AICA	5	
PICA	5	
Unidentified artery	4	
Cochlear + AICA	1	
Vertebral	2	
Superior cerebellar	2	
AICA + PICA	1	
Vein		8
Artery and vein		4
Total		38

AICA, anterior inferior cerebellar artery; PICA, posterior inferior cerebellar artery.

TABLE 238-5 Eighth Cranial Nerve Dysfunction

	Results of Operation			
Symptoms	Relieved	Mild Improvement	Recurred or No Relief	Worse
Vertigo and tinnitus	13	0	6	1
Vertigo	6	1	0	0
Tinnitus	5	0	6	0
Total	24	1	12	1

TABLE 238-6 Eighth Cranial Nerve Dysfunction

Complications

Temporary
   Epidural hematoma
   Paresis of cranial nerve VI
   Paresis of cranial nerve X
   Aseptic meningitis
Permanent
   Internuclear ophthalmoplegia and worsening of vertigo
   Deterioration of hearing

fluid pressure may be elevated. There are usually white blood cells and an elevated protein value present. A Gram's stain shows no bacteria. A culture is performed. The pressure, if elevated, is dropped slowly to normal. A single dose of adrenal cortical steroids is given, and the patient usually improves dramatically. The headache occasionally occurs after discharge. The patient and the patient's physician should be warned of this possibility and arrangements made for lumbar puncture, etc., if such should occur.

The other late problem that may occur is a delayed Bell's palsy. This has happened eight or nine times in our series of over 400 operations and has always been incomplete and self-limited.

Advances in monitoring have made a substantial difference in morbidity. The major morbidity early in the series was loss of hearing in the ipsilateral ear.[10,11,13–15] Using intraoperative BSEP monitoring and, more recently, direct auditory monitoring, we have found that lateral-to-medial retraction of the cerebellum causes abnormalities of the evoked potentials and presumably is a cause of hearing loss. Further, we have not infrequently noted the presence of preoperative mild hearing loss at 2000 dB on the side of HFS[21] as a result of compression of the auditory system by the same blood vessel causing the HFS, which is relieved by MVD.

All the implants that we have used have been found wanting for one reason or another. Shredded Teflon felt is superior to the others except for the delayed headache problem, which has been more common with its use than with the material used previously and which is fortunately self-limited. We have not had a wound infection or case of meningitis in our MVD patients since initiating the perioperative antibiotic regimen of Malis in late 1979.[16] MVD is the only definitive treatment of HFS. The procedure is of low morbidity, negligible mortality, and offers excellent quality of life.

References

1. Briani S, Ammannati F: Patologia dei nervi cranici da compressione vasale diretta. Riv Neurobiol 24:285–310, 1978.
2. Campbell E, Keedy C: Hemifacial spasm: A note on the etiology in two cases. J Neurosurg 4:342–347, 1947.
3. Cushing H: Strangulation of the nervi abducentes by lateral branches of the basilar artery in cases of brain tumour. Brain 33:204–235, 1910.
4. Gardner WJ: The mechanism of tic douloureux. Trans Am Neurol Assoc 78:168–173, 1953.
5. Gardner WJ: Concerning the mechanism of trigeminal neuralgia and hemifacial spasm. J Neurosurg 19:947–958, 1962.
6. Gardner WJ, Sava GA: Hemifacial spasm: A reversible pathophysiologic state. J Neurosurg 19:240–247, 1962.
7. Grundy BL, Jannetta PJ, Lina A, Procopio P, Boston JR: BAEP monitoring during cerebellopontine angle surgery. Anesthesiology 55:A127, 1981 (abstr).
8. Grundy BL, Lina A, Procopio PT, Jannetta PJ: Reversible evoked potential changes with retraction of the eighth cranial nerve. Anesth Analg 60:835–838, 1981.
9. Hankinson HL, Wilson CB: Microsurgical treatment of hemifacial spasm. West J Med 124:191–193, 1976.
10. Jannetta PJ: Microsurgical exploration and decompression of the facial nerve in hemifacial spasm. Curr Top Surg Res 2:217–220, 1970.
11. Jannetta PJ: The cause of hemifacial spasm: Definitive microsurgical treatment at the brainstem in 31 patients. Trans Am Acad Ophthalmol Otolaryngol 80:319–322, 1975.
12. Jannetta PJ: Neurovascular cross-compression in patients with hyperactive dysfunction symptoms of the eighth cranial nerve. Surg Forum 26:467–469, 1975.
13. Jannetta PJ: Neurovascular compression in cranial nerve and systemic disease. Ann Surg 192:518–525, 1980.
14. Jannetta PJ: Hemifacial spasm. Neurology and Neurosurgery, Update Series. 3:8, 1982.
15. Jannetta PJ, Abbasy M, Maroon JC, Ramos FM, Albin MS: Etiology and definitive microsurgical treatment of hemifacial spasm: Operative techniques and results in 47 patients. J Neurosurg 47:321–328, 1977.
16. Malis LI: Prevention of neurosurgical infection by intraoperative antibiotics. Neurosurgery 5:339–343, 1979.
17. Maroon JC: Hemifacial spasm: A vascular cause. Arch Neurol 35:481–483, 1978.
18. Møller AR, Jannetta PJ: Comparison between intracranially recorded potentials from the human auditory nerve and scalp recorded auditory brainstem responses (ABR). Scand Audiol 11:33–40, 1982.
19. Møller AR, Jannetta PJ: Monitoring auditory functions during cranial nerve microvascular decompression operations by direct recording from the eighth nerve. J Neurosurg 59:493–499, 1983.
20. Møller AR, Jannetta P, Bennett MH, Møller MB: Intracranially recorded responses from the human auditory nerve: New insights into the origin of brain stem evoked potentials (BSEPs). Electroencephalogr Clin Neurophysiol 52:18–27, 1981.
21. Møller M, Jannetta PJ, Møller A: Vascular compression of the eighth nerve in vertigo and tinnitus (in press).
22. Møller MB, Møller AR, Jannetta PJ: Brainstem auditory evoked potentials in patients with hemifacial spasm. Laryngoscope 92:848–852, 1982.
23. Petty PG, Southby R: Vascular compression of lower cranial nerves: Observations using microsurgery, with particular reference to trigeminal neuralgia. Aust NZ J Surg 47:314–320, 1977.
24. Rhoton AL Jr: Microsurgical neurovascular decompression for trigeminal neuralgia and hemifacial spasm. J Fla Med Assoc 65:425–428, 1978.
25. Schultze F: Linksseitiger Facialiskrampf in Folge eines Aneurysma der Arteria vertebralis sinistra. Virchows Arch [Pathol Anat] 65:385–391, 1875.
26. Scoville WB: Hearing loss following exploration of cerebellopontine angle in the treatment of hemifacial spasm. J Neurosurg 31:47–49, 1969.

SECTION E

Miscellaneous

239

Techniques of Diagnostic Nerve and Muscle Biopsies

Edward S. Connolly

Nerve Biopsy

Nerve biopsies are helpful in the diagnosis of periarteritis nodosa, amyloidosis, leprosy, metachromatic leukodystrophy, Krabbe's disease, ataxia-telangiectasia, and in conditions in which the peripheral nerve is palpably enlarged. Less information is gained in acute or subacute distal symmetrical polyneuropathies of toxic or metabolic origin.

The neurosurgeon is frequently asked by neurology colleagues to provide specimens of peripheral nerves for both light and electron microscopy studies. Frequently, a muscle specimen is also desired. In picking a nerve for biopsy, it is important to pick one that can be tested electrically and be shown to be affected by the neuropathy, that is constant in location and readily accessible, that is either a pure sensory or a pure motor nerve, and that is sufficiently long to obtain an adequate biopsy specimen. The two nerves that are most commonly biopsied are the sural nerve and the anterior tibial or deep peroneal nerve. The sural nerve is the ideal sensory nerve for biopsy purposes. Since the neurological impairment in peripheral neuropathies is greatest distally in the lower extremities, the sural nerve is usually involved and it can be easily tested electrically. Its position is constant and its superficial location and long length without branching lends itself to biopsy. In those patients in whom there is marked sensory loss in the distribution of the sural nerve, a total resection is done and in those who have normal sensation, a fascicular biopsy, as suggested by Dyck and Lofgren,[2] can be performed. In those with purely motor neuropathy in whom a motor nerve is desired, one can perform a lateral fascicular biopsy of the deep peroneal nerve or, if the nerve is shown electrically to be present, a biopsy of the accessory deep peroneal nerve, which innervates the extensor digitorum brevis muscle.[3] These biopsies may be done on both hospitalized patients and outpatients and are usually carried out under local anesthesia with 1% lidocaine or its equivalent.

Operative Technique for Sural Nerve Biopsy

The patient is positioned in the lateral decubitus position, slightly inclined toward the prone position, with the operative side up and the underneath leg flexed. A pillow is placed between the knees and a sandbag is placed underneath the upper foot to be operated upon. The lateral aspect of the leg is shaved if necessary and then prepped with povidone-iodine scrub followed by povidone-iodine solution. A skin-marking pencil is used to mark an incision just lateral and parallel to the achilles tendon, beginning 1 cm proximal to the lateral malleolus and extending proximally for 8 cm. This area then is infiltrated with 1% lidocaine.

The sural nerve lies just superficial to the deep fascia, almost always in close association with the lesser saphenous vein. Branching of the nerve trunk occurs in most cases near the distal end of the incision but the nerve is a single, 1-mm-diameter trunk at its proximal end. The nerve is composed of 5 to 14 bundles of nerve fibers, which often are grossly apparent and help to distinguish the nerve from sclerotic veins in this location. Another helpful distinction is that veins branch more nearly at right angles than do nerves. Once the nerve trunk is identified, sharp dissection with a minimum of traction should be practiced in dissecting free the nerve from the adjacent tissues. Loupe magnification, 2½×, is a helpful adjunct.

Section of the nerve trunk is performed with a very sharp instrument, preferably a razor blade, with a wooden tongue depressor as the cutting block. Severing the nerve usually causes a jolt of pain in the lateral part of the foot, so the patient must be warned before the section is performed. We have found it useful to block the nerve trunk itself with a small amount of lidocaine a few millimeters proximal to the intended site prior to severing the nerve. The proximal section is always done first in order to render the distal section painless. For most purposes, a 3- to 4-cm length of nerve suffices. The proximal section should be performed so that following it the proximal nerve stump will retract above the level of the skin incision and will not be involved in the healing of the wound. Ligation of the proximal end has not been found necessary. Hemostasis is best obtained by using microtip bipolar coagulation.

The biopsy specimen should be laid out on a piece of sterile stiff paper or cardboard (a standard 3 × 5 index card is suitable), straightened, slightly stretched with a minimum of handling, and allowed to adhere for approximately 1 min. Excess cardboard or paper is trimmed away and the specimen, backing and all, is immersed in the fixative.

An interrupted mattress skin closure using 4-0 nylon or some other monofilament suture is recommended. An elastic roll pressure dressing may then be applied. The patient may be up and ambulatory the same day. Sitting with the leg in a dependent position for long periods of time should be discouraged. Sutures should be left in place for 10 to 14 days.[1] If one desires to try to prevent hypesthesia of the lateral aspect of the foot and heel, a fascicular biopsy of the nerve can best be carried out by using the operative microscope, approximately half of the fascicular bundle being spared. The distal exposed fascicles can be lightly coagulated with microbipolar coagulation to seal the ends.

Operative Technique for Lateral Fascicular Biopsy of the Deep Peroneal Nerve and for Biopsy of the Accessory Deep Peroneal Nerve

The patient is placed in the same lateral decubitus position as with the sural nerve biopsy with the biopsy side up, the knee on the down side flexed, and with a pillow between the legs. The lower aspect of the thigh and the upper aspect of the calf are then shaved, prepped with povidone-iodine scrub followed by povidone-iodine solution, and draped in sterile fashion. An incision is marked on the skin superior and posterior to the fibular head and curved around behind and beneath the fibular head, swinging forward and down just lateral to the tibia for exposure to the deep peroneal nerve.

The common peroneal nerve is exposed as it curves about the fibular head and is followed distally to where it gives off its first branch, a recurrent sensory branch to the knee joint; the second or middle branch, the deep peroneal; and the third, most lateral branch, the musculocutaneous nerve. By using the operative microscope, a fascicular biopsy can be carried out, approximately 3 cm of nerve tissue being obtained. The use of a nerve stimulator may be helpful if there is a question about what branch is going to the extensor digitorum brevis. One or two fascicles should be sufficient for diagnosis.

If it is shown electrically that the patient has an accessory deep peroneal nerve, it is preferable to take this nerve since it can be removed through the same incision as a sural nerve biopsy specimen. It is found passing along the posterior border of the peroneus brevis muscle and travels with that tendon as it goes posterior to the lateral malleolus to enter the foot. A nerve stimulator can demonstrate innervation to the extensor digitorum brevis.

It is important in all nerve biopsies to inform the patient that a deficit may result from the biopsy and that the biopsy is strictly for diagnostic purposes and has no therapeutic purpose. One also has to warn the patient that a neuroma may occur. In my experience, however, the incidence of painful neuroma formation is less than 1 percent.

Muscle Biopsy

A muscle biopsy is often desirable and may be requested in combination with a peripheral nerve biopsy. By using either the sural nerve biopsy incision or the deep peroneal or accessory deep peroneal nerve biopsy incision, it is easy to obtain an associated muscle biopsy of the gastrocnemius muscle.

The fascia of the muscle is incised in a longitudinal fashion over approximately a 3-cm length. Then an approximately 5-mm-diameter fascicle of muscle is dissected in a longitudinal fashion. When this has been done, a ligature of 2-0 silk is passed about the fascicle of muscle and tied proximally; the procedure is repeated distally. A sterile tongue blade is passed underneath the muscle and the muscle is cut with a razor blade just above the proximal ligature and just below the inferior ligature, after the two ligatures have been tied securely to the tongue blade to prevent shortening of the muscle bundle. The specimen attached to the tongue blade is inserted into isotonic saline solution for 20 min and then placed in formaldehyde. (A double-ended muscle clamp can be used instead of the sutures and tongue blade for the removal and fixation of the muscle specimen.) Hemostasis at the cut ends of the muscle is achieved with bipolar coagulation. The fascia of the muscle is loosely closed with 4-0 sutures to prevent a muscle hernia, and the rest of the incision is closed in the usual manner.

References

1. Asbury AK, Connolly ES: Sural nerve biopsy: Technical note. J Neurosurg 38:391–392, 1973.
2. Dyck PJ, Lofgren EP: Method of fascicular biopsy of human peripheral nerve for electrophysiologic and histologic study. Mayo Clin Proc 41:778–784, 1966.
3. Lambert EH: The accessory deep peroneal nerve: A common variation in innervation of extensor digitorum brevis. Neurology 19:1169–1176, 1969.

240
Nontraumatic Brachial Plexopathy

E. Wayne Massey

General Clinical Features

Nontraumatic plexopathies account for approximately 50 percent of all lesions of the brachial plexus. Traumatic causes of such neuropathy have been described in an earlier chapter, as has the anatomy of the brachial plexus. Some general clinical features are important to summarize. Most plexus lesions are incomplete. They are characterized by combinations of weakness, muscle atrophy, alteration in muscle stretch reflexes, sensory changes, and sometimes sympathetic dysfunction. Pain due to brachial plexus lesions is usually constant and quite often severe. It is usually localized above the elbow, aggravated by arm movement, and accompanied by a variable degree of weakness. Weakness without pain or sensory disturbance can be the presenting manifestation of plexopathy associated with tumor or following inoculations. When sensory impairment occurs, it is usually patchy and sometimes associated with hyperesthesia or dysesthesia. Muscle atrophy may occur rapidly. Fasciculations are uncommon. Complications such as joint contractures and causalgic pain may occur.

An *upper plexus lesion* involves the fifth and sixth cervical roots or upper trunk and is the most common type of involvement. Muscle weakness includes the deltoid, biceps, brachioradialis, brachialis, and sometimes the infra- and supraspinatus and subcapularis muscles. Sensation is often unaffected or may involve the lateral aspect of the shoulder (circumflex nerve). Occasionally the phrenic nerve is involved.

A *middle plexus lesion* involves weakness of the triceps and extensor muscles supplied by the middle trunk. Involvement is similar to that of primary derangements of the C7 root and the radial nerve. A sensory deficit may be present on the radial aspect of the dorsum of the hand. Muscle weakness involves the C7-innervated muscles but spares the brachioradialis, which is supplied by the C6 nerve root.

A *lower plexus lesion* involves the C8 and T1 roots or the lower trunk and causes paralysis of the flexors of the forearm and the intrinsic hand muscles. Sensory alteration includes involvement of the posterior medial arm, mid forearm, and ulnar aspect of the hand. A Horner's syndrome may occur if the first thoracic root is involved.

Occasionally the entire plexus is involved, which results in a paralyzed extremity. This is extremely rare in a cryptogenic, nontraumatic brachial plexus neuropathy. Lesions of the lateral cord cause weakness of the musculocutaneous nerve and lateral head of the median nerve. A lesion of the medial cord produces weakness of the muscles innervated by the ulnar nerve and the medial head of the median nerve. A posterior cord lesion produces weakness of the deltoid and extensors of the wrists and fingers due to dysfunction of the axillary and radial nerves.

Types of Nontraumatic Brachial Plexopathy

Neuralgic Amyotrophy (Cryptogenic Brachial Plexopathy)

Many names have been used for this entity, including *acute brachial radiculitis, localized neuritis of the shoulder girdle, neuralgic amyotrophy, acute shoulder neuritis, paralytic brachial neuritis,* and *brachial plexus neuropathy.*[9] It is also called the Parsonage-Turner syndrome.[11]

Brachial plexus neuropathy is an adequate descriptive term and refers to a well-defined, relatively common clinical entity with a fairly typical pattern of symptoms and signs. It must be differentiated from acute cervical root disease, spinal cord tumor, systemic polyneuropathy, and anterior horn cell disease.

Brachial plexus neuropathy usually has a rapid onset of severe, often nocturnal, pain, accompanied by or shortly followed by muscle weakness. It occurs in both males and females but is twice as common in males and is most frequent in the third to seventh decades. The pain may involve the shoulder, arm, forearm, and hand, but if the lesion is predominantly in the upper plexus, the pain does not extend below the elbow. Arm movement may exacerbate the pain and neck traction often aggravates the symptoms. The pain usually subsides after several weeks when the weakness becomes most marked. Weakness is confined to the shoulder girdle in about 50 percent of the patients with cryptogenic brachial plexopathy. The axillary and suprascapular nerves are most commonly affected. Rarely, complete limb paralysis is seen. Bilateral involvement may occur but is never complete and rarely symmetrical. Diaphragmatic paralysis may occur. The lack of radicular features of the pain and the absence of exacerbation on neck movement suggest that the nerve roots are not involved.

Electromyographic evidence of plexus or of other nerve involvement outside the affected limb may be present. Widespread slowing of motor conduction has been reported in some cases.[10] Other laboratory tests, including cerebrospinal fluid analysis, immunologic studies, and measurements of the sedimentation rate, are usually normal. Biopsy of the cutaneous branch of the radial nerve has been shown to reveal axonal degeneration.[10]

Cryptogenic brachial plexopathy is presumed to be due to a viral infection, an allergic reaction to an infectious proc-

1909

ess, or a toxin.[6] In 25 percent of the patients, a history of an antecedent upper respiratory illness may be obtained. Some epidemiological studies have suggested that the Coxsackie virus[9] and the Epstein-Barr virus[7] may be responsible for the etiology in some cases.

Treatment is largely symptomatic and must be individualized. Oral steroid or ACTH administration may reduce the pain but probably does not alter the course of the disease. Strong pain medication may be required in the acute stages of the illness. No other specific therapy is recommended except for rest of the arm. As the pain subsides, an appropriate range of motion exercises should be instituted. Physical therapy and splinting may be required in some patients.

The prognosis for cryptogenic brachial plexus lesions is excellent. Patients with severe muscle weakness and atrophy may recover completely, with 80 percent of patients recovering within 2 years after the onset of symptoms and 90 percent recovering by the end of 3 years, regardless of the duration of the acute course.[10] Accurate diagnosis at the beginning is therefore essential. Recovery is slightly less in bilateral cases. A poor prognosis is suggested when: (1) severe and prolonged recurrences of pain are encountered (2) no improvement is seen by 3 months; or (3) complete plexus or isolated lower plexus lesions are present.[9]

Recurrences are rare, are usually are less severe than the initial occurrence, and occur in less than 5 percent of patients. Residual deficits are minimal in the majority of patients. However, although muscle function is regained, many patients have residual atrophy present in the shoulder girdle muscles, particularly the supraspinatus and infraspinatus muscles. When pain in the upper back continues several months after the onset, it may be caused by persistent winging of the scapula (Fig. 240-1), and a surgical aid to support the scapula may be necessary.

Postinoculation Plexopathy

Following an injection of a foreign serum or vaccine, diffuse polyneuropathy or isolated brachial plexus involvement may occur.[4] This usually is not accompanied by a generalized manifestation of serum sickness. It has followed inoculations with tetanus antitoxin and diphtheria antiserum and inoculations against streptococci, pneumococci, gonococci, and anthrax and Clostridium bacilli.[9] Severe pain occurs, followed by wasting and weakness of the musculature, usually of the upper trunk. No correlation can be made between the site of inoculation and localization of the plexopathy. Despite the similarity of the immune to the nonimmune form of brachial plexopathy, the interval between pain and onset of weakness frequently is significantly shorter in the immune cases.

Plexopathy Associated with Systemic or Toxic Factors

Rarely, the brachial plexus is involved by direct extension of a local septic focus. Plexopathy may also occur following infection of distant organs such as the gallbladder, tonsils, or teeth or following a generalized infection such as tuberculosis, syphilis, infectious mononucleosis, or toxoplasmosis.

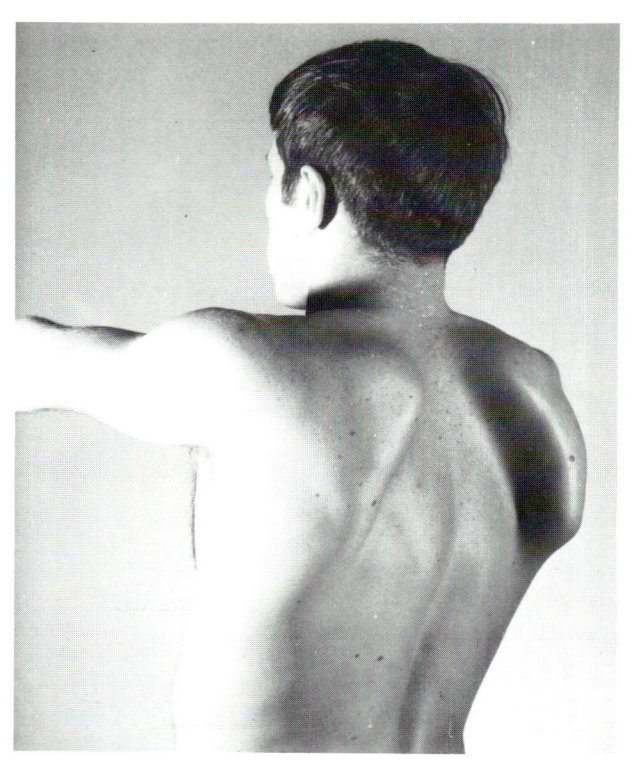

Figure 240-1 Patient with scapular winging due to a cryptogenic lesion of the long thoracic nerve.

Many mononeuropathies have been described following a generalized infection.[14]

Collagen vascular disease may cause mononeuritis multiplex involving one upper extremity and simulate a plexus lesion. Diabetes mellitus may produce a brachial plexopathy particularly involving the circumflex (axillary) nerve.

Toxic effects on the brachial plexus can occur in heroin addicts following intravenous administration, producing a painless monoparesis probably due to a direct toxic or hypersensitivity reaction.

Tumors Involving the Brachial Plexus

Primary tumors of the brachial plexus are rare and usually benign. These can be neurilemmomas or neurofibromas. They are usually isolated and encapsulated tumors. Some present with a firm mass in the supraclavicular area. These tumors are rarely cystic and vary in size.

Metastatic tumors to the brachial plexus may present with symptoms and signs similar to those of cryptogenic brachial plexopathy.[5] Most commonly these tumors are from the breast or lung, often by direct extension. Malignant lymphomas may also compress the plexus. Unbearable pain is the rule with malignant lesions. Radiation therapy may be helpful in some cases but often results in later complications. Surgical intervention is usually for palliation, as detailed dissection is most difficult.

Several characteristics may help to differentiate the clinical presentation of neoplastic versus radiation plexopathy.[5] Pain occurs four times more commonly in tumor patients. Tumors more often involve the lower trunk (72 percent) and radiation injuries the upper plexus (78 percent).[5] Horner's syndrome is more common with tumors. Lymphedema is seen more in radiation injury. If symptoms occur within 1 year of radiation therapy with doses exceeding 6000 R, radiation damage is more likely. Therefore painless upper trunk lesions with lymphedema suggest radiation injury, and painful lower trunk lesions with Horner's syndrome imply tumor infiltration.[5]

In a large series of brachial plexus lesions due to cancer, CT scanning was of some benefit in diagnosis.[1] Roentgenography of the cervical spine, myelography, bone scanning, and electromyography may also be helpful.

Fatty tumors may involve the brachial plexus, which results in complete atrophy of the nerve plexus with infiltration of fatty tissue without malignant cells. The exact etiology of this is unknown. Solitary fibrosis, dysplasia, aneurysm, or bone cyst are rare but may cause compression of the neurovascular structures of the plexus.

Radiation or Electrical Injury Involving the Brachial Plexus

Radiation damage to the brachial plexus occurs in patients following radiation therapy for breast cancer or head and neck tumors. Months or years may pass following irradiation before symptoms occur. Brachial pain may be the initial symptom followed by progressive weakness, atrophy, and sensory loss. However, many cases occur without pain, as indicated previously. Skin discoloration, subcutaneous induration, and lymphedema in the radiated field may be evident.

A CT scan may show a soft tissue mass with or without local bone destruction or epidural extension if a metastatic tumor is present.[5] In radiation fibrosis the CT scan may show distortion of normal tissue planes without a discrete mass. However, although CT scanning provides a useful guide for surgical exploration, it does not definitively differentiate tumor infiltration from radiation fibrosis.[1] In radiation plexopathy, electromyography sometimes will aid when an irritable motor unit is present.

In general, surgical neurolysis of the plexus is of minimal benefit. Pain and sensory loss may respond to neurolysis better than motor dysfunction.[9]

Brachial plexus involvement may occur following electrical injuries. Atrophic paralysis of the upper extremity is a late manifestation, probably due to the direct effect of the current.

Isolated Mononeuropathy of the Plexus

Isolated involvement of the long thoracic nerve of Bell supplying the serratus anterior muscle may be due to the wearing of a knapsack or rucksack or to a similar traumatic cause.[2] It has been reported following serum injections or during systemic infection and is a very common residual deficit of cryptogenic brachial plexopathy. On clinical evaluation, the scapula moves upward and laterally with forward flexion of the arm or with pressure on the hyperextended arm (Fig. 240-1). This may actually go unnoticed in the initial stages.

Isolated involvement of the suprascapular nerve causes atrophy of the supraspinatus and infraspinatus muscles. It may follow infection, such as malaria, and has been reported after traumatic exercise. The suprascapular nerve is often involved in combination with other nerves in cryptogenic lesions.

Isolated involvement of the musculocutaneous nerve causes weakness of the biceps brachii, coracobrachialis, and brachialis muscles with sensory involvement of the lateral cutaneous nerve of the forearm. This may follow a systemic illness such as pneumonia, influenza, tuberculosis, or malaria but usually follows a fracture of the humerus.

The axillary nerve may be involved, which causes weakness of the deltoid and teres minor muscles, following smallpox vaccination, dysentery, malaria, or barbiturate or carbon monoxide poisoning, in addition to traumatic or cryptogenic causes.

Lesions of the dorsal scapular nerve, subscapular nerve, or thoracodorsal nerve usually occur in combination with nerve involvement elsewhere in the plexus.

Heredofamilial Plexopathy

Many cases of familial plexopathy have been reported and several families have been described. In one family of 119 individuals, 24 members covering five generations had single or multiple attacks of acute brachial plexopathy associated with excruciating shoulder pain, severe weakness and atrophy, and incomplete sensory involvement. These were unilateral or bilateral. The roles of genetic and environmental factors are not clear.[8,9]

Several features of heredofamilial brachial plexopathy are distinct from those of cryptogenic plexus neuropathy. Lower cranial nerve involvement and isolated mononeuropathies of other extremities occur in some patients. Associated peculiar physiognomy, including syndactyly and dwarfism, have been reported.[3] Involvement of the lumbosacral plexus and recurrent laryngeal nerve may occur. Sometimes recurrent attacks are associated with pregnancy or the puerperium[12]; cryptogenic brachial plexopathy seldom occurs in pregnancy.

Generally, the course of the heredofamilial brachial plexopathy is benign and self-limiting, with full functional recovery. Partial recovery, with persistent mild residual deficits, occurs in some.

Thoracic Outlet Syndrome

The brachial plexus may be compressed along with the subclavian vessels at the superior aperture of the thorax. This is discussed in detail in another chapter.

Double Crush Syndrome

For an unknown reason, some individuals experience a "double crush" involving the median nerve and either a cervical radiculopathy or brachial plexus involvement. This may have its onset with trauma-causing whiplash from an auto accident but is quite frequently cryptogenic.[13] The par-

References

1. Cascino TL, Kori SH, Krol G, Foley KM: Brachial plexopathy in cancer patients: Diagnostic usefulness of CT scans. Neurology (NY) 32(2):A74, 1982.
2. Daube JR: Rucksack paralysis. JAMA 208:2447–2452, 1969.
3. Gardner JH, Maloney W: Hereditary brachial and cranial neuritis genetically linked with ocular hypotelorism and syndactyly. Neurology 18:278, 1968.
4. Gathier JC, Bruyn GW: Peripheral neuropathies following the administration of heterologous immune sera: A critical evaluation. Psychiatr Neurol Neurochir 71:351–371, 1968.
5. Kori SH, Foley KM, Posner JB: Brachial plexus lesions in patients with cancer: 100 cases. Neurology (NY) 31:45–50, 1981.
6. Magee KR, DeJong RN: Paralytic brachial neuritis: Discussion of clinical features with review of 23 cases. JAMA 174:1258–1262, 1960.
7. Massey EW, Pleet AB, Brannon WL Jr: Epstein-Barr virus in acute nontraumatic mononeuropathies. Milit Med 146:780–782, 1981.
8. Taylor RA: Heredofamilial mononeuritis multiplex with brachial predilection. Brain 83:113–137, 1960.
9. Tsairis P: Brachial plexus neuropathies, in Dyck PJ, Thomas PK, Lambert EH (eds): *Peripheral Neuropathy*. Philadelphia, Saunders, 1975, pp 659–681.
10. Tsairis P, Dyck PJ, Mulder DW: Natural history of brachial plexus neuropathy: Report on 99 patients. Arch Neurol 27:109–117, 1972.
11. Turner JWA, Parsonage MJ: Neuralgic amyotrophy (paralytic brachial neuritis) with special reference to prognosis. Lancet 2:209–212, 1957.
12. Ungley CC: Recurrent polyneuritis in pregnancy and puerperium affecting three members of family. J Neurol Psychopathol 14:15–26, 1933.
13. Upton ARM, McComas AJ: The double crush in nerve-entrapment syndromes. Lancet 2:359–362, 1973.
14. Wartenberg R: Neuritis of the cervical and brachial plexus, in Wartenberg R: *Neuritis, Sensory Neuritis, Neuralgia; A Clinical Study with Review of the Literature*. London, Oxford University Press, 1958, pp 85–99.

241

Surgical Sympathectomy

Janet W. Bay
Donald F. Dohn

Surgery of the sympathetic nervous system constitutes a minor portion of the training for and practice of modern day neurosurgery. Many of the indications for sympathectomy utilized earlier in this century (e.g., hypertension) have been eclipsed by improvements in medical therapy as well as by an increased understanding of the pathophysiology of the disease states treated (e.g., spasticity, transient cerebral ischemia). Nevertheless, sympathectomy remains in the therapeutic armamentarium of the neurosurgeon as a uniquely effective treatment for a number of distressing disorders (Table 241-1).

Attention was first drawn to sympathectomy as a clinically useful tool late in the nineteenth century.[5] Jaboulay and later Jonnesco reported early favorable results with sympathectomy for the diverse ailments due to vascular insufficiency of the leg, for epilepsy, and for goiter. Further interest in sympathectomy as a means of treating vasospastic conditions was stimulated by the work of Hunter and Royle in the 1920s.[5] In the United States, Adson was among the first to advocate sympathectomy to treat Raynaud's disease as well as hyperhidrosis.[1] Although early enthusiasm for sympathectomy has waned, several solid indications remain. In this chapter we will focus on current indications and selected techniques for surgical sympathectomy.

General Anatomical Considerations

The sympathetic division of the autonomic nervous system is that portion which equips the body to respond maximally during crisis conditions.[9,11] Such reflexes, which prepare the individual for "fight or flight," include pupillary dilata-

TABLE 241-1 Indications for Sympathectomy

Past	Present
Spasticity	Causalgia
Hypertension	Essential hyperhidrosis
Angina pectoris	Shoulder-hand syndrome
Transient cerebral ischemia	Vascular occlusive states
Epilepsy	Raynaud's disease
Exophthalmic goiter	Visceral pain (pancreatic carcinoma, chronic pancreatitis)
Migraine	
Glaucoma	

Surgical Sympathectomy

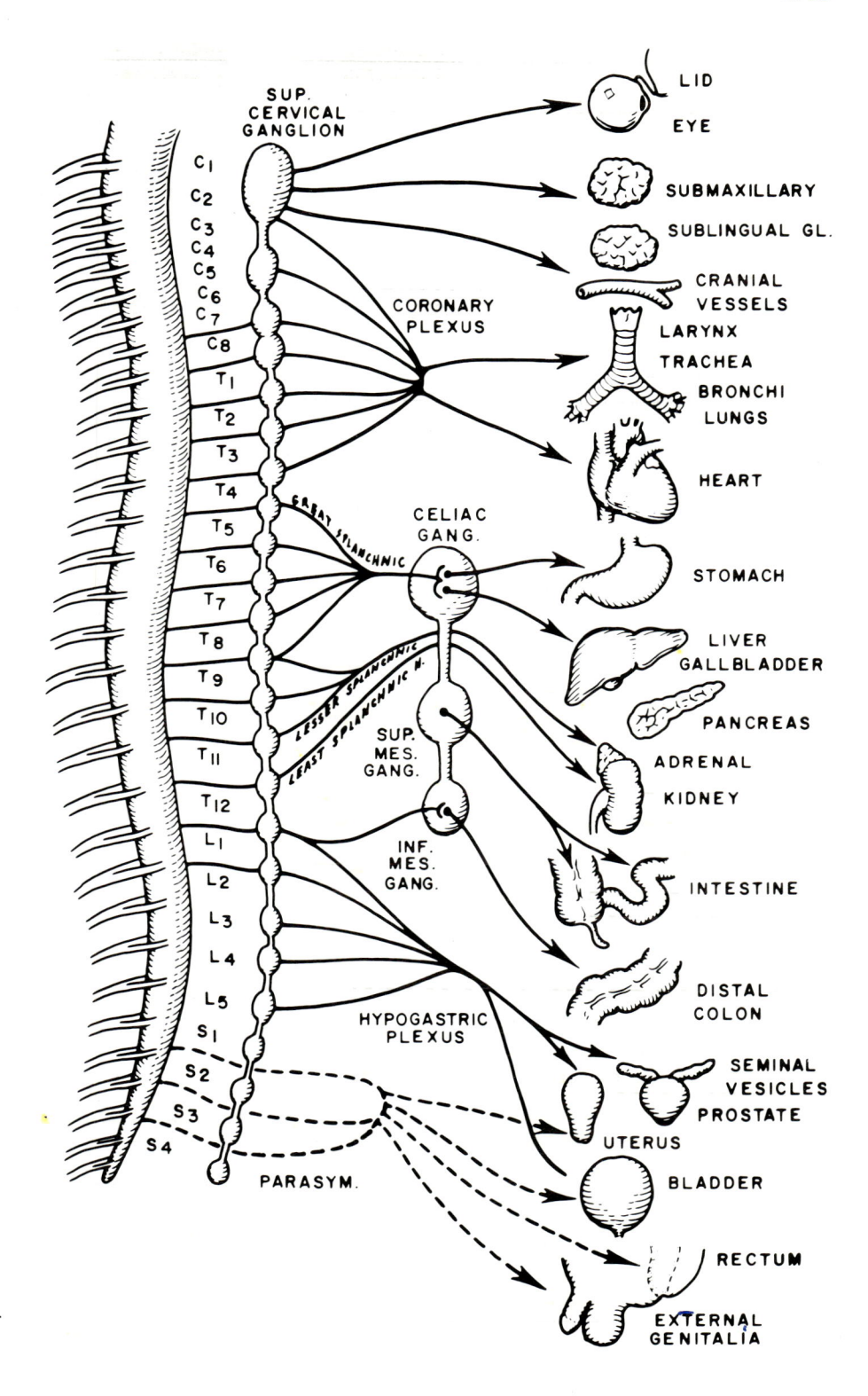

Figure 241-1 Diagram of the sympathetic outflow of the autonomic nervous system.

tion, deepened respirations, increased heart rate, and cutaneous vasoconstriction.

The sympathetic outflow of the central nervous system is composed of two symmetrical ganglionated cords extending from the skull base to the coccyx along the anterolateral aspects of the vertebral bodies (Fig. 241-1). The eight original cervical ganglia fuse to form the superior cervical, middle cervical, and inferior cervical ganglia. The inferior cervical ganglion, located at the C7 vertebral body, frequently fuses with the first thoracic ganglion to form the cervicothoracic (stellate) ganglion. The ganglia are segmentally arranged in the thoracic, lumbar, and sacral areas.

The sympathetic ganglia receive preganglionic fibers from the spinal cord (intermediolateral nucleus) via the ventral roots of all of the thoracic and the upper two lumbar nerves. The sympathetic fibers leave the ventral roots via the white rami communicantes to enter the sympathetic trunk. Such fibers are destined either for the paravertebral sympathetic ganglia or the prevertebral ganglia. The prevertebral ganglia are ganglionated masses located on the visceral branches of the aorta. These include the celiac, superior mesenteric, and inferior mesenteric ganglia (Fig. 241-1). From either the paravertebral or prevertebral ganglia, postganglionic fibers are distributed to the various organs innervated (e.g., blood vessels, sweat glands, lungs, heart, and visceral organs).

Sympathetic Denervation of the Upper Extremities

Indications

Sympathetic denervation of the arm should be considered for treatment of major causalgia, essential hyperhidrosis, and upper limb ischemia caused by a variety of vasospastic and vascular occlusive conditions.

Causalgia is characterized by burning pain, aggravated by light tactile stimuli or temperature change.[2] The onset of the pain is typically soon after partial injury to a mixed peripheral nerve, most commonly the median (or sciatic). The response is dramatic to sympathetic blockade via stellate ganglion injection under a local anesthetic. The adequacy of the block is judged by the production of an ipsilateral Horner's syndrome as well as by the increased temperature of the involved limb. Occasionally a series of stellate blocks will provide permanent pain relief. If not, surgical sympathectomy should be considered.

Sympathectomy has also been recommended for a number of other post-traumatic painful states including *minor causalgia, sympathetic dystrophy,* and *Sudeck's atrophy.*[2] The results in this diverse group of patients are not as favorable as with major causalgia, although stellate blocks may be useful in selecting proper operative candidates.[2,6]

Essential hyperhidrosis is an idiopathic condition characterized by markedly excessive sweating, which is most pronounced in the hands but also sometimes involves the feet and axillae. The diagnosis is easily made by history and examination of the patient. The condition may represent an occupational handicap as well as a source of social embarrassment. Mild cases may be treated with local drying agents or anticholinergic drugs. Such therapy is inadequate in severe cases. The most effective and permanent therapy for severe hyperhidrosis is surgical sympathectomy.[1,4,6]

Sympathectomy has been recommended for a variety of vascular disorders since the turn of the century.[4,5] Obviously, ischemia caused by an embolus must be treated by embolectomy. However, sympathectomy is indicated in certain patients with symptoms caused by distal embolization or arteriosclerotic occlusive disease.[3,4] The beneficial effects of sympathectomy for *Raynaud's disease* have been well described.[3,4] Although the clinical picture of digital vasospasm with resultant cold-induced pallor, pain, and numbness has been well characterized, there remains confusion between Raynaud's phenomenon (secondary) and Raynaud's disease (primary).[4] The phenomenon may occur with a number of underlying systemic diseases and the diagnosis of primary Raynaud's disease should not be reached until underlying causal disease has been excluded.

Surgical Technique

A great variety of surgical techniques have been described for sympathetic denervation of the upper extremities.[1-4,7,8] Approaches to the lower cervical and upper thoracic sympathetic chain include the supraclavicular, transaxillary, anterior transpleural (thoracotomy), and several posterior thoracic operations, including through paramedian and oblique incisions as well as costotransversectomy via a midline thoracic incision.[4] The extent of sympathetic resection has been variable, with some surgeons thinking that the entire stellate ganglion must be removed for complete denervation. Early experience with sympathectomies in the 1940s suggested that removal of the second thoracic ganglion alone provided complete and permanent denervation of the upper extremity, and our experience has reaffirmed this.[4,7]

Although the supraclavicular and transaxillary approaches to the T2 ganglion have been widely used, we have employed as our standard procedure a posterior midline incision allowing access for a one-stage bilateral costotransversectomy and ganglionectomy[4] (Fig. 241-2). This approach has the advantages of bilateral exposure, adequate visualiza-

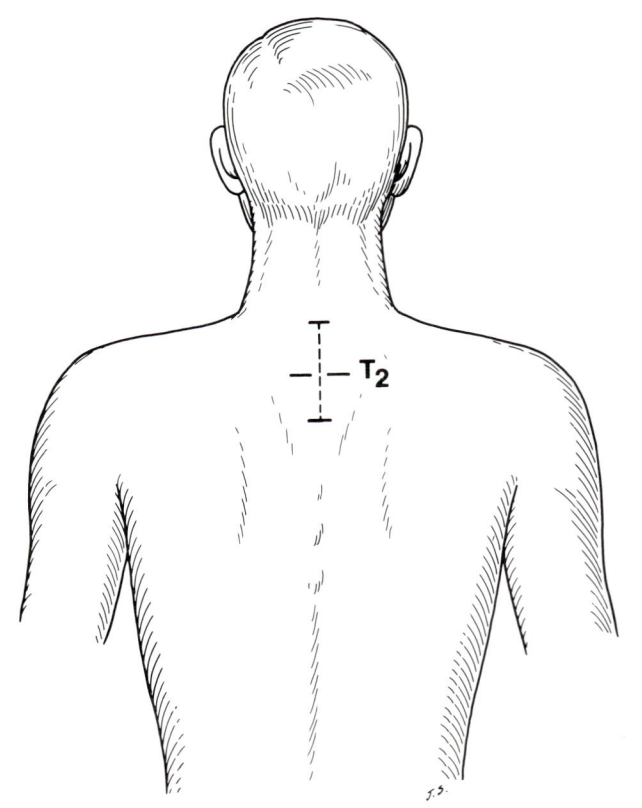

Figure 241-2 Incision for posterior upper dorsal sympathectomy (From Dohn and Sava.[4])

tion of the ganglia, and low incidence of complications such as Horner's syndrome or pneumothorax.

The patient is operated upon in the sitting position, with the initial exposure identical to that of a thoracic laminectomy. The T3 transverse process must be exposed bilaterally and identified via an intraoperative x-ray film. A costotransversectomy of T3 is then carried out with Kerrison punches. During the bone removal, careful dissection is necessary to avoid pleural injury or inadvertent removal of a portion of the sympathetic chain. Once the chain has been identified and isolated with a long hook (Smithwick), the T2 ganglion is dissected sharply from the overlying second thoracic nerve by sectioning of the rami communicantes. Fiberoptic illumination and loupe magnification are invaluable in this portion of the procedure. If easily exposed, the T3 ganglion is removed as well. Surgical clips are placed on the chain above and below the resected ganglion (Fig. 241-3). Hemostasis is obtained with bipolar coagulation and the field is flooded with saline to check for an occult pleural tear. Should the pleura be opened, a 12F catheter is placed within the pleural space and fascial closure performed. Air is aspirated through the catheter as it is removed, with positive ventilatory pressure applied by the anesthetist.

Hospital stay following surgery is typically 5 to 7 days, with return to work or school within 1 month.

Surgical Results and Complications

Excellent immediate results from sympathectomy by the various approaches mentioned above have been reported for causalgia, chronic distal occlusive disease, Raynaud's disease, and essential hyperhidrosis.[1-4] Pain relief is quite consistent in properly selected patients with major causalgia, and in patients with ischemia there is relief of pain, healing of skin lesions, and at times reversal of trophic changes. Long-term follow-up studies have been most frequent in hyperhidrosis, with continued relief of symptoms noted for many years.[4]

Our surgical results and complications with bilateral T2 ganglionectomy for hyperhidrosis reported in 1978 are rep-

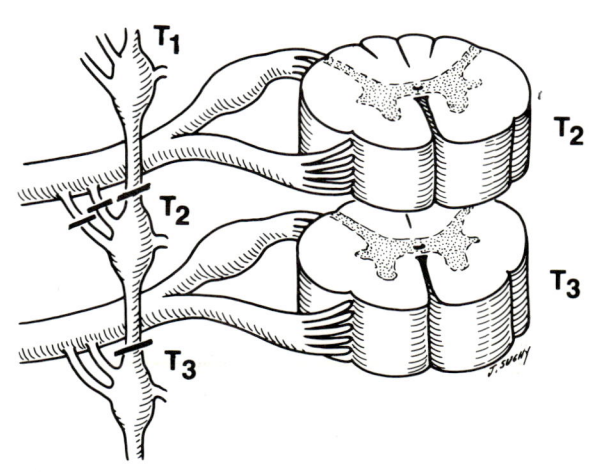

Figure 241-3 Extent of sympathectomy (From Dohn and Sava.[4])

resentative.[4] Of 100 patients, 87 had complete relief of palmar hyperhidrosis, 9 had incomplete (75 percent) relief or an undesirable side effect, and 4 had a poor result as defined by no relief of sweating, a major side effect, or recurrence of hyperhidrosis. Ninety-seven patients felt that the operation was a success. Complications occurred in six patients with intercostal neuralgia, three with minor wound infections, one with a pneumothorax, and one with empyema. One patient developed a transient CSF leak and one a Horner's syndrome. Compensatory sweating occurred in 44 patients but was usually a minor, self-limited problem.

Thoracic Splanchnicectomy and Sympathectomy

Indications

Splanchnicectomy is primarily indicated for pancreatic pain of malignant origin.[10] This procedure has been advised for the pain of chronic pancreatitis as well. Although it may be helpful in selected cases, long-term results have been disappointing. Hardy's group of patients, who were often addicted to narcotics preoperatively, tended to develop new chronic incisional pain and once again required narcotics for relief.[6]

Selection of appropriate candidates for splanchnicectomy from a group of patients with pancreatic cancer pain requires a careful pain history and at times a splanchnic block.[10] Abdominal or back pain with radicular features suggests involvement of parietal somatic nerves and is a contraindication to splanchnicectomy. If doubt exists, diagnostic splanchnic blocks utilizing local anesthetic agents can be performed. Unfortunately, a diagnostic block can be technically difficult to achieve and the results may further confuse the issue.

Surgical Technique

Visceral afferent fibers from the pancreas travel through the greater splanchnic nerve after traversing the celiac ganglion (Fig. 241-1). The pancreas receives bilateral innervation from the greater and lesser splanchnic nerves.[9] The lower thoracic and upper lumbar sympathetic ganglia may be involved as well.[10] Although successful unilateral denervation procedures for pancreatic pain have been reported in small numbers of cases, it would seem that a bilateral approach would be required.[10] The extent of sympathetic resection necessary is controversial and many surgical approaches to the splanchnic nerves have been described, including the unilateral supradiaphragmatic approach, the subdiaphragmatic approach, and combinations of these.[6,10]

Our preference has been excision of the sympathetic chains and the greater, lesser, and least splanchnic nerves bilaterally from T9 down to the diaphragm. This is accomplished via a technique adapted from the surgical splanchnicectomy described by Peet in 1935.[10]

The patient is operated upon in the prone position on a laminectomy frame. Separate paramedian incisions, 4 to

5 in. in length and centered over the eleventh rib (Fig. 241-4), are made four finger breadths from the midline. After dissection through the latissimus dorsi and sacrospinalis muscles, the eleventh rib is exposed and the proximal 4 in. resected. Access to the extrapleural space is facilitated by making this resection as medial as possible although the head of the rib need not be disarticulated. The exposure is widened by blunt dissection and the lung retracted with a malleable retractor.

The sympathetic chain is then identified running across the costovertebral articulations ventral to the head of each rib. The chain is dissected from the diaphragm below to the T9 ganglion above. During this dissection the splanchnic nerves will be identified ventral to the ganglionated sympathetic chain. The greater splanchnic nerve is large, often 2.0 mm in diameter, and must be removed. The lesser and the least splanchnic nerves are anatomically more variable and may be represented by several smaller nerves. All the splanchnic nerves identified along with the sympathetic chain are then excised between surgical clips (Fig. 241-5). If there is difficulty locating the splanchnic nerves along the vertebral body, the retracted pleural surface should be examined carefully as the nerves may be adherent. The entire process is aided by headlight illumination and loupe magnification. At the completion of the resection, the wound is flooded with saline and pleural tears are searched for. If a hole is identified, a 12F red rubber catheter is inserted into the pleural space and closure is carried out around it. It is removed under suction at the termination of the procedure while the lung is being fully expanded with positive pressure ventilation.

Surgical Results and Complications

Of patients with pancreatic cancer and back or abdominal pain, 70 percent have obtained excellent relief from the above procedure,[10] 14 percent were partially relieved, and in 16 percent the operation achieved nothing. Some of the failures were explained by direct invasion of the abdominal wall or somatic nerves by the carcinoma. Of those patients with good initial relief, 23 percent noted some recurrence or increase in pain, although usually not severe. This occurred

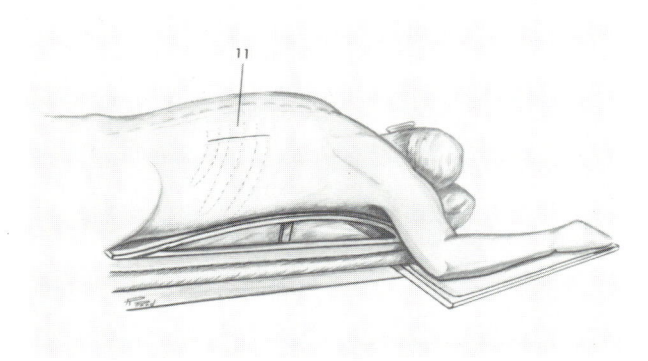

Figure 241-4 Paramedian incision for right thoracic splanchnicectomy and sympathectomy (From Sadar and Hardy.[10])

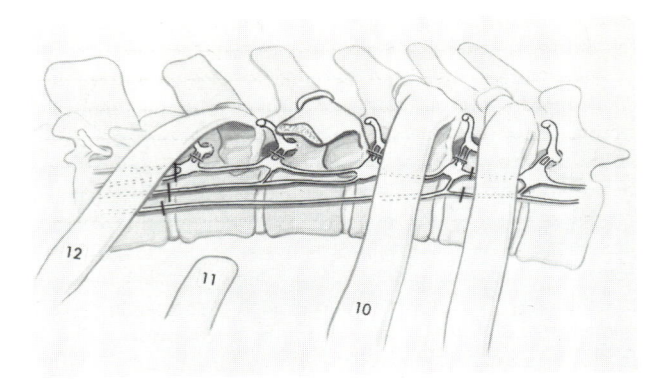

Figure 241-5 Optimal extent of resection of the sympathetic chain and splanchnic nerves (From Sadar and Hardy.[10])

more commonly with long-term survivors (average 11 months).

Pleural tears may occur, but symptomatic pneumothorax requiring chest tube placement is quite rare. Wound infection and even empyema are potential problems in this group of nutritionally depleted patients. Operative mortality in a group of patients on whom both splanchnicectomy and laparotomy for primary treatment of the pancreatic cancer were performed under the same anesthesia was 7 percent.[10]

Lumbar Splanchnicectomy

Indications

The principal indication for lumbar sympathectomy is causalgia of the lower extremity, a rare peacetime affliction.[2,6,8] It is also useful in the treatment of distal occlusive arteriosclerotic vascular disease with resultant ischemic rest pain and skin ulcers of the lower extremity.[8] Although the operation may be considered for hyperhidrosis of the lower extremity, the extensive nature of this bilateral operation and the risk of sexual dysfunction in males limits its application in this disease.

Lumbar sympathetic blocks may be performed preoperatively in an attempt to relieve causalgic pain and select proper operative candidates.[8] Unfortunately, this requires three separate injection sites to block the L1-3 ganglia and is considerably more difficult technically than a stellate block. The degree of blockage obtained is variable and the results are difficult to interpret.

Surgical Technique

Resection of the second and third lumbar sympathetic ganglia has been found to be adequate to denervate the lower extremity in the majority of individuals.[8,9] In some patients with causalgic pain involving the thigh, removal of the L1 and even the T12 ganglion has been necessary.[6]

There are several approaches to the lumbar sympathetic chain, including the retroperitoneal flank approach or the abdominal approach.[8] Although the transabdominal approach allows simultaneous bilateral sympathectomies, good exposure, and excellent vascular control, the prolonged postoperative ileus, intra-abdominal adhesions, and incisional pain counterbalance these advantages. Therefore, most surgeons employ the flank approach via a transverse or oblique incision.[6,8,9]

The patient is operated upon in the lateral jackknife position with the incision extending obliquely from the anterior-superior iliac crest superiorly and laterally to the tip of the twelfth rib. The external oblique, internal oblique, and transversalis muscles are opened in the direction of their fibers. The peritoneum is dissected bluntly from the lateral abdominal wall and retracted anteriorly. Dissection is continued along the anterior surface of the quadratus lumborum and iliacus muscles, with gentle retraction of the kidney and ureter anteriorly. Care must be taken to avoid injury to the ureter throughout the procedure. The sympathetic chain can be identified between the psoas muscle and the vertebral bodies.

On the right side, lumbar bridging veins may obscure the chain as they drain into the vena cava. Careful coagulation or clipping with mobilization of the vena cava may be necessary for adequate visualization. On the left side, the aorta lies anteromedial to the chain, which makes dissection somewhat easier. Once the ganglionated chain is palpated on the vertebral bodies, it is dissected free and elevated with a blunt nerve hook. At least two ganglia are excised between surgical clips. Any tears in the peritoneum are repaired and a multilayered wound closure carried out.

Surgical Results and Complications

Although extensive civilian experience with sympathectomy of the lower extremity for causalgia has not been reported, excellent initial results have generally been obtained.[2,6,8]

Complications include wound infection, prolonged incisional pain, ureteral damage, and damage to the major vascular structures encountered. Excision of the L1 ganglia bilaterally in males must be avoided to prevent permanent sexual dysfunction.[6,8]

References

1. Adson AW, Craig WM, Brown GE: Essential hyperhidrosis cured by sympathetic ganglionectomy and trunk resection. Arch Surg 31:794–806, 1935.
2. Bergan JJ, Conn J Jr: Sympathectomy for pain relief. Med Clin North Am 52:147–159, 1968.
3. Dale WA, Lewis MR: Management of ischemia of the hand and fingers. Surgery 67:62–79, 1970.
4. Dohn DF, Sava GM: Sympathectomy for vascular syndromes and hyperhidrosis of the upper extremities. Clin Neurosurg 25:637–650, 1978.
5. Greenwood B: The origins of sympathectomy. Med Hist 11:165–169, 1967.
6. Hardy RW: Surgery of the sympathetic nervous system, in Schmidek HH, Sweet WH (eds): *Operative Neurosurgical Techniques*. New York, Grune & Stratton, 1982, pp 1045–1061.
7. Hyndman OR, Wolkin J: Sympathectomy of the upper extremity. Arch Surg 45:145–155, 1942.
8. Kleinert HE, Norberg H, McDonough JJ: Surgical sympathectomy—upper and lower extremity, in Omer GE Jr, Spinner M (eds): *Management of Peripheral Nerve Problems*. Philadelphia, Saunders, 1980, pp 285–302.
9. Pick J: *The Autonomic Nervous System: Morphological, Comparative, Clinical, and Surgical Aspects*. Philadelphia, Lippincott, 1970.
10. Sadar ES, Hardy RW Jr: Thoracic splanchnicectomy and sympathectomy for relief of pancreatic pain, in Cooperman AM, Hoerr SO (eds): *Surgery of the Pancreas: A Text and Atlas*. St Louis, Mosby, 1978, pp 141–152.
11. Truex RC, Carpenter MB: *Human Neuroanatomy*. Baltimore, Williams & Wilkins, 1969, pp 216–235.